Vascular and Interventional

R A D I O L O G Y

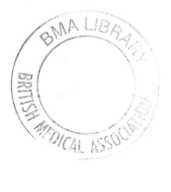

Vascular and Interventional
RADIOLOGY
SECOND EDITION

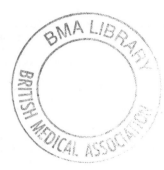

Karim Valji, MD

Professor of Radiology
University of California, San Diego

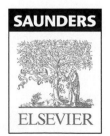

SAUNDERS

ELSEVIER

SAUNDERS
ELSEVIER

1600 John F. Kennedy Boulevard
Suite 1800
Philadelphia, Pennsylvania 19103-2899

VASCULAR AND INTERVENTIONAL RADIOLOGY   ISBN-13: 978-0-7216-0621-7
Second Edition   ISBN-10: 0-7216-0621-0

NOTICE

Knowledge and best practice in this field are constantly changing. As new research and experience
broaden our knowledge, changes in practice, treatment and drug therapy may become necessary or
appropriate. Readers are advised to check the most current information provided (i) on procedures
featured or (ii) by the manufacturer of each product to be administered, to verify the recommended
dose or formula, the method and duration of administration, and contraindications. It is the responsibility of the practitioner, relying on his or her own experience and knowledge of the patient, to make
diagnoses, to determine dosages and the best treatment for each individual patient, and to take all
appropriate safety precautions. To the fullest extent of the law, neither the Publisher nor the Editor
assumes any liability for any injury and/or damage to persons or property arising out of or related to
any use of the material contained in this book.

Library of Congress Cataloging-in-Publication Data
Valji, Karim.
   Vascular and interventional radiology / Karim Valji.—2nd ed.
      p. ; cm.
   Includes bibliographical references and index.
   ISBN-13: 978-0-7216-0621-7
   ISBN-10: 0-7216-0621-0
      1. Blood-vessels—Interventional radiology. 2. Interventional radiology.
   3. Angiography. I. Title.
      [DNLM: 1. Vascular Diseases—radiography. 2. Diagnostic Imaging—methods.
   3. Radiography, Interventional—methods. WG 500 V173v 2006]
   RD598.5.V26   2006
   616.1'307572—dc22

                                                              2006041722

Acquisitions Editor: Allan Ross
Marketing Manager: Emily Christie

Printed in the United States of America

Last digit is the print number   9 8 7 6 5 4 3 2 1

To Eric
and again
to Matthew and Andrea,
who make it all worthwhile

and to
the memory of my father

Contributors

HORACIO B. D'AGOSTINO, MD
Professor and Chairman
Department of Radiology
Louisiana State University Health Sciences Center
Shreveport, Louisiana

EDUARDO GONZALEZ TOLEDO, MD, PhD
Professor and Director of Neuroradiology
Department of Radiology
Louisiana State University Health Sciences Center
Shreveport, Louisiana

DENISSE HURVITZ, MD
Associate Professor and Director of Breast Imaging
Department of Radiology
Louisiana State University Health Sciences Center
Shreveport, Louisiana

THOMAS B. KINNEY, MD
Professor of Radiology
University of California, San Diego
San Diego, California

GREGORY M. LIM, MD
Staff Radiologist
San Mateo Division of Marin Radiology Group
Novato, California

LINDA NALL, MD
Professor and Vice Chairman of Radiology
Department of Radiology
Louisiana State University Health Sciences Center
Shreveport, Louisiana

STEVEN B. OGLEVIE, MD
Chief of Interventional Radiology
Hoag Memorial Hospital Presbyterian
Newport Beach, California

GERANT RIVERA-SANFELIZ, MD
Assistant Professor of Radiology
University of California, San Diego
San Diego, California

ANNE C. ROBERTS, MD
Professor of Radiology and Chief, Division of Vascular
and Interventional Radiology
University of California, San Diego
San Diego, California

STEVEN C. ROSE, MD
Professor of Radiology,
University of California, San Diego
San Diego, California

GUILLERMO P. SANGSTER, MD
Associate Professor
Department of Radiology
Louisiana State University Health Sciences Center
Shreveport, Louisiana

Preface

In the seven years since the first edition of *Vascular and Interventional Radiology* was published, the field of interventional radiology (IR) has seen significant changes in procedures, practice, and philosophy. Many new techniques and refinements of old ones were widely adopted. There is finally widespread (although not universal) acceptance that IR is a true clinical specialty and not simply a procedure-driven referral service. As such, all practitioners must possess a thorough understanding of the pathology and pathophysiology of the disease processes at hand and an appreciation of the relative merits of various alternative therapies. Just as important, they must be willing to assume the primary role in both pre-procedure evaluation *and* long-term clinical follow-up. The incorporation of IR procedures into the arenas of cardiology, vascular surgery, and nephrology (among others) is a testament to the efficacy of many of these techniques and the important benefits afforded to patients. Finally, IR now impacts so many areas of medical practice that even purely diagnostic radiologists must have some familiarity with the available procedures and expected outcomes in order to suggest these options to referring physicians and best serve their patients. An updated version of the original text is thus long overdue.

Again, the book aims to cover the entire spectrum of vascular and nonvascular interventional procedures in a practical, concise, and balanced fashion. Neurointerventional procedures (which are usually learned by trainees in separate rotations) have not been included. Although all of the primary authors are (or were) affiliated with UCSD, a narrow institutional slant was purposely avoided. The structure and style of the second edition is identical to the first. The introductory chapters provide a foundation for interventional radiology practice, including the essential elements of patient care, basic interventional techniques, and the pathology of vascular diseases. The second and third sections are divided into chapters that cover diagnosis and intervention in each of the major arterial and venous vascular beds (with the exception of the head and heart) and nonvascular interventional procedures organized by organ system and procedure type. Principles of disease pathogenesis and natural history, individual interventional methods and outcomes, and comparison with other treatment modalities are emphasized. Many interventional procedures are described in some detail, but in fact the "craft" of interventional radiology can and should only be learned by extensive hands-on training from experienced practitioners.

This edition is somewhat longer than the first, but it was purposely kept to a manageable size. Unlike more comprehensive reference texts, the book can easily be read cover-to-cover. Every chapter has been thoroughly updated to include all of the essential interventional techniques that have arisen or matured since the first edition was written. There are now over 1300 illustrations, almost half of them new. Outdated cut-film angiograms have been replaced with digital images wherever possible. CT and MR angiography and duplex sonography, now the cornerstones of vascular imaging, are given much greater emphasis; diagnostic angiography is only discussed and illustrated to the extent that it may be encountered during routine practice. References have been thoroughly updated. The citations are extensive but not exhaustive; they should direct the reader to the most important current (and classic or historic) papers covering each topic.

As before, the book was written primarily for trainees in diagnostic radiology and vascular and interventional radiology. It should also serve as a comprehensive review of the current state of the field for practicing interventional radiologists and as a reference source for occasional consultation. Finally, the text will be of value to physicians in other specialties who have an interest in performing selected IR procedures; however, it can only supplement (and certainly not replace) extensive formal training in these subjects.

Karim Valji, MD

Acknowledgments

I am privileged to work with an exceptional group of colleagues in interventional radiology at the University of California, San Diego (UCSD). They all enthusiastically contributed to this project with new or revised chapters for the book, and many of the illustrations come from cases they performed. Lynne Olson at UCLA provided more superb artwork. Gabriella Iussich, MD, created many of the CT and MR reconstructions that have become so vital in vascular imaging diagnosis. As with the first edition, the IR technologists continued to hunt for "cool" cases to include in the book. I am indebted to my editors, Allan Ross and Todd Hummel, and their team at Elsevier/Saunders for their encouragement and support throughout the writing and publication process and to Peggy Gordon for a superb job in book production.

The diagnostic radiology residents and interventional radiology fellows at UCSD were the impetus for the first edition of the text, and their enthusiastic response to that book inspired me to revise it. As we academic physicians progress in our careers, it is these trainees who keep us young, fresh, and inspired.

Karim Valji, MD

Contents

SECTION I

GENERAL PRINCIPLES

1

Patient Evaluation and Care

During the past three decades, the field of vascular and interventional radiology has developed into a mature discipline, and the interventionalist has evolved from consultant to clinician. The increased scope and complexity of interventional procedures demand that the practicing interventionalist master myriad technical skills and possess extensive knowledge of pharmacology, sedation and anesthesia, and clinical management of patients. A successful and safe outcome often depends as much on preprocedure and postprocedure care as it does on performance of the case itself. Although the nuances of patient care vary from one institution to the next, the principles are universal.

■ PREPROCEDURE CARE

Patient Referral and Contact

For simple diagnostic and interventional procedures (e.g., vascular access placement), patient referral without direct contact between physicians may be appropriate. For more complex procedures or difficult cases, a discussion between the interventionalist and the referring physician ensures that the appropriate procedure is performed, the risks for the particular patient are appreciated, and the likely outcome is understood.

The interventionalist should review the medical history and all pertinent diagnostic tests and imaging studies before contacting the patient. The initial conversation between the patient and the physician is vitally important and, if possible, should take place before the day of the procedure. The goals of this discussion are to establish rapport with the patient, review the history, explain the procedure in detail, and reduce the patient's anxiety.

History and Physical Examination

Case review with the referring physician does not replace a personal evaluation of the patient by the interventionalist. A review of all available, pertinent imaging studies is critical. The interview and chart review include several components (Box 1-1). One should be confident that there are appropriate indications for the procedure based on criteria established in the medical literature or by the Society of Interventional Radiology.[1] The interventionalist should identify risk factors that may require a delay or modification of the proposed procedure or an alternative therapy (Boxes 1-2 through 1-4).[2] Sedation and analgesia requirements should be determined. Most procedures on adults are performed with moderate sedation under the supervision of the operating physician.

BOX 1-1 ■ Evaluation of the Patient

History of current problem
Pertinent medical and surgical history
Review of organ systems
  Cardiac
  Pulmonary
  Renal
  Hepatic
  Hematologic (e.g., coagulopathy, hypercoagulable state)
  Endocrine (e.g., diabetes)
History of allergies
Current medications
Directed physical examination

BOX 1-2 ■ Risk Factors for Contrast Material Reactions

Previous allergic reaction to contrast agent
Other drug allergy
Asthma
Reaction to skin allergens

BOX 1-3 ■ **Risk Factors for Contrast-Induced Nephropathy**

Preexisting renal dysfunction (serum creatinine > 1.2–1.5 mg/dL)
Diabetes
Dehydration
Large contrast dose
Advanced age
Nephrotoxic drugs
Solitary kidney
Uric acid > 8.0 mg/dL

However, it may be necessary to consult an anesthesiologist about regional anesthesia (e.g., epidural) or general anesthesia for extremely painful procedures (e.g., biliary tract dilation), for patients who are uncooperative or medically unstable, or for patients with a history of chronic narcotic use.

A directed physical examination is performed. For angiographic procedures, the interventionalist should evaluate the following parameters:

■ The proposed puncture site for contraindications to use (e.g., groin infection, common femoral artery aneurysm, overlying hernia, fresh incision, recent injury)
■ All extremity pulses, using a Doppler probe when necessary
■ The status of the extremities (e.g., color, perfusion, presence of swelling, ulceration)
■ Bilateral arm blood pressures and upper extremity pulses when a high brachial artery puncture is planned

Hypercoagulable (thrombophilic) states are an uncommon but important risk factor for vascular thrombosis and can be associated with significant complications from diagnostic and therapeutic vascular procedures.[3-7] The major hereditary and acquired disorders are listed in Chapter 3 (see Box 3-5). These conditions should be suspected when thrombosis occurs in young patients, at atypical sites, in the absence of underlying vascular disease, with familial tendency, or with apparent resistance to anticoagulants.

BOX 1-4 ■ **Risk Factors for Bleeding from Vascular and Interventional Procedures**

Thrombocytopenia
Anticoagulant medications
Liver disease
History of bleeding diathesis
Malignant hypertension
Malnutrition
Hematologic malignancy
Splenomegaly
Disseminated intravascular coagulation
Selected chemotherapeutic agents

Informed Consent

It is the obligation of the physician performing any medical procedure to explain the intervention to the patient, to the parent of a minor patient, or to a legal representative or the closest relative if the patient is mentally incompetent.[8,9] For emergent procedures on patients with an altered mental status, the "implied consent" doctrine is considered to be in force, and obtaining consent is unnecessary. To give informed consent, the patient must understand the reasons for undergoing the procedure, the risks and benefits, the consequences of refusing the procedure, and alternative therapies. To avoid "exceeding" consent during the case, the discussion also should include possible interventions (e.g., thrombolysis, angioplasty, or stent placement in patients undergoing angiography for evaluation of peripheral vascular disease).

Informed consent is both a legal and medical concept. In the United States, some states have adopted a "prudent patient" standard that is based on the information a patient needs to make a decision regarding medical care. Other states use a standard based on the information that a "prudent physician" in the community would have discussed for such a procedure.[8,9] Informed consent should include a discussion of the various elements of each case:

■ Access, including the risk of hematoma, pseudoaneurysm, arteriovenous fistula, thrombosis, and dissection for vascular cases
■ Catheter or guidewire manipulation en route to and at the site of angiography or intervention (e.g., risk of bleeding, embolization, dissection, perforation, thrombosis, arrhythmias, stroke)
■ Contrast agents, including allergic reactions and nephrotoxicity
■ Sedatives and analgesics (e.g., respiratory depression, hypotension)
■ Other medications that may be required during or after the procedure (e.g., anticoagulants)

The complications of angiographic procedures are outlined in Table 1-1.[1,10,11] As a rough guide, the overall incidence of major complications (Box 1-5) after the most common

---

TABLE 1-1 COMPLICATIONS AFTER DIAGNOSTIC ANGIOGRAPHIC PROCEDURES

Complication	Estimated Frequency (%)
Minor puncture site hematoma or bleeding	2–10
Major puncture site hematoma (requiring treatment)	0.2–2.0
Other puncture site complications (e.g., dissection, pseudoaneurysm, arteriovenous fistula)	<2
Thrombosis or distal embolization	<1
Contrast-induced renal dysfunction	
Transient	0.2–1.4
Chronic dialysis	<0.1
Contrast material reactions (LOCM)	
Moderate	0.2–0.4
Severe	0.04
Other systemic complications (e.g., cardiac, neurologic)	<2
Death	<0.05

LOCM, low osmolar iodinated contrast materials.

interventional procedures (e.g., diagnostic arteriography, vascular access placement, inferior vena cava filter placement, percutaneous biopsy) should be no more than 1% to 2%.[1,12] Patients with established risk factors are more likely to suffer adverse events related to bleeding, thrombosis, renal dysfunction, or allergic reactions to contrast agents. The risks for specific diagnostic and interventional procedures are discussed in later chapters.

In addition to having the patient sign a consent form, a preprocedure note stating that informed consent was obtained must be included in the medical record. Some practitioners list all common and serious risks of the procedure, but others prefer to be less specific. The note also includes a brief medical history, indications for the procedure, directed physical examination, and results of relevant laboratory tests.

Laboratory Testing

The purpose of preprocedure laboratory testing is to minimize risk by detecting and correcting abnormalities, altering the technique as needed, or canceling the case and choosing a safer treatment. Preprocedure testing may be routine (screening) or selective (directed).[13] Indiscriminate preprocedure testing has proved to be of little value in virtually every medical and surgical study.[14,15] However, *selective* testing is worthwhile before vascular and interventional procedures. Screening is probably not warranted in otherwise healthy patients younger than 40 years of age. Testing is certainly advisable in the elderly and those with predisposing risk factors. The evaluation focuses primarily on renal function and coagulation status. Laboratory tests performed within 1 to 2 months are valid if there has been no change in the clinical condition or risk factors. Certain procedures require other routine screening (e.g., electrocardiography before pulmonary angiography).

Renal Function

Contrast-induced nephropathy is marked by a significant rise in the serum creatinine level (by 0.5 mg/dL or 25% of baseline) 1 to 3 days after intravascular administration and by resolution at 7 to 10 days. This (usually) transient renal dysfunction is related to direct toxic effects on the kidney by oxygen free radicals or ischemia of the renal medulla.[16] In the general population, the overall risk of contrast-induced nephropathy after diagnostic angiography is low (about 0.2% to 1.4%).[1] The risk increases to about 5% in patients with preexisting mild renal dysfunction and up to 50% in patients with severe renal insufficiency and diabetes. Nonetheless, only a small fraction of patients who suffer this complication require long-term hemodialysis. Serum creatinine concentration may not accurately reflect actual renal function, particularly in cachectic or elderly patients.

The only widely accepted measure to prevent contrast-induced renal dysfunction is hydration with IV saline for 6 to 12 hours before and several hours after angiographic procedures. In addition, several other approaches should be considered:

■ Low osmolar iodinated contrast materials (LOCM) are safer than high osmolar contrast materials (HOCM) in patients with preexisting renal dysfunction.[17-20] HOCM are now rarely used for intravascular use. Isosmolar iodinated agents (e.g., iodixanol) may further reduce risk.[21]
■ Limit the total volume of iodinated contrast material given.
■ Carbon dioxide or limited volumes of gadolinium-based agents may replace or supplement standard iodinated contrast in some situations (see Chapter 2).
■ Magnetic resonance angiography should be considered as an alternative to catheter-based angiography.
■ Several pharmacologic regimens have recently shown promise in reducing the likelihood of contrast-induced nephropathy (see below).

Coagulation and Hematologic Parameters

The overall incidence of significant bleeding from vascular and interventional procedures is low. The risk varies with the likelihood of traversing a major arterial or venous branch and with the ability to detect or control bleeding when it occurs. For this reason, the need for screening depends on the type of procedure being performed:

■ For diagnostic and most therapeutic vascular procedures, the frequency of major bleeding complications is less than 1%.[1] Routine assessment of coagulation parameters is unnecessary, but patients with risk factors for bleeding should be evaluated (see Box 1-4).
■ With thrombolytic therapy, the increased risk of local or remote bleeding (e.g., intracranial hemorrhage) supports routine testing.
■ Many nonvascular interventional procedures (e.g., deep large-core biopsy, fluid drainage, nephrostomy, biliary drainage) may cause bleeding at inaccessible sites, and testing is done routinely. Other procedures (e.g., small-gauge superficial biopsy) may not require screening tests. However, severe or fatal hemorrhage has been reported even with apparently low-risk procedures (e.g., thoracentesis, vascular access placement).

Coagulation testing includes several measurements[22]:

Routine

■ Prothrombin time (PT)
■ Activated partial thromboplastin time (PTT)
■ Platelet count
■ International normalized ratio (INR).[23] The INR standardizes the variability in responsiveness of different thromboplastin assays to warfarin anticoagulation. In most patients, the target therapeutic range for INR is 2.0 to 3.0.

Selective Studies

■ Bleeding time in patients with suspected qualitative platelet dysfunction or with minimal elevation of the PT or PTT
■ Fibrinogen before planned thrombolytic procedures (optional)
■ Hemoglobin and hematocrit in patients who will undergo deep, large-bore biopsy, drainage, or thrombolysis procedures

Commonly accepted thresholds for defining a coagulopathy in interventional procedures are outlined in Table 1-2.[24]

Patient Preparation

Diet and Hydration

Oral intake restrictions before interventional procedures must comply with institutional guidelines for moderate sedation. Typically, patients are limited to clear liquids within 8 hours and made NPO within 2 hours of the expected start time to avoid nausea and vomiting occasionally caused by contrast agents and sedatives.[25] For inpatients who will receive significant volumes of intravascular contrast, overnight IV hydration should be considered (e.g., half-normal saline at 1 mL/kg/hr). Outpatients are encouraged to drink plenty of fluids. IV fluids should be ordered in consultation with the referring physician, particularly for patients with cardiac or renal disease.

Medications

Patients are instructed to take their regular medications on the day of the procedure, with certain exceptions:

■ Insulin-dependent diabetic patients may take their usual insulin doses for early morning cases or reduce

their morning dose by one half for midday cases to avoid hypoglycemia. Non–insulin-dependent diabetics may withhold the drug until after the procedure.[26] Blood glucose monitoring during the procedure may be advisable.
■ Diabetic patients taking the oral hypoglycemic *metformin (Glucophage)* are at a very small risk for severe lactic acidosis if contrast-induced renal failure occurs after an angiographic procedure *when preexisting renal dysfunction is present*.[27] For elective studies, metformin should be withheld for 48 hours before and 48 hours after the case. The drug is resumed after obtaining a new serum creatinine.
■ Antihypertensive medications should be taken. Diuretics may be withheld from patients undergoing angiography.
■ When feasible, *heparin* is stopped for 2 to 6 hours before interventional procedures and restarted 1 to 6 hours afterward.
■ *Warfarin* may be withheld for several days before elective procedures, during which time the patient is switched to heparin. If the PT or INR is mildly elevated on the day of the study, infusion of fresh-frozen plasma should be considered.
■ Low-molecular-weight heparin compounds (e.g., *enoxaparin [Lovenox]*) and potent oral antiplatelet agents (e.g., *clopidogrel [Plavix]* and *ticlopidine [Ticlid]*) will generally not alter standard coagulation tests. Studies in coronary interventions have failed to show a significant added risk when these agents are being administered.[28] However, there is little data on their effect during noncoronary interventions. Some practitioners favor discontinuation of the drugs for 5 to 10 days before elective, high-risk procedures.
■ *Aspirin* or another antiplatelet agent often is started on the day before possible vascular recanalization procedures (e.g., angioplasty, thrombolysis, stent placement).
■ Preprocedure sedation (e.g., *lorazepam [Ativan]*, 0.5 to 2.0 mg PO) is favored by some interventionalists.

Contrast Reaction Pretreatment

For the most part, LOCM have completely replaced HOCM for intravascular use. The frequency of mild and moderate contrast material reactions is significantly reduced by using LOCM. The safest approach to patients with a history of moderate to severe reactions in whom other alternative methods are not acceptable (e.g., magnetic resonance angiography, carbon dioxide angiography) is premedication *and* use of LOCM. However, so-called "breakthrough reactions" may occur despite these measures.[29]

The standard prophylactic regimen[30,31] includes two agents:

■ Steroids: 32 to 50 mg PO of prednisone given 12 hours and 2 hours before the procedure (mandatory)
■ Histamine receptor (H_1) blocker: 25 to 50 mg PO of diphenhydramine (Benadryl) given 2 hours before the procedure (optional)

TABLE 1-2	SAFETY THRESHOLDS FOR COAGULATION PARAMETERS

Parameter	Threshold
Prothrombin time (PT)	<3 s from control
Partial thromboplastin time (PTT)	<6 s from control
International normalized ratio (INR)	<1.6–1.8
Platelet count (normal INR/PTT)	>50,000/mm³
Platelet count (abnormal INR/PTT)	>50–100,000/mm³
Bleeding time	<8 min

Prevention of Contrast-Induced Nephropathy

N-acetylcysteine (Mucomyst) is an antioxidant that acts as a scavenger of oxygen free radicals and inhibitor of certain proteins implicated in kidney damage from iodine-based contrast media. Dosing protocols vary, but typically patients receive 600 mg PO twice a day on the day before, day of, and day after the procedure. Several randomized, controlled studies have shown its efficacy when used in addition to IV hydration, although some reports have failed to show any additional benefit.[32-36] In fact, serum creatinine may even drop below levels achieved with simple hydration. The agent may be more effective when smaller volumes of contrast material are given.[35]

Fenoldopam (Corlopam) is a dopamine-1 agonist approved by the U.S. Food and Drug Administration (FDA) for treatment of severe, refractory hypertension. There is some evidence that the drug also may limit the risk of contrast-induced nephropathy, although large, controlled trials are lacking.[37-39] The drug is given as an IV infusion at 0.1 µg/min beginning 2 to 4 hours before and continuing 4 to 6 hours after contrast is given.

Sodium bicarbonate infusion (154 mEq/L as 3 mL/kg/hr bolus for 1 hour before contrast administration, followed by 1 mL/kg/hr for 6 hours afterward) was found to be more effective than saline hydration in prevention of contrast nephropathy in patients with some degree of renal dysfunction undergoing cardiac catheterization.[40]

Theophylline is an antagonist of adenosine, which has been implicated in contrast-related nephropathy by a vasoconstrictor effect leading to reduced glomerular filtration. A number of reports have identified a substantial renal protective effect of theophylline in patients.[41,42] The drug is given orally or as an IV infusion (200 mg) several hours before the procedure.

Prophylactic Antibiotics

Antibiotic prophylaxis is primarily used for procedures in which infected tissues or colonized mucosal surfaces may be traversed. Surgical practice dictates that antibiotics are given within 2 hours of the procedure. Supplemental doses may be required for long cases. In some situations, antibiotics should be continued for several days afterward (e.g., biliary drainage).[43,44]

In few areas of interventional radiology is there more controversy than the indications for and selection of antibiotics for prophylaxis. The preferred drugs for antibiotic coverage vary widely among physicians and institutions. General guidelines have been described, but each group should establish protocols in conjunction with infectious disease colleagues.[43-45]

Antibiotics are generally used in the following cases:

- All biliary procedures
- Genitourinary procedures (with noted exceptions)
- Drainage of suspected abscess collections
- Therapeutic vascular procedures leading to tissue ablation (e.g., chemoembolization, tumor devascularization)
- Transjugular intrahepatic portosystemic shunt (TIPS) procedure
- Endograft placement

Prophylactic antibiotics are generally **not** indicated in the following cases:

- Routine angiographic procedures
- Urinary tract tube changes and checks in patients with intact immune systems
- Clear fluid aspirations (e.g., renal cyst)

Use of prophylactic antibiotics is controversial in the following cases:

- Placement of implanted vascular access devices
- Hemodialysis access treatment
- Intravascular stent placement
- Thrombolysis procedures
- Non-neoplastic embolization procedures
- Gastrostomy

Patients with prosthetic heart valves, history of bacterial endocarditis, or valvular abnormalities require coverage for *Enterococcus* species during urinary, gastrointestinal, biliary, and abscess drainage procedures.

Correction of Coagulopathies

Treatment of coagulation abnormalities is outlined in Table 1-3.[22,24,46] PT/INR prolongation commonly results from warfarin therapy, liver disease, vitamin K deficiency, or disseminated intravascular coagulopathy. Prolongation of the PTT is most often seen with heparin therapy. Qualitative platelet defects may be present in patients with uremia or consumptive coagulopathies.

TABLE 1-3   CORRECTION OF COAGULATION ABNORMALITIES

Parameter	Treatment
Prothrombin time or international normalized ratio	Withhold warfarin, start heparin, withhold before procedure Fresh-frozen plasma (FFP), 2–4 bags or 10–15 mL/kg Vitamin K, 1–3 mg (IV); may be repeated after 6–8 hr
Partial thromboplastin time	Withhold heparin 2–6 hr before procedure FFP, 2–4 bags or 10–15 mL/kg
Platelet count	Platelet transfusion (10 units to increase count by 50,000–100,000/mm³)
Bleeding time	Cryoprecipitate (0.2 bag/kg) Desmopressin (DDAVP), 0.4 µg/kg over 30 min Platelet transfusion

Some agents, such as platelets, fresh-frozen plasma, or desmopressin, should be given just before the cases. Other regimens, such as withholding warfarin, require a delay of the procedure. The effect of oral antiplatelet and non-steroidal anti-inflammatory agents on bleeding time usually is small. However, some practitioners withhold these drugs for 5 to 10 days before elective nonvascular procedures that involve insertion of very-large-bore catheters or needles.

■ INTRAPROCEDURE CARE

Radiation Safety

The radiation dose to the patient can be minimized by limiting fluoroscopy time, careful beam collimation, and use of lead shields. As more complex interventional procedures have developed over the last decade, there is now evidence that some procedures cause significant radiation exposure and a real risk of skin injury.[47-50] Transient skin damage may occur after a dose of 2 Gy. Permanent damage usually requires doses above 5 Gy.[50] The procedures with greatest risk include TIPS, embolization, intravascular stent placement, and uterine artery embolization. Dose data should be recorded for all interventional radiology (IR) procedures, ideally as peak skin dose. Unfortunately, fluoroscopy time is a relatively poor measure of actual skin dose. Doses should be carefully monitored for the higher risk cases or when multiple sequential procedures are performed.

Interventionalists are at particular risk for excessive radiation exposure over their lifetimes. Radiation monitoring badges must be worn at all times. The major complications of long-term radiation exposure in this group include cataracts, thyroid cancer, and hematologic malignancies. Operators should protect themselves by use of protective clothing, such as body aprons, thyroid shields, and leaded glasses, and by other methods, such as beam collimation, use of last image hold, and use of moveable leaded barriers during fluoroscopy and manual acquisition of digital images.[51] Appropriate tube angulation can greatly reduce radiation exposure to the arm during nonvascular procedures.

Infectious Disease Precautions

The risk of transmission of blood-borne pathogens from physician to patient during vascular and interventional procedures is vanishingly small. However, the risk of transmission from patient to operator is very real.[52-54] In particular, transmission of hepatitis B or C virus and human immunodeficiency virus (HIV) is of particular concern to health care workers.

Because of the potentially grave consequences of these infections, universal precautions should be followed, as mandated in the United States by the Occupational Safety and Health Administration. These precautions include use of surgical gowns, masks, protective eyewear, and two pairs of gloves. Gloves should be changed every few hours during long procedures and whenever glove integrity is breeched.[55]

A secure place for all sharp objects is kept on the interventional table. Needles are never recapped with a gloved hand alone. If a needle stick does occur, the occupational safety department should be consulted immediately. Prophylactic treatment for possible HIV infection should begin within 1 hour of exposure.

Patient Monitoring

The interventionalist should note the baseline vital signs before the procedure begins. Patients undergo continuous cardiac monitoring, continuous pulse oximetry, and cuff blood pressure measurement every 5 to 10 minutes, depending on the patient's condition. The nurse should record the respiratory rate, degree of sedation, and overall patient status every 5 to 10 minutes throughout the case. Oxygen is given by nasal cannula or face mask to maintain the oxygen saturation above about 90% to 92%.

Fluid Management

The type and rate of IV fluid infusion are based on preexisting conditions (e.g., diabetes, renal failure, congestive heart failure) and the volume of intravascular contrast material being given. As a general rule, fluids are run at about 1 mL/kg/hr. One study found that the incidence of renal dysfunction after angiography was lower with vigorous saline hydration alone than with the use of mannitol or furosemide to induce diuresis after the procedure.[56] A Foley catheter is placed for patient comfort and to monitor urine output during long or complex procedures.

Sedation and Analgesia

Patients undergoing vascular and interventional radiologic procedures always experience some anxiety and pain, but the degree of discomfort may not reflect the invasiveness of the procedure. Perhaps the most important (and sometimes neglected) method to reduce anxiety and pain is reassurance. Patients can tolerate an invasive procedure more easily when the interventionalist and other personnel show genuine concern for the patient's fears and discomfort and alert the patient to each sensation he or she is about to experience as the case proceeds.

The goals of sedation during interventional procedures are relief of pain, anxiolysis, partial amnesia, and control of patient behavior. In most cases, these goals can be met with *moderate (conscious) sedation*, in which the patient is calm, drowsy, and may even close his eyes but is responsive to verbal commands and able to protect his reflexes and airway.[57,58] *Deep sedation* (in which protective reflexes are lost) and *general anesthesia* are required for some interventional procedures but should be administered only by an anesthesiologist or a physician specially trained in these techniques.

The standard analgesic and sedative agents employed during vascular and interventional procedures are narcotics, benzodiazepines, and neuroleptic tranquilizers. A wide variety of agents can be used to produce moderate sedation. One of the most popular combinations is midazolam and fentanyl.[58,59]

Midazolam (Versed) is a short-acting benzodiazepine that acts on GABA receptors to cause central nervous system depression (including anxiolysis and antegrade amnesia). It is metabolized by the liver. The onset of action is 2 to 4 minutes, and the duration of action is about 45 to 60 minutes. The standard initial dose is 0.5 to 2.0 mg IV. Additional doses are given every 3 to 5 minutes to achieve the desired level of sedation. The optimal dose often is lower in patients with small body mass, advanced age, liver or cardiopulmonary disease, baseline hypotension, or a depressed level of consciousness. The major side effects of midazolam are respiratory depression and apnea.

Fentanyl (Sublimaze) is a short-acting narcotic opioid analgesic that also is metabolized by the liver. Its onset of action is 2 to 4 minutes, and the duration of action is about 30 to 60 minutes. The initial and incremental IV dose is 25 to 50 μg. Larger doses may be required in patients with a history of chronic narcotic use or abuse. Major side effects include vasovagal reactions, dysphoria, and respiratory depression.

After the initial doses are given, additional doses are generally required every 3 to 10 minutes to maintain a continuous level of comfort. The interventional nurse must work closely with the interventionalist to achieve a steady but safe level of sedation and analgesia throughout the procedure. Particularly high-risk comorbid conditions include advanced age, obesity, chronic obstructive lung disease, coronary artery disease, hepatic or renal insufficiency, and history of drug addiction.

The primary signs of overmedication are a drop in oxygen saturation and respiratory depression. Some patients exhibit a delayed or profound reaction to even small doses of these agents. Oxygen administered by nasal cannula or face mask should be given if the oxygen saturation falls below 90%. A discussion of pediatric sedation is beyond the scope of this chapter but has been the subject of numerous reviews.[60]

Treatment of Adverse Events and Reactions

Fortunately, adverse reactions during interventional procedures are relatively infrequent. Successful management of these events depends on recognizing problems

---

BOX 1-7 ■ Intraprocedural Hypoxia/Respiratory Depression

Overmedication with sedatives/analgesics
Pulmonary embolism (including air embolism)
Congestive heart failure
Pneumothorax
Aspiration

---

quickly, acting promptly, and employing basic resuscitative efforts:

- Continuous patient monitoring
- Protecting the patient's airway
- Securing the intravenous line and administering fluid replacement as needed
- Giving supplemental oxygen
- Calling for assistance early

Some of the more common clinical scenarios are outlined in Boxes 1-6 through 1-9. Management of specific events are discussed below.

Reaction to Sedatives and Analgesics

The most common symptoms of overdosage are hypoxia and respiratory depression. Less commonly, patients exhibit nausea, vomiting, hypotension, bradycardia, agitation, or confusion. Hypoxia alone can usually be managed by supplemental oxygen, a jaw thrust to maintain the airway, and withholding additional sedatives. Nausea and vomiting respond to a variety of antiemetic agents, including 2.5 to 10 mg IV of *prochlorperazine (Compazine)*.

Patients with profound respiratory depression or hypotension should receive supplemental oxygen, airway maintenance, and antagonists to the offending drugs. *Naloxone (Narcan)* is an opiate antagonist. The initial dose of 0.2 to 0.4 mg given by IV push may be repeated every 2 to 3 minutes. *Flumazenil (Romazicon)* is a benzodiazepine antagonist. The initial dose of 0.2 mg given by IV push may be repeated up to a total dose of 3 mg. Continued administration of these agents may be needed to treat overmedication.

BOX 1-6 ■ Intraprocedural Hypotension

Overmedication with sedatives/analgesics
Bleeding
Sepsis
Contrast or drug reaction
Myocardial infarction
Pulmonary embolism (including air embolism)

BOX 1-8 ■ Intraprocedural Altered Mental Status

Sedative/analgesic medication
Hypoglycemia
Anxiety
Vasovagal reaction
Bleeding/hypovolemia
Hypoxia
Stroke
Myocardial infarction or dysrhythmia

Vasovagal Reaction

Symptoms include hypotension with **bradycardia**, nausea, and diaphoresis. Immediate treatment includes elevation of the legs, rapid infusion of IV fluids, and administration of atropine. *Atropine* is a muscarinic, cholinergic blocking agent that affects the heart, bronchial and intestinal smooth muscle, central nervous system, secretory glands, and iris.[61] The initial dose is 0.5 to 1.0 mg IV, which may be repeated every 3 to 5 minutes up to a total dose of 2.5 mg. Major side effects include confusion, dry mouth, blurred vision, and bladder retention. The drug can be reversed with 1 to 4 mg IV of *physostigmine*.

Hypertension

The most common causes of hypertension during interventional procedures are uncontrolled baseline hypertension, withholding routine antihypertensive medications, anxiety or pain, bladder distention, and hypoxia. Most patients become normotensive after sedatives and analgesics are given. The major risks of sustained hypertension are local bleeding after removal of an angiographic catheter or remote bleeding in patients undergoing treatment with anticoagulants or fibrinolytic agents. If severe hypertension persists, several drugs should be considered.[62]

Sublingual *nifedipine* (10 mg) was once considered the first-line agent for several reasons, including its rapid onset of action (5 to 10 minutes). Because of scattered reports of life-threatening hypotension associated with this drug, many practitioners have turned to the nonselective beta blocker *labetalol*. This agent is given intravenously in 5 to 10 mg increments up to 20 mg. The action is rapid (5 to 10 minutes) and prolonged (3 to 6 hours). Labetalol should be avoided in patients with asthma or congestive heart failure. Other agents to consider in patients with refractory hypertension are metoprolol, esmolol, and nitroglycerin paste. Oral *clonidine* (initial dose 0.1 to 0.2 mg PO) may be useful in the postprocedure period.

Bleeding

When tachycardia and hypotension occur without other explanation, bleeding from the puncture site or by inadvertent laceration of major vessels should be considered. Often, this bleeding will be undetectable by observation alone. Rapid infusion of fluid should be started, a blood count and type and cross obtained, and assessment of potentially damaged structures considered (e.g., CT scan).

Mild Contrast Agent Reaction

Patient reassurance should be the first step in the treatment of all contrast reactions, regardless of severity.[63,64] Mild contrast reactions produce urticaria or nausea and vomiting. These symptoms may presage a more severe reaction. Nausea and vomiting usually occur with the first dose of contrast material and are self-limited. Persistent symptoms may be treated with an intravenous antiemetic, such as *prochlorperazine* 2.5 to 10 mg or *droperidol* 0.625 to 1.25 mg. Many interventionalists have observed that mild contrast reactions are less common with intra-arterial injections than intravenous injections, and specific therapy is rarely needed.

Hives usually require no direct treatment. If itching is bothersome or the rash is widespread, intravenous administration of the H_1 receptor–blocking agent *diphenhydramine (Benadryl)* (12.5 to 25 mg) may be helpful. Intravenous administration of 300 mg of the H_2 antagonist *cimetidine (Tagamet)* may be added if diphenhydramine is incompletely effective.

Moderate Contrast Agent Reaction

Moderate reactions to contrast are manifested by mild bronchospasm or wheezing, mild facial or laryngeal edema, or isolated hypotension with tachycardia. Patients being treated with beta-adrenergic blocking agents may not become tachycardiac. Bronchospasm should be treated with supplemental oxygen, an inhaled bronchodilator such as *metaproterenol (Alupent)*, and *subcutaneous* administration of 0.1 mg of a *1:1000* concentration of epinephrine, which may be repeated every 15 minutes. Some practitioners also give 100 mg of methylprednisolone *(Solu-Medrol)* intravenously. Isolated hypotension and tachycardia should be treated with leg elevation, rapid infusion of IV fluids (normal saline or Ringer's lactate), and 10 to 20 μg/kg/min of *dopamine* (as needed). Fluid overload should be avoided.

Severe Contrast Agent Reaction

Life-threatening reactions to contrast are fortunately very rare. They are manifested by severe bronchospasm or laryngospasm and profound hypotension. These events require prompt, aggressive treatment with supplemental oxygen, rapid IV fluid infusion, and *IV* administration of 0.1 mg of a *1:10,000* concentration of epinephrine. The dose may be repeated every 2 to 3 minutes.

Epinephrine must be given with care in patients with cardiac dysrhythmias, coronary artery disease, or those undergoing treatment with nonselective beta-adrenergic blocking agents (e.g., propranolol). Patients who are poor candidates for epinephrine or have refractory hypotension may be treated with 300 mg IV of cimetidine. These reactions may progress to complete cardiovascular collapse.

Hypoglycemia

Diabetic patients receiving insulin or oral hypoglycemic agents may become hypoglycemic during the procedure. Symptoms may include mental confusion, agitation, tremors, seizures, and cardiac arrest (which is rare). If hypoglycemia is suspected, an infusion of 5% to 10% dextrose should be started and the blood glucose level should be checked. If symptoms are severe or the serum glucose level is very low, one ampule (50 mL) of 50% dextrose given by IV push is indicated.

Dysrhythmias

Cardiac dysrhythmias that develop during interventional procedures usually are caused by guidewire or catheter manipulation in the heart or by metabolic problems such as hypoxia, hypercarbia, electrolyte imbalances, or myocardial ischemia. Mechanically induced dysrhythmias usually revert after repositioning the guidewire. Sustained dysrhythmias should be treated in consultation with a cardiologist or physician with experience in such situations.

Paroxysmal supraventricular tachycardia usually reverts with *adenosine*, which slows the sinus rate and atrioventricular node conduction velocity.[65] The initial dose is 6 mg given by rapid IV push; a 12-mg dose may be required if there is no response after several minutes. The onset of action is immediate, and transient asystole (<5 seconds) should be expected.

An alternative to adenosine is the calcium channel blocking agent *verapamil*; a dose of 0.1 mg/kg is given by slow IV push. This drug should be avoided in patients with conduction abnormalities or those who are taking beta-adrenergic blocking agents.

Ventricular tachycardia (VT), when caused by guidewire manipulation in the heart, usually is transient and reverts with a chest thump or asking the patient to cough. Asymptomatic sustained VT is treated with *lidocaine*, which affects neuronal membranes by blocking sodium ion channels. The initial dose is 3 to 4 mg/kg given IV over 20 to 30 minutes followed by an infusion at 1 to 4 mg/min. The onset of action is immediate. Major side effects include confusion, seizures, and cardiopulmonary depression. Symptomatic VT requires cardioversion (1 to 50 watt-sec) followed by *amiodarone* infusion (150 mg in 100 mL dextrose given over 10 minutes).

Sepsis

Bacteremia is a concern during nonvascular procedures, particularly those that involve manipulation of abscesses or the biliary and urinary systems.[66] Fever, chills, or rigors are common; frank septic shock occurs much less frequently. Broad spectrum antibiotics should be started immediately if they have not already been given. Rigors usually respond to 25 to 50 mg IV of *meperidine* (Demerol). Hypotension from sepsis can be initially managed with IV saline boluses and a 10 to 20 mcg/kg/min infusion of *dopamine*.

Seizures

Seizures may be idiopathic or a reaction to drugs given during the procedure (e.g., contrast agents). Treatment includes protection of the patient's airway and body, supplemental oxygen, and 5 to 10 mg IV of *diazepam* (Valium), given as needed.

Air Embolism

This event is a rare occurrence during vascular access placement.[67] Most patients remain asymptomatic but hypoxia and hypotension can occur. Although some experts advocate placing the patient in a left lateral decubitus position to prevent air from entering the right ventricular outflow tract, by the time the event is detected by fluoroscopy, air has usually migrated into the pulmonary arteries. Air embolism is rarely fatal. Treatment usually is supportive, including supplemental oxygen, IV fluids, and continuous patient monitoring.

Cardiopulmonary Arrest

Cardiorespiratory collapse may result from the patient's underlying condition (e.g., massive pulmonary embolus, multiorgan failure) or some aspect of the procedure itself (e.g., contrast agent reaction, oversedation). Regardless of the cause, basic life support maneuvers must be started immediately, including alerting a code team, establishing an airway, and beginning cardiopulmonary resuscitation.

■ POSTPROCEDURE CARE

Catheter Removal

Catheters are withdrawn immediately after vascular and interventional procedures unless ongoing intervention is necessary (e.g., overnight thrombolysis, abscess drainage). Before removing an angiographic catheter, the status of the puncture site and distal extremity should be assessed. Hypertension should be controlled beforehand. The risk of hemorrhagic complications can be reduced in patients who have received heparin during the procedure if catheter removal is delayed until the activated clotting time (ACT) falls into the high-normal range.

Specific details of puncture site compression and use of compressive dressings or arterial closure devices are considered in Chapter 2. In general, sufficient digital compression is applied directly at, above, and below the puncture site to stop bleeding but maintain blood flow. Pressure is applied for 10 to 20 minutes or until bleeding has stopped. Closure of jugular vein punctures is facilitated by elevating the patient's head. If a hematoma is present after the procedure, it should be marked on the skin and documented in the patient's chart.

Patient Monitoring

Postprocedure monitoring is similar to the routine used during the procedure. After arterial catheterization, the puncture site and distal pulses should be checked throughout the observation period: every 15 minutes for 1 hour, every 30 minutes for the next hour, and every hour thereafter. The length of outpatient monitoring varies with the type of procedure. Generally, patients are observed for 30 to 90 minutes after the last dose of sedatives or analgesics is given and until institutional discharge criteria are met. After diagnostic femoral or brachial arteriography, a 4- to 6-hour observation period is routine (unless a closure device is used). After diagnostic femoral or jugular venography, a 2- to 4-hour observation period is common.

Orders

Patient orders should include the following information:

- *Activity*: The patient is kept on bed rest until the monitoring period is completed.
- *Pain control*: Immediate postprocedure analgesia is primarily accomplished with oral and parenteral opioids (e.g., morphine, hydromorphone [Dilaudid], fentanyl, meperidine [Demerol], codeine, and hydrocodone [Vicodin]).[68]
- *Diet*: After sedatives and analgesics wear off, patients can be given liquids or a soft solid meal.
- *Hydration*: IV hydration usually is continued throughout the postprocedure period if intravascular contrast was given. IV access should be maintained while the patient recovers from moderate sedation.
- *Vital signs and access site checks*: Monitoring usually is done every 15 minutes for the first hour and then tapered over the observation period.

Management of Acute Complications

Identification and management of delayed complications of various vascular and interventional procedures are considered in detail in Chapter 2. The most common acute angiographic complications are described here.

Puncture site bleeding or hematoma in most cases produces firm swelling directly around the access site. Treatment includes local compression and correction of precipitating factors (e.g., coagulopathy, hypertension). If the patient has received heparin and hemostasis cannot be achieved in a reasonable period, *protamine sulfate* can be used to reverse anticoagulation.[69] By itself, protamine is a weak anticoagulant; 10 mg of protamine neutralizes 1000 units of heparin. A typical IV dose of 20 to 40 mg is injected *slowly* over 10 minutes. Rapid injection can produce profound hypotension, bradycardia, flushing, and dyspnea. Patients with a history of fish allergy, previous protamine therapy, or treatment with protamine-containing insulin (e.g., NPH, isophane insulin) are at increased risk for anaphylactic reactions and should not receive the drug.

Patients with an enlarging hematoma or postprocedure hypotension should be followed with serial hematocrits. Consultation with a vascular surgeon is warranted in most cases. Occasionally, occult bleeding into the retroperitoneal space or thigh may occur, but the patient presents only with hypotension or a decreased hematocrit. In this case, CT scanning may be helpful to localize the bleeding.[70] A marked drop in hematocrit or massive hematoma may require blood transfusion, surgical evacuation, or both.

Arterial occlusion can be produced by thrombosis or dissection at the puncture site. Femoral or brachial artery occlusion is suspected by a loss of distal pulses or the development of ischemic symptoms. Angiography of the affected limb should be performed.

Distal clot embolization usually results from a clot that formed on the catheter or punctured artery. These emboli

---

BOX 1-10 ■ Discharge Criteria after Vascular and Interventional Procedures

Stable vital signs with no respiratory depression
Alert and oriented
Able to drink, void, and ambulate
Minimal residual pain
Minimal nausea
No bleeding at access site
Discharge with competent adult

---

often are silent. Some cases of asymptomatic embolization may be treated conservatively with observation and anticoagulation. A patient with a threatened limb should undergo diagnostic arteriography.

Cholesterol embolization is a rare complication that results from disruption of an atherosclerotic plaque by manipulation of catheters or guidewires.[71] Cholesterol microemboli are showered into distal vascular beds, including those of the legs, kidneys, or bowel. Patients develop severe leg pain and a reddish, netlike pattern on the lower abdomen and legs *(livedo reticularis)*, but the pedal pulses remain intact. Renal failure is common, and the mortality rate is high.

Discharge Instructions and Follow-up

Several criteria should be met before discharge of outpatients after vascular and interventional procedures (Box 1-10). Patients should receive written instructions about care of the access or puncture site, catheter exit site, or external catheter. Postprocedure antibiotics or medications (if any), treatment of postprocedure pain, and warning signs of complications and how to deal with them (including a physician or nurse contact) are discussed with the patient. A responsible adult should accompany the patient home and preferably stay with him or her until the following day.

Performing an interventional procedure often entails a commitment to follow-up and long-term care of the patient, including daily rounds for inpatients or periodic outpatient visits. A follow-up appointment should be scheduled to evaluate the results of therapy, identify complications, and determine the need for further intervention.

REFERENCES

1. Sacks D, McClenny TE, Cardella JF, Lewis CA: Society of Interventional Radiology clinical practice guidelines. J Vasc Interv Radiol 2003;14 (9 Pt 2):S199.
2. Kandarpa K, Aruny JE, eds: Handbook of Interventional Radiologic Procedures. Boston, Philadelphia, Lippincott Williams & Wilkins, 2001:3.
3. Perler BA: Hypercoagulability and the hypercoagulability syndromes. AJR Am J Roentgenol 1995;164:559.
4. Insko EK, Haskal ZJ: Antiphospholipid syndrome: patterns of life-threatening and severe recurrent vascular complications. Radiology 1997;202:319.
5. Caprini JA, Glase CJ, Anderson CB, et al: Laboratory markers in the diagnosis of venous thromboembolism. Circulation 2004;109(Suppl 1):I4.

6. Perler BA: Review of hypercoagulability syndromes: what the interventionalist needs to know. J Vasc Interv Radiol 1991;2:183.
7. Crowther MA, Kelton JG: Congenital thrombophilic states associated with venous thrombosis: a qualitative overview and proposed classification system. Ann Intern Med 2003;138:128.
8. Berlin L: Informed consent. AJR Am J Roentgenol 1997;169:15.
9. Reuter SR: An overview of informed consent for radiologists. AJR Am J Roentgenol 1987;148:219.
10. Egglin TKP, O'Moore PV, Feinstein AR, et al: Complications of peripheral arteriography: a new system to identify patients at increased risk. J Vasc Surg 1995;22:787.
11. Katzenschlager R, Ugurluoglu A, Ahmadi A, et al: Incidence of pseudoaneurysm after diagnostic and therapeutic angiography. Radiology 1995;195:463.
12. Arepally A, Oechsle D, Kirkwood S, et al: Safety of conscious sedation in interventional radiology. Cardiovasc Intervent Radiol 2001;24:185.
13. Murphy TP, Dorfman GS, Becker J: Use of preprocedure tests by interventional radiologists. Radiology 1993;186:213.
14. Johnson H, Knee-Ioli S, Butler TA, et al: Are routine preoperative laboratory screening tests necessary to evaluate ambulatory surgical patients? Surgery 1988;104:639.
15. Kaplan EB, Sheiner LB, Boeckmann AJ, et al: The usefulness of preoperative laboratory screening. JAMA 1985;253:3576.
16. Curhan GC: Prevention of contrast nephropathy. JAMA 2003;289:606.
17. Ellis JH, Cohan RH, Sonnad SS, Cohan NS: Selective use of radiographic low-osmolality contrast media in the 1990s. Radiology 1996; 200:297.
18. Barrett BJ, Carlisle EJ: Metaanalysis of the relative nephrotoxicity of high- and low-osmolality iodinated contrast media. Radiology 1993;188:171.
19. Rudnick RR, Goldfarb S, Wexler L, et al: Nephrotoxicity of ionic and nonionic contrast media in 1196 patients: a randomized trial. The Iohexol Cooperative Study. Kidney Int 1995;47:254.
20. Katholi RE, Taylor GJ, Woods WT, et al: Nephrotoxicity of nonionic low-osmolality versus ionic high-osmolality contrast media: a prospective double blind randomized comparison in human beings. Radiology 1993;186:183.
21. Aspelin P, Aubry P, Fransson S-G, et al: Nephrotoxic effects in high-risk patients undergoing angiography. N Engl J Med 2003;348:491.
22. Payne CS: A primer on patient management problems in interventional radiology. AJR Am J Roentgenol 1998;170:1169.
23. Hirsh J, Poller L: The international normalized ratio: a guide to understanding and correcting its problems. Arch Intern Med 1994;154:282.
24. Barth KH, Matsumoto AH: Patient care in interventional radiology: a perspective. Radiology 1991;178:11.
25. Gross JB, Bailey PL, Caplan RA, et al: Practice guidelines for sedation and analgesia by non-anesthesiologists. Anesthesiology 1996;84:459.
26. Hirsch IB: Management of the diabetic patient. J Vasc Interv Radiol 1996;7(Suppl):79.
27. Nawaz S, Cleveland T, Gaines PA, Chan P: Clinical risk associated with contrast angiography in metformin treated patients: a clinical review. Clin Radiol 1998;53:342.
28. Bhatt DL, Lee BI, Castarella PJ, et al: Safety of concomitant therapy with eptifibatide and enoxaparin patients undergoing percutaneous coronary intervention: results of the Coronary Revascularization Using Integrilin and Single Bolus Enoxaparin Study. J Am Coll Cardiol 2003;41:20.
29. Freed KS, Leder RA, Alexander C, et al: Breakthrough adverse reactions to low-osmolar contrast media after steroid premedication. AJR Am J Roentgenol 2001;176:1389.
30. Thomsen HS, Morcos SK, Contrast Media Safety Committee of the European Society of Urogenital Radiology (ESUR): Prevention of generalized reactions to CM. Acad Radiol 2002;9(Suppl 2):S433.
31. Wittbrodt ET, Spinler SA: Prevention of anaphylactoid reactions in high-risk patients receiving radiographic contrast media. Ann Pharmacother 1994;28:236.
32. Shyu K-G, Cheng J-J, Kuan P: Acetylcysteine protects against acute renal damage in patients with abnormal renal function undergoing a coronary procedure. J Am Coll Cardiol 2002;40:1383.
33. Tepel M, van der Giet M, Schwarzfeld C, et al: Prevention of radiographic-contrast agent-induced reductions in renal function by acetylcysteine. N Engl J Med 2000;343:180.
34. Kay J, Chow WH, Chan TM, et al: Acetylcysteine for prevention of acute deterioration of renal function following elective coronary angiography and intervention. A randomized controlled trial. JAMA 2003;289:553.
35. Briguori C, Manganelli F, Scarpato P, et al: Acetylcysteine and contrast agent-associated nephrotoxicity. J Am Coll Cardiol 2002;40:298.
36. Diaz-Sandoval LJ, Kosowsky BD, Losordo DW: Acetylcysteine to prevent angiography-related renal tissue issue (the APART trial). Am J Cardiol 2002;89:356.
37. Hunter D: Fenoldopam: a dopamine 1 receptor agonist in the prevention of renal injury associated with the administration of intravascular contrast. J Vasc Interv Radiol 2000;11:396.
38. Madyoon H, Croushore L, Weaver D, et al: Use of fenoldopam to prevent radiocontrast nephropathy in high-risk patients. Catheter Cardiovasc Interv 2001;53:341
39. Allaqaband S, Tumuluri R, Malik AM, et al: Prospective, randomized study of N-acetylcysteine, fenoldopam, and saline for prevention of radiocontrast-induced nephropathy. Catheter Cardiovasc Interv 2002;57:279.
40. Merten GJ, Burgess WP, Gray LV, et al: Prevention of contrast-induced nephropathy with sodium bicarbonate: a randomized controlled trial. JAMA 2004;291:2328.
41. Erley CM, Duda SH, Rehfuss D, et al: Prevention of radiocontrast-media-induced nephropathy in patients with pre-existing renal insufficiency by hydration in combination with the adenosine antagonist theophylline. Nephrol Dial Transplant 1999;14:1146.
42. Huber W, Ilgmann K, Page M, et al: Effect of theophylline on contrast material-induced nephropathy in patients with chronic renal insufficiency: controlled, randomized double-blinded study. Radiology 2002;223:772.
43. Ryan JM, Ryan BM, Smith TP: Antibiotic prophylaxis in interventional radiology. J Vasc Interv Radiol 2004;15:547.
44. McDermott VG, Schuster MG, Smith TP: Antibiotic prophylaxis in vascular and interventional radiology. AJR Am J Roentgenol 1997;169:31.
45. Dravid VS, Gupta A, Zegel HG, et al: Investigation of antibiotic prophylaxis usage for vascular and non-vascular interventional procedures. J Vasc Interv Radiol 1998;9:401.
46. Development Task Force of the College of American Pathologists: Practice parameter for the use of fresh-frozen plasma, cryoprecipitate, and platelets. JAMA 1994;271:777.
47. Wagner LK, McNeese MD, Marx MV, et al: Severe skin reactions from interventional fluoroscopy: case report and review of the literature. Radiology 1999;213:773.
48. Miller DL, Balter S, Cole PE, et al: Radiation doses in interventional radiology procedures: The RAD-IR study. Part I: Overall measures of dose. J Vasc Interv Radiol 2003;14:711.
49. Miller DL, Balter S, Cole PE, et al: Radiation doses in interventional radiology procedures: The RAD-IR study. Part II: Skin dose. J Vasc Interv Radiol 2003;14:977.
50. Marx MV: The radiation dose in interventional radiology: knowledge brings responsibility. J Vasc Interv Radiol 2003;14:947.
51. Marx MV, Niklason L, Mauger EA: Occupational radiation exposure to interventional radiologists: a prospective study. J Vasc Intervent Radiol 1992;3:597.
52. Hansen ME, Miller GL III, Redman HC, et al: HIV and interventional radiology: a national survey of physician attitudes and behaviors. J Vasc Intervent Radiol 1993;4:229.
53. Hansen ME, Miller GL III, Redman HC, et al: Needle-stick injuries and blood contacts during invasive radiologic procedures: frequency and risk factors. AJR Am J Roentgenol 1993;160:1119.
54. Baffoy-Fayard N, Maugat S, Sapoval M, et al: Potential exposure of hepatitis C virus through accidental blood contact in interventional radiology. J Vasc Interv Radiol 2003;14:173.
55. Hansen ME, McIntire DD, Miller GL III: Occult glove perforations: frequency during interventional radiologic procedures. AJR Am J Roentgenol 1992;159:131.
56. Solomon R, Werner C, Mann D, et al: Effects of saline, mannitol, and furosemide on acute decreases in renal function induced by radiocontrast agents. N Engl J Med 1994;331:1416.
57. Skehan SJ, Malone DE, Buckley N, et al: Sedation and analgesia in adult patients: evaluation of a staged-dose system based on body weight for use in abdominal interventional radiology. Radiology 2000;216:653.
58. Martin ML, Lennox PH: Sedation and analgesia in the interventional radiology department. J Vasc Interv Radiol 2003;14:1119.
59. Cragg AH, Smith TP, Berbaum KS, et al: Randomized double-blind trial of midazolam/placebo and midazolam/fentanyl for sedation and analgesia in lower-extremity angiography. AJR Am J Roentgenol 1991;157:173.
60. Fisher DM: Sedation of pediatric patients: an anesthesiologist's perspective. Radiology 1990;175:613.
61. McEvoy GK, ed: AHFS Drug Information 2002. Bethesda, Md, American Society of Health-System Pharmacists, 2002:1215.

62. Waybill MM, Waybill PN: A practical approach to hypertension in the 21st century. J Vasc Interv Radiol 2002;14:961.

63. Bush WH, Swanson DP: Acute reactions to intravascular contrast media: types, risk factors, recognition, and specific treatment. AJR Am J Roentgenol 1991;157:1153.

64. Thomsen HS, Bush WH Jr: Adverse effects of contrast media: incidence, prevention, and management. Drug Saf 1998;19:313.

65. Roden DM: Antiarrhythmic drugs. In: Hardman JG, Limbird LE, eds. Goodman and Gilman's Pharmacological Basis of Therapeutics, 10th ed. New York, McGraw-Hill, 2001:953.

66. Smith TP, Ryan JM, Niklason LE: Sepsis in the interventional radiology patient. J Vasc Interv Radiol 2004;15:317.

67. Vesely T: Air embolism during insertion of central venous catheters. J Vasc Interv Radiol 2001;12:1291.

68. Hatsiopoulou O, Cohen RI, Lang EV: Postprocedure pain management of interventional radiology patients. J Vasc Interv Radiol 2003;14:1373.

69. McEvoy GK, ed: AHFS Drug Information 2002. Bethesda, Md, American Society of Health-System Pharmacists, 2002:1453.

70. Trerotola SO, Kuhlman JE, Fishman EK: Bleeding complications of femoral catheterization: CT evaluation. Radiology 1990;174:37.

71. Bashore TM, Gehrig T: Cholesterol emboli after invasive cardiac procedures. J Am Coll Cardiol 2003;42:217.

2

Standard Angiographic and Interventional Techniques

▪ VASCULAR ACCESS

Anesthesia

A local anesthetic is given at the start of every vascular/ interventional procedure. The preferred agent is 1% or 2% lidocaine (Xylocaine), which inhibits sodium channels involved in the conduction of nerve impulses. An intradermal skin wheal is made with a 25-gauge needle. The deeper subcutaneous tissues are anesthetized with a long 22- or 25-gauge needle. Intravascular injection must be avoided by intermittent aspiration. The pain from lidocaine is largely caused by the low pH of commercially available preparations. Admixing the drug with sodium bicarbonate (1 mL of 1 mEq/mL $NaHCO_3$ solution in 10 mL of 1% lidocaine) diminishes the discomfort.[1] Patients with a lidocaine allergy may receive a procaine-based anesthetic (e.g., 1% chloroprocaine).[2] As an alternative, anesthesia can be achieved with a solution of diphenhydramine (Benadryl) with epinephrine (e.g., 0.2 mL epinephrine 1:1000 plus 10 mg Benadryl with saline to make a 10 mL solution).[3]

Retrograde Femoral Artery Catheterization

In 1953, Sven Ivar Seldinger first described the method for percutaneous arterial catheterization involving a needle, guidewire, and catheter.[4] The common femoral artery (CFA) is the safest and simplest arterial access route because it is large, superficial, usually disease free, and can be compressed against the femoral head to close the puncture. However, this approach should be avoided when the patient has a CFA aneurysm, local infection, overlying bowel, or a fresh incision. Within several weeks after placement, synthetic grafts in the groin also may be accessed safely using a single-wall needle.

When the skin is punctured over the bottom of the femoral head and the needle is angled at 45 degrees, the needle usually enters the CFA at its midpoint (Fig. 2-1). The inguinal crease is an imprecise landmark for skin puncture. If the puncture is low (into the superficial femoral artery [SFA] or deep femoral artery [DFA]), the risk of thrombosis, pseudoaneurysm, or arteriovenous fistula formation is significantly increased.[5,6] If the puncture is too high (into the external iliac artery above the inguinal ligament), the risk of

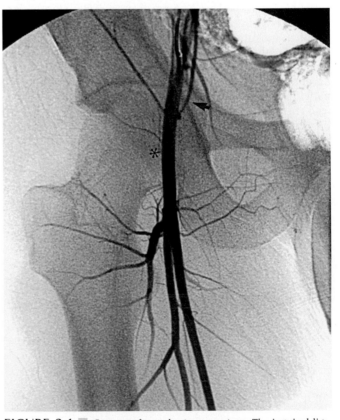

FIGURE 2-1 ▪ Common femoral artery puncture. The inguinal ligament is demarcated by the inferior epigastric artery *(arrow)*. The ideal arterial entry site is indicated by the *asterisk*.

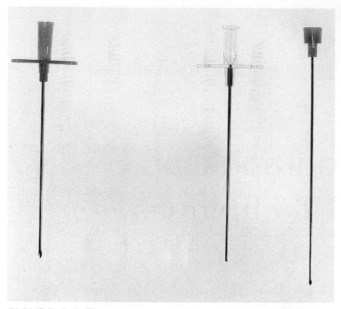

FIGURE 2-2 ■ Needles for vascular catheterization. The single-wall needle *(left)* has a sharp beveled edge. The Seldinger-type needle with stylet *(right)* can also be used for most arterial catheterization procedures.

retroperitoneal or intraperitoneal bleeding is increased. The bony landmarks for the inguinal ligament—a line running from the anterior superior iliac spine to the pubic tubercle—provide only a rough approximation.[7,8]

After selecting a skin entry site with fluoroscopy and applying local anesthesia, a small, superficial skin nick is made directly over the arterial pulse. A clamp is used to dissect the subcutaneous tissues. The course of the artery is palpated while an 18-gauge needle is advanced at a 45-degree angle toward the femoral head (Fig. 2-2). It is safer to use a 21-gauge micropuncture needle set in coagulopathic patients (Fig. 2-3). Many practitioners now prefer a single-wall entry into the vessel. However, because single-wall needles have a beveled tip, the tip may be partially subintimal despite brisk pulsatile blood return. Particular caution should be taken during guidewire insertion. If double-wall technique is used, the stylet is removed after bone is reached, and additional lidocaine is injected. The hub of the needle is depressed and then slowly withdrawn until pulsatile blood returns.

Slow return of dark blood usually is a sign of venous entry; the site is then compressed and a more lateral puncture is made.

A 0.035- or 0.038-inch Bentson or other floppy-tipped guidewire is carefully inserted and advanced under fluoroscopy. Resistance to passage usually means that the tip of the needle is partially subintimal, up against the sidewall, or abutting common femoral or iliac artery plaque. The wire should *never* be forced. A small change in needle position (e.g., medial to lateral, shallow to steep angle, slight withdrawal) usually allows the wire to pass; if not, contrast can be injected to identify the reason for resistance. If the guidewire still cannot be advanced, the needle is removed, compression is applied for about 5 minutes, and the artery is repunctured. Occasionally, the guidewire enters the deep iliac circumflex artery rather than the external iliac artery (Fig. 2-4). In this case, it is withdrawn and redirected.

After the guidewire is advanced to the abdominal aorta, a dilator is placed and then exchanged for an angiographic catheter (Fig. 2-5). If the iliac arteries are severely diseased, it may be easier and safer to first place a dilator in the external iliac artery and then negotiate a hydrophilic guidewire into the aorta.

A pulsatile artery may be surprisingly hard to puncture if the skin nick is malpositioned, the artery is unusually mobile, underlying disease exists, or vasospasm follows repeated puncture attempts. In these situations, the operator should consider making a second skin nick directly over the arterial pulse or at a slightly higher location, waiting until a strong pulse has returned, or using the opposite groin. When access is difficult or the femoral pulse is diminished, the artery can be punctured by using real-time sonographic guidance or fluoroscopic landmarks (e.g., medial edge of the femoral head, arterial calcification) (Fig. 2-6).[9,10] In fact, it is sometimes possible to catheterize the abdominal aorta even in the face of iliac artery occlusion if some flow can be detected by ultrasound in the CFA and a dilator and hydrophilic guidewire are used to negotiate the occlusion.

Catheter advancement often is difficult in patients with marked obesity, heavily diseased arteries, or a scarred groin. In this case, placement of a stiff or super-stiff guidewire, overdilation of the access site by 1 French size, or use of a stiff, tapered catheter (e.g., van Andel) may be helpful.

The puncture site is examined immediately after the catheter is inserted. Mild oozing usually stops after several minutes of gentle compression. A vascular sheath is placed

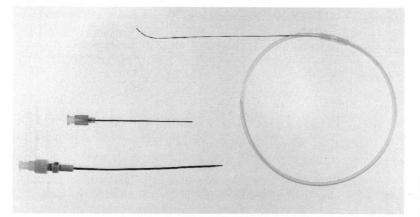

FIGURE 2-3 ■ Micropuncture access set with a 21-gauge needle, a 0.018-inch steerable guidewire, and a 4-French transitional dilator.

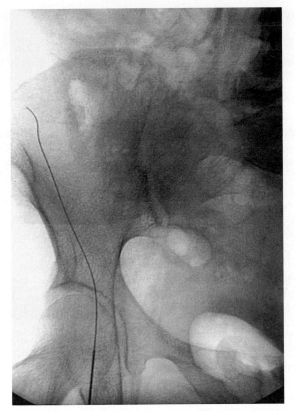

FIGURE 2-4 ■ The guidewire has entered the deep iliac circumflex artery. Notice that the needle enters the common femoral artery over the middle of the femoral head.

for persistent oozing or hematoma formation (see Fig. 2-5). If the pulse has diminished, an angiogram of the iliac and common femoral artery is obtained immediately. If the catheter has occluded a critical stenosis, heparin is given, and the obstruction is treated with angioplasty.

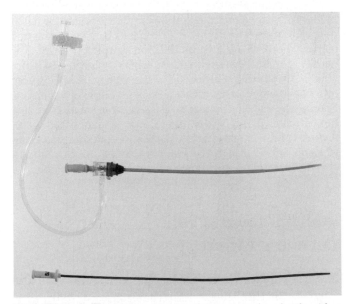

FIGURE 2-5 ■ Vascular access catheters: vascular sheath with a sidearm and inner dilator *(top)* and a tapered dilator *(bottom)*.

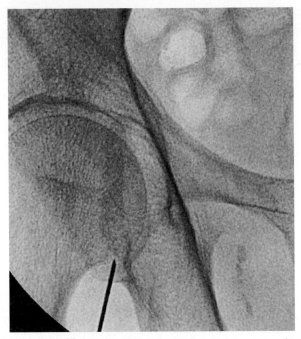

FIGURE 2-6 ■ Calcification in the wall of a pulseless common femoral artery is used to guide needle placement.

Antegrade Femoral Artery Catheterization

Antegrade (downhill) puncture of the CFA is occasionally required for infrainguinal procedures. The skin puncture is made over the top of the femoral head to enter the middle of the CFA below the inguinal ligament (see Fig. 2-1).[11] In obese patients, it is helpful to tape the pannus onto the abdomen. A steep needle angle (>45 to 60 degrees) should be avoided because catheters and sheaths may be difficult to insert or may kink after placement. Many practitioners prefer to use a single-wall needle.

The guidewire often enters the DFA. Access into the SFA[12-14] is accomplished in several ways:

- Replace the entry wire with an angled, steerable hydrophilic wire, which can often be manipulated into the SFA.
- Place an angled catheter into the DFA, mark the skin entry site with a clamp, and then slowly withdraw the catheter while injecting contrast. After the catheter tip is in the CFA, it can be directed medially and a steerable guidewire can be advanced into the SFA.
- Withdraw the guidewire into the needle, redirect the needle toward the opposite arterial wall, and readvance the wire.

High Brachial (Axillary) Artery Catheterization

Upper brachial or axillary artery catheterization is less desirable than CFA access because it is associated with a higher rate of debilitating complications and is more uncomfortable and awkward for the patient and physician. Indications for this route include:

- Absent femoral pulses or known aortic occlusion
- Recanalization of steeply downgoing mesenteric or renal arteries
- Treatment of obstructions in upper extremity arteries
- History of cholesterol embolization from prior retrograde aortic catheterization

The high brachial artery is preferred over the axillary or mid-brachial artery because complications occur less frequently.[15] The right arm is avoided because of the greater risk of embolic stroke with the catheter crossing all three arch vessels. However, if the brachial systolic blood pressure is significantly lower on the left (>20 mm Hg), suggesting significant left subclavian artery disease, the right side is used.

The arm is abducted. Entry is made over the proximal humeral shaft below the axillary fold (Fig. 2-7). Many interventionalists prefer to use a single-wall needle and real-time sonographic guidance. The artery is fixed in position by compressing it along its length or trapping it between the thumb and index finger. The needle is advanced at a 45-degree angle.

Often, the guidewire will enter the ascending thoracic aorta. With an angled or pigtail catheter in the aortic arch, a hydrophilic guidewire can be negotiated into the descending thoracic aorta.

Femoral Vein Catheterization

Before performing common femoral vein (CFV) catheterization, available lower extremity venous sonograms are reviewed

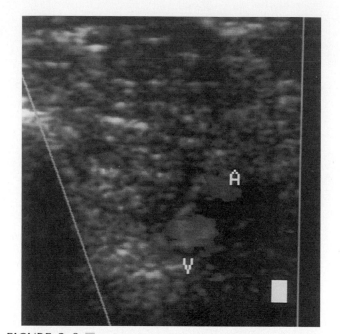

FIGURE 2-8 ■ Left common femoral vein (V) deep to the common femoral artery (A) is identified by color Doppler sonography.

to determine vessel patency. The CFV usually lies 0.5 to 1.5 cm medial to the CFA. The skin entry is made just medial to the arterial pulse and just below the bottom of the femoral head. In some patients, the vein is just medial and deep to the artery (Fig. 2-8).[16] A single-wall needle is preferred to avoid unknowingly passing through the artery before entering the vein. Otherwise, an arteriovenous fistula could result.[17]

Some practitioners use a 21-gauge micropuncture needle and ultrasound guidance to minimize the risk of arterial puncture, especially in coagulopathic patients. A saline-filled syringe with connecting tubing is attached to the needle. Cooperative patients are asked to perform a Valsalva maneuver to dilate the vein. The artery is palpated continuously. The needle is advanced with intermittent aspiration and should be redirected if transmitted pulsations from the artery are felt at the needle hub. Sometimes, the tip coapts both vein walls and pierces the back wall without blood return on entry. The needle is then slowly withdrawn while aspiration is maintained. After blood returns freely, the guidewire is advanced into the inferior vena cava (IVC), and a dilator is placed. Frequently, the wire tip meets resistance in a small ascending lumbar vein. If the guidewire is floppy, it may be advanced further until it buckles into the IVC. Repeated unsuccessful attempts at CFV puncture usually signify venous thrombosis, chronic disease, or an abnormally positioned vein.

Internal Jugular Vein Catheterization

Internal jugular (IJ) vein access is required for certain procedures (e.g., transjugular intrahepatic portosystemic shunt [TIPS] creation, IVC filter insertion with bilateral femoral or IVC thrombus) and preferred for other interventions

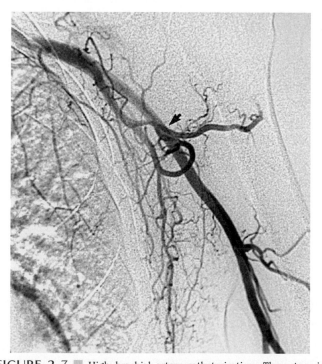

FIGURE 2-7 ■ High brachial artery catheterization. The artery is punctured over the proximal humeral shaft to enter below the axillary-brachial artery junction *(arrow)*.

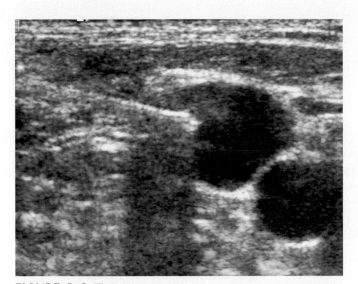

FIGURE 2-9 ■ Right internal jugular vein entry under sonographic guidance in the transverse plane. Needle enters from lateral approach, carotid artery is medial to the vein.

(e.g., vascular access placement, internal spermatic vein embolization, transvenous liver biopsy). In most cases, the right IJ vein is chosen over the left.

The vein is entered above the clavicle using direct sonographic guidance in a transverse plane to avoid arterial puncture or pneumothorax (Fig. 2-9).[18] The needle is advanced from a lateral approach or directly superior to the vein. A micropuncture set can be used to minimize trauma to the artery if it is accidentally pierced. Entry into the venous system is confirmed by following the course of the guidewire advanced into the right atrium.

Axillary/Subclavian Vein Catheterization

Subclavian vein access to the central venous system is discouraged over IJ catheterization for several reasons. Stenosis or occlusion is more frequent after placement of subclavian vein catheters.[19] The risk of pneumothorax is increased also. Finally, bleeding is more difficult to control if the subclavian artery is inadvertently entered or venous access is lost. If this route must be used, puncture should always be made with sonographic guidance. The preferred point of entry is the central axillary vein at the level of the coracoid process. The axillary/subclavian artery is first identified with ultrasound coursing just superior to the vein. With real-time guidance in a longitudinal plane, a micropuncture needle is used for venous entry (see Fig. 16-8).

Arterial Closure Devices

Manual compression of catheterization puncture sites has been the standard hemostatic technique for more than 50 years. However, this method requires additional operator time and rather prolonged patient immobilization afterward. Gaining hemostasis in anticoagulated patients or after large sheaths have been placed can be problematic. Arterial closure devices are meant to reduce time to ambulation while allowing effective and safe vascular closure, even in the face of anticoagulation.[20-24] Three categories of devices are currently in use:

■ Placement of collagen or creation of a collagen plug external to the punctured artery (e.g., VasoSeal, AngioSeal, and Duett devices) (Figs. 2-10 through 2-12)

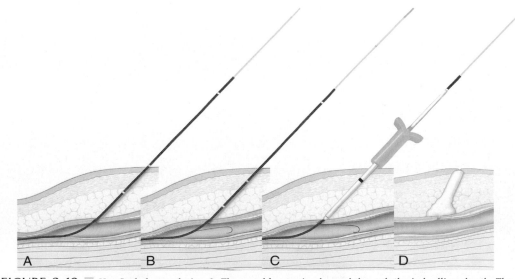

FIGURE 2-10 ■ VasoSeal closure device. **A,** The vessel locator is advanced through the indwelling sheath. The sheath is removed, and the locator is withdrawn until a green marker appears. **B,** The outer aspect is advanced until the green line appears on the inner silver aspect of the device. The entire device is then retracted until tension is felt. **C,** The tissue dilator is inserted until the white marker on the arterial locator is seen. The blue sheath is then inserted until the hub is at the level of the blue marker on the dilator. The entire device except the outer sheath is removed. **D,** The collagen cartridge in injected into the sheath and plunger advanced until resistance is felt. The sheath is retracted until the plunger is seated. Moderate manual pressure is then applied. (From Hoffer EK, Bloch RD: Percutaneous arterial closure devices. J Vasc Interv Radiol 2003;14:865. Reprinted with permission.)

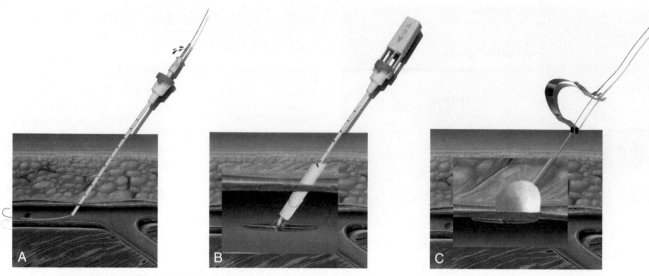

FIGURE 2-11 ■ AngioSeal closure device. **A,** The indwelling sheath is placed over a guidewire with the locator/sheath assembly. The locator is withdrawn until blood flow stops. It is then readvanced 2 cm to 3 cm into the artery. **B,** The locator and wire are withdrawn, and the closure device is inserted completely into the sheath. The anchor is deployed by partial withdrawal of the proximal portion of the device. The entire assembly is then withdrawn until resistance is felt. **C,** As the sheath is withdrawn further out of the skin, the tamper tube is seen. The tamper is advanced with tension on the stay suture, which may be cut immediately. (From Hoffer EK, Bloch RD: Percutaneous arterial closure devices. J Vasc Interv Radiol 2003;14:865. Reprinted with permission.)

■ Suture-mediated closure devices (e.g., Perclose Closer and Prostar, Xpress devices) (Fig. 2-13)
■ External patches that accelerate coagulation (e.g., Syvek patch, Clo-sur, D-stat Dry Patch)

No one device has been found to be superior to the others, although the collagen-mediated products are not effective for larger defects (e.g., >8 to 9 French). Device failure or conversion to manual compression is uncommon (<15% of cases). There is convincing evidence that most of these devices will significantly reduce time to hemostasis and time to ambulation, particularly in anticoagulated patients.[20] Overall, the frequency of complications is no different from manual compression. Nonetheless, routine use of these devices is controversial for several reasons:

■ The list of exclusionary criteria for many of these devices is long and includes peripheral vascular disease,

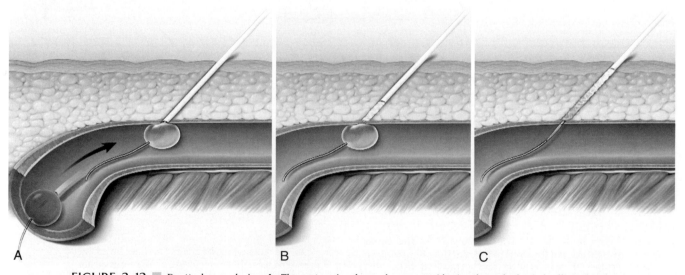

FIGURE 2-12 ■ Duett closure device. **A,** The system is advanced over a guidewire through the indwelling sheath. **B,** After the balloon is inflated, the catheter is withdrawn until resistance is felt. During slow withdrawal of the sheath, the procoagulant material is slowly injected through the sheath sidearm along the course of the tract. **C,** After the balloon is deflated, catheter and wire are removed. The site is compressed manually for about 5 minutes. (From Hoffer EK, Bloch RD: Percutaneous arterial closure devices. J Vasc Interv Radiol 2003;14:865. Reprinted with permission.)

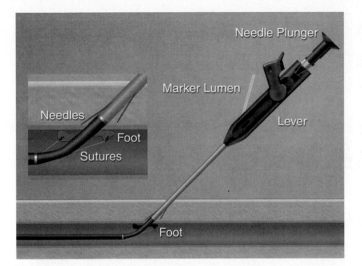

FIGURE 2-13 ■ Closure device. The indwelling sheath is exchanged over a guidewire for the device. When blood flow is noted through the marker lumen, the lever is raised to deploy the foot. The assembly is withdrawn until resistance is felt. With depression of the plunger, paired needles pierce the arterial wall and then the foot with suture attached. By withdrawing the plunger, the suture and needles exit the device. The lever is then lowered to close the foot. With partial withdrawal of the device, the freed sutures are tied, the device removed, and the knot cinched to secure the arteriotomy. (From Hoffer EK, Bloch RD: Percutaneous arterial closure devices. J Vasc Interv Radiol 2003;14:865. Reprinted with permission.)

uncontrolled hypertension, puncture outside the CFA, small caliber artery (<5 mm), existing hematoma, and double wall puncture. In addition, collagen-based catheters should not be used if closure is delayed, early repeat puncture is anticipated, or operation in the groin is planned.

■ Certain complications, albeit rare, are somewhat exclusive to these devices. Local thrombosis or embolization of the AngioSeal anchor or part of the collagen plug has been reported, as has device failure requiring operative removal. Most important, the presence of a foreign body adjacent to or in the artery increases the possibility (albeit remote) of local infection, which often requires surgical treatment and can be life-threatening.

Most interventionalists reserve closure devices for specific cases, such as large sheath size and patients requiring ongoing anticoagulation. Administration of IV antibiotics and fresh preparation of the access site are recommended.

Complications

The overall risk of a major complication after diagnostic arteriography is less than 2%.[25] For a particular case, however, the risk depends on the type of procedure, coexisting risk factors, and experience of the operator.[26-28] The most common complications of femoral artery catheterization are outlined in Table 2-1. Specific complications of interventional procedures are considered in subsequent chapters.

Minor bleeding or hematoma formation occurs in less than 10% of femoral artery catheterization procedures. Major bleeding requiring transfusion or surgical evacuation

TABLE 2-1	COMPLICATIONS OF FEMORAL ARTERY CATHETERIZATION

Type	Frequency (%)
Minor bleeding or hematoma	6–10
Major hemorrhage requiring therapy	<1
Pseudoaneurysm	1–6
Arteriovenous fistula	0.01
Occlusion (thrombosis or dissection)	<1
Perforation or extravasation	<1
Distal embolization	<0.10

is much less common (<1%). Blood may collect in the thigh, groin, retroperitoneum, or, rarely, the peritoneal space. Retroperitoneal hemorrhage should be suspected in a patient with an unexplained drop in hematocrit, hypotension, or flank pain (Fig. 2-14).

Catheterization-related pseudoaneurysms are relatively uncommon with proper technique; arteriovenous fistulas are rare (Fig. 2-15).[28,29] Most small (<2 cm) pseudoaneurysms will close spontaneously. Large or persistent lesions require treatment (see below). Femoral artery thrombosis or occlusion usually is caused by dissection, spasm, or pericatheter clot (Figs. 2-16 and 2-17). Cholesterol embolization from traumatic disruption of an atherosclerotic plaque is a rare but potentially devastating complication of arteriography (see Chapter 1).[30]

Other potential adverse events include nausea and vomiting, vasovagal reactions, and contrast media–related reaction or nephropathy. Cardiac events (e.g., arrhythmias, angina, heart failure) and neurologic events (e.g., seizures, femoral nerve injury, stroke) also can occur during angiography.[31]

The reported frequency of complications from axillary or brachial artery catheterization varies widely, from 2% to 24%.[15,32-35] Thrombosis and pseudoaneurysm formation are

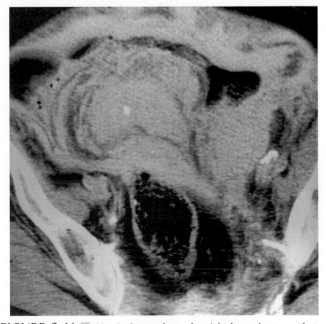

FIGURE 2-14 ■ Massive hemorrhage after right femoral artery catheterization seen on axial CT scan.

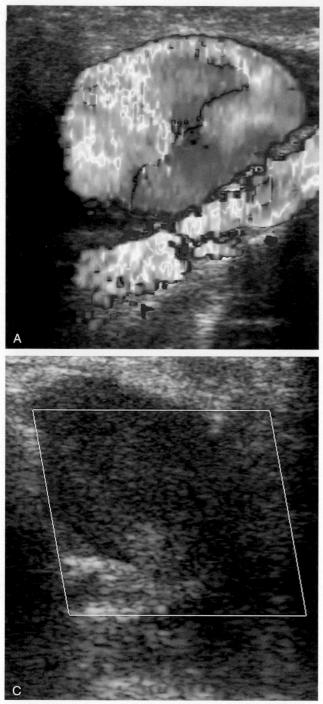

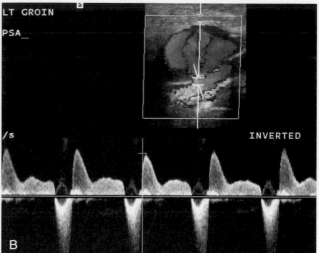

FIGURE 2-15 ▪ Postcatheterization femoral artery pseudoaneurysm treated with thrombin injection. **A,** Color Doppler ultrasound shows large pseudoaneurysm contiguous with superficial femoral artery. **B,** Waveform analysis reveals classic "to-and-fro" flow in the neck of the pseudoaneurysm. **C,** Following percutaneous thrombin injection, flow in the pseudoaneurysm has been abolished.

more common with this approach than with retrograde CFA catheterization (see Fig. 7-14). Distal neuropathy is a distinct but fortunately uncommon sequela of brachial artery puncture. Because the axillary and proximal brachial arteries run in a tight fascial sheath along with the median and ulnar nerves, even small hematomas can cause nerve compression. Sensory or motor neuropathy is reported in about 2% to 7% of patients who undergo this procedure.[32-36] The deficit is more likely to become permanent if early surgical decompression is not accomplished as soon as the problem is suspected. The other devastating neurologic complication of retrograde brachial artery catheterization is cerebral embolization of pericatheter clot, which has been reported in up to 4% of cases.[33]

Treatment of Postcatheterization Pseudoaneurysms and Arteriovenous Fistulas

Ultrasound-guided compression repair is effective in many cases of postcatheterization pseudoaneurysms.[37,38] In this

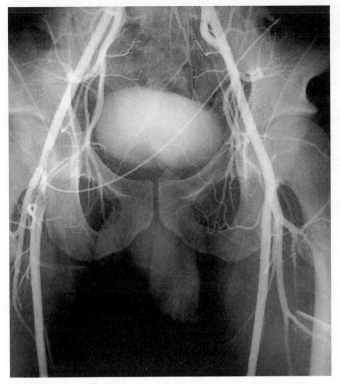

FIGURE 2-16 ■ Thrombus and vasospasm associated with a low puncture into the right superficial femoral artery.

technique, the ultrasound transducer is used to compress the neck of the pseudoaneurysm while flow is maintained in the SFA (Fig. 2-18). Patients are then kept on bed rest for 4 to 6 hours. Follow-up sonography is required to confirm permanent thrombosis. Pseudoaneurysm closure is successful in about 75% to 85% of cases. However, the method is painful (usually requiring moderate sedation), time-consuming, and sometimes ineffective, particularly in patients receiving anticoagulation.[39] Compression repair is not advised when flow in the neck cannot be obliterated or for lesions located above the inguinal ligament.

Percutaneous ultrasound-guided thrombin injection has become the first-line treatment for angiographic-related pseudoaneurysms in many institutions.[39-41] The procedure is quick, relatively painless, and highly effective. After excluding an arteriovenous fistula and using real-time ultrasound guidance, a 22-gauge needle is inserted into the body of the pseudoaneurysm away from the neck (see Fig. 2-15). Bovine thrombin (1000 units/mL) is injected into the lesion over 5 to 10 seconds. Most pseudoaneurysms require less than 1000 units for complete thrombosis. Clot formation is monitored with color Doppler imaging. The success rate is greater than 90%, even in the face of anticoagulation. Treatment is more problematic with complex pseudoaneurysms.[40] A failed first attempt should be repeated. However, the patient and operator should be aware that prior exposure to thrombin (topical or otherwise) can lead to antibody formation and the small risk of anaphylactic reaction. Although complications are rare, limb-threatening embolization or downstream thrombosis has been reported.[42] The technique also has been used to treat postcatheterization brachial artery pseudoaneurysms.[43]

Arteriovenous fistulas are much less common than pseudoaneurysms after femoral artery catheterization (Fig. 2-19). Many fistulas will close spontaneously. Operative repair is recommended if they persist for more than 2 months, double or more in size, or become symptomatic.[44] Covered stents have been used to treat such fistulas, but subsequent arterial occlusion is reported in a minority of cases.[44,45]

BASIC ANGIOGRAPHIC AND INTERVENTIONAL TOOLS

Catheters and Guidewires

The interventionalist can choose from a vast assortment of commercially available guidewires and catheters. Selection of suitable materials can be learned only through hands-on training and experience.

The primary characteristics of guidewires are length, diameter, tip configuration, torqueability, stiffness, and composition. Standard guidewires are made of a stainless steel coil wrapped tightly around an inner mandril that tapers at the working end of the wire. A central safety wire filament is incorporated also to prevent complete separation if the wire breaks. Hydrophilic guidewires are extremely useful in diseased or tortuous vessels. Standard guidewire diameters are 0.035 and 0.038 inch. Finer-gauge wires (e.g., 0.014 and 0.018 inch) are available for use with microcatheters or small-caliber needles. Standard guidewire lengths are 125 cm and 145 cm. A long (260-cm) exchange wire may be needed for selective catheter changes. The more commonly used guidewires are outlined in Table 2-2.

Angiographic and interventional catheters are made of polyurethane, polyethylene, nylon, or Teflon. Many catheters are wire braided for extra torqueability. Others are coated with a hydrophilic polymer to improve trackability. Catheters vary in length, diameter, and the presence of side holes. Outer catheter diameter is designated by French size (3 French = 1 mm).

Several types of catheters are available:

- *Straight catheters* come in many shapes (Fig. 2-20). Nonbraided catheters can be reshaped by heating them under a steam jet.
- *Reverse-curve catheters*, in which the tip is advanced into a vessel by catheter withdrawal at the groin, are available in many designs (Fig. 2-21). Although these catheters are quite versatile, they must first be reformed after insertion into the aorta or IVC (Fig. 2-22).[46] Some straight catheters can also be manipulated into a reverse-curve shape by formation of a Waltman loop (Fig. 2-23).[47]
- *Pigtail-type catheters* are used for angiography in large vessels and for drainage procedures (urinary, biliary, fluid collections) (Fig. 2-24). Angiographic catheters have multiple side holes along the distal shaft that produce a tight bolus of contrast while avoiding subintimal dissection from contrast exiting the endhole alone. Drainage catheters have side holes in the distal shaft or the pigtail loop, which is formed and secured by tightening a string attached to the tip, running within the lumen of the

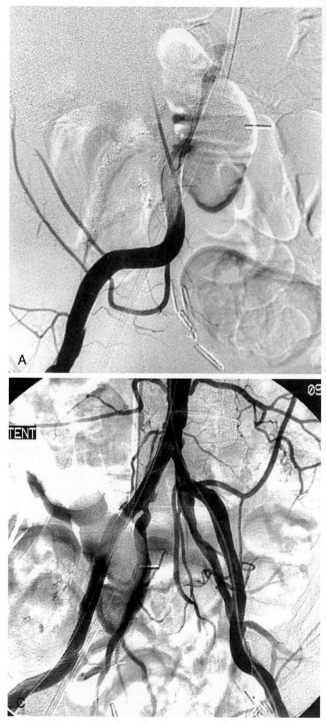

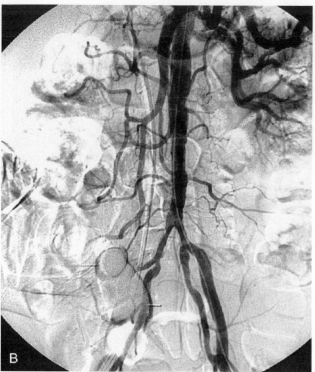

FIGURE 2-17 ■ Right iliac artery and aortic dissection from retrograde femoral artery catheterization. **A,** Injection from the right external iliac artery shows a dissection with a thin channel of contrast in the false lumen. **B,** Aortogram from the left common femoral artery shows narrowing of the distal abdominal aorta and right common iliac artery and complete occlusion of the right external iliac artery. **C,** A guidewire was placed across the aortic bifurcation and through the true lumen into the right external iliac artery. The entire segment was reopened with a Wallstent.

catheter, and exiting the catheter hub (Cope loop). The loop is designed to prevent catheter dislodgement.

■ *Sheaths* are thin-walled valved supporting catheters placed when there is persistent oozing or hematoma at the access site, multiple catheter exchanges are expected, a prolonged procedure is anticipated, or vascular intervention is planned (see Fig. 2-5). Contrast can be injected through the side arm around guidewires or nonocclusive catheters. Vascular and peel-away sheaths also are useful in nonvascular interventional procedures for maintaining access, placement of multiple guidewires,

and other reasons. Generally, true outer sheath diameter is two sizes larger than the stated French size.

■ *Guiding catheters* allow safer or more secure passage of devices into vessels (e.g., renal artery stent placement or coil embolization of pulmonary arteriovenous malformations). These catheters usually are inserted through larger sheaths at the vascular access site.

■ *Microcatheters* are placed through standard angiographic catheters to allow entry into small or tortuous arteries. They are guided by small-caliber (e.g., 0.014 to 0.018 inch) steerable guidewires.

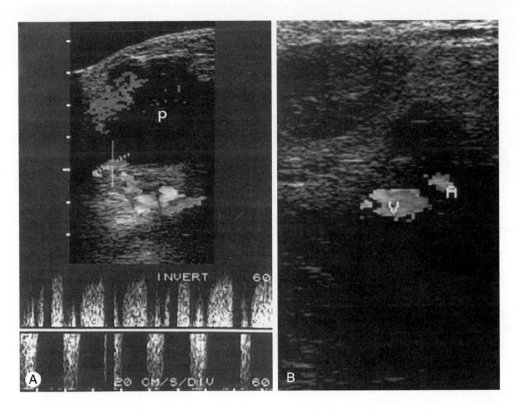

FIGURE 2-18 ■ Ultrasound-guided compression repair of a postcatheterization pseudoaneurysm. **A,** Color Doppler sonogram shows a large pseudoaneurysm (p) arising from the left common femoral artery with classic "to-and-fro" flow at the aneurysm neck. **B,** After 30 minutes of compression of the neck, the pseudoaneurysm has thrombosed. Flow is maintained in the femoral artery (A) and vein (V).

Pressure Measurements

Intravascular pressure monitoring is primarily used to determine the hemodynamic significance of stenoses, assess the results of revascularization procedures, and diagnose pulmonary artery or portal venous hypertension. A pressure gradient is far more accurate than multiple angiographic images for proving the significance of a vascular stenosis.[48] Hemodynamic measurements must be obtained with meticulous attention to detail to minimize artifacts.

The pressure gradient across a stenosis in a tube with flowing fluid is defined by *Poiseuille's law:*

$$\Delta P = \frac{8\eta Q L}{\pi r^4}$$

In the equation, ΔP = pressure gradient, Q = blood flow, L = length of the stenosis, η = blood viscosity, and r = radius. In medium-sized arteries, blood flow is unchanged until the luminal diameter is reduced by 50%, which corresponds to a cross-sectional area reduction of 75% (Fig. 2-25). Blood flow falls precipitously as the diameter stenosis approaches 75% (about a 95% reduction in cross-sectional area).

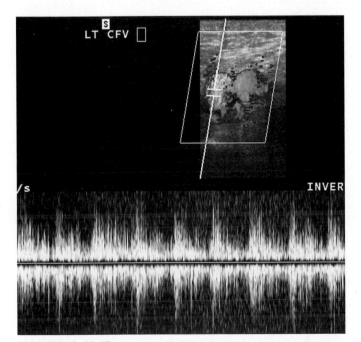

FIGURE 2-19 ■ Postcatheterization femoral artery arteriovenous fistula. Transverse color Doppler sonography shows pulsatile flow in the left common femoral vein.

TABLE 2-2 COMMONLY USED GUIDEWIRES

Type	Function
Bentson and floppy-tipped wires	Standard access wire
Hydrophilic wires (e.g., Terumo wire)	Use in tortuous or diseased vessels
Extra stiff wires (e.g., Amplatz)	Insertion of larger devices or within long tracts
Exchange wires	Exchange of long angiographic catheters or devices or remote distance from access
Tapered wires (e.g., TAD wire)	Placement of devices into sensitive territories
Low-profile steerable wires	Use in microcatheters for selective catheterization

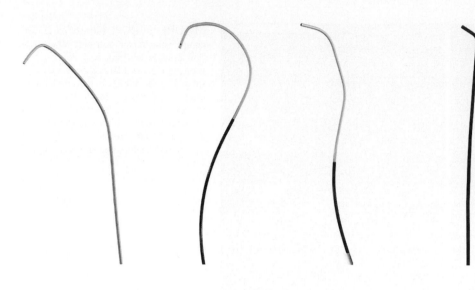

FIGURE 2-20 ■ Basic straight angiographic catheters. **Left to right,** spinal, cobra, headhunter, and angled shapes.

The relationship between flow reduction and luminal diameter becomes more complex with diffuse disease or tandem lesions. Pressure gradients are affected by blood flow. For example, as the peripheral arterial resistance in the legs drops with exercise, the magnitude (and therefore the clinical significance) of proximal pressure gradients increases.

The thresholds used to define a significant arterial pressure gradient are controversial. Resting systolic and mean gradients from 5 to 34 mm Hg have been suggested.[49-51] Absolute or relative gradients after flow augmentation (intra-arterial injection of a vasodilator) are favored by some experts. As a general rule, a resting systolic gradient of 10 mm Hg or greater is considered significant in the arterial system. In the central veins, a focal gradient of greater than 2 to 3 mm Hg can be flow limiting.

Pressure gradients are most accurate when simultaneous measurements are obtained from endhole catheters on either side of a stenosis. However, often it is more practical to use a single catheter to measure a "pullback pressure" across the lesion. With this method, however, the gradient may be spuriously elevated if the diameters of the catheter and vessel are similar (such as arteries ≤5 mm in diameter).

Contrast Agents

Standard contrast materials used for vascular and interventional procedures are iodinated organic compounds. The most commonly used materials are listed in Table 2-3.

- *Ionic monomeric agents* have a single triply iodinated benzene ring and form salts in plasma.
- *Ionic dimeric agents* (e.g., ioxaglate) contain twice the number of iodine atoms per molecule.
- *Nonionic monomeric agents* are less toxic because of lower osmolality, nondissociation in solution, and increased hydrophilicity.

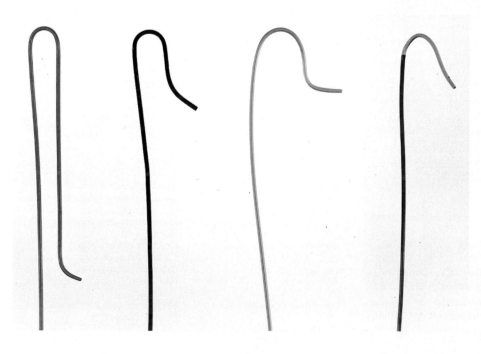

FIGURE 2-21 ■ Basic reverse-curve catheters. **Left to right,** Bookstein, Simmons (sidewinder), Shetty, and visceral hook.

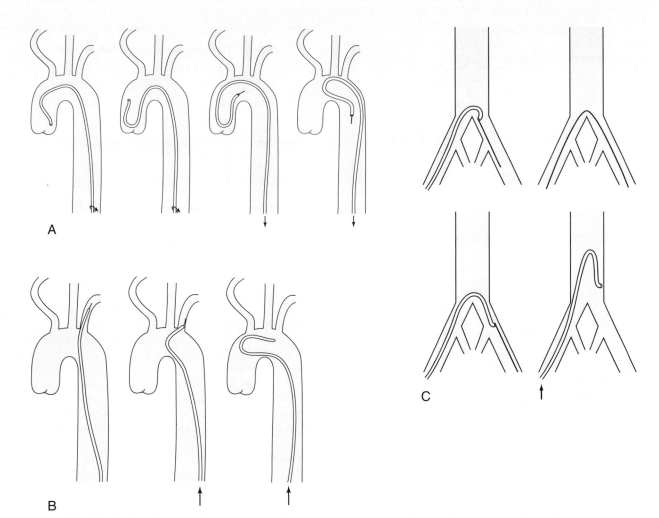

FIGURE 2-22 ■ Methods for reforming a Simmons catheter. (Adapted from Kadir S: Diagnostic Angiography. Philadelphia, WB Saunders, 1986:74.)

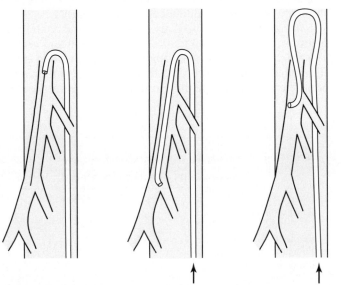

FIGURE 2-23 ■ Method for forming a Waltman loop. (From Kadir S: Med Radiogr Photog 1981;57:22. Reprinted courtesy of Eastman Kodak Company.)

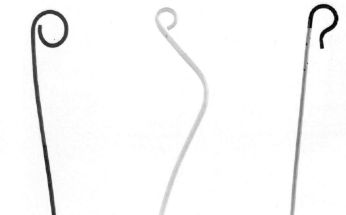

FIGURE 2-24 ■ High-flow catheters. **Left to right,** pigtail, Grollman, and modified pigtail.

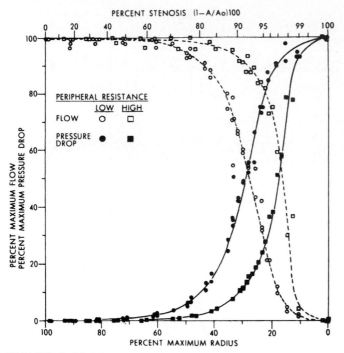

FIGURE 2-25 ■ Relationship between arterial blood flow (*y* axis), cross-sectional area reduction (upper *x* axis), and luminal diameter (lower *x* axis). (From Sumner DS: Hemodynamics and diagnosis of arterial disease: basic techniques and applications. In: Rutherford RB, ed. Vascular Surgery, 3rd ed. Philadelphia, WB Saunders, 1989:24.)

■ *Nonionic dimeric agents* are isosmolar (or nearly so) with plasma and are the least toxic of the available materials.

Iodinated contrast agents can produce several systemic effects after intravascular administration (Box 2-1).[52-54] The severity of these alterations depends largely on the osmolality of the material. At similar iodine concentrations, low osmolar contrast materials (LOCM) (i.e., ionic dimers and nonionic agents) have a significantly lower osmolality (600 to

TABLE 2-3   COMMONLY USED IODINATED CONTRAST AGENTS

Generic Name	Trade Name
Ionic Agents	
Iothalamate	Conray
Diatrizoate	Renografin
	Angiovist
	Hypaque
	MD
Ioxaglate	Hexabrix
Nonionic Agents	
Iopamidol	Isovue
Ioversol	Optiray
Iohexol	Omnipaque
Iopromide	Ultravist
Ioxilan	Oxilan
Iodixanol	Visipaque
Iotrolan	Isovist

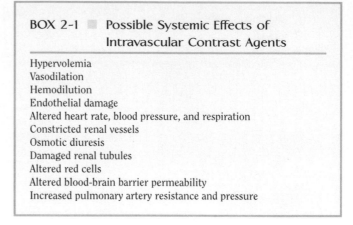

BOX 2-1 ■ Possible Systemic Effects of Intravascular Contrast Agents

Hypervolemia
Vasodilation
Hemodilution
Endothelial damage
Altered heart rate, blood pressure, and respiration
Constricted renal vessels
Osmotic diuresis
Damaged renal tubules
Altered red cells
Altered blood-brain barrier permeability
Increased pulmonary artery resistance and pressure

800 mOsm/kg) than high osmolar contrast materials (HOCM) (ionic monomers) (1400 to 2000 mOsm/kg). Iodixanol (Visipaque) is the only isosmolar agent (290 mOsm/kg) currently available in the United States.

In most centers, nonionic agents are chosen for all intravascular applications. Minor side effects, such as nausea, vomiting, and local pain, are much less common with these drugs.[55] The incidence of minor or moderate contrast reactions also is reduced with LOCM; however, the frequency of severe or fatal reactions may not be significantly different. For certain procedures (such as pulmonary, bronchial, or spinal arteriography), nonionic agents are mandatory to avoid potentially devastating complications. There are only small differences in imaging quality among the various agents at the same iodine concentration,[55-57] and the safety and efficacy of the various nonionic agents are similar.[58] However, one study has suggested that the isosmolar agent iodixanol causes fewer cases of contrast-induced nephropathy.[59] At centers in which cost issues are of particular concern, an argument can be made for selective use of nonionic material (Box 2-2).[60]

In patients with renal dysfunction or a history of life-threatening allergy, two alternative contrast agents should be considered. Use of these media may limit or completely eliminate the need for iodinated contrast material.

Carbon dioxide has been used extensively as a contrast agent for digital imaging in a variety of arterial and venous beds (Fig. 2-26).[61-66] The gas rapidly dissolves in blood and is eliminated from the lung less than 30 seconds after injection. There is no risk of allergic reaction or nephrotoxicity.

BOX 2-2 ■ Selective Indications for Low Osmolality Contrast Material

Allergic history (e.g., contrast or drug reactions, asthma)
Renal insufficiency
Cardiopulmonary instability
Cardiac disease
Pulmonary hypertension
Children
Age > 60 years
Dehydration
Specific applications (e.g., pulmonary or bronchial arteriography)

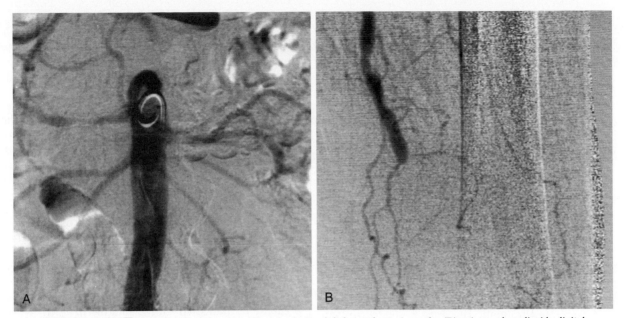

FIGURE 2-26 ▪ Abdominal aortography (**A**) and selective left femoral arteriography (**B**) using carbon dioxide digital subtraction technique.

An airtight system of reservoir bag, tubing, and syringes is constructed to purge a delivery syringe of room air and substitute instrument grade CO_2. For abdominal aortography or inferior venacavography, a 60-mL syringe is required. The catheter is then primed with the gas before rapid injection. Commercially available injectors also may be used. Some patients experience discomfort with injection, and the quality of images is clearly inferior to those obtained with iodinated contrast. In addition, complications can arise from gas trapping and "vapor lock," especially in the pulmonary artery, abdominal aortic aneurysms, and the inferior mesenteric artery. The agent cannot be used in arteries above the diaphragm because of the risk of intracerebral embolization.

Gadolinium-based contrast material also is used for digital angiography and injection of the urinary and biliary systems.[67-69] At standard doses, the drug is almost completely nontoxic. Anaphylactic reactions are exceedingly rare. However, worsening of renal function has been reported, particularly when volumes exceed maximum recommended doses (0.3 to 0.4 mmol/kg).[68,70,71] Some critics argue that gadolinium-based agents are not less nephrotoxic when used at concentrations comparable to iodine-based agents.[71] This limits the total injected volume to less than 70 mL in most adults. The lower osmolality preparations should be used for extremity arteriography. Owing to the higher K edge of gadolinium compared with iodine, image quality is improved at higher kilovolt peaks (i.e., >90 kVp). Images are inferior to those obtained with iodinated contrast, largely because of the much lower concentration of the drug. In some cases, image quality is superior to CO_2-based studies.[72]

Pharmacologic Adjuncts

A variety of drugs are widely used during or after diagnostic and therapeutic vascular procedures.

Antiplatelet Agents

Aspirin (acetylsalicylic acid) inhibits platelet aggregation by irreversibly inactivating cyclooxygenase, a critical enzyme in the production of thromboxane A_2.[73,74] Aspirin also may limit intimal hyperplasia after balloon angioplasty through its anti-inflammatory properties. The drug is rapidly absorbed from the stomach, and platelet function is inhibited within 1 hour of ingestion. Aspirin prolongs the bleeding time without significantly affecting other coagulation parameters. Patients often are maintained on a daily dose of 80 to 325 mg for several months after recanalization procedures.

Thienopyridines (clopidogrel [Plavix] and *ticlopidine [Ticlid])* are more potent oral antiplatelet agents that inhibit the binding of adenosine diphosphate to platelet receptors, thus preventing platelet-fibrinogen binding and glycoprotein GP IIb/IIIa–mediated platelet aggregation.[75-77] The standard doses are Plavix 75 mg daily and Ticlid 250 mg twice daily. All patients with symptomatic peripheral arterial disease are candidates for long-term therapy to limit associated myocardial infarction, stroke, or vascular death. These agents also show promise in preventing restenosis after angioplasty, stent insertion, or bypass graft placement.[77] Potential complications include bleeding, neutropenia, and thrombocytopenia (particularly with ticlopidine).

Cilostazol (Pletal) is a phosphodiesterase-III inhibitor that has antiplatelet, antithrombotic, smooth muscle antiproliferative, and vasodilatory effects.[78,79] There is abundant evidence that chronic therapy (50 to 100 mg PO twice daily) increases exercise ability and overall quality of life in patients with intermittent claudication. The agent appears to be more effective than *pentoxifylline (Trental)* in this regard. Significant drug interactions can occur with certain cytochrome P450 inhibitors (e.g., diltiazem, erythromycin, and omeprazole).

GP IIb/IIIa inhibitors are a relatively new class of potent cell receptor antagonists that act on the final common pathway to platelet aggregation. While interplatelet binding is inhibited, platelet attachment to subendothelial elements is maintained. Although these parenteral drugs have been used extensively in patients with coronary artery disease, there is little published experience with their use for non-coronary applications.[80-82] As such, these agents should *not* be used routinely but instead reserved for selected cases (e.g., slow response to thrombolytic agents, thrombophilic states, need for rapid revascularization, infrageniculate interventions [Table 2-4]). It is important to reduce heparin and fibrinolytic drug doses and carefully monitor platelet levels (which can fall precipitously during treatment).

Antithrombin Agents

Heparin is a polyanionic protein that binds with antithrombin III and other plasma proteins.[83] The heparin-antithrombin III complex inhibits clot formation by inactivating thrombin and other coagulation factors. Because thrombin is the critical enzyme in clot formation (see Fig. 3-11), heparin is a potent antithrombotic agent. However, it has no effect against fibrin-bound thrombin. The drug is cleared in two phases. Rapid initial clearance by indiscriminate binding to plasma proteins and endothelial cells is followed by slower clearance by the kidneys. The biologic half-life varies widely among patients, but it is roughly 1 hour at typical therapeutic doses (5000 units IV bolus followed by 500 to 1500 units/hr infusion).

Because heparin pharmacokinetics are unpredictable, anticoagulation monitoring is mandatory. During vascular procedures, the antithrombotic effect can be followed with the activated clotting time (ACT), which measures whole blood clotting.[84] Normal and therapeutic ranges are specific to each device. The activated partial thromboplastin time (PTT) is used to monitor short-term anticoagulation. The therapeutic range is 1.5 to 2.5 times the control value. One protocol for adjusting heparin doses based on the PTT was proposed by Hirsh and Fuster.[83] Patients who are extremely resistant to heparin may require titration by direct heparin assay or treatment with low-molecular-weight heparin agents (see below).[85]

The major complications of heparin therapy are bleeding, heparin-induced thrombocytopenia, and osteopenia (with chronic use). The risk of bleeding is a function of drug dose, concomitant use of thrombolytic agents, recent surgery or trauma, baseline coagulation status, kidney function, and age. The heparin effect can be reversed with *protamine* (see Chapter 1).

Low-molecular-weight heparin agents (LMWHs) have more predictable and persistent anticoagulant activity than unfractionated heparin.[85-87] This class of drugs include *enoxaparin (Lovenox), dalteparin (Fragmin), reviparin,* and *tinzaparin (Innohep).* The agents cause inhibition of factor X_a and thrombin. They have little effect on standard coagulation parameters (i.e., international normalized ratio [INR] and PTT) and monitoring is generally not required. With a half-life of about 3 to 5 hours, they can be given once or twice daily by subcutaneous injection. LMWHs are becoming the standard prophylactic regimen in prevention of deep venous thrombosis (e.g., before major orthopedic or abdominal surgery) and are replacing the heparin/Coumadin sequence for treatment of acute deep venous thrombosis. As yet, there is no proven benefit of these drugs in patients undergoing peripheral or renal artery recanalization. Bleeding is the major adverse event with use.

Direct thrombin inhibitors (bivalirudin [Angiomax], argatroban, and lepirudin [Refludan]) are recombinant or synthetic agents that unlike heparin act on both free and circulating thrombin and do not require antithrombin III for activity.[88-90] The anticoagulative effect is much more predictable than with unfractionated heparin. While they are used widely during coronary interventions, experience in other vascular beds is limited. However, these drugs are clearly indicated in the setting of heparin-induced thrombocytopenia.

Warfarin (Coumadin) is an antithrombotic agent that inhibits vitamin K–dependent liver synthesis of the proenzymes for coagulation factors II, VII, IX, and X.[91] Its primary use in interventional radiology is maintaining patency of recanalized arteries, veins, bypass grafts, and vascular access devices. Warfarin has a half-life of 36 to 42 hours. A full anticoagulative effect is not achieved until 3 to 7 days after therapy is started. Drug monitoring and reversal are discussed in Chapter 1. A wide variety of medications can potentiate or inhibit the anticoagulant effect of warfarin.

Antispasmodic Agents

Vasodilators are sometimes used during vascular procedures to prevent or relieve vasospasm and to augment arterial flow.[92,93] The most commonly used agent is the direct smooth muscle relaxant *nitroglycerin* (100 to 200 µg IA or IV), which has a half-life of 1 to 4 minutes. The calcium channel blocker *verapamil* can be used also. Verapamil and other calcium channel blockers are contraindicated in patients with elevated intracranial pressure and certain cardiac conditions. Adverse effects include hypotension, tachycardia, and nausea; these reactions are uncommon with standard doses.

TABLE 2-4   GP IIb/IIIa PLATELET INHIBITOR AGENTS

Agent	Structure	Half-life	Dose
Abciximab (ReoPro)	Monoclonal antibody	8–12 hr	Bolus 0.25 mg/kg Infuse 0.125 µg/kg/min × 12 h
Eptifibatide (Integrilin)	Synthetic peptide	2.5 hr	Bolus 180 µg/kg t = 0,10 min Infuse 2.0 µg/kg/min 18–24 h
Tirofiban (Aggrastat)	Nonpeptide tyrosine	2 hr	Bolus 0.10 µg/kg Infuse 0.15 µg/min 18–24 hr

■ VASCULAR INTERVENTIONAL TECHNIQUES

Balloon Angioplasty

Percutaneous transluminal balloon angioplasty (PTA) remains the first-line minimally invasive technique for treatment of stenoses in the vascular, biliary, and urinary systems (Fig. 2-27). PTA was conceived by Dotter and Judkins, who first used sequential dilators to open an occluded superficial femoral artery.[94] Gruentzig is credited with the development of balloon angioplasty catheters that are the basis of the current method.[95] In many situations, PTA is performed in conjunction with stent placement to obtain optimal results (see below).

Mechanism of Action

Inflation of an angioplasty balloon in a stenotic artery causes desquamation of endothelial cells, splitting or dissection of the atherosclerotic plaque and adjacent intima, and stretching of the media and adventitia.[96,97] There is virtually no compression of the plaque itself. This controlled stretch injury increases the cross-sectional area of the vascular lumen. Platelets and fibrin cover the denuded surface immediately. Over the next several weeks, reendothelialization of the intima occurs and the artery remodels. Clinically significant restenosis is caused by prolific neointimal hyperplasia and/or major vascular remodeling (e.g., recoil) that is largely an inflammatory response to the injury (see Chapter 3). On the other hand, PTA of venous stenoses stretches the entire vein wall usually without causing a frank tear.

Patient Selection

The specific indications for PTA are considered in later chapters. Angioplasty should be performed only when a vascular obstruction is hemodynamically significant, reopening the vessel is likely to improve the patient's symptoms or clinical condition, and other treatment options are less attractive.

Angioplasty *alone* is less effective or relatively unsafe in the following situations:

- ■ Stenosis adjoining an aneurysm (owing to higher risk for rupture)
- ■ Bulky, polypoid atherosclerotic plaque (owing to higher risk for distal embolization)
- ■ Diffuse disease (Fig. 2-28)
- ■ Long-segment stenosis or occlusion
- ■ Impaired pain sensation

Technique

The important factors in catheter selection are balloon diameter, balloon length, profile (a function of shaft size and balloon material), peak inflation pressure, and trackability:

- ■ The shortest balloon that will span the lesion is chosen. However, if the balloon is too short and not centered precisely, it may be squeezed away from the stenosis during inflation ("watermelon seed effect").
- ■ For most arteries and veins, better results are obtained with *slight* overdilation. However, it is prudent to start with smaller diameter balloons and upsize as needed.
- ■ Atherosclerotic plaques yield with inflation pressures of 5 to 10 atm. Venous and graft stenoses may require much higher pressures (18 to ≥24 atm).
- ■ The relative importance of catheter profile and trackability depends on the vessel being treated.

Pharmacologic adjuncts are critical to the vascular angioplasty procedure:

- ■ Aspirin or a thienopyridine platelet inhibitor is given beforehand to prevent postangioplasty thrombosis and for several months thereafter to limit restenosis.
- ■ Heparin (or a direct thrombin inhibitor) usually is administered immediately before crossing the obstruction,

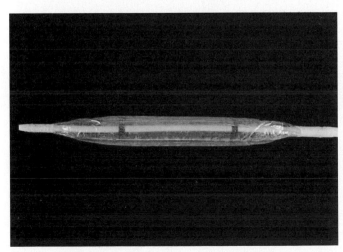

FIGURE 2-27 ■ Balloon angioplasty catheter.

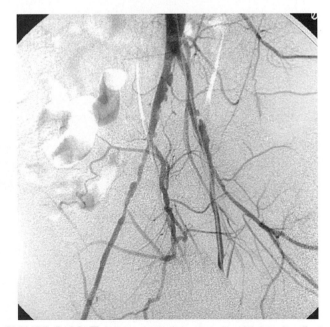

FIGURE 2-28 ■ Balloon angioplasty alone is unlikely to be effective for diffuse disease in the right common and external iliac arteries.

continued for the duration of the procedure, and, in some cases, continued afterward to prevent thrombosis (e.g., with small vessels, poor runoff, or slow flow).

◼ Vasodilators are used to prevent or relieve angioplasty-induced vasospasm, which is especially problematic in the renal, mesenteric, infrapopliteal, and upper extremity arteries.

Placement of a vascular sheath can simplify post-PTA angiograms and minimize vessel trauma during removal of the deflated balloon.

With an angiographic catheter or the balloon catheter itself near the stenosis, the lesion is crossed with a guidewire (Fig. 2-29). Stenoses in veins and large arteries can be crossed safely with a variety of guidewires. Steerable, tapered wires with very floppy tips may be used to traverse critical lesions or those more prone to dissection. Road-mapping often is helpful. Forceful guidewire manipulation can convert a stenosis into a dissection or occlusion (Fig. 2-30).

The balloon is advanced across the stenosis. A stiff guidewire with a soft flexible tip or a lower-profile device may be tried if the catheter will not pass easily. With the balloon centered over the obstruction, it is inflated with dilute contrast material manually with a 10-mL syringe or with an inflation device. A wire is maintained through the end hole to prevent the rigid catheter tip from injuring the vessel as the balloon inflates. The "waist" produced by an atherosclerotic stenosis yields suddenly as the plaque cracks.

Venous stenoses usually open more gradually. Optimal inflation parameters (number, duration, and pressure) are not firmly established. However, two to three inflations of 30 to 120 seconds usually are necessary to ensure that the lumen has been completely expanded. Venous stenoses may require multiple, prolonged inflations to achieve an acceptable result.

Most patients feel mild discomfort during balloon inflation. If the patient complains of severe pain, the balloon should be deflated and a smaller one used. If pain persists after deflation, vessel rupture must be excluded by contrast injection while maintaining guidewire access. In this rare circumstance, the balloon is reinflated across the tear to stop the bleeding and a vascular surgeon is consulted. If prolonged balloon inflation does not close the leak in an artery or central vein, placement of a covered stent or urgent operative repair is necessary.

It is standard teaching that a guidewire should be left across the lesion while the deflated balloon is withdrawn. However, many interventionalists "abandon" stenoses in large arteries and veins. If a small-caliber (e.g., 0.018-inch) guidewire is left in place, angiography can be performed through a 5-French catheter around the guidewire using a hemostatic valve. If a sheath or guiding catheter is being used, contrast injections are made around a standard 0.035-inch guidewire.

An angiogram of the treated vessel is obtained in several projections, in some cases along with a pressure gradient. A technically successful result is defined as a residual luminal diameter stenosis of less than 30% or a minimal pressure

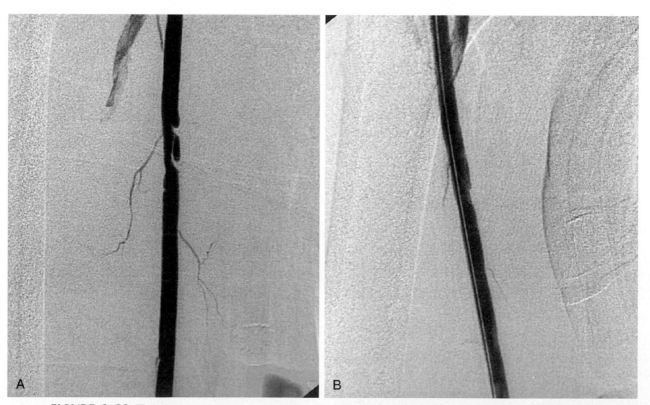

FIGURE 2-29 ◼ Balloon angioplasty of eccentric right superficial femoral artery stenosis (**A**) produces a widely patent vessel (**B**).

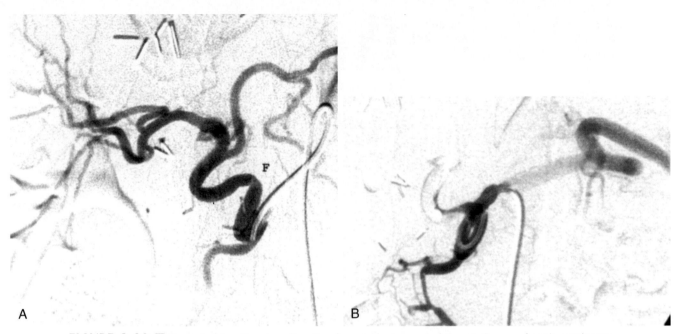

FIGURE 2-30 ■ Transplant hepatic artery dissection from guidewire manipulation. **A,** Common hepatic arteriogram shows a bandlike mural flap at the arterial anastomosis (F). **B,** After attempted guidewire advancement, arteriogram in oblique projection shows flow-limiting dissection beyond the anastomosis.

gradient (arterial < 5 to 10 mm Hg systolic). An inadequate result may occur for several reasons:

- *Large dissection.* Minor dissection is an expected result of balloon angioplasty. However, large, flow-limiting dissections can threaten the outcome of angioplasty. If repeated prolonged balloon inflation fails to tack down the flap, stent placement should be considered.
- *Elastic recoil.* Some stenoses (particularly in veins) may fully dilate with balloon inflation but return to their stenotic form after deflation. In many cases, stent placement is required to maintain patency.
- *Resistant stenoses.* Some lesions fail to dilate even with multiple, prolonged, high-pressure inflations. In this case, use of larger balloons or cutting balloons (see below) should be considered.

If the results are suboptimal or the risk of rethrombosis is significant (e.g., transplant artery stenosis) and heparin infusion must be continued, use of an arterial closure device should be considered. Otherwise, the heparin infusion is stopped. When the ACT has fallen into the high-normal range (typically <200 seconds), the sheath is removed. In some cases, heparin is restarted and continued for 24 to 48 hours to prevent early rethrombosis.

Results and Complications

The effectiveness of PTA depends on many factors. As a rule, the best results are obtained with short, solitary, concentric, noncalcified stenoses with good outflow. For arterial stenoses, the procedure is technically successful in greater than 90% of patients.[98-101] Long-term results vary widely for different vascular beds. The overall complication rate is about 10% (Box 2-3). Major complications that require specific therapy occur in about 2% to 3% of cases.

Vessel occlusion (1% to 7% of procedures) can result from acute thrombosis, dissection, or vasospasm (Fig. 2-31). An intravenous bolus of heparin and an intra-arterial vasodilator should be given immediately. Repeat angioplasty or stent placement is performed to tack down a dissection. Local infusion of a fibrinolytic agent will dissolve most acute thrombi.

Distal embolization occurs after 2% to 5% of arterial angioplasty procedures. Emboli are composed of fresh lysable thrombus, old organized thrombus, or unlysable atherosclerotic plaque. Treatment options include anticoagulation alone (for insignificant emboli), local thrombolytic infusion, percutaneous aspiration, or surgical embolectomy.

Cutting balloons with microthin longitudinal blades running along the balloon surface have been used to treat stenoses that are resistant to even high-pressure balloons.[102-104]

BOX 2-3 ■ Complications of Vascular Balloon Angioplasty

Access site complications (see Table 2-1)
Thrombosis
Vessel rupture
Distal embolization
Flow-limiting dissecton
Pseudoaneurysm
Guidewire perforation
Acute renal failure

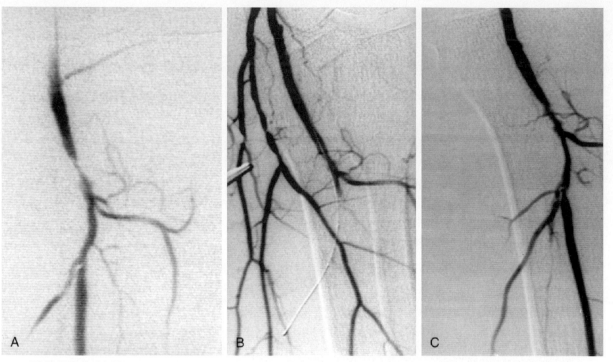

FIGURE 2-31 ▪ Acute postangioplasty occlusion. **A,** Tight stenoses are present in the distal left popliteal artery and proximal peroneal artery. **B,** After angioplasty with a 3-mm balloon, the vessel is completely occluded. The tip of the guidewire is in the left posterior tibial artery. **C,** After a heparin bolus, 200 μg of intra-arterial nitroglycerin, and repeat angioplasty, the vessel has reopened.

The primary applications of these devices are resistant lesions in hemodialysis grafts and arterial bypass grafts.

Atherectomy Devices

Unlike balloon angioplasty catheters, atherectomy devices actually remove diseased material from stenotic arteries and veins. Their initial popularity waned because long-term results were no better and in some cases worse than with balloon angioplasty or stent placement.[105,106] Significantly higher complication rates with certain atherectomy devices have been reported in some series. Despite these discouraging results, several atherectomy catheters are still on the market and others are in development, largely to handle failures of angioplasty.[107-111]

Uncovered Metallic Stents

Mechanism of Action

Stents maintain luminal patency by providing a rigid scaffold that compresses atherosclerotic disease, neointimal hyperplasia, or dissection flaps and also limits or prevents remodeling and elastic recoil. In addition, alterations in wall shear stress imposed by the stent may retard the process of neointimal hyperplasia (see Chapter 3). Thinning of the media is a consistent feature of stented arteries.[112,113]

Immediately after vascular stent insertion, a layer of fibrin coats the luminal surface.[112] Intraprocedural anticoagulation prevents immediate thrombosis of the device. Over several weeks, this thin layer of clot is replaced by fibromuscular tissue. Eventual reendothelialization of the stented vessel protects it from late thrombosis.

Patient Selection

Uncovered (bare) stents are used in several vascular disorders:

- Primary treatment of coronary, iliac, and renal artery obstructions
- Immediate or long-term failures of balloon angioplasty (arterial and venous)
- Complications of angioplasty or catheterization procedures (e.g., dissection)

Contraindications to uncovered stent placement include:

- Stenosis resistant to balloon angioplasty (absolute)
- Arterial rupture after angioplasty (absolute)
- Adjacent to an aneurysm (relative)
- Impaired pain sensation (relative)

Stent Selection

A wide variety of stents is available for vascular and nonvascular recanalization, and new stents come on the market every year (Fig. 2-32).[114-118] Most stents enter the U.S. market labeled for use in the biliary or tracheobronchial system,

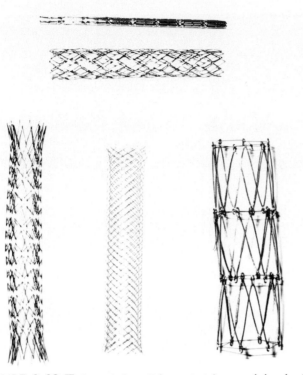

FIGURE 2-32 ■ Stent designs: Palmaz stent in expanded and collapsed forms (**top**), nitinol stent (**bottom left,** Bard Inc., Covington, Ga.), Wallstent (**bottom center,** Boston Scientific, Natick, Mass.), and Gianturco-Rösch Z stent (**bottom right,** Cook, Inc., Bloomington Ind.).

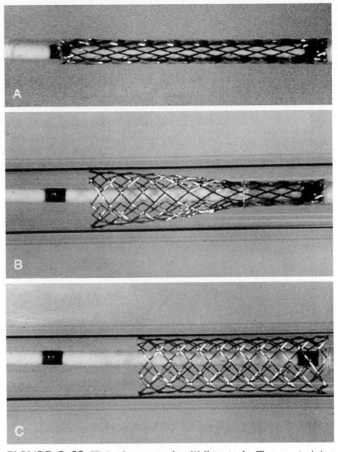

FIGURE 2-33 ■ Deployment of a Wallstent. **A,** The constraining membrane covers the compressed stent. **B,** The membrane is partially withdrawn. If necessary, the stent can be pulled back in the vessel, or the stent can be recovered by the constraining membrane. **C,** The stent is completely deployed. (Courtesy of Schneider [USA] Inc., Minneapolis, Minn.)

although off-label use in the vascular system is the standard of practice with many of these devices. Only the Palmaz stent, Wallstent, and SMART stent are currently approved by the U.S. Food and Drug Administration (FDA) for iliac artery placement. The most important properties of these devices are longitudinal flexibility, elastic deformation (tendency to return to nominal diameter), plastic deformation (tendency to maintain diameter imposed by external forces), radial and hoop strength, composition, metallic surface area, radiopacity, shortening with deployment, and magnetic resonance compatibility.

Self-expanding stents are compressed onto a catheter and deployed by uncovering a constraining sheath or membrane (Fig. 2-33). Most are composed of nitinol (a nickel/titanium alloy) or the metallic alloy Elgiloy. The final diameter of the stent is a function of the outward elastic load of the stent and the inward forces of elastic wall recoil or extrinsic compression. For peripheral vascular use, nominal diameters are 4 to 24 mm for placement through 5- to 12-French sheaths. Stents are oversized by 1 to 2 mm to ensure firm vessel apposition and prevent migration. As a rule, these devices are more flexible and trackable than balloon-expandable stents. When the route to the lesion is tortuous or steeply angled (such as over the aortic bifurcation), these stents may be easier to use than some balloon-expandable ones. Segmented nitinol stents may be more appropriate in vessels that change diameter (e.g., common to external iliac artery) since they are more likely to appose the entire arterial wall.

Balloon-expandable stents are premounted or self-mounted on angioplasty balloons in a compressed state and then deployed by balloon inflation. Most of these devices are composed of stainless steel, giving them significant hoop strength. Balloon-expandable stents then retain the diameter imposed by the angioplasty balloon. They have almost no elastic deformity but considerable plastic deformity.[119] Therefore, they should not be used at sites prone to significant external compression (e.g., superficial arm veins, subclavian vein at the costoclavicular ligament, adductor canal in the leg, around joints).[120] For peripheral vascular use, stent diameters range from 4 to 12 mm placed through 5- to 10-French introducers. Stent placement is very precise and shortening is minimal. These stents are particularly useful for calcified or fibrous lesions and sites prone to elastic recoil. If the balloon ruptures during expansion, rapid injection of a large volume of saline usually causes sufficient balloon distention to release the stent. If the stent embolizes during placement, it may be deployed in another location or in some cases retrieved.[121,122]

Drug-eluting stents are designed to prevent restenosis after recanalization.[123-125] Compounds that inhibit smooth muscle cell proliferation are introduced into a polymer that is bonded to the stent and slowly released into the arterial wall. Despite the theoretical benefits of these devices, there is no substantial evidence to date that they are more effective in peripheral arteries than uncovered stents.

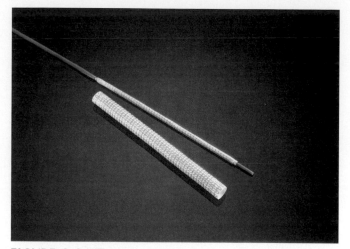

FIGURE 2-34 ■ Viabahn covered stent in constrained and open configurations. (Courtesy of W. L. Gore & Associates.)

Relative advantages of balloon-expandable and self-expanding stents are summarized in Box 2-4.

Common Technical Points

Anticoagulants and antiplatelet agents are given during vascular stent placement. Postprocedure anticoagulation is used selectively.

Several general principles apply to vascular stent placement:

■ Choose a device slightly larger in diameter than the normal vessel and longer than the diseased segment to ensure good wall apposition and prevent stent migration (see Fig. 15-26).
■ In arteries, always use a sheath and/or guiding catheter to protect the stent and vessel during transit to the site.
■ Cover the entire obstruction. Residual disease at the mouth of a stent can promote acute thrombosis or restenosis.
■ Be certain tandem stents are well overlapped. Gaps that develop between stents predispose to restenosis.
■ Generally avoid stent placement at joints and at sites where surgery may be necessary (e.g., common femoral artery, distal renal artery).

Covered Stents

Covered stents are metallic devices lined on the luminal and/or abluminal surface with a thin layer of synthetic graft material (Fig. 2-34). The metallic scaffold is made of nitinol, Elgiloy, or stainless steel. The fabric is polyethylene terephthalate (PET) (Wallgraft), polytetrafluoroethylene (PTFE) (aSpire, Hemobahn, Viabahn or Viatorr, Jostent), or dacron (Cragg Endopro System). The presence of the impermeable (or semipermeable) material seals the lumen and prevents neointimal proliferation in the stented segment. They are widely used for TIPS creation and for exclusion of aneurysms and pseudoaneurysms, vascular rupture, and arteriovenous fistulas.[126-128] Covered stents also are useful in malignant gastrointestinal obstructions and possibly in some infrainguinal arterial applications.

Enzymatic Thrombolysis

Patient Selection

Thrombolysis refers to any procedure that removes clot from the vascular system, including enzymatic fibrinolysis, mechanical thrombectomy, and thromboaspiration. Thrombolysis is primarily indicated for treatment of acute occlusion of hemodialysis grafts, iliac and infrainguinal arteries, bypass grafts, central venous catheters, upper extremity arteries, central upper or lower veins unresponsive to anticoagulation, and central pulmonary arteries.[129] Thrombolysis is an acceptable therapy when the anticipated technical and long-term outcome is comparable to that of surgical treatment, revascularization can be accomplished quickly enough to avoid irreversible ischemia, and the risks of the procedure are reasonable. Contraindications to enzymatic fibrinolysis are outlined in Box 2-5.[129]

Thrombolytic Agents

Enzymatic thrombolysis is accomplished with one of several fibrinolytic agents.[130] The key enzyme in clot dissolution is *plasmin*, a nonspecific serine protease that degrades fibrin and circulating fibrinogen and releases a variety of fibrin degradation products. Plasmin is inhibited by several circulating antiplasmins. The precursor of plasmin is plasminogen, which is cleaved by naturally occurring or exogenous *plasminogen activators*. These agents are the basis for thrombolytic therapy.[131-133] The various drugs are characterized by differences in half-life, *fibrin affinity* (ability to bind fibrin), and *fibrin specificity* (preferential activation of fibrin [clot]-bound plasminogen). Plasminogen activators are inactivated by inhibitors such as PAI-1.

Streptokinase (SK) is a naturally occurring polypeptide derived from group C streptococci. A streptokinase-plasminogen complex converts a second molecule of plasminogen to plasmin. The biologic half-life of streptokinase is about 23 minutes.[134] Antibodies present from prior streptococcal infection or streptokinase treatment may preclude use of the drug. For this among other reasons, SK is rarely used in clinical practice.

Urokinase (UK, Abbokinase) is a double-chain polypeptide originally derived from cultures of human fetal kidney cells. The half-life of UK is about 16 minutes. Unlike SK, UK is a direct plasminogen activator and is not antigenic. For many years, UK was the thrombolytic agent of choice. It is no longer manufactured in the United States.

Recombinant tissue–type plasminogen activator (t-PA, alteplase, Activase) is a naturally occurring serine protease produced by endothelial cells. The drug is manufactured by recombinant DNA techniques. Its biologic half-life is about 6 minutes. t-PA is a weak plasminogen activator in the absence of fibrin. Its activity is enhanced about 1000-fold in the presence of fibrin. However, fibrin specificity is dose-dependent.

Reteplase (r-PA, Retavase) is a recombinant mutant form of t-PA in which the finger domain of the molecule is removed (decreasing fibrin specificity and possibly enhancing diffusion into thrombus) along with epidermal growth factor and kringle 1 domains (increasing half-life to about 13 to 16 minutes). Unlike UK and t-PA, reteplase has not been the subject of multiple, large clinical trials to establish its relative efficacy and safety in noncoronary vessels.[81]

Tenecteplase (TNK) is a relatively new variant of t-PA formed by removal of the T, N, and K domains. The agent has markedly enhanced fibrin specificity and increased resistance to PAI-1. Its half-life is about 20 to 24 minutes.

With currently accepted dosing regimens, the safety and efficacy of these agents is similar. No one drug has been proven superior to the others. Theoretical advantages of each agent with regard to limiting systemic effects and associated bleeding complications have not entirely borne out in clinical practice.

Technique

Systemic administration is only used for acute coronary thrombosis, acute ischemic stroke, and pulmonary embolism.

Catheter-directed thrombolysis is done by one of several methods[135-138]:

- Intra-arterial infusion
  - Stepwise infusion (gradual advancement of endhole catheter)
  - Graded infusion (high to lower dose)
- Intrathrombic infusion
  - Continuous infusion
  - Lacing with a bolus dose followed by continuous infusion
  - Pulse-spray pharmacomechanical thrombolysis (PSPMT)

The concept of high-dose intrathrombic infusion thrombolysis is based on the technique described by McNamara and Fischer.[136] PSPMT is a method for accelerated clot dissolution developed by Bookstein and colleagues in which concentrated fibrinolytic agent is injected directly into clot as a high-pressure spray through a catheter with many side holes (Fig. 2-35).[137,139] Direct intrathrombic infusion seems to shorten the time for lysis and may limit systemic effects of the drug.

Oral antiplatelet agents are administered before and after thrombolysis to help limit restenosis. An antithrombin agent (heparin or direct thrombin inhibitor) is given during and occasionally after the procedure to limit pericatheter thrombus, acute rethrombosis, or post-PTA occlusion. The standard heparin dose is a 5000-unit IV bolus followed by

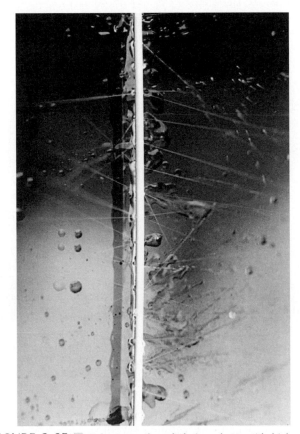

FIGURE 2-35 ■ Pulse-spray thrombolysis catheter with high-pressure fluid spray.

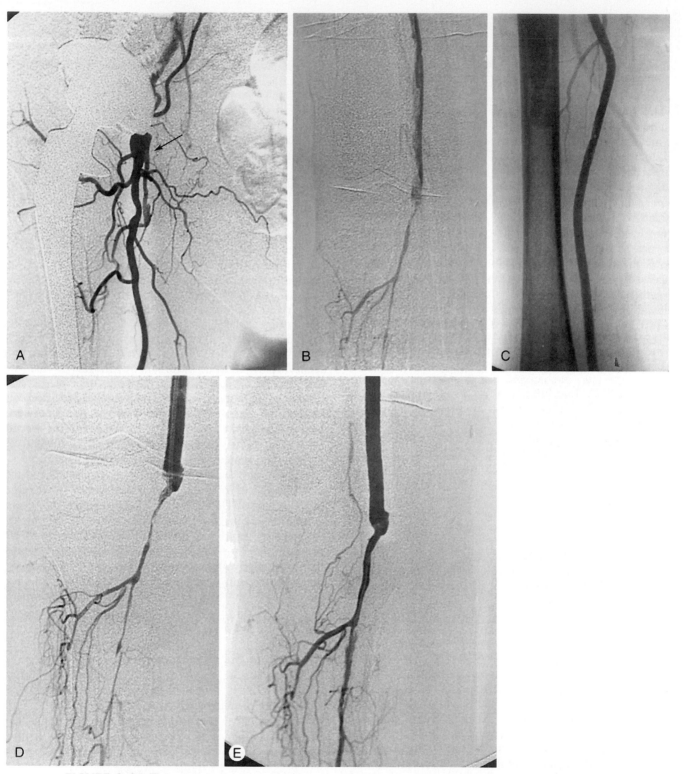

FIGURE 2-36 ■ Combined pulse-spray and infusion thrombolysis of an occluded femoropopliteal bypass graft. **A,** The graft is occluded at its origin *(arrow)*. **B,** After pulse-spray thrombolysis with 250,000 IU of urokinase, significant clot lysis has occurred. **C,** After overnight infusion with urokinase, the body of the graft is almost entirely free of clot. **D,** A long stenosis in the distal popliteal artery and tibioperoneal trunk is revealed. **E,** After balloon angioplasty, the graft outflow is significantly improved.

TABLE 2-5 FIBRINOLYTIC AGENT DOSING REGIMENS

Agent	Infusion Dose	Maximum Bolus	Maximum Dose	Heparin Dose
Urokinase	240→120K IU/hr (graded) 60–120K IU/hr (constant)	125–250K IU	Not established	Full
Alteplase	0.5–1.0 mg/hr 0.001–0.02 mg/kg/hr	10 mg	40 mg	Half or low
Reteplase	0.25–1.0 U/hr	2-5 U	20 U	Half or low

infusion at about 1000 units/hr (with urokinase) or 500 units/hr (with t-PA and derivatives). However, some practitioners prefer to administer only low-dose heparin (50 to 100 units/hr) through the indwelling access sheath. The standard dose of bivalirudin is 0.75 mg/kg IV bolus followed by 1.75 mg/kg/hr infusion.

The occlusion is first crossed with a guidewire from an antegrade or retrograde approach after diagnostic arteriography (Fig. 2-36). Hydrophilic guidewires are particularly useful for this purpose. If the occlusion cannot be crossed (guidewire traversal test), thrombolysis is much less likely to be successful.[140] However, a short trial of fibrinolytic agent infusion to "soften" the clot may be warranted. Infusion is done with an endhole catheter, a multiside hole catheter with tip-occluding wire, or through a coaxial infusion wire.[141] Ideally, the entire thrombus is bathed in the thrombolytic solution. Rough dosing guidelines for peripheral arteries and veins are given in Table 2-5.[130-132,142]

The patient is monitored for bleeding complications and reperfusion in an intensive care or intermediate care unit. The heparin drip is then adjusted by monitoring the PTT every 4 to 6 hours during infusion to maintain at 40 to 60 seconds (with t-PA) or 80 to 100 seconds (with urokinase). Fibrinogen levels can be checked periodically; the risk of hemorrhage may increase when the serum level falls below 100 to 150 mg/dL, in which case the infusion usually is stopped.[143,144] Angiograms are repeated at 4- to 12-hour intervals to assess the degree of lysis and to adjust doses and catheter position. When lysis is complete or near complete (>90% to 95%), underlying disease is treated with angioplasty, stents, or both. Arterial thrombolysis usually is accomplished in less than 24 hours. Venous lysis may require much more time.

If clot dissolution is unusually sluggish or rethrombosis occurs, several factors should be considered. Inadequate anticoagulation is corrected by increasing the heparin dose. In small vessels, vasospasm may be present and is aggressively treated with vasodilators. Consideration should be given to starting an IV GP IIb/IIIa inhibitor infusion to inactivate platelets.

After thrombolysis, residual disease often is found in the vessel wall (atherosclerotic plaque, intimal hyperplasia) or the lumen (organized clot, fibrin- and platelet-rich [white] clot, embolus composed of one or more of these elements). Mural plaque or intimal hyperplasia is treated with angioplasty and sometimes stent placement (see Fig. 2-36). Percutaneous aspiration, mechanical thrombectomy, or operative removal may be required for residual luminal disease resistant to thrombolytics. Angioplasty of such material can cause fragmentation and embolization. At the end of the procedure, a completion angiogram is obtained to document vessel patency and search for occult downstream emboli, which should be treated by local fibrinolytic infusion through a microcatheter.

Results and Complications

Immediate and long-term results of enzymatic thrombolysis are discussed in later chapters. The important complications of the procedure are outlined in Table 2-6.[129-132,145-149]

Hemorrhage can occur at the access site, regions of altered vascular integrity (e.g., recent vascular punctures, fresh graft anastomoses), or remote sites (e.g., retroperitoneum, brain, gastrointestinal tract). Bleeding may occur for several reasons. Circulating plasminogen activator can deplete plasminogen activator inhibitors and generate unbound plasmin. As antiplasmins are exhausted, a systemic "lytic state" can result. t-PA and its derivatives are less likely to degrade unbound fibrinogen. But because they are more fibrin-specific than urokinase, they may preferentially dissolve hemostatic plugs at remote sites of minor trauma and cause major bleeding (e.g., intracranial hemorrhage).

Total thrombolytic dose and overall infusion time have some bearing on bleeding risk, but the relationship is not linear. In some studies, significant fibrinogen depletion is strongly associated with increased risk for major hemorrhage, but in other studies it is not.[132,143,144] In many cases, bleeding is the result of excessive anticoagulation, not the fibrinolytic agent itself.

Distal embolization is detected in about 10% of peripheral arterial revascularization procedures and does not seem to be influenced by the thrombolytic method. An attempt should be made to lyse distal clot by advancing a small-caliber infusion catheter directly to the embolus. Unlysable clot may be left in place or removed surgically, depending on the nature of the occlusion and the condition of the patient.

TABLE 2-6 COMPLICATIONS OF ENZYMATIC THROMBOLYSIS

Complication	Frequency (%)
Minor puncture site bleeding	5–25
Major bleeding requiring transfusion or surgery	3–7
Distal embolization	2–15
Pericatheter thrombosis	
Reperfusion syndrome	
Compartment syndrome	
Drug reactions	
Vessel or graft extravasation	

Complications directly related to revascularization of the extremities include *reperfusion syndrome* and *compartment syndrome*. Revascularization of a nonsalvageable necrotic limb can release lactic acid, myoglobin, and other substances that may lead to acute renal failure and cardiovascular instability. Bleeding into the treated or untreated limb may significantly elevate muscular compartment pressures and require fasciotomy.

Mechanical Thrombectomy

Percutaneous thrombectomy devices are emerging as an attractive alternative or adjunct to enzymatic thrombolysis (Fig. 2-37). These devices are designed to be faster and safer than enzymatic thrombolysis. Potential disadvantages include the increased risk of vessel injury or distal embolization, and device cost. Existing thrombectomy catheters can

---

BOX 2-6 ■ **Mechanical Thrombectomy Devices**

Clot Maceration and Aspiration
Arrow-Trerotola percutaneous thrombectomy device (PTD)
AngioJet/Xpeedior
Hydrolyser
Oasis
Gelbfish Endovac
Thrombex PMT
Prolumen

Clot Pulverization
Helix device
Cragg brush
Castaneda brush

---

be classified by their mechanism of action (Box 2-6).[150-158] With the exception of one device, mechanical thrombectomy catheters are currently approved by the FDA for use only in hemodialysis grafts (see Chapter 17).

The primary application of these catheters is treatment of thrombosed hemodialysis fistulas and grafts. In this setting, immediate and long-term results are comparable to those with enzymatic lysis. There is limited published experience with these devices for acute arterial or venous occlusions.[150] Technical success ranges from 50% to 90%, with no clear advantage of any particular device. Adjunctive enzymatic lysis often is needed to complete thrombus removal. Bleeding complications are not completely eliminated (up to 10% to 15% in some series). The rate of distal embolization ranges from 5% to 15%. Vessel perforation or dissection is reported in 5% to 12% of cases. Finally, device failure is an occasional problem with some catheters.

Embolotherapy

Patient Selection

Transcatheter embolization is used for several reasons:

■ To stop or prevent bleeding
■ To destroy tissue (e.g., neoplasms)
■ To occlude vascular abnormalities (e.g., arteriovenous malformations, varicoceles)

For the treatment of hemorrhage, the goal of embolotherapy is to reduce flow to the bleeding site enough to allow endogenous clotting while maintaining collateral perfusion to neighboring tissue (Fig. 2-38). For tissue obliteration or vascular malformation occlusion, the goal is to completely eliminate perfusion to or outflow from the target site (including potential collaterals) while preserving nearby tissue (see Figs. 6-55 and 10-33). Embolization has several advantages over surgery.[159-161] Vital structures are not damaged en route to the bleeding site or organ, tissue loss is minimized by limiting occlusion to target vessels, and the risks associated with an operation are avoided.

The decision to perform embolotherapy is based on several factors, including the risks of embolization, the feasibility and efficacy of alternative procedures, and the experience of

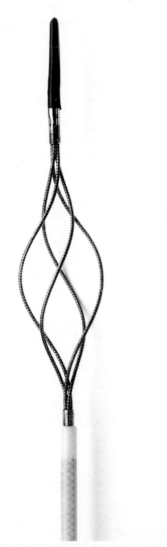

FIGURE 2-37 ■ Arrow-Trerotola mechanical thrombectomy device (Courtesy Arrow, Inc.).

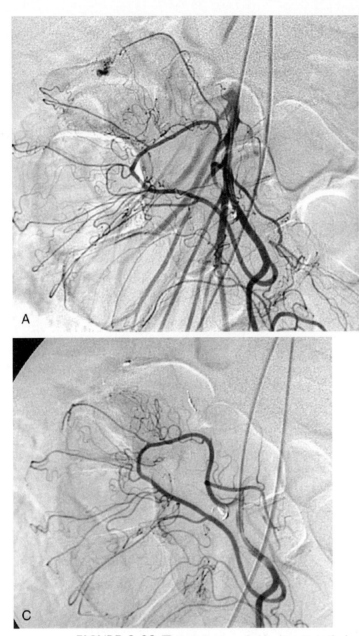

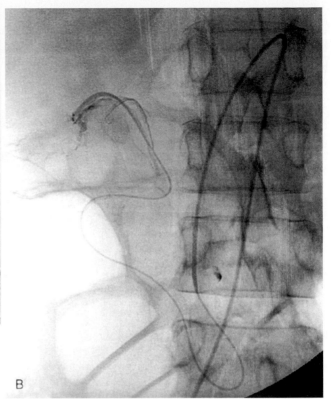

FIGURE 2-38 ■ Embolization of a bleeding site in the hepatic flexure of the colon. **A,** Extravasation from a vasa recta arising from the middle colic branch of the superior mesenteric artery. **B,** A 3-French microcatheter was placed through the long Bookstein catheter directly into the branch feeding the bleeding site. **C,** After placement of two microcoils, extravasation has stopped. Perfusion to adjacent bowel has been maintained.

the operator. Beforehand, a thorough angiographic evaluation is needed to define the bleeding site or abnormality, the path to the target, and the state of existing and potential collateral vessels.

Technique

A vascular sheath is placed to maintain access in case the delivery catheter becomes occluded with embolic material. Delivery catheters must not have side holes through which embolic material can escape. In some cases, the diagnostic catheter can be advanced without difficulty. Otherwise, a coaxial microcatheter can be inserted and directed to the

target site using a steerable guidewire. The outer catheter should be secured in a stable position. With this approach, superselective embolization is possible at almost any site in the body.

A wide assortment of embolic agents are available for vascular occlusion (Table 2-7).

The selection of an agent for embolotherapy is based on the particular goals of vascular occlusion:

■ *Temporary or permanent occlusion.* Permanent occlusion is generally required for progressive diseases (e.g., tumors, inflammatory processes). Temporary occlusion is appropriate for self-limited processes (e.g., traumatic lesions).

TABLE 2-7   COMMONLY USED EMBOLIC AGENTS

Material	Vascular Occlusion
Permanent	
Macrocoils	P
Microcoils	P
Polyvinyl alcohol (PVA) particles	D
Microspheres	D
Alcohol	P, D
Ethanolamine oleate	P, D
Detachable balloon	P
Avitene	P, D
Glue	P, D
Onyx	P, D
Temporary	
Gelfoam pieces	P
Occlusion balloon catheter	P
Thrombin	P

P, proximal; D, distal.

■ *Proximal or distal embolization.* Embolization into or around small arteries or beyond venules is used to stop flow through a vessel when remaining collateral vessels will not compromise the result (e.g., pseudoaneurysms, traumatic extravasation). Distal embolization at the arteriolar or capillary level is needed to destroy tissue or stop flow through a vessel when new collateral vessels could lead to recurrence of the problem (e.g., tumor ablation, bronchial artery bleeding, arteriovenous malformation).

Coils are used for permanent vascular occlusion. Macrocoils are made of guidewire material with polyester threads attached to promote thrombosis (Fig. 2-39). They are available in a variety of lengths, diameters (2 to 15 mm), and shapes for use with standard 5-French (0.035- or 0.038-inch) nonhydrophilic catheters. The unwound coil preloaded in a metal tube is pushed into the catheter and then deployed with a guidewire or a brisk fluid pulse. Before inserting the coil, it is prudent to test whether the catheter tip will back away when the guidewire is advanced alone or saline pulse is made.

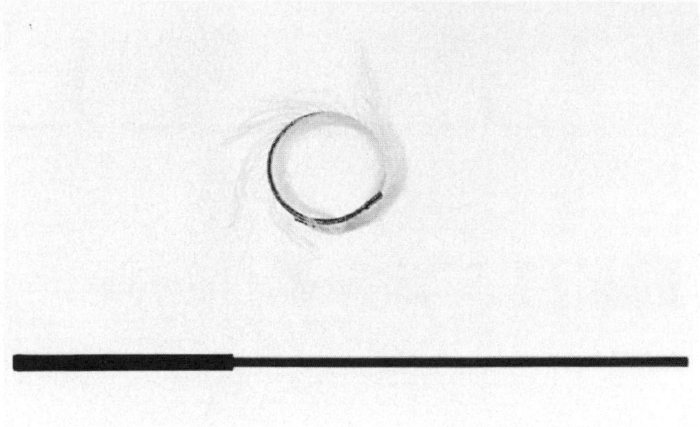

FIGURE 2-39 ■ Macrocoil with loader.

Microcoils are made for passage through microcatheters. They come preloaded in a plastic delivery device (Fig. 2-40). A wide variety of shapes and sizes are available. Conventional microcoils are less thrombogenic than macrocoils and should be used with Gelfoam (see below). Newer microcoils are more thrombogenic, and more radiopaque because they are made of platinum wire.

Coil selection is primarily based on the diameter and length of the vessel to be occluded. The nominal coil diameter should be slightly larger than the target vessel. If the coil is too small, it can migrate distally or proximally, with potentially disastrous results (e.g., through a pulmonary arteriovenous malformation into the brain). If the coil is too large, it may unravel proximally and obstruct nontarget branches or even embolize to a distant site. Although more costly and complicated to use, detachable coils are released only after the coil is situated in the proper location and can be removed if the position is suboptimal. Once a large coil is secured in the vessel, additional coils of the same or smaller size are densely packed in front of it to make a "nest." Gelatin sponge often is used along with coils to promote rapid thrombosis.

Gelfoam is a surgical hemostatic sponge that expands on contact with fluids. It is an extremely versatile embolic agent used for temporary vascular occlusion (Fig. 2-41). The occluded segment may recanalize within several days to

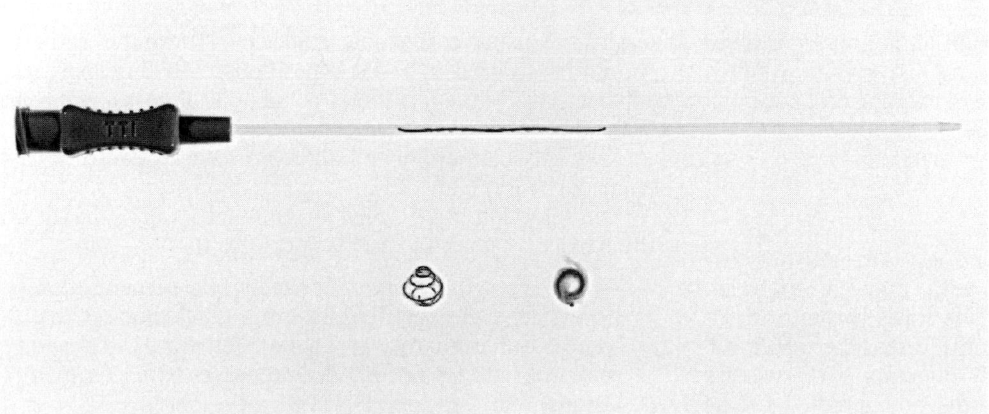

FIGURE 2-40 ■ Microcoils with unwound coil in a plastic loader.

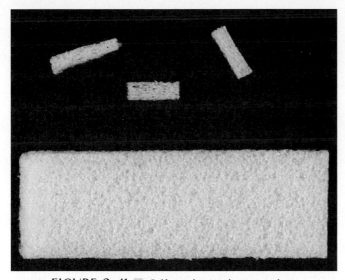

FIGURE 2-41 ■ Gelfoam sheet and cut torpedoes.

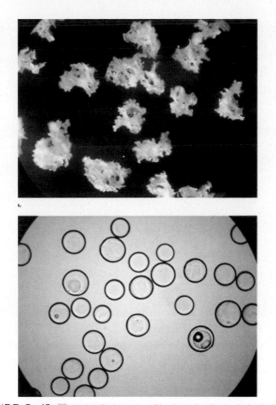

FIGURE 2-43 ■ Magnified image of hydrated polyvinyl alcohol particles (**top**) and tris-acryl gelatin microspheres (**bottom**). (From Andrews RT, Binkert CA: Relative rates of blood flow reduction during transcatheter arterial embolization with tris-acryl gelatin microspheres or polyvinyl alcohol: quantitative comparison in a swine model. J Vasc Interv Radiol 2003;14:1311. Reprinted with permission.)

months after placement. Gelfoam sheets are cut into "torpedoes" or small pledgets tailored to the embolic needs and catheter size. Larger pieces are delivered individually with a tuberculin syringe suspended in dilute contrast material. Smaller pieces may be suspended in fluid and injected as a slurry in small increments until the blood column is static. Overzealous injection can cause reflux of material. Gelfoam powder (100 to 200 μm) also has been used for small vessel embolization, but the risk of distal ischemia is significant.

Polyvinyl alcohol (PVA) particles occlude small arteries and arterioles (50 to 2500 μm) (Fig. 2-42). PVA causes an inflammatory reaction in the vessel wall. These particles tend to aggregate within the vessel lumen and occasionally do not provide complete or permanent vascular occlusion (Fig. 2-43). The agent, which expands on contact with fluid, is commercially available in narrow size ranges (e.g., 300 to 500 μm).

For delivery, the material is suspended in dilute contrast, mixed immediately before injection in a three-way stopcock system, and infused *slowly* under fluoroscopic guidance. After each aliquot is given, contrast is injected to assess flow. Dilute suspensions of small particles (<500 to 700 μm) pass easily through most microcatheters.

Tris-acryl gelatin microspheres (Embospheres) and *PVA microspheres (Contour SE Microspheres)* are spherical particles that cause relatively permanent occlusion.[162] Owing to their uniform size and inability to clump, they are easier to deliver through microcatheters (see Fig. 2-43). These agents have been used in a variety of vascular beds with good clinical results, although there is some concern that the risk of ischemia or infarction is increased with microspheres compared with PVA particles of comparable size due to more distal vascular occlusion or escape through arteriovenous shunts.[163,164]

Absolute ethanol is an extremely toxic liquid embolic agent that causes permanent occlusion from the point of entry. It is a particularly dangerous agent and should be handled with great care. Alcohol completely denatures proteins in the vessel wall, causing a painful inflammatory reaction that can extend into the perivascular spaces and injure adjacent tissues, vessels, and nerves. The alcohol volume is estimated by first injecting contrast until the desired level of vascular filling is achieved. In the arterial system, the liquid may be delivered through the lumen of an inflated occlusion

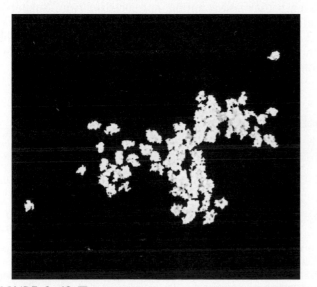

FIGURE 2-42 ■ Polyvinyl alcohol particles (1000 μm to 1500 μm) in a dry state.

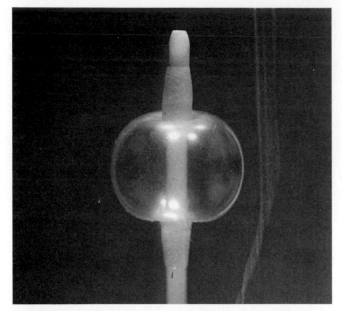

FIGURE 2-44 ■ The balloon occlusion catheter can be used as a temporary occlusive device or to avoid reflux during delivery of certain embolic agents.

balloon to prevent reflux (Fig. 2-44; see also Fig. 8-42). Patients should be warned that moderate to intense pain may follow embolization. In many cases, general or epidural anesthesia is required for the procedure and aggressive analgesia used afterward.

Ethylene vinyl alcohol copolymer (Onyx) is a nonadhesive liquid embolic agent that is gaining popularity particularly in neurovascular interventions. Catheters are prefilled with a small volume of dimethyl sulfoxide (DMSO) to prevent precipitation of the drug. The delivery system must be compatible with DMSO, which can dissolve many plastic catheters. Onyx, which is radiopaque, is then slowly injected to endpoint. Outside the brain, it has been used in treating arteriovenous malformations and endoleaks after endovascular aneurysm repair.[165,166]

Microfibrillar collagen (Avitene) produces an intense inflammatory reaction and immediate thrombosis in large and small vessels. The occlusion is effectively permanent. The fibrils are suspended in dilute contrast and injected slowly in small increments. The catheter should be flushed between injections to prevent blockage.

Cyanoacrylates (glues) are liquid adhesives and versatile embolic agents.[167] Glues provide effectively permanent occlusion and cause acute inflammatory changes in treated vessels. Their liquid nature allows them to penetrate into the nidus of arteriovenous malformations (AVMs), thus effecting the most optimal treatment. Several derivatives exist; in the United States, *n-butyl cyanoacrylate (n-BCA, Trufill)* is currently approved for use in cranial arteriovenous malformations. The primary noncranial application is also for AVMs, but glues have been used in a variety of other settings, including aneurysms and pseudoaneurysms, aortobronchial fistulas, varicocele treatment, and gastrointestinal bleeding.[167-170]

Cyanoacrylates solidify on contact with ionic surfaces (e.g., blood). Therefore, the delivery system is purged with dextrose before and after injection and great care must be taken to avoid any contact with blood or saline before injection. The glue is admixed with Ethiodol to provide radiopacity and to control the time for polymerization (cyanoacrylate to oil ratio of 1:1 to 1:4 corresponding to solidification interval of about 1 to 4 seconds). The volume of agent (usually 0.1 to 0.5 mL) is estimated by several test injections of contrast through the microcatheter placed just proximal to the AVM nidus. The complex details of the technique (estimating injection volume and rate, preparation of the mixture, avoidance of contact with blood, saline, or polycarbonate syringes, proper purging of the entire system with dextrose, agent delivery and dextrose flush, and immediate withdrawal of the microcatheter to avoid gluing the tip to the vessel) demand considerable expertise and experience.

Ethanolamine oleate and *sodium morrhuate* are fatty acid–based sclerosing agents used primarily for endoscopic treatment of gastroesophageal varices and transcatheter embolization of gastric varices.[171] Sodium morrhuate also is indicated for sclerotherapy of varicose veins. They cause a mild inflammatory reaction that ultimately leads to vessel fibrosis and occlusion. Both agents have been used for transvenous treatment of intestinal varices in portal hypertension and for venous malformations.

Results and Complications

With available microcatheter systems, embolotherapy is technically successful in more than 90% of attempts. Immediate and long-term results for specific applications are considered in later chapters.

The major risks of transcatheter embolization are ischemia of adjacent tissue and nontarget embolization. Ischemia can be minimized by careful placement of embolic material. Nontarget embolization is avoided by patience and meticulous technique during the procedure.

Postembolization syndrome is a frequent occurrence after embolization. The symptoms usually begin immediately or within 24 hours of embolization, and consist of fever, nausea and vomiting, and localized pain. Supportive care usually is successful, including antipyretics, antiemetics, and analgesia (sometimes requiring patient-controlled anesthesia [PCA]). Patients should be carefully evaluated for infection or evidence of infarction.

REFERENCES

1. Bancroft JW, Benenati JF, Becker GJ, et al: Neutralized lidocaine: use in pain reduction in local anesthesia. J Vasc Interv Radiol 1992;3:107.
2. McEvoy GK, ed: Chloroprocaine Hydrochloride. AHFS Drug Information 98. Bethesda, Md, American Society of Health-System Pharmacists, 1998:2661.
3. Bartfield JM, Jandreau SW, Raccio-Robak N: Randomized trial of diphenhydramine versus benzyl alcohol with epinephrine as an alternative to lidocaine local anesthesia. Ann Emerg Med 1998;32:650.
4. Seldinger SI: Catheter replacement of the needle in percutaneous arteriography. Acta Radiol 1953;39:368.
5. Illescas FF, Baker ME, McCann R, et al: CT evaluation of retroperitoneal hemorrhage associated with femoral arteriography. AJR Am J Roentgenol 1986;146:1289.

6. Altin RS, Flicker S, Naidech HJ: Pseudoaneurysm and arteriovenous fistula after femoral artery catheterization: association with low femoral punctures. AJR Am J Roentgenol 1989;152:629.

7. Grier D, Hartnell G: Percutaneous femoral artery puncture: practice and anatomy. Br J Radiol 1990;63:602.

8. Rupp SB, Vogelzang RL, Nemcek AA Jr, et al: Relationship of the inguinal ligament to pelvic radiographic landmarks: anatomic correlation and its role in femoral arteriography. J Vasc Interv Radiol 1993;4:409.

9. Jaques PF, Mauro MA, Keefe B: US guidance for vascular access. J Vasc Interv Radiol 1992;3:427.

10. Millward SF, Burbridge BE, Luna G: Puncturing the pulseless femoral artery: a simple technique that uses palpation of anatomic landmarks. J Vasc Interv Radiol 1993;4:415.

11. Spijkerboer AM, Scholten FG, Mali WP, van Schaik JP, et al: Antegrade puncture of the femoral artery: morphologic study. Radiology 1990;176:57.

12. Sacks D, Summers TA: Antegrade selective catheterization of femoral vessels with a 4- or 5-F catheter and safety wire. J Vasc Interv Radiol 1991;2:325.

13. Saddekni S, Srur M, Cohn DJ, et al: Antegrade catheterization of the superficial femoral artery. Radiology 1985;157:531.

14. Bishop AF, Berkman WA, Palagallo GL: Antegrade selective catheterization of the superficial femoral artery using a moveable core guide wire. Radiology 1985;157:548.

15. Gaines PA, Reidy JF: Percutaneous high brachial aortography: a safe alternative to the translumbar approach. Clin Radiol 1986;37:595.

16. Baum PA, Matsumoto AH, Teitelbaum GP, et al: Anatomic relationship between the common femoral artery and vein: CT evaluation and clinical significance. Radiology 1989;173:775.

17. Grassi CJ, Bettman MA, Rogoff P, et al: Femoral arteriovenous fistula after placement of a Kimray-Greenfield filter. AJR Am J Roentgenol 1988;151:681.

18. Troianos CA, Kuwik RJ, Pasqual JR, et al: Internal jugular vein and carotid artery anatomic relation as determined by ultrasonography. Anesthesiology 1996;85:43.

19. Trerotola SO, Kuhn-Fulton J, Johnson MS, et al: Tunneled infusion catheters: increased incidence of symptomatic venous thrombosis after subclavian versus internal jugular venous access. Radiology 2000;217:89.

20. Hoffer EK, Bloch RD: Percutaneous arterial closure devices. J Vasc Interv Radiol 2003;14:865.

21. Balzer JO, Scheinert D, Diebold T, et al: Postinterventional transcutaneous suture of femoral artery access sites in patients with peripheral arterial occlusive disease: a study of 930 patients. Catheter Cardiovasc Interv 2001;53:174.

22. Duda SH, Wiskirchen J, Erb M, et al: Suture mediated percutaneous closure of antegrade femoral arterial access sites in patients who have received full anticoagulation therapy. Radiology 1999;210:47.

23. Koreny M, Riedmuller E, Nikfardjam M, et al: Arterial puncture closing devices compared with standard manual compression after cardiac catheterization: systematic review and meta-analysis. JAMA 2004;291:350.

24. Carey D, Martin JR, Moore CA, et al: Complications of femoral artery closure devices. Catheter Cardiovasc Interv 2001;52:3.

25. Singh H, Cardella JF, Cole PE, et al. Quality improvement guidelines for diagnostic arteriography. J Vasc Interv Radiol 2003;14(9 Pt 2):S283.

26. Egglin TK, O'Moore PV, Feinstein AR, et al: Complications of peripheral arteriography: a new system to identify patients at increased risk. J Vasc Surg 1995;22:787.

27. Darcy MD, Kanterman RY, Kleinhoffer MA, et al: Evaluation of coagulation tests as predictors of angiographic bleeding complications. Radiology 1996;198:741.

28. Katzenschlager R, Ugurluoglu A, Ahmadi A, et al: Incidence of pseudoaneurysm after diagnostic and therapeutic angiography. Radiology 1995;195:463.

29. Toursarkissian B, Allen BT, Petrinec D, et al: Spontaneous closure of selected iatrogenic pseudoaneurysms and arteriovenous fistulae. J Vasc Surg 1997;25:803.

30. Fukumoto Y, Tsutsui H, Tsuchihasi M, et al: The incidence and risk factors of cholesterol embolization syndrome, a complication of cardiac catheterization: a prospective study. J Am Coll Cardiol 2003;42:211.

31. Jarosz JM, McKeown B, Reidy JF: Short-term femoral nerve complications following percutaneous transfemoral procedures. J Vasc Interv Radiol 1995;6:351.

32. Lipchik EO, Sugimoto H: Percutaneous brachial artery catheterization. Radiology 1986;160:842.

33. Gagliardi JM, Batt M, Avril G, et al: Neurologic complications of axillary and brachial catheter arteriography in atherosclerotic patients: predictive factors. Ann Vasc Surg 1990;4:546.

34. Gritter KJ, Laidlaw WW, Peterson NT: Complications of outpatient transbrachial intraarterial digital subtraction angiography: work in progress. Radiology 1987;162:125.

35. Chitwood RW, Shepard AD, Shetty PC, et al: Surgical complications of transaxillary arteriography: a case-control study. J Vasc Surg 1996;23:844.

36. Smith DC, Mitchell DA, Peterson GW, et al: Medial brachial fascial compartment syndrome: anatomic basis of neuropathy after transaxillary arteriography. Radiology 1989;173:149.

37. Eisenberg L, Paulson EK, Kliewer MA, et al: Sonographically guided compression repair of pseudoaneurysms: further experience from a single institution. AJR Am J Roentgenol 1999;173:1567.

38. Coley BD, Roberts AC, Fellmeth BD, et al: Postangiographic femoral artery pseudoaneurysms: further experience with US guided compression repair. Radiology 1995;194:307.

39. Morgan R, Belli A-M: Current treatment methods for postcatheterization pseudoaneurysms. J Vasc Interv Radiol 2003;14:697.

40. Krueger K, Zaehringer M, Soehngen F-D, et al: Femoral pseudoaneurysms: management with percutaneous thrombin injections—success rates and effects on systemic coagulation. Radiology 2003;226:452.

41. Sheiman RG, Brophy DP: Treatment of iatrogenic femoral pseudoaneurysms with percutaneous thrombin injection: experience in 54 patients. Radiology 2001;219:123.

42. Sadiq S, Ibrahim W: Thromboembolism complicating thrombin injection of femoral artery pseudoaneurysm: management with intraarterial thrombolysis. J Vasc Interv Radiol 2001;12:633.

43. Sheiman RG, Brophy DP, Perry LJ, et al: Thrombin injection for the repair of brachial artery pseudoaneurysms. AJR Am J Roentgenol 1999;173:1029.

44. Ruebben A, Tettoni S, Muratore P, et al: Arteriovenous fistulas induced by femoral artery catheterization: percutaneous treatment. Radiology 1998;209:729.

45. Thalhammer C, Kirchherr AS, Uhlich F, et al: Postcatheterization pseudoaneurysms and arteriovenous fistulas: repair with percutaneous implantation of endovascular covered stents. Radiology 2000;214:127.

46. Silberstein M, Tress BM, Hennessy O: Selecting the right technique to reform a reverse curve catheter (Simmons style): critical review. Cardiovasc Intervent Radiol 1992;15:171.

47. Waltman AC, Courey WR, Athanasoulis C, et al: Technique for left gastric artery catheterization. Radiology 1973;109:732.

48. Tetteroo E, van Engelen AD, Spithoven JH, et al: Stent placement after iliac angioplasty. Comparison of hemodynamic and angiographic criteria. Radiology 1996;201:155.

49. Bonn J: Percutaneous vascular intervention: value of hemodynamic measurements. Radiology 1996;201:18.

50. Kinney TB, Rose SC: Intraarterial pressure measurements during angiographic evaluation of peripheral vascular disease: techniques, interpretation, applications, and limitations. AJR Am J Roentgenol 1996;166:277.

51. Archie JP Jr: Analysis and comparison of pressure gradients and ratios for predicting iliac stenosis. Ann Vasc Surg 1994;8:271.

52. Morcos SK, Thomsen HS: Adverse reactions to iodinated contrast media. Eur Radiol 2001;11:1267.

53. Bush WH, Swanson DP: Acute reactions to intravascular contrast media: types, risk factors, recognition, and treatment. AJR Am J Roentgenol 1991;157:1153.

54. McClennan BL: Ionic and non-ionic iodinated contrast media: evolution and strategies for use. AJR Am J Roentgenol 1990;155:225.

55. Krouwels MM, Overbosch EH, Guit GL: Iohexol vs. ioxaglate in lower extremity angiography: a comparative randomized double-blind study in 80 patients. Eur J Radiol 1996;22:133.

56. Lawrence V, Matthai W, Hartmare S: Comparative safety of high-osmolality and low-osmolality radiographic contrast agents: report of a multidisciplinary working group. Invest Radiol 1992;27:2.

57. Druy EM, Bettman MA, Jeans W: A double-blind study of iopromide 300 for peripheral arteriography. Results of a multi-institutional comparison of iopromide with iohexol and iopamidol. Invest Radiol 1994;29(Suppl):S102.

58. Faykus MH Jr, Cope C, Athanasoulis C, et al: Double-blind study of the safety, tolerance, and diagnostic efficacy of iopromide as compared

with iopamidol and iohexol in patients requiring aortography and visceral angiography. Invest Radiol 1994;29(Suppl):S98.

59. Aspelin P, Aubry P, Fransson SG, et al: Nephrotoxic effects in high risk patients undergoing angiography. N Engl J Med 2003;348:491.

60. Ellis JH, Cohan RH, Sonnad SS, et al: Selective use of radiographic low-osmolality contrast media in the 1990s. Radiology 1996;200:297.

61. Eschelman DJ, Sullivan KL, Bonn J, et al: Carbon dioxide as a contrast agent to guide vascular interventional procedures. AJR Am J Roentgenol 1998;171:1265.

62. Caridi JG, Hawkins IF Jr: CO_2 digital subtraction angiography: potential complications and their prevention. J Vasc Interv Radiol 1997;8:383.

63. Kerns SR, Hawkins IF Jr: Carbon dioxide digital subtraction angiography: expanding applications and technical evolution. AJR Am J Roentgenol 1995;164:735.

64. Caridi JG, Hawkins IF Jr, Klioze SD, et al: Carbon dioxide digital subtraction angiography: the practical approach. Tech Vasc Interv Radiol 2001;4:57.

65. Oliva VL, Denbow N, Therasse E, et al: Digital subtraction angiography of the abdominal aorta and lower extremities: carbon dioxide versus iodinated contrast material. J Vasc Interv Radiol 1999;10:723.

66. Diaz LP, Pabon IP, Garcia JS, et al: Assessment of CO_2 arteriography in arterial occlusive disease of the lower extremities. J Vasc Interv Radiol 2000;11:163.

67. Kaufman JA, Geller SC, Waltman AC: Renal insufficiency: gadopentetate dimeglumine as a radiographic contrast agent during peripheral vascular interventional procedures. Radiology 1996;198:579.

68. Spinosa DJ, Kaufman JA, Hartwell GD, et al: Gadolinium chelates in angiography and interventional radiology: a useful alternative to iodinated contrast media for angiography. Radiology 2002;223:319.

69. Kaufman JA, Geller SC, Bazari H, et al: Gadolinium based contrast agents as an alternative at vena cavography in patients with renal insufficiency: early experience. Radiology 1999;21:280.

70. Gemery J, Idelson B, Reid S, et al: Acute renal failure after arteriography with a gadolinium-based contrast agent. AJR Am J Roentgenol 1998;171:1277.

71. Nyman U, Elmståhl B, Leander P, et al: Are gadolinium-based contrast media really safer than iodinated media for digital subtraction angiography in patients with azotemia? Radiology 2002;223:311.

72. Brown DB, Pappas JA, Vedantham S, et al: Gadolinium, carbon dioxide, and iodinated contrast material for planning inferior vena cava filter placement: a prospective trial. J Vasc Interv Radiol 2003;14:1017.

73. Kereiakes DJ: Adjunctive pharmacotherapy before percutaneous coronary intervention in non-ST-elevation acute coronary syndromes: the role of modulating inflammation. Circulation 2003;108(16 Suppl 1):III22.

74. Goodnight SH: Aspirin therapy for cardiovascular disease. Curr Opin Hematol 1996;3:355.

75. Easton JD: Evidence with antiplatelet therapy and ADP-receptor antagonists. Cerebrovasc Dis 2003;16(Suppl 1):20.

76. Cannon CP, CAPRIE investigators: Effectiveness of clopidogrel versus aspirin in preventing acute myocardial infarction in patients with symptomatic atherothrombosis (CAPRIE trial). Am J Cardiol 2002;90:760.

77. Hiatt WR: Pharmacologic therapy for peripheral arterial disease and claudication. J Vasc Surg 2002;36:1283.

78. Chapman TM, Goa KL: Cilostazol: a review of its use in intermittent claudication. Am J Cardiovasc Drugs 2003;3:117.

79. Kambayashi J, Liu Y, Sun B, et al: Cilostazol as a unique antithrombotic agent. Curr Pharm Des 2003;9:2289.

80. Schweizer J, Kirch W, Koch R, et al: Use of abciximab and tirofiban in patients with peripheral arterial occlusive disease and arterial thrombosis. Angiology 2003;54:155.

81. Ouriel K, Castaneda F, McNamara T, et al: Reteplase monotherapy and reteplase/abciximab combination therapy in peripheral arterial occlusive disease: results from the RELAX trial. J Vasc Interv Radiol 2004;15:229.

82. Shlansky-Goldberg R: Platelet aggregation inhibitors for use in peripheral vascular interventions: what can we learn from the experience in the coronary arteries? J Vasc Interv Radiol 2002;13:229.

83. Hirsh J, Fuster V: Guide to anticoagulant therapy. Part I: Heparin. Circulation 1994;89:1449.

84. Simko RJ, Tsung FF, Stanek EJ: Activated clotting time versus activated partial thromboplastin time for therapeutic monitoring of heparin. Ann Pharmacother 1995;29:1015.

85. Fedullo PF, Tapson VF: Clinical practice. The evaluation of suspected pulmonary embolism. N Engl J Med 2003;349:1247.

86. Raskob GE, Hirsch J: Controversies in timing of the first dose of anticoagulant prophylaxis against venous thromboembolism after major orthopedic surgery. Chest 2003;124(6 Suppl):379S.

87. Gulba D: Differentiation of low molecular weight heparins in acute coronary syndromes: an interventionalist's perspective. Semin Thromb Hemost 1999;25(Suppl 3):123.

88. Kaplan KL: Direct thrombin inhibitors. Expert Opin Pharmacother 2003;4:653.

89. Shammas NW: Complications in peripheral vascular interventions: emerging role of direct thrombin inhibitors. J Vasc Interv Radiol 2005;16(2 Pt 1):165.

90. Allie DE, Lirtzman MD, Wyatt CH, et al: Bivalirudin as a foundation anticoagulant in peripheral vascular disease: a safe and feasible alternative for renal and iliac interventions. J Invasive Cardiol 2003;15:334.

91. Hirsh J, Fuster V: Guide to anticoagulant therapy. Part 2: Oral anticoagulants. Circulation 1994;89:1469.

92. Kandarpa K: Commonly used medications. In: Kandarpa K, Aruny JE, eds. Handbook of Interventional Radiologic Procedures. Boston, Little Brown, 1996:397.

93. Stoeckelhuber BM, Suttmann I, Stoeckelhuber M, et al: Comparison of the vasodilating effects of nitroglycerin, verapamil, and tolazoline in hand angiography. J Vasc Interv Radiol 2003;14:749.

94. Dotter CT, Judkins MP: Transluminal treatment of arteriosclerotic obstruction. Circulation 1964;30:654.

95. Gruentzig A, Hopff H: Perkutane Rekanalisation chronischer arterieller Verschluesse mit einem neuen Dilatationskatheter. Dtsch Med Wochenschr 1974;99:2502.

96. Castaneda-Zuniga WR, Formanek A, Tadavarthy M, et al: The mechanism of balloon angioplasty. Radiology 1980;135:565.

97. Block PC, Baughman KL, Pasternak RC, et al: Transluminal angioplasty: correlation of morphologic and angiographic findings in an experimental model. Circulation 1980;61:778.

98. Rosenfield K, Schainfeld R, Isner JM: Percutaneous revascularization in peripheral arterial disease. Curr Prob Cardiol 1996;21:7.

99. Johnston KW, Rae M, Hogg-Johnston SA, et al: Five-year results of a prospective study of percutaneous transluminal angioplasty. Ann Surg 1987;206:403.

100. Anand S, Creager M: Peripheral arterial disease. Clin Evid 2002;7:79

101. Society of Interventional Radiology Standards of Practice Committee: Guidelines for percutaneous transluminal angioplasty. J Vasc Interv Radiol 2003;14(9 Pt 2):S209.

102. Engelke C, Morgan RA, Belli AM: Cutting balloon percutaneous transluminal angioplasty for salvage of lower limb arterial bypass grafts: feasibility. Radiology 2002;223:106.

103. Engelke C, Sandhu C, Morgan RA, et al: Using 6-mm cutting balloon angioplasty in patients with resistant peripheral artery stenosis: preliminary results. AJR Am J Roentgenol 2002;179:619.

104. Vorwerk D, Adam G, Muller-Leisse C, et al: Hemodialysis fistulas and grafts: use of cutting balloons to dilate venous stenoses. Radiology 1996;201:864.

105. Tielbeek AV, Vroegindeweij D, Buth J, et al: Comparison of balloon angioplasty and Simpson atherectomy for lesions in the femoropopliteal artery: angiographic and clinical results of a prospective randomized trial. J Vasc Interv Radiol 1996;7:837.

106. McLean GK: Percutaneous peripheral atherectomy. J Vasc Interv Radiol 1993;4:465.

107. Dolmatch BL, Gray RJ, Horton KM, et al: Treatment of anastomotic bypass graft stenosis with directional atherectomy: short-term and intermediate-term results. J Vasc Interv Radiol 1995;6:105.

108. Zeller T, Frank U, Burgelin K, et al: Initial experience with percutaneous atherectomy in the infragenicular arteries. J Endovasc Ther 2003;10:987.

109. Zeller T, Frank U, Burgelin K, et al: Early experience with rotational thrombectomy device for treatment of acute and subacute infra-aortic arterial occlusions. J Endovasc Ther 2003;10:322.

110. Mueller-Huelsbeck S, Jahnke T: Peripheral arterial applications of percutaneous thrombectomy. Tech Vasc Interv Radiol 2003;6:22.

111. Yoffe B, Yavnel L, Altshuler A, et al: Preliminary experience with the Xtrak debulking device in the treatment of peripheral occlusions. J Endovasc Ther 2002;9:234.

112. Palmaz JC: Intravascular stents: tissue-stent interactions and design considerations. AJR Am J Roentgenol 1993;160:613.

113. Fontaine AB, Spigos DG, Eaton G, et al: Stent-induced intimal hyperplasia: are there fundamental differences between flexible and rigid stent designs? J Vasc Interv Radiol 1994;5:739.

114. Leung DA, Spinosa DJ, Hagspiel KD, et al: Selection of stents for treating iliac arterial occlusive disease. J Vasc Interv Radiol 2003;14:137.

115. Palmaz JC: Balloon-expandable intravascular stent. AJR Am J Roentgenol 1988;150:1263.

116. Martin EC, Katzen BT, Benenati JF, et al: Multicenter trial of the Wallstent in the iliac and femoral arteries. J Vasc Interv Radiol 1995;6:843.

117. Strecker E-P, Boos IBL, Hagen B: Flexible tantalum stents for the treatment of iliac artery lesions: long-term patency, complications, and risk factors. Radiology 1996;199:641.

118. Furui S, Sawada S, Kuramoto K, et al: Gianturco stent placement in malignant caval obstruction: analysis of factors for predicting the outcome. Radiology 1995;195:147.

119. Lossef SV, Lutz RL, Mundorf J, et al: Comparison of mechanical deformation properties of metallic stents with use of stress-strain analysis. J Vasc Interv Radiol 1994;5:341.

120. Bjarnason H, Hunter DW, Crain MR, et al: Collapse of a Palmaz stent in the subclavian vein. AJR Am J Roentgenol 1993;160:1123.

121. Saeed M, Knowles HJ Jr, Brems JJ, et al: Percutaneous retrieval of a large Palmaz stent from the pulmonary artery. J Vasc Interv Radiol 1993;4:811.

122. Sanchez RB, Roberts AC, Valji K, et al: Wallstent misplaced during transjugular placement of an intrahepatic portosystemic shunt: retrieval with a loop snare. AJR Am J Roentgenol 1992;159:129.

123. Duda SH, Poerner TC, Wiesinger B, et al: Drug-eluting stents: potential applications for peripheral arterial occlusive disease. J Vasc Interv Radiol. 2003;14:291.

124. Duda SH, Bosiers M, Lammer J: Sirolimus-eluting versus Bare Nitinol Stent for obstructive superficial femoral artery disease: the SIROCCO II trial. J Vasc Interv Radiol 2005;16:331.

125. Holmes DR, Leon MB, Moses JW, et al: Analysis of 1-year clinical outcomes in the SIRIUS trial: a randomized trial of a sirolimus-eluting stent versus a standard stent in patients at high risk for coronary restenosis. Circulation 2004;109:634.

126. Saxon RR, Coffman JM, Gooding JM, et al: Long-term Results of ePTFE stent-graft versus angioplasty in the femoropopliteal artery: single center experience from a prospective, randomized trial. J Vasc Interv Radiol 2003;14:303.

127. Hausegger KA, Karnel F, Georgieva B, et al: Transjugular intrahepatic portosystemic shunt creation with the Viatorr expanded polytetralfluoroethylene covered stent graft. J Vasc Interv Radiol 2004;15:239.

128. Baltacioglu F, Cimsit NC, Cil B, et al: Endovascular stent-graft applications in iatrogenic vascular injuries. Cardiovasc Intervent Radiol 2003;26:434.

129. Valji K, Bookstein JJ: Thrombolysis: clinical applications. In: Baum S, Pentecost MJ, eds. Abrams' Angiography: Interventional Radiology. Boston, Little Brown, 1997:132.

130. Razavi MK, Lee DS, Hofmann LV: Catheter-directed thrombolytic therapy for limb ischemia: current status and controversies. J Vasc Interv Radiol 2004;15:13.

131. Semba CP, Bakal CW, Calis KA, et al: Alteplase as an alternative to urokinase. J Vasc Interv Radiol 2000;11:279.

132. Valji K: Evolving strategies for thrombolytic therapy of peripheral vascular occlusion. J Vasc Interv Radiol 2000;11:411.

133. Ouriel K: Comparison of safety and efficacy of the various thrombolytic agents. Rev Cardiovasc Med 2002;3(Suppl 2):S17.

134. Margaglione M, Grandone E, DiMinno G: Mechanisms of fibrinolysis and clinical use of thrombolytic agents. Prog Drug Res 1992;39:197.

135. Ouriel K, Shortell CK, DeWeese JA, et al: A comparison of thrombolytic therapy with operative revascularization in the initial treatment of acute peripheral arterial ischemia. J Vasc Surg 1994;19:1021.

136. McNamara TO, Fischer JR: Thrombolysis of peripheral arteries and bypass grafts: improved results using high dose urokinase. AJR Am J Roentgenol 1985;144:769.

137. Bookstein JJ, Fellmeth B, Roberts A, et al: Pulsed-spray pharmacomechanical thrombolysis: preliminary clinical results. AJR Am J Roentgenol 1989;152:1097.

138. Valji K, Bookstein JJ, Roberts AC, et al: Pulse-spray pharmacomechanical thrombolysis of thrombosed hemodialysis grafts: long-term experience and comparison of original and current techniques. AJR Am J Roentgenol 1995;164:1495.

139. Valji K, Roberts AC, Davis GB, et al: Pulsed spray thrombolysis of arterial and bypass graft occlusions. AJR Am J Roentgenol 1991;156:617.

140. Ouriel K, Shortell CK, Azodo MV, et al: Acute peripheral arterial occlusion: predictors of success in catheter-directed thrombolytic therapy. Radiology 1994;193:561.

141. Hicks ME, Picus D, Darcy MD, et al: Multilevel infusion catheter for use with thrombolytic agents. J Vasc Interv Radiol 1991;2:73.

142. Benenati J, Shlansky-Goldberg R, Meglin A, et al: Thrombolytic and antiplatelet therapy in peripheral vascular disease with use of reteplase and/or abciximab. J Vasc Interv Radiol 2001;12:796.

143. The STILE investigators. Results of a prospective randomized trial evaluating surgery versus thrombolysis for ischemia of the lower extremity. The STILE trial. Ann Surg 1994;220:251.

144. Earnshaw JJ, Westby JC, Gregson RHS, et al: Local thrombolytic therapy of acute peripheral arterial ischaemia with tissue plasminogen activator: a dose ranging study. Br J Surg 1988;75:1196.

145. Semba CP, Murphy TP, Bakal CW, et al: Thrombolytic therapy with use of alteplase (rt-PA) in peripheral arterial occlusive disease: review of the clinical literature. J Vasc Interv Radiol 2000;11:149.

146. Durham JD, Geller SC, Abbott WM, et al: Regional infusion of urokinase into occluded lower extremity bypass grafts: long-term clinical results. Radiology 1989;172:83.

147. LeBlang SD, Becker GJ, Benenati JF, et al: Low dose urokinase regimen for the treatment of lower extremity arterial and graft occlusions: experience in 132 cases. J Vasc Interv Radiol 1992;3:475.

148. McNamara TO, Bomberger RA, Merchant RF: Intra-arterial urokinase as the initial therapy for acutely ischemic lower limbs. Circulation 1991;83(Suppl):106.

149. Working party on thrombolysis in the management of limb ischemia: Thrombolysis in the management of lower limb peripheral arterial occlusion—a consensus document. J Vasc Interv Radiol 2003;14 (9 Pt 2):S337.

150. Haskal ZJ: Mechanical thrombectomy devices for the treatment of peripheral arterial occlusions. Rev Cardiovasc Med 2002;3(Suppl 2):S45.

151. Kasirajan K, Haskal ZJ, Ouriel K: The use of mechanical thrombectomy devices in the management of acute peripheral arterial occlusive disease. J Vasc Interv Radiol 2001;12:405.

152. Uflacker R, Strange C, Vujic I: Massive pulmonary embolism: preliminary results of treatment with the Amplatz thrombectomy device. J Vasc Interv Radiol 1996;7:519.

153. Rilinger N, Goerich J, Scharrer-Pamler R, et al: Short-term results with use of the Amplatz thrombectomy device in the treatment of acute lower limb occlusions. J Vasc Interv Radiol 1997;8:343.

154. Overbosch EH, Pattynama PMT, Aarts HJ, et al: Occluded hemodialysis shunts: Dutch multicenter experience with the Hydrolyser catheter. Radiology 1996;201:485.

155. Sarac TP, Hilleman D, Arko FR, et al: Clinical and economic evaluation of the Trellis thrombectomy device for arterial occlusions: preliminary analysis. J Vasc Surg 2004;39:556.

156. Turmel-Rodrigues L, Sapoval M, Pengloan J, et al: Manual thromboaspiration and dilation of thrombosed dialysis access: mid-term results of a simple concept. J Vasc Interv Radiol 1997;8:813.

157. Sharafuddin MJ, Kadir S, Joshi SJ, et al: Percutaneous balloon-assisted aspiration thrombectomy of clotted hemodialysis access grafts. J Vasc Interv Radiol 1996;7:177.

158. Beyssen B, Sapoval M, Emmerich J, et al: Acute femoro-popliteal ischemia—new therapeutic approach: respective role of thromboaspiration and in situ thrombolysis. Chirurgie 1996;121:127.

159. Lee BB, Do YS, Yakes W, et al: Management of arteriovenous malformations: a multidisciplinary approach. J Vasc Surg 2004;39:590.

160. DiSegni R, Young AT, Tadavarthy SM, et al: Vascular embolotherapy. Part 1. Embolotherapy: agents, equipment, and techniques. In: Castaneda-Zuniga WR, ed. Interventional Radiology, 3rd ed. Baltimore, Williams & Wilkins, 1997:29.

161. Coldwell DM, Stokes KR, Yakes WF: Embolotherapy: agents, clinical applications, and techniques. Radiographics 1994;14:623.

162. Siskin GP, Dowling K, Virmani R, et al: Pathologic evaluation of a spherical polyvinyl alcohol embolic agent in a porcine renal model. J Vasc Interv Radiol 2003;14:89.

163. Pelage J-P, LeDref O, Beregi J-P, et al: Limited uterine artery embolization with tris-acryl gelatin microspheres for uterine fibroids. J Vasc Interv Radiol 2003;14:15.

164. Brown KT: Fatal pulmonary complication after arterial embolization with 40-120 μm tris-acryl gelatin microspheres. J Vasc Interv Radiol 2004;15:197.

165. Martin ML, Dolmatch BL, Fry PD, et al: Treatment of type II endoleak with Onyx. J Vasc Interv Radiol 2001;12:629.
166. Castaneda F, Goodwin SC, Swischuk JL, et al: Treatment of pelvic arteriovenous malformations with ethylene vinyl alcohol copolymer (Onyx). J Vasc Interv Radiol 2002;13:513.
167. Pollak JS, White RI: The use of cyanoacrylate adhesives in peripheral embolization. J Vasc Interv Radiol 2001;12:907.
168. Yamakado K, Nakatsuka A, Tanaka N, et al: Transcatheter arterial embolization of ruptured pseudoaneurysms with coils and n-butyl cyanoacrylate. J Vasc Interv Radiol 2000;11:66.
169. Hiraki T, Mimura H, Kanazawa S, et al: Transcatheter embolization of an aortobronchial fistula with n-butyl cyanoacrylate. J Vasc Interv Radiol 2002;13:743.
170. Kim BS, Do HM, Razavi M: N-butyl cyanoacrylate glue embolization of splenic artery aneurysms. J Vasc Interv Radiol 2004;15:91.
171. Kiyosue H, Mori H, Matsumoto S, et al: Transcatheter obliteration of gastric varices: Part 2. Strategy and techniques based on hemodynamic features. Radiographics 2003;23:921.

3

Pathogenesis of Vascular Diseases

ARTERIES

Normal Structure

Human arteries are composed of three layers (Fig. 3-1). The *intima* consists of a single layer of endothelial cells lining the vessel lumen and a thin subendothelial matrix.[1] The endothelium has a variety of critical functions.[2] It controls hemostasis by acting as a barrier between circulating blood and the thrombogenic subendothelial layer and by secreting antithrombogenic substances such as the platelet inhibitor prostacyclin I_2. Endothelial cells can indirectly alter vessel caliber when changes in blood oxygen tension, pressure, or flow are detected. The endothelium produces and responds to a variety of factors that are vital to arterial repair after injury.

The *media* is separated from the intima by the *internal elastic lamina*. The layer is primarily composed of collagen, elastin, and smooth muscle cells arranged in longitudinal and circumferential bundles. *Elastic arteries* (i.e., aorta, aortic arch vessels, iliac and pulmonary arteries) propel blood forward because dense layers of elastin allow these vessels to expand during systole and contract during diastole.[3] In the smaller-caliber *muscular arteries,* smooth muscle cells predominate, and the circumferential orientation of the cells allows the lumen to dilate or constrict in response to various stimuli.

The *adventitia* is composed of a fibrocellular matrix that includes fibroblasts, collagen, and elastin. In some vessels, an *external elastic lamina* separates the media from this outer layer. Sympathetic nerves penetrate into the vessel wall and can alter smooth muscle tone in the media. A fine network of blood vessels, the *vasa vasorum,* supplies the adventitia of larger arteries and provides nutrients to this layer and the outer media. The intima and inner media are nourished by diffusion from the lumen.

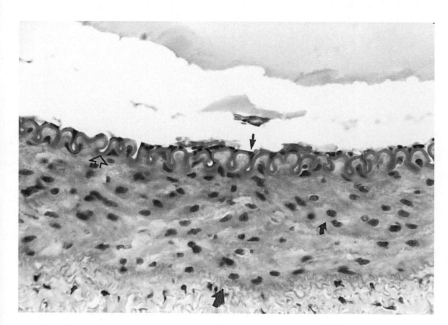

FIGURE 3-1 ▪ Photomicrograph of a normal artery (hematoxylin and eosin stain, original magnification ×40). A single layer of endothelial cells *(small arrow)* lines the internal elastic lamina *(open arrow)*. The media is primarily made up of smooth muscle cells *(curved arrow)*. The external elastic lamina *(large arrow)* separates the media from the adventitia.

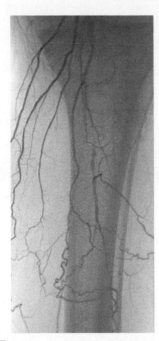

FIGURE 3-2 ■ Enlarged collateral vessels bypass a distal left superficial femoral and popliteal artery occlusion from a gunshot wound.

Small arteries become *arterioles*, which are 40 to 200 μm in diameter. Arterioles lead into capillary networks. Direct arteriovenous shunts exist in some vascular beds. These connections allow diversion of blood away from certain parts of the body in physiologic and pathologic states, such as shunting blood from the skin and extremities in a hypotensive patient.

Functional Disorders

Arterial tone and luminal diameter are regulated by several mechanisms[3]:

- Endothelial cells release smooth muscle vasodilators (e.g., nitric oxide [NO]) or vasoconstrictors (e.g., endothelin).
- Vasomotor nerves act through neurotransmitters such as norepinephrine and acetylcholine.
- Circulating agents (e.g., angiotensin II and vasopressin) also affect vascular tone.

Vasodilation is seen primarily in low-resistance systems, such as arteriovenous fistulas, arteriovenous malformations,

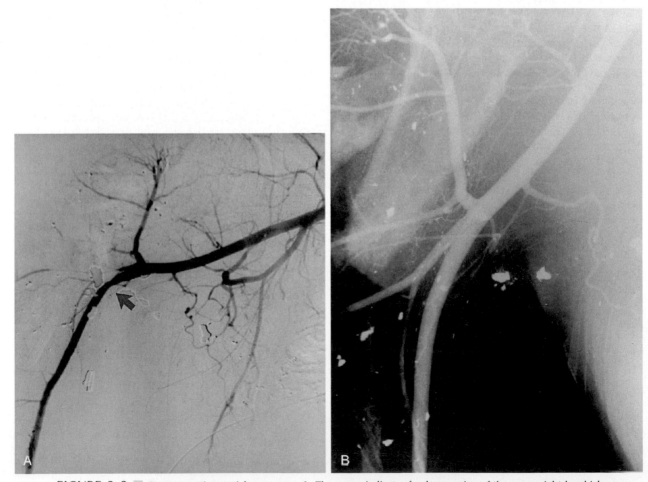

FIGURE 3-3 ■ Posttraumatic arterial vasospasm. **A,** The *arrow* indicates focal narrowing of the upper right brachial artery. **B,** A follow-up arteriogram obtained 3 days later shows complete resolution of spasm.

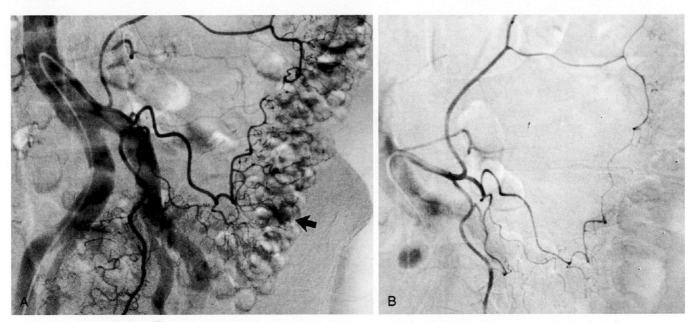

FIGURE 3-4 ■ Vasopressin-induced vasospasm. **A,** Inferior mesenteric arteriogram shows extravasation in the left colon. **B,** After infusion of vasopressin, the vessels are diffusely constricted and the bleeding has stopped.

and hypervascular tumors, and in collateral circulations (Fig. 3-2). Vasoconstriction usually is the result of vascular trauma or low-flow states (Fig. 3-3). Ingestion or infusion of certain drugs (e.g., vasopressin, dopamine, epinephrine) also can lead to vasospasm (Fig. 3-4). *Raynaud's disease* is a functional disorder primarily affecting the small arteries of the hands and feet in which intermittent vasospasm is caused by external stimuli (see Chapter 7).[4] The hallmark of vasospasm is resolution over time or relief with vasodilators.

Arterial "standing" or "stationary" waves are an arteriographic curiosity that may be confused with functional vasospasm (Fig. 3-5).[5] Although their precise cause is unknown, this temporary oscillating pattern may sometimes be related to high-pressure contrast injection into a high-resistance vascular bed.

Atherosclerosis

Atherosclerosis is the most common disease affecting the vascular system and is the leading cause of morbidity and mortality in the Western world. It develops as a result of an *inflammatory reaction* and a *response to lipid storage* in the arterial wall.[6] The various risks factors for the disease (see below) may act as triggers for inflammation. The common inciting event is endothelial injury mediated through the immune system. The damaged endothelium allows lipoproteins and monocytes to enter the subendothelial space and produce "fatty streaks" composed largely of foam cells.[7] A variety of factors is generated in response to this process. These substances cause medial smooth muscle cells to migrate to and then proliferate in the intima. Overproduction of collagen, elastin, and proteoglycans gives the lesion a fibrotic character. With time, medial thinning, cellular necrosis, and plaque calcification and degeneration occur (Fig. 3-6). Ultimately, plaque fracture, ulceration, hemorrhage, or thrombosis may

occur. The inflammatory process appears to participate in every stage of the disease.

A number of risk factors for atherosclerosis have been identified (Box 3-1). However, these conditions do not account for all cases of the disease. There is growing evidence that several other markers for the development of

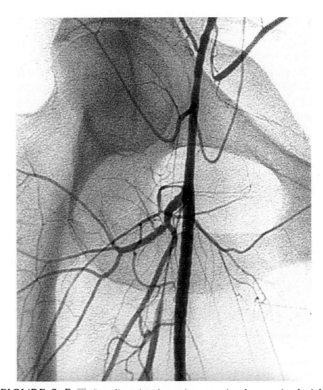

FIGURE 3-5 ■ Standing (stationary) waves in the proximal right superficial femoral artery. These appear as subtle periodic oscillations in the lumen contour.

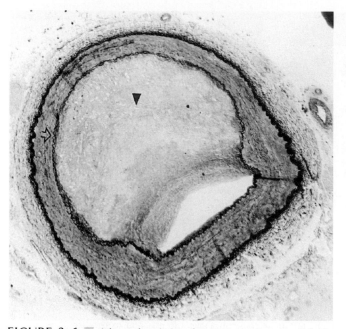

FIGURE 3-6 ▪ Atherosclerosis in a human coronary artery (elastin stain, original magnification ×20). An advanced acellular intimal plaque markedly narrows the vessel lumen. Multiple cholesterol clefts *(arrowhead)* are seen. The internal elastic lamina *(open arrow)* is relatively intact. (Specimen courtesy of Ahmed Shabaik, MD.)

atherosclerosis exist (Box 3-2).[8] C-reactive protein, fibrinogen, and lipoprotein (a) are all acute phase reactants that increase markedly in the presence of an inflammatory state. Elevated levels of the amino acid homocysteine are associated with a significant risk of arterial and venous thrombosis. All four factors may be predictive of the progression of atherosclerosis both in asymptomatic patients and in those with established disease.

Atherosclerosis produces symptoms through blood flow reduction, thrombotic occlusion, plaque ulceration with distal embolization, and rarely by penetration into the media. Plaques can cause mild to severe irregularity of the wall or smooth, concentric narrowing (Fig. 3-7). A protruding plaque can mimic a luminal filling defect (Fig. 3-8). Significant atherosclerosis is most commonly seen at branch points and at certain anatomic sites, including the coronary arteries, carotid artery bifurcation, infrarenal abdominal aorta, and lower extremity arteries. Most affected

---

BOX 3-2 ▪ Emerging Risk Factors or Markers of Atherosclerosis

C-reactive protein
Lipoprotein (a)
Fibrinogen
Homocysteine

---

patients have diffuse disease at many sites. Arterial luminal narrowing has several causes, although atherosclerosis is the most common (Box 3-3).

Neointimal Hyperplasia and Restenosis

Neointimal hyperplasia is the "scar" produced by arteries (and veins) in response to significant vessel injury or altered hemodynamics. While it has certain features in common with atherosclerosis, it is a different pathophysiologic process. When caused by endovascular or surgical maneuvers (e.g., balloon angioplasty or stent placement), neointimal hyperplasia is triggered by clot formation and wall stretching at the site of injury.[9,10] Over several days, monocytes and lymphocytes infiltrate the thrombus, which is partially resorbed. Growth factors released from smooth muscle cells, macrophages, and platelets cause smooth muscle cell proliferation and migration to form a thickened intima (Figs. 3-9 and 3-10). This process is complete within 3 to 6 months after injury.[11] As with atherosclerosis, there is emerging evidence that inflammation plays a central role in neointimal hyperplasia and restenosis.[12] In one study, C-reactive protein levels were strong predictors of the extent of restenosis after peripheral artery angioplasty.[13]

The degree of luminal narrowing (restenosis) after angioplasty or stent placement depends on the exuberance of the neointimal hyperplastic response and the extent of arterial (or venous) remodeling. Negative remodeling, which may be due to elastic recoil of the vessel or progressive thickening of the adventitia, can be partially limited by placement of a stent.

BOX 3-1 ▪ Established Risk Factors for Atherosclerosis

Smoking
Hypertension
Hyperlipidemia
Age
Family history
Obesity
Diabetes

BOX 3-3 ▪ Causes of Arterial Luminal Narrowing

Atherosclerosis
Intimal hyperplasia
Vasospasm
Low-flow state
Dissection
Neoplastic or inflammatory encasement
Vasculitis
Extrinsic compression
Fibromuscular dysplasia

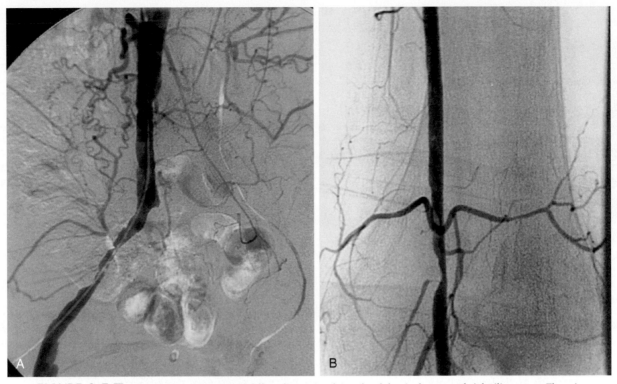

FIGURE 3-7 ▨ Atherosclerosis. **A,** Typical diffuse disease involving the abdominal aorta and right iliac artery. There is also thrombotic occlusion of the left iliac and right internal iliac arteries. **B,** Focal eccentric narrowing of the popliteal artery.

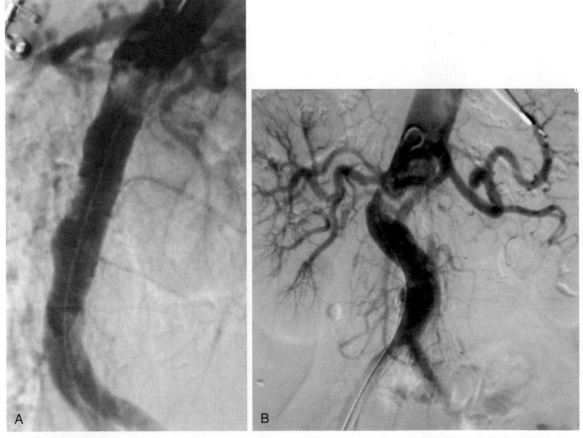

FIGURE 3-8 ▨ **A,** Lateral abdominal aortogram shows apparent embolus in the mid-abdominal aorta. **B,** Frontal image shows that the defect is a large polypoid plaque arising from the left side of the aorta.

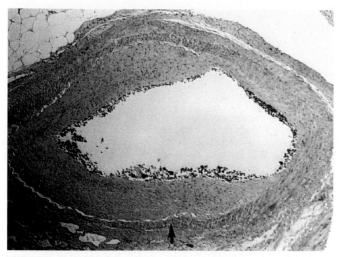

FIGURE 3-9 ■ Intimal hyperplasia in a human renal artery (hematoxylin and eosin stain, original magnification ×40). The concentric thickening of the intima can be identified along with smooth muscle cells, fibroblasts, and matrix material. The internal elastic lamina *(arrow)* denotes the boundary between intima and media. (Specimen courtesy of Ahmed Shabaik, MD.)

Thrombosis

The ingredients for thrombosis are platelets and other cellular blood elements, coagulation proteins, and an abnormal endothelium (Fig. 3-11). Clot formation begins with platelet adhesion and aggregation on the subendothelial surface.[14] Platelets release substances that further promote platelet aggregation, such as adenosine diphosphate and thromboxane A_2. The endothelium may be deficient in producing several antithrombotic substances, including plasminogen activators, thrombin inactivators, and certain prostacyclins. Activation of the intrinsic or extrinsic coagulation pathway leads to the generation of *thrombin*, which is the critical enzyme needed for conversion of fibrinogen to fibrin. A complex thrombus is formed from platelets, red blood cells, and white blood cells enmeshed within a fibrin matrix. Portions of the clot are relatively rich in red blood cells ("red clot"). Other parts, especially at the proximal edge of an arterial occlusion, are poor in red blood cells and relatively rich in fibrin or platelets ("white clot").

Thrombosis occurs in the presence of vessel injury, slow flow, or a hypercoagulable state (i.e., *Virchow's triad*). In most cases, thrombi form at sites of preexisting disease (e.g., atherosclerosis, intimal hyperplasia) or acute trauma (see Figs. 3-2 and 3-7). However, clot also may form in the presence of an hereditary or acquired hypercoagulable (thrombophilic) state in the absence of underlying vascular disease (e.g., in situ thrombosis).[15-17]

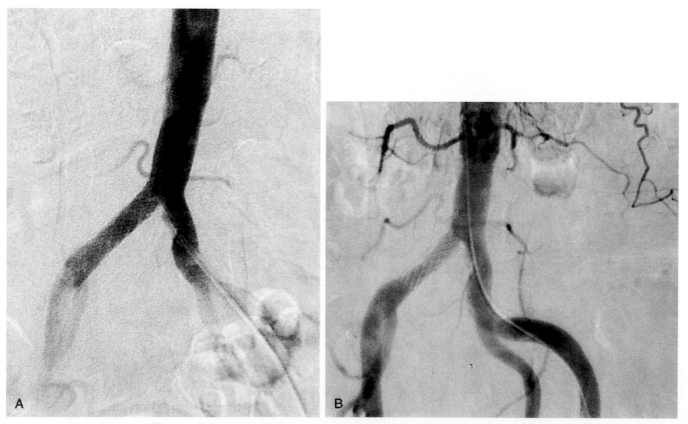

FIGURE 3-10 ■ Intimal hyperplasia. **A,** Initial arteriogram following angioplasty and stent placement in the right common iliac artery. **B,** A follow-up arteriogram obtained months later shows intimal hyperplasia in the stented segment.

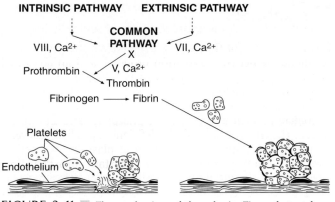

INTRINSIC PATHWAY   EXTRINSIC PATHWAY

COMMON PATHWAY

VIII, Ca²⁺   VII, Ca²⁺

X

Prothrombin   V, Ca²⁺

Thrombin

Fibrinogen ⟶ Fibrin

Platelets

Endothelium

FIGURE 3-11 ■ The mechanism of thrombosis. Tissue factors from vessel injury activate the extrinsic pathway. The damaged vessel wall itself activates the intrinsic pathway through factors XII, XI, and IX.

In addition to thrombosis, arterial occlusion has several other causes (Box 3-4).

Thrombophilia

There is a variety of hereditary and acquired disorders that predispose to venous and/or arterial thrombosis in the absence of other risk factors for clot formation (Box 3-5). While the risk for thrombosis is much higher with the relatively rare hereditary factor deficiency states, the disorders of increased activity are much more common. All of these conditions can cause venous thrombosis. Arterial thrombosis is particularly associated with heparin-induced thrombocytopenia and hyperhomocysteinemia.

Antiphospholipid syndrome includes a primary form and a type associated with systemic lupus erythematosus or other collagen vascular diseases. The common autoantigen is beta-2-glycoprotein I. The diagnosis requires elevated levels of *lupus anticoagulant* (which prolongs the partial thromboplastin time) or IgG/IgM *anticardiolipin antibodies*. This syndrome is one of the most common causes of thrombophilia.[18]

Antithrombin deficiency is an uncommon disorder in which the enzyme that inactivates thrombin and several other coagulation factors is deficient or relatively inactive. The condition usually is inherited as an autosomal dominant disease. Over 50% of patients with this disorder will develop

---

BOX 3-4 ■ Causes of Arterial Occlusion

Thrombosis
Embolism
Dissection
Trauma
Neoplastic invasion
Extrinsic compression
Vasculitis
Functional defect (e.g., drug-induced)

BOX 3-5 ■ Major Thrombophilia Disorders

Largely Hereditary
Activated protein C resistance (factor V Leiden)
Antithrombin deficiency
Protein S deficiency
Protein C deficiency
Prothrombin regulatory sequence mutation
Elevated factors VIII, IX, and Xi
Dysfibrinogenemia
Hyperhomocysteinemia

Largely Acquired
Antiphospholipid syndromes
Malignancy-associated hypercoagulability
Heparin-induced thrombocytopenic thrombosis
Polycythemia vera
Pregnancy
Estrogen therapy
Thrombocytosis

---

thrombosis before the age of 60. Acquired forms also have been described, notably in women taking oral contraceptives.

Protein C is an enzyme that inactivates factors Va and VIIIa in the coagulation cascade. *Protein S* is a required cofactor in this process. Congenital or acquired deficiency of either protein, as occurs in advanced liver disease or human immunodeficiency virus infection, can lead to a hypercoagulable state.[19]

Factor V Leiden is a single amino acid alteration on the factor V molecule that causes activated protein C resistance. Factor V Leiden is perhaps the most common coagulation abnormality detected in patients studied for hypercoagulability, although the risk for thrombosis in an individual patient is small.

Heparin-induced thrombocytopenia is triggered by heparin-dependent antiplatelet antibodies. Binding of this antibody, platelet factor 4, and heparin on the cell surface activates the platelets. However, thrombocytopenia with vascular thrombosis occurs in fewer than 1% of patients treated with heparin. The disorder has been reported after therapy with various heparin sources, doses, and routes of administration. When bleeding or thrombosis occurs, all heparin products must be stopped and replaced with oral warfarin or direct thrombin inhibitors.

Malignancy-associated hypercoagulability (Trousseau's syndrome) is caused by a thromboplastin-like substance that triggers the coagulation cascade. Affected patients are prone to deep or superficial venous thrombosis, arterial thromboembolism, or bleeding (Fig. 3-12). Hypercoagulability is particularly common with lung and gastrointestinal tract malignancies. The platelet count may be depressed, and the prothrombin and partial thromboplastin times prolonged.

Embolism

An embolus is any material that passes through the circulation and eventually lodges in a downstream vessel.

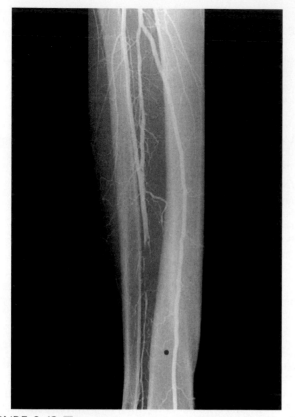

FIGURE 3-12 ■ In situ thrombosis in the tibial arteries of a patient with metastatic melanoma and severe thrombocytosis.

Macroembolism and microembolism of the arterial circulation have numerous causes (Box 3-6).

Macroemboli usually are clots that originate from the heart or a central artery. Atherosclerotic plaque also can fragment and obstruct peripheral arteries. Emboli tend to lodge at arterial bifurcations or at sites of preexisting disease. After the embolic event occurs, the distal arteries constrict, and thrombus propagates proximally and distally to the level of the next large collateral branches. It may be

---

BOX 3-6   ■   Sources of Arterial Emboli

Heart
    Left atrial or ventricular thrombus
    Endocardial vegetations
    Atrial myxoma
Thrombus superimposed on vascular disease (including aneurysms)
Atherosclerotic plaque
Catheterization procedures
    Catheter-related thrombus
    Plaque disruption
    Gas bubbles
Foreign bodies
    Catheter or wire fragments
    Gunshot pellets
Paradoxical emboli from the venous circulation

BOX 3-7   ■   Angiographic Signs of Acute Arterial Embolism

Meniscus or filling defect
Mild or absent diffuse vascular disease
Lack of contralateral disease in extremity arteries
Poorly developed collateral circulation
Emboli at other sites

---

impossible to differentiate thrombotic from embolic occlusions by imaging, although an acute embolus has several classic angiographic features (Box 3-7 and Fig. 3-13). Real or apparent luminal filling defects are seen also with intimal flaps, protruding atherosclerotic plaques, inflow defects, and rarely with intraluminal tumor (Figs. 3-14 through 3-16; see also Fig. 3-8). An arterial *inflow defect* is caused by unopacified blood entering an artery beyond an obstruction through a collateral vessel.

Microemboli are seen in patients with ulcerated, protruding atherosclerotic plaques. Platelet-fibrin deposits can be released spontaneously into the distal circulation from a site of underlying disease.[20] Cholesterol crystals (100 to 200 µm) also may shower into the distal circulation from a plaque.[21] Spontaneous release of small atheroemboli cause the *blue toe* (or *blue finger*) syndrome. However, the event may be associated with surgical manipulation, catheterization procedures, or treatment with anticoagulants or fibrinolytic agents.[22] Widespread embolization into the legs, kidneys, head, or intestinal tract can result in acute renal failure, stroke, profound lower extremity or intestinal ischemia, and even death (see Chapter 1).

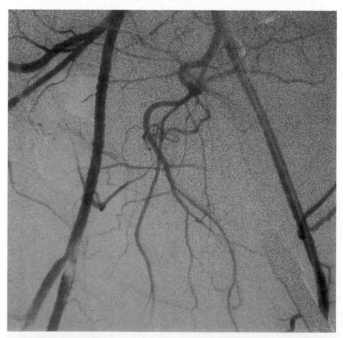

FIGURE 3-13 ■ Acute embolus to the right common/superficial femoral artery. Note absence of other vascular disease, normal left common femoral artery, and lack of significant collateral circulation. Also note incidental finding of standing waves in the right external iliac artery.

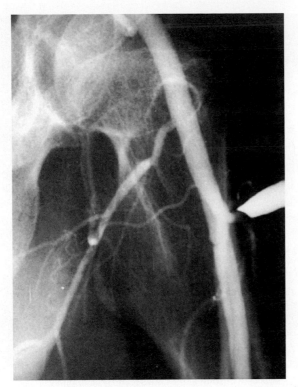

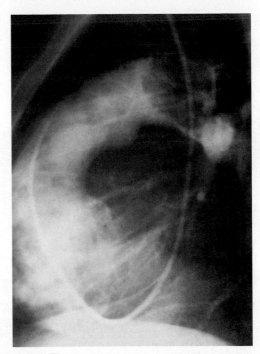

FIGURE 3-16 ■ Main pulmonary artery sarcoma seen on a lateral right ventriculogram.

FIGURE 3-14 ■ Traumatic intimal flap in the medial left superficial femoral artery.

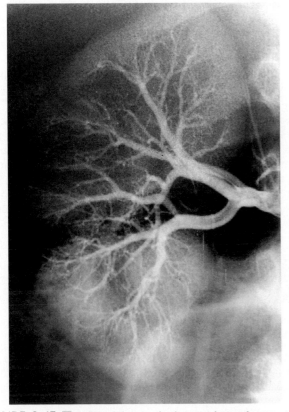

FIGURE 3-15 ■ Inflow defect in the lower pole renal artery trunk caused by unopacified blood from a collateral vessel entering the artery beyond a proximal stenosis.

Aneurysms and Arterial Dilation

An aneurysm is defined as focal or diffuse dilation of an artery by more than 50% of its normal diameter.[23] In a *true aneurysm,* all three layers of the arterial wall are dilated but remain intact (Fig. 3-17). Degenerative (atherosclerosis-associated) aneurysms fall into this category. In a *false aneurysm* (i.e., pseudoaneurysm), one or more layers of the arterial wall are disrupted (Fig. 3-18). Blood may be contained by the outer adventitia and surrounding supportive tissue. Trauma and infectious, neoplastic, or inflammatory masses typically produce pseudoaneurysms. True aneurysms usually are *fusiform* (i.e., diffuse dilation involving the entire circumference of an artery) and false aneurysms usually are *saccular* (i.e., focal dilation involving part of the circumference of an artery), but these morphologic features are not always diagnostic of the actual pathology.

True and false aneurysms have a variety of causes (Box 3-8). *Degenerative aneurysms* are the most common. Although atherosclerosis and degenerative aneurysms are linked and often coexist, the two conditions are distinct disorders.[24] Degenerative aneurysms form because of inflammatory damage to the vessel wall and hemodynamic forces that produce remodeling.[25,26] A variety of reactive oxygen species activate matrix metalloproteinases (MMP) that cause thinning of the media. These reactive oxygen species are probably liberated as part of an inflammatory process.

The most common sites for degenerative aneurysms are the infrarenal abdominal aorta, descending thoracic aorta, and common iliac artery. Aneurysms of the popliteal, common femoral, brachiocephalic, and subclavian arteries are less common. Imaging features include diffuse arterial dilation, intimal calcification, and sometimes intraluminal

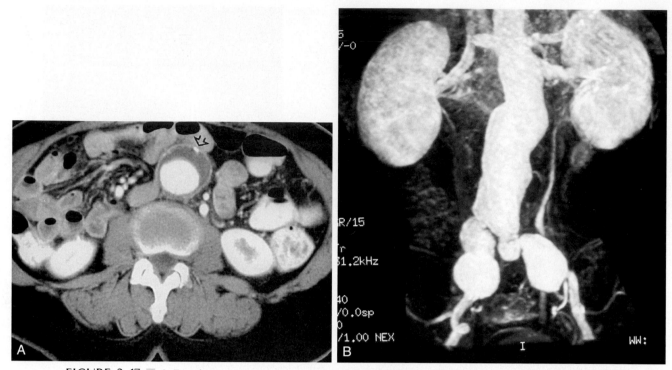

FIGURE 3-17 ■ **A,** True degenerative aneurysm of the abdominal aorta with dilation of the entire aortic wall, luminal thrombus, and intimal calcification *(open arrow).* **B,** Maximum intensity projection gadolinium MR angiogram shows large infrarenal true abdominal aortic aneurysm with extension to both iliac arteries.

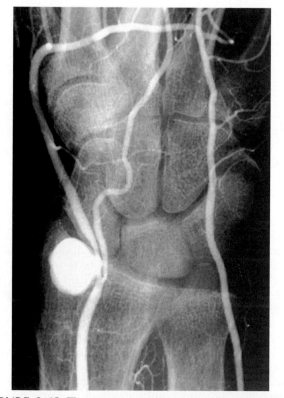

FIGURE 3-18 ■ A saccular pseudoaneurysm of the distal radial artery developed after removal of a radial artery line. (From Roberts AC, Kaufman JA, Geller SC: Angiographic assessment in peripheral vascular disease. In: Strandness DE Jr, Van Breda A, eds. Vascular Diseases: Surgical and Interventional Therapy. Philadelphia, Churchill Livingstone, 1994:218.)

clot (see Fig. 3-17). Mural thrombus, which is common at most sites except the thoracic aorta, can obstruct branch vessels and give the lumen a smooth appearance. If clot is present, angiography can underestimate the size or even mask the existence of an aneurysm (see Fig. 5-14).

Infectious (mycotic) aneurysms are caused by localized infection of the arterial wall.[27,28] They result from inoculation of a preexisting aneurysm or from infection and progressive dilation of a previously normal artery. The infection can arise through seeding of the artery from the lumen or vasa vasorum, invasion from a neighboring infection, or from penetrating trauma. Infectious aneurysms are typically saccular, occur at unusual sites, and can be multiple (see Figs. 4-31 and 5-30). They are most commonly seen in the aorta, visceral, and lower extremity arteries. In addition to

BOX 3-8 ■ Causes of Arterial Aneurysms

Atherosclerosis-associated degeneration
Trauma
Infection
Inflammation
Neoplastic invasion
Vasculitis
Chronic dissection
Connective tissue disorders
Congenital

bacterial infections, tuberculous arteritis may cause an aneurysm to form.[29]

Traumatic pseudoaneurysms result from blunt trauma (e.g., deceleration injury), criminal penetrating trauma, and medical procedures (e.g., catheterization, surgical repair) (see Fig. 3-18 and 4-21). Like infectious aneurysms, they usually are saccular and eccentric and often occur in the absence of other vascular disease.

The potential complications of aneurysms and pseudoaneurysms include rupture, thrombosis, distal embolization of mural clot, and compression or erosion of adjacent organs. The frequency of each of these complications varies with the type of aneurysm and its location. Aneurysm expansion is governed by *Laplace's law* (wall tension = pressure × radius). The larger the aneurysm, the more rapid is the rate of expansion and the greater the likelihood of rupture.

Several forms of arterial dilation may be confused with an aneurysm:

■ *Arterial ectasia* is the age-related change that causes arteries to become dilated, tortuous, and lengthened (Fig. 3-19). Ectasia is particularly common in the thoracic aorta, abdominal aorta, and iliac and splenic arteries.
■ *Arteriomegaly* is the diffuse enlargement of a long arterial segment (Fig. 3-20). It occurs most frequently in the iliac and femoropopliteal vessels. The underlying pathology may be elastin deficiency within the media.[30]
■ *Compensatory dilation* of inflow arteries occurs in high-flow states such as arteriovenous malformations and fistulas, hemodialysis grafts, and hypervascular tumors.
■ *Post-stenotic dilation* results from turbulence beyond a site of significant arterial narrowing (Fig. 3-21).

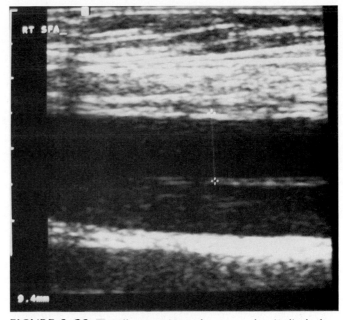

FIGURE 3-20 ■ Diffuse arteriomegaly seen on longitudinal ultrasound. The right superficial femoral artery diameter (normally 5 to 6 mm) is 9 to 10 mm throughout its entire course.

Dissection

Arterial dissection is a separation of layers of the vessel wall, usually between the intima and media or within the media. In most cases, an *intimal tear* initially connects the natural arterial lumen *(true lumen)* with the intramural channel

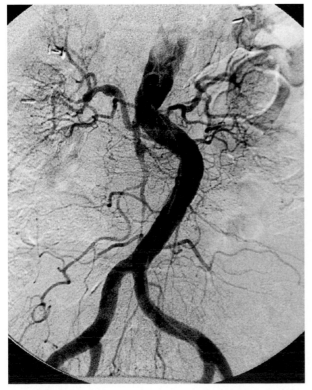

FIGURE 3-19 ■ Ectasia of the aorta and iliac arteries in an elderly patient.

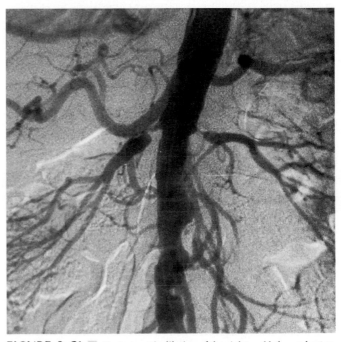

FIGURE 3-21 ■ Post-stenotic dilation of the right and left renal arteries beyond bilateral ostial stenoses.

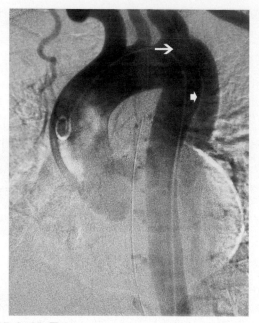

FIGURE 3-22 ■ Dissection of the descending thoracic aorta *(arrowhead)* extending into the left subclavian artery *(arrow)*. Note delayed opacification of the laterally based false lumen.

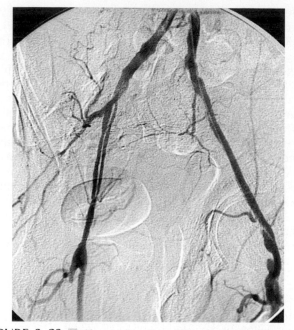

FIGURE 3-23 ■ Chronic dissection of the right external iliac artery with a double-barrel lumen from a prior catheterization procedure.

(false lumen) (Fig. 3-22).[31] An exit tear may later reconnect the false and true lumens and permit blood to flow freely through both channels. Branches along the course of the dissection can be fed by either lumen. Occasionally, the dissection is completely isolated from the lumen (i.e., *intramural hematoma*; see Fig. 4-34).[32] The most common causes of aortic dissection are long-standing hypertension, chronic degeneration of the media, and trauma.

The major complications of dissection are rupture and ischemia. Rupture through the adventitia often occurs at the site of the intimal tear. Ischemia results from obstruction of a branch vessel by the intimal flap or from slow flow in a branch fed by the nondominant lumen. In some cases, the false channel enlarges and compresses the true lumen. Left untreated, the false lumen can rupture, persist (chronic dissection), enlarge, or thrombose (Fig. 3-23).

Vasculitis

The hallmark of vasculitis is inflammation (and sometimes necrosis) of the blood vessel wall (Box 3-9). The acute phase often is marked by constitutional symptoms and an elevated erythrocyte sedimentation rate. In the chronic phase, the effects of vascular damage, such as arterial narrowing, thrombosis, or necrosis with aneurysm formation, become apparent.[33,34] The affected sites and severity of disease vary widely among the various disorders. Vasculitis should always be considered when obstructive or aneurysmal vascular disease is atypical (e.g., with a young patient or unusual location, distribution, or appearance).

Takayasu's arteritis is a chronic, inflammatory vasculitis of large elastic arteries.[35,36] An autoimmune process has been implicated. In the acute phase, the adventitia and

media are infiltrated with T cells, monocytes, and granulocytes. Destruction and progressive fibrosis of the entire vessel wall lead to luminal narrowing or dilation. The disease primarily affects the aorta, its major branches, and the pulmonary arteries. Several classification schemes have been devised to categorize the distribution of disease.[37] In most patients, the thoracic and/or abdominal aorta and some of their principal branches (i.e., arch, renal, mesenteric, or iliac arteries) are involved. The pulmonary arteries are affected in many cases.

Takayasu's arteritis is most commonly seen in Japan, China, Southeast Asia, India, and South Africa. However, it is being diagnosed more frequently in Western countries, particularly Mexico.[36] There is a strong female predilection,

---

BOX 3-9 ■ Major Vasculitides with Vascular Imaging Manifestations

Large vessel (aorta and primary branches)
   Takayasu's arteritis
   Giant cell arteritis
Medium and small vessel (named arteries and their branches)
   Buerger's disease
   Polyarteritis nodosa
   Kawasaki disease
HLA-B27–related diseases (e.g., rheumatoid arthritis)
Other connective tissue disorders
   Marfan syndrome
   Behçet's disease
   Ehlers-Danlos syndrome
   Systemic lupus erythematosis
   Scleroderma

and most patients present as teenagers or young adults. There is some controversy regarding the optimal clinical/imaging criteria required to make the diagnosis. However, most schemes involve some combination of appropriate demographic, clinical, and imaging features. Clinical symptoms and signs in the chronic phase include upper extremity (and occasionally lower extremity) ischemia, arm blood pressure discrepancies, renovascular hypertension, cerebral ischemia, headaches, mesenteric ischemia, and angina. Aortic dilation (usually proximal) and aortic narrowing (usually distal) are characteristic (Fig. 3-24).[38,39] Smooth, long stenoses or complete occlusions of the proximal portions of the major aortic branches also are typical (see Fig. 4-28). Arterial obstructions are treated when the patient has end-organ ischemia, such as renovascular hypertension or arm "claudication." Aneurysm rupture is unusual, and operative treatment of asymptomatic aneurysms is rarely indicated.

Giant cell arteritis, or *temporal arteritis,* is related to but distinct from Takayasu's arteritis.[36,40] The pathologic findings are similar, with early T-lymphocyte, histiocyte, and giant cell vessel infiltration and late narrowing or thrombosis of medium-sized arteries. The precise etiology is unknown, but autoimmune, genetic, and hormonal factors have been implicated. However, the chronic symptoms and vascular distribution are different from Takayasu's arteritis. Many of those afflicted are of Scandinavian descent. It is virtually never seen in patients younger than 50 years of age, and women are affected more commonly than men. Acute symptoms include fever, polymyalgia rheumatica, and scalp tenderness; headaches; and, rarely, visual loss may follow. The typical imaging findings are long, smooth stenoses or occlusions, particularly in the external carotid artery and its branches or the distal subclavian artery.[41] Lesions are sometimes difficult to differentiate from atherosclerosis. Aortic aneurysms have been described also. The diagnosis is confirmed by temporal artery biopsy.

Buerger's disease, or *thromboangiitis obliterans,* is a vasculitis affecting small and medium-sized arteries and veins. The disease begins as an occlusive inflammatory thrombus with little involvement of the vessel wall.[42,43] With time, the clot becomes organized and the wall fibrotic. Affected vascular segments are separated by essentially normal vessels. Unlike most other vasculitides, the disease usually is confined to the extremities; involvement of mesenteric branches and other sites is rare.[44] Buerger's disease attacks the lower and upper extremity arteries in 90% and 50% of cases, respectively. A superficial (or sometimes deep) thrombophlebitis occurs in up to 40% of patients.

The cause of Buerger's disease is unknown, although an immunologic abnormality has been postulated. Virtually all patients are smokers. Although the disease is historically associated with young Jewish men of Ashkenazi descent, it is being recognized more frequently in other populations, in women, and in older patients.[43] It is a common cause of peripheral vascular disease in smokers younger than 40 years of age. On imaging studies, the arteries above the elbow and knee are relatively disease free. Abrupt occlusions of distal arteries with skip areas are seen along with tortuous ("corkscrew") collateral vessels (Fig. 3-25; see also Fig. 6-19). These findings usually are present also in asymptomatic limbs. Diagnosis is important for prognostic reasons. Patients must be counseled about the likelihood of amputation if there is continued exposure to tobacco.

Polyarteritis nodosa (PAN) is a necrotizing vasculitis of small- and medium-sized arteries.[45] Certain infections, such as hepatitis B, are clearly associated with the disease, but in many cases, the cause is unknown. An almost identical form of arteritis has been described in drug abusers.[46] PAN affects the kidneys, intestinal tract, spleen, liver, and occasionally the hands and feet.[47] Multiple small aneurysms, with or without stenoses and occlusions of distal arteries, are characteristic (Fig. 3-26). The finding of multiple microaneurysms is almost pathognomonic, although a similar appearance has been described for other diseases such as drug abuse, Sjögren's syndrome, and Wegener's granulomatosis.[48] CT scans may show renal or perirenal hematomas and focal thickening of the bowel wall.

Connective tissue disorders may cause an arteritis.[49,50] With few exceptions (see below), clinical vasculitis is not a prominent feature of these diseases. The affected sites vary widely (Fig. 3-27). Rheumatoid arthritis and other HLA-B27–related disorders can cause inflammation in the aortic root with aortic regurgitation; aneurysm formation is rare. Systemic lupus erythematosus can produce symptomatic small vessel arteritis in the lung, kidneys, intestinal tract, or digits.

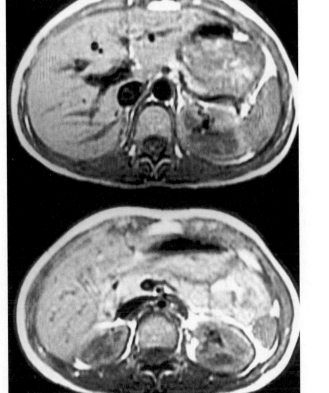

FIGURE 3-24 ■ Takayasu's arteritis of the abdominal aorta by MR imaging. The caliber of the upper abdominal aorta is normal *(top).* Narrowing of the aortic lumen and concentric thickening of the aortic wall are seen in the middle abdomen *(bottom).*

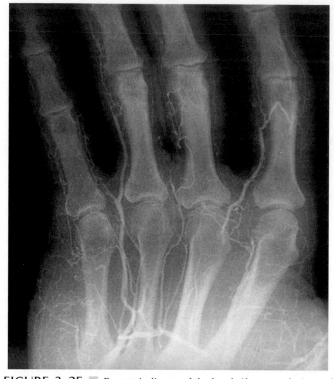

FIGURE 3-25 ■ Buerger's disease of the hand. Abrupt occlusions of multiple digital arteries are seen, but the intervening vessels are relatively normal.

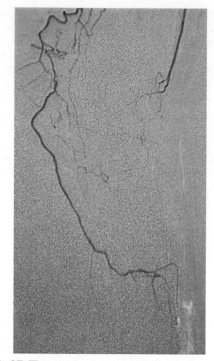

FIGURE 3-27 ■ Scleroderma vasculitis in the left foot of a young patient with no other risk factors for vascular disease. Note occlusion of distal tibial and pedal vessels.

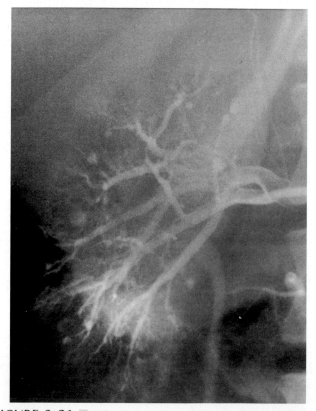

FIGURE 3-26 ■ Polyarteritis nodosa of the right kidney with multiple microaneurysms of distal intrarenal vessels.

Ehlers-Danlos syndrome is a rare set of distinct genetic disorders of collagen production.[51] More than nine types have been described, and many feature hyperextensibility of the joints and thin skin. Type IV disease, in which there is a defect in type III collagen, has characteristic vascular features. Spontaneous arterial ruptures, aneurysms, and severe angiographic complications are seen with this form of the syndrome (Fig. 3-28).

Behçet's disease is a rare connective tissue disorder marked by oral and genital ulcers, uveitis, and skin lesions.[52,53] Panvasculitis (arterial or venous) is a major feature of the disease in a minority of patients, particularly young men. The involved vessels show a severe cellular inflammatory reaction that ultimately scars the entire wall and may lead to aneurysm formation or vascular occlusion. Characteristic findings include superficial venous thrombosis, inferior vena cava (IVC) thrombosis with Budd-Chiari syndrome, aortic aneurysms, pulmonary artery aneurysms, and brachiocephalic arterial obstructions.

Kawasaki disease (mucocutaneous lymph node syndrome) is a necrotizing vasculitis of unknown origin that primarily afflicts young children.[54] Coronary artery aneurysms, myocarditis, and coronary artery stenoses are the major cardiovascular manifestation of the disorder. Peripheral aneurysms also have been reported.

Radiation arteritis can develop in arteries of any size after high-dose radiotherapy. In large- and medium-sized

luminal narrowing, irregular mural plaques, or complete occlusion (Fig. 3-29).

Fibromuscular Dysplasia

Fibromuscular dysplasia is a group of related *noninflammatory* disorders that produce arterial narrowing and small aneurysms.[56,57] The cause is unknown, but genetic, hormonal, and mechanical stress factors have been postulated. Fibromuscular dysplasia occurs most often in the renal arteries. Less common sites include the carotid artery, external iliac artery, and mesenteric arteries.[58,59] Up to six distinct pathologic subtypes have been described (see Table 8-3). The medial fibroplasia type is the most common. Medial smooth muscle cells are largely replaced by fibrous tissue and extracellular matrix. These thickened segments alternate with regions of severe thinning of the media. The effect on the lumen is alternating aneurysms and focal stenoses (string of beads) (Fig. 3-30). The less common forms of fibromuscular dysplasia, such as perimedial fibroplasia and intimal fibroplasia, may produce smooth and tapered stenosis, focal bandlike narrowing, dissection, or aneurysms without stenoses.

Segmental Arterial Mediolysis

This exceedingly rare disease of unknown etiology results from destruction of arterial medial smooth muscle cells and eventual replacement by fibrin and granulation tissue.[60] Over time, extension to the entire arterial wall can produce multiple spontaneous dissections and/or aneurysms. It has

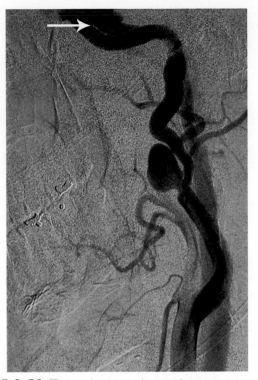

FIGURE 3-28 ■ Saccular internal carotid artery aneurysm in a patient with Ehlers-Danlos syndrome. Also note a carotid-cavernous fistula *(arrow).*

arteries, radiation can cause periarterial fibrosis, intimal atherosclerotic-like changes, or fibrotic occlusion.[55] Radiation-induced arterial disease usually presents 5 or more years after therapy. Angiography may reveal smooth

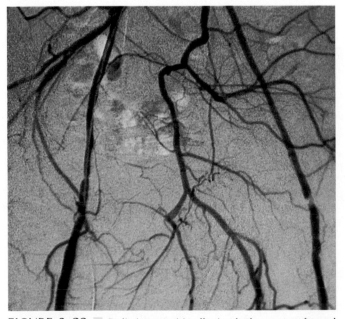

FIGURE 3-29 ■ Radiation arteritis affecting both common femoral arteries in a patient who underwent radiation therapy for cervical cancer seven years prior. Note absence of other vascular disease.

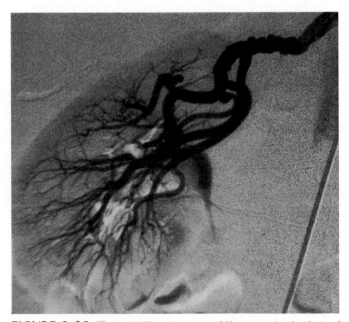

FIGURE 3-30 ■ Medial fibroplasia type of fibromuscular dysplasia of the distal right renal artery.

been postulated that segmental arterial mediolysis is related to fibromuscular dysplasia. The disorder primarily affects mesenteric, renal, and coronary arteries.[61,62]

Extrinsic Compression

The lumen of an artery can be narrowed by a variety of extrinsic sources, including inflammatory masses, tumors, hematomas or other fluid collections, musculoskeletal structures, and external compression (Fig. 3-31).

■ ARTERIES AND VEINS

Neoplasms

Primary vascular tumors are rare, and sarcomas of the aorta, pulmonary artery, or IVC account for most of them (see Fig. 3-16).[63] Most tumors of the aorta and pulmonary artery are intimal sarcomas that produce large luminal masses; angiosarcomas are less common (see Fig. 12-36). Most IVC tumors are leiomyosarcomas (see Fig. 14-27).

Extravascular benign and malignant tumors produce several effects on neighboring vessels.[64] These patterns of hypervascularity, neovascularity, vascular displacement, and vascular invasion may be seen alone or in combination.

Hypervascularity occurs because neoplasms require abundant blood supply for significant growth. Tumors liberate several substances, including tumor angiogenesis factors, that induce formation of new blood vessels. These "tumor vessels" are blood channels and spaces devoid of smooth muscle cells.[65,66] The angiographic hallmark of these

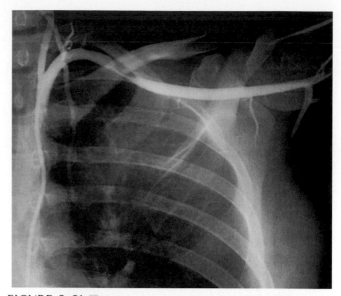

FIGURE 3-31 ■ Extrinsic compression of the left subclavian artery in the costoclavicular space with the arm in abduction, causing thoracic outlet syndrome.

changes is *neovascularity,* which is characterized by increased number of small, bizarrely formed arterial branches that have alternating dilated and narrowed segments and an angulated course. Other features of hypervascular tumors include enlargement of the feeding artery, an increased number of small arteries, dense contrast opacification of the mass (tumor blush*),* filling of enlarged vascular spaces (pools or lakes) and, occasionally, arteriovenous shunting (Fig. 3-32). The classic hypervascular tumors include renal cell carcinoma, hepatocellular carcinoma, choriocarcinoma, endocrine tumors, and leiomyosarcoma.

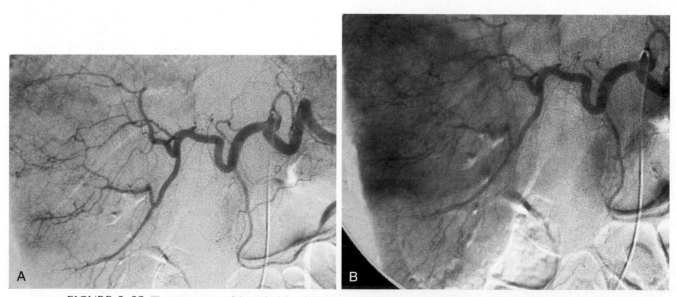

FIGURE 3-32 ■ **A,** Hepatoma of the right lobe of the liver produces hypervascularity and neovascularity in the arterial phase of the celiac angiogram. Note displacement of branches around the large mass. **B,** Later phase shows inhomogeneous tumor stain.

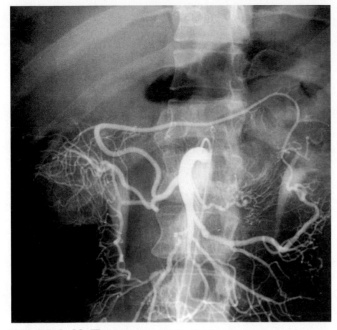

FIGURE 3-33   Encasement of the distal superior mesenteric artery by a duodenal adenocarcinoma.

Vascular invasion is another characteristic of some tumors. Many solid neoplasms show little blood vessel proliferation. Instead, they are infiltrative or scirrhous and compress, encase, or completely occlude adjacent arteries or veins (Fig. 3-33). Usually it is impossible to differentiate these changes from those caused by an inflammatory mass. Invasive

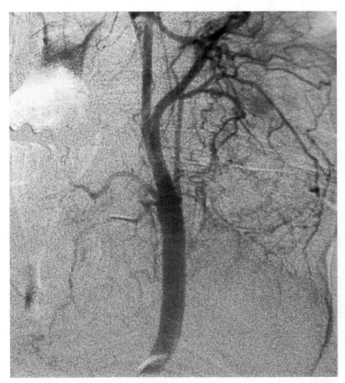

FIGURE 3-34   Branches of the left external carotid artery are displaced around a large metastatic mass from cutaneous melanoma.

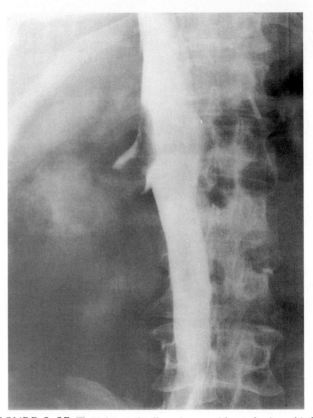

FIGURE 3-35   Right renal cell carcinoma with renal vein and inferior vena cava invasion.

tumors include adenocarcinomas of the intestinal tract, pancreatic adenocarcinoma, breast carcinoma, and most lung cancers (see Fig. 12-35).

Vascular displacement occurs during malignant growth. Some tumors primarily displace neighboring arteries or veins (Fig. 3-34). Mild hypervascularity or neovascularity may be seen in some of these cases.

Intravascular venous invasion is characteristic of a few malignancies, most notably hepatocellular carcinoma and renal cell carcinoma (Fig. 3-35; see also Fig. 10-30). At angiography, fine tumor vessels are occasionally seen within the thrombus.

Inflammatory Disorders

Every acute inflammatory process increases blood flow to the site and causes dilation of feeding arteries, hypervascularity, and parenchymal stain that can mimic a hypervascular tumor (Fig. 3-36). Chronic inflammatory masses, such as pancreatic pseudocysts, can displace, encase, occlude, or rupture into blood vessels (Fig. 3-37).

Arteriovenous Communications

Development of the capillary system between arterioles and venules occurs through capillary network, retiform, and

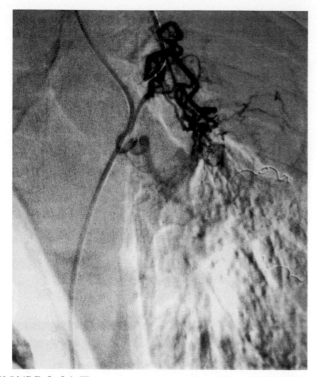

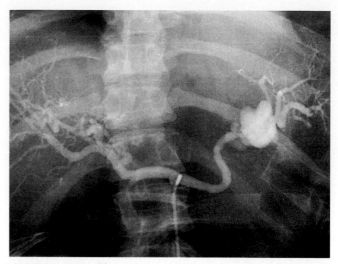

FIGURE 3-37 ■ Pancreatic pseudocyst erosion into the splenic artery with pseudoaneurysm formation.

FIGURE 3-36 ■ Pulmonary aspergillosis infection of the left upper lobe causes hypervascularity and enlargement of collateral vessels from a branch of the left internal thoracic artery.

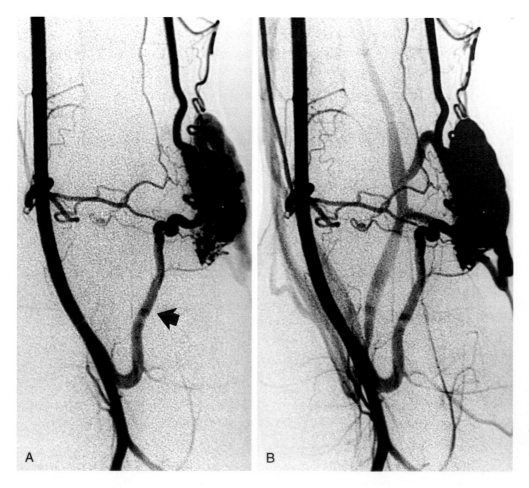

FIGURE 3-38 ■ Arteriovenous malformation of the left upper arm. **A,** The malformation is primarily fed by the radial recurrent artery *(arrowhead)* and branches of the deep brachial artery. **B,** Early and rapid venous filling occurs during the arterial phase of the angiogram.

gross differentiation stages. Direct communications between arteries and veins without an interposed capillary network can be normal or pathologic. Vascular malformations and tumors have been classified by the revised system of Mulliken.[67]

Vascular malformations are congenital lesions that occur during the retiform stage of development.[68,69] These anomalies have no proliferating cells and enlarge slowly and continuously over a patient's lifetime. They are classified as simple (capillary, lymphatic, venous, and arterial) or combined (e.g., arteriovenous malformation). Cutaneous and mucosal lesions are typically red or violet. Many are associated with an underlying clinical syndrome. Vascular malformations are most frequently located in the extremities, head, neck, and pelvis, but they may be seen in any organ in the body. Arteriovenous malformations are characterized by marked dilation of the feeding vessels, hypervascularity, numerous arteriovenous connections around the nidus of the malformation, early venous filling, and rapid venous washout (Fig. 3-38). Venous malformations have slightly dilated or nondilated inflow arteries, variable flow patterns, and large venous spaces.

Vascular tumors include *hemangiomas*, which are superficial *(capillary)* or deep *(cavernous)*, and others entities (e.g., *angiosarcoma, hemangiopericytoma*). Benign lesions are small at birth, proliferate over time, and usually involute during young adulthood. They may be cutaneous or found in internal organs, including the brain, liver, spleen, pancreas, and kidneys. *Capillary* hemangiomas are in a growth phase; *cavernous* hemangiomas are in a quiescent stage and characterized by large vascular channels. They are marked by normal-caliber feeding vessels and early filling of vascular spaces that persists through the venous phase of a vascular imaging study (Fig. 3-39).

Telangiectasias are focal lesions composed of dilated arterioles, capillaries, and venules. They are typically found on the skin and mucous membranes but can be seen also in visceral organs. *Hereditary hemorrhagic telangiectasia* (Osler-Weber-Rendu syndrome) is an autosomal dominant

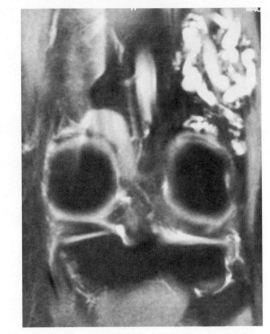

FIGURE 3-39 ■ Hemangioma lateral to the distal left femur seen on gadolinium-enhanced MR angiogram. Note enlarged, tortuous venous spaces.

disorder in which telangiectasias are present on the lips and mouth and in the intestinal tract, liver, spleen, lung, and brain (Fig. 3-40).[70]

Arteriovenous fistulas are almost always acquired direct connections between an artery and neighboring vein. Most arteriovenous fistulas are caused by trauma. Color Doppler sonography or MR angiography can identify the site of communication along with the enlarged feeding artery and early and rapid filling of the draining vein (Fig. 3-41). Arteriovenous fistulas can close spontaneously or enlarge over time. Patients often are asymptomatic but may present

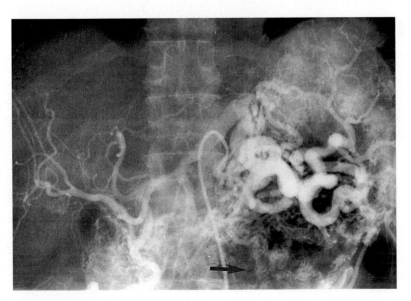

FIGURE 3-40 ■ Multiple telangiectasias of the stomach *(arrow)* in a patient with hereditary hemorrhagic telangiectasia.

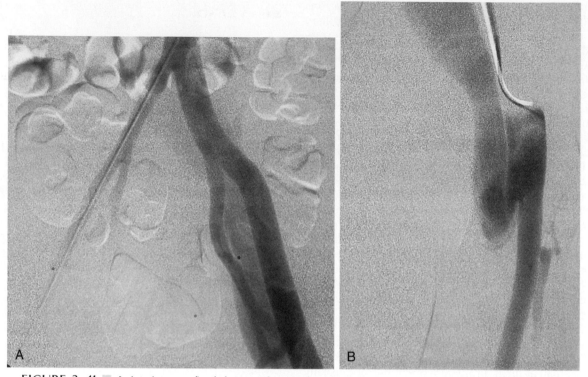

FIGURE 3-41 ■ **A,** Arteriovenous fistula between the superficial femoral artery and vein after femoral artery catheterization. Note the marked enlargement of the left iliac arteries compared with the right side. **B,** Selective injection in the left common femoral artery in oblique projection identifies the site of communication.

with local symptoms, distal ischemia (from a steal phenomenon), or high-output heart failure. Very rarely, the fistulas are congenital.[71]

Arteriovenous shunts are normally present in many vascular beds. These physiologic shunts sometimes become quite prominent (Fig. 3-42).[72] They may be seen also in certain disease states, such as cirrhosis and in hypervascular tumors (Fig. 3-43).

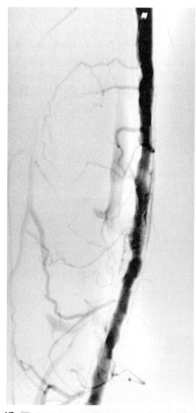

FIGURE 3-42 ■ Prominent arteriovenous shunts after balloon angioplasty of the superficial femoral artery in a patient with peripheral vascular disease.

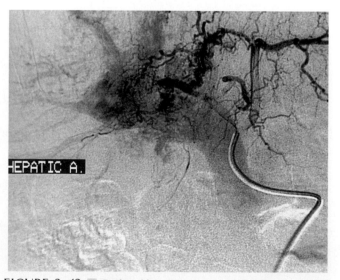

FIGURE 3-43 ■ Profound hepatic arterioportal shunting in a patient with cirrhosis and hepatocellular carcinoma.

Vascular Injury

Arteries and veins can be damaged for a variety of reasons. Penetrating injuries may be caused by sharp objects, gunshot wounds, bone fragments, or medical procedures.[73] Gunshot wounds produce vascular injury by direct penetration or when a vessel is stretched by the temporary cavitation effect of a moving bullet.[74]

Blunt arterial trauma is typically caused by rapid deceleration, moving objects, crush injuries, or falls from a height. Deceleration injuries result from sudden compression of the vessel or from shearing or twisting forces. Bone fracture or joint dislocation also can cause blunt arterial damage. Hemorrhage or edema into a confined space, such as the anterior tibial compartment of the calf, can result in a *compartment syndrome* that can compromise the arterial circulation in the extremity.[75]

The wide spectrum of traumatic arterial injuries includes intimal flaps, intraluminal thrombus, complete tear with extravasation or thrombosis, dissection, arteriovenous fistula, pseudoaneurysm formation, vasospasm, intramural hematoma, or extrinsic compression from hematoma (Fig. 3-44; see also Figs. 3-3, 3-14, 3-18, 3-23, and 3-41).[76] Rarely, bullets or gunshot pellets embolize within the arterial or venous circulation. Venous injuries are also common with penetrating injuries but rarely require imaging evaluation.

Invasion by neighboring inflammatory or neoplastic masses is another cause of vascular injury. Disruption of an artery causes frank extravasation or a pseudoaneurysm.

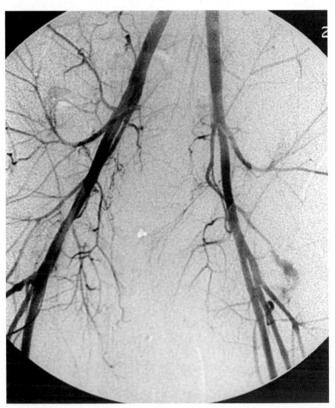

FIGURE 3-44 ▪ Extravasation from the left inferior gluteal artery after pelvic trauma from a motor vehicle accident.

▪ VEINS

Normal Structure and Function

Veins are composed of intima, media, and adventitia, but unlike arteries, there is less distinction among these layers.[1] Veins are thinner, less elastic, and more compliant than arteries. Venous valves are bicuspid leaflets that direct blood flow toward the heart. They are typically located near venous tributaries, at which point a slight bulge above the valve attachments is seen. The numerous valves in medium-sized veins of the extremities become less frequent as the veins move centrally. With the exception of the eustachian valve below the right atrium, the superior and inferior vena cavae are valveless.

Systemic venous blood is propelled centrally by several forces, including extrinsic compression (e.g., the muscular "calf pump"), changes in intrathoracic and intraabdominal pressure, and venous tone. Venous hemodynamics in the legs and arms are discussed in Chapters 13 and 15. The fall in intrathoracic pressure during inspiration increases blood flow from the IVC to the heart. The rise in intrathoracic or intra-abdominal pressure during expiration or a Valsalva maneuver reduces blood flow from the abdomen into the thorax.

Venospasm

Functional venous narrowing usually is caused by minor injury, including manipulation during angiographic procedures. The cardinal feature of venospasm is resolution with time. Spasm may also respond to vasodilating agents.

Venous Thromboembolic Disease

Venous thrombosis occurs through a complex process involving cellular blood elements, coagulation proteins, and the vascular wall. Clot is more likely to form in the setting of vessel wall injury, stasis of blood, or a hypercoagulable state (i.e., Virchow's triad). Low-flow states occur with intrinsic or extrinsic vein obstruction, immobilization, operative procedures, heart failure, or venous insufficiency.[77] Several hereditary and acquired disorders predispose to hypercoagulability (see Box 3-5).

Fresh thrombus produces an intraluminal filling defect (Fig. 3-45). At sonography, the clot also alters normal vein compressibility and flow phasicity caused by reflected atrial or respiratory activity. Thrombus should not be confused with unopacified blood (inflow defect) or overlying bowel gas (Fig. 3-46).

The fate of an acute venous clot depends on the site of thrombosis, any underlying thrombophilic factors, and anticoagulant or thrombolytic treatment[78,79]:

- *Embolization.* Left untreated, lower or upper extremity clots may embolize to the lung.
- *Progression.* Less than 30% of untreated calf vein thrombi will progress centrally.

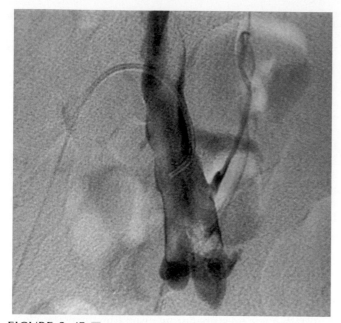

FIGURE 3-45 ■ Acute thrombosis of the left common iliac vein seen with selective catheterization from the right common femoral vein.

■ *Resolution.* In the superficial and deep veins of the leg, clot may lyse completely and leave vein walls and valves intact. At other sites (e.g., upper extremity veins, portal venous system, hepatic veins, IVC), complete resolution is less common.

■ *Recanalization.* In some cases, partial lysis occurs, leaving thickened vein walls, luminal narrowing, and damaged, incompetent valves (Fig. 3-47).

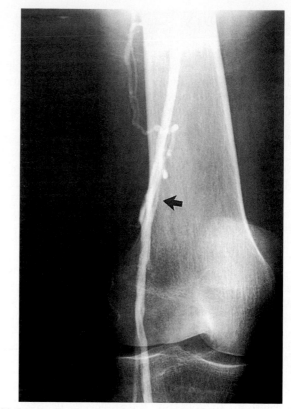

FIGURE 3-47 ■ Recanalization of occluded popliteal and superficial femoral veins results in diffuse irregular luminal narrowing and webs *(arrow)* and incompetent perforating veins.

■ *Chronic occlusion.* If the clot becomes organized, chronic occlusion results. This is the usual case in upper extremity and mesenteric veins. Long-term symptoms depend on the adequacy of collateral channels (Fig. 3-48).

Rarely, malignancies invade neighboring veins and produce tumor thrombus that mimics bland clot (see Fig. 3-35).

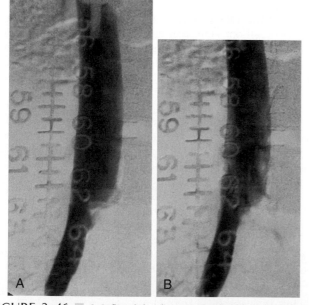

FIGURE 3-46 ■ **A,** Inflow defect from unopacified blood from the left iliac vein on inferior venacavography. The hallmark of this finding is change over the course of the injection (**B**).

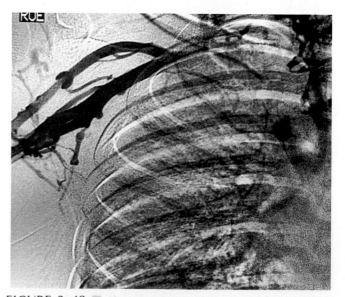

FIGURE 3-48 ■ Chronic occlusion of the right subclavian vein was caused by previous vascular access placement.

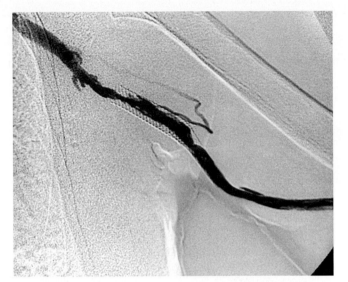

FIGURE 3-49 ■ Intimal hyperplasia within a Wallstent placed in the outflow vein of a hemodialysis access graft.

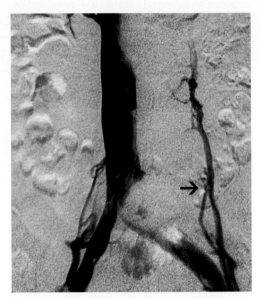

FIGURE 3-51 ■ Extrinsic compression of the left common iliac vein and inferior vena cava proven by CT scan. Note filling of collateral ascending lumbar veins *(arrow)*, proving the hemodynamic significance of this compression.

The most susceptible veins are the portal, renal, and hepatic veins and the IVC.

Neointimal Hyperplasia

Neointimal hyperplasia is the reaction of veins to acute injury or chronic hemodynamic changes. Clinically, the disease is seen most often in venous bypass grafts and the outflow veins of hemodialysis grafts (Fig. 3-49). The thickened intima is composed almost entirely of smooth muscle cells with little connective tissue matrix.[80] For this reason, these lesions

tend to be more elastic and more resistant to balloon dilation than comparable arterial stenoses.

Varices and Aneurysms

A *varix* is a dilated, tortuous vein. Varices occur at many sites in the body, including superficial leg, rectal, intestinal, gonadal, and renal veins. They result from chronically elevated pressure in the venous circulation from any cause (Fig. 3-50). The clinical sequelae include ulceration, bleeding, thrombosis, pain, and cosmetic deformity.

Venous aneurysms are quite rare.[81] Most are true aneurysms with an intact vein wall. Common sites are the internal jugular vein, superior vena cava, portal vein, IVC, and popliteal vein. False aneurysms usually are posttraumatic lesions. Venous aneurysms of the neck and thorax usually are asymptomatic. Abdominal venous aneurysms may result in pain,

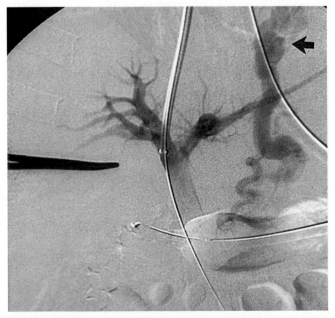

FIGURE 3-50 ■ Gastroesophageal varices *(arrow)* fill from a direct portal vein injection in a patient with portal hypertension.

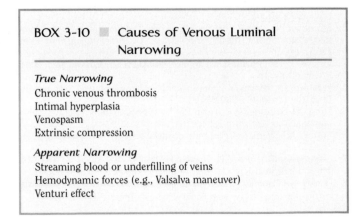

BOX 3-10 ■ Causes of Venous Luminal Narrowing
True Narrowing
Chronic venous thrombosis
Intimal hyperplasia
Venospasm
Extrinsic compression
Apparent Narrowing
Streaming blood or underfilling of veins
Hemodynamic forces (e.g., Valsalva maneuver)
Venturi effect

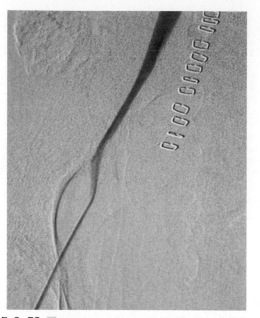

FIGURE 3-52 ■ Apparent narrowing of the inferior right iliac vein illustrates the Venturi effect.

bleeding, or thrombosis. Lower extremity venous aneurysms are complicated by thrombosis or pulmonary embolism.

Extrinsic Compression

The lumen of veins can be narrowed by inflammatory masses, tumors, hematomas or other fluid collections, fibromuscular bands, and external compression (Fig. 3-51). Real or apparent venous narrowing can have other causes (Box 3-10). Coaptation of vein walls during rapid contrast injection through an endhole catheter is caused by the Venturi effect (increased velocity of high-pressure contrast jet causing a reduction in neighboring pressure and associated coaptation of compliant vein walls) (Fig. 3-52).

REFERENCES

1. Fawcett DW: Blood and lymph vascular systems. In: Fawcett DW, ed. Bloom and Fawcett, A Textbook of Histology. New York, Chapman & Hall, 1994:368.
2. Shireman PK, Pearce WH: Endothelial cell function: biologic and physiologic functions in health and disease. AJR Am J Roentgenol 1996; 166:7.
3. Aird WC: Endothelium as an organ system. Crit Care Med 2004; 32(Suppl):S271.
4. Fraenkel L: Raynaud's phenomenon: epidemiology and risk factors. Curr Rheumatol Rep 2002;4:123.
5. Long CD, Santora TA, Fairman RM, et al: Stationary arterial wave phenomena. Ann Vasc Surg 1994;8:195.
6. Ross R: Atherosclerosis: an inflammatory disease. N Engl J Med 1999; 340:115.
7. Landmesser U, Hornig B, Drexler H: Endothelial function: a critical determinant in atherosclerosis? Circulation 2004;109(Suppl 1):I127.
8. Hackam DG, Anand SS: Emerging risk factors for atherosclerotic vascular disease. A critical review of the evidence. JAMA 2003;290:932.
9. Olson NE, Chao S, Lindner V, et al: Intimal smooth muscle cell proliferation after balloon catheter injury. Am J Pathol 1992;140:1017.
10. Schwartz RS, Henry TD: Pathophysiology of coronary artery restenosis. Rev Cardiovasc Med 2002;3(Suppl 5):S4.
11. Rajagopal V, Rockson SG: Coronary restenosis: a review of mechanisms and management. Am J Med 2003;115:547.
12. McCowan TC, Eidt JF: Angioplasty, C-reactive protein, and the patient at risk. Radiology 2003;227:314.
13. Schillinger M, Exner M, Mlekusch W, et al: Endovascular revascularization below the knee: 6-month results and predictive value of C-reactive protein. Radiology 2003;227:419.
14. Benditt EP, Schwartz SM: Blood vessels. In: Rubin E, Farber JL, eds. Essential Pathology, 3rd ed. Philadelphia, Lippincott Williams & Wilkins, 2000:245.
15. Crowther MA, Kelton JG: Congenital thrombophilic states associated with venous thrombosis: a qualitative overview and proposed classification system. Ann Intern Med 2003;138:128.
16. Lockshin MD, Erkan D: Treatment of the antiphospholipid syndrome. N Engl J Med 2003;349:1177.
17. Perler BA: Review of hypercoagulability syndromes: what the interventionalist needs to know. J Vasc Interv Radiol 1991;2:183.
18. Insko EK, Haskal ZJ: Antiphospholipid syndrome: patterns of life-threatening and severe recurrent vascular complications. Radiology 1997;202:319.
19. Stahl CP, Wideman CS, Spira TJ, et al: Protein S deficiency in men with long-term human immunodeficiency virus infection. Blood 1993; 81:1801.
20. Applebaum RM, Kronzon I: Evaluation and management of cholesterol embolization and blue toe syndrome. Curr Opin Cardiol 1996;11:533.
21. Bashore TM, Gehrig T: Cholesterol emboli after invasive cardiac procedures. J Am Coll Cardiol 2003;42:217.
22. Fukumoto Y, Tsutsui H, Tsuchihasi M, et al: The incidence and risk factors of cholesterol embolization syndrome, a complication of cardiac catheterization: a prospective study. J Am Coll Cardiol 2003; 42:211.
23. Johnston KW, Rutherford RB, Tilson MD, et al: Suggested standards for reporting on arterial aneurysms. J Vasc Surg 1991;13:452.
24. Reed D, Reed C, Stemmermann G, et al: Are aortic aneurysms caused by atherosclerosis? Circulation 1992;85:205.
25. Miller FJ: Aortic aneurysms. It's all about the stress. Arterioscler Thromb Vasc Biol 2002;22:1948.
26. Annabi B, Shedid D, Ghosn P, et al: Differential regulation of matrix metalloproteinase activities in abdominal aortic aneurysms. J Vasc Surg 2002;35:539.
27. Hsu RB, Tsay YG, Wang SS, et al: Surgical treatment for primary infected aneurysm of the descending thoracic aorta, abdominal aorta, and iliac arteries. J Vasc Surg 2002;36:746.
28. Pasic M: Mycotic aneurysm of the aorta: evolving surgical concept. Ann Thorac Surg 1996;61:1053.
29. Long R, Guzman R, Greenberg H, et al: Tuberculous mycotic aneurysm of the aorta: review of published medical and surgical experience. Chest 1999;115:522.
30. Lawrence PF, Wallis C, Dobrin PB, et al: Peripheral aneurysms and arteriomegaly: is there a familial pattern? J Vasc Surg 1998;28:599.
31. Khan IA, Nair CK: Clinical, diagnostic, and management perspectives of aortic dissection. Chest 2002;122:311.
32. O'Gara PT, DeSanctis RW: Acute aortic dissection and its variants. Towards a common diagnostic and therapeutic approach. Circulation 1995;92:1376.
33. Parums DV: The arteritides. Histopathology 1994;25:1.
34. Hunder G: Vasculitis: diagnosis and therapy. Am J Med 1996; 100(Suppl):2A.
35. Kerr GS: Takayasu's arteritis. Rheum Dis Clin North Am 1995;21:1041.
36. Johnston SL, Lock RJ, Gompels MM: Takayasu arteritis: a review. J Clin Pathol 2002;55:481.
37. Moriwaki R, Noda M, Yajima M, et al: Clinical manifestations of Takayasu arteritis in India and Japan—a new classification of angiographic findings. Angiology 1997;48:369.
38. Matsunaga N, Hayashi K, Sakamoto I, et al: Takayasu arteritis: protean radiologic manifestations and diagnosis. Radiographics 1997;17:579.
39. Yamato M, Lecky JW, Hiramatsu K, et al: Takayasu arteritis: radiographic and angiographic findings in 59 patients. Radiology 1986;161:329.
40. Nordborg E, Nordborg C: Giant cell arteritis: epidemiological clues to its pathogenesis and an update on its treatment. Rheumatology 2003; 42:413.

41. Stanson AW: Roentgenographic findings in major vasculitic syndromes. Rheum Clin North Am 1990;16:293.
42. Olin JW: Thromboangiitis obliterans (Buerger's disease). N Engl J Med 2000;343:864.
43. Olin JW, Young JR, Graor RA, et al: The changing clinical spectrum of thromboangiitis obliterans (Buerger's disease). Circulation 1990; 82(Suppl IV):IV3.
44. Kobayashi M, Kurose K, Kobata T, et al: Ischemic intestinal involvement in a patient with Buerger disease: case report and literature review. J Vasc Surg 2003;38:170.
45. Ha HK, Lee SH, Rha SE, et al: Radiologic features of vasculitis involving the gastrointestinal tract. Radiographics 2000;20:779.
46. Citron BP, Halpern M, McCarron M, et al: Necrotizing angiitis associated with drug abuse. N Engl J Med 1970;283:1003.
47. Jee KN, Ha HK, Lee IJ, et al: Radiologic findings of abdominal polyarteritis nodosa. AJR Am J Roentgenol 2000;174:1675.
48. Hoffman GS, Kerr GS, Leavitt RY, et al: Wegener granulomatosis: an analysis of 158 patients. Ann Intern Med 1992;116:488.
49. Kerr HE, Sturrock RD: Clinical aspects, outcome assessment, disease course, and extraarticular features of spondyloarthropathies. Curr Opin Rheumatol 1999;11:235.
50. Bacon PA, Carruthers DM: Vasculitis associated with connective tissue disorders. Rheum Clin North Am 1995;21:1077.
51. Freeman RK, Swegle J, Sise MJ: The surgical complications of Ehlers-Danlos syndrome. Am Surgeon 1996;62:869.
52. Tunaci A, Berkmen YM, Goekmen E: Thoracic involvement in Behçet's disease: pathologic, clinical, and imaging features. AJR Am J Roentgenol 1995;164:51.
53. Park JH, Chung JW, Joh JH, et al: Aortic and arterial aneurysms in Behçet disease: management with stent-grafts—initial experience. Radiology 2001;220:745.
54. Chung CJ, Stein L: Kawasaki disease: a review. Radiology 1998;208:25.
55. Modrall JG, Sadjadi J: Early and late presentations of radiation arteritis. Semin Vasc Surg 2003;16:209.
56. Stanley JC: Pathogenesis of arterial fibrodysplasia. In: White RA, Hollier LH, eds. Vascular Surgery: Basic Science and Clinical Correlations. Philadelphia, Lippincott, 1994:143.
57. Begelman SM, Olin JW: Fibromuscular dysplasia. Curr Opin Rheumatol 2000;12:41.
58. Furie DM, Tien RD: Fibromuscular dysplasia of arteries of the head and neck: imaging findings. AJR Am J Roentgenol 1994;162:1205.
59. Yamaguchi R, Yamaguchi A, Isogai M, et al: Fibromuscular dysplasia of the visceral arteries. Am J Gastroenterol 1996;91:1635.
60. Slavin RE, Saeki K, Bhagavan B, et al: Segmental arterial mediolysis: a precursor to fibromuscular dysplasia? Mod Pathol 1995;8:287.
61. Soulen MC, Cohen DL, Itkin M, et al: Segmental arterial mediolysis: angioplasty of bilateral renal artery stenoses with 2-year imaging follow-up. J Vasc Interv Radiol 2004;15:763.
62. Ryan JM, Suhocki PV, Smith TP: Coil embolization of segmental arterial mediolysis of the hepatic artery. J Vasc Interv Radiol 2000; 11:865.
63. Burke AP, Virmani R: Sarcomas of the great vessels: a clinicopathologic study. Cancer 1993;71:1761.
64. Reuter SR, Redman HC, Cho KJ, eds: Tumors. In: Gastrointestinal Angiography, 3rd ed. Philadelphia, WB Saunders, 1986:128.
65. Weidner N: Tumor angiogenesis: review of current applications in tumor prognostication. Semin Diagn Pathol 1993;10:302.
66. Folkman J: Role of angiogenesis in tumor growth and metastasis. Semin Oncol 2002;29(Suppl 16):15.
67. Enjolras O, Mulliken JB: Vascular tumors and malformations (new issues). Adv Dermatol 1997;13:375.
68. Konez O, Burrows PE: Magnetic resonance of vascular anomalies. Magn Reson Imaging Clin N Am 2002;10:363.
69. Dubois J, Garel L: Imaging and therapeutic approach of hemangiomas and vascular malformations in the pediatric age group. Pediatr Radiol 1999;19:879.
70. Guttmacher AE, Marchuk DA, White RI Jr: Hereditary hemorrhagic telangiectasia. N Engl J Med 1995;333:918.
71. Doehlemann C, Hauser M, Nicolai T, et al: Innominate artery enlargement in congenital arteriovenous fistula with subsequent tracheal compression and stridor. Pediatr Cardiol 1995;16:287.
72. Vallance R, Quin RO, Forrest H: Arteriovenous shunting complicating occlusive atherosclerotic peripheral vascular disease. Clin Radiol 1986;37:389.
73. Ben-Menachem Y: Exploratory and interventional angiography in severe trauma: present and future procedure of choice. Radiographics 1996;16:963.
74. Hollerman JJ, Fackler ML, Coldwell DM, et al: Gunshot wounds: 1. Bullets, ballistics, and mechanisms of injury. AJR Am J Roentgenol 1990;155:685.
75. Ulmer T: The clinical diagnosis of compartment syndrome of the lower leg: are clinical findings predictive of the disorder? J Orthop Trauma 2002;16:572.
76. Scalea TM, Sclafani S: Interventional techniques in vascular trauma. Surg Clin North Am 2001;81:1281.
77. Hull RD, Pineo GF: Venous thrombosis. In: Loscalzo J, Creager MA, Dzau VJ, eds. Vascular Medicine: A Textbook of Vascular Biology and Disease, 2nd ed. Boston, Little, Brown, 1996:1051.
78. Fraser JD, Anderson DR: Deep venous thrombosis: recent advances and optimal investigation with US. Radiology 1999;211:9.
79. Kearon C: Natural history of venous thromboembolism. Circulation 2003;107(23 Suppl 1):I22.
80. Allaire E, Clowes AW: Endothelial cell injury in cardiovascular surgery: the intimal hyperplastic response. Ann Thorac Surg 1997;63:582.
81. Calligaro KD, Ahmad S, Dandora R, et al: Venous aneurysms: surgical indications and review of the literature. Surgery 1995;117:1.

SECTION II

VASCULAR DIAGNOSIS AND INTERVENTION

4

Thoracic Aorta

ARTERIOGRAPHY

Thoracic aortography usually is performed from the femoral artery approach. Some angiographers use a high right brachial artery route in patients requiring aortography for possible aortic dissection if the femoral pulses are diminished. In patients with a history of catheterization-related cholesterol embolization, angiography is sometimes performed from a brachial approach to avoid recurrent embolization. When studying patients with suspected traumatic aortic injury, the arch should be traversed with a guidewire; advancing a formed pigtail catheter into a traumatic pseudoaneurysm can be lethal.[1] A pigtail or similarly shaped catheter is placed about 2 cm above the aortic valve to avoid catheter recoil into the left ventricle during rapid contrast injection. A steep right posterior oblique projection is standard. Additional projections are obtained as needed.

ANATOMY

Development

In the fetus, two paired blood vessels (dorsal and ventral aortae) form in the chest.[2] The ventral aortae merge into the aortic sac, which forms parts of the ascending aorta, aortic arch, and pulmonary trunk. The left dorsal aorta becomes the descending thoracic aorta. Six pairs of branchial arches connect the two vascular channels (Fig. 4-1 and Table 4-1). The normal left aortic arch develops when the right arch involutes beyond the origin of the right subclavian artery. The remaining portion of the right arch becomes the brachiocephalic (innominate) artery.

Normal Anatomy

The aortic valve is composed of three leaflets that form the three *sinuses of Valsalva:* right, left, and posterior or noncoronary (Fig. 4-2).[3] The *right* and *left coronary arteries* arise from their respective sinuses. Beyond the sinus segment, the ascending aorta courses anteriorly and superiorly. This segment is enclosed within the fibrous pericardium. In adults, its mean diameter is 3.5 cm.[4] The aorta then passes over the main pulmonary artery and left main stem bronchus. The *brachiocephalic, left common carotid,* and *left subclavian arteries* arise in turn from the upper surface of the aortic arch.

Just beyond the take-off of the left subclavian artery, the aorta narrows slightly at the *aortic isthmus.* It then widens slightly beyond this point at the *aortic spindle* (Fig. 4-3).

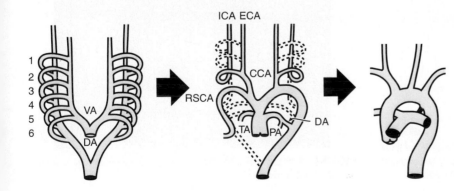

FIGURE 4-1 ■ Embryologic development of the thoracic aorta. The numbers in the first panel refer to the branchial arches. CCA, common carotid artery; DA, dorsal aortae; DA, ductus arteriosus; ECA, external carotid artery; ICA, internal carotid artery; PA, pulmonary artery; RSCA, right subclavian artery; TA, thoracic aorta; VA, ventral aortae. (Adapted from Langman J: Medical Embryology, 3rd ed. Baltimore, Williams & Wilkins, 1975:235.)

TABLE 4-1   FATE OF EMBRYOLOGIC AORTIC AND
             BRANCHIAL VESSELS

Embryologic Vessel	Neonatal Vessel
Ventral aorta (upper)	External carotid artery
Dorsal aorta (upper)	Internal carotid artery
Branchial arch 1	Maxillary artery
Branchial arch 2	Hyoid and stapedial arteries
Branchial arch 3	Carotid arteries
Branchial arch 4	Aortic arch
Branchial arch 5	Involutes
Branchial arch 6	Pulmonary artery, ductus arteriosus
7th intersegmental artery	Subclavian artery

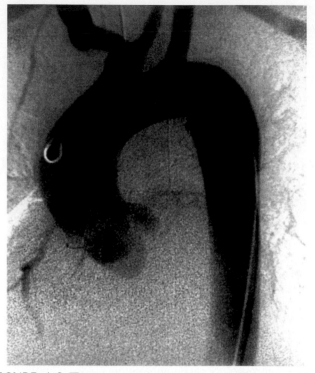

The *ligamentum arteriosum,* a remnant of the ductus arteriosus, tethers the aorta to the left pulmonary artery at the isthmus. In some cases, a shallow, smooth, symmetric outpouching persists: the ductus diverticulum, or "ductus bump" (Fig. 4-4).

The descending thoracic aorta runs in front of the spine. In adults, its mean diameter is 2.5 cm.[4] Nine pairs of *posterior intercostal arteries* (levels 3 through 11) arise from the descending aorta. The first and second posterior intercostal arteries are supplied by the superior intercostal artery,

FIGURE 4-3 ■ The common origin of the brachiocephalic and left common carotid arteries is called the bovine arch. Just beyond the left subclavian artery, the aorta narrows slightly (aortic isthmus) and then widens (aortic spindle).

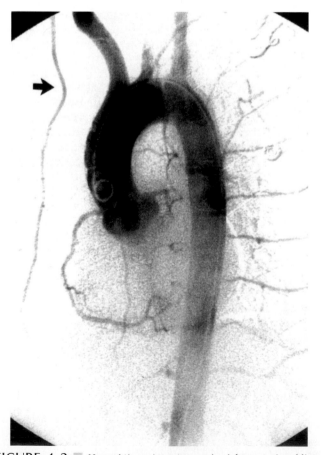

FIGURE 4-2 ■ Normal thoracic aortogram in right posterior oblique projection. There is prominent filling of the Right coronary artery, right internal thoracic artery *(arrow),* and posterior intercostal arteries.

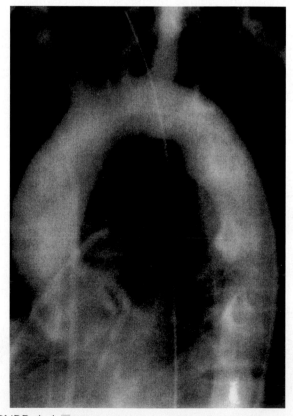

FIGURE 4-4 ■ Normal thoracic aortogram demonstrates a prominent ductus diverticulum.

which arises from the costocervical branch of the subclavian artery. The subcostal arteries take off at the level of the 12th ribs. One or more *bronchial arteries* supply each lung and originate as separate branches or bronchointercostal trunks at the fourth to sixth thoracic level (see Chapter 12). Numerous small vessels that supply the chest wall, mediastinum, esophagus, spinal cord, and pericardium are rarely seen during aortography.

Variant Anatomy

Congenital anomalies of the thoracic aorta can be explained by abnormal evolution of the dorsal and ventral aortae and the branchial arches using the double aortic arch system proposed by Edwards (Box 4-1).[5,6] The aorta, pulmonary artery, and anomalous branches may form *vascular rings* that compress the trachea or esophagus. Aortic arch variants often are associated with congenital cardiac anomalies.

A common origin of the brachiocephalic and left common carotid arteries or origin of the left common carotid artery from the root of the brachiocephalic artery (i.e., *bovine arch*) is reported in 1% to 22% of the population (see Fig. 4-3).[7] Other unusual branching patterns also exist.[7] Take-off of the left vertebral artery directly from the arch is an uncommon variant (Fig. 4-5). Separate origin of the right subclavian and common carotid arteries from the arch is rare.

An *aberrant right subclavian artery* is the most common aortic arch malformation of clinical significance, with a reported frequency of 0.4% to 2%.[8] This anomaly results from involution of the embryonic aortic segment between the right subclavian and right common carotid arteries. The right subclavian artery becomes the last branch of the aortic arch (Fig. 4-6). It usually passes behind the trachea and esophagus to reach the right side of the chest. The vessel may indent the posterior surface of the esophagus, but patients rarely have symptoms. The aberrant artery often arises from a dilated portion of the most distal remnant of the right aortic arch, the so-called *diverticulum of Kommerell* (Fig. 4-7).

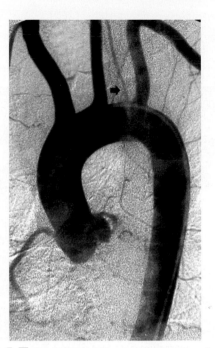

FIGURE 4-5 ■ Origin of the left vertebral artery from the aortic arch *(arrow).*

Right aortic arch with aberrant left subclavian artery is the most common of the several types of right aortic arch, occurring in 0.05% to 0.1% of the population.[5] It results from involution of the left aortic arch between the left common and left subclavian arteries with persistence of the embryologic right arch. The order of aortic arch branching is therefore left carotid artery, right carotid artery, right subclavian artery, and left subclavian artery. The arch passes over the right main stem bronchus and descends on either side of the spine (Fig. 4-8). Despite the presence of a vascular ring, respiratory and esophageal symptoms are rare. About 5% to 10% of patients have associated congenital heart disease.

Right aortic arch with mirror-image branching imposes a branch order of left brachiocephalic artery, right common carotid artery, and right subclavian artery. The descending thoracic aorta is virtually always to the right of the spine. Some form of congenital heart disease is present in 90% to 95% of patients, including tetralogy of Fallot, truncus arteriosus, double-outlet right ventricle, and transposition of the great vessels. About one third of patients with tetralogy of Fallot have a right aortic arch, usually of this type. Although the vascular ring created by the right arch and ligamentum arteriosum produces tracheal or esophageal compression, patients usually have no symptoms.

Coarctation of the aorta occurs in 0.02% to 0.06% of the population.[5] The obstruction takes the form of a discrete, bandlike narrowing at or beyond the attachment of the ligamentum arteriosum *(postductal coarctation).* This anomaly should not be confused with *fetal coarctation,* which produces diffuse narrowing of the aortic arch and hypoplasia of left heart chambers *(preductal coarctation).* Coarctation is associated with bicuspid aortic valve, patent ductus arteriosus, ventricular septal defect, and Turner's syndrome. Coarctation usually is discovered in a child or young adult with upper extremity hypertension, diminished lower extremity pulses,

---

BOX 4-1 ■ **Congenital Anomalies of the Thoracic Aorta**

Aberrant right subclavian artery
Right aortic arch
    Aberrant left subclavian artery
    Mirror-image branching
Aberrant left brachiocephalic artery
Isolated left subclavian artery
Coarctation of the aorta
Pseudocoarctation
Cervical aortic arch
Double aortic arch
Circumflex aorta
Double dorsal aortic arch
Persistence of the fifth aortic arch

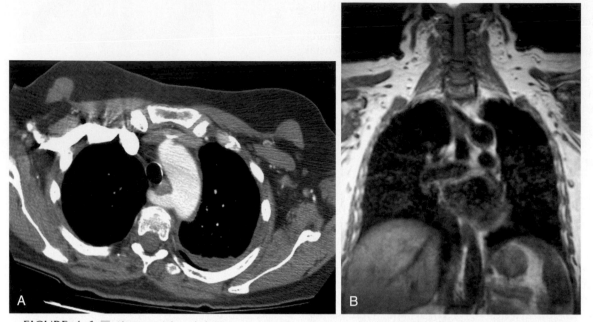

FIGURE 4-6 ▪ Aberrant right subclavian artery. **A,** The artery runs posterior to the trachea and esophagus on CT angiography. **B,** Aberrant vessel arises as the last branch of the aortic arch on black-blood MR image. (Courtesy of Eric Goodman, MD, San Diego.)

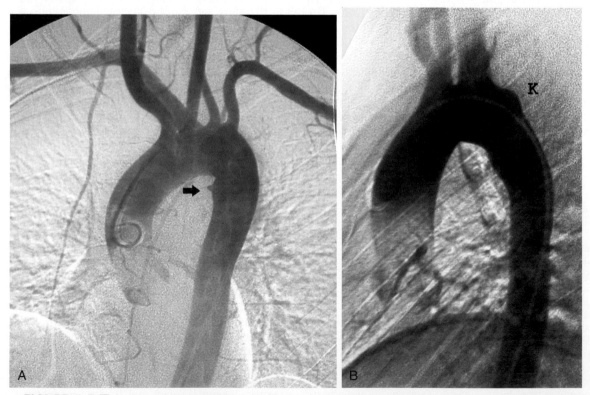

FIGURE 4-7 ▪ **A,** Aberrant right subclavian artery on arch aortography in the left anterior oblique projection. Also note bronchial artery diverticulum *(arrow)*. **B,** Aberrant subclavian artery arises from a diverticulum of Kommerell (K) in lateral projection.

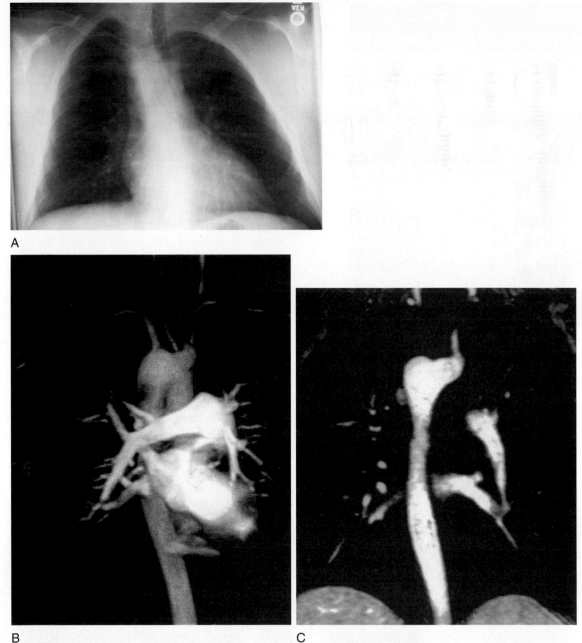

A

B   C

FIGURE 4-8 ▪ Right aortic arch with aberrant left subclavian artery. **A,** Chest radiograph shows right-sided aorta displacing the trachea to the left. **B,** Coronal three-dimensional MR angiography with cine breath-hold technique shows the right aortic arch. **C,** The left subclavian artery is the final branch of the aortic arch and arises from a large diverticulum.

or heart failure. To bypass the stenosis, blood flows from the anterior intercostal branches of the internal thoracic arteries retrograde into the posterior intercostal branches of the descending aorta. Enlargement and tortuosity of the intercostal arteries cause pressure erosion on the undersurface of the third through ninth ribs (rib notching).

The characteristic findings of coarctation are severe, discrete narrowing around the aortic isthmus, dilation of the ascending aorta, and enlarged internal thoracic and intercostal arteries (Fig. 4-9).[9] Operative treatment of aortic coarctation is by direct resection with end-to-end anastomosis or by patch aortoplasty.[10] Balloon angioplasty has been used as an alternative to surgery.[11] Long-term results are generally good, but restenosis or aneurysm formation at the angioplasty site occurs in about 20% of patients. Use of intravascular stents may improve on these results.[12]

Pseudocoarctation of the aorta is a congenital elongation of the thoracic aorta with a discrete kink at the aortic isthmus.[5] Although it may look similar to a true aortic coarctation, pseudocoarctation produces no pressure gradient across the kink and has no collateral circulation (Fig. 4-10). Occasionally, aneurysms form adjacent to the aortic twist.

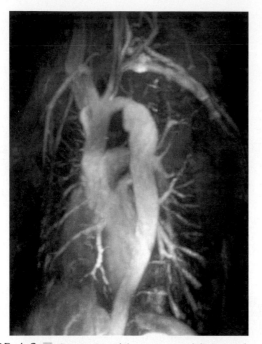

FIGURE 4-9 ■ Coarctation of the aorta on gadolinium-enhanced MR angiography. There is discrete narrowing of the aorta beyond the left sub-clavian artery with significant post-stenotic aortic dilation. (Courtesy of Eric Goodman, MD, San Diego.)

■ MAJOR DISORDERS

Atherosclerosis

Atherosclerosis is the most common disease affecting the thoracic aorta, but usually it is silent. Complete athero-sclerotic obstruction of the thoracic aorta does not occur. Plaques cause symptoms when fragments embolize into the brain or peripheral circulation. Emboli usually arise from "protruding" plaques with a mobile component that is probably overlying thrombus.[13] Most of these plaques are located in the aortic arch and descending thoracic aorta. In one study, about one third of patients with such atheromas suffered distal embolization within 1 year.[14] In addition to stroke, peripheral atheroembolism may occur. Cholesterol crystals shower into the distal circula-tion (spontaneously or after aortic manipulation) and result in renal insufficiency, bowel ischemia, or blue toe syndrome.[15]

Suspected thoracic aortic atherosclerosis in patients with unexplained stroke or peripheral embolization normally is studied by transesophageal echocardiography (TEE).[16] Occasionally, CT or MR imaging is used to confirm suspicious lesions.[17] The disease produces an irregular contour to the aortic lumen, typically in the arch or distal aorta (Fig. 4-11). Rarely, ulcerated plaque penetrates into the aortic wall (see below). Other causes for narrowing of the aortic lumen include dissection (with encroachment by the false lumen) and arteritis.

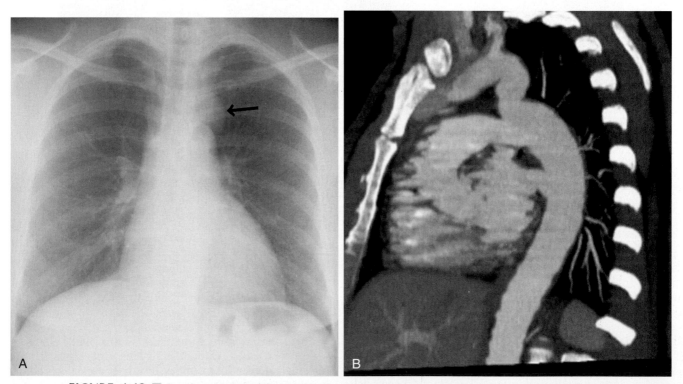

FIGURE 4-10 ■ Pseudocoarctation of the aorta. **A,** Chest radiograph shows a rounded density *(arrow)* superior to the aortic knob. **B,** Oblique parasagittal reformatted CT angiogram shows marked kinking of the descending thoracic aorta but no discrete stenosis. (Courtesy of Eric Goodman, MD, San Diego.)

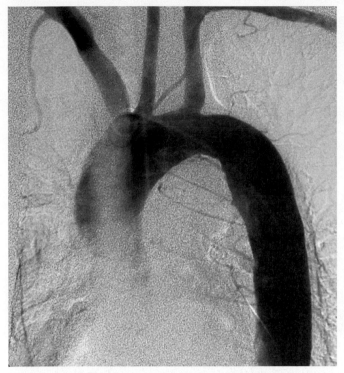

FIGURE 4-11 ■ Diffuse aortic atherosclerosis seen at arch aortography.

Degenerative Aneurysms

Etiology and Natural History

Thoracic aortic aneurysms (TAAs) and pseudoaneurysms are caused by a variety of disorders (Box 4-2). The classic features of several types of thoracic aneurysms are summarized in Table 4-2. The pathologic and imaging features of the uncommon forms are considered in later sections.

About 75% of TAAs are degenerative (so-called atherosclerotic aneurysms). Degenerative aneurysms form because of inflammatory damage to the vessel wall and hemodynamic forces that produce remodeling.[18,19] A variety of reactive oxygen species activate matrix metalloproteinases that cause thinning of the medial layer. These reactive oxygen

---

BOX 4-2 ■ Causes of Thoracic Aortic Aneurysms

Degeneration (atherosclerosis-associated)
Cystic medial degeneration
Trauma
Chronic dissection
Infection (bacterial, syphilitic, tuberculous)
Connective tissue disorder
Marfan syndrome
Ehlers-Danlos syndrome
Behçet's disease
Vasculitis (see Box 4-5)
Congenital (sinus of Valsalva aneurysm)

TABLE 4-2   CLASSIC APPEARANCE OF THORACIC AORTIC ANEURYSMS

Type	Features
Degenerative	Fusiform aneurysm of the descending aorta with atherosclerotic changes
Posttraumatic	Saccular pseudoaneurysm at the aortic isthmus
Bacterial	Saccular, eccentric aneurysm at an unusual site
Marfan syndrome	Aneurysm of aortic root and tubular segment (sinotubular ectasia)
Syphilitic	Saccular ascending aortic aneurysm sparing the aortic root
Takayasu's arteritis	Wall thickening and enhancement
	Diffuse fusiform dilation of the ascending aorta with branch stenoses or occlusions
Post-stenotic	Dilation beyond an obstruction (e.g., aortic stenosis, coarctation)

---

species are probably liberated as part of an inflammatory process. Most degenerative aneurysms involve the descending aorta; about 5% are thoracoabdominal.[20] The most common cause of **isolated** ascending aortic aneurysms is cystic medial degeneration, in which diminished quantities of elastin and smooth muscle cells are found in the media.[21]

Compared with abdominal aortic aneurysms, the natural history of thoracic aneurysms is less well understood. The most feared complication is rupture. Based on *Laplace's law* (wall stress = pressure × radius), the most important predictor of rupture is aneurysm size. The risk is low if the aneurysm is less than 5 cm in diameter, unless the rate of expansion exceeds about 1 cm/yr.[22] After a TAA reaches 5 to 6 cm in diameter, the likelihood of rupture goes up substantially, and elective repair is indicated.[23,24] Descending TAAs are sometimes watched until they reach about 7 cm in diameter because of concern about surgical complications, particularly spinal cord ischemia. The risk of rupture is greater for thoracoabdominal aneurysms than for comparably sized aneurysms confined to the chest.

Clinical Features

Most affected patients are elderly. Many are asymptomatic at the time the aneurysm is discovered on a routine chest radiograph or CT scan obtained for unrelated reasons. Symptoms, which usually are caused by compression of adjacent organs by the enlarging aorta, include dysphagia, respiratory complaints, superior vena cava syndrome, and hoarseness from compression on the recurrent laryngeal nerve. Some patients with intact aneurysms complain of chest or back pain. Symptoms are common after the aneurysm has ruptured. They include chest pain, hypotension, massive hemoptysis, hematemesis, and dyspnea from leakage into the pleural space.

Imaging

Chest Radiography. Plain chest radiographs usually show enlargement of the ascending aorta, descending aorta, or both. A massive aneurysm can erode the vertebral bodies or sternum. Atelectasis can result from compression of the airways. A left pleural effusion suggests the possibility of rupture.

Transesophageal Echocardiography. TEE can detect and size TAA.[25] However, TEE is less valuable for aneurysm staging, evaluation of adjacent structures, or postoperative surveillance.

Computed Tomography. Helical CT is a standard tool for the diagnosis of suspected thoracic aortic aneurysms, surveillance of known aneurysms, and detection of aneurysm rupture.[26] Aneurysm size and extent, presence of mural thrombus, and associated atherosclerotic disease are well depicted by CT. Multiplanar reformatting and shaded-surface display images provide exquisite views of the aneurysm, its relationship to adjacent structures (e.g., compression of the pulmonary artery), and involvement of arch vessels.[27]

Magnetic Resonance Imaging. MR imaging is probably the best modality for studying TAA in stable patients. With essentially no risk to the patient, gadolinium-enhanced MR angiography can characterize the entire extent of the aneurysm, its effect on neighboring organs, branch vessel involvement, the aortic valve, and the heart (Fig. 4-12).[9,28,29] Several features can differentiate degenerative aneurysms from other types (see Table 4-2). Sometimes, the cause cannot be determined. Postoperative evaluation of TAA usually is done with MR imaging.[30]

Treatment

Surgical Therapy. The primary treatment for TAAs is operative.[31] As a rule, they are repaired when the diameter exceeds 5 to 6 cm or the patient is symptomatic.[21] The standard

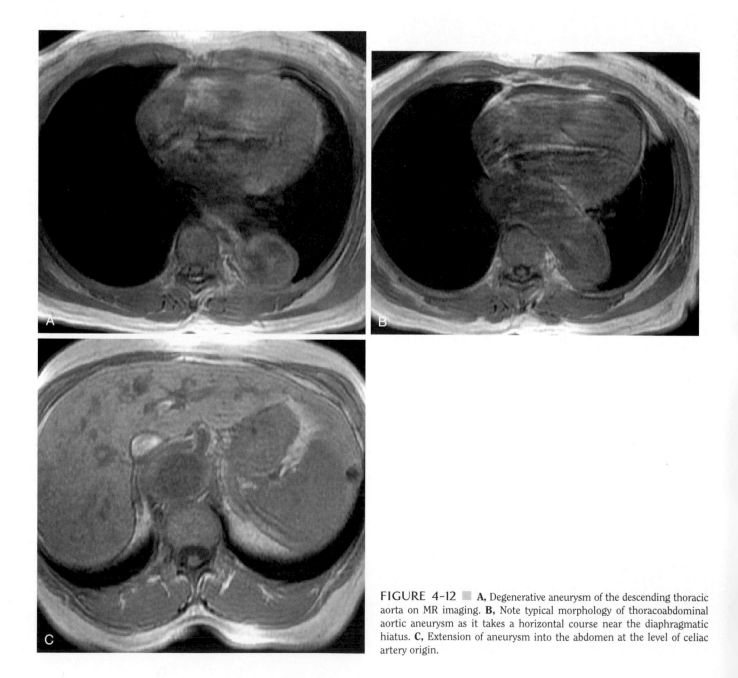

FIGURE 4-12 ■ **A,** Degenerative aneurysm of the descending thoracic aorta on MR imaging. **B,** Note typical morphology of thoracoabdominal aortic aneurysm as it takes a horizontal course near the diaphragmatic hiatus. **C,** Extension of aneurysm into the abdomen at the level of celiac artery origin.

procedure is to replace the diseased segment with a Dacron graft. Major complications include stroke, myocardial infarction, and renal failure. Paraplegia is another devastating complication (particularly associated with thoracoabdominal aneurysm repair) caused by ligation of branches to the spinal artery. The frequency of spinal cord injury is less than 15% with the use of intraoperative maneuvers such as distal perfusion, hypothermia, and monitoring of evoked potentials. Preoperative spinal arteriography may be useful in this setting to allow reimplantation of major spinal artery branches.[32] The mortality rate for elective repair is less than that for emergent repair (9% versus 22%).[33]

Endovascular Therapy. Stent-grafts are used as an alternative to surgical repair to treat selected high-risk patients with degenerative thoracic aortic aneurysms.[34-37] First-generation homemade grafts were constructed with synthetic vascular graft fabric attached to one of several uncovered stents. At present, several devices are undergoing approval by the U.S. Food and Drug Administration (FDA). All require a femoral artery cutdown for placement due to their large size (20 to 27 French). The Excluder stent-graft (W. L. Gore and Associates) has a nitinol skeleton covered with thin polytetrafluoroethylene graft fabric. The device requires both proximal and distal necks of 15 to 20 mm for proper sealing of the aneurysm. For several reasons, it is simpler to use in long aneurysms. The Talent stent-graft (Medtronic/AVE) is composed of a nitinol stent covered by polyester with bare metal ends which may cross side branches such as the left subclavian artery. The device and delivery system are more flexible than the Excluder, allowing for placement through tortuous arterial systems. In cases in which the proximal neck is short, placement across the left subclavian artery can be combined with operative left carotid to left subclavian bypass.

Technical success and immediate aneurysm thrombosis is noted in over 90% of cases with very low mortality rates (Fig. 4-13). With limited follow-up, endoleak (usually type I, occurring at the attachment sites) occurs in less than 5% of patients (see Chapter 5). Uncommon complications include stroke and paraplegia from exclusion of side branches feeding the spinal cord. However, early access-related complications are a significant drawback to this technology. Late problems include proximal and distal endoleaks, aneurysm development at the edges of the device, stent-graft movement or kinking, and aneurysm rupture.

Dissection

Etiology and Natural History

An aortic dissection is a longitudinal split in the media of the aortic wall. In most cases, an *intimal tear* connects this medial channel with the aortic lumen. Dissections confined to the aortic wall are *intramural hematomas* (see below).

The pathogenesis of aortic dissection is not entirely understood. Dissections are generally attributed to hemodynamic effects such as long-standing hypertension or to abnormalities of the media that often are congenital (Box 4-3).[38] In the former group, the pathologic basis for dissection is unclear; only mild medial degeneration is seen histologically. In the latter group, degeneration of medial smooth muscle, elastin,

and collagen matrix can be identified. It is unknown why pregnant women are at greater risk for dissection, although hemodynamic stress factors and hormonal effects have been postulated. Illicit drug use (particularly with cocaine or methamphetamines) is being recognized as an increasingly frequent cause of acute dissection.[39] Rarely, aortic dissection is caused by trauma (e.g., deceleration injury, catheterization procedures).[40]

Regardless of the underlying pathology, the inciting event usually is an intimal tear. Sometimes, the dissection begins spontaneously within the aortic wall, possibly from rupture of the vasa vasorum. The intimal tear connects the lumen in direct continuity with the aortic valve *(true lumen)* with the channel of blood in the media *(false lumen)*. In as many as 13% of cases, the dissection is confined to the wall, and no intimal tear is identified at autopsy.[41] The dissection propagates distally, proximally, or in both directions as blood under high pressure enters the false channel. Blood flow in the false lumen usually is slower than in the true lumen. The false channel, however, can become quite large and compress the true lumen. The dissection usually stops at an aortic branch or atherosclerotic plaque. In many cases, it extends to the aortic bifurcation or beyond.

The location and extent of the dissection has important implications for treatment and prognosis. The DeBakey and Stanford classifications are illustrated in Figure 4-14. Stanford type A dissections, which usually begin with a tear just above the aortic valve and *always* involve the ascending aorta, account for about two thirds of cases. Type B dissections, which usually begin with a tear just beyond the origin of the left subclavian artery and *only* involve the descending aorta, account for the remaining cases. Occasionally, a dissection that begins at this site extends distally and proximally toward the aortic valve.

Complications of aortic dissection are the result of complete *rupture* (often at the site of the intimal tear) or *ischemia*. Rupture, which often is fatal, can occur from the ascending aorta into the pericardium, from the aortic arch into the mediastinum, or from the descending aorta into the mediastinum or left pleural space. In about one half of patients with type A dissection, aortic regurgitation follows damage to the aortic root. If the intimal flap obstructs a major aortic branch or flow is diminished in the true or false channel supplying an organ, ischemia can result. Over time, untreated dissections can persist (i.e., chronic dissection), enlarge, thrombose, or rupture. *Chronic dissections* are those that have been present for more than 2 weeks. Late complications of untreated chronic dissections include aneurysm formation and delayed ischemic events.

Clinical Features

Men have aortic dissections about twice as frequently as women. Most patients are more than 50 years of age and have one or more risk factors for dissection (see Box 4-3).[42] Hypertension is present in about three fourths of patients and is even more common in patients with type B dissection. The classic symptom is the sudden onset of searing chest or back pain. Patients also may present with a stroke, renal failure or hypertension, mesenteric ischemia, lower extremity ischemia, or even paraplegia from obstruction of spinal artery branches of the descending aorta.

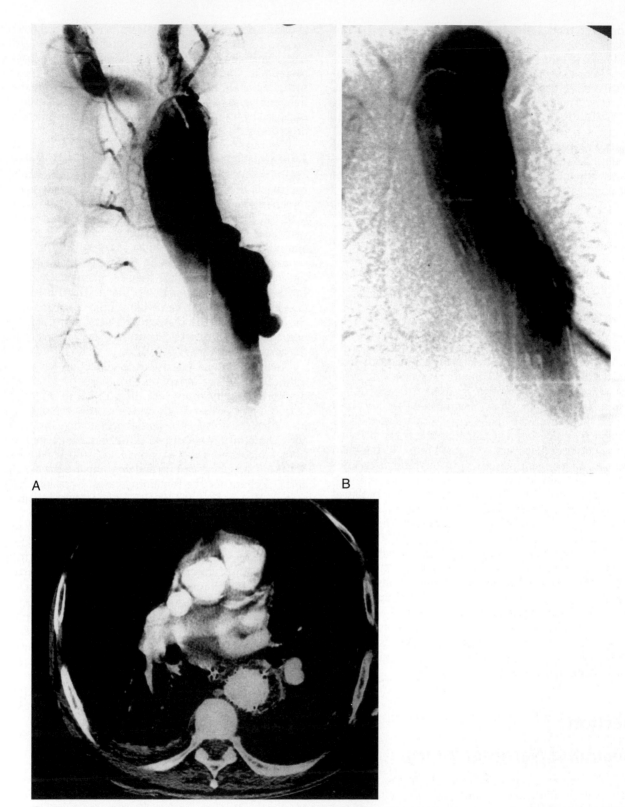

A

B

C

FIGURE 4-13 ■ Stent-graft repair of a thoracic aortic aneurysm. **A,** The anteroposterior aortogram shows a saccular aneurysm of the descending thoracic aorta. **B,** A stent-graft was placed under imaging guidance, and the aneurysm has been excluded. **C,** Exclusion of the aneurysm with thrombosis outside the graft is confirmed on a follow-up CT scan. (Courtesy of John Kaufman, MD, Portland, Ore.)

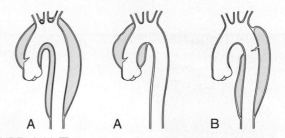

FIGURE 4-14 ■ Classification for aortic dissection. Figures (from left to right) correspond to DeBakey types I, II, and III, and the Stanford classification (A or B) is stated for each. (Adapted from Kadir S: Diagnostic Angiography. Philadelphia, WB Saunders, 1986:141.)

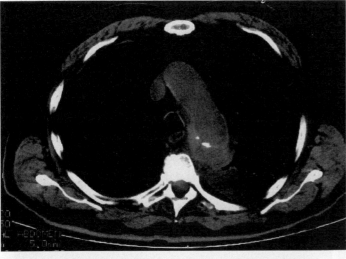

A

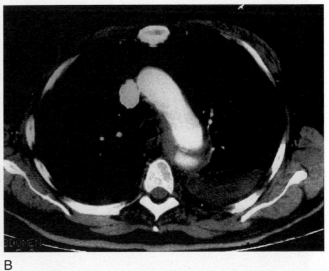

B

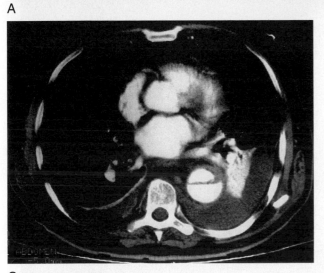

C

FIGURE 4-15 ■ Stanford type B aortic dissection is revealed by CT imaging. **A,** The noncontrast scan shows marked displacement of intimal calcification from the outer posterior aortic wall at the distal aortic arch and reveals a left pleural effusion. **B,** The contrast scan shows a dissection flap with diminished enhancement of the posterior false lumen. **C,** The dissection continues into the descending thoracic aorta. The false lumen is larger than the true lumen.

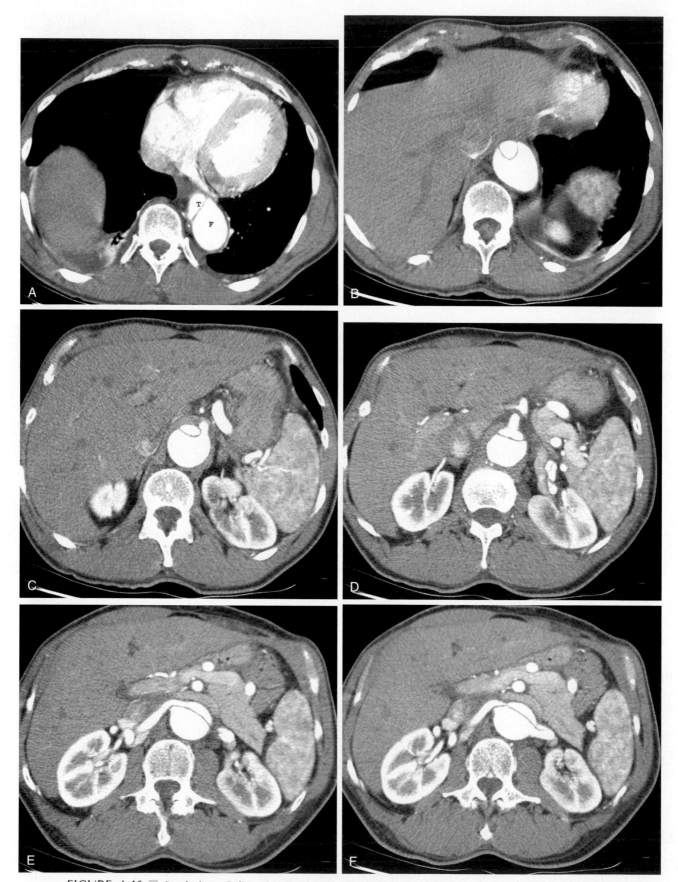

FIGURE 4-16 ■ Stanford type B dissection (**A, B**) with extension into the abdominal aorta seen with CT angiography (T, true lumen; F, false lumen). Note relationship of lumens to celiac (**C**), superior mesenteric (**D**), right renal (**E**), and left renal arteries into which the dissection flap extends (**F**). The dissection continued down both iliac arteries to the groin (not shown).

Imaging

Imaging studies are used for detection, preoperative assessment, and postoperative evaluation of aortic dissections.[43] The surgeon requires the following information to guide therapy:

- Extent of dissection (stage)
- Entry (and reentry) site
- Location of true and false lumens and relationship of major aortic branches to each
- Evidence of rupture
- Existence of aortic insufficiency

Chest Radiography. Plain radiographs of the chest may point to the diagnosis of aortic dissection. The most common findings are an increase in size of the thoracic aorta, a double aortic arch contour, widening of the mediastinal silhouette, pleural effusion, and tracheal shift.[44,45] The classic plain film sign is displacement of intimal calcification from the outer edge of the aortic knob by more than 6 mm. This finding is moderately specific but rarely seen. A completely normal chest radiograph does not exclude the diagnosis.

Computed Tomography. CT is widely used for evaluation of acute aortic dissection.[26,45,46] It is extremely accurate for detection and staging. CT is readily available, relatively non-invasive, and able to accommodate critically ill patients. Scans reveal an intimal flap separating two lumens, often with different enhancement patterns (Fig. 4-15). Other possible findings are dilation of the aorta, compression of the true lumen by the false lumen, thrombosis of the false lumen, mediastinal hematoma, and pleural or pericardial effusion. A localized dissection must be differentiated from an intramural hematoma or a penetrating aortic ulcer (see below).

It is important to distinguish the true lumen from the false lumen. The true lumen is the one in continuity with the aortic valve. The most reliable features of the true lumen are outer wall calcification and eccentric flap calcification (see Fig 4-15).[46] The false lumen usually has a larger cross-sectional area and an acute angle between the flap and the outer aortic wall (Fig. 4-16). In most type B aortic dissections, the false lumen is posterior/lateral to the true lumen in the chest and then spirals down the aorta in a somewhat unpredictable fashion.

Magnetic Resonance Imaging. Gadolinium-enhanced MR angiography also is extremely accurate for diagnosing and staging aortic dissection.[29] The risks of iodinated contrast material are avoided. Aortic branch vessels, the aortic valve, and the heart can be evaluated with MR imaging. Its major limitations are longer scanning times and difficulties with monitoring critically ill patients. Both axial black-blood sequences and reformatted gadolinium-enhanced MR angiography are used.[9,28,29] Cine imaging will help detect aortic insufficiency. MR images can identify an intimal flap and different signal intensities in the true and false lumens caused by variations in blood flow or by clot (Fig. 4-17; see also Fig. 5-28). Noncommunicating dissection (i.e., intramural hematoma) can usually be differentiated from a communicating dissection with slow flow.

Transesophageal Echocardiography. TEE is performed with multiplanar color flow Doppler techniques.[25,47] The procedure can be performed at the bedside in less than

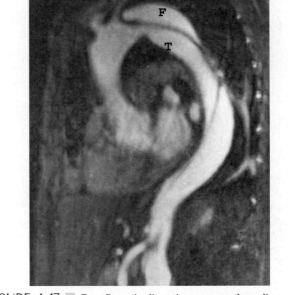

FIGURE 4-17 ■ Type B aortic dissection seen on three-dimensional MR angiography in oblique sagittal plane (T, true lumen; F, false lumen). The dissection spirals down into the abdominal aorta.

30 minutes with the patient under moderate sedation. TEE is favored by cardiologists because it is fast and convenient. Besides identifying an intimal flap, TEE also can detect aortic insufficiency and extension of dissection into the coronary arteries. It is extremely sensitive but somewhat less specific than CT and MR imaging.

Angiography. Aortography was once the primary method for preoperative diagnosis of aortic dissection but now is rarely necessary. Aortography is more risky and less sensitive than cross-sectional techniques in the detection of acute dissection. It often misses the diagnosis of intramural hematoma or chronic dissection with thrombosis of the false lumen.

Special care should be taken to avoid extending or over-injecting the false lumen if it is entered during catheterization, which should be suspected when the guidewire cannot pass easily to the aortic valve or when blood flow in the channel is sluggish. Abdominal or pelvic arteriography usually is needed to follow the dissection to the level of reentry.

A lucent flap between the true and false lumens is diagnostic (Fig. 4-18; see also Fig. 3-22). Delayed filling and slow washout of the false lumen are characteristic. The true lumen may be narrowed by an expanding false channel. The relationship of branch vessels to the two lumens should be established.

Choice of Imaging Modality. Multiplanar TEE, helical CT, and MR angiography have similar accuracy in the diagnosis of aortic dissection.[28,47-49] The optimal approach to the patient with suspected or known dissection depends on the relative availability of equipment, condition of the patient, and capability of operators.

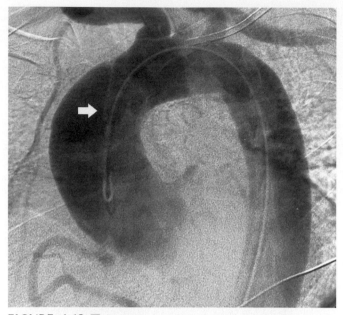

FIGURE 4-18 ■ Stanford type A dissection on arch aortography in the right posterior oblique projection. An intimal tear is seen in the proximal ascending aorta *(arrow).*

Treatment

Surgical Therapy. Management of patients with acute aortic dissection depends on the location and extent of the dissection, existence of complications, and the general health of the patient. There is a consensus that most patients with Stanford type A dissection should undergo repair with graft placement or primary obliteration of the false lumen.[21,50] The aortic valve is replaced when necessary. Patients with type B dissection are first treated medically with blood pressure control. Repair is performed if there is a complication (e.g., renal failure, mesenteric ischemia), rapid expansion, or impending rupture signaled by continuing pain or hypotension. Chronic dissections usually are treated when the aortic diameter exceeds 6 cm or the patient has symptoms.

Transcatheter Therapy. Endovascular methods have been developed to treat ischemic complications of aortic dissection, particularly when they involve the kidney, intestines, or lower extremities.[51,52] An uncovered stent can be used to tack down an intimal flap extending into a branch vessel and to reopen the artery. When ischemia is caused by slow flow through the aortic lumen supplying an aortic branch, balloon fenestration or aortic stent-graft placement can relieve symptoms. To perform *aortic fenestration,* a large-caliber needle within a protective cannula is used to puncture through the intimal flap from one lumen to the other. The hole is then widened with an angioplasty balloon (Fig. 4-19). Fenestration equalizes pressures in the two lumens and improves flow to ischemic organs.

Both homemade and commercially available stent-grafts have recently been used to successfully treat acute and chronic aortic dissections.[37,53-55] The primary objective is to seal the entry tear and eliminate flow in the false lumen. Stent-grafts may be inappropriate in patients with difficult access due to highly calcified or tortuous vessels, or large aortic diameter. Treatment of chronic dissections can be more difficult because of the development of multiple entry flaps or predominance of the false lumen.

Follow-up Imaging

All patients with aortic dissection, whether treated medically or surgically, need routine follow-up examinations to evaluate the dissection (or graft) and to detect complications.[56,57] The surgeon or interventionalist is concerned about several issues:

- Patency of the graft
- Status of the false lumen (e.g., persistent flow, extension, expansion, thrombosis)
- Degree of aortic insufficiency

The most common late problems are pseudoaneurysm formation at graft anastomoses and aneurysmal expansion of the false lumen.[58] Residual flow in the false lumen is common after operation.

Trauma

Etiology and Natural History

Motor vehicle accidents are responsible for most thoracic aortic injuries by rapid deceleration of a passenger or pedestrian. Other cases are caused by falls from a height, crush injuries, and penetrating wounds.[59] Deceleration injuries usually result in an intimal or transmural tear (rupture), which is instantly fatal in about 80% to 90% of cases.[60] Dissection is an unusual result of such trauma. Rarely, the injury produces an aortic intramural hematoma or complete transection with thrombosis. Immediate survival is possible if the rupture is contained by periadventitial tissues to form a fragile pseudoaneurysm.

The most widely held explanation for these injuries is that relatively fixed and mobile parts of the aorta experience unequal forces at the moment of impact. These forces, which may be caused by traction, torsion, shearing, or compression, lacerate the aortic wall.[59,60] An alternative theory is that sudden compression of the thoracic aorta between the spine and anterior bony structures (sternum and ribs) causes the tear.[61] None of these theories has been proven.

Aortic rupture can occur at any site or at multiple sites.[62,63] In about 90% of initial survivors, the tear is located at the aortic isthmus just beyond the left subclavian artery. Less commonly, the aortic root, origins of the arch vessels, or lower descending aorta is injured.

The mortality rate for aortic rupture is almost 95% if left untreated, and many of these patients die within the first 24 hours after injury. Untreated survivors develop a chronic pseudoaneurysm that often is silent for decades.[60,63] These cases often come to medical attention as incidental findings on chest radiographs or CT scans.

Clinical Features

The violence of the accident may not correlate with the likelihood of aortic injury. Clinical symptoms and signs are not particularly helpful in screening patients. For these reasons,

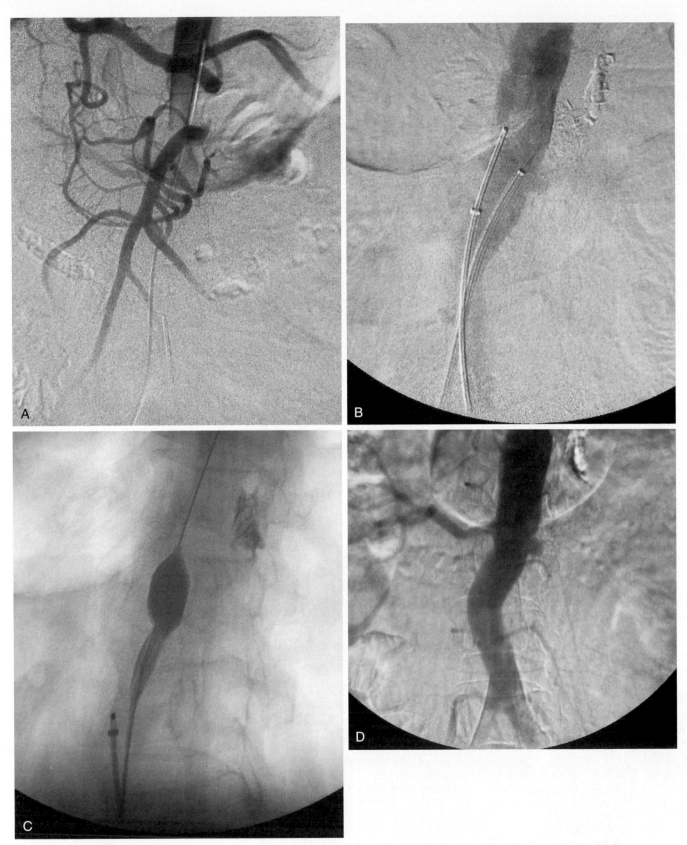

FIGURE 4-19 ■ Balloon fenestration of a type B aortic dissection. **A,** Abdominal aortography shows right and left common femoral artery (CFA) catheters lying in the true lumen, which feeds the celiac and superior mesenteric arteries with poor flow to the right renal artery and none to the left. **B,** Intravascular ultrasound introduced from the left CFA, Rosch-Uchida TIPS set introduced from the right CFA. Puncture was made posterolaterally and proven to be intraluminal. **C,** Angioplasty with 18-mm balloon is performed. **D,** Repeat angiography shows improved flow to the right renal artery and equivalent flow in both aortic lumens.

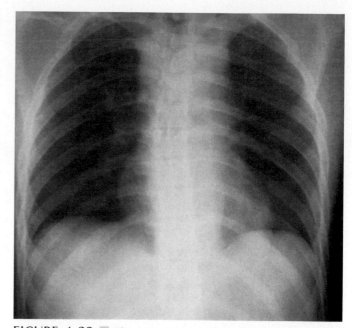

FIGURE 4-20 ■ The supine chest radiograph of a patient with a traumatic aortic tear shows marked widening of the mediastinum and loss of the normal aortic knob.

every patient with the appropriate "mechanism of injury" is suspect. Because the consequence of missing an aortic injury is so grave, imaging studies are used liberally.

Imaging

Chest Radiography. A plain radiograph is obtained for every patient with significant chest trauma. Radiographs are most useful with the patient in an upright position, although this is rarely feasible. A ruptured aorta produces a host of findings (Box 4-4).[59,64-66] The most sensitive signs are widening of the superior mediastinum (ultimately a subjective call), indistinctness of the aortic arch contour, and loss of the descending aortic shadow (Fig. 4-20). However, these findings are not particularly specific to aortic injury and may be seen in a patient with an intact aorta. Some of the other signs, such as tracheal deviation and paraspinal line displacement, are relatively insensitive but fairly specific for aortic injury. Fewer than 1% to 2% of patients with normal chest radiographs are subsequently found to have an aortic laceration.[66]

Computed Tomography. The early rationale for screening trauma patients with chest CT was that the force needed to rupture the aorta would invariably be associated with mediastinal bleeding. A "clean" mediastinum without fluid,

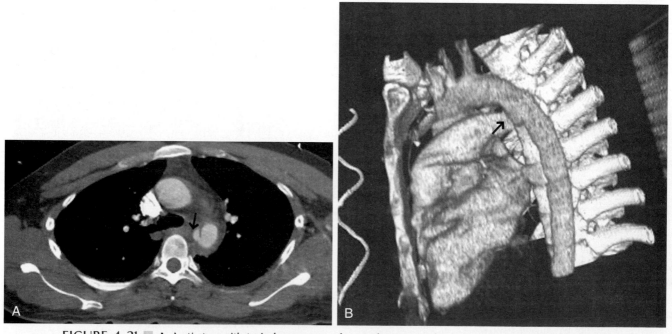

FIGURE 4-21 ■ **A,** Aortic tear with typical appearance of a pseudoaneurysm *(arrow)* just beyond the left subclavian artery on axial CT angiogram. Also note increased para-aortic density from mediastinal blood. **B,** Shaded surface displayed reformatted image demonstrates pseudoaneurysm.

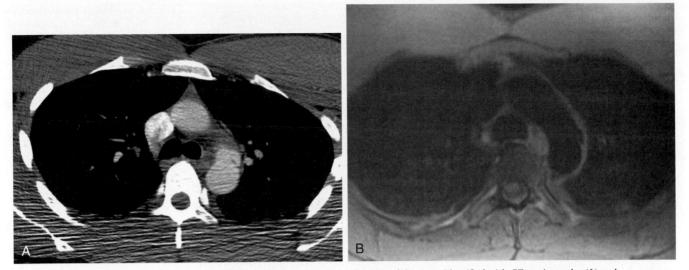

FIGURE 4-22 ■ Subtle traumatic aortic flap on the lateral aspect of the aorta identified with CT angiography (**A**) and confirmed with black-blood MR imaging (**B**).

aortic deformity, or artifact would essentially exclude an aortic injury and eliminate the need for aortography. The sensitivity of CT for detecting thoracic aortic damage approaches 100%.[66-70] However, the false-positive rate based on the presence of mediastinal blood alone is substantial because of artifacts and bleeding without an accompanying aortic injury.

Multidetector, helical techniques now permit a specific diagnosis of aortic rupture in most cases. CT has replaced aortography as the primary imaging study in this setting. In recent studies, helical CT was 100% sensitive and about 80% to 96% specific in detecting an actual site of aortic injury in large populations of trauma patients.[62,70,71] In addition to indirect signs of bleeding, direct signs include intraluminal flaps, pseudoaneurysm, irregular contour, dissection, or intramural hematoma (Figs. 4-21 through 4-23). Particular care must

be taken to identify abnormalities at the origins of the arch vessels.

Aortography. Although catheter arteriography was considered the gold standard for the diagnosis of aortic trauma, it is only employed when CT is uninterpretable or inconclusive. Guidewire hang-up, particularly near the aortic isthmus, may be the first indication of an aortic tear. Aortography is then performed below this level with a small contrast injection to avoid further damage to the vessel (Fig. 4-24).[1] The entire thoracic aorta, from the aortic valve to the diaphragmatic hiatus and including the arch

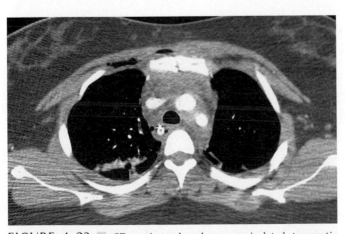

FIGURE 4-23 ■ CT angiography shows an isolated traumatic pseudoaneurysm of the origin of the brachiocephalic/left carotid artery (bovine arch) following a motor vehicle accident. A sternal fracture is present.

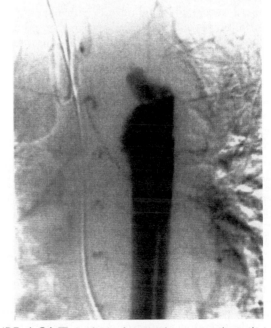

FIGURE 4-24 ■ Guidewire hang-up in a traumatic aortic tear. The wire would not pass easily into the aortic arch. The digital aortogram below this site using 20 mL of contrast material shows the injury.

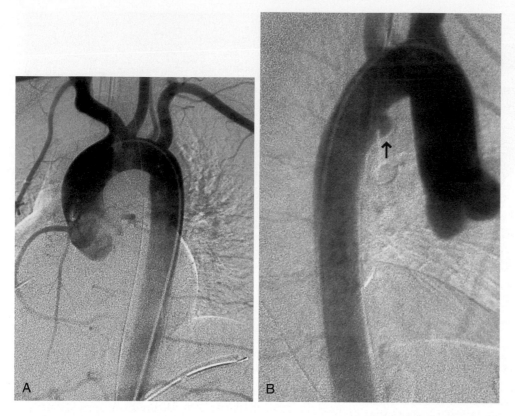

FIGURE 4-25   ■   Occult traumatic aortic injury. **A,** The initial right posterior oblique aortogram showed no definite injury. A bovine arch is present. The left vertebral artery arises directly from the aorta. **B,** The shallow left posterior oblique aortogram shows an abnormal outpouching of the proximal descending thoracic aorta *(arrow).*

vessels must be imaged. Aortography is always done in **at least** two views to exclude the diagnosis, typically a steep right posterior oblique projection and an orthogonal left posterior oblique or frontal projection. Subtle tears or intimal flaps can easily be missed on a single view (Fig. 4-25). For cases of penetrating trauma, the initial aortogram is done in a projection that is parallel to the trajectory of the bullet or stab wound.

The usual aortographic finding is an irregular outpouching of the aorta just beyond the left subclavian artery (Fig. 4-26). These contained pseudoaneurysms can take on a variety of shapes and sizes. Less often, injury produces an intimal flap, dissection (usually Stanford type B), arch vessel pseudoaneurysm or intimal flap, or, rarely, complete transection (Fig. 4-27).[72] Free extravasation is rare. Chronic traumatic pseudoaneurysms can be saccular or fusiform, and the wall often is heavily calcified.

Several entities can mimic an acute aortic injury[73,74]:

■ The ductus diverticulum occurs at the usual site for deceleration injury. However, this normal variant usually has smooth, continuous edges with the aorta, no associated intimal flap, and rapid washout of contrast (see Fig. 4-4).

■ An infundibulum of an aortic branch (usually left subclavian or bronchointercostal artery) can be mistaken for an injured segment. This error is avoided by noticing its smooth, symmetric, conical margins and association with a normal vessel (see Fig. 4-7).

■ In elderly patients, ulcerated atherosclerotic plaque or a focal degenerative aneurysm may be impossible to differentiate from an acute traumatic injury.

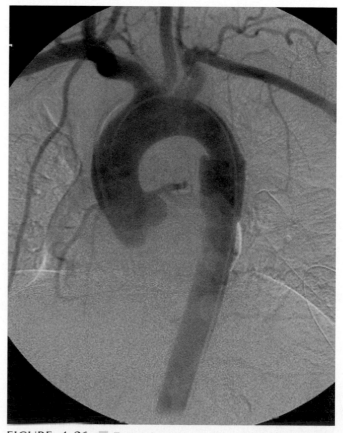

FIGURE 4-26   ■   Traumatic rupture at the aortic isthmus on right posterior oblique arch aortography.

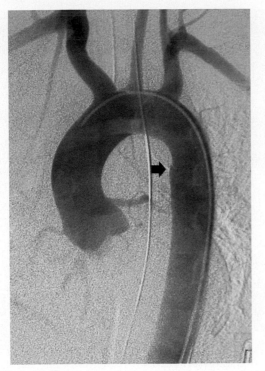

FIGURE 4-27 ■ Subtle intimal flap in the upper descending thoracic aorta *(arrow)* from a deceleration injury (proven at operation).

■ The normal widening of the aortic spindle should not be confused with a traumatic pseudoaneurysm (see Fig. 4-3).

Other Modalities. Trauma surgeons have great interest in the use of *TEE* for diagnosing suspected aortic injuries.[75] TEE is fast and can be performed at the bedside. However, some blind spots exist, the procedure is highly operator dependent, and there is a risk (albeit small) of serious complications. *Intravascular ultrasound* has the ability to detect most of the typical findings of acute aortic injury.[76] However, its accuracy has yet to be proven in large clinical series. Its primary role is to confirm suspicious findings when CT or catheter angiography is equivocal.[77] In general, *MR imaging* is not suitable for this clinical situation (except to confirm other equivocal studies) because of the patient's unstable condition (see Fig. 4-22).

Treatment

Surgical Therapy. Traditionally, all acute traumatic aortic injuries were repaired emergently with primary resection or graft placement.[78] Recent trends in trauma care have allowed more elective operation for patients with severe intracranial injury or at high risk for thoracic surgery. Small intimal flaps may be managed medically with vigorous imaging follow-up. Chronic pseudoaneurysms usually require surgical treatment.

Transcatheter Therapy. Endovascular stent-grafts have been used successfully in selected high-risk patients with acute and chronic posttraumatic pseudoaneurysms (see earlier).[34,35,37,53,55,79]

■ OTHER DISORDERS

Vasculitis

Several forms of vasculitis affect the aorta and its branches (Box 4-5; see also Chapter 3).[80-82] Most of them produce dilation of the proximal aorta, obstructions of large aortic branches, or both.

Takayasu's arteritis is a chronic, inflammatory vasculitis of large elastic arteries (see Chapter 3).[83-85] It primarily affects the aorta, its major branches, and the pulmonary arteries. Chest radiographs may show irregularity of the contour of the descending thoracic aorta, linear calcification in the aortic wall, ectasia of the aortic arch, or cardiomegaly. CT and MR imaging will demonstrate variable patterns of enhancement in the early stages of the disease.[86,87] In the chronic stages, typical imaging findings include aortic dilation or irregularity, narrowing of the descending aorta, long stenoses or occlusions of arch vessels, wall thickening, calcifications, mural thrombi, and, rarely, aortic insufficiency or dissection (Fig. 4-28).

In the chronic phase of the disease, branch obstructions are treated if there is end-organ ischemia (e.g., arm "claudication"). Surgical bypass was the standard therapy.[88] Balloon angioplasty is now an attractive alternative. Angioplasty is effective and safe for descending thoracic and abdominal aortic stenoses, and restenosis is uncommon.[89,90] Intravascular stents have been used as an adjunct to angioplasty.[91] For best results, surgery or percutaneous therapy should be delayed until the acute constitutional symptoms have subsided. Expanding aneurysms usually require operative repair.

Giant cell (temporal) arteritis is a vasculitis of large- and medium-sized arteries.[92] The disease has some features in common with Takayasu's arteritis but is a distinct entity (see Chapter 3). Significant aortic disease, such as aneurysm, annular dilation, or aortic insufficiency, is relatively uncommon. Involved aortic branches have long, smooth stenoses alternating with normal segments. These findings, along with the distribution of disease, differentiate giant cell arteritis from atherosclerosis.

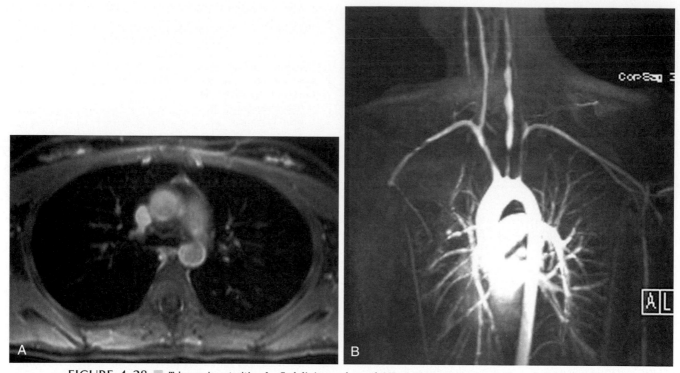

FIGURE 4-28 ■ Takayasu's arteritis. **A,** Gadolinium-enhanced MR angiogram shows aortic wall thickening and enhancement. **B,** Maximum intensity projection image shows long, smooth left common carotid artery (CCA) and left subclavian and right subclavian artery stenoses with dilation of the upper left CCA.

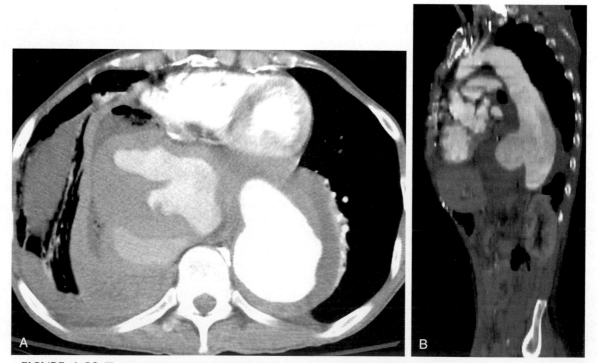

FIGURE 4-29 ■ HIV-related arteritis. **A,** The disease causes diffuse dilation of the descending thoracic aorta along with a large saccular aneurysm on transverse CT angiography and oblique sagittal reformatted image (**B**).

Collagen-vascular disorders, particularly those linked to the HLA-B27 antigen, occasionally produce aortitis.[93] Acute inflammation followed by fibrotic scarring occurs in the sinotubular portion of the ascending aorta and may extend into the ventricular septum and mitral valve apparatus. Aortic regurgitation can result; dilation of the aortic root is unusual.

HIV-related arteritis is well known to affect medium- and small-caliber vessels. However, a rarer form of large vessel arteritis can cause solitary or multiple aneurysms in the aorta and its major branches.[94,95] The disease produces a leukocytoclastic reaction in the vasa vasorum and periadventitial tissues along with chronic inflammation. The aneurysms often are saccular in appearance (Fig 4-29).

Inherited Connective Tissue Disorders

Several inherited diseases are responsible for noninflammatory degeneration of the aortic wall leading to aneurysm formation, dissection, or rupture. These disorders include Marfan syndrome, Ehlers-Danlos syndrome, Behçet's disease, osteogenesis imperfecta, and hereditary annuloaortic ectasia.[96,97]

Marfan syndrome is a rare autosomal dominant disorder that affects the aorta, heart, eyes (ectopia lentis), and skeleton.[98] The underlying defect is an abnormality of microfibrils in elastic tissue throughout the body.[99] Cardiovascular complications occur in more than 50% of patients. Cystic medial degeneration and elastic fiber fragmentation weaken the aortic wall. These changes result in aortic root dilation with aortic ectasia, aortic insufficiency, aneurysm formation, or dissection. Aortic dilation in Marfan syndrome usually is confined to the aortic root, producing *sinotubular ectasia* with a characteristic "tulip bulb" appearance (Fig. 4-30).

Ehlers-Danlos syndrome is a rare set of distinct genetic disorders of collagen production.[100] More than nine types have been described, and many feature hyperextensibility of the joints and thin skin. Type IV disease, in which there is a defect in type III collagen, has characteristic vascular features. Spontaneous arterial ruptures, aneurysms, and severe angiographic complications are seen with this form of the syndrome.

Infectious Aortitis

Bacterial aortitis is caused by seeding of an aortic lesion such as atherosclerotic plaque or a preexisting aneurysm, septic embolization into the aortic vasa vasorum, transmural spread from an adjacent infection, or penetrating trauma. The inflamed wall can form an infected (mycotic) aneurysm or pseudoaneurysm.[101] Although infectious aneurysms are rare, the aorta and femoral artery are the most commonly affected sites. The usual pathogens are *Salmonella* species and *Staphylococcus aureus.*[102] *Tuberculous aortitis*

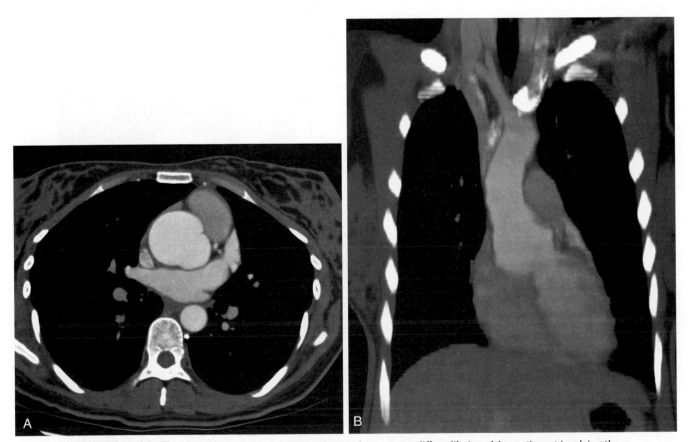

FIGURE 4-30 ■ Marfan syndrome. **A,** Axial CT angiogram demonstrates diffuse dilation of the aortic root involving the aortic sinuses. **B,** Coronal maximum intensity projection shows fusiform aortic root dilation with characteristic "tulip bulb" appearance. (Courtesy of Eric Goodman, MD, San Diego.)

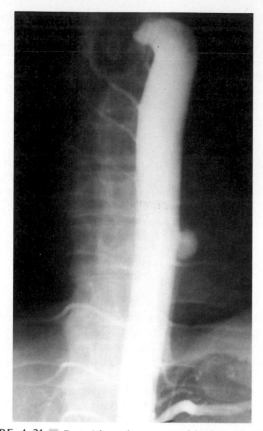

FIGURE 4-31 ■ Bacterial pseudoaneurysm of the descending thoracic aorta in an intravenous drug abuser.

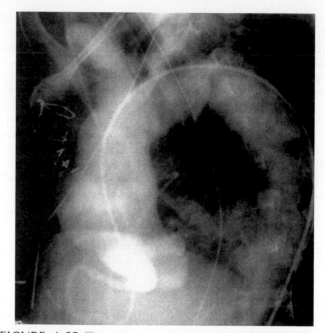

FIGURE 4-32 ■ Syphilitic aortic aneurysm. The dilation is saccular and spares the aortic root.

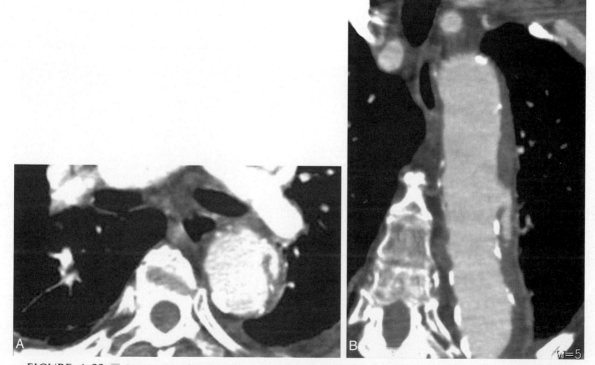

FIGURE 4-33 ■ Penetrating atherosclerotic ulcer of the descending thoracic aorta. **A,** Transverse CT angiogram shows ulcerated lesion penetrating the aortic wall. **B,** Coronal reformatted image demonstrates longitudinal extension of the ulcer in a diffusely diseased and calcified aorta.

may develop from lymphangitic spread or contiguous extension of disease in the chest. Some patients have localized pain, fever, and positive blood cultures. With this clinical picture, the presence of an uncalcified, smooth, eccentric saccular aneurysm is diagnostic (Fig. 4-31).

Syphilitic aortitis has been largely eradicated in most parts of the world. About 10% of patients with long-standing, untreated tertiary syphilis develop cardiovascular disease.[103] Damage to the arterial wall occurs when *Treponema* spirochetes invade the vasa vasorum of the aorta during the early stages of infection. Occlusion of these vessels weakens the aortic wall, predisposing the area to aneurysm formation. When atherosclerotic plaques develop in diseased areas, the intima takes on a "tree bark" appearance. The proximal portion of the aorta is the most extensively involved, leading to aortic dilation with mural calcification, aortic insufficiency, coronary artery stenosis, or frank aneurysm formation. Aneurysms usually are saccular and typically spare the aortic sinuses (Fig. 4-32). This feature differentiates them from aneurysms in Marfan syndrome.

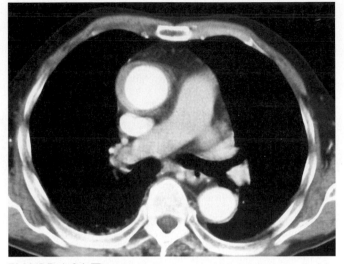

FIGURE 4-34 ■ Intramural hematoma of the right lateral wall of the ascending aorta on CT angiogram.

Penetrating Aortic Ulcer

Rarely, an ulcerated atherosclerotic aortic plaque penetrates into the media and forms a longitudinal hematoma in the vessel wall.[104,105] With time, a pseudoaneurysm may develop, or frank rupture may occur. Penetrating ulcers often are found in the lower descending thoracic or upper abdominal aorta but may occur anywhere. As with aortic dissection, the patient is typically elderly and hypertensive. Most patients are asymptomatic, but some complain of sudden onset of back pain.

The diagnosis is made by CT, MR, or TEE.[106,107] The descending thoracic aorta often is diffusely dilated. Displaced intimal calcification and a focal ulcerated plaque with underlying mural hematoma are seen (Fig. 4-33).[108] Pleural or mediastinal fluid may be present. Many asymptomatic lesions fail to enlarge, but some will display slowly progressive aortic dilation, pseudoaneurysm formation, distal embolization, and uncommonly fatal rupture.

Most patients are treated with antihypertensive medications. Surgery or stent-graft placement is performed in selected cases, including ascending aortic involvement, large ulcer diameter or depth, persistent pain, expansion, or rupture. Percutaneous coil embolization of the ulcer has been described also.[109]

Intramural Hematoma

In this disorder, a localized hematoma develops spontaneously in the wall of the aorta from rupture of the vasa vasorum without an intimal tear or overlying atherosclerotic plaque.[110-112] Intramural hematoma represents a type of noncommunicating aortic dissection. It can progress to frank dissection or rupture. Intramural hematoma is being diagnosed more frequently with the widespread use of cross-sectional imaging in patients with aortic disease. The clinical picture is similar to that of aortic dissection, with sudden onset of chest or back pain in a middle-aged to elderly, hypertensive patient. Classically, intramural hematoma occurs in the descending thoracic aorta (type B), but some reports show a significant frequency in the ascending aorta (type A).[111]

Intramural hematoma usually is detected by CT or MR imaging, which shows a crescentic mural hematoma of medium to high density or signal intensity (depending on clot age) extending over a length of the thoracic aorta (Fig. 4-34).[113] There is no intimal flap nor flow within the collection. Intramural hematoma must be differentiated from other diseases that cause mural thickening, such as aortitis, atherosclerotic plaque, and mural thrombus.

Intramural hematoma usually is treated by blood pressure management alone regardless of location. Surgery or stent-graft insertion usually is reserved for patients with expansion of the hematoma or progression to frank dissection, which occurs in about one third of cases.[112]

REFERENCES

1. LaBerge JM, Jeffrey RB: Aortic lacerations: fatal complications of thoracic aortography. Radiology 1987;165:367.
2. Collins P, ed: Embryology and development. In: Williams PL, Bannister LH, Berry MM, et al, eds. Gray's Anatomy, 38th ed. New York, Churchill Livingstone, 1995:312.
3. Gabella G, ed: Cardiovascular system. In: Williams PL, Bannister LH, Berry MM, et al, eds. Gray's Anatomy, 38th ed. New York, Churchill Livingstone, 1995:1505.
4. Aronberg DJ, Glazer HS, Madsen K, et al: Normal thoracic aortic diameters by computed tomography. J Comput Assist Tomogr 1984;8:247.
5. Hougen TJ: Congenital anomalies of the aortic arch. In: Lindsay J Jr, ed. Diseases of the Aorta. Philadelphia, Lea & Febiger, 1994:19.
6. Vogt FM, Goyen M, Debatin JF: MR angiography of the chest. Radiol Clin North Am 2003;41:29.
7. Kadir S: Regional anatomy of the thoracic aorta. In: Kadir S, ed. Atlas of Normal and Variant Angiographic Anatomy. Philadelphia, WB Saunders, 1991:19.
8. Freed K, Low VH: The aberrant subclavian artery. AJR Am J Roentgenol 1997;168:481.
9. Ho VB, Prince MR: Thoracic MR aortography: imaging techniques and strategies. Radiographics 1998;18:287.

10. Backer CL, Paape K, Zales VR, et al: Coarctation of the aorta. Repair with polytetrafluoroethylene patch aortoplasty. Circulation 1995;92(Suppl II):II132.

11. Mack G, Burch GH, Sahn DJ: Coarctation of the aorta. Curr Treat Options Cardiovasc Med 1999;1:347.

12. Tyagi S, Singh S, Mukhopadhyay S, et al: Self- and balloon-expandable stent implantation for severe native coarctation of aorta in adults. Am Heart J 2003;146:920.

13. Kronzon I, Tunick PA: Atheromatous disease of the thoracic aorta: pathologic and clinical implications. Ann Intern Med 1997;126:629.

14. Tunick PA, Rosenzweig BP, Katz ES, et al: High risk for vascular events in patients with protruding aortic atheromas: a prospective study. J Am Coll Cardiol 1994;23:1085.

15. Bashore TM, Gehrig T: Cholesterol emboli after invasive cardiac procedures. J Am Coll Cardiol 2003;42:217.

16. Kronzon I, Tunick PA: Transesophageal echocardiography as a tool in the evaluation of patients with embolic disorders. Prog Cardiovasc Dis 1993;36:39.

17. Tunick PA, Krinsky GA, Lee VS, et al: Diagnostic imaging of thoracic aortic atherosclerosis. AJR Am J Roentgenol 2000;174:1119.

18. Miller FJ: Aortic aneurysms. It's all about the stress. Arterioscler Thromb Vasc Biol 2002;22:1948.

19. Annabi B, Shedid D, Ghosn P, et al: Differential regulation of matrix metalloproteinase activities in abdominal aortic aneurysms. J Vasc Surg 2002;35:539.

20. Svensjö S, Bengtsson H, Bergqvist D: Thoracic and thoracoabdominal aortic aneurysm and dissection: an investigation based on autopsy. Br J Surg 1996;83:68.

21. Kouchoukos NT, Dougenis D: Surgery of the thoracic aorta. N Engl J Med 1997;336:1876.

22. Hirose Y, Hamada S, Takamiya M, et al: Aortic aneurysms: growth rates measured with CT. Radiology 1992;185:249.

23. Dapunt OE, Galla JD, Sadeghi AM, et al: The natural history of thoracic aortic aneurysms. J Thorac Cardiovasc Surg 1994;107:1323.

24. Cambria RA, Gloviczki P, Stanson AW, et al: Outcome and expansion rate of 57 thoracoabdominal aortic aneurysms managed nonoperatively. Am J Surg 1995;170:213.

25. Blanchard DG, Kimura BJ, Dittrich HC, et al: Transesophageal echocardiography of the aorta. JAMA 1994;272:546.

26. Quint LE, Francis IR, Williams DM, et al: Evaluation of thoracic aortic disease with the use of helical CT and multiplanar reconstructions: comparison with surgical findings. Radiology 1996;201:37.

27. Castaner E, Andreu M, Gallardo X, et al: CT in nontraumatic acute thoracic aortic disease: typical and atypical features and complications. Radiographics 2003;23:S93.

28. Tatli S, Lipton MJ, Davison BD, et al: MR imaging of aortic and peripheral vascular disease. Radiographics 2003;23:S59.

29. Prince MR, Narasimham DL, Jacoby WT, et al: Three-dimensional gadolinium-enhanced MR angiography of the thoracic aorta. AJR Am J Roentgenol 1996;166:1387.

30. Kawamoto S, Bluemke DA, Traill TA, et al: Thoracoabdominal aorta in Marfan syndrome: MR imaging findings of progression of vasculopathy after surgical repair. Radiology 1997;203:727.

31. Lawrie GM, Earle N, DeBakey ME: Evolution of surgical techniques for aneurysms of the descending thoracic aorta: twenty-nine years experience with 659 patients. J Cardiac Surg 1994;9:648.

32. Savader SJ, Williams GM, Trerotola SO, et al: Preoperative spinal artery localization and its relationship to postoperative neurologic complications. Radiology 1993;189:165.

33. Coady MA, Rizzo JA, Hammond GL, et al: What is the appropriate size criterion for resection of thoracic aortic aneurysms? J Thorac Cardiovasc Surg 1997;113:476.

34. Dake MD: Endovascular stent-graft management of thoracic aortic diseases. Eur J Radiol 2001;39:42.

35. Cambria RP, Brewster DC, Lauterbach SR, et al: Evolving experience with thoracic aortic stent graft repair. J Vasc Surg 2002;35:1129.

36. Taylor PR, Gaines PA, McGuinness CL, et al: Thoracic aortic stent-grafts—early experience from two centers using commercially available devices. Eur J Endovasc Surg 2001;22:70.

37. Czermak BV, Waldenberger P, Perkmann R, et al: Placement of endovascular stent-grafts for emergency treatment of acute disease of the descending thoracic aorta. AJR Am J Roentgenol 2002;179:337.

38. Larson EW, Edwards WD: Risk factors for aortic dissection: a necropsy study of 161 cases. Am J Cardiol 1984;53:849.

39. Gotway MB, Marder SR, Hanks DK, et al: Thoracic complications of illicit drug use: an organ system approach. Radiographics 2002;22:S119.

40. Sakamoto I, Hayashi K, Matsunaga N, et al: Aortic dissection caused by angiographic procedures. Radiology 1994;191:467.

41. O'Gara PT, DeSanctis RW: Acute aortic dissection and its variants: towards a common diagnostic and therapeutic approach. Circulation 1995;92:1376.

42. Spittell PC, Spittell JA Jr, Joyce JW, et al: Clinical features and differential diagnosis of aortic dissection: experience with 236 cases (1980 through 1990). Mayo Clin Proc 1993;68:642.

43. Cigarroa JE, Isselbacher EM, DeSanctis RW, et al: Diagnostic imaging in the evaluation of suspected aortic dissection. N Engl J Med 1993;328:35.

44. Jagannath AS, Sos TA, Lockhart SH, et al: Aortic dissection: a statistical analysis of the usefulness of plain chest radiographic findings. AJR Am J Roentgenol 1986;147:1123.

45. Fisher ER, Stern EJ, Godwin JD II, et al: Acute aortic dissection: typical and atypical imaging features. Radiographics 1994;14:1263.

46. LePage MA, Quint LE, Sonnad SS, et al: Aortic dissection: CT features that distinguish true lumen from false lumen. AJR Am J Roentgenol 2001;177:207.

47. Laissy J-P, Blanc F, Soyer P, et al: Thoracic aortic dissection: diagnosis with transesophageal echocardiography versus MR imaging. Radiology 1995;194:331.

48. Nienaber CA, von Kodolitsch Y, Nicolas V, et al: The diagnosis of thoracic aortic dissection by noninvasive imaging procedures. N Engl J Med 1993;328:1.

49. Sommer T, Fehske W, Holzknecht N, et al: Aortic dissection: a comparative study of diagnosis with spiral CT, multiplanar transesophageal echocardiography, and MR imaging. Radiology 1996;199:347.

50. Glower DD, Speier RH, White WD, et al: Management and long-term outcome of aortic dissection. Ann Surg 1991;214:31.

51. Slonim SM, Nyman U, Semba CP, et al: Aortic dissection: percutaneous management of ischemic complications with endovascular stents and balloon fenestration. J Vasc Surg 1996;23:241.

52. Vedantham S, Picus D, Sanchez LA, et al: Percutaneous management of ischemic complications in patients with type B aortic dissection. J Vasc Interv Radiol 2003;14:181.

53. Hoffer EK, Karmy-Jones R, Bloch RD, et al: Treatment of acute thoracic aortic injury with commercially available abdominal aortic stent-grafts. J Vasc Interv Radiol 2002;13:1037.

54. Sailer J, Peloschek P, Rand T, et al: Endovascular treatment of aortic type B dissection and penetrating ulcer using commercially available stent-grafts. AJR Am J Roentgenol 2001;177:1365.

55. Bortone AS, Schena S, D'Agostino D, et al: Immediate versus delayed endovascular treatment of post-traumatic aortic pseudoaneurysms and type B dissections: retrospective analysis and premises to the upcoming European trial. Circulation 2002;106(Suppl I):234.

56. Deutsch HJ, Sechtem U, Meyer H, et al: Chronic aortic dissection: comparison of MR imaging and transesophageal echocardiography. Radiology 1994;192:645.

57. Masani ND, Banning AP, Jones RA, et al: Follow-up of chronic thoracic aortic dissection: comparison of transesophageal echocardiography and magnetic resonance imaging. Am Heart J 1996;131:1156.

58. DeBakey ME, McCollum CH, Crawford ES, et al: Dissection and dissecting aneurysms of the aorta: twenty-year follow-up of five hundred twenty-seven patients treated surgically. Surgery 1982;92:1118.

59. Creasy JD, Chiles C, Routh WD, et al: Overview of traumatic injury of the thoracic aorta. Radiographics 1997;17:27.

60. Parmley LF, Mattingly TW, Manion WC, et al: Non-penetrating traumatic injury of the aorta. Circulation 1958;17:1086.

61. Crass JR, Cohen AM, Motta AO, et al: A proposed new mechanism of traumatic aortic rupture: the osseous pinch. Radiology 1990;176:645.

62. Patel NH, Stephens KE, Mirvis SE, et al: Imaging of acute thoracic aortic injury due to blunt trauma: a review. Radiology 1998;209:335.

63. Fisher RG, Hadlock F, Ben-Menachem Y: Laceration of the thoracic aorta and brachiocephalic arteries by blunt trauma: report of 54 cases and review of the literature. Radiol Clin North Am 1981;19:91.

64. Gundry SR, Williams S, Burney RE, et al: Indications for aortography. Radiography after blunt chest trauma: a reassessment of the radiographic findings associated with traumatic rupture of the aorta. Invest Radiol 1983;18:230.

65. Mirvis SE, Bidwell JK, Buddemeyer EU, et al: Value of chest radiography in excluding traumatic aortic rupture. Radiology 1987;163:487.

66. White CS, Mirvis SE: Pictorial review: Imaging of traumatic aortic injury. Clin Radiol 1995;50:281.

67. Hunink MG, Bos JJ: Triage of patients to angiography for detection of aortic rupture after blunt chest trauma: cost-effectiveness analysis of using CT. AJR Am J Roentgenol 1995;165:27.

68. Gavant ML, Flick P, Menke P, et al: CT aortography of thoracic aortic rupture. AJR Am J Roentgenol 1996;166:955.

69. Mirvis SE, Shanmuganathan K, Miller BH, et al: Traumatic aortic injury: diagnosis with contrast-enhanced thoracic CT—five-year experience at a major trauma center. Radiology 1996;200:413.

70. Dyer DS, Moore EE, Mestek MF, et al: Can chest CT be used to exclude aortic injury? Radiology 1999;213:195.

71. Parker MS, Matheson TL, Rao AV, et al: Making the transition: the role of helical CT in the evaluation of potentially acute thoracic aortic injuries. AJR Am J Roentgenol 2001;176:1267.

72. Fisher RG, Sanchez-Torres M, Thomas JW, et al: Subtle or atypical injuries of the thoracic aorta and brachiocephalic vessels in blunt thoracic trauma. Radiographics 1997;17:835.

73. Morse SS, Glickman MG, Greenwood LH, et al: Traumatic aortic rupture: false-positive aortographic diagnosis due to atypical ductus diverticulum. AJR Am J Roentgenol 1988;150:793.

74. Fisher RG, Sanchez-Torres M, Whigham CJ, et al: "Lumps" and "bumps" that mimic acute aortic and brachiocephalic vessel injury. Radiographics 1997;17:825.

75. Smith MD, Cassidy JM, Souther S, et al: Transesophageal echocardiography in the diagnosis of traumatic rupture of the aorta. N Engl J Med 1995;332:356.

76. Uflacker R, Horn J, Phillips G, et al: Intravascular sonography in the assessment of traumatic injury of the thoracic aorta. AJR Am J Roentgenol 1999;173:665.

77. Lee DE, Arslan B, Quieroz R, et al: Assessment of inter- and intraobserver agreement between intravascular US and aortic angiography of thoracic aortic injury. Radiology 2003;227:434.

78. Fabian TC, Richardson JD, Croce MA, et al: Prospective study of blunt aortic injury: Multicenter Trial of the American Association for the Surgery of Trauma. J Trauma 1997;42:374.

79. Fattori R, Napoli G, Lovato L, et al: Indications for, timing of, and results of catheter-based treatment of traumatic injury to the aorta. AJR Am J Roentgenol 2002;179:603.

80. Yacoe ME, Dake MD: Development and resolution of systemic and coronary artery aneurysms in Kawasaki disease. AJR Am J Roentgenol 1992;159:708.

81. Tunaci A, Berkmen YM, Gokmen E: Thoracic involvement in Behçet's disease: pathologic, clinical, and imaging features. AJR Am J Roentgenol 1995;164:51.

82. Hunder G: Vasculitis: diagnosis and therapy. Am J Med 1996;100(Suppl 2A):37S.

83. Choe YH, Han B-K, Koh E-M, et al: Takayasu's arteritis: assessment of disease activity with contrast-enhanced MR imaging. AJR Am J Roentgenol 2000;175:505.

84. Yamada I, Nakagawa T, Himeno Y, et al: Takayasu arteritis: evaluation of the thoracic aorta with CT angiography. Radiology 1998;209:103.

85. Matsunaga N, Hayashi K, Sakamoto I, et al: Takayasu arteritis: protean radiologic manifestations and diagnosis. Radiographics 1997;17:579.

86. Park JH, Chung JW, Im JG, et al: Takayasu arteritis: evaluation of mural changes in the aorta and pulmonary artery with CT angiography. Radiology 1995;196:89.

87. Yamada I, Numano F, Suzuki S: Takayasu arteritis: evaluation with MR imaging. Radiology 1993;188:89.

88. Giordano JM, Leavitt RY, Hoffman G, et al: Experience with surgical treatment of Takayasu's disease. Surgery 1991;109:252.

89. Tyagi S, Kaul UA, Nair M, et al: Balloon angioplasty of the aorta in Takayasu's arteritis: initial and long-term results. Am Heart J 1992;124:876.

90. Rao SA, Mandalam KR, Rao VR, et al: Takayasu arteritis: initial and long term follow-up in 16 patients after percutaneous transluminal angioplasty of the descending thoracic and abdominal aorta. Radiology 1993;189:173.

91. Bali HK, Bhargava M, Jain AK, et al: De novo stenting of descending thoracic aorta in Takayasu arteritis: intermediate-term follow-up results. J Invasive Cardiol 2000;12:612.

92. Nordborg E, Nordborg C: Giant cell arteritis: epidemiological clues to its pathogenesis and an update on its treatment. Rheumatology 2003;42:413.

93. Townend JN, Emery P, Davies MK, et al: Acute aortitis and aortic incompetence due to systemic rheumatologic disorders. Int J Cardiol 1991;33:253.

94. Chetty R, Batitang S, Nair R: Large artery vasculopathy in HIV positive patients: another vasculitic enigma. Hum Pathol 2000;31:374.

95. Woolgar JD, Ray R, Maharaj K, et al: Colour Doppler and grey scale ultrasound features of HIV-related vascular aneurysms. Br J Radiol 2002;75:884.

96. Moriyama Y, Nishida T, Toyohira H, et al: Acute aortic dissection in a patient with osteogenesis imperfecta. Ann Thorac Surg 1995;60:1397.

97. Tunaci A, Berkmen YM, Gokmen E: Thoracic involvement in Behçet's disease: pathologic, clinical, and imaging features. AJR Am J Roentgenol 1995;164:51.

98. Gott VL, Laschinger JC, Cameron DE, et al: The Marfan syndrome and the cardiovascular surgeon. Eur J Cardiothorac Surg 1996;10:149.

99. Hollister DW, Godfrey M, Sakai LY, et al: Immunohistologic abnormalities of the microfibrillar-fiber system in the Marfan syndrome. N Engl J Med 1990;323:152.

100. Freeman RK, Swegle J, Sise MJ: The surgical complications of Ehlers-Danlos syndrome. Am Surgeon 1996;62:869.

101. Malouf JF, Chandrasekaran K, Orszulak TA: Mycotic aneurysms of the thoracic aorta: a diagnostic challenge. Am J Med 2003;115:489.

102. Oz MC, McNicholas KW, Serra AJ, et al: Review of *Salmonella* mycotic aneurysms of the thoracic aorta. J Cardiovasc Surg 1989;30:99.

103. Jackman JD Jr, Radolf JD: Cardiovascular syphilis. Am J Med 1989;87:425.

104. Harris JA, Bis KG, Glover JL, et al: Penetrating atherosclerotic ulcers of the aorta. J Vasc Surg 1994;19:90.

105. Welch TJ, Stanson AW, Sheedy PF II, et al: Radiologic evaluation of penetrating aortic atherosclerotic ulcer. Radiographics 1990;10:675.

106. Kazerooni EA, Bree RL, Williams DM: Penetrating atherosclerotic ulcers of the descending thoracic aorta: evaluation with CT and distinction from aortic dissection. Radiology 1992;183:759.

107. Quint LE, Williams DM, Francis IR, et al: Ulcerlike lesions of the aorta: imaging features and natural history. Radiology 2001;218:719.

108. Levy JR, Heiken JP, Gutierrez FR: Imaging of penetrating atherosclerotic ulcers of the aorta. AJR Am J Roentgenol 1999;173:151.

109. Williams DM, Kirsh MM, Abrams GD: Penetrating atherosclerotic aortic ulcer with dissecting hematoma: control of bleeding with percutaneous embolization. Radiology 1991;181:85.

110. Robbins RC, McManus RP, Mitchell RS, et al: Management of patients with intramural hematoma of the thoracic aorta. Circulation 1993;88(5 part 2):II1.

111. Ganaha F, Miller DC, Sugimoto K, et al: Prognosis of aortic intramural hematoma with and without penetrating aortic ulcer: a clinical and radiological analysis. Circulation 2002;106:342.

112. Kaji S, Akasaka T, Horibata Y, et al: Long-term prognosis of patients with Type A aortic intramural hematoma. Circulation 2002;106(Suppl I):248.

113. Murray JG, Manisali M, Flamm SD, et al: Intramural hematoma of the thoracic aorta: MR image findings and their prognostic implications. Radiology 1997;204:349.

5

Abdominal Aorta

■ AORTOGRAPHY

Abdominal aortography is performed using a 4- or 5-French catheter with a pigtail or similar configuration. To properly evaluate the renal artery origins, the side holes of the catheter are positioned at the L1-L2 level. When visualization of the celiac and superior mesenteric arteries is necessary, higher catheter placement (above the T12 level) is required. Lateral projections are sometimes used to supplement frontal images in order to study the orifices of the mesenteric arteries and disease that may predominate on the anterior or posterior aortic walls. Particular care should be taken when catheterizing the abdominal aorta in patients known to have aneurysms or severe atherosclerotic disease to avoid dislodging mural thrombus or plaque.

■ ANATOMY

Development

In the embryo, the abdominal aorta is formed from the right and left dorsal aortae.[1] Numerous ventral splanchnic branches of the aorta supply the primitive digestive tract. These channels are eventually reduced to the celiac artery, superior mesenteric artery (SMA), and inferior mesenteric artery (IMA). Lateral splanchnic branches supply organs arising from the mesonephric ridge, giving rise to the inferior phrenic, adrenal, renal, and gonadal arteries. Four sets of somatic arterial branches develop into the intersegmental lumbar arteries.

Normal Anatomy

The *abdominal aorta* begins at the diaphragmatic hiatus.[2] The vessel runs in front of the spine and to the left of the *inferior vena cava* (IVC) until it bifurcates into the *common iliac arteries* at about the L4 vertebra. The normal caliber of

the abdominal aorta increases with age; at the renal hila, its mean diameter varies from about 1.5 cm in women in the fourth decade of life to about 2.0 cm in men in the eighth decade.[3,4]

The abdominal aorta has three ventral branches (Figs. 5-1 and 5-2). The *celiac artery* arises at the T12-L1 level. It can

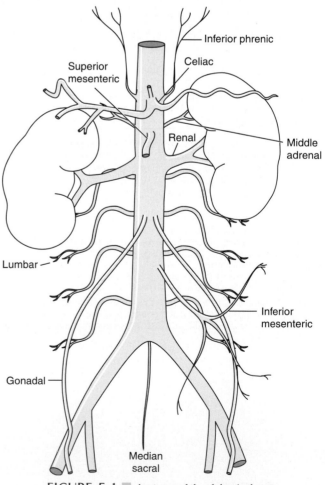

FIGURE 5-1 ■ Anatomy of the abdominal aorta.

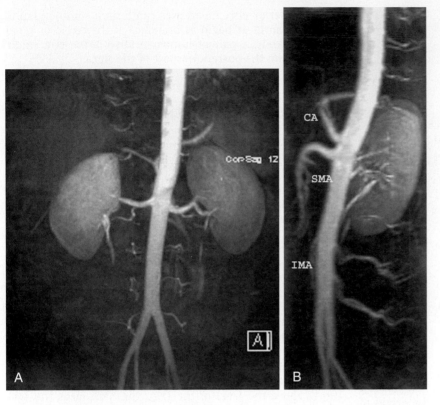

FIGURE 5-2 ■ Normal MR angiogram of the abdominal aorta in frontal (**A**) and lateral (**B**) projections. Ventral branches: CA, celiac artery; IMA, inferior mesenteric artery; SMA, superior mesenteric artery.

initially take a forward, upward, or downward course. The *SMA* takes off at the L1-L2 level about 1 cm below the celiac axis. The *IMA* originates at the L3-L4 level, typically on the left anterolateral surface of the aorta.

The paired *inferior phrenic arteries* usually arise immediately above the celiac artery. They course superolaterally toward the central tendon of the hemidiaphragms, where they bifurcate. Paired *middle adrenal arteries* take off from the aorta adjacent to the SMA to provide partial blood supply to the adrenal glands. The *renal arteries* originate just below or at the level of the SMA. The *gonadal (testicular* or *ovarian) arteries* are paired vessels that arise from the anterolateral surface of the aorta just below the main renal arteries.

Four pairs of *lumbar arteries* exit the posterolateral aspect of the aorta. There are extensive anastomoses between these vessels, the lower intercostal arteries (superiorly), and the iliolumbar, deep iliac circumflex, and gluteal vessels (inferiorly). The *median sacral artery* takes off posteriorly just above the aortic bifurcation and descends toward the coccyx.

The smaller somatic and splanchnic vessels (i.e., inferior phrenic, middle adrenal, gonadal, and median sacral arteries) are not always seen on routine abdominal aortograms. In a patient with an enlarged aorta or sluggish flow, the IMA may not opacify with a mid-abdominal aortic injection because of layering of contrast in the posterior (dependent) portion of the distal aortic lumen.

Variant Anatomy

Congenital anomalies of the abdominal aorta are rare. However, anomalies of the primary branches are common.

Multiple renal arteries are present in about 25% to 35% of the population.[5-8] Although most accessory arteries are found just below the main renal artery, they may arise proximal to the main trunk or as far distally as the iliac artery (Fig. 5-3).

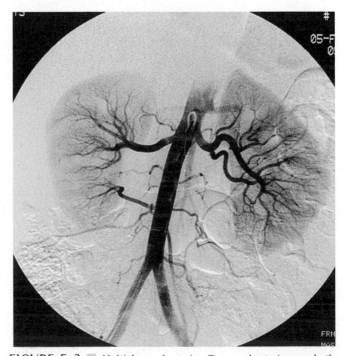

FIGURE 5-3 ■ Multiple renal arteries. Two renal arteries supply the right kidney.

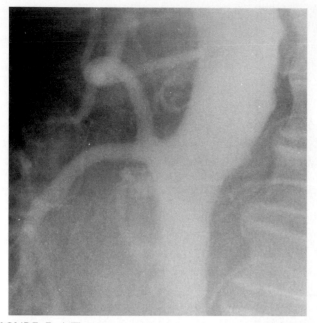

FIGURE 5-4 ■ Celiomesenteric artery variant on a lateral abdominal aortogram.

Persistence of the embryonic ventral connection between the celiac artery and SMA with regression of the origin of one of these vessels leads to the rare *celiomesenteric artery* (Fig. 5-4; see also Fig. 9-3).[9] The hepatic, left gastric, or splenic arteries may have a separate origin from the aorta (Fig. 5-5).

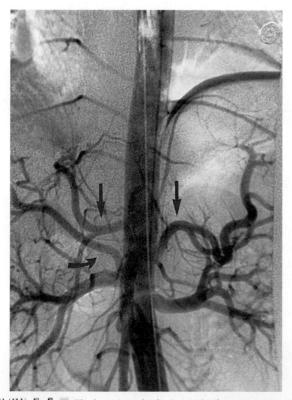

FIGURE 5-5 ■ The hepatic and splenic arteries have separate origins from the abdominal aorta *(straight arrows)*. Notice the right hepatic artery replaced to the superior mesenteric artery *(curved arrow)*.

The inferior phrenic arteries can form a common trunk from the aorta or begin as branches of the celiac or renal artery.[2] Rarely, a pair of lumbar arteries arise as a single branch from the posterior aspect of the aorta.

Collateral Circulation

With severe narrowing or complete occlusion of the abdominal aorta, several parietal and visceral collateral pathways divert blood flow around the obstructed segment. The chief **parietal** collateral routes are from the intercostal, subcostal, and lumbar arteries to the iliolumbar, lateral sacral, and superior gluteal branches of the internal iliac artery and to the deep and superficial iliac circumflex branches of the external iliac artery (Fig. 5-6). With the former system, blood flows in a retrograde direction through the internal iliac artery to feed the external iliac artery. Interconnections between the lumbar arteries help to support this collateral network. A pathway also exists from the superior epigastric artery (terminal branch of the internal thoracic artery) to the inferior epigastric artery that joins the common femoral artery.

The SMA and IMA are important **visceral** conduits when the abdominal aorta is obstructed. With occlusion of the aorta **above** the level of the IMA, the SMA feeds the IMA through the middle colic and marginal arteries, which then connect with branches of the internal iliac artery through the rectal network (Fig. 5-7). With occlusion of the abdominal aorta **below** the IMA origin, the rectal collateral network (between the superior rectal branch of the IMA and the middle and inferior rectal branches of the internal iliac artery) may be an important collateral route. In cases of short-segment aortic stenosis involving the SMA, the so-called *meandering mesenteric artery* can fill the SMA from the IMA circulation (see Fig. 9-15).[10]

■ MAJOR DISORDERS

Atherosclerosis

Atherosclerosis is the most common disease affecting the abdominal aorta (Figs. 5-8 and 5-9). This condition is considered as part of lower extremity peripheral vascular disease in Chapter 6.

Abdominal Aortic Aneurysms

Etiology

An abdominal aortic aneurysm (AAA) is defined as a localized dilation of the vessel by 50% or more of its normal diameter (when the wall-to-wall diameter is ≥3 cm in adults).[11] Most AAAs are infrarenal; about 7% to 12% are suprarenal or *juxtarenal* (extending ≤1 cm from the renal arteries).[12,13] About 20% of AAAs extend into one or both common iliac arteries. The incidence of AAA has risen

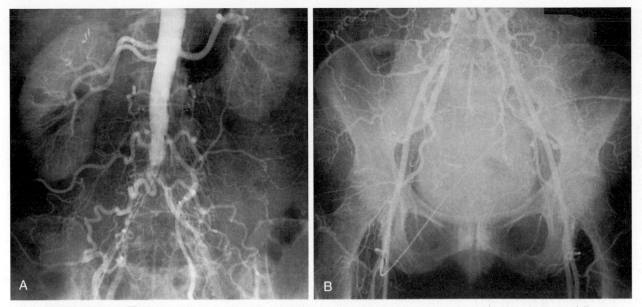

FIGURE 5-6 ▪ Distal aortic occlusion below the inferior mesenteric artery origin. The occlusion was successfully traversed from the right common femoral artery. Collateral flow courses primarily from the enlarged lumbar and inferior mesenteric arteries (**A**), through the internal iliac artery branches, and then into the external iliac arteries (**B**).

significantly during the last 50 years, and this phenomenon cannot be attributed entirely to earlier detection or aging of the population.[14,15]

The cause of the common *degenerative* form of AAA is under intense study.[16] Although atherosclerosis is present in more than 90% of patients with AAA, it is no longer thought to be the principal cause of the disease. It is notable that many patients with AAA do not have significant obstructive atherosclerotic disease of the iliac or femoral arteries.

Abnormalities of wall structure are probably a major factor in aneurysm formation. Degenerative AAAs form because of inflammatory damage to the vessel and hemodynamic forces that produce remodeling.[16,17] Increased levels of matrix metalloproteinases elaborated from smooth muscle cells result in macrophage infiltration and subsequent thinning of elastin in the media.[18,19]

The predilection for the **infrarenal** abdominal aorta is probably a consequence of hemodynamic factors. Increased wall stress exists in this portion of the abdominal aorta

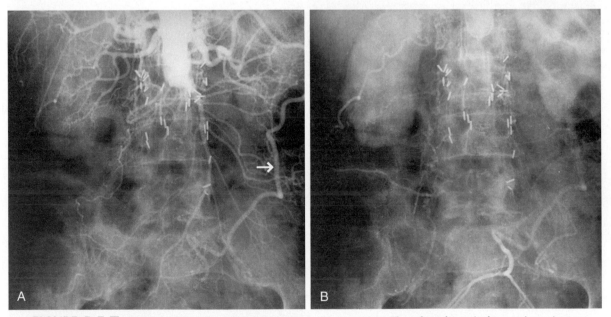

FIGURE 5-7 ▪ Aortic occlusion above the inferior mesenteric artery origin. The enlarged marginal artery *(arrow)* seen in the early-phase arteriogram (**A**) feeds the superior rectal artery seen in the late-phase arteriogram (**B**). This route is a major collateral pathway into the pelvis and lower extremities.

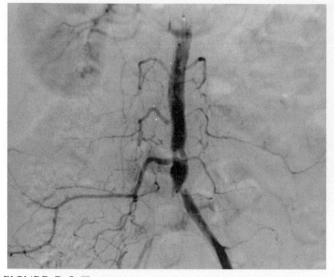

FIGURE 5-8 ■ Atherosclerosis of the distal abdominal aorta and occlusion of the right common iliac artery. The focal aortic plaque has a weblike appearance.

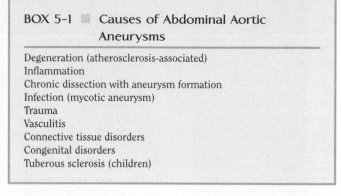

BOX 5-1 ■ **Causes of Abdominal Aortic Aneurysms**

Degeneration (atherosclerosis-associated)
Inflammation
Chronic dissection with aneurysm formation
Infection (mycotic aneurysm)
Trauma
Vasculitis
Connective tissue disorders
Congenital disorders
Tuberous sclerosis (children)

Natural History

The most common and feared complication of AAA is **rupture**. The likelihood of this event is governed by *Laplace's law* (wall stress = pressure × radius). Rupture is thus mainly a function of aneurysm size. Although the typical growth rate of AAA is estimated at about 3 to 4 mm/yr, the rate of expansion is unpredictable in a particular patient, and the growth rate is not completely linear.[22,23] Expansion accelerates as the aneurysm grows, though periods of stability are observed.

Nonetheless, numerous studies have shown that the risk of AAA rupture increases substantially when the diameter is greater than **5 cm**; for example, the 5-year risk of rupture of untreated AAAs of 5 cm or larger is at least 25%.[23,24]

because of decreased wall compliance, tapering of the vessel, and reflected pressure waves during diastole from the high resistance in the peripheral vessels.[20] Although most AAAs are degenerative, a small percentage of patients develop aortic dilation for other reasons (Box 5-1).[21]

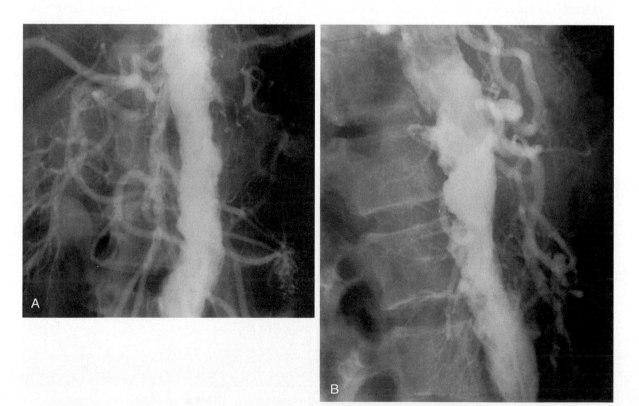

FIGURE 5-9 ■ Atherosclerosis of the abdominal aorta. The anteroposterior projection (**A**) underestimates the extent of disease, which is most severe on the posterior wall (**B**).

Elective repair of smaller asymptomatic aneurysms does not appear to be beneficial relative to the attendant risks.

More than 60% of patients with rupture do not survive to reach medical care, and the mortality rate with emergent surgery can exceed 75%.[25,26] When rupture occurs, the tear usually starts in the posterior or lateral wall of the aorta, with bleeding into the retroperitoneal space. Less often, the rupture penetrates the anterior wall, sometimes leading to hemorrhage into the peritoneal cavity.

Other sequelae of AAA include distal embolization, thrombosis, and aortocaval fistula. The latter complication occurs in fewer than 1% of patients with AAA.[27]

Clinical Features

AAAs occur at least four times more frequently in men than in women.[26,28] Other risk factors include advancing age, white race, hypertension, cigarette smoking, and a family history of AAA.

Most patients are asymptomatic at the time the aneurysm is detected by physical examination or more often by imaging studies obtained for screening or unrelated problems. A rapidly expanding aneurysm may produce abdominal or back pain. Less than one fourth of cases present with AAA rupture, which may be suggested by the presence of abdominal or back pain, a pulsatile abdominal mass, and hypotension. Occasionally, patients have symptoms caused by extrinsic compression of adjacent organs, aneurysm thrombosis, distal embolization, or dissection. A patient with an aortocaval fistula may exhibit pain, a pulsatile abdominal mass, continuous abdominal bruit or thrill, congestive heart failure, lower extremity edema, or hematuria.

Pretreatment Imaging

The purpose of imaging studies is detection and staging of the AAA, surveillance of small aneurysms, preprocedure assessment, postprocedure evaluation, and diagnosis of rupture.

Sonography. Sonography is the chief tool for detecting, sizing, and monitoring AAAs (Fig. 5-10). The technique is almost 100% sensitive for aneurysm diagnosis. Sonography also is highly accurate in determining aneurysm size, the presence of mural thrombus, and associated abdominal pathology. Sonography is less accurate in determining the cranial and caudal extent of the aneurysm, the relationship to and number of renal arteries, and the presence of iliofemoral arterial disease.

Computed Tomography. CT is the key modality for pre- and postprocedure assessment of patients with AAA.[29-35] CT also is useful in following aneurysm growth in patients who cannot be imaged adequately with sonography. Strict pre- and postcontrast protocols must be carefully followed. Multiplanar reconstructions and shaded-surface display renderings also are very useful in planning repair.

The typical AAA is a fusiform dilation of the infrarenal abdominal aorta (Fig. 5-11). Intimal calcification and mural thrombus are common. If the aneurysm is saccular or eccentric without calcification or adjacent aortic disease, or is present in a young patient, uncommon causes should be considered (see Box 5-1).

Magnetic Resonance Imaging. MR imaging also is used in pre- and postprocedure assessment of patients with AAA.[36-41] Evaluation of stent-grafts with low magnetic susceptibility is feasible with MR angiography.[42] Complete evaluation generally includes an initial T1-weighted spin-echo sequence; dynamic gadolinium-enhanced, three-dimensional gradient-echo sequence; and sagittal and axial two-dimensional time-of-flight sequences (Fig 5-12).

Angiography. Catheter angiography is only used prior to endovascular stent-graft placement (see below). A complete evaluation includes frontal and lateral (or steep oblique) images along with rotational or multiplanar pelvic angiography (Fig. 5-13).

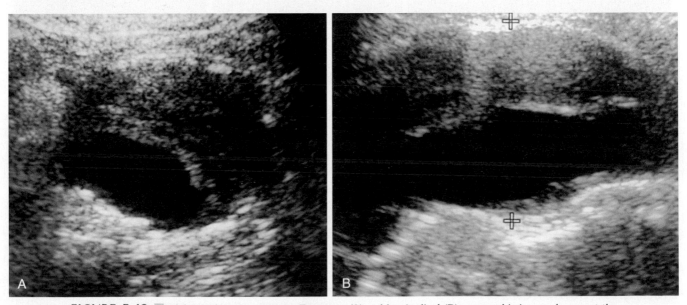

FIGURE 5-10 ■ Abdominal aortic aneurysm. Transverse (**A**) and longitudinal (**B**) sonographic images document the size of the aneurysm and show extensive eccentric luminal thrombus.

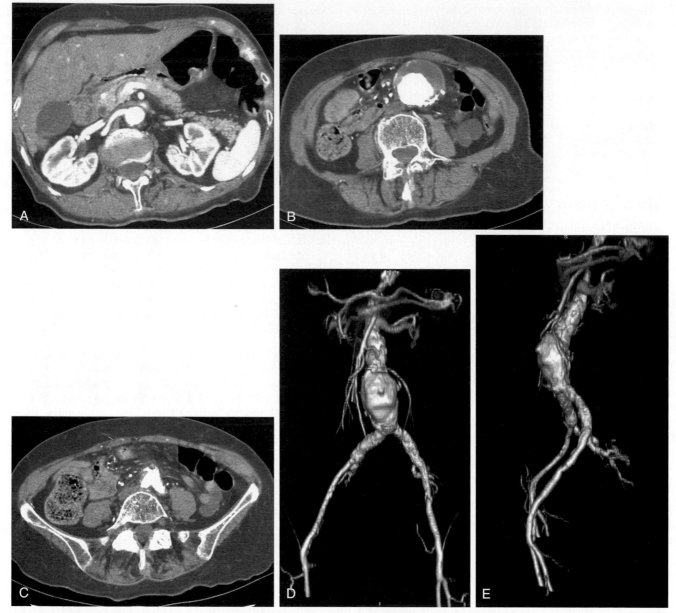

FIGURE 5-11 ■ Infrarenal abdominal aortic aneurysm on CT angiography. Axial images show aneurysm beginning below the renal arteries (**A**), with large volume of mural thrombus and intimal calcification (**B**) and no involvement of the common iliac artery origins (**C**). Shaded surface display reconstructions in frontal (**D**) and lateral (**E**) projections nicely demonstrate the aneurysm, relationship to branch vessels, and status of the iliac arteries.

The presence of mural thrombus may produce a sharp, straight border to the aortic lumen and occlusion of the inferior mesenteric or lumbar arteries. A large volume of mural thrombus within an aneurysm can cause apparent narrowing of the aortic lumen (Fig. 5-14).

Flow from the middle colic branch of the SMA to the marginal artery of Drummond or arc of Riolan and then into the IMA distribution is indirect but good evidence for occlusion or severe stenosis of the IMA (see Fig. 5-14).

Imaging of Abdominal Aortic Aneurysm Complications

CT is the best modality for evaluating patients with suspected *AAA rupture*.[43-46] CT often identifies other abdominal or pelvic pathology when the aneurysm has not leaked. Acute aneurysm rupture produces strandlike soft tissue density sometimes with high attenuation in the retroperitoneum adjacent to the aneurysm (often posteriorly) due to extravasation (Fig. 5-15). It usually is difficult to pinpoint the exact site of rupture.

Other entities can mimic acute aneurysm leak, including chronic rupture, perianeurysmal fibrosis from an inflammatory aneurysm (see below), lymphadenopathy, unopacified duodenum, and spontaneous retroperitoneal hemorrhage (Fig. 5-16). Rarely, CT fails to detect a very small leak. Several CT findings have been described as suggestive of impending aortic rupture, including a high-attenuation crescent sign within or between luminal thrombus and the aortic wall.[43]

The diagnosis of *aortocaval fistula* is made by sonography, CT angiography, or MR angiography (Fig. 5-17).

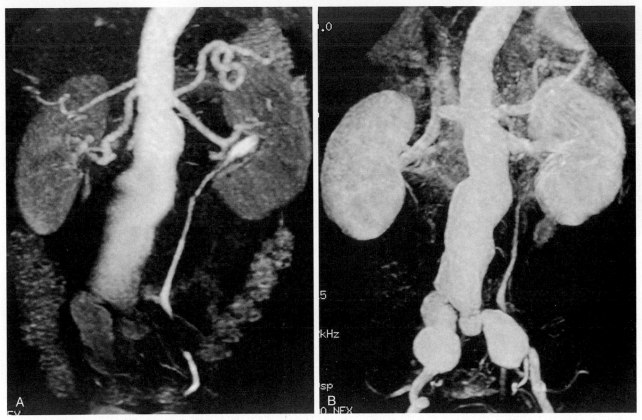

FIGURE 5-12 ■ Infrarenal abdominal aortic aneurysm on coronal gadolinium-enhanced MR angiography maximum intensity projection image shows renal artery vasculature and celiac artery branches (**A**) and delineates the aneurysm with extension to both common iliac arteries (**B**).

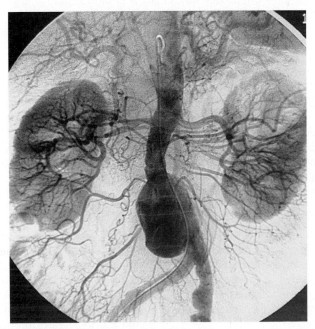

FIGURE 5-13 ■ Infrarenal abdominal aortic aneurysm by catheter angiography.

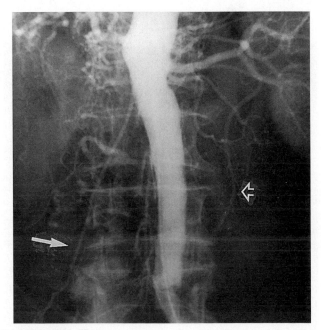

FIGURE 5-14 ■ Abdominal aortic aneurysm with luminal narrowing from mural thrombus. The smooth, straight luminal border and absence of branch vessels suggest the presence of an aneurysm. No mural calcification was seen. The inferior mesenteric artery is occluded, and there is collateral flow to the left colon from the superior mesenteric artery through the arc of Riolan *(arrowhead)*. Notice the right gonadal artery *(arrow)*.

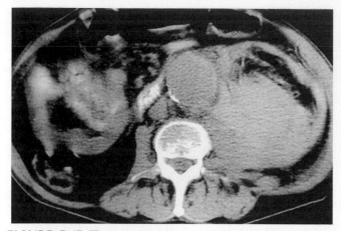

FIGURE 5-15 ■ Acute rupture of an abdominal aortic aneurysm (AAA). The CT scan shows inhomogeneous, irregular, high-attenuation soft tissue density in the left retroperitoneum that is contiguous with the AAA.

The communication most frequently develops between the distal aorta and IVC. In the absence of AAA, aortocaval fistula is either spontaneous or secondary to infection or trauma.[47,48] Stent-grafts have been used to manage these rare lesions.[49]

Treatment

The purpose of intervention is to prevent rupture by excluding the dilated vessel(s) from the circulation. There is general agreement among vascular surgeons that asymptomatic AAA larger than 5 cm in transverse wall-to-wall diameter should be repaired electively and that smaller asymptomatic

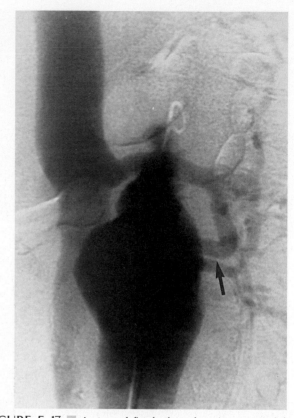

FIGURE 5-17 ■ Aortocaval fistula through a circumaortic left renal vein. Injection above the infrarenal abdominal aortic aneurysm demonstrates filling of the aneurysm, followed by filling of a retroaortic segment of the circumaortic left renal vein *(arrow)* and subsequent filling of the main left renal vein and inferior vena cava.

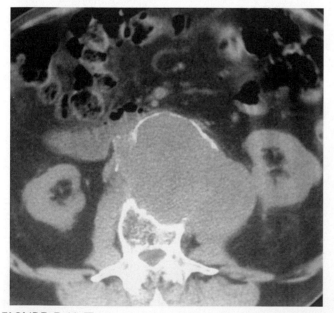

FIGURE 5-16 ■ Chronic rupture of an abdominal aortic aneurysm. Note well-defined soft tissue density continuous with the abdominal aortic aneurysm, which has eroded the adjacent vertebra.

aneurysms be routinely followed by imaging studies.[24,25] Small AAAs are considered for repair if they are symptomatic (causing pain, tenderness, or distal embolization) or enlarging rapidly (>5 mm/6 months).

Of course, the benefits of watchful waiting with imaging surveillance must be weighed against the operative mortality rate for elective open AAA repair (≤5%) and the high mortality rate associated with ruptured AAAs (50% to 75%).[25,26,50] Risk factors for rupture include female gender, advanced age, and continued smoking. The indications for open versus endovascular repair are evolving. Endovascular AAA repair (EVAR) with a stent-graft should certainly be considered in patients with advanced age, significant operative risk, or a hostile abdomen.[51] EVAR has been used also in selected patients with acute rupture.[52]

Open Surgical Therapy

Imaging. For open repair, several factors are particularly important to the surgeon (Box 5-2). The relationship of the neck of the aneurysm to the renal and mesenteric arteries is critical because it influences the operative approach, placement of the proximal aortic clamp, and the need for arterial reconstruction. For example, a juxtarenal AAA necessitates suprarenal aortic cross-clamping.

Extension of the aneurysm into the iliac arteries or occlusive iliofemoral disease requires placement of a bifurcated graft. The presence of a horseshoe kidney necessitates an altered surgical approach and reimplantation of multiple renal arteries.

Technique. The aneurysm is approached through an abdominal or retroperitoneal incision.[53] Synthetic graft material is used to bypass the aneurysm. Even when the aneurysm is located well below the renal arteries, the proximal end-to-end anastomosis is made near the renal arteries to prevent recurrent disease in the infrarenal aorta. If the aneurysm ends above the bifurcation and the common iliac arteries are relatively disease free, a tube graft to the aortic bifurcation may be inserted. Otherwise, a bifurcated graft to the common femoral (or iliac) artery is placed. Reimplantation of the IMA is performed if collateral flow appears insufficient to maintain viability of the left colon. The aneurysm sac is then wrapped around the graft to avoid contact with the bowel, which can lead to infection or fistula formation. Open AAA repair is a major operation, leading to several days in an intensive care unit, a hospital stay of 5 to 10 days, and up to 2 months for recovery.

Complications. Early complications after AAA repair include myocardial infarction, bleeding, renal failure, left colon ischemia, impotence, and paraplegia. Delayed complications include graft infection, anastomotic pseudoaneurysm formation, limb occlusion, graft rupture, and aortoenteric fistula.

Graft infection occurs after less than 2% of open AAA repair procedures.[54] Infections in the groin often are symptomatic and may be treated in some cases with intravenous antibiotics and debridement. Abdominal or pelvic infections may be difficult to diagnose. Graft infection usually is evaluated by CT and/or radionuclide white blood cell scanning. Signs of infection on CT include fluid density adjacent to the graft or air within the graft.[55] Unfortunately, these findings may not be distinguishable from the normal appearance of the postoperative graft 2 to 3 months after operation.[56] Graft infections generally require takedown and extra-anatomic bypass. Recently, however, primary conduit replacement or insertion of cryopreserved allograft have been studied by some groups.[57,58]

Anastomotic pseudoaneurysms develop in about 5% of aortoiliac reconstruction procedures.[59,60] Pseudoaneurysms can appear many years after surgery. They occur more frequently at the distal anastomosis than at the aortic end of the graft (see Fig. 6-44). Pseudoaneurysms can lead to graft thrombosis, rupture, or distal embolization. When distal anastomotic pseudoaneurysms grow to more than 2 cm in diameter, graft interposition is recommended.

Aortoenteric fistula is observed in about 1% of cases of aortoiliac graft placement.[61,62] The fistula between the bowel (usually duodenum) and the prosthetic material is almost always a result of graft infection. Most patients present with gastrointestinal bleeding, fever, or both. A "herald" bleed may occur, presaging a massive hemorrhage. A few patients show signs of graft infection but have no intestinal tract bleeding. CT is the standard imaging tool in suspected cases (Fig. 5-18). In addition to identifying perigraft fluid and gas in the graft, findings may include thickening of small bowel adjacent to the graft and exchange of contrast material between the small bowel and graft.

Endovascular Abdominal Aortic Aneurysm Repair

In 1991, Juan Parodi and co-workers reported the first endovascular placement of a homemade stent-graft in a human for treatment of AAA.[63] This seminal paper ushered in a period of intense investigation and rapid evolution of this remarkable alternative to the traditional operation. The anticipated advantages of endovascular repair over open operation (decreased blood loss and morbidity and mortality, shorter hospital stay, and speedier recovery) have largely been realized. However, the need for secondary procedures and lifelong surveillance, and the risk (albeit small) of late rupture are still limitations of currently available devices.

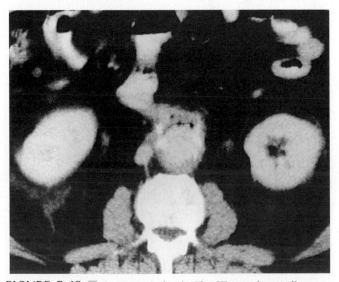

FIGURE 5-18 ■ Aortoenteric fistula. The CT scan shows a linear gas collection in the aortic graft wall contiguous with the transverse portion of the duodenum.

Patient Selection. The indications for EVAR are evolving, but they are based primarily on anatomic factors, comorbid conditions, and patient preference. Some patients cannot undergo EVAR based on strict anatomic criteria (see below). Elderly patients and those at particularly high risk for open repair and general anesthesia often are ideal candidates. Frankly, however, the enthusiasm for this procedure is partly driven by patient demand for a less invasive and morbid approach to this life-threatening condition.

Preprocedure Imaging. Patient and device selection, and preprocedure planning demand high-quality noncontrast CT and CT angiography (with multiplanar reformatted images) followed by catheter angiography (including biplane aortography and pelvic arteriography in multiple projections (Box 5-3 and Fig. 5-19).[64,65]

Technique. Currently, there are three devices approved by the U.S. Food and Drug Administration for treatment of AAA (Table 5-1 and Fig. 5-20).

■ The *AneuRx* endograft (Medtronic AVE, Santa Rosa, Calif.) is composed of a self-expanding nitinol stent incorporated into polyester fabric.

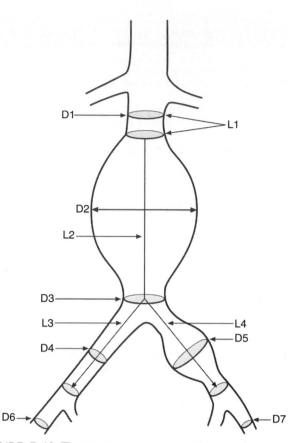

FIGURE 5-19 ■ Critical measurement before endovascular stent-graft placement for abdominal aortic aneurysm. D1, proximal aneurysm neck; D2, maximum aneurysm diameter; D3, distal aneurysm neck; D4 and D5, right and left common iliac artery diameters; D6 and D7, right and left external iliac artery diameters; L1, neck between renal arteries and aneurysm; L2, aneurysm length; L3 and L4, length of right and left common iliac arteries. (Adapted from Rydberg J, Kopecky KK, Lalka SG, et al: Stent grafting of abdominal aortic aneurysms: pre- and post-operative evaluation with multislice helical CT. J Comput Assist Tomogr 2001;25:580, with permission.)

BOX 5-3 ■ Criteria for Patient and Device Selection for EVAR

Aorta
Diameter at renal arteries
Disease (thrombus, atheroma, or calcification) at proximal attachment site (may affect seal)
Length (>15 mm) and diameter (18–28 mm) of proximal neck
Distance from lowest renal artery to iliac bifurcations
Status of mesenteric arteries (effect of covering the inferior mesenteric artery)
Status of main and accessory renal arteries (may affect proximal landing site)
Status of all branch vessels (lumbar, inferior mesenteric, median sacral arteries)
Aneurysm diameter and length (for follow-up assessment) and location of thrombus
Identification of rupture or inflammation
Angulation (<60 degrees) (affects ability to place device, seal abdominal aortic aneurysm, or prevent migration)
Diameter at bifurcation (small size may impinge on graft)

Common Iliac Aarteries
Diameters (>7.5 mm)
Landing site length (>20 mm), diameter (<20 mm), and angulation
Concomitant disease (thrombus, calcium, atheroma, or aneurysm) (may affect seal or selection of landing site)
Tortuosity

Distal Arteries
External iliac artery length, diameter (usually >7 mm), angulation and disease (to assess distal landing site or to accommodate delivery system)
Internal iliac artery disease (pre-EVAR embolization may be required)
Common femoral artery disease and diameter
Overall required length from proximal to distal anastomosis

■ The *Excluder* device (W. L. Gore and Associates, Flagstaff, Ariz.) is manufactured by winding a single nitinol wire around the outside of ultra-thin polytetrafluoroethylene.
■ The *Zenith* endograft (Cook, Inc., Bloomington, Ind.) is made of three parts: an aortic component and two separate iliac artery components. Stainless steel Z-stents are bonded to a polyester skin. A bare anchoring stent with barbs (which extends 26 mm above the covered portion) allows suprarenal aortic fixation.

A host of experimental devices also are under investigation. The details of EVAR are beyond the scope of this text (Fig. 5-21), but it is perhaps the most challenging endovascular procedure in practice today. It requires extensive experience in arterial catheter and guidewire manipulation; knowledge of a wide variety of angioplasty balloon catheters, stents (covered and uncovered), and other angiographic tools; and thorough familiarity with imaging guidance for interventions. The patient is given prophylactic antibiotics

TABLE 5-1	FDA-APPROVED STENT-GRAFTS FOR ABDOMINAL AORTIC ANEURYSMS		
Factor	**AneuRx**	**Excluder**	**Zenith**
Design	2-piece, bifurcated	2-piece, modular	3-piece, modular
Diameters	20–28 mm	23–28.5 mm	22–32 mm
Lengths	13.5–16.5 cm	14–18 cm	7.4–12.2 cm
Iliac limb diameter	12–16 mm	12–20 mm	8–24 mm
Aortic sheath	22 French	18 French	20 or 24 French
Iliac sheath	16–18 French	12 French	14 French

and full anticoagulation with heparin. The procedure must be performed in a room with state-of-the-art digital imaging capability and sterile operating room conditions. General, epidural, or deep anesthesia is achieved under the direction of a dedicated anesthesiologist. Surgical cutdown is performed on the common femoral arteries. Many patients can be discharged from the hospital the next day if there is no evidence of bleeding, infection, or bowel ischemia.

Sometimes, the endograft must be extended down into the external iliac artery because of concomitant aneurysm, extreme tortuosity, or short landing zone in the common iliac artery or the presence of an internal iliac artery aneurysm. In this situation (about 20% of cases), collateral flow through the ipsilateral internal iliac artery (from the contralateral vessel or lumbar or IMA collaterals) may continue to pressurize the aneurysm after the stent-graft is placed.

Internal iliac artery embolization is commonly performed before EVAR to avoid this type II endoleak (see below).[66-69] Either simultaneous bilateral or staged unilateral occlusion is acceptable. A cobra or long reverse curve catheter is directed into the main internal iliac artery from an ipsilateral or contralateral approach. The embolic material of choice is stainless steel or platinum coils, supplemented by large Gelfoam pieces as needed. An oversized coil is first deposited, followed by additional coils to create an occlusive "nest." The goal is obstruction and marked reduction in flow; complete cessation of antegrade flow is not necessary.[70]

This procedure, when performed properly, is highly effective in preventing subsequent endoleak related to the internal iliac artery. The downside is the risk of pelvic ischemia, which can present later as buttock claudication or impotence (about 25% of cases), bladder or colonic ischemia, or, rarely, nerve injury. These symptoms may be transient. The most important technical factor in preventing ischemic complications is occlusion of the main internal iliac artery trunk **proximal** to the bifurcation into anterior and posterior divisions.[68,69]

Results. The immediate and long-term results of stent-graft repair for AAA are outlined in Table 5-2.[52,71-76] There is convincing evidence that procedural blood loss, hospital stay, major adverse events, and 30-day mortality are reduced with EVAR compared with open repair.[77,78] The lingering questions are durability and cost-effectiveness with respect to secondary procedures (to treat endoleak and limb thrombosis), risk of aneurysm rupture, and management of aneurysm expansion. Persistent endoleak seems to predispose to aneurysm growth (though not necessarily rupture).

Complications. The primary long-term problems are endoleak and endotension (see below), graft limb thrombosis, and device migration, angulation, and kinks. Less common events include aortoenteric fistula, bleeding, separation of components, hook fracture, infection, graft degeneration, perigraft stenosis, and occlusion of important branch vessels (Table 5-2). Limb occlusions have been treated with open bypass or thrombolytic therapy.[79]

Follow-up Imaging and Secondary Procedures. With the currently available devices, lifelong periodic imaging follow-up is necessary to identify changes in aneurysm size, persistent aneurysm sac pressurization, and device migration. Routine surveillance (with triple phase CT angiography and plain abdominal radiographs in multiple projections) is typically done at 1, 3, and 6 months postprocedure and yearly thereafter. Color Doppler ultrasound and MR angiography have been evaluated in this regard, but these imaging techniques are generally inferior for a number of reasons. Catheter angiography usually is reserved for patients with suspected endoleak (see below). Factors evaluated on follow-up are outlined in Box 5-4.

Endoleak implies persistent blood flow into an AAA sac after EVAR. There is a standard classification system for these potential failures of the technique (Table 5-3). Endoleaks may only be apparent on delayed images from CT angiography. Catheter angiography may allow more accurate categorization of the **type** of endoleak.[80,81]

Type I and *type III endoleaks* require immediate treatment (Figs. 5-22 and 5-23). Grafts are salvaged by balloon dilation of leaky attachment sites or insertion of a stent-graft cuff or uncovered stent. Rarely, conversion to open repair is necessary. *Type IV endoleak* is typically seen just after placement and usually is self-limited.

Type II endoleak is by far the most common. In this situation, blood flows in a retrograde direction from an aortic side branch (e.g., internal iliac artery branch) into the aneurysm sac via lumbar, inferior mesenteric, accessory renal, or median sacral arteries (Figs. 5-24 and 5-25). **Simple** type II endoleaks involve a single vessel that provides inflow during systole and outflow during diastole. **Complex** type II endoleaks result from multiple inflow and outflow vessels.

Type II endoleaks are detected after about 10% to 20% of procedures. Management is controversial. About one third will close spontaneously. Most experts believe that **persistent** endoleaks (even those without associated AAA enlargement) require repair because of the continued pressurization of the aneurysm sac and risk for rupture.[82-84]

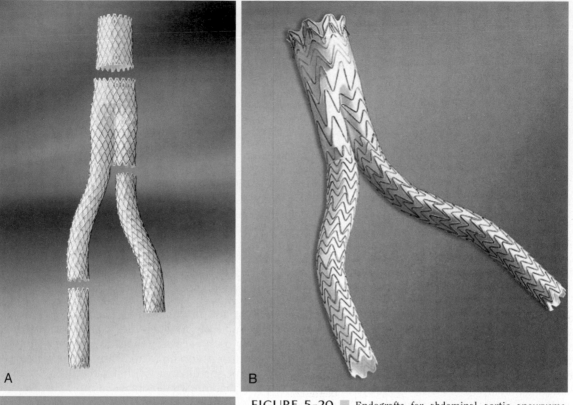

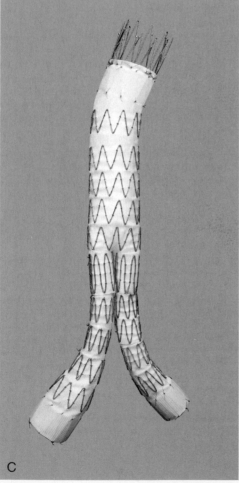

FIGURE 5-20 ■ Endografts for abdominal aortic aneurysms. **A,** AneuRx endograft. **B,** Excluder device. **C,** Zenith endograft. (**A,** Courtesy of Medtronic Vascular; **B,** Courtesy of W. L. Gore and Associates; **C,** Courtesy of Cook, Inc.)

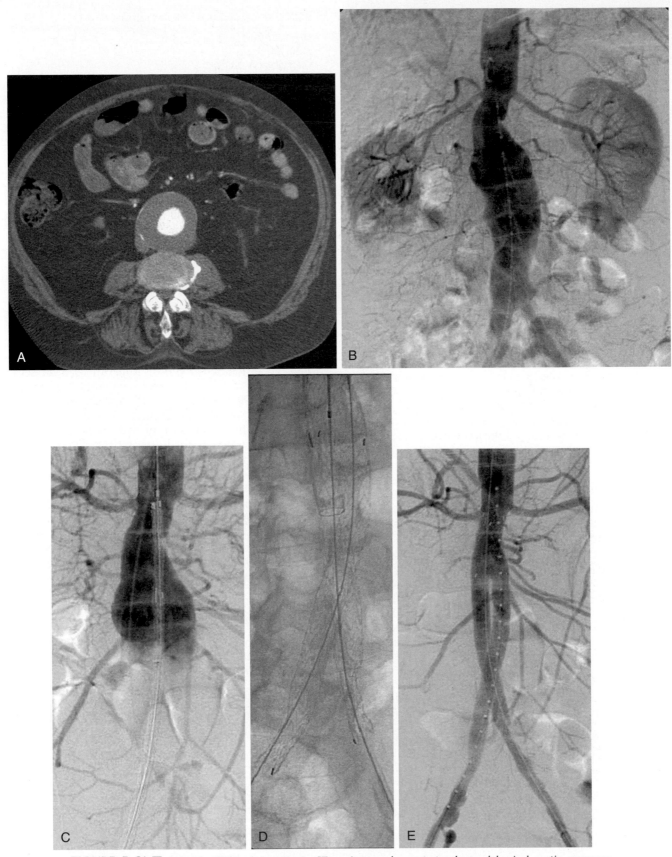

FIGURE 5-21 ■ Steps in EVAR placement. **A,** CT angiogram demonstrates large abdominal aortic aneurysm. **B,** Marking pigtail catheter used for measurements at catheter angiography. **C,** Placement of device prior to expansion of proximal neck. **D,** Stent-graft secured in place. **E,** Final catheter angiogram shows proper placement and no evidence of endoleak.

Continued

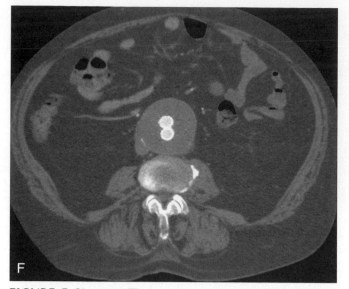

FIGURE 5-21 *Cont'd* ■ **F,** Postprocedure angiogram demonstrates stent-graft without endoleak. (Courtesy of Gerant Rivera-Sanfeliz, San Diego, Calif.)

Some interventionalists will not treat type II endoleaks if the aneurysm is shrinking.

Simple type II endoleaks may be closed successfully by transarterial embolization (see Fig. 5-24). However, complex lesions treated in this fashion are bound to recur.[85] Therefore, direct percutaneous translumbar embolization of the aneurysm sac is necessary.[86] With the patient prone and following analysis of the CT angiogram, a 19-gauge sheath-needle or micropuncture system is inserted about one hand breadth from the midline toward the left lateral border of the spine from the left flank (or right flank if a transcaval approach is deemed necessary). Once the aneurysm sac is entered, the pressure is measured and the sac is embolized with coils and/or cyanoacrylate (Fig. 5-26).

Endotension (type V "endoleak") refers to aneurysm growth after EVAR with persistent pressurization of the sac without evidence for endoleak.[87] Aspiration of the residual sac often yields a serous fluid, suggesting that "ultrafiltration" through the fabric may be occurring in some instances. Aneurysm rupture is theoretically possible.

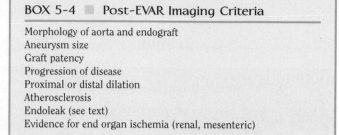

Endovascular methods may be used to treat this condition, and open repair is rarely necessary. Future modifications in graft material may ultimately prevent this perplexing, though fortunately uncommon, problem.

Occlusive Disease

Etiology

Complete occlusion of the abdominal aorta can present as an acute or chronic condition. The most common cause of **chronic** occlusion is thrombosis superimposed on severe atherosclerosis of the distal abdominal aorta and common iliac arteries. The *Leriche syndrome* describes such patients with buttock and thigh claudication, impotence, thigh muscle atrophy, and diminished femoral pulses.[88] Thrombosis also may occur in the setting of less common entities that narrow the aorta (Box 5-5).

The major reasons for **acute** abdominal aortic occlusion are outlined in Box 5-6.[89,90] About 50% to 65% of cases result from embolism.[90,91] Thrombosis of AAAs often results from disruption of mural thrombus followed by distal embolization.[92] In many cases, distal aortic occlusion propagates back toward the level of the renal arteries or SMA. The ultimate level of the occlusion is distributed about evenly above and below the origin of the IMA.

Clinical Features

Most patients with chronic aortic occlusion have a long history of smoking. Symptoms and signs depend largely on whether the occlusion is acute or chronic. Patients with acute occlusion may have sudden onset of bilateral lower extremity rest pain, absent pulses, cool and mottled skin, and neurologic deficits. Prior episodes of myocardial

TABLE 5-2 OUTCOMES OF ENDOVASCULAR ABDOMINAL AORTIC ANEURYSM REPAIR

Technical success	98–100%
Major adverse events	4–14%
Access complications	6–14%
30-day overall mortality	1–4%
Endoleak rate at 2 yr	10–20%
Device migration	2%
Limb occlusion/kink	3–11%
Secondary procedures at 2 yr	11–14%
Aneurysm expansion	12–19%
Aneurysm shrinkage (1 yr)	15–67%
Conversions (early and late)	<5%
Aneurysm rupture	~1%/yr
2 yr survival	>85%

TABLE 5-3 ENDOLEAK CLASSIFICATION

Type	Definition
I	Attachment leak or failure
II	Retrograde branch flow into aneurysm sac
III	Device deterioration or dehiscence
IV	Graft porosity
V	Endotension

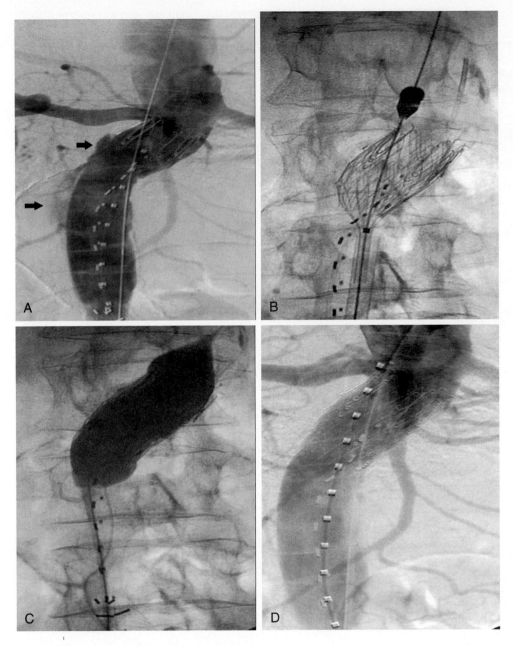

infarction or cardiac dysrhythmias are common. Patients with chronic occlusion usually complain of severe, progressive, bilateral leg claudication, along with impotence in some men. Distal leg pulses often are diminished or absent. However, with good collateral circulation, weak femoral pulses may be palpable in patients with complete long-standing occlusion.

Imaging

Some vascular surgeons question the need for preoperative imaging in patients with suspected acute aortic occlusion.[91] Acute and chronic occlusions are imaged with CT or MR angiography. When catheter arteriography is performed

(usually because endovascular treatment is contemplated), a high left brachial artery approach is recommended. However, it may be possible to enter the femoral artery using ultrasound guidance and traverse the occlusion with a hydrophilic guidewire, even with faint or absent pulses (see Fig. 5-6). The catheter should be advanced carefully into the abdominal aorta to within several centimeters of the site of occlusion.

Chronic occlusion invokes an extensive collateral circulation (see Figs. 5-6 and 5-7). A filling defect in the aorta indicates acute embolism or in situ thrombosis (Fig. 5-27). Involvement of the renal or mesenteric arteries should be sought. Rarely, extension of a thoracic aortic dissection causes acute abdominal aortic occlusion.

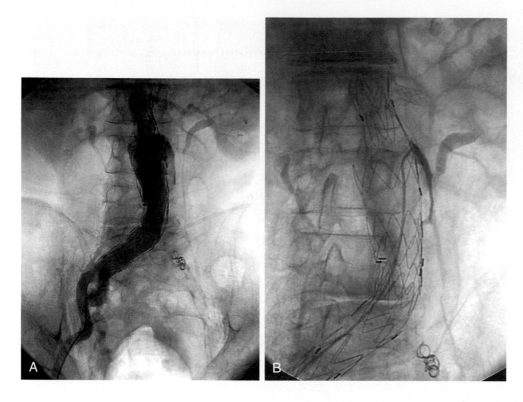

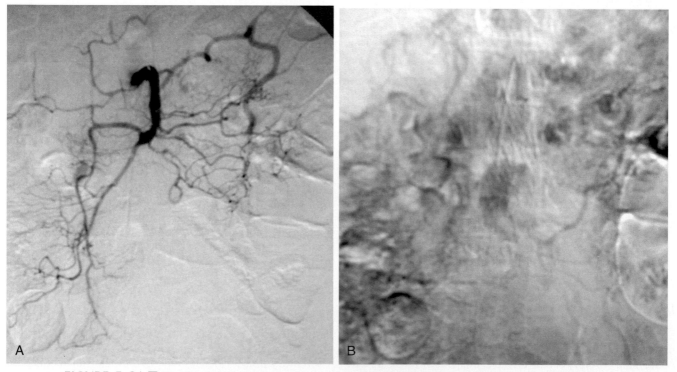

FIGURE 5-24 ■ Type II endoleak with transarterial embolization. A, Superior mesenteric arteriogram. B, Late phase of study shows leak into aneurysm sac through inferior mesenteric artery collaterals.

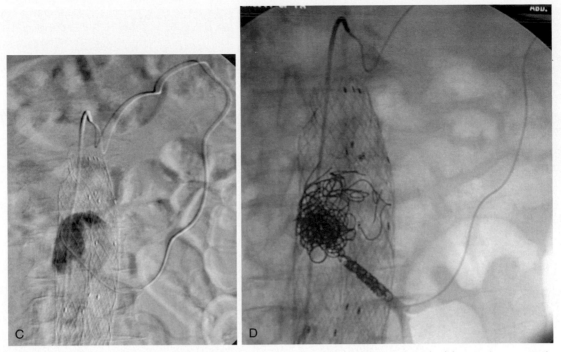

FIGURE 5-24 *Cont'd* ▪ **C,** Coaxial microcatheter was directed from the middle colic branch of the superior mesenteric artery through the inferior mesenteric artery and into the aneurysm sac. **D,** Exclusion of collateral leak with multiple coils. (Courtesy of William Stavropoulos, Philadelphia, Pa.)

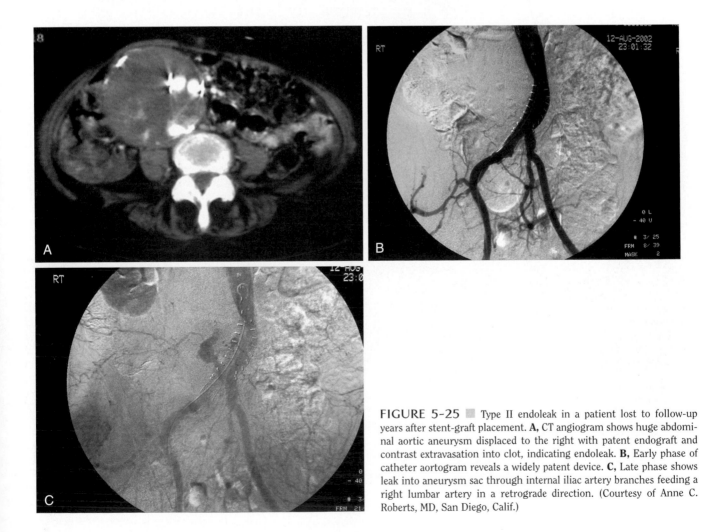

FIGURE 5-25 ▪ Type II endoleak in a patient lost to follow-up years after stent-graft placement. **A,** CT angiogram shows huge abdominal aortic aneurysm displaced to the right with patent endograft and contrast extravasation into clot, indicating endoleak. **B,** Early phase of catheter aortogram reveals a widely patent device. **C,** Late phase shows leak into aneurysm sac through internal iliac artery branches feeding a right lumbar artery in a retrograde direction. (Courtesy of Anne C. Roberts, MD, San Diego, Calif.)

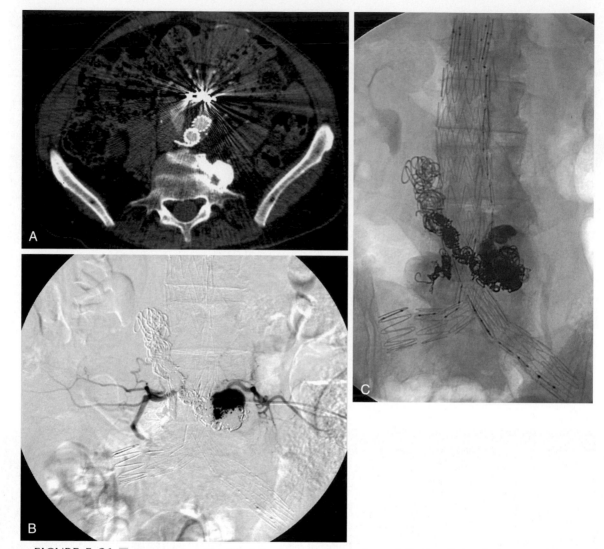

FIGURE 5-26 ■ Recurrent type II endoleak treatment by translumbar embolization. Patient had type II endoleak treated 2 years prior. **A,** CT angiogram shows persistent leak into aneurysm sac. **B,** Following translumbar catheter placement, there is antegrade filling of bilateral lumbar arteries. **C,** Multiple coils and n-butyl cyanoacrylate were used to fill the sac. (Courtesy of William Stavropoulos, Philadelphia, Pa.)

BOX 5-5 ■ Causes of Abdominal Aortic Narrowing

Atherosclerosis
Dissection
Aneurysm with mural thrombus
Takayasu's arteritis
Congenital coarctation syndromes
   Neurofibromatosis
   Congenital rubella
   Williams' syndrome
   Tuberous sclerosis
Middle aortic syndrome
Radiation aortitis

BOX 5-6 ■ Causes of Acute Occlusion of the Abdominal Aorta

Embolism (usually cardiac source)
Thrombosis superimposed on atherosclerotic disease
Thrombosis of abdominal aortic aneurysm
Trauma
Iatrogenic injury (e.g., catheterization)
Thrombophilic state
Dissection
Extrinsic compression

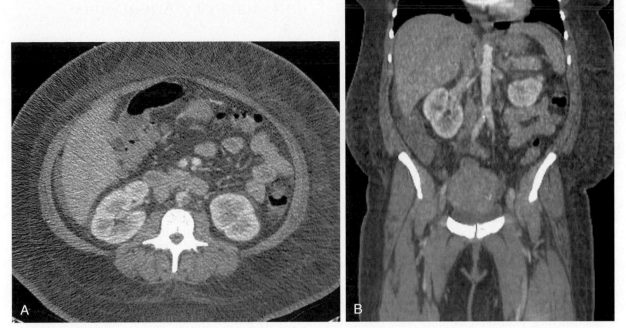

FIGURE 5-27 ■ Embolus to the abdominal aorta. Axial (**A**) and reformatted (**B**) CT angiogram images show a filling defect on left lateral wall of the distal abdominal aorta.

Treatment

Surgical Therapy. The mortality rate for patients with acute aortic occlusion is greater than 50%.[91] Patients with embolic aortic occlusion are treated with embolectomy in many cases.[90,91] For acute or chronic thrombotic occlusion, aortobifemoral bypass grafting is the procedure of choice.

Endovascular Therapy. Interventional radiology has a role in the management of chronic aortic occlusion, particularly when disease is isolated to the distal portion of the abdominal aorta.[93-95] Thrombolysis (to lyse fresh thrombus), angioplasty, and intravascular stent placement have been used successfully in selected cases (see Chapter 6). However, long-term patency in large series of patients has not been established.

Dissection

Dissection of the abdominal aorta almost always results from extension of a thoracic aortic dissection. Rare causes of isolated abdominal aortic dissection include trauma, catheterization, and spontaneous dissection.[96] With cross-sectional imaging, an intimal flap is seen with differential flow signal or density in the true and false lumens. The true aortic lumen may appear tapered or narrowed because of expansion of the false lumen (Fig. 5-28). Progressive enlargement of the false lumen of a chronic aortic dissection can produce an aneurysm.

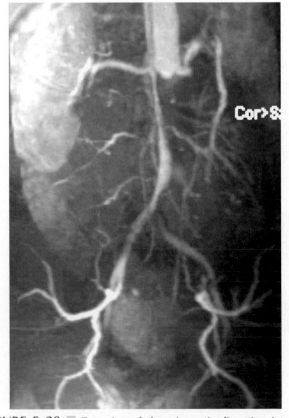

FIGURE 5-28 ■ Extension of thoracic aortic dissection into the abdominal aorta with thrombosis of the false lumen on the left side of the vessel as seen on maximum intensity projection MR angiogram.

■ OTHER DISORDERS

Trauma

Injury to the abdominal aorta occurs from accidental, criminal, or iatrogenic penetrating trauma and, less commonly, from blunt trauma.[97-99] Penetrating injuries occur more frequently to the abdominal aorta than to the thoracic aorta. The most common causes of blunt trauma are motor vehicle accidents and crush injuries. Injury to the abdominal aorta accounts for 10% to 15% of aortic injuries seen from such accidents.[97-99] However, few patients survive to reach medical care. When the vascular injury is minor (e.g., an intimal flap), patients may have no ischemic symptoms. Signs of major abdominal aortic injury include diminished pulses or a reduction in ankle-brachial indices. Associated lumbar spine fractures are characteristic.

Unstable patients with penetrating or blunt trauma usually go immediately to exploratory laparotomy without imaging studies. Those with abdominal trauma who are hemodynamically stable usually undergo CT scanning. The findings may include a discrete intimal flap, dissection, intramural hematoma, penetrating tear, pseudoaneurysm, complete transection with acute thrombosis, and aortocaval fistula.[97-102] In the absence of AAA, *aortocaval fistula* usually is the result of blunt or penetrating injury or lumbar disk surgery.[101]

The mortality rate from abdominal aortic injury is greater than 75% and is higher for suprarenal injuries.[97-99] The usual treatment is operation with aortic reconstruction or bypass graft placement. Endovascular techniques have been used to treat selected patients. In particular, balloon fenestration of dissections, stent insertion, or stent-graft placement has been used successfully.[103,104]

Injury to abdominal aortic branches is considered in the related chapters. Injury to lumbar arteries should be suspected in any patient with blunt abdominal or pelvic trauma and evidence for significant retroperitoneal bleeding (see Chapter 6).

Inflammatory Aneurysms

Inflammatory AAAs are caused by cellular infiltration of the media and adventitia of the abdominal aorta, leading to marked thickening of the vessel and a dense, periadventitial fibrotic reaction.[105] The precise cause is unknown, but the disorder may involve an immune-related reaction to material within the aortic wall. Genetic factors also have been implicated, including a relationship to the human leukocyte antigen molecule and autoimmune diseases.[106] Others have suggested that these aneurysms can begin as conventional degenerative AAAs with contained leak.

In one report, inflammatory aneurysms accounted for about 3% of all AAAs, although some studies suggest a greater frequency.[107,108] The disease also can affect the duodenum, small bowel, IVC, and ureters.[109] Aortic fistulas are more common (but rupture less common) than with degenerative AAA.[110] Patients may have fever and an elevated erythrocyte sedimentation rate during the acute phase of the illness. Abdominal or back pain is more common in patients with inflammatory aneurysms than in those with degenerative AAA.

On CT or MR imaging, the diagnosis is suggested by a smooth, confluent rind of enhancing soft tissue around the anterior and lateral margins of the aorta (Fig. 5-29).[111-113] The posterior border of the aorta often is spared. These features usually allow differentiation from aortic rupture, metastatic disease, or lymphadenopathy (see Figs. 5-15 and 5-16). Detection of disease in adjacent organs is important before surgery.

There is controversy regarding the role of corticosteroids and the optimal timing of surgery in patients with inflammatory aneurysms. However, aneurysm repair appears to halt (and even reverse) the inflammatory process.

Infectious Aneurysms

Infectious (mycotic) aneurysms or pseudoaneurysms are caused by local seeding of diseased vessel wall (usually

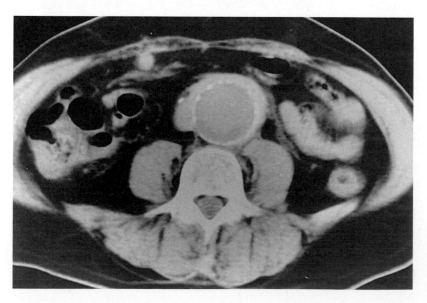

FIGURE 5-29 ■ Inflammatory abdominal aortic aneurysm. CT scan shows the aortic aneurysm with an enhancing rind of soft tissue around the anterolateral portion of the aorta.

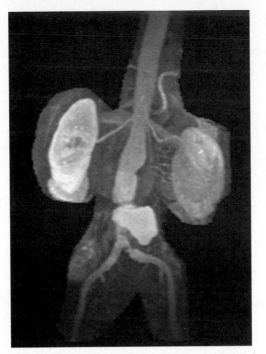

FIGURE 5-30 ■ Mycotic aneurysm of the distal abdominal aorta on gadolinium-enhanced MR angiogram.

atherosclerotic plaque), seeding through the vasa vasorum, direct invasion from an adjacent infection (e.g., *Mycobacterium tuberculosis*), or penetrating trauma. Among the more common offending organisms are *Staphylococcus aureus* and *Salmonella* species.[114] The thoracoabdominal and abdominal aorta are more commonly affected than the thoracic aorta. Unfortunately, the classic symptoms and signs of fever, abdominal pain, pulsatile

mass, and elevated white blood cell count are seen in only a few cases. Most patients are intravenous drug abusers, alcoholics, or are immunocompromised.

The diagnosis is made by cross-sectional imaging. The typical finding is a saccular, eccentric aneurysm, usually with little or no adjacent aortic disease (Fig. 5-30).[115] Enhancing periaortic soft tissue density may be seen before aneurysm growth occurs. Multiple aneurysms are common. Patients are treated vigorously with antibiotics. Early operation is recommended in most cases, usually with prosthetic graft placement or ligation and extra-anatomic bypass grafting.[116] Stent graft placement also has been tried.[117]

Penetrating Aortic Ulcer and Intramural Hematoma

These two uncommon but important entities are considered in Chapter 4.

Vasculitis

Takayasu's arteritis is an inflammatory vasculitis affecting large- and medium-sized elastic arteries. Details of this unusual entity are considered in Chapters 3 and 4. The typical patient is young and female, usually of Asian or Central American descent. The abdominal aorta and its branches are involved in about two thirds of cases (see Fig. 3-24).[118-120] The most common imaging finding is smooth narrowing of the abdominal aorta, which may be focal, segmental, or diffuse; rarely, complete obstruction occurs (Fig. 5-31A). Associated narrowing of the proximal portions of the renal,

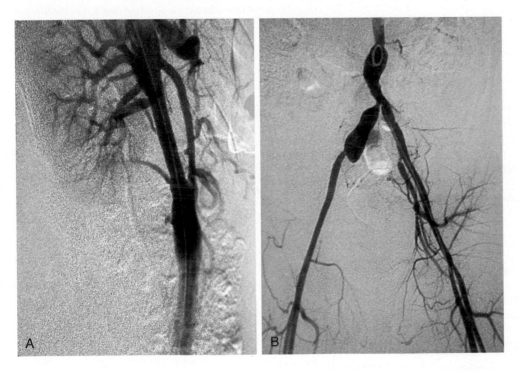

FIGURE 5-31 ■ Takayasu's arteritis. **A,** Typical smooth long-segment infrarenal aortic narrowing in a 7-year-old girl (lateral projection of abdominal aortogram). **B,** Atypical aortic and iliac artery aneurysms in another young girl.

mesenteric, or iliac arteries is common. Conversely, fusiform aneurysms of the aorta (usually suprarenal) and branch vessels are occasionally seen (Fig. 5-31B). Most lesions remain stable after the disease becomes chronic.

Radiation arteritis may develop in large or small blood vessels. In large- and medium-sized arteries, high-dose radiotherapy can induce periarterial fibrosis, intimal atherosclerotic-like changes with mural thrombus formation, or frank fibrotic occlusion.[121] Radiation-induced arterial disease usually becomes apparent 5 or more years after therapy. Imaging reveals smooth narrowing of the affected vessel, irregular atherosclerotic-like lesions, or complete occlusion.[121,122]

HIV-related arteritis is well known to affect medium- and small-caliber vessels. However, a rarer form of large vessel arteritis can produce solitary or multiple aneurysms in the aorta and its major branches.[123] The disease provokes a leukocytoclastic reaction in the vasa vasorum and periadventitial tissues along with chronic inflammation. The aneurysms often are saccular in appearance (see Fig 4-29).

Coarctation Syndromes

Several disorders associated with *congenital coarctation syndromes,* including *neurofibromatosis, Williams syndrome, congenital rubella,* and *tuberous sclerosis,* can affect the abdominal aorta and its major branches.[124-127] Vascular involvement in neurofibromatosis is uncommon; when present, stenoses of the aorta and branch vessels (particularly the renal arteries) or arterial aneurysms are found. Narrowing of large- and medium-caliber vessels results from proliferation of neurofibromas or ganglioneuromatous tissue within the vascular wall.[124,125] Williams syndrome is a congenital disorder that includes infantile hypercalcemia, supravalvular aortic stenosis, elfin facies, and developmental delays.

This rare and diverse group of patients usually presents with hypertension as children or young adults. Imaging findings include smooth narrowing of the proximal or mid-abdominal aorta, narrowing of the proximal renal arteries in almost all cases, and stenoses of the superior mesenteric or celiac artery with enlarged collateral vessels (see Fig. 8-50).

Middle aortic syndrome (or atypical coarctation) produces narrowing of the mid-abdominal aorta and its major branches. Despite extensive research, there is still controversy about the relationships between middle aortic syndrome, Takayasu's arteritis, and the congenital coarctation syndromes. Some experts believe that middle aortic syndrome is simply a subtype of Takayasu's arteritis and that the features in this subgroup of patients are found in the spectrum of patients with nonspecific aortoarteritis. Other investigators believe that these entities are distinct, although perhaps related, diseases.[126] It may differ from Takayasu's arteritis in its lack of geographic predilection, younger age at presentation (first and second decades of life), noninflammatory pathology, and lack of an acute febrile phase. Surgical revascularization is the standard treatment. Stent placement has been used in this setting, but the durability of such an approach in this young population is unknown.[128,129]

REFERENCES

1. Collins P, ed: Embryology and development. In: Williams PL, Bannister LH, Berry MM, et al, eds. Gray's Anatomy, 38th ed. New York, Churchill Livingstone, 1995:318.
2. Gabella G, ed: Cardiovascular system. In: Williams PL, Bannister LH, Berry MM, et al, eds. Gray's Anatomy, 38th ed. New York, Churchill Livingstone, 1995:1547.
3. da Silva ES, Rodrigues AJ Jr, Castro de Tolosa EM, et al: Variation of infrarenal aortic diameter: a necropsy study. J Vasc Surg 1999; 29:920.
4. Horejs D, Gilbert PM, Burstein S, et al: Normal aortoiliac diameters by CT. J Comput Assist Tomogr 1988;12:602.
5. Shokeir AA, el-Diasty TA, Nabeeh A, et al: Digital subtraction angiography in potential live-kidney donors: a study of 1000 cases. Abdom Imaging 1994;19:461.
6. Gupta A, Tello R: Accessory renal arteries are not related to hypertension risk: a review of MR angiography data. AJR Am J Roentgenol 2004;182:1521.
7. Platt JF, Ellis JH, Korobkin M, et al: Helical CT evaluation of potential kidney donors: findings in 154 subjects. AJR Am J Roentgenol 1997;169:1325.
8. Rankin SC, Jan W, Koffman CG: Noninvasive imaging of living related kidney donors: evaluation of CT angiography and gadolinium enhanced MR angiography. AJR Am J Roentgenol 2001;177:349.
9. Kalra M, Panneton JM, Hofer JM, et al: Aneurysm and stenosis of the celiomesenteric trunk: a rare anomaly. J Vasc Surg 2003;37:679.
10. Inoue Y, Iwai T, Endo M: Determining variations in colonic circulation during aortic surgery. Cardiovasc Surg 1997;5:626.
11. Johnston KW, Rutherford RB, Tilson MD, et al: Suggested standards for reporting on arterial aneurysms. J Vasc Surg 1991;13:452.
12. Johnston KW, Scobie TK: Multicenter prospective study of nonruptured abdominal aortic aneurysms. I. Population and operative management. J Vasc Surg 1988;7:69.
13. Nypaver TJ, Shepard AD, Reddy DJ, et al: Repair of pararenal abdominal aortic aneurysms: an analysis of operative management. Arch Surg 1993;128:803.
14. Melton LJ 3rd, Bickerstaff LK, Hollier LH, et al: Changing incidence of abdominal aortic aneurysms: a population-based study. Am J Epidemiol 1984;120:379.
15. Reitsma JB, Pleumeekers HJ, Hoes AW, et al: Increasing incidence of aneurysms of the abdominal aorta in The Netherlands. Eur J Vasc Endovasc Surg 1996;12:446.
16. Daugherty A, Cassis LA: Mechanisms of abdominal aortic aneurysm formation. Curr Atheroscler Rep 2002;4:222.
17. Miller FJ: Aortic aneurysms. It's all about the stress. Arterioscler Thromb Vasc Biol 2002;22:1948.
18. Annabi B, Shedid D, Ghosn P, et al: Differential regulation of matrix metalloproteinase activities in abdominal aortic aneurysms. J Vasc Surg 2002;35:539.
19. Longo GM, Xiong W, Greiner TC, et al: Matrix metalloproteinases 2 and 9 work in concert to produce aortic aneurysms. J Clin Invest 2002; 110:613.
20. Goldstone J: Aneurysms of the aorta and iliac arteries. In: Moore WS, ed. Vascular Surgery. A comprehensive review. Philadelphia, WB Saunders, 1993:401.
21. Jost CJ, Gloviczki P, Edwards WD, et al: Aortic aneurysms in children and young adults with tuberous sclerosis: report of two cases and review of the literature. J Vasc Surg 2001;33:639.
22. Kurvers H, Veith FJ, Lipsitz EC, et al: Discontinuous, staccato growth of abdominal aortic aneurysms. J Am Coll Surg 2004;199:709.
23. Brady AR, Thompson SG, Fowkes FG, et al: Abdominal aortic aneurysm expansion: risk factors and time intervals for surveillance. Circulation 2004;110:16.
24. Mortality results for randomised controlled trial of early elective surgery or ultrasonographic surveillance for small abdominal aortic aneurysms. The UK Small Aneurysm Trial Participants. Lancet 1998; 352:1649.
25. Lederle FA, Wilson SE, Johnson GR, et al: Immediate repair compared with surveillance of small abdominal aortic aneurysms. N Engl J Med 2002;346:1437.
26. Singh K, Bonaa KH, Jacobsen BK, et al: Prevalence of and risk factors for abdominal aortic aneurysms in a population-based study: The Tromso Study. Am J Epidemiol 2001;154:236.

27. Bednarkiewicz M, Pretre R, Kalangos A, et al: Aortocaval fistula associated with abdominal aortic aneurysm: a diagnostic challenge. Ann Vasc Surg 1997;11:464.

28. Vardulaki KA, Walker NM, Day NE, et al: Quantifying the risks of hypertension, age, sex and smoking in patients with abdominal aortic aneurysm. Br J Surg 2000;87:195.

29. Rydberg J, Kopecky KK, Lalka SG, et al: Stent grafting of abdominal aortic aneurysms: pre- and postoperative evaluation with multislice helical CT. J Comput Assist Tomogr 2001;25:580.

30. Armerding MD, Rubin GD, Beaulieu CF, et al: Aortic aneurysmal disease: assessment of stent-graft treatment—CT versus conventional angiography. Radiology 2000;215:138.

31. Bromley PJ, Kaufman JA: Abdominal aortic aneurysms before and after endograft implantation: evaluation by computed tomography. Tech Vasc Interv Radiol 2001;4:15.

32. Costello P, Gaa J: Spiral CT angiography of abdominal aortic aneurysms. Radiographics 1995;15:397.

33. Gomes MN, Davros WJ, Zeman RK: Preoperative assessment of abdominal aortic aneurysm: the value of helical and three-dimensional computed tomography. J Vasc Surg 1994;20:367.

34. Raptopoulos V, Rosen MP, Kent KC, et al: Sequential helical CT angiography of aortoiliac disease. AJR Am J Roentgenol 1996;166:1347.

35. Van Hoe L, Baert AL, Gryspeerdt S, et al: Supra- and juxtarenal aneurysms of the abdominal aorta: preoperative assessment with thin-section spiral CT. Radiology 1996;198:443.

36. Thurnher SA, Dorffner R, Thurnher MM, et al: Evaluation of abdominal aortic aneurysm for stent-graft placement: comparison of gadolinium-enhanced MR angiography versus helical CT angiography and digital subtraction angiography. Radiology 1997;205:341.

37. Persson A, Dahlstrom N, Engellau L, et al: Volume rendering compared with maximum intensity projection for magnetic resonance angiography measurements of the abdominal aorta. Acta Radiol 2004; 45:453.

38. Lookstein RA, Goldman J, Pukin L, et al: Time-resolved magnetic resonance angiography as a noninvasive method to characterize endoleaks: initial results compared with conventional angiography. J Vasc Surg 2004;39:27.

39. Prince MR, Narasimham DL, Stanley JC, et al: Gadolinium-enhanced magnetic resonance angiography of abdominal aortic aneurysms. J Vasc Surg 1995;21:656.

40. Petersen MJ, Cambria RP, Kaufman JA, et al: Magnetic resonance angiography in the preoperative evaluation of abdominal aortic aneurysms. J Vasc Surg 1995;21:891.

41. Holland GA, Dougherty L, Carpenter JP, et al: Breath-hold ultrafast three-dimensional gadolinium-enhanced MR angiography of the aorta and the renal and other visceral abdominal arteries. AJR Am J Roentgenol 1996;166:971.

42. Insko EK, Kulzer LM, Fairman RM, et al: MR imaging for the detection of endoleaks in recipients of abdominal aortic stent-grafts with low magnetic susceptibility. Acad Radiol 2003;10:509.

43. Mehard WB, Heiken JP, Sicard GA: High-attenuation crescent in abdominal aortic aneurysm wall at CT: sign of acute or impending rupture. Radiology 1992;185(P):321.

44. Fillinger MF, Racusin J, Baker RK, et al: Anatomic characteristics of ruptured abdominal aortic aneurysm on conventional CT scans: implications for rupture risk. J Vasc Surg 2004;39:1243.

45. Lederle FA, Johnson GR, Wilson SE, et al: Rupture rate of large abdominal aortic aneurysms in patients refusing or unfit for elective repair. JAMA 2002;287:2968.

46. Bhalla S, Menias CO, Heiken JP: CT of acute abdominal aortic disorders. Radiol Clin North Am 2003;41:1153.

47. Torigian DA, Carpenter JP, Roberts DA: Mycotic aortocaval fistula: efficient evaluation by bolus-chase MR angiography. J Magn Reson Imaging 2002;15:195.

48. Rajmohan B: Spontaneous aortocaval fistula. J Postgrad Med 2002;48:203.

49. Lau LL, O'Reilly MJ, Johnston LC, et al: Endovascular stent-graft repair of primary aortocaval fistula with an abdominal aortoiliac aneurysm. J Vasc Surg 2001;33:425.

50. Crawford ES, Saleh SA, Babb JW 3rd, et al: Infrarenal abdominal aortic aneurysm: factors influencing survival after operations performed over a 25-year period. Ann Surg 1981;193:699.

51. Brewster DC, Cronenwett JL, Hallett JW Jr, et al: Guidelines for the treatment of abdominal aortic aneurysm. Report of a subcommittee of the Joint Council of the American Association for Vascular Surgery and Society for Vascular Surgery. J Vasc Surg 2003;37:1106.

52. Towne JB: Endovascular treatment of abdominal aortic aneurysms. Am J Surg 2005;189:140.

53. Cambria RP, Brewster DC, Abbott WM, et al: Transperitoneal versus retroperitoneal approach for aortic reconstruction: a randomized, prospective study. J Vasc Surg 1990;11:314.

54. O'Hara PJ, Hertzer NR, Beven EG, et al: Surgical management of infected abdominal aortic grafts: review of a 25-year experience. J Vasc Surg 1986;3:725.

55. O'Hara PJ, Borkowski GP, Hertzer NR, et al: Natural history of periprosthetic air on computerized axial tomographic examination of the abdomen following abdominal aortic aneurysm repair. J Vasc Surg 1984;1:429.

56. Qvarfordt PG, Reilly LM, Mark AS, et al: Computerized tomographic assessment of graft incorporation after aortic reconstruction. Am J Surg 1985;150:227.

57. Calligaro KD, Veith FJ, Yuan JG, et al: Intra-abdominal aortic graft infection: complete or partial graft preservation in patients at very high risk. J Vasc Surg 2003;38:1199.

58. Noel AA, Gloviczki P, Cherry KJ Jr, et al: Abdominal aortic reconstruction in infected fields: early results of the United States cryopreserved aortic allograft registry. J Vasc Surg 2002;35:847.

59. Van den Akker PJ, Brand R, van Schilfgaarde R, et al: False aneurysms after prosthetic reconstructions for aortoiliac obstructive disease. Ann Surg 1989;210:658.

60. Dennis JW, Littooy FN, Greisler HP, et al: Anastomotic pseudoaneurysms. A continuing late complication of vascular reconstructive procedures. Arch Surg 1986;121:314.

61. Cendan JC, Thomas JB 4th, Seeger JM: Twenty-one cases of aortoenteric fistula: lessons for the general surgeon. Am Surg 2004;70:583.

62. Busuttil SJ, Goldstone J: Diagnosis and management of aortoenteric fistulas. Semin Vasc Surg 2001;14:302.

63. Parodi JC, Palmaz JC, Barone HD: Transfemoral intraluminal graft implantation for abdominal aortic aneurysms. Ann Vasc Surg 1991;5:491.

64. Rydberg J, Kopecky KK, Johnson MS, et al: Endovascular repair of abdominal aortic aneurysms: assessment with multislice CT. AJR Am J Roentgenol 2001;177:607.

65. Geller SC: Imaging guidelines for abdominal aortic aneurysm repair with endovascular stent grafts. J Vasc Interv Radiol 2003;14:S263.

66. Lee CW, Kaufman JA, Fan C-M, et al: Clinical outcome of internal iliac artery occlusions during endovascular treatment of aorto-iliac aneurysmal disease. J Vasc Interv Radiol 2000;11:567.

67. Razavi MK, DeGroot M, Olcott C, et al: Internal iliac artery embolization in the stent graft treatment of aortoiliac aneurysms: analysis of outcomes and complications. J Vasc Interv Radiol 2000;11:561.

68. Soulen MC, Fairman RM, Baum RA: Embolization of the internal iliac artery: still more to learn. J Vasc Interv Radiol 2000;11:543.

69. Engelke C, Elford J, Morgan RA, et al: Internal iliac artery embolization with bilateral occlusion before endovascular aortoiliac aneurysm repair—clinical outcome of simultaneous and sequential intervention. J Vasc Interv Radiol 2002;13:667.

70. Heye S, Nevelsteen A, Maleux G: Internal iliac artery coil embolization in the prevention of potential type 2 endoleak after endovascular repair of abdominal aortoiliac and iliac artery aneurysms: effect of total occlusion versus residual flow. J Vasc Interv Radiol 2005;16:235.

71. Zarins CK, AneuRx Clinical Investigators: The US AneuRx Clinical Trial: 6-year clinical update 2002. J Vasc Surg 2003;37:904.

72. Ouriel K, Clair DG, Greenberg RK, et al: Endovascular repair of abdominal aortic aneurysms: device-specific outcome. J Vasc Surg 2003; 37:991.

73. Greenberg RK, Chuter TA, Sternbergh WC 3rd, et al: Zenith AAA endovascular graft: intermediate-term results of the US multicenter trial. J Vasc Surg 2004;39:1209.

74. Kibbe MR, Matsumura JS: Excluder Investigators: The Gore Excluder US multi-center trial: analysis of adverse events at 2 years. Semin Vasc Surg 2003;16:144.

75. Criado FJ, Fairman RM, Becker GJ, et al: Talent LPS AAA stent graft: results of a pivotal clinical trial. J Vasc Surg 2003;37:709.

76. Prinssen M, Verhoeven EL, Buth J, et al: A randomized trial comparing conventional and endovascular repair of abdominal aortic aneurysms. N Engl J Med 2004;351:1607.

77. Adriaensen ME, Bosch JL, Halpern EF, et al: Elective endovascular versus open surgical repair of abdominal aortic aneurysms: systematic review of short-term results. Radiology 2002;224:739.

78. Greenhalgh RM, Brown LC, Kwong GP, et al: Comparison of endovascular aneurysm repair with open repair in patients with abdominal

aortic aneurysm (EVAR trial 1), 30-day operative mortality results: randomised controlled trial. Lancet 2004;364:843.

79. Erzurum VZ, Sampram ES, Sarac TP, et al: Initial management and outcome of aortic endograft limb occlusion. J Vasc Surg 2004;40:419.

80. Stavropoulos SW, Baum RA: Imaging modalities for the detection and management of endoleaks. Semin Vasc Surg 2004;17:154.

81. Armerding MD, Rubin GD, Beaulieu CF, et al: Aortic aneurysmal disease: assessment of stent-graft treatment—CT versus conventional angiography. Radiology 2000;215:138.

82. Veith FJ, Baum RA, Ohki T, et al: Nature and significance of endoleaks and endotension: summary of opinions expressed at an international conference. J Vasc Surg 2002;35:1029.

83. Baum RA, Stavropoulos SW, Fairman RM, et al: Endoleaks after endovascular repair of abdominal aortic aneurysms. J Vasc Interv Radiol 2003;14(Pt 1):1111.

84. Faries PL, Cadot H, Agarwal G, et al: Management of endoleak after endovascular aneurysm repair: cuffs, coils, and conversion. J Vasc Surg 2003;37:1155.

85. Baum RA, Carpenter JP, Stavropoulos SW, et al: Treatment of type 2 endoleaks after endovascular repair of abdominal aortic aneurysms: comparison of transarterial and translumbar techniques. J Vasc Surg 2002;35:23.

86. Baum RA, Cope C, Fairman RM, et al: Translumbar embolization of type 2 endoleaks after endovascular repair of abdominal aortic aneurysms. J Vasc Interv Radiol 2001;12:111.

87. Schwartz LB, Baldwin ZK, Curi MA: The changing face of abdominal aortic aneurysm management. Ann Surg 2003;238:S56.

88. Leriche R, Morel A: The syndrome of thrombotic obliteration of the aortic bifurcation. Ann Surg 1948;127:193.

89. Hirose H, Takagi M, Hashiyada H, et al: Acute occlusion of an abdominal aortic aneurysm—case report and review of the literature. Angiology 2000;51:515.

90. Tapper SS, Jenkins JM, Edwards WH, et al: Juxtarenal aortic occlusion. Ann Surg 1992;215:443.

91. Dossa CD, Shepard AD, Reddy DJ, et al: Acute aortic occlusion: a 40-year experience. Arch Surg 1994;129:603.

92. Patel H, Krishnamoorthy M, Dorazio RA, et al: Thrombosis of abdominal aortic aneurysms. Am Surgeon 1994;60:801.

93. Pilger E, Decrinis M, Stark G, et al: Thrombolytic treatment and balloon angioplasty in chronic occlusion of the aortic bifurcation. Ann Intern Med 1994;120:40.

94. Ballard JL, Taylor FC, Sparks SR, et al: Stenting without thrombolysis for aortoiliac occlusive disease: experience in 14 high-risk patients. Ann Vasc Surg 1995;9:453.

95. Nyman U, Uher P, Lindh M, et al: Primary stenting in infrarenal aortic occlusive disease. Cardiovasc Intervent Radiol 2000;23:97.

96. Farber A, Wagner WH, Cossman DV, et al: Isolated dissection of the abdominal aorta: clinical presentation and therapeutic options. J Vasc Surg 2002;36:205.

97. Naude GP, Back M, Perry MO, et al: Blunt disruption of the abdominal aorta: report of a case and review of the literature. J Vasc Surg 1997;25:931.

98. Demetriades D, Theodorou D, Murray J, et al: Mortality and prognostic factors in penetrating injuries of the aorta. J Trauma 1996;40:761.

99. Michaels AJ, Gerndt SJ, Taheri PA, et al: Blunt force injury of the abdominal aorta. J Trauma 1996;41:105.

100. Meghoo CA, Gonzalez EA, Tyroch AH, et al: Complete occlusion after blunt injury to the abdominal aorta. J Trauma 2003;55:795.

101. Davidovic LB, Kostic DM, Cvetkovic SD, et al: Aorto-caval fistulas. Cardiovasc Surg 2002;10:555.

102. Berthet JP, Marty-Ane CH, Veerapen R, et al: Dissection of the abdominal aorta in blunt trauma: endovascular or conventional surgical management? J Vasc Surg 2003;38:997.

103. Marin ML, Veith FJ, Panetta TF, et al: Transluminally placed endovascular stented graft repair for arterial trauma. J Vasc Surg 1994;20:466.

104. Fontaine AB, Nicholls SC, Borsa JJ, et al: Seat belt aorta: endovascular management with a stent-graft. J Endovasc Ther 2001;8:83.

105. Rasmussen TE, Hallett JW Jr: Inflammatory aortic aneurysms. A clinical review with new perspectives in pathogenesis. Ann Surg 1997;225:155.

106. Haug ES, Skomsvoll JF, Jacobsen G, et al: Inflammatory aortic aneurysm is associated with increased incidence of autoimmune disease. J Vasc Surg 2003;38:492.

107. Leseche G, Schaetz A, Arrive L, et al: Diagnosis and management of 17 consecutive patients with inflammatory abdominal aortic aneurysm. Am J Surg 1992;164:39.

108. Di Marzo L, Sapienza P, Bernucci P, et al: Inflammatory aneurysm of the abdominal aorta. A prospective clinical study. J Cardiovasc Surg (Torino) 1999;40:407.

109. Illig KA, Green RM: Diagnosis and management of the "difficult" abdominal aortic aneurysm: pararenal aneurysms, inflammatory aneurysms, and horseshoe kidney. Semin Vasc Surg 2001;14:312.

110. Tambyraja AL, Murie JA, Chalmers RT: Ruptured inflammatory abdominal aortic aneurysm: insights in clinical management and outcome. J Vasc Surg 2004;39:400.

111. Iino M, Kuribayashi S, Imakita S, et al: Sensitivity and specificity of CT in the diagnosis of inflammatory abdominal aortic aneurysms. J Comput Assist Tomogr 2002;26:1006.

112. Wallis F, Roditi GH, Redpath TW, et al: Inflammatory abdominal aortic aneurysms: diagnosis with gadolinium enhanced T1-weighted imaging. Clin Radiol 2000;55:136.

113. Tennant WG, Hartnell GG, Baird RN, et al: Radiologic investigation of abdominal aortic aneurysm disease: comparison of three modalities in staging and the detection of inflammatory change. J Vasc Surg 1993;17:703.

114. Chan FY, Crawford ES, Coselli JS, et al: In situ prosthetic graft replacement for mycotic aneurysm of the aorta. Ann Thorac Surg 1989;47:193.

115. Macedo TA, Stanson AW, Oderich GS, et al: Infected aortic aneurysms: imaging findings. Radiology 2004;231:250.

116. Muller BT, Wegener OR, Grabitz K, et al: Mycotic aneurysms of the thoracic and abdominal aorta and iliac arteries: experience with anatomic and extra-anatomic repair in 33 cases. J Vasc Surg 2001;33:106.

117. Koeppel TA, Gahlen J, Diehl S, et al: Mycotic aneurysm of the abdominal aorta with retroperitoneal abscess: successful endovascular repair. J Vasc Surg 2004;40:164.

118. Matsunaga N, Hayashi K, Sakamoto I, et al: Takayasu arteritis: protean radiologic manifestations and diagnosis. Radiographics 1997;17:579.

119. Choe YH, Han B-K, Koh E-M, et al: Takayasu's arteritis: assessment of disease activity with contrast-enhanced MR imaging. AJR Am J Roentgenol 2000;175:505.

120. Mandalam KR, Joseph S, Rao VRK, et al: Aortoarteritis of abdominal aorta: an angiographic profile in 110 patients. Clin Radiol 1993;48:29.

121. Chuang VP: Radiation-induced arteritis. Semin Roentgenol 1994;29:64.

122. Israel G, Krinsky G, Lee V: The "skinny aorta." Clin Imaging 2002; 26:116.

123. Chetty R, Batitang S, Nair R: Large artery vasculopathy in HIV-positive patients: another vasculitic enigma. Hum Pathol 2000;31:374.

124. Criado E, Izquierdo L, Lujan S, et al: Abdominal aortic coarctation, renovascular, hypertension, and neurofibromatosis. Ann Vasc Surg 2002;16:363.

125. Welch TJ, McKusick MA: Cardiovascular case of the day: case 1: abdominal coarctation due to neurofibromatosis. AJR Am J Roentgenol 1993;160:1313.

126. Connolly JE, Wilson SE, Lawrence PL, et al: Middle aortic syndrome: distal thoracic and abdominal coarctation, a disorder with multiple etiologies. J Am Coll Surg 2002;194:774.

127. Flynn PM, Robinson MB, Stapleton FB, et al: Coarctation of the aorta and renal artery stenosis in tuberous sclerosis. Pediatric Radiol 1984;14:337.

128. Siwik ES, Perry SB, Lock JE: Endovascular stent implantation in patients with stenotic aortoarteriopathies: early and medium-term results. Catheter Cardiovasc Interv 2003;59:380.

129. Brzezinska-Rajszys G, Qureshi SA, Ksiazyk J, et al: Middle aortic syndrome treated by stent implantation. Heart 1999;81:166.

6

Pelvic and Lower Extremity Arteries

ARTERIOGRAPHY

Pelvic arteriography is performed from common femoral artery access with a pigtail or similarly shaped catheter placed at the aortic bifurcation. Even with diminished or absent femoral pulses, catheterization is sometimes possible using real-time ultrasound guidance and a steerable hydrophilic guidewire. A retrograde high brachial artery (or very rarely, translumbar) puncture is made if femoral access is not possible. Some interventionalists prefer the brachial route in patients who have suffered cholesterol embolization during prior retrograde femoral artery catheterization procedures. Axillofemoral grafts can be evaluated by directly puncturing the graft as it passes over the ribs.

When an iliac artery is occluded, multiple ipsilateral lumbar arteries can serve as major collaterals into the pelvis; in this situation, the catheter side holes are positioned slightly below the renal arteries to opacify these vessels. In patients with peripheral vascular disease (PVD), bilateral, 25- to 30-degree oblique pelvic arteriograms often are needed to thoroughly assess iliac artery disease and to lay out the iliac and femoral artery bifurcations. The **left** posterior oblique projection opens the left iliac and right femoral bifurcations; the **right** posterior oblique projection opens the opposite bifurcations.

Bilateral lower extremity arteriography ("run-off" study) is done with the pigtail just above the aortic bifurcation. Serial images are obtained down to the feet. If only one leg needs to be examined, it is usual practice to catheterize the contralateral groin and direct a cobra or similarly shaped catheter over the aortic bifurcation (see Chapter 2). If a pigtail catheter is already in place, it can be gently unwound on the bifurcation and replaced with a straight catheter (see Fig. 2-22). A long, reverse-curve catheter simplifies entry into internal iliac artery branches (see Fig. 2-21).

When the tibial or pedal arteries are poorly seen on the initial angiogram, they often are better seen by advancing a catheter into the superficial femoral artery and first injecting an intra-arterial vasodilator (e.g., 100 to 200 µg of nitroglycerin). In patients with a history of severe contrast allergy or renal insufficiency, alternative noninvasive imaging should be attempted. If catheter angiography is required prior to treatment, both gadolinium-based agents and carbon dioxide can be used exclusively, or they can be supplemented with small volumes of iodinated contrast (see Chapter 2).[1-4]

ANATOMY

Development

In the embryo, the lower extremities are supplied by the axial artery, which arises from the sciatic branch of the internal iliac artery.[5] This vessel ends in a plantar network in the developing foot. The femoral artery, which runs along the ventral aspect of the limb, is the continuation of the external iliac artery; it joins the axial artery at the knee to form the popliteal artery. The posterior tibial and peroneal arteries originate from the axial artery below the knee and run along the dorsal aspect of the calf. The anterior tibial artery takes off from the lower popliteal artery and courses along the ventral aspect of the calf. The superficial femoral artery eventually becomes the dominant vessel to the lower leg. The deep femoral artery arises near the bottom of the femoral head. Most of the axial artery regresses before birth; normally, the only remnants are portions of the inferior gluteal, popliteal, and peroneal arteries.

Normal Anatomy

The abdominal aorta divides into the *common iliac arteries* at the L4-L5 level (Figs. 6-1A and 6-2).[6] The common iliac arteries lie in front of the iliac veins and the inferior vena cava. They usually have no major branches; rarely, they give off aberrant iliolumbar or accessory renal arteries.

127

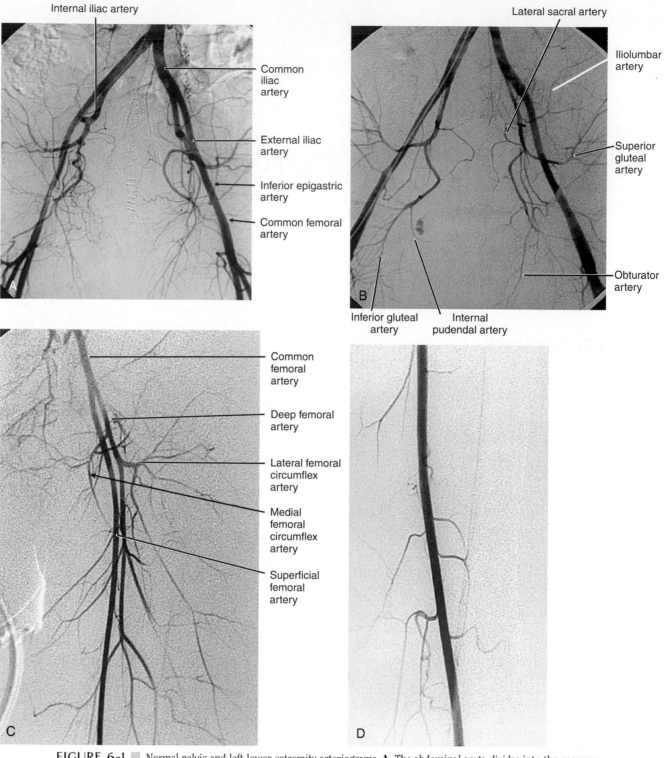

FIGURE 6-1 ■ Normal pelvic and left lower extremity arteriograms. **A,** The abdominal aorta divides into the common iliac arteries at the L4-L5 level. **B,** The branching pattern of the internal iliac artery varies. **C,** The common femoral artery divides into the superficial femoral artery (SFA) and deep femoral artery near the bottom of the femoral head. **D,** The SFA passes down the anteromedial aspect of the thigh, dives into the flexor muscle compartment, and runs through the adductor (Hunter's) canal.

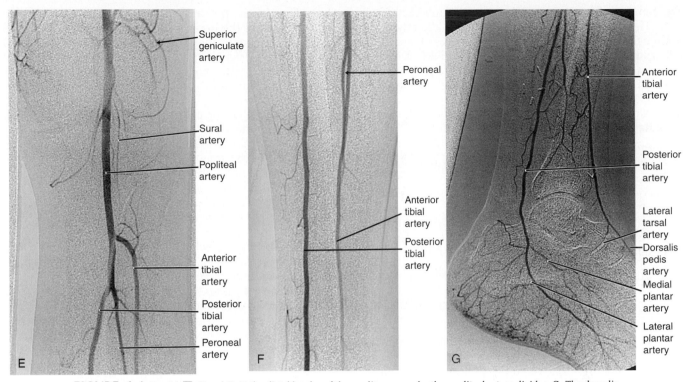

FIGURE 6-1 *Cont'd* ■ **E** and **F,** At the distal border of the popliteus muscle, the popliteal artery divides. **G,** The dorsalis pedis artery gives off medial and lateral tarsal branches. The posterior tibial artery gives off medial and lateral plantar branches.

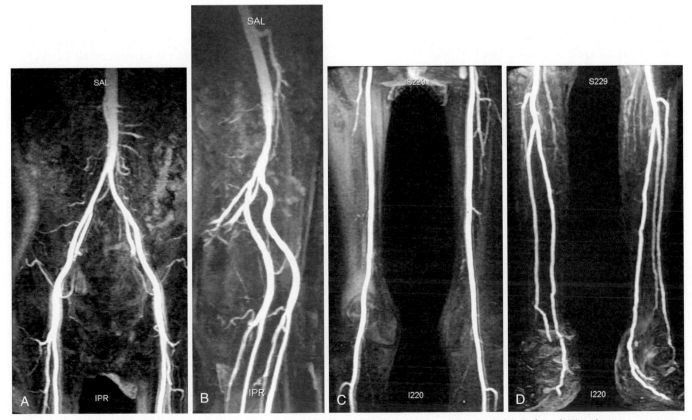

FIGURE 6-2 ■ Pelvic and lower extremity maximum intensity projection MR angiogram. Pelvis in frontal (**A**) and near lateral (**B**) views. Thigh (**C**) and calf (**D**) in frontal view. The right anterior tibial artery is occluded in the upper calf.

The common iliac artery divides near the lumbosacral junction. The *external iliac artery* continues directly to the groin behind the inguinal ligament. This vessel also has no major branches. The *internal iliac artery* takes off medially and posteriorly. At the superior edge of the greater sciatic foramen, it usually divides into anterior and posterior trunks. The branching pattern of the internal iliac artery is quite variable (Fig. 6-1B). Classically, the major branches of the **anterior division** are the

- *Obturator artery*
- *Internal pudendal artery,* which supplies the external genitalia and rectum (see Fig. 11-13)
- *Inferior gluteal artery,* which nourishes muscles of the thigh and buttocks and the sciatic nerve
- *Visceral arteries,* which supply the bladder, rectum, and uterus or prostate through the superior and inferior vesicular, middle rectal, and uterine or prostatic arteries (see Fig. 11-17). They may be hard to identify on a routine pelvic arteriogram.

The major branches of the **posterior division** of the internal iliac artery are the

- *Iliolumbar artery,* which takes off **laterally** to supply the lumbar muscles
- *Lateral sacral artery,* which takes off **medially** toward the sacral foramina
- *Superior gluteal artery,* which is the largest branch of the division and feeds the gluteal muscles

At the junction of the external iliac and common femoral arteries (which corresponds to the inguinal ligament), the inferior epigastric artery arises medially (see Fig. 2-1). It runs alongside the rectus abdominis muscle before communicating with the superior epigastric branch of the internal thoracic (mammary) artery. The deep iliac circumflex artery takes off laterally and superiorly (see Fig. 2-3).

The *common femoral artery* (CFA) courses over the femoral head encased in the femoral sheath along with the femoral vein (medial or posteromedial) and the femoral nerve (lateral). Branches of the CFA include the superficial epigastric artery, superficial circumflex iliac artery (laterally), and external pudendal artery (medially); all of these are inconsistently seen by angiography.

The CFA divides into the *superficial femoral artery* (SFA) and *deep femoral artery* (DFA) or *profunda femoris artery* near the bottom of the femoral head (Fig. 6-1C). A "high" bifurcation is occasionally seen. The DFA takes off laterally and posteriorly. Its major branches are the lateral circumflex femoral, medial circumflex femoral, and four or so pairs of perforating arteries.

The SFA passes down the anteromedial aspect of the thigh, dives into the flexor muscle compartment, and runs through the adductor (Hunter's) canal (Fig. 6-1D). The SFA then becomes the *popliteal artery,* which lies posterior to the femur (surrounded by the heads of the gastrocnemius muscle) and deep to the popliteal vein. Its major muscular branches are the sural arteries and paired superior, middle, and inferior geniculate arteries, all of which form an anastomotic network around the knee.

At the distal border of the popliteus muscle, the popliteal artery divides. The *anterior tibial artery* arises laterally, pierces the interosseous membrane, and then runs in front of the lower tibia (Fig. 6-1E and F). It passes over the ankle onto the dorsum of the foot to become the *dorsalis pedis artery.* The *tibioperoneal trunk* is the direct continuation of the popliteal artery and bifurcates just beyond its origin into the posterior tibial and peroneal arteries. The *posterior tibial artery* runs posteriorly and medially in the flexor compartment. *The peroneal artery* runs between the posterior and anterior tibial arteries near the fibula. It is a small-caliber vessel unless functioning as a collateral in the face of tibial artery obstruction. In the distal calf, its perforating and communicating branches may join the anterior and posterior tibial arteries, respectively. Above the ankle, the artery divides into two calcaneal branches ("fish tail") that have anastomoses with the distal tibial arteries.

A network of malleolar arteries interconnect the tibial arteries above the ankle.[7] The dorsalis pedis artery gives off *medial* and *lateral tarsal branches* (Fig. 6-1G). The posterior tibial artery passes behind the medial malleolus, where it divides into *medial* and *lateral plantar arteries.* The plantar arch is formed by the dominant lateral plantar branch of the posterior tibial artery and the distal dorsalis pedis artery. Smaller secondary arches are created by other branches of the distal tibial arteries. Metatarsal arteries arise primarily from the plantar arch.

Variant Anatomy

The most commonly observed branching variations of the internal iliac artery involve anomalous origin of a major muscular branch (e.g., obturator, inferior gluteal, or superior gluteal artery) from another major branch of either division.

The *persistent sciatic artery* is a rare anomaly (about 0.1% of the population) in which the embryologic sciatic artery remains the dominant inflow vessel to the leg.[8,9] The aberrant vessel comes off the internal iliac artery, passes through the greater sciatic foramen, and lies deep to the gluteus maximus muscle (Fig. 6-3). Above the knee, it joins the popliteal artery. The SFA usually is hypoplastic or absent. The anomaly is occasionally bilateral. Because of its relatively superficial location in the ischial region, the sciatic artery is prone to intimal injury or aneurysm formation.

Very rare femoral artery variants include the *saphenous artery* and *duplication of the SFA.* Anomalies of the DFA are common, including a posterior or even medial origin of the main DFA trunk and separate origins of the medial and lateral circumflex femoral branches.[10]

Tibial artery anomalies are present in about 3% to 10% of the population.[11-13] The variants often are bilateral. The most common anomalies are high bifurcation or true trifurcation of the popliteal artery, common origin of the anterior tibial and peroneal arteries, and hypoplasia or absence of the anterior or posterior tibial artery (Fig. 6-4). In the last case, the artery is normal at its origin but gradually tapers in the mid- to distal calf without discrete termination. A major branch of the peroneal artery often reforms the absent vessel above the ankle, resulting in normal pedal pulses.

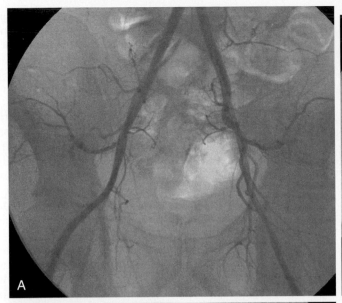

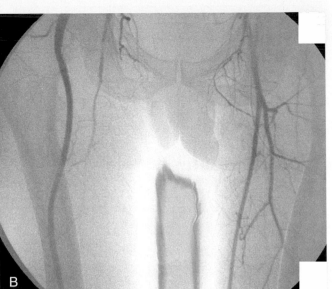

FIGURE 6-3 ■ Persistent right sciatic artery. **A,** The anomalous vessel arises from the internal iliac artery and passes through the greater sciatic foramen. The vessel continues down the leg behind the femur (**B**) and later joins the normal popliteal artery (**C**). The superficial femoral artery fills in a retrograde fashion due to proximal obstruction.

Collateral Circulation

The pelvis and lower extremities have rich and complex systems of collateral circulation that maintain blood flow to the leg when proximal arteries are obstructed. The major routes are formed by branches of the internal iliac, deep femoral, and popliteal arteries (Fig. 6-5):

■ Common iliac artery obstruction: ipsilateral lumbar or contralateral lateral sacral branches to the deep iliac circumflex or the internal iliac artery (allowing retrograde flow into the external iliac artery)
■ Internal iliac artery obstruction: inferior mesenteric artery to the inferior gluteal branches through the rectal network, lumbar to the iliolumbar arteries, DFA to the gluteal arteries through femoral circumflex branches
■ External iliac artery obstruction: posterior division of the internal iliac artery branches to the CFA through the deep iliac circumflex artery, anterior division of the internal iliac artery branches to circumflex femoral branches of DFA, transpelvic collaterals
■ SFA obstruction: Collaterals depend on the site and length of the obstruction. The DFA is the main conduit to the lower leg, with lateral femoral circumflex and perforating branches supplying branches of the distal SFA and popliteal arteries.
■ DFA obstruction: internal iliac artery branches to medial and lateral circumflex femoral branches of the DFA

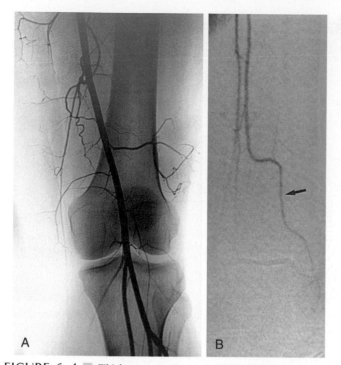

FIGURE 6-4 ■ Tibial artery variants. **A,** High bifurcation of the popliteal artery, with common origin of the anterior tibial and peroneal arteries. **B,** Absence of the right posterior tibial artery, which is reformed distally by a congenitally enlarged branch of the peroneal artery *(arrow)*.

- Popliteal artery obstruction: geniculate and sural collateral network
- Tibial artery obstruction: The peroneal artery is the principal collateral channel with anterior or posterior tibial artery obstruction.

■ MAJOR DISORDERS

Chronic Lower Extremity Ischemia

Etiology

Obstructive disease of the pelvic and lower extremity arteries is one of the most frequent clinical problems encountered by interventionalists. A variety of disorders is responsible for lower extremity PVD (Box 6-1). However, the vast majority of cases result from atherosclerotic stenoses, superimposed thrombosis, or embolism. The cardinal feature is that blood flow to the pelvis or legs is significantly reduced with exercise or at rest.

By a wide margin, atherosclerosis is the most common disease affecting the lower extremity arteries. Smoking and diabetes are the biggest risk factors, followed by long-standing hypertension and lipid disorders (Box 6-2).[14,15] The pathophysiology of atherosclerosis and the emerging significance of certain inflammatory markers in progression and response to treatment are discussed in Chapter 3.[14,16]

Atherosclerosis is typically diffuse and bilateral. There is a predilection for clinically significant disease in the distal aorta, common and external iliac arteries, distal SFA, and tibial arteries. The frequency of disease as the SFA passes through the adductor canal may be related to constant flow turbulence caused by extrinsic compression from the adductor magnus muscle and fascia at this site.[17] Atherosclerotic plaques cause symptoms by impeding blood flow to the leg, inducing thrombotic occlusion, or through embolization of clot or plaque fragments.

Diabetes produces intimal atherosclerotic obstructions and medial calcification (i.e., Mönckeberg's medial sclerosis). Extensive tibial and pedal artery disease is characteristic; the aortoiliac and femoropopliteal segments are relatively spared. Arterial obstructions tend to be more severe than in patients with atherosclerosis, and the collateral circulation often is less effective. For these reasons, nonhealing ulcers, gangrene, and amputation are more common in this population.

Macroemboli usually are thrombi that originate from the heart. In fewer than 25% of cases, clot or plaque fragments break off from aneurysms or atherosclerotic surfaces in the proximal arteries.[18] Emboli usually lodge at branch points or sites of underlying disease. *Microemboli* are composed of platelet-fibrin deposits or cholesterol crystals arising from atherosclerotic plaques or aneurysms. These particles may be released spontaneously or during operative manipulation or catheterization. Microemboli can lead to "blue toe syndrome" or an acute cholesterol embolization event (see Chapter 3).

Clinical Features

At least 50% of patients with PVD are asymptomatic or have atypical symptoms; only 10% or so will ultimately develop chronic limb ischemia at rest.[14] Chronic peripheral arterial occlusive disease is unusual before age 40. Men are affected more frequently than women. Most patients have one or more risk factors for disease (see Box 6-2).

Sometimes, the initial symptom is *intermittent claudication,* which is characterized by predictable and reproducible muscle pain or fatigue with exercise (especially walking on an incline) that is invariably relieved by rest. The pain does not resolve with continued leg exercise. Symptoms are felt in the calf, thigh, or buttock and correspond to some extent with the level of arterial obstruction. Unfortunately, a variety of disorders (including musculoskeletal and neurologic disorders [e.g., spinal stenosis] and chronic compartment syndrome) often is confused with true claudication.[19,20]

With progression of disease (and in a minority of patients), the collateral circulation may become insufficient to prevent muscle ischemia even at rest despite maximum peripheral vasodilation. *Rest pain,* which affects the **foot,** is made worse with leg elevation and is relieved with dependency (such as dangling the limb off a bed). As the obstructions become more severe, ischemic ulcers often develop at sites of skin breakdown, particularly in diabetic patients with peripheral neuropathy. Gangrene may set in and ultimately require amputation. The severity of chronic limb ischemia often is graded according to the scale of Rutherford and Becker (Table 6-1).[21]

Physical signs include dependent rubor, leg coolness, delayed capillary refill (>1 second), and trophic changes

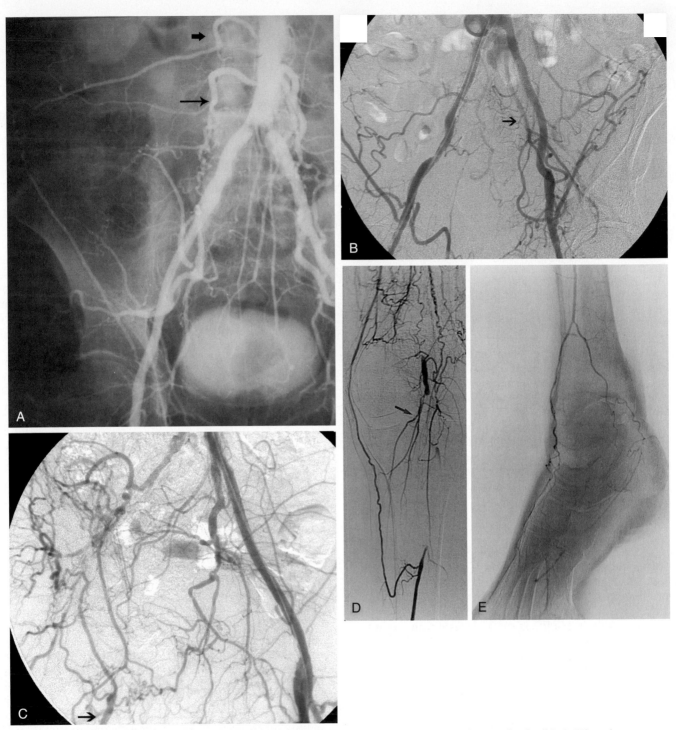

FIGURE 6-5 ■ Collateral patterns in cases of lower extremity arterial obstructions (see text for details). **A,** Bilateral common iliac artery obstructions. The enlarged 3rd lumbar artery *(short arrow)* feeds the deep iliac circumflex artery. The enlarged 4th lumbar artery *(long arrow)* supplies branches of the right internal iliac artery. **B,** Bilateral internal iliac artery occlusions. In addition to distal external iliac/common femoral collaterals, the enlarged inferior mesenteric artery *(arrow)* contributes to internal iliac artery branches. **C,** Right external iliac artery occlusion with reconstitution of the proximal deep femoral artery *(arrow).* **D,** Left femoropopliteal and proximal tibial artery occlusions. Deep femoral branches reconstitute a short segment of the mid-popliteal artery, which supplies sural collaterals *(arrow)* into the calf. The posterior tibial artery is reconstituted in the mid-calf. **E,** Posterior and anterior tibial artery occlusion, with the peroneal artery reconstituting the distal vessels in the foot.

TABLE 6-1   RUTHERFORD-BECKER CLASSIFICATION OF PERIPHERAL VASCULAR DISEASE

Grade	Category	Symptoms
0	0	None
I	1	Mild claudication
I	2	Moderate claudication
I	3	Severe (lifestyle-limiting) claudication
II	4	Rest pain
III	5	Nonhealing ulcers, focal gangrene
III	6	Major tissue loss

(e.g., hair loss over the lower legs, thin shiny skin, nail thickening). With advanced PVD, ulcers and gangrenous changes occur. The peripheral pulses (i.e., femoral, popliteal, dorsal pedis, and posterior tibial) usually reflect the severity and location of disease. Nonpalpable peripheral pulses should be examined with a Doppler probe. A venous signal may be pulsatile but vanishes with compression by the transducer.

Patients with *blue toe syndrome* complain of relatively acute onset of painful, bluish-colored toes on one or both feet.[22] The symptoms often resolve but may recur and occasionally lead to tissue loss. The peripheral pulses often are intact.

Natural History

PVD is a remarkably slowly progressive disease. More than 50% of patients show no worsening of initial symptoms; no more than about 10% require revascularization within 5 years of presentation.[14] However, atherosclerosis is a systemic vascular disease, and this population has a high risk of mortality after the diagnosis of PVD is made, largely from coronary artery disease or stroke (i.e., 30% at 5 years, 50% at 10 years).[14] Almost every patient who suffers from severe limb ischemia (rest pain or gangrene) is dead within a decade.

Noninvasive Testing

Noninvasive vascular studies are employed to confirm the diagnosis of PVD in patients with equivocal history or physical findings, to determine the severity and level of obstructions, to follow the progression of disease, and to monitor surgical and percutaneous therapy. The most commonly used tests are segmental blood pressure measurements and plethysmography (pulse-volume recording).

To obtain *segmental blood pressures*, cuffs are sequentially inflated around the upper thigh, lower thigh, calf, ankle, and toe. The systolic pressure at each location is divided by the systolic brachial arterial pressure to yield an index (e.g., *ankle-brachial index* [ABI]). Several sets of guidelines have been established to interpret these indexes.[14,23,24] The ankle-brachial index is highly accurate (>95%) in detection of PVD.[14] It should correlate with the diagnosis and staging of disease:

- Greater than 1.4: noncompressible vessels, likely to have significant PVD
- 0.91 to 1.3: no significant obstructive disease
- 0.41 to 0.90: claudication (grade I)
- Less than 0.40: limb-threatening ischemia (grade II or III)

A drop of 20 to 30 mm Hg between levels (or comparing legs at the same level) indicates a significant stenosis or occlusion (Fig. 6-6A). Abnormal values at the upper thigh, lower thigh, calf, and ankle reflect obstructions in the aortoiliac segments, SFA, femoropopliteal segment, and tibial arteries, respectively (Fig. 6-6B). However, the correlation is not always precise; for example, proximal femoral artery disease can mimic aortoiliac disease.

Calcified or noncompressible arteries (as found in patients with diabetes or chronic renal failure) falsely elevate pressure measurements and can lead to underestimation of disease severity. In these cases, toe pressure measurements are more accurate. The toe index is normally greater than 0.60. An absolute toe pressure of greater than 30 mm Hg is generally required for wound healing.

Segmental pressure measurements after exercise can detect occult disease in patients with suggestive symptoms and a normal study at rest (Fig. 6-6C). While walking on an inclined treadmill, ankle and brachial pressure measurements are periodically recorded. A fall in ankle pressure is diagnostic of obstructive arterial disease.

Plethysmography employs changes in leg volume to reflect overall perfusion of the limb.[23] With mild or moderate PVD, digital or segmental pulse volume tracings are

FIGURE 6-6 ■ Segmental blood pressure measurements. **A,** Abnormal left upper thigh index (0.88) in a patient with left leg claudication. The angiogram showed a tight left common iliac artery stenosis. **B,** Bilateral drop in lower thigh pressures in a patient with bilateral leg claudication. Notice dampening of the normal waveform at this level. Angiography showed bilateral occlusions of the superficial femoral arteries. **C,** After exercise, the ankle pressures dropped abnormally in a patient with bilateral calf claudication and normal resting segmental pressures. The angiogram demonstrated bilateral tibial artery disease.

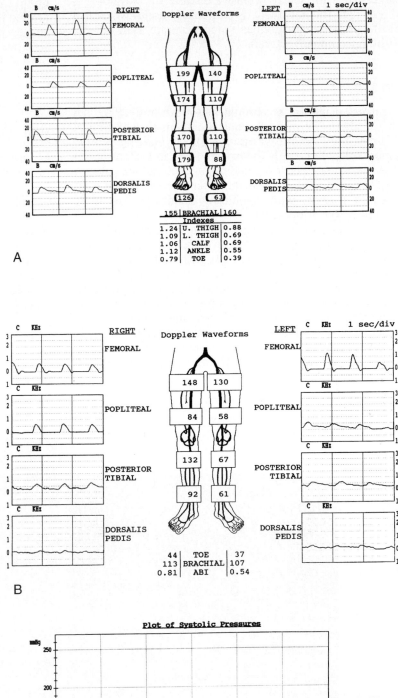

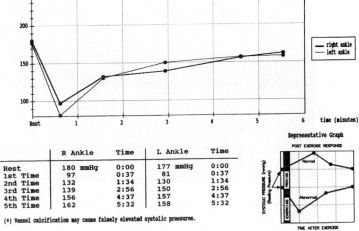

dampened; with severe occlusive disease, the waveform is almost flat. This technique is particularly useful when segmental pressure measurements are inaccurate, as in patients with noncompliant arteries.

Imaging

A correct diagnosis of chronic lower extremity PVD can almost always be made through a combination of clinical findings and noninvasive testing. Direct imaging is used almost solely to identify the nature, sites, and extent of disease in patients whose symptoms warrant endovascular or surgical treatment. In general, intervention is only indicated in patients with significant claudication or more severe degrees of ischemia.

Atherosclerosis is typically diffuse, bilateral, and often strikingly symmetric. Patients with claudication usually have single-level disease; patients with rest pain or more severe ischemia have multilevel disease. Clinically relevant lesions includes hemodynamically significant stenoses (as measured by pressure gradients or luminal diameter reduction of >50%), diffuse long-segment atherosclerosis, thrombotic occlusions, and ulcerated or exophytic plaques. Plaques may be characterized as focal or long, calcified or noncalcified, concentric or eccentric, and smooth or ulcerated.

Color Doppler Sonography. Color Doppler sonography is favored in some laboratories for arterial mapping to depict and grade arterial stenoses and occlusions. The technique is sensitive ($\approx$80% to 90%) and quite specific ($\approx$95%).[23] The normal Doppler spectral pattern in these high-resistance arteries is triphasic, with rapid forward flow in systole followed by brief reversal of flow in early diastole. Peak systolic (and sometimes end-diastolic) velocities are more than doubled at sites of significant stenosis. The waveform is dampened downstream from an obstruction.

Magnetic Resonance Angiography. MR angiography has revolutionized the evaluation of patients with PVD.[25,26] When properly performed, these studies can provide images almost comparable in quality and form to conventional catheter angiography with none of the associated risks (see Fig. 6-2). The sensitivity and specificity of state-of-the-art MR angiography approaches or exceeds 95% (Figs. 6-7 and 6-8).[26-29]

MR angiography is clearly advantageous for patients with a history of anaphylactic reaction to iodinated contrast material or preexisting renal insufficiency. MR angiography is obviously contraindicated in certain groups (e.g., those with pacemakers, intracranial clips, severe claustrophobia). Each institution must develop its own protocol for routine imaging of patients with PVD, and software and hardware are constantly evolving. Currently, many centers do the entire

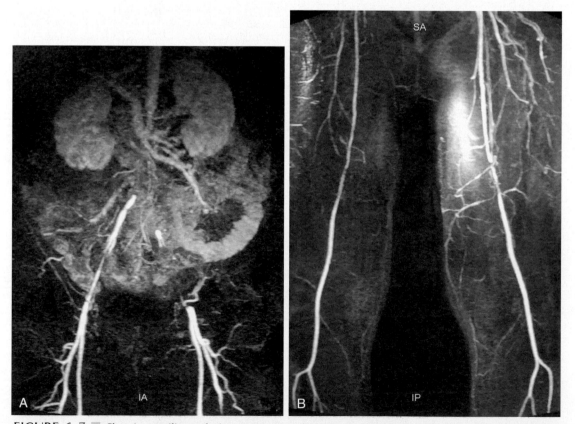

FIGURE 6-7 ■ Chronic aortoiliac occlusion on maximum intensity projection MR angiogram of the pelvis (**A**) and thigh (**B**). There is complete occlusion of the distal aorta, proximal right common iliac artery, and left common and external iliac arteries. The right external iliac artery is diseased. Diffuse right superficial femoral artery (SFA) disease with a tight mid left SFA stenosis is present.

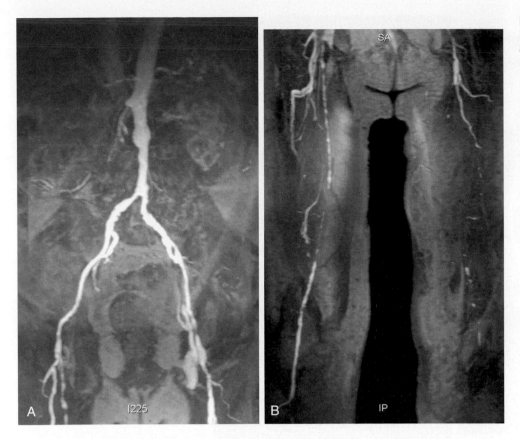

FIGURE 6-8 ■ Acute occlusion of left deep femoral to below knee popliteal artery bypass graft. History of a right nephrectomy and left renal artery stent (**A**). MR angiogram shows a small infrarenal abdominal aortic aneurysm. The right renal artery is occluded. The proximal left renal artery is obscured by the stent. Proximal portions of both common iliac arteries are stenotic. **B,** The bypass graft is thrombosed; a stenosis is seen in the left common femoral artery. The right superficial femoral artery (SFA) is diffusely diseased, and the left SFA is occluded.

examination with time-resolved two-dimensional (2-D) MR angiography from the knees to the feet (to minimize venous contamination), followed by three-dimensional (3-D) bolus-chase (three station) MR angiography.[30,31] The gadolinium injections and imaging acquisitions are coordinated such that the imaging interval is centered around the time of peak gadolinium concentration. Initial unenhanced 2-D time-of-flight acquisitions can be helpful in evaluating the calf and pedal vessels, but add substantial time to the exam.

In addition to inspecting the maximum intensity projections in multiple planes, it is crucial to review source data to confirm findings. Box 6-3 explains some of the potential artifacts with 2-D time-of-flight and gadolinium-enhanced 3-D MR angiography (see Fig. 6-8).[32,33]

Computed Tomographic Angiography. The development of multidetector helical CT scanners has now made this modality an important tool in evaluation of a wide variety of vascular diseases, including PVD (Fig. 6-9). These scanners produce images with extremely high resolution, require less contrast material, and allow rapid imaging.[34,35] Settings vary with the equipment and manufacturer. A typical protocol for a 16-channel scanner would be 0.625 to 1.25 mm cuts, with pitch of 1.75, and overlap every 0.5 to 0.8 mm. Total contrast volume is about 175 mL.

The sensitivity and specificity with state-of-the-art technology is about 95% compared with catheter digital angiography.[36-40] The major pitfalls of CT angiography for PVD include pulsation artifacts (which are minimized with cardiac gating), contrast bolus mistiming, calcified vessels, and the presence of metallic objects (e.g., stents, coils) (Fig. 6-10).

Angiography. Catheter arteriography remains the gold standard for evaluation of patients with symptomatic PVD. In practice, however, it is only requested when endovascular revascularization is being contemplated or when the results of noninvasive vascular imaging is equivocal. The procedure includes the following components:

■ Abdominal aortography
■ Bilateral lower extremity run-off study (Fig. 6-11)

BOX 6-3 ■ Artifacts with Magnetic Resonance Imaging in Peripheral Vascular Disease

Gadolinium-Enhanced Magnetic Resonance Angiography
Overestimation of stenoses
Motion artifact
Signal loss due to calcium and metallic objects
Venous contamination

Two-Dimensional Time-of-Flight Imaging
In-plane flow due to proton saturation
Turbulent flow due to dephasing of proton spins
Reverse flow (e.g., arterial loops and reconstituted arteries from the inferior saturation band)
"Venetian blind" effect from diastolic reversal of flow
"Stair stepping" in arteries running in an oblique plane
Pulsatility ghosts from phase decoding
Patient or bowel motion
Magnetic susceptibility artifacts (prosthetic joint, stents, clips)

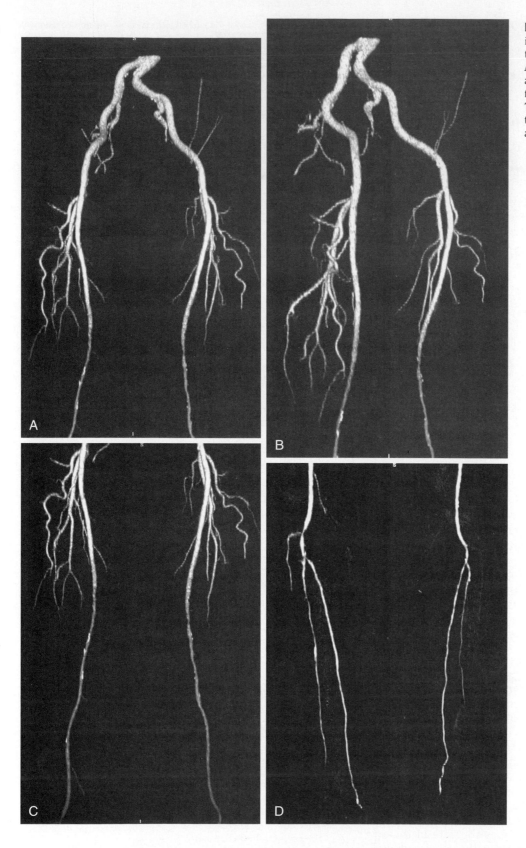

FIGURE 6-9 ■ Pelvic and extremity arteries at CT angiography, including the pelvis (**A** and **B**), thigh (**C**), and calf (**D**). A kink is noted in the left common iliac artery. Diffuse bilateral mid–superficial femoral artery (SFA) disease is present. There are right distal popliteal and tibioperoneal trunk stenoses. Neither anterior tibial artery is opacified.

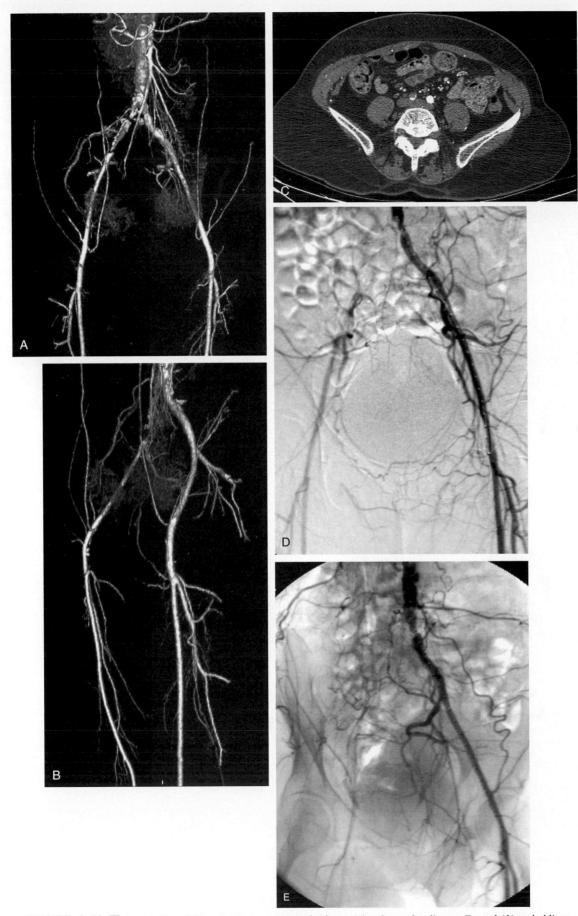

FIGURE 6-10 ■ Correlation of CT and catheter angiography for peripheral vascular disease. Frontal (**A**) and oblique (**B**) shaded surface display CT reconstructions suggest complete right common iliac artery occlusion and moderate left common iliac artery stenosis. The former is confirmed on review of axial images (**C**). Note that significant calcification partially obscures the occlusion on reformatted images. The findings were confirmed on a catheter angiogram in frontal (**D**) and left posterior oblique (**E**) projections.

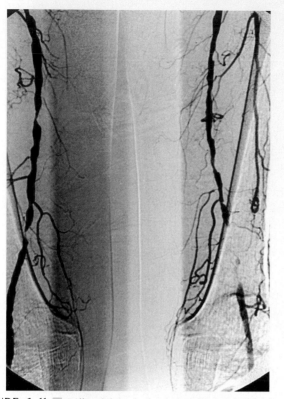

FIGURE 6-11 ▓ Diffuse bilateral atherosclerosis of superficial femoral arteries and short occlusion of the distal left SFA.

- Bilateral oblique pelvic arteriography
- Selective arteriography (sometimes in multiple projections or after intra-arterial vasodilator injection) to evaluate equivocal findings
- Measurement of pressure gradients in the aorta and iliac arteries to determine the significance of moderate or suspicious stenoses (>5 to 10 mm Hg systolic)

If the angiogram is performed through the CFA on the less symptomatic leg, groin complications do not interfere with surgical bypass procedures, catheter occlusion of a stenotic iliac artery is less likely, and antegrade puncture can be performed on the affected leg. On the other hand, immediate access to iliac artery stenoses is available if the angiogram is performed on the side with diminished femoral pulses.

Visualization of the arterial supply to the foot is mandatory because current vascular surgical techniques allow bypass to the pedal arteries. Measurement of aortoiliac pressure gradients after vasodilator injection is particularly important in patients with claudication or before infrainguinal bypass graft placement (Fig. 6-12). The drop in peripheral vascular resistance and resulting increase in flow that occurs with exercise or after graft placement increase the significance of proximal stenoses (see Chapter 2).

Certain points in the interpretation of lower extremity run-off studies are important:

- The only sign of an eccentric plaque along the posterior or anterior wall of an artery may be a relative dilution of the contrast column. Multiple projections or pressure gradients often are required to outline such lesions (Fig. 6-13).

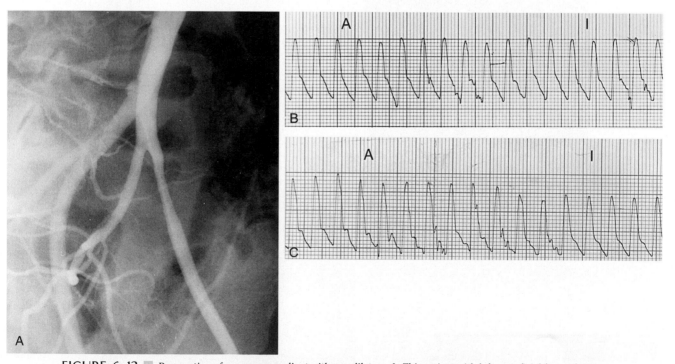

FIGURE 6-12 ▓ Provocation of a pressure gradient with vasodilators. **A,** This patient with left superficial femoral artery occlusion and a moderate left external iliac artery stenosis is about to undergo infrainguinal bypass graft placement. **B,** No pressure gradient was found between the aorta (A) and external iliac artery (I) with the initial pullback method. **C,** After intra-arterial injection of 25 mg of tolazoline, the repeat pullback pressure measurement showed a systolic gradient of 20 mm Hg that warranted treatment.

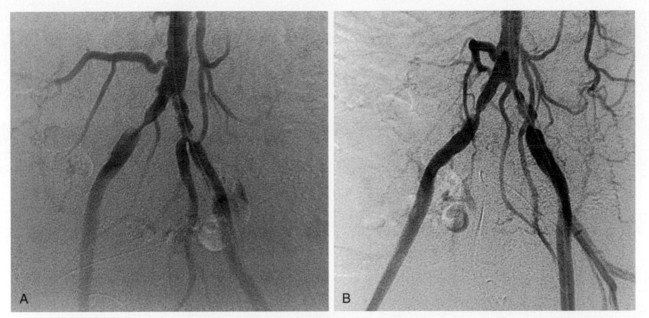

FIGURE 6-13 ■ Eccentric atherosclerotic plaque. **A,** The left posterior oblique pelvic arteriogram shows right iliac stenosis and only moderate disease of the left common iliac artery. Note the enlarged right lumbar artery indicating the significance of the right-sided disease. **B,** The right posterior oblique projection shows the true severity of the left-sided disease.

■ Uncalcified aneurysms may go undetected if the lumen is lined with thrombus or the aneurysm is completely thrombosed (Fig. 6-14).

■ The length of an occlusion can be overestimated if collateral backfilling of the patent segment of the artery is not followed on delayed images.

■ In addition to thrombotic occlusion, nonopacification of arteries can result from inadequate filling (especially

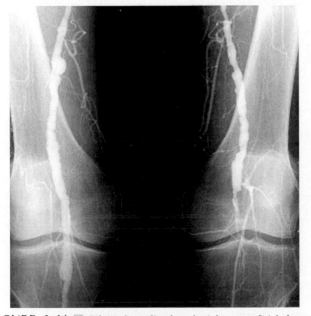

FIGURE 6-14 ■ Bilateral popliteal and right superficial femoral artery aneurysms. Dilation of the right popliteal artery is hidden by mural thrombus. The left popliteal artery aneurysm is completely occluded.

the tibial and pedal arteries) or congenital absence (see Fig. 6-4). Visualization of distal tibial vessels may be improved with selective studies after intra-arterial vasodilator injection (Fig. 6-15).

■ Luminal filling defects may be caused by emboli, in situ thrombosis, inflow defects (unopacified blood entering the contrast column), plaques seen en face, or dissection flaps (Fig. 6-16; see also Figs. 3-12, 3-14, and 3-15).

■ Occasionally, luminal narrowing has other causes than atherosclerosis (Box 6-4 and Fig. 6-17).

■ Diabetics are prone to severe disease of the infrapopliteal arteries with relative sparing of proximal vessels (Fig. 6-18).

■ The presence of atypical clinical or angiographic features should raise the possibility of other causes for PVD (Box 6-5).

■ Infrapopliteal disease with relative sparing of proximal arteries in a young to middle-aged smoker may suggest Buerger's disease (Fig. 6-19).

■ The pressure gradient across a stenosis proximal to a distal obstruction will be underestimated until downstream flow is reestablished.

Treatment

Medical Therapy

Most patients with PVD respond to conservative therapy without the need for any type of imaging or intervention. The goals are to stabilize or reduce lower extremity symptoms and prevent other cardiovascular events (such as myocardial infarction or stroke). The interventionalist must work aggressively with the patient to accomplish these goals (Box 6-6).[14]

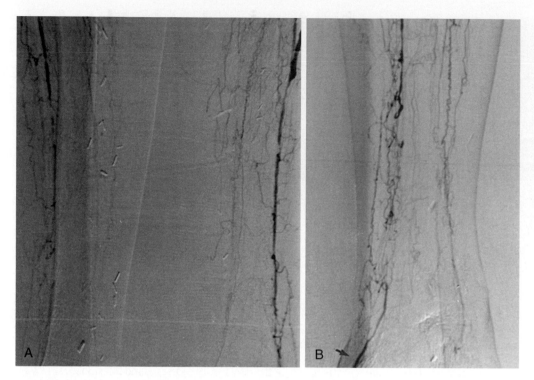

FIGURE 6-15 ■ Enhanced opacification of tibial arteries after vasodilator injection. **A,** The initial run-off study fails to identify a target vessel for bypass graft placement in a patient with right leg rest pain. **B,** After a catheter was advanced into the right external iliac artery and 12.5 mg of tolazoline was injected, the repeat arteriogram showed a patent dorsal pedis artery at the ankle *(arrow).*

Endovascular Therapy[41]

Revascularization is clearly indicated for patients with lifestyle-limiting claudication or limb-threatening ischemia. The primary goals are improved quality of life and limb salvage. Some interventionalists will offer endovascular therapy in patients with moderate claudication because the risk of the procedure is relatively low. However, this approach must be weighed against the possibility that neointimal hyperplasia at the treatment site may accelerate the obstructive process or that a complication might occur that could worsen the patient's symptoms, perhaps necessitating an unplanned operation.

Selection of patients for endovascular rather than surgical therapy depends on a variety of patient factors and the site and nature of disease. For almost all arterial segments, results are better with patients suffering from claudication than those with critical limb ischemia. A rigorous analysis

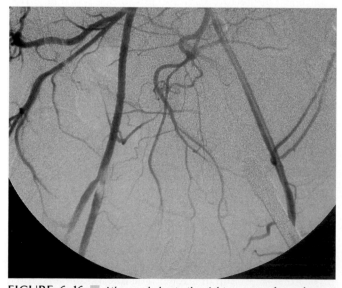

FIGURE 6-16 ■ Atheroembolus to the right common femoral artery bifurcation in a patient with acute right leg ischemia. This material was removed by simple operation at the groin. Also note the standing waves in the right external iliac artery.

BOX 6-4 ■ Causes of Lower Extremity Arterial Narrowing

Fixed Causes
Atherosclerosis
Neointimal hyperplasia
Trauma
Vasculitis
    Buerger's disease
    Irradiation
    Collagen vascular diseases
Extrinsic compression (e.g., popliteal artery entrapment)
Fibromuscular dysplasia
Endofibrosis

Functional Causes
Hypotension
Traumatic vasospasm
Catheterization
Vasospastic drugs (e.g., vasopressin, ergots, methysergide)
Raynaud's disease
Standing waves

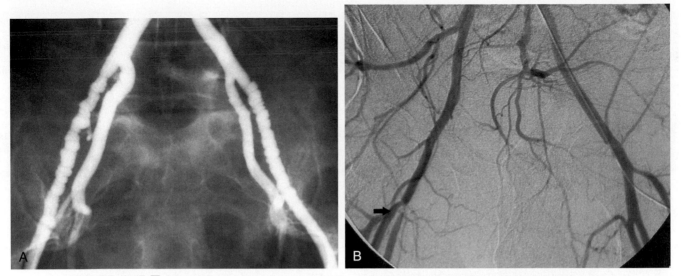

FIGURE 6-17 ■ Unusual causes of peripheral vascular disease. **A,** Fibromuscular dysplasia of both external iliac arteries. **B,** Puncture site neointimal hyperplasia at the origin of the right superficial femoral artery after cardiac catheterization *(arrow)*. Notably, no other vascular disease is seen.

has suggested that angioplasty is more cost-effective than exercise therapy in patients with intermittent claudication.[42]

There are some minor differences between the widely recognized TransAtlantic Inter-Society Consensus (TASC) working group and the Society of Interventional Radiology (SIR) recommendations (Table 6-2).[43,44] Angioplasty is clearly the first-line therapy for categories 1 and 2 lesions (Table 6-3); although immediate and long-term success are less impressive, angioplasty (and possibly stent placement) are reasonable in selected category 3 lesions. Some lesions should virtually never be addressed by angioplasty (category 4).

The common steps in percutaneous revascularization are considered in detail in Chapter 2. Selection criteria, specific technical features, and outcomes at various sites are discussed below. Perhaps in no other area of interventional radiology are reports of the efficacy of a procedure more disparate and confusing. Radiologic series have focused primarily on technical success and patency rates. To properly compare these procedures with surgical treatment, however, these modalities must be evaluated in terms of durable clinical improvement in ischemic symptoms, limb salvage, and survival. The outcomes provided in Table 6-4 are **rough** estimates based on the very widely reported patency rates; they are meant only to guide case selection and to educate patients and referring physicians.

It is interesting to note that arterial angioplasty and stent placement provoke an inflammatory response in all patients. This response is marked by serum elevations of C-reactive protein and fibrinogen (among other factors) and is more intense after femoropopliteal percutaneous transluminal balloon angioplasty (PTA) than carotid or iliac artery PTA; this phenomenon may partly explain the increased frequency

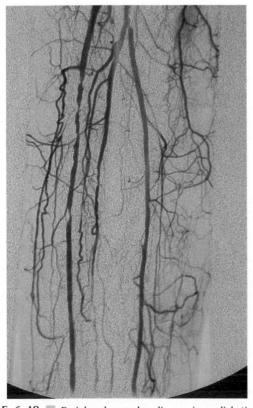

FIGURE 6-18 ■ Peripheral vascular disease in a diabetic patient. Severe diffuse right tibial artery lesions with relatively mild disease proximally (not shown).

BOX 6-5 ■ Suspicious Signs of Unusual Causes for Peripheral Vascular Disease

Age < 40 years
No risk factors for atherosclerosis or thromboembolism
Isolated, unilateral disease
Disease at unusual sites (e.g., common femoral artery)

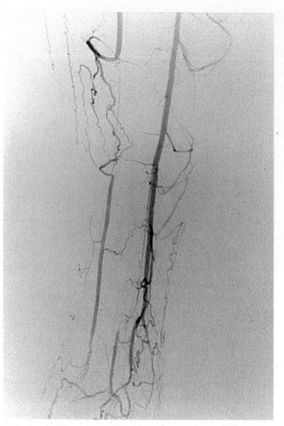

FIGURE 6-19 ■ Buerger's disease in a 45-year-old smoker. An arteriogram of the right calf shows abrupt occlusions of the tibial arteries with relatively normal intervening segments and tortuous corkscrew collaterals.

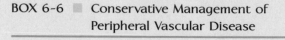

BOX 6-6 ■ Conservative Management of Peripheral Vascular Disease

(Supervised) exercise therapy
Smoking cessation
Dietary modifications (for weight and cholesterol control)
Blood glucose control in diabetics
Blood pressure control
Statin therapy for hypercholesterolemia
Daily antiplatelet therapy (aspirin, clopidogrel)

aorta and hypoplastic iliofemoral arteries).[48] The traditional therapy was surgical endarterectomy or bypass grafting. Balloon angioplasty and intravascular stents are now used with considerable success (Fig. 6-20). Single or dual balloons may be required for adequate dilation.

Although these lesions often are approached with some trepidation because the theoretical risk of rupture is greater than at other sites due to the large diameter of the aorta, angioplasty is remarkably safe, effective, and durable (see Table 6-4).[49-54] Intravascular stents are used for failures of angioplasty and for large exophytic lesions that are more likely to shower emboli with balloon dilation. As in many vascular beds, clinical restenosis is predicted by smaller aortic diameter. Primary hemodynamic patency at 10 years with PTA alone is close to 50%.

Aortic Occlusion. This relatively uncommon form of PVD is typically seen in a somewhat younger population, most of whom smoke (see Fig. 6-7).[55] Symptoms of bilateral claudication (and impotence in men) are common (*Leriche's syndrome*). Relative sparing of distal arteries is characteristic. The particular risk of an untreated infrarenal aortic occlusion is proximal propagation of clot leading to renal or mesenteric artery thrombosis. Standard treatment is aortobifemoral bypass grafting with endarterectomy, axillobifemoral grafting, or thoracoaortic femoral grafting.

of clinical restenosis at this site.[45] The risk of restenosis also may be associated with higher pre- and postprocedure levels of C-reactive protein.[46,47]

Abdominal Aortic Stenosis. Isolated atherosclerotic abdominal aortic stenoses are relatively uncommon. They are seen more frequently in middle-aged women who smoke and in patients with *hypoplastic aortic syndrome* (small

TABLE 6-2   GUIDELINES FOR PERIPHERAL PERCUTANEOUS TRANSLUMINAL ANGIOPLASTY (PTA)

Site	*Category 1*	*Category 2*	*Category 3*	*Category 4*
Aorta	Isolated < 2 cm stenosis	Isolated 2–4 cm stenosis	Longer segment stenosis with significant aortic disease	Occlusions and stenoses associated with aneurysm
Iliac artery	Concentric, noncalcified stenoses < 3 cm	3–5 cm stenoses or calcified eccentric < 3 cm stenoses	5–10 cm stenoses or occlusions < 5 cm	More severe lesions or extensive disease requiring surgery
Femoropopliteal artery	<3 cm lesions not at SFA origin or distal popliteal solitary stenosis < 1 cm	3–10 cm lesions, calcified or tandem lesions < 3 cm tandem or trifurcation stenoses < 1 cm	Lesions between categories 2 and 4	Complete SFA or popliteal occlusions
Tibial artery			1–4 cm stenoses or 1–2 cm occlusions	Occlusions > 2 cm or diffuse disease

Category 1: PTA procedure of choice; Category 2: PTA suitable, sometimes with adjunctive surgery; Category 3: treatable with PTA but with modest results, indicated in some situations (poor operative risk, no bypass material); Category 4: PTA generally not advisable.
SFA, superficial femoral artery.
From Society of Interventional Radiology Standards of Practice Committee: Guidelines for percutaneous transluminal angioplasty. J Vasc Interv Radiol 2003; 14(9 Pt 2):S209.

TABLE 6-3	IDEAL CONDITIONS FOR BALLOON ANGIOPLASTY OF LOWER EXTREMITY ARTERIES

Lesion Characteristics	Patient Characteristics
Short	Nondiabetic
Concentric	Milder degrees of ischemia
Noncalcified	
Solitary	
Nonocclusive	
Large vessel	
Continuous in-line run-off	

Reconstruction with intravascular stents is sometimes feasible, but long-term results have not been established.[56]

Iliac Artery Stenosis. Balloon angioplasty with or without stent placement is the accepted therapy for most iliac artery obstructions (Fig. 6-21; see also Table 6-2).[43,44] The role of stents in iliac artery stenosis is controversial. Stents are clearly indicated for failures of angioplasty, including:

■ Residual pressure gradient (>5 to 10 mm Hg systolic) or residual luminal stenosis (>30%)
■ Flow-limiting dissection flap
■ Immediate elastic recoil
■ Subacute restenosis

Stents are used also to remodel polypoid plaques, particularly in patients with blue toe syndrome. Many practitioners favor stent placement for almost all iliac artery stenoses. However, the existing literature suggests that short- and long-term success and cost-effectiveness are maximized by **selective** stent placement for failures of iliac artery balloon angioplasty.[57-59]

Predilation with a balloon catheter ensures that the lumen can be fully expanded and that the appropriate balloon and stent size is chosen to avoid vessel rupture. In reality, many operators perform primary stent placement to expedite the procedure and theoretically decrease the risk of distal embolization of plaque fragments.

If a stent is placed up to the aortic bifurcation, some interventionalists also stent or angioplasty the contralateral iliac artery regardless of the extent of disease ("kissing stents" or "kissing balloons"; Fig. 6-22) to avoid occlusion or extension of a dissection from the ipsilateral treatment site. However, there is no good evidence to support this approach.[60] Notably, the internal iliac artery will remain patent in most cases when a stent is placed across its origin.

The 3-year patency of balloon angioplasty for iliac artery stenoses is about 65% to 70%.[58,61] Five-year patency with stents for iliac artery stenoses is upward of 70% to 82%[62-65] Eight- to ten-year primary patency rates of iliac artery stents (including occlusions) have been reported at 46% to 74%.[66,67] Secondary patency rates at 3 years approach 95% with most devices. A wide variety of stents is used for iliac artery lesions (see Chapter 2). Although no single device has proven most effective or durable, there is growing evidence that nitinol devices are associated with better long-term results.[68-76]

The most commonly reported predictors of long-term patency are male gender, abstinence from smoking, common iliac artery location, large arterial (stent) diameter, patent outflow arteries, short lesion length, and complete covering of the diseased segment.[66,77,78] For example, patency rates for common versus external iliac artery angioplasty and stent placement at 5 years in one study were 76% and 56%, respectively.[79] This response may be related to the smaller size of the vessel and the fact that hip flexion causes arterial angulation in this region (not around the CFA as commonly thought).[80]

Complications (most of which are minor) occur in about 10% of cases and include puncture site injury or hematoma, acute stent thrombosis, distal embolization, stent dislodgment, pseudoaneurysm formation, and vessel rupture. If restenosis occurs, balloon angioplasty (with or without additional stent placement) usually is successful in relieving the narrowing.[69,70]

Iliac Artery Occlusion. Endovascular therapy is an acceptable alternative to surgery for some unilateral common or external iliac artery occlusions (see Table 6-2). However, patients with bilateral severe iliac disease are best managed operatively. Balloon angioplasty alone is not sufficient to treat most complete occlusions unless they are very short. Immediate and long-term results are clearly better after stent placement. On theoretical grounds, thrombolysis should dissolve lysable clot and decrease the risk of distal embolization.[81] Nonetheless, it is common practice to eliminate this step and proceed directly to primary stent placement once the obstruction is crossed.[82]

TABLE 6-4	RESULTS OF TRANSCATHETER THERAPY FOR CHRONIC PERIPHERAL VASCULAR DISEASE

Site and Disease	Therapy	Technical Success (%)	1-Year Patency (%)	3-Year Patency (%)	5-Year Patency (%)
Abdominal aortic stenosis	Angioplasty	70	60	50	50
Iliac stenosis	Angioplasty	95	75–80	65–70	
Iliac stenosis	Stent	98	90	75–80	70–80
Iliac occlusion	Stent	80	70	60	
Femoropopliteal stenosis	Angioplasty	95	70	50	50
Femoropopliteal occlusion	Angioplasty	80	50	40	35
Femoropopliteal lesions	Stent (older)	98	50–60	40	
Femoropopliteal lesions	Stent (nitinol)	98	75–85	70–75	
Tibial obstruction*	Angioplasty	60–90	50–80		

*Two-year limb salvage of 60% to 80%.

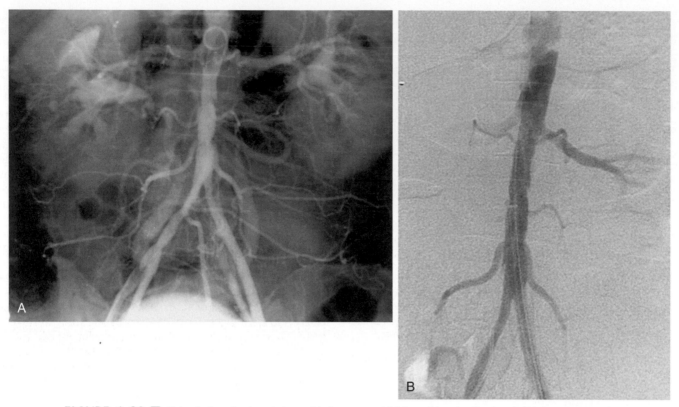

FIGURE 6-20 ■ Abdominal aortic stenosis in an elderly woman with bilateral leg claudication. **A,** Tandem stenoses of the infrarenal aorta are associated with a systolic pressure gradient of 30 mm Hg. **B,** The pressure gradient was reduced to 5 mm Hg after balloon angioplasty.

Although an ipsilateral groin approach is more direct, most stents can be advanced and deployed over the aortic bifurcation from the opposite groin unless the occlusion extends up to the bifurcation. Rarely, a high brachial artery approach is necessary. The occlusion is crossed with a steerable hydrophilic guidewire (Fig. 6-23). If the guidewire can be advanced only from the contralateral groin, the tip can be snared from the ipsilateral CFA and pulled through the sheath. An angiographic catheter is then placed in a retrograde direction for stent placement. Stents may be inserted even if guidewire passage is partially subintimal, provided the wire reenters the lumen before reaching the aorta. Stents are deposited along the entire length of the occlusion, incorporating adjacent segments of significant atherosclerotic disease. As a rule, stents are not placed beyond the upper CFA.

Revascularization of iliac artery occlusions is somewhat less successful than iliac artery stenoses (see Table 6-4).[74,78] However, the difference is largely attributable to cases in which the occlusion cannot be traversed with a guidewire. Thus, following a technically successful procedure, long-term patency rates are about 15% higher than published figures. The overall complication rate is about 10%. The frequency of distal embolization is about 2% to 5% whether or not thrombolysis is performed.[64,65,75,82-85] Stent-graft devices may ultimately improve on these results.[86]

Internal Iliac Artery Stenosis. Occasionally, proximal internal iliac artery stenoses cause isolated buttock claudication or contribute to impotence.[87] Balloon angioplasty has been used successfully to relieve such lesions.

Common Femoral Artery Obstruction. Isolated CFA obstruction is unusual without a history of injury (e.g., catheterization) (see Fig. 6-17B). Most CFA stenoses and occlusions are best treated surgically (e.g., endarterectomy), because the operation is simple, requires only local anesthesia and moderate sedation, and is more lasting than angioplasty.

Deep Femoral Artery Stenosis. Given the ease and durability of endarterectomy for focal proximal DFA disease, angioplasty is not often used at this site (Fig. 6-24). However, it has been performed successfully with moderately good long-term results.[88-90] It may be more useful in relieving rest pain than healing ulcers.[91]

Femoropopliteal Artery Stenosis. Unlike the iliac artery, SFA stenoses are at least three times less common in clinical practice than occlusions. Balloon angioplasty is first-line treatment for certain femoropopliteal lesions in patients with disabling claudication or more severe symptoms (see Table 6-2 and Fig. 2-29).[43,44,92,93] As technology improves, this procedure also is being offered to patients with lesser degrees of exercise-induced leg ischemia.

Femoropopliteal angioplasty is less durable than femoropopliteal bypass grafting (5-year primary patency rates of 25% to 55% versus 80%, respectively).[93-100] Long-term patency is better with simple category 1 lesions, absence of diabetes, and in-line tibial run-off.[99] Limb salvage rates in patients with grade III or IV ischemia are about 60% at 5 years.[101] Adverse events are observed in about 10% of

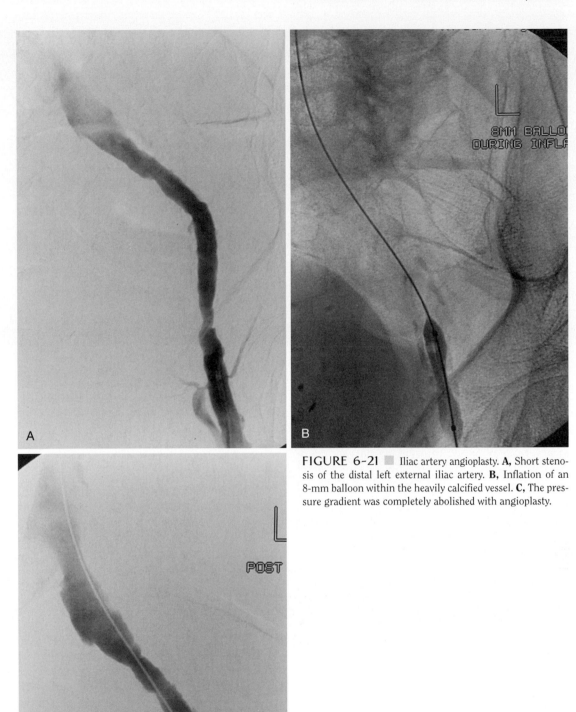

FIGURE 6-21 ■ Iliac artery angioplasty. **A,** Short stenosis of the distal left external iliac artery. **B,** Inflation of an 8-mm balloon within the heavily calcified vessel. **C,** The pressure gradient was completely abolished with angioplasty.

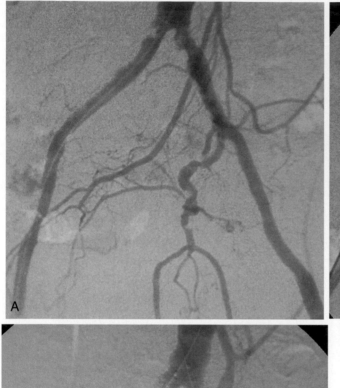

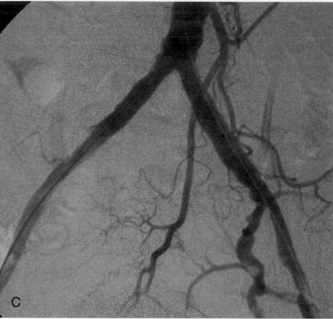

FIGURE 6-22 ■ "Kissing stents" for proximal bilateral iliac artery disease. **A,** Eccentric plaque is seen in the right common iliac artery with moderate disease in the left common iliac artery. **B,** Nitinol SMART stents have been advanced from both groins and will be deployed simultaneously. **C,** Both lumens are widely patent after stent insertion.

procedures, although surgical repair is only required about 2% of the time.[93]

It is not entirely clear why the results of femoropopliteal balloon angioplasty are so disappointing. Proposed theories include the large atherosclerotic burden typically present in this long vascular segment and hemodynamic factors related to bending and shortening of the vessel with leg motion and extrinsic compression at the adductor canal. Because femoropopliteal artery disease is so common and results of angioplasty are modest, numerous strategies have been pursued to improve outcomes. All of these measures are aimed at reducing the extent of neointimal hyperplasia and/or limiting progression of atherosclerosis. So far, no ideal technique has been discovered.

Cutting angioplasty balloons are useful when a lesion is resistant to balloon dilation.[102] However, there is no evidence as yet that these devices improve long-term patency.

Cryoplasty involves balloon dilation combined with delivery of cold thermal energy.[103] Liquid nitrous oxide (rather than diluted contrast material) is used to inflate the balloon to no more than eight atmospheres. As the agent rapidly assumes a gaseous state, a local −10°C heat sink is created. This procedure induces smooth muscle cell apoptosis (programmed cell death), which inhibits neointimal hyperplasia and restricts arterial elasticity by thermal effects on collagen and elastin. Experimental work also suggests that cryoplasty has no significant effect on normal arteries or the reendothelialization process. Only scant follow-up

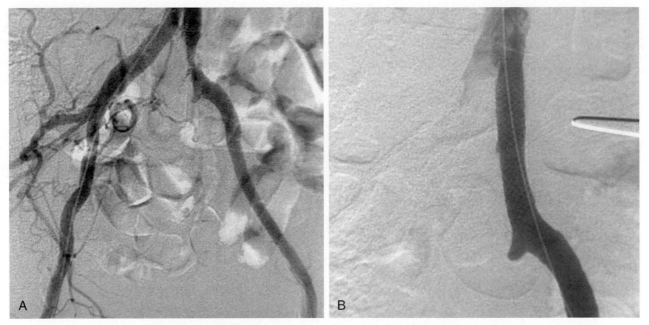

FIGURE 6-23 ■ **A** and **B,** Primary left common iliac artery stent placement.

data are available, but sonographic patency at 9 months in one series was 70%.[103]

Femoropopliteal artery stent placement has received considerable attention given the outstanding results in other vascular beds. Stents are definitely useful for salvage

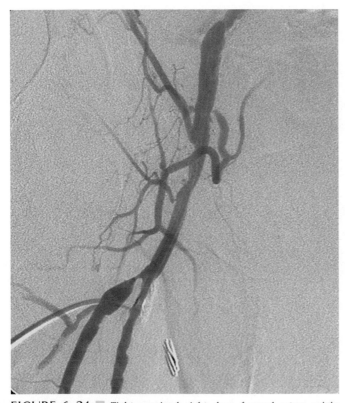

FIGURE 6-24 ■ Tight proximal right deep femoral artery origin stenosis with post-stenotic dilation.

of angioplasty failures (e.g., elastic recoil, flow-limiting dissection) (Fig. 6-25).[63,104] However, results of routine bare stent placement at this site have been mixed (Fig. 6-26). Much of the improvement noted with older stents is secondary to improved technical success.[105,106] Results may be slightly better with more complex lesions or in patients with critical limb ischemia (e.g., 43% versus 65% at 3 years).[107] However, there is encouraging evidence that outcome is improved with **nitinol** stents, particularly for angioplasty salvage (e.g., patency of 75% to 86% at 1 year and 78% at 3 years).[108-111] One vexing problem with some nitinol stents is a significant risk of stent fracture when multiple overlapping devices are placed.

Stent-grafts (covered stents) also have been used for femoropopliteal artery recanalization. It is clear that Dacron-covered stents are worse than angioplasty alone because of the intense inflammatory reaction they induce.[112] Polytetrafluoroethylene (PTFE)-covered stents are an entirely different story. These devices include the *Viabahn* (formerly *Hemobahn*) *stent* (W. L. Gore and Associates, Flagstaff, Ariz.), the *aSpire stent* (Vascular Architects, San Jose, Calif.), and the *Fluency stent* (C. R. Bard, Inc., Covington, Ga.) (see Fig. 2-34); however, none are yet approved for this indication in the United States by the Food and Drug Administration (FDA).

Careful selection of balloon and stent size is important; the graft should be slightly oversized but dilated to actual arterial diameter. This approach may prevent the transient thigh pain noted afterward in a small percentage of patients. In addition, complete coverage of diseased artery appears to be important. Most patients receive aspirin and/or clopidogrel before and for months after the procedure. Results have been mixed so far. In three studies, Viabahn stents achieved patency rates of 78% and 79% at 1 year and 87% at 2 years for femoropopliteal stenoses.[113-115] In another study, a 72% graft occlusion rate was observed, and abscess formation occurred in one patient.[116]

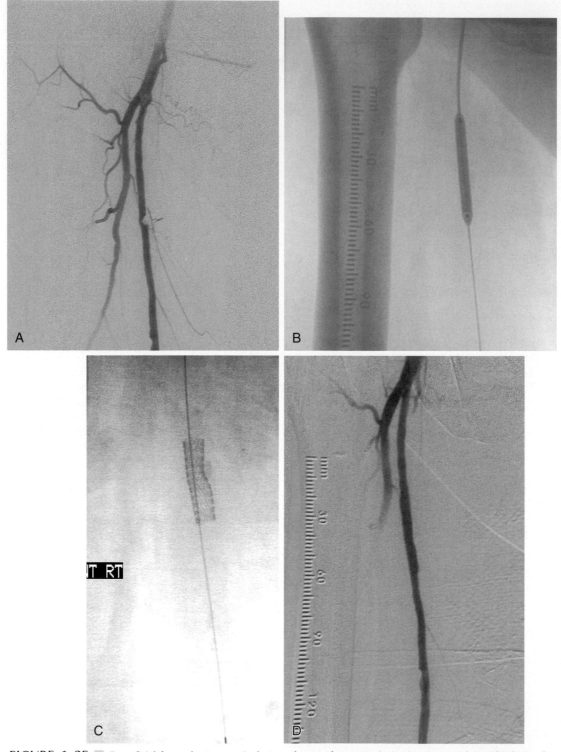

FIGURE 6-25 ■ Superficial femoral artery angioplasty and stent placement. **A,** Angiogram reveals an idea lesion for angioplasty. **B,** Although the balloon inflated completely, follow-up angiogram showed elastic recoil (not shown). **C,** Nitinol SMART stent deposited to limit remodeling. **D,** Widely patent artery afterward.

Drug-eluting stents show dramatic benefit in the coronary circulation where clinically significant restenosis has almost been eliminated. A polymer matrix is bonded to the stent. The matrix allows controlled release of an agent chosen to retard the process of neointimal hyperplasia. The principal drugs in use today are *sirolimus* (a lipophilic macrocyclic drugs with immunosuppressive and antibiotic activity) and *paclitaxel* (a lipophilic diterpenoid that inhibits cell function by microtubule stabilization, thus preventing smooth muscle cell proliferation and migration).[117] Other agents under study include tacrolimus, dexamethasone, actinomycin D, and batimastat. The currently available

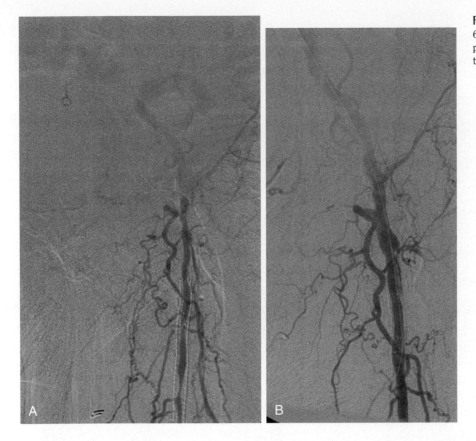

FIGURE 6-26 ■ Exuberant diffuse restenosis 6 months after left superficial femoral artery stent placement (**A**). After angioplasty with a 5-mm balloon, the luminal diameter is markedly improved (**B**).

devices on the U.S. market are the CYPHER stent (Cordis Corp), the TAXUS stent (Boston Scientific, Inc.), and the Zilver PTX stent (Cook, Inc.). So far, drug-eluting stents have not shown much promise in femoropopliteal artery obstructions.[118,119]

Atherectomy devices have a long history in peripheral arterial interventions. Although directional (Simpson) atherectomy (along with many other catheters) had some limited applications (e.g., resistant stenoses, removal of large intimal flaps), they were no better and perhaps worse than balloon angioplasty in most instances.[120,121] Investigations are still under way to find a device that works in the femoropopliteal segment.

The Silverhawk catheter (Fox Hollow) is approved by the FDA for use in peripheral arteries. The joint on the working end of the catheter presses an open metallic container onto the vessel wall. A rotating blade shaves plaque (or neointimal hyperplasia) from the artery and deposits it into the container for removal (Figs. 6-27 and 6-28).[122,123]

Brachytherapy (endovascular radiation therapy) also has been touted as a means to limit the restenosis process in femoropopliteal obstructions, but data at present are scant.[124-126]

Femoropopliteal Artery Occlusion. Focal occlusions (<2 to 3 cm) are treated with balloon angioplasty alone.[43,44,93] While early reports with stainless steel and Elgiloy stents were disappointing, many interventionalists now use nitinol bare stents or PTFE-covered stents to optimize results for more complex lesions (Fig. 6-29).[86,108,109,114] Sometimes, a

short course thrombolysis is performed to dissolve lysable clot. Nitinol stents should certainly be considered for initial or late angioplasty failures.[107,127] PTFE stent-grafts may further improve on these results (primary patency at 1 and 2 years of 79% and 74%, respectively).[113,115]

Mechanical revascularization devices (e.g., Amplatz thrombectomy catheter) have excellent technical success in some series, but long-term patency is modest or unreported.[128]

Subintimal angioplasty is advocated by some experts for treating long-segment femoropopliteal artery occlusions.[129-133] This novel technique usually is reserved for patients with high operative risk, critical limb ischemia, or no suitable vein conduit. A distal target vessel that allows in-line run-off must be present. Access is gained through the contralateral or ipsilateral CFA, or antegrade or retrograde from the popliteal artery. The optimal entry (diseased) and exit (nondiseased) points are determined. With an angled angiographic catheter wedged at the diseased upper arterial segment, an 0.035-inch angled hydrophilic guidewire is directed subintimally. A small loop is formed with the wire; a reinforced, hydrophilic catheter is then advanced to the loop, and the entire unit is run down the subintimal space until the planned exit site is reached. The lumen is then reentered with the wire tip, a step which sometimes requires a reentry needle. The entire channel is widened with an angioplasty balloon; stents are used selectively as needed. The reported overall success and 1-year limb salvage rates are about 75%.

There are two major risks from subintimal angioplasty. To prevent bleeding should transmural perforation occur,

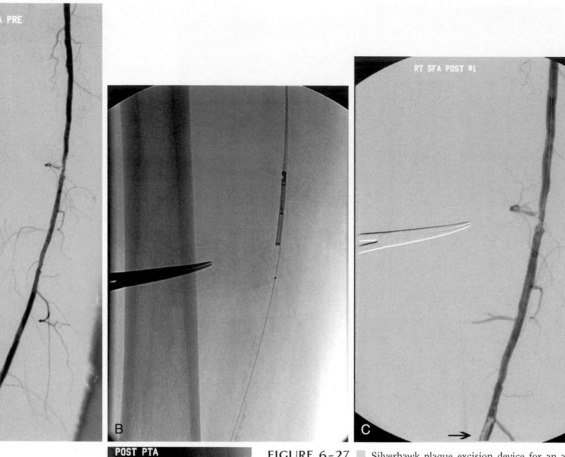

FIGURE 6-27 ■ Silverhawk plaque excision device for an atherosclerotic superficial femoral artery (SFA) lesion. **A,** Focal stenosis is seen in the mid-SFA. **B,** Silverhawk device in place. **C,** Luminal diameter is improved, but an embolus is evident in the distal SFA *(arrow)*. **D,** In addition, the peroneal artery (the only patent vessel to the foot) is now obstructed. **E,** Following a short course of thrombolysis and angioplasty, the artery is still diseased but adequate flow has been reestablished. (Courtesy of David Lopresti, MD, San Diego, Calif.)

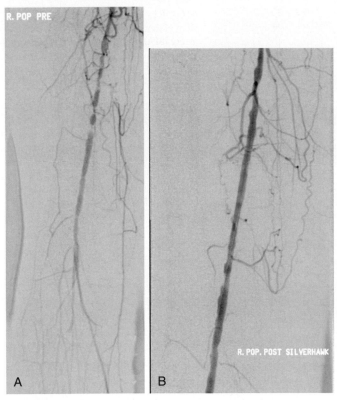

FIGURE 6-28 ■ Silverhawk atherectomy device for superficial femoral artery in-stent restenosis. **A,** Diffuse in-stent neointimal hyperplasia is demonstrated. **B,** The vessel is widely patent after treatment. (Courtesy of David Lopresti, MD, San Diego, Calif.)

full anticoagulation is delayed until the channel is created. Rarely, coil embolization of the tract is necessary. In addition, worsening of ischemia may result from occlusion of important collateral branches if the procedure is not successful.

Tibial Artery Obstruction. Infrapopliteal angioplasty is almost always performed for limb salvage (Fig. 6-30). Even short-term patency may be sufficient to allow healing of an ischemic ulcer or amputation site or to avoid amputation altogether. However, tibial angioplasty is not particularly effective when in-line run-off (continuous flow to the pedal arch) is not reestablished or when heroic procedures are performed on patients with severe, widespread infrapopliteal disease because they are poor surgical candidates.[134]

Technical success can be anticipated for most stenotic lesions (see Table 6-4).[134-137] Outcomes are clearly better for stenoses than occlusions (patency at 1 year, 68% versus 48%, respectively).[137] Repeat angioplasty should be considered before operative bypass in patients who develop restenosis. Liberal use of heparin is important to maintain vessel patency after angioplasty. Intraprocedural intra-arterial vasodilators may prevent or limit vessel spasm. Major complications occur in up to 14% of cases.

There has been some recent interest in the use of mechanical atherectomy devices to assist or replace standard balloon dilation when treating tibial artery disease.[138]

Complications. Although most angioplasty and stent procedures are uncomplicated, several problems can arise.

For residual stenosis greater than 30%, a higher pressure or larger diameter balloon may help, provided the patient does not complain of severe pain with balloon inflation. If the balloon inflates fully but elastic recoil occurs, a stent can be inserted in iliac or femoral lesions (see Fig. 6-25). A stent should **not** be placed if the "waist" on the balloon cannot be eliminated.

Vasospasm is most frequently a problem during angioplasty below the knee (Fig. 6-31). Spasm may be largely prevented by giving intra-arterial nitroglycerin (100 to 200 µg) immediately before dilation. If severe spasm occurs, more heparin is administered immediately (as needed) to prevent occlusion. Spasm usually resolves with an intra-arterial vasodilator and time.

For a flow-limiting dissection flap in the iliac and femoropopliteal arteries, a stent should be placed. For smaller vessels, the balloon may be reinflated for a short time to "tack down" the flap.

Repeat angioplasty is performed for acute thrombosis immediately after angioplasty (see Fig. 2-31). If the occlusion is long, a brief trial of thrombolytic therapy followed by repeat angioplasty and stent placement often is successful.

For arterial rupture, the balloon is advanced across the torn artery and reinflated. Some ruptures close with this maneuver. If not, placement of a covered stent or surgical repair is mandatory.

Surgical Therapy

For *aortoiliac occlusions,* surgical options include an aortobifemoral bypass graft (AFB), extra-anatomic graft, or (rarely) endarterectomy.[139] When the external iliac artery is patent, the distal anastomosis is made in an end-to-side fashion to the CFA to maintain perfusion to the pelvis and left colon (Fig. 6-32). Extra-anatomic conduits include axillobifemoral, axillofemoral, and femorofemoral grafts (Fig. 6-33). These grafts are preferred in patients with unilateral iliac disease, high surgical risk, severe scarring from multiple prior vascular procedures, abdominal or groin infections, or chronic occlusion of one limb of an AFB. The 5-year patency of an AFB placed for occlusive disease is 85% to 95%.[139] Complications of aortoiliac grafts are discussed in a later section.

Infrainguinal occlusions not amenable to endovascular therapy are treated with a bypass graft. Autologous vein and synthetic material (e.g., PTFE) are used for **above-knee** femoropopliteal grafts for SFA disease. Distal bypass grafts for **below-knee** femoropopliteal, tibial, and pedal grafts are constructed with vein. *Reversed saphenous vein grafts* are created by ligating all major tributaries of the vessel, harvesting the graft, and then reversing it so that blood can flow through the valves. *In situ saphenous vein grafts* are constructed by ligating all main tributaries of the dissected vein, anastomosing the proximal and distal ends to the appropriate arteries, and destroying the valves with an endoluminal valvulotome to permit antegrade flow. When the ipsilateral saphenous vein is not suitable or available, the options are to use short or accessory saphenous veins, the contralateral great saphenous vein, or superficial upper arm vein. Composite grafts can be made from autologous vein and PTFE. A critical step in preoperative planning is to identify a target vessel for distal bypass.

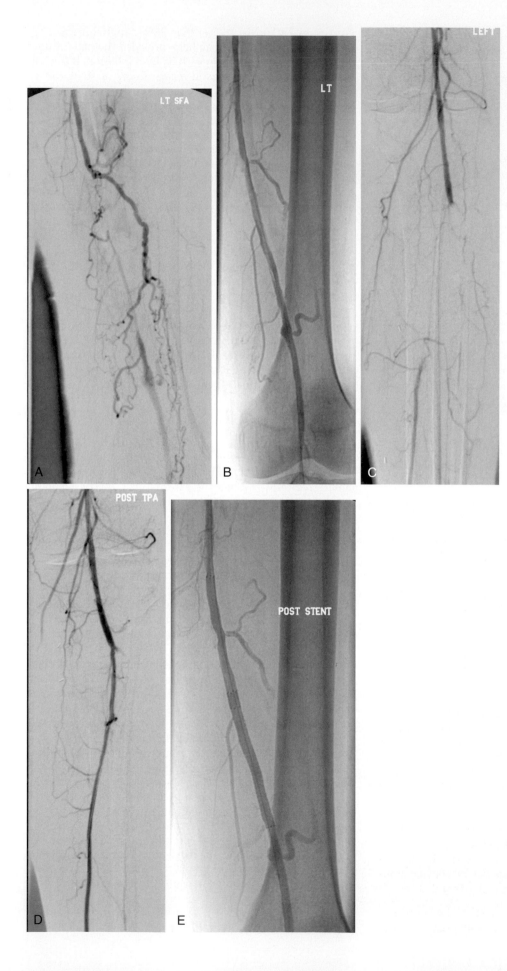

FIGURE 6-29 ■ Angioplasty and stent placement for a left superficial femoral artery (SFA) occlusion. **A,** Distal SFA occlusion. Note that the actual length of the obstruction is relatively short because of backfilling from the collateral circulation. **B,** After 5-mm balloon angioplasty, a long dissection flap is seen. **C,** Embolic occlusion of the tibioperoneal trunk and anterior tibial artery has occurred. **D,** After angioplasty, flow in the peroneal artery has been reestablished. **E,** Following placement of two overlapping SMART Control stents, the artery is widely patent. (Courtesy of David Lopresti, MD, San Diego, Calif.)

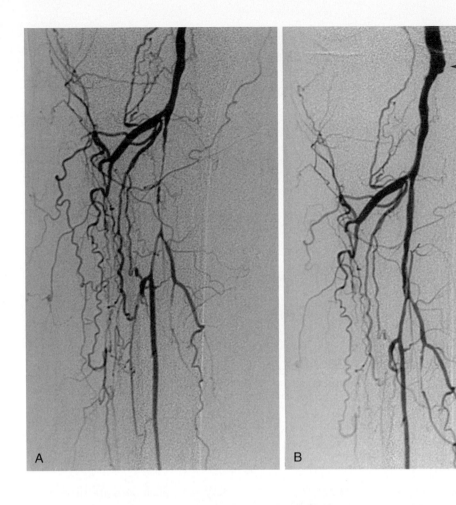

FIGURE 6-30 ■ Severe infrapopliteal disease in a patient with a nonhealing right foot ulcer and patent femoropopliteal graft. **A,** The tibioperoneal trunk has critical stenoses, and the posterior and anterior tibial arteries are occluded proximally. **B,** A 2.5-mm angioplasty balloon was used to reestablish continuous run-off to the foot through the peroneal artery. Notice the below-knee distal graft anastomosis *(arrow)*.

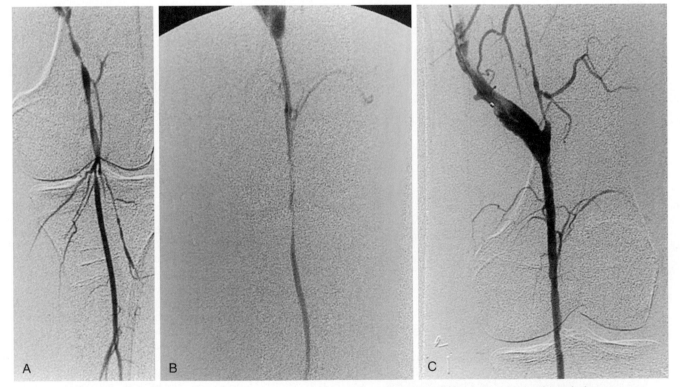

FIGURE 6-31 ■ Vasospasm after balloon angioplasty. **A,** Tight stenoses of the popliteal artery are just beyond a bypass graft anastomosis. **B,** Severe vasospasm occurred after initial angioplasty with a 4-mm balloon. **C,** The vasospasm resolved with additional heparin, intra-arterial nitroglycerin (200 μg), and time.

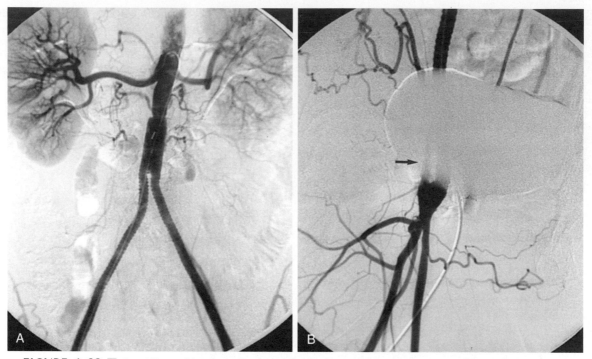

FIGURE 6-32 ■ Aortobifemoral bypass graft. **A,** An end-to-end proximal anastomosis is established to the infrarenal aorta. **B,** An end-to-side common femoral anastomosis allows retrograde flow up the patent external iliac artery *(arrow)* to supply the pelvis.

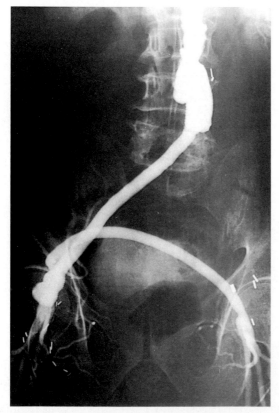

FIGURE 6-33 ■ A right-to-left femorofemoral cross-over graft is placed for occlusion of the left limb of an aortobifemoral bypass graft.

Ideally, the selected artery has continuous in-line run-off to the pedal arch.

The overall 5-year primary patency of above-knee femoropopliteal bypass grafts is about 60%.[140] More than 70% to 80% of in situ saphenous vein grafts are patent 5 years after placement.[141] Outcomes are less favorable with prosthetic material and poor with umbilical vein conduit.[142] Good results are expected with distal pedal bypass procedures if patients are properly selected, with 3-year patency and limb salvage rates of about 60% and 90%, respectively.[143,144]

Acute Lower Extremity Ischemia

Etiology

The most frequent causes of acute lower extremity ischemia are embolization, thrombosis of diseased native arteries, and occlusion of bypass grafts (Box 6-7).[145] Most emboli arise from the heart in patients with left atrial or ventricular dilation, dysrhythmias, coronary artery disease, valvular heart disease, left ventricular aneurysm, or left atrial myxoma. Less often, clot or plaque debris from a proximal artery embolizes distally.[146] Immediately after the embolic event, distal arteries become vasospastic. Clot then propagates proximally or distally to the next large collateral branch. The extent of collateral circulation largely determines the degree of limb ischemia. If blood flow is inadequate and revascularization is delayed, the result may be muscle or skin necrosis and nerve injury.

Microemboli consist of minute atheromatous material from ulcerated plaques or aneurysms, cholesterol crystals, fibrin-platelet deposits, or cellular thrombi (Chapter 3).[147,148] The source usually is the aorta or iliac arteries.[149,150] *Cholesterol embolization syndrome* is an acute, life-threatening event usually caused by catheterization or aortic manipulation. *Blue toe syndrome* is a more subacute or chronic condition resulting from spontaneous embolization of microemboli.[22,151] Recurrent embolic showers are the rule, resulting in necrosis and tissue loss in about 60% of cases.

Acute thrombotic occlusion usually is superimposed on underlying disease in a native artery or bypass graft. If blood flow has been compromised long enough for collateral channels to develop, the patient may present with chronic symptoms rather than sudden onset of ischemia. In situ thrombosis without underlying disease virtually always occurs in patients with a thrombophilic state (see Chapter 3 and Box 3-5).

Clinical Features

By convention, acute lower extremity ischemic symptoms are less than 2 weeks in duration. A history of cardiac disease, atrial dysrhythmias, claudication, or bypass graft placement usually is given. The patient presents with a "cold leg" that is painful, pale or cyanotic, and numb. Profound sensory loss, muscle weakness, or paralysis can indicate irreversible ischemia. The pulse examination will help identify the level of arterial obstruction. The classic presentation of cholesterol embolization syndrome is the acute development of a painful, white, marbled extremity *(livido reticularis)*, often accompanied by acute renal failure or mesenteric ischemia.

Imaging

Computed Tomographic and Magnetic Resonance Angiography. In many cases, the surgeon can make the diagnosis and predict the level of disease based on the physical exam and vascular laboratory studies. In this situation, immediate operation without preprocedure imaging may be appropriate. Otherwise, CT or MR angiography is used to confirm the diagnosis and determine the operative or endovascular strategy.

Catheter Angiography. In patients with acute infrainguinal bypass graft occlusion, the diagnostic arteriogram usually is done from the contralateral groin (Fig. 6-34). However, if recent imaging studies document normal aortoiliac inflow, direct antegrade CFA puncture on the affected side can simplify thrombolysis and subsequent angioplasty, provided there is sufficient purchase to enter the artery below the inguinal ligament and select the graft. Thrombosed AFBs usually are studied through a high left brachial artery approach.

Embolism may be impossible to differentiate from acute thrombosis, although certain angiographic features are characteristic (Fig. 6-35; see also Box 3-7). Most macroemboli lodge in the femoral or popliteal artery. Total occlusion can hide an unusual cause for thrombosis, such as a popliteal artery aneurysm (see Fig. 6-14). In situ thrombosis often appears as wormlike filling defects that simulate emboli (see Fig. 3-12).

In patients with microembolization syndromes, proximal atherosclerotic disease (particularly shaggy, ulcerated

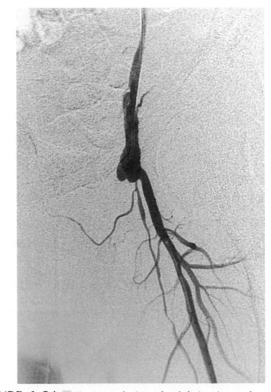

FIGURE 6-34 ■ Acute occlusion of a left in situ saphenous vein femoropopliteal bypass graft that was placed to remedy superficial femoral artery occlusion. Notice the residual graft "nipple" at the bottom of the common femoral artery. Antegrade puncture on this side for recanalization would be difficult because of the short distance between the external iliac artery and graft origin.

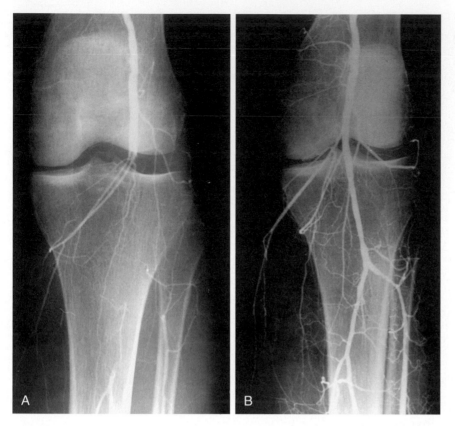

FIGURE 6-35 ■ Thrombolysis of a left popliteal artery embolus. **A,** The occlusion begins at the knee joint and extends to the proximal tibial arteries. **B,** After pulse-spray thrombolysis with 500,000 units of urokinase, the vessel is completely recanalized. Mild disease or spasm is detected at the origin of the anterior tibial artery. (From Bookstein JJ, Valji K: Pulse-spray pharmacomechanical thrombolysis: updated clinical and laboratory observations. Semin Intervent Radiol 1992;9:174.)

plaques) or aneurysms usually are found in the abdominal aorta, iliac arteries, or SFA (Fig. 6-36). Aortic disease often is most severe along the posterior wall (see Fig. 5-9). Rarely, the thoracic aorta is a source of lower extremity microemboli. It is sometimes impossible to determine which lesion is responsible. Although a continuous channel usually exists between the presumed embolic source and the feet, microemboli can pass through collateral beds around major arterial obstructions.

Treatment

Medical Therapy

Some patients with embolic occlusions respond to anticoagulation alone and do not require revascularization. Blue toe syndrome is initially treated with aspirin or clopidogrel and long-term anticoagulation. More definitive therapy is required if symptoms recur or worsen.

Endovascular Therapy

Enzymatic thrombolysis, mechanical thrombectomy, and thromboaspiration are used to treat many acute lower extremity arterial occlusions (see Fig. 2-36).[152-159] Clot lyses easily because it is relatively fresh; fibrinolytic agents also can dissolve small vessel thrombus that would be inaccessible to surgical removal. In some cases, thrombolysis and angioplasty provide definitive treatment without the need for operation. With embolic occlusions, however, enzymatic thrombolysis

cannot lyse the nidus if it is composed of organized clot or plaque material. There is also the remote possibility that systemic effects of the fibrinolytic agent might lyse more clot from the original embolic source. Nonetheless, most embolic occlusions respond favorably (see Fig. 6-35).

Patient Selection. Thrombolytic therapy has proven effective in patients with limb-threatening ischemia and an acute occlusion (<14 days old) in native arteries and bypass grafts.[160,161] It is sometimes valuable in cases of subacute thrombosis when endovascular therapy is safer than open operation. As a rule, it has no proven value in chronic lower extremity arterial occlusions (>6 months old).

Patients are screened for contraindications to therapy, including risks from thrombolytic agents, anticoagulants, and contrast material (see Boxes 1-2, 1-3, 1-4, and 2-5). Patients with irreversible ischemia in which tissue loss or nerve damage are inevitable (marked sensory and motor loss with **inaudible** venous Doppler signal) should **not** undergo thrombolysis to avoid a reperfusion syndrome. If thrombolysis can be accomplished with alacrity, patients with an immediately threatened limb (some motor/sensory loss but **audible** venous Doppler signal) are sometimes candidates. Any patient with suspected infected thrombus requires operative removal to prevent sepsis. Finally, success is much more likely if a guidewire can be negotiated through the entire occlusion before beginning lytic therapy.[162]

Technique. The details of catheter-directed thrombolysis are discussed in Chapter 2. Strict adherence to recent guidelines for fibrinolytic agent dosing is necessary to avoid

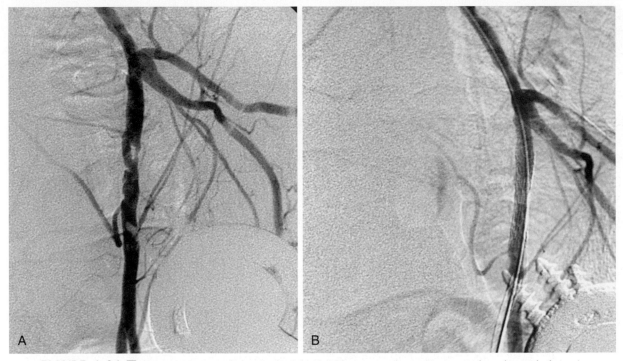

FIGURE 6-36 ■ Iliac artery stent placement for left-sided blue toe syndrome. **A,** A complex, ulcerated plaque is detected in the distal left external iliac artery. **B,** Primary stent placement was done to remodel and cover the plaque to prevent recurrent microembolization.

undue bleeding complications.[155-159,163-165] Based on current dosing guidelines (see Table 2-5), no particular fibrinolytic agent has been convincingly shown to be more effective or safe.[166-169]

Antiplatelet and antithrombin agents play an important role during this procedure. Recently, there has been some enthusiasm for use of potent intravenous glycoprotein IIb-IIIa platelet inhibitor agents to improve the efficacy and speed of lysis (see Chapter 2).[170-174] However, the safety of these drugs in this setting has not been established. Some reports have described increased bleeding events and faster lysis but no substantial advantage in terms of efficacy. Therefore, many interventionalists reserve these agents for specific circumstances (e.g., slow response to fibrinolytic agents, presence of a thrombophilic state, need for rapid revascularization, and below-knee thrombolysis). If they are used, anticoagulant and fibrinolytic doses should be adjusted downward, and platelet counts should be monitored periodically. Sudden and profound thrombocytopenia can occur with some of these drugs.

Many interventionalists start with bolus or pulse-spray injection using a multi–side hole catheter to accelerate the lytic process (Fig. 6-37). The infusion is continued while the patient is carefully monitored for local or remote bleeding (e.g., headache or altered mental status) and the condition of treated extremity. Most centers monitor hematocrit, partial thromboplastin time, and fibrinogen levels every 4 to 6 hours. If the fibrinogen drops below about 100 to 150 mg/dL, drug infusion is slowed or stopped. Transient worsening of ischemic symptoms is common as clot lyses and small emboli shower distally. In most cases, thrombolysis

should still be continued. The patient is reevaluated every 6 to 12 hours by angiography for progression of lysis.

When the clot burden is less than 5%, any underlying stenoses are treated with angioplasty and/or stent placement. Drug infusion is continued when significant thrombus remains; if substantial lysis has not occurred with 24 hours, further therapy usually is fruitless. Angiography of the distal arteries is always performed to identify subclinical emboli that may need treatment.

Mechanical thrombectomy catheters (see Box 2-6) are popular also as primary or adjunctive treatment for acute lower extremity arterial occlusions.[41,155,175-178] These devices have the potential to shorten procedure times and reduce bleeding complications. Potential disadvantages include direct vessel injury, distal embolization, and the cost of the devices. There is very limited published experience with these catheters in this setting. They often are employed as adjuncts to enzymatic fibrinolytic therapy or in patients with a contraindication to the latter. Aspiration thrombectomy is especially popular among European interventionalists as first-line treatment for acute arterial occlusions.[179]

Some cases of acute arterial ischemia are managed solely with angioplasty and stent placement when the expected clot burden is minimal (Fig. 6-38).

Results. Technical success is achieved in about 75% to 85% of attempts. The procedure fails because of inability to traverse the obstruction, the presence of organized clot, inadequate anticoagulation, a thrombophilic state, or poor run-off. Thrombolysis is comparable to surgery in terms of both limb salvage and mortality.[160,161,180,181] In patients

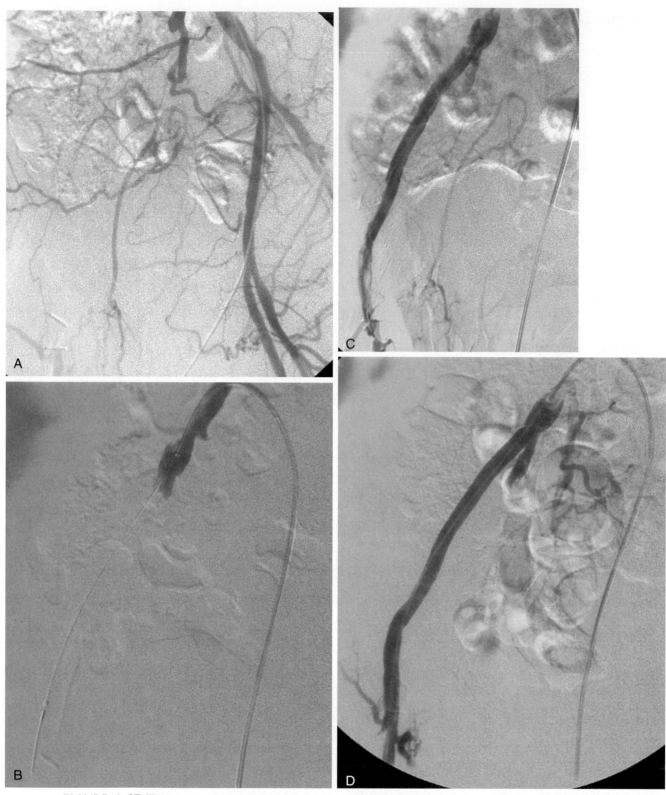

FIGURE 6-37 ▪ Iliac artery thrombolysis for acute ischemic symptoms. **A,** Right posterior oblique pelvic angiogram shows complete occlusion of a graft from the right external iliac artery to the deep femoral artery. **B,** A guiding sheath was placed over the aortic bifurcation and the occlusion crossed with an angled hydrophilic guidewire. A pulse-spray catheter with multiple side slits spans the lesion. **C,** After 35 minutes of periodic injection of recombinant tissue–type plasminogen activator (t-PA) to a dose of 4 mg, there is substantial lysis. **D,** Following overnight infusion of t-PA at 0.5 mg/hr, the graft is widely patent.

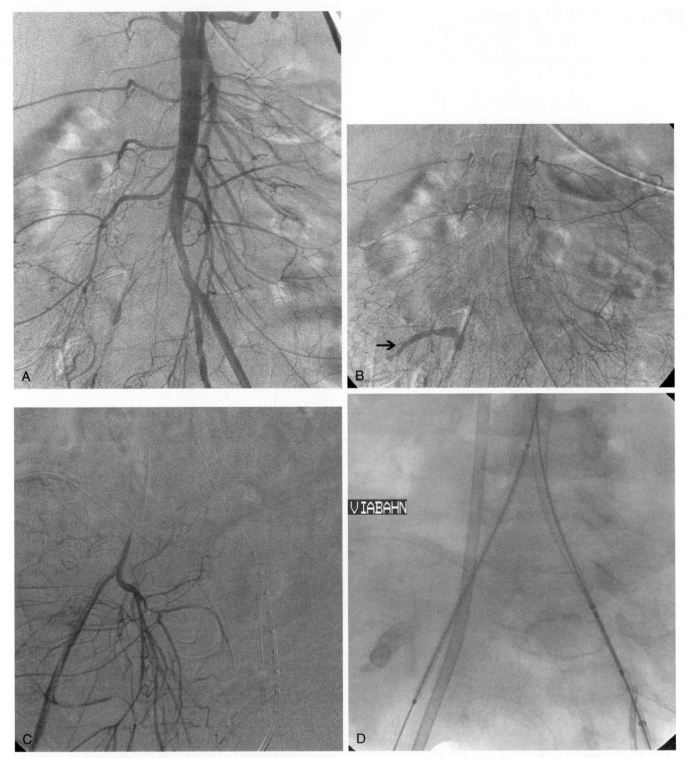

FIGURE 6-38 ▇ Bilateral stent placement for iliac artery dissection and rupture. The patient had just undergone attempted blind temporary hemodialysis catheter insertion into the right common femoral vein. **A,** Catheter pelvic arteriogram shows complete right iliac artery occlusion probably secondary to traumatic dissection, with the flap extending to the left common iliac artery origin. **B,** Late phase shows actual rupture of the right iliac artery with extravasation *(arrow).* **C,** The dissection is crossed from an ipsilateral approach. **D,** In a retrograde fashion, a Viabahn covered stent was positioned on the right and an uncovered Wallstent on the left (partially deployed).   *Continued*

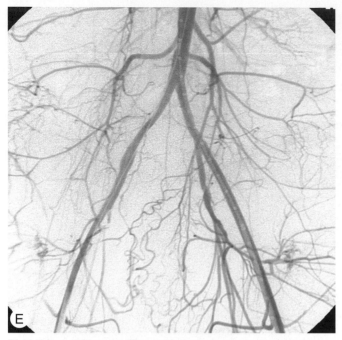

FIGURE 6-38 *Cont'd* ■ **E,** Both stents have been deployed; the vessels are recanalized, and the leak has been sealed.

suffering from microembolization syndromes, balloon angioplasty, directional atherectomy, and stents have been used to remodel, remove, or cover the embolic surface and prevent recurrent microembolization (see Fig. 6-36).[151,182]

Complications. The most important adverse events from lower extremity thrombolytic therapy are outlined in Table 2-6. Major complications are relatively frequent in some series. However, 30-day mortality is mostly related to underlying cardiac disease, which is common in this population. Other problems include pericatheter thrombosis, reperfusion syndrome, drug reaction, and vessel or graft extravasation. Causes of bleeding are multifactorial and include a systemic "lytic state" from fibrinogen depletion, lysis of hemostatic plugs (e.g., in the brain) by fibrin-specific agents, effects of anticoagulants or antiplatelet agents, and patient-related factors.

Surgical Therapy

For acute thromboembolic occlusions, revascularization involves Fogarty balloon thromboembolectomy or bypass grafting. Significant mortality is associated with operative treatment in this population. The surgical approach to patients with atheroembolism is removal or exclusion of the offending source by endarterectomy or bypass grafting.[150]

Arterial Bypass Graft Failure

Etiology

Early complications of an *aortobifemoral bypass graft* include occlusion, bleeding, colonic ischemia, and spinal cord ischemia. Late complications include infection, pseudoaneurysm formation, partial or complete thrombosis, and aortoenteric fistula (see Fig. 5-18). Acute graft thrombosis often is the result of an operative error and is treated with reoperation. Late graft thrombosis is caused by neointimal hyperplasia at graft anastomoses, progressive atherosclerosis, pseudoaneurysm formation, or infection.

Early or subacute *infrainguinal bypass graft failure* has several causes:

- Scarred vein segments
- Anastomotic strictures
- Retained valve cusps (in situ grafts)
- Clamp injury
- Nonligated venous tributaries that divert flow from the graft ("arteriovenous" fistulas)

The major reasons for late infrainguinal graft failure are graft stenosis from neointimal hyperplasia, progression of atherosclerosis, and poor run-off. About one half of the obstructions develop within the graft, and the remainder occur at the anastomoses or within native arteries.[183]

Clinical Features

Most patients with acute graft occlusion present with sudden onset of ischemic symptoms (i.e., "cold leg"). Unfortunately, less than 50% of cases of graft dysfunction with impending failure are symptomatic.

Imaging

Noninvasive Screening. Routine surveillance of infrainguinal venous bypass grafts is necessary to identify conditions that may lead to complete graft occlusion. Screening involves periodic measurement of the ABI and color Doppler sonography of the graft.[23,184,185] Imaging studies are obtained when one or more of the following criteria are met:

- A fall in ABI by 0.15 to 0.20, or 10%
- Peak systolic velocity of less than 40 to 45 cm/second in the body of the graft
- Peak systolic velocity at a stenosis greater than 300 cm/second
- Systolic velocity ratio greater than 2–3 at the site of a suspected stenosis versus adjacent graft

Surveillance programs have extended the longevity of infrainguinal venous bypass grafts; conduits are much more durable after detected stenoses are treated than after thrombosed grafts are repaired.[183,186]

Cross-sectional Techniques. Multidetector row CT angiography and MR angiography are at least as accurate as color Doppler sonography for screening.[39,187,188] Because of the longer procedure time and greater expense, however, they usually are reserved for more complex cases. On the other hand, MR and CT angiography provide more thorough evaluation of the inflow and outflow vessels, sometimes obviating the need for catheter angiography before operation (see Fig. 6-8).

Catheter Angiography. The findings with a failing or occluded bypass graft include complete thrombosis, focal or long segment stenoses, clamp injuries, arteriovenous fistulas (AVFs), retained valve cusps, anastomotic native arterial stenoses, pseudoaneurysms, and poor distal run-off (Figs. 6-39 through 6-44; see also Fig. 6-34).

Treatment

Endovascular Therapy

Most bypass graft–related stenoses respond initially to balloon angioplasty.[189,190] Although less than half are patent at 1 year, some interventionalists still attempt angioplasty for focal lesions because the risk is low and some studies have reported more encouraging results (see Figs. 6-40 and 6-42).[191] If antegrade puncture of an infrainguinal graft is not feasible, angioplasty is done from the opposite groin with the aid of a guiding catheter placed over the aortic bifurcation. Multiple, prolonged balloon inflations may be required to dilate these strictures. Lesions resistant to conventional balloon dilation are tackled with cutting balloons or even atherectomy.[192] Some AVFs may be closed with embolotherapy. Atherectomy catheter also can be used to obliterate retained valves.[193]

The role of thrombolysis for clotted arterial bypass grafts is controversial.[194,195] Although revascularization is initially successful in more than 90% of cases, long-term results are dismal (20% to 60% patency at 1 year).[194-197] However, these results are not much worse than those for surgical thrombectomy and revision.[198] Although some graft characteristics may be associated with a better outcome (e.g., age > 1 year, a correctable lesion, good run-off), no factor or combination of factors is consistently shown to predict long-term success.[195] Thrombolysis is performed using infusion or pulse-spray techniques (see Chapter 2 and Fig. 2-36). After thrombolysis, underlying lesions are treated with balloon angioplasty or a limited operation.

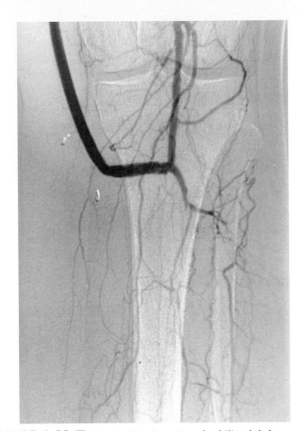

FIGURE 6-39 ■ Sonographic detection of a failing left femoropopliteal bypass graft. Sonography showed diffuse decreased velocities in the range of 20 to 30 cm/sec. The angiogram shows a widely patent graft and anastomoses but almost no distal run-off.

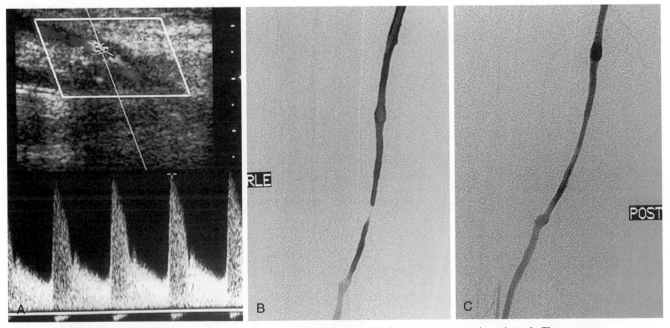

FIGURE 6-40 ■ Stenosis of an in situ saphenous vein bypass graft in an asymptomatic patient. **A,** The sonogram detected overall diminished velocities (13 to 28 cm/sec) but a markedly increased velocity (512 cm/sec) in the middle thigh. **B,** A critical intragraft stenosis was discovered. **C,** It was treated successfully with a 4-mm balloon.

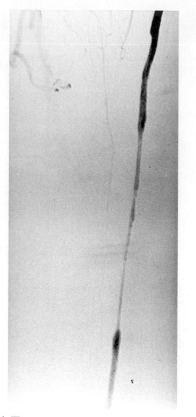

FIGURE 6-41 ■ Long-segment fibrosis of a right saphenous vein infrainguinal bypass graft.

Surgical Therapy

Failing grafts are repaired with a patch graft or graft extension. Retained valves are obliterated with an endoluminal valvulotome. Clotted grafts require surgical thrombectomy and revision or complete graft replacement. The 2-year patency rate for the former approach is less than 40%.[194,198]

Aneurysms

Etiology

Most pelvic and lower extremity artery aneurysms are degenerative true or iatrogenic false aneurysms (Box 6-8). Degenerative (atherosclerosis-associated) aneurysms occur most often in the iliac artery, popliteal artery, and CFA.[199,200] True aneurysms of the SFA, DFA, and infrapopliteal artery are relatively unusual (see Fig. 6-14).[201] Individuals with CFA and popliteal artery aneurysms often have aneurysms at other sites.

The iliac artery is considered aneurysmal when the diameter exceeds 2 cm. Common iliac artery aneurysms often are extensions of abdominal aortic aneurysms (see Fig. 5-12). In one series, the relative frequency of isolated common, internal, and external iliac aneurysms was 89%, 10%, and 1%, respectively (Fig. 6-45).[202] The major risk from common iliac artery aneurysms is rupture, which is unlikely until the vessel becomes larger than 3 cm. Conversely, popliteal artery aneurysms are prone to thrombosis or distal embolization.

Most false aneurysms of lower extremity arteries are posttraumatic (e.g., postcatheterization femoral artery pseudoaneurysms). Although some of these lesions close

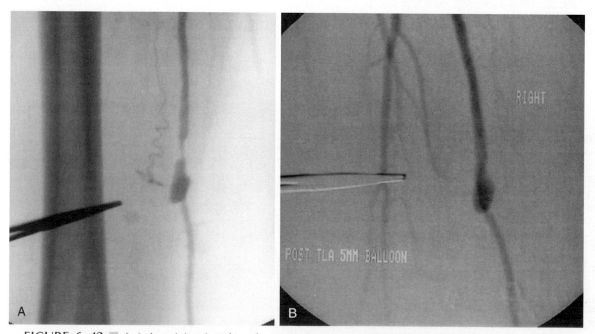

FIGURE 6-42 ■ **A,** A clamp injury just above the proximal anastomosis of a composite vein graft and an anastomotic pseudoaneurysm are evident. **B,** Balloon angioplasty was used to treat the graft stenosis.

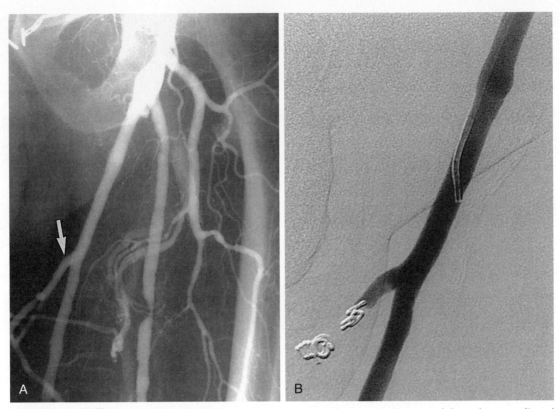

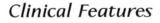

FIGURE 6-43 ■ Arteriovenous graft fistula. **A,** The left in situ saphenous vein bypass graft has a large, nonligated tributary *(arrow)*. **B,** A 5-French catheter was advanced into the tributary from the contralateral groin and used to embolize the branch.

spontaneously, expansion and rupture is a significant concern. Infectious (mycotic) aneurysms can occur at any site but are most often seen in the iliac and common femoral arteries.[203] The offending organism usually is a *Salmonella* or *Staphylococcus* species. Pseudoaneurysms at graft anastomoses often are a consequence of indolent infection.[204]

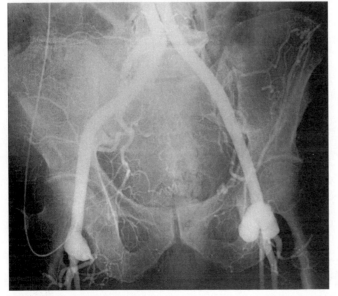

FIGURE 6-44 ■ Pseudoaneurysms of the distal anastomoses of an aortobifemoral bypass graft.

Clinical Features

Many patients with iliac artery aneurysms are asymptomatic. In particular, internal iliac artery aneurysms often are silent until they rupture.[202,205] Warning symptoms are related to compression of adjacent structures or (rarely) fistulization with a pelvic organ. Up to one third of popliteal artery aneurysms are unsuspected at the time of diagnosis.[206] Degenerative CFA aneurysms may present with local swelling and pain or

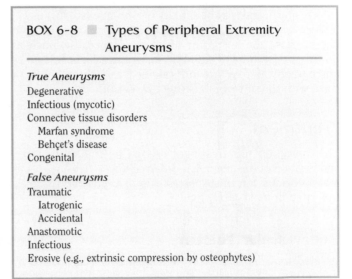

BOX 6-8 ■ Types of Peripheral Extremity Aneurysms

True Aneurysms
Degenerative
Infectious (mycotic)
Connective tissue disorders
    Marfan syndrome
    Behçet's disease
Congenital

False Aneurysms
Traumatic
    Iatrogenic
    Accidental
Anastomotic
Infectious
Erosive (e.g., extrinsic compression by osteophytes)

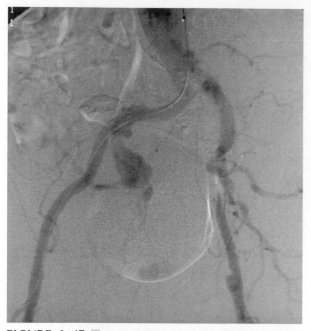

FIGURE 6-45 ■ Isolated right internal iliac artery aneurysm.

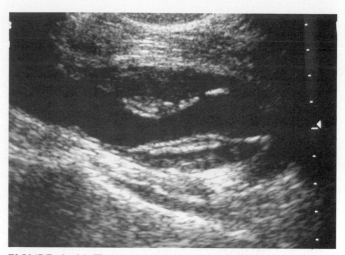

FIGURE 6-46 ■ Popliteal artery aneurysm on longitudinal sonogram. Note the extensive mural thrombus that actually narrows the lumen.

evidence for distal embolization; a substantial number of patients are asymptomatic. Catheterization-related pseudoaneurysms can produce a pulsatile, expanding mass. Classically, patients with mycotic aneurysms have fever, local tenderness, and a risk factor for bacteremia (e.g., intravenous drug abuse).

Imaging

Cross-sectional Techniques. For aneurysm detection and surveillance, MR or CT imaging is used for the iliac arteries and color Doppler sonography for the infrainguinal arteries (Figs. 6-46 and 6-47).[207,208] Sonography is essentially 100% accurate in the diagnosis of postcatheterization pseudoaneurysms. These lesions are characterized by swirling color flow in the aneurysm sac and to-and-fro flow at the aneurysm neck (see Fig. 2-15).

Catheter Angiography. Degenerative aneurysms are typically fusiform and may be solitary or multiple (see Fig. 6-45). Aneurysms that are saccular, eccentric, or atypical in location should raise the suspicion of an unusual cause, such as infection or trauma (Fig. 6-48). Aneurysms can be missed by angiography if they are noncalcified and thrombosed or lined with mural thrombus (see Fig. 6-14).

Treatment

The indications for treatment depend on the nature, size, and location of the aneurysm. Internal iliac artery aneurysms are notorious for unsuspected rupture; elective repair is indicated in most cases.

Endovascular Therapy

Isolated internal iliac artery aneurysms can be treated by iliac artery embolization and femorofemoral bypass or by

exclusion of the aneurysm through distal embolization of the vessel and placement of a covered stent over its origin.[209,210] Distal embolization is necessary to prevent aneurysm backfilling through pelvic collaterals. Stent-grafts and covered stents also have been used to treat common iliac and popliteal artery aneurysms, but long-term results are unknown; unlike operative bypass, late thrombosis may be a significant problem.[211-213] Many femoral artery pseudoaneurysms close spontaneously.[214] Treatment of postcatheterization pseudoaneurysms is described in Chapter 2.[215,216]

Surgical Therapy

Iliac and CFA aneurysms are excluded with a bypass graft. Postcatheterization femoral artery pseudoaneurysms are operated only if percutaneous thrombin injection or ultrasound-guided neck compression fails and the aneurysm continues to expand. Because popliteal artery aneurysms are prone to thrombosis or embolization, elective repair (usually with bypass grafting) is indicated in almost all cases.

Pelvic Trauma

Etiology

Because the internal iliac artery and its branches run close to the bony and ligamentous structures of the pelvis, they are frequently injured during severe blunt pelvic trauma from motor vehicle accidents, falls from a height, and crush accidents. About 10% of patients with pelvic fractures have persistent arterial bleeding that requires embolotherapy. The mechanism of injury in this subgroup often is severe anteroposterior compression (with diastasis of the symphysis pubis, pubic rami fractures, and sacroiliac joint disruption) or lateral compression (with sacral and pubic rami fractures).[217,218]

Clinical Features

Most patients with pelvic arterial hemorrhage are hypotensive and have extensive multiorgan injury. Survival depends

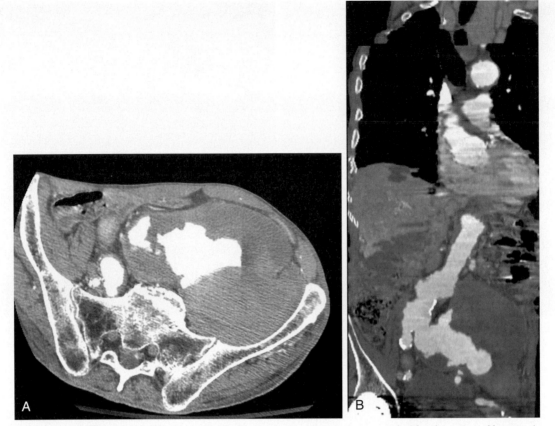

FIGURE 6-47 ■ Ruptured left common iliac artery aneurysm. The patient presented with pelvic pain and hypotension. Transverse (**A**) and reformatted coronal (**B**) CT images show a massive aneurysm with ill-defined hyperattenuation in the thrombus, indicating active extravasation.

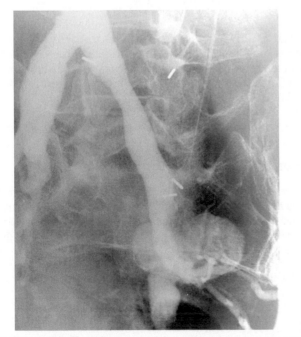

FIGURE 6-48 ■ Infectious aneurysms of the left external iliac artery.

on prompt angiographic evaluation and treatment before attending to less significant problems. The decision to proceed with angiography is based on the hemodynamic response to resuscitation and evidence for contrast extravasation on CT. However, elderly patients have a significant likelihood of arterial bleeding even when they are hemodynamically stable.[219]

Imaging

Computed Tomography. CT scans will delineate pelvic fractures and associated hematomas. If bleeding is very brisk, extravasation of contrast may point to the bleeding site.

Angiography. Evaluation includes pelvic and bilateral internal iliac arteriography.[220] The entire pelvis must be visualized, including the femoral regions. If no bleeding source is found, abdominal (or thoracic aortography) should be considered to search for other sources (e.g., lumbar or splenic artery).

Arterial hemorrhage is marked by extravasation of contrast (Fig. 6-49). Additional findings include abrupt vessel occlusion and severe tapering from vasospasm or extrinsic compression. Care must be taken not to mistake bowel activity, hypervascularity, or "road dirt" for a bleeding site. The most commonly injured vessels are the superior gluteal and internal pudendal arteries.

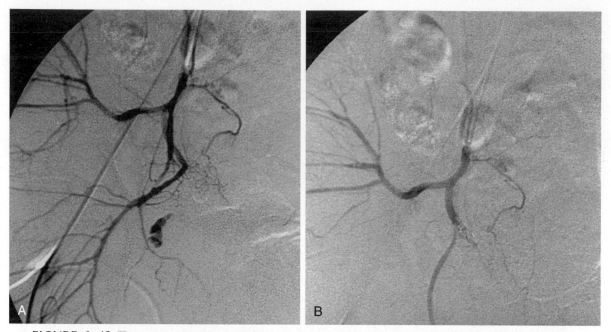

FIGURE 6-49 ■ Arterial bleeding from a pelvic injury due to a motor vehicle accident. The initial pelvic arteriogram (see Fig. 6-1B) showed extravasation. **A,** The bleeding is coming from the right internal pudendal artery. **B,** The vessel was occluded with Gelfoam pledgets and coils. No further bleeding was seen from either side of the pelvis.

Treatment

Venous and minor arterial bleeding often stop with time or external fixation of the pelvis. Surgery should be avoided, because it is almost impossible to find the bleeding vessels at operation and because it releases the tamponading effect of the hematoma below the pelvic peritoneum.

Endovascular Therapy

Embolization is the primary therapy for traumatic pelvic arterial hemorrhage.[219-221] If the patient is exsanguinating and massive extravasation is seen, bleeding must be stopped with alacrity by rapidly depositing stainless steel coils, Gelfoam, or both in the proximal internal iliac artery. In most situations, however, there is time for selective embolization of the damaged artery(ies). If multiple bleeding sites are found, "scatter embolization" with small Gelfoam pieces often is appropriate. Some interventionalists embolize truncated or narrowed arteries without extravasation on the grounds that hemorrhage may have come or may resume from these injured vessels. If no significant abnormalities of iliac artery branches are noted, the lumbar arteries are studied (Fig. 6-50).

Angiography reveals extravasation in about 50% of patients with pelvic trauma who are studied. A significant fraction of patients with initially negative studies but evidence for continued bleeding will exhibit bleeding at repeat angiography.[221]

Both internal iliac arteries are injected after embolization to confirm that hemorrhage has stopped and that collateral branches are not reconstituting the bleeding vessel. Even bilateral internal iliac artery embolization is well tolerated; the collateral circulation usually is sufficient to prevent ischemia of the pelvic organs. Sexual dysfunction (which is

frequent after pelvic fractures) is probably related to the injury itself rather than embolization.[222]

Lower Extremity Trauma

Etiology

Lower extremity arteries are subject to injury from penetrating objects, blunt trauma, medical procedures (e.g., catheterization), and bone fractures or joint dislocations.[223] Postcatheterization abnormalities include pseudoaneurysm or AVF formation, dissection, and thrombosis. Any long bone fracture can damage a major artery; posterior knee dislocations are a classic cause of popliteal artery injury.

Clinical Features

Some patients have symptoms that strongly predict a clinically significant arterial injury (hard signs), including active bleeding, diminished distal pulses, expanding or pulsatile hematoma, neurological deficit, or evidence for distal ischemia (see Box 7-4).[224,225] Other patients have less convincing findings, namely *proximity* of the injury to a major artery, small hematoma, or unexplained hypotension. AVFs may become apparent long after the traumatic event.

Imaging

Because only a small percentage of patients with lower extremity trauma have arterial damage that requires repair, they must be screened for arteriography or surgical exploration based on the physical examination findings and quick,

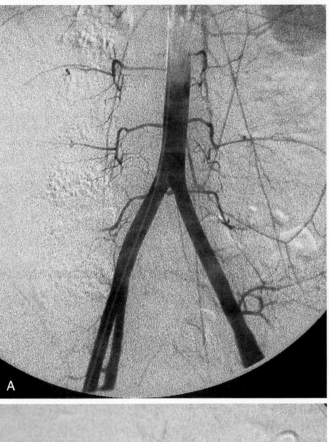

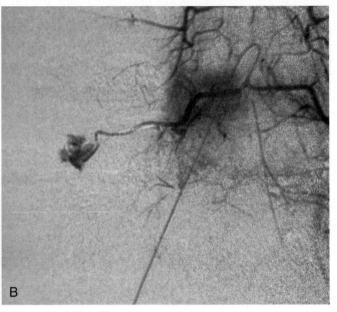

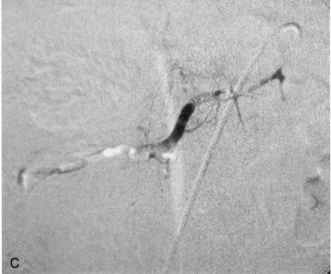

FIGURE 6-50 ■ Lumbar artery embolization for pelvic trauma. **A,** Pelvic arteriogram reveals truncation of the right fourth lumbar artery. Neither selective internal iliac artery study showed extravasation or abnormal vessels. **B,** Shetty catheter was used to engage the common L4 trunk; active bleeding is evident. **C,** The vessel was embolized to stasis with Gelfoam torpedoes via a selective microcatheter.

noninvasive tests. After decades in which exploratory surgery and arteriography were routine procedures in this setting, there has been a gradual shift to more careful selection of patients for invasive evaluation. Some trauma centers still consider injury in proximity to a major vessel a valid reason for arteriography. However, several studies have shown that the frequency of arterial injuries that require surgical intervention in the absence of hard signs is only 0 to 3%.[225-228] In one widely used algorithm, patients with intact distal pulses, an ABI greater than 1.00, and no hard signs are managed conservatively. Well-accepted indications for arteriography include[225,229]

■ Abnormal ABI (<1.0) or color Doppler ultrasound

■ Blunt or penetrating trauma with hard signs
■ Penetrating trauma in the setting of a shotgun injury, projectile path that follows a major artery for a long distance, history of PVD, or extensive limb injury
■ Postoperative evaluation
■ Delayed diagnosis

There is a short therapeutic window (about 6 to 8 hours) between acute injury and the possibility of permanent nerve injury due to ischemia; therefore, definitive imaging (or operation) must proceed without delay.

Noninvasive Imaging. Color Doppler sonography is a standard tool for detecting iatrogenic lower extremity arterial injuries.[230] Sonography also is extremely useful for identifying venous injuries, which can be a major source of morbidity and will go undetected by angiography.[231] Recently, CT angiography has shown some promise in this setting.[232]

Angiography. The spectrum of findings includes intimal tears, intraluminal thrombus, vasospasm, intramural hematoma, dissection, transection with or without thrombosis, vessel deviation, AVF, pseudoaneurysm, and slow flow (which can be seen with a compartment syndrome) (Figs. 6-51 through 6-54; see also Figs. 2-15 through 2-17, and 3-14).

Treatment

Surgical Therapy

Major injury to a named artery is managed by direct repair or bypass graft placement using autologous vein or prosthetic material. Isolated tibial artery injuries are sometimes left alone. Many trauma surgeons simply observe minor vascular injuries such as nonocclusive intimal flaps, intramural hematomas, small (<1 cm) pseudoaneurysms, and small asymptomatic AVFs.[224,233] These lesions usually have a benign course.

Endovascular Therapy

Embolotherapy is used to treat large pseudoaneurysms, AVFs, or extravasation from minor arterial branches. The neck of a pseudoaneurysm or AVF must be completely excluded from the circulation (distally and proximally) to prevent backfilling from collateral vessels (see Fig. 6-54).

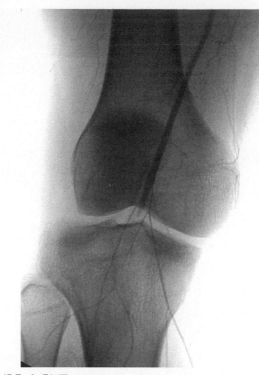

FIGURE 6-51 ■ Complete popliteal artery occlusion after posterior knee dislocation.

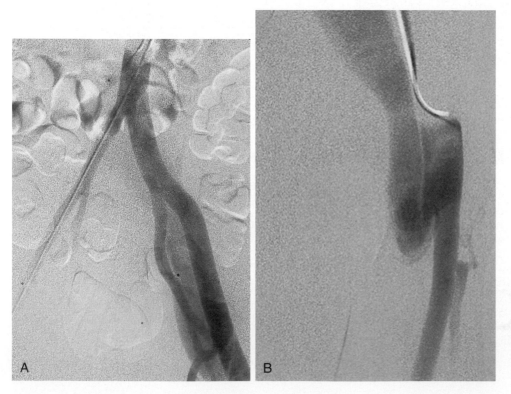

FIGURE 6-52 ■ Arteriovenous fistula after cardiac catheterization. **A,** Pelvic arteriogram shows torrential flow up the left iliac vein early in the arterial injection. Notice the marked enlargement of the left iliac artery from chronically increased flow. **B,** Selective catheterization documents the site of the fistula in the upper superficial femoral artery.

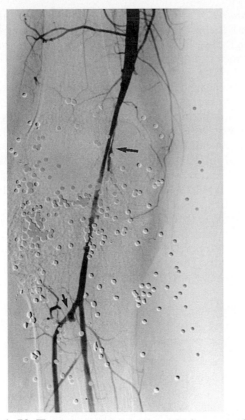

FIGURE 6-53 ▪ A shotgun blast to the right knee caused diffuse spasm or intramural hematoma in the popliteal artery, a focal dissection *(long arrow)*, and an anterior tibial artery pseudoaneurysm *(short arrow)*.

Gelfoam pieces and coils are the most commonly used agents. Stent-grafts have been effective in closing major arterial pseudoaneurysms and AVFs that would not be amenable to embolotherapy.[234]

▪ OTHER DISORDERS

Dissection

Lower extremity arterial dissection most often results from extension of an abdominal aortic dissection or a medical procedure such as catheterization (see Figs. 2-17 and 3-23).

Vasculitis and Related Disorders

Buerger's disease (thromboangiitis obliterans) is a rare systemic inflammatory disorder affecting small- and medium-sized arteries and veins (see Chapter 3).[235-237] Large arteries (proximal to the tibial vessels) usually are spared. The disease involves the lower extremity in 90% of cases; the upper extremity is affected in about 50%. It is a common cause of PVD in smokers (usually male) younger than 40 years of age. Patients complain of symptoms of distal ischemia and Raynaud's phenomenon. The classic angiographic features are abrupt occlusions of tibial and pedal arteries with normal intervening segments, tortuous "corkscrew" collaterals, and relative sparing of proximal arteries (see Fig. 6-19).

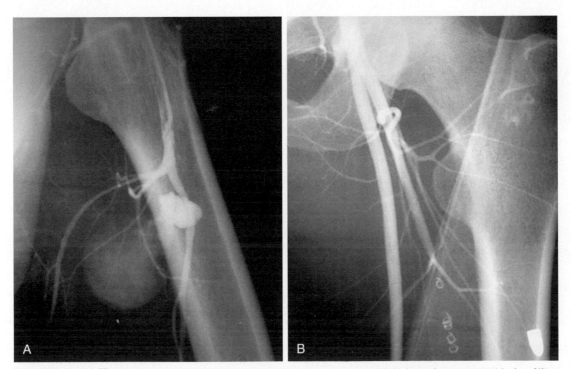

FIGURE 6-54 ▪ Traumatic deep femoral artery pseudoaneurysm. **A,** A large, bilobed pseudoaneurysm with slow filling of the larger cavity arises from a muscular branch of the deep femoral artery. **B,** The pseudoaneurysm was excluded by placing coils distal and proximal to the aneurysm neck.

If the patient continues to smoke, gangrene and amputation may result. If the patient stops smoking, stabilization and some improvement in symptoms can be expected. Pharmacologic treatment with the prostacyclin analogue iloprost is effective in some cases. Thrombolytic therapy has had mixed results.[238] Surgical options include sympathectomy, bypass grafting (when feasible), and, ultimately, amputation.

Vasospasm of the lower extremity arteries is seen with a variety of disorders (see Box 6-4 and Figs. 2-16, 6-31, and 6-53). Functional arterial narrowing also occurs when proximal arteries are obstructed. Chronic use or abuse of certain vasospastic agents can cause ischemic symptoms, diminished pulses, and occasionally gangrene.[239] The characteristic finding of drug-induced vasospasm is bilateral, symmetric, abrupt narrowing of the iliac, femoral, or popliteal arteries that resolves after discontinuation of the drug. Vasospasm from any source is partially or completely relieved with vasodilators, removal of the causative factor, and time.

Standing waves are periodic oscillations in an arterial segment that are occasionally seen during lower extremity arteriography (see Fig. 6-16). The regular, corrugated appearance should not be confused with other entities. This unusual phenomenon may be related to the physiology of flow in this particular vascular bed.[240]

Fibromuscular dysplasia is a set of related disorders in which noninflammatory fibrotic tissue proliferates in one or more layers of the arterial wall (see Chapter 3). It is an uncommon cause of renal artery stenosis; it is a rare cause of carotid or iliac artery disease.[241] The medial fibroplasia type of fibromuscular dysplasia produces a "string of beads" appearance, with alternating constriction and dilation of the vessel (see Fig. 6-17A).

Radiation arteritis can develop years after high-dose radiotherapy for pelvic malignancy (see Chapter 3 and Fig. 3-29).[242] Patients with preexisting PVD are more susceptible to radiation arteritis. The typical angiographic findings are focal or diffuse stenoses and occlusions within the radiation field.

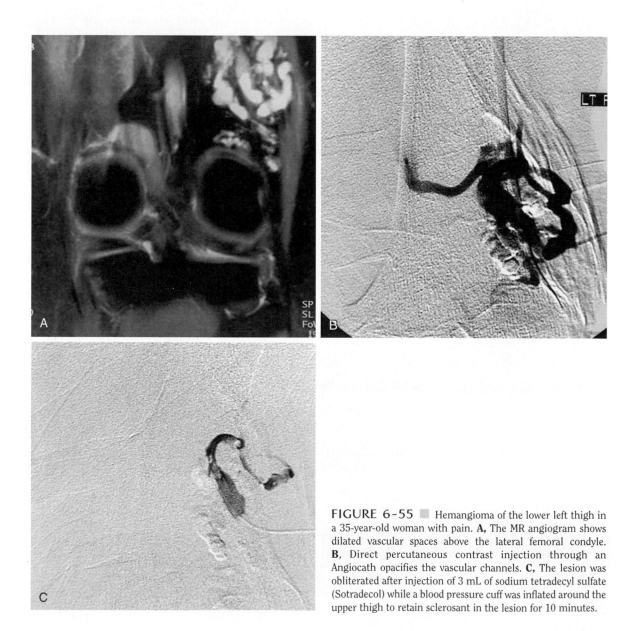

FIGURE 6-55 ■ Hemangioma of the lower left thigh in a 35-year-old woman with pain. **A,** The MR angiogram shows dilated vascular spaces above the lateral femoral condyle. **B,** Direct percutaneous contrast injection through an Angiocath opacifies the vascular channels. **C,** The lesion was obliterated after injection of 3 mL of sodium tetradecyl sulfate (Sotradecol) while a blood pressure cuff was inflated around the upper thigh to retain sclerosant in the lesion for 10 minutes.

Arteriovenous Communications

Congenital arteriovenous malformations (AVMs) are rare, but the pelvis and legs are among the most commonly affected sites. Lower extremity lesions include classic AVMs and *hemangiomas* (see Chapter 3).[243] Patients usually present as children or young adults with an enlarging leg mass associated with pain, limb hypertrophy, varices, or a thrill or bruit over the lesion. Color Doppler sonography and MR imaging are the primary tools for diagnosis and staging of suspected extremity AVMs (Fig. 6-55).[244-246] Angiography (arteriography or direct lesion puncture) is reserved for embolotherapy or operative planning.

Arterial-type AVMs have markedly dilated feeding vessels, hypervascularity, pooling of contrast within the nidus of the malformation, and early, rapid venous washout (Fig. 6-56). Occasionally, a highly vascular soft tissue or bony tumor will have a similar appearance. *Hemangiomas* appear as large, amorphous, vascular spaces with relatively normal inflow arteries and slow venous washout (see Fig. 6-55).

It is exceedingly difficult to completely eradicate lower extremity AVMs. Invasive therapy should only be undertaken to relieve pain, bleeding, ulceration, severe deformity, or high-output cardiac failure. When feasible, the treatment of choice is embolotherapy by an intra-arterial route or by direct percutaneous puncture (see Chapter 2).[247-250] Embolization is performed in stages to limit nontarget tissue loss. The theoretical goal is to permanently obliterate the nidus. Proximal embolization must be strictly avoided.

Depending on the subtype of AVM (e.g., arterial, venous), the agents of choice are absolute alcohol, cyanoacrylates (glue), microparticles or microspheres, and ethylene vinyl alcohol copolymer (Onyx).[249-251] Unfortunately, amputation is ultimately required for some lower extremity high-flow AVMs, even after multiple aggressive percutaneous treatment sessions.[247] For hemangiomas and venous malformations,

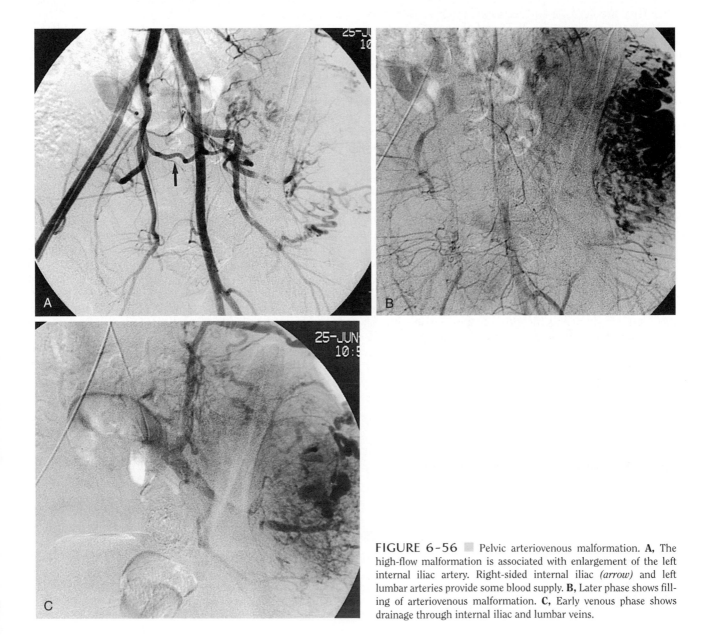

FIGURE 6-56 ▪ Pelvic arteriovenous malformation. **A,** The high-flow malformation is associated with enlargement of the left internal iliac artery. Right-sided internal iliac *(arrow)* and left lumbar arteries provide some blood supply. **B,** Later phase shows filling of arteriovenous malformation. **C,** Early venous phase shows drainage through internal iliac and lumbar veins.

direct injection with a sclerosing agent (such as absolute alcohol) can be extremely effective.[248]

Pelvic AVMs include true congenital AVMs (often arising from the uterus) and acquired lesions (from gestational trophoblastic disease, prior surgery, tumor, or other causes) (see Chapter 11).[251,252] These malformations, which are typically seen in young to middle-aged women, cause pelvic pain, vaginal bleeding, spontaneous abortion, and (occasionally) congestive heart failure. Congenital lesions are supplied by numerous vessels, including branches of the internal iliac, ovarian, and inferior mesenteric arteries. Acquired lesions may be supplied entirely by the uterine arteries. Surgical resection is only possible in some cases and often requires hysterectomy. Embolotherapy is more effective for palliation and may allow preservation of the uterus. A variety of embolic agents has been tried, including polyvinyl alcohol, absolute alcohol, and Gelfoam.

AVFs in the lower extremity are almost always caused by accidental or iatrogenic trauma (see Fig. 6-52). Physiologic *arteriovenous shunts* are present throughout most vascular beds.[253] They are occasionally seen during lower extremity angiography in patients with PVD and after angioplasty of arterial stenoses (see Fig. 3-42).

Popliteal Artery Disorders

The popliteal artery is affected by a unique set of diseases, some of which are seen in relatively young patients (Box 6-9).

Popliteal artery aneurysms are almost always degenerative. About one half of these lesions are bilateral, and about one third of patients have coexistent abdominal aortic aneurysms.[206,207,254] The disorder is almost exclusively seen in elderly men, and one fourth to one third of them have no symptoms at presentation. The major complications are thrombosis, distal embolization, and extrinsic compression of the popliteal vein or tibial nerve. Rupture is uncommon.[255]

Most popliteal artery aneurysms are detected by physical examination and confirmed with sonography. Imaging studies show intimal calcification, fusiform widening of the artery, and mural thrombus (see Figs. 6-14 and 6-46).[256] The disease usually spares the distal popliteal artery. If the aneurysm is completely thrombosed, it may be unsuspected by arteriography unless mural calcification or displacement of geniculate branches is noted. Because of the significant risk of thrombosis or distal embolization, elective surgical bypass is performed in most patients. Endovascular stent-grafts also have been used.

Adventitial cystic disease is a rare condition in which mucin collects in the adventitial layer of the popliteal artery and rarely in other vessels (femoral, axillary, iliac, and forearm arteries).[257-259] It is most typically seen in young to middle-aged men who complain of sudden onset of popliteal fossa pain and claudication. The precise cause of this disorder is unknown, although it may arise from the adjacent joint capsule, nerve, or tendon. As the cysts grow and coalesce, they can eventually rupture and narrow (or occlude) the arterial lumen.

The diagnosis is made with color Doppler sonography or CT or MR angiography.[256,260,261] The radiographic appearance is that of smooth, eccentric, extrinsic ("hourglass") narrowing of the upper popliteal artery (Fig. 6-57). Stenosis may progress to complete occlusion. Standard treatment is cyst evacuation (with or without patching) or primary resection. The safety or effectiveness of balloon angioplasty has not been proven.

Popliteal artery entrapment results from an abnormal relationship between the popliteal artery and the gastrocnemius (or less often, the popliteus) muscle, causing arterial compression.[262,263] Entrapment is bilateral in about one third of patients. Men are affected far more often than women, and many of them are athletes. In a significant percentage of the general population, transient narrowing or occlusion of the popliteal artery by muscles in the normally positioned "soleal sling" can occur, particularly with active plantar flexion.[264]

Three or four distinct anatomic subtypes have been described.[261,262] Most commonly, the artery deviates medially behind a normally positioned medial head of the gastrocnemius muscle (type I) or around an abnormally positioned muscle bundle (type II). The popliteal vein is not usually affected. Popliteal entrapment can be diagnosed with a variety of imaging modalities. Typical findings include narrowing and medial (or occasionally lateral) deviation of the midportion of the popliteal artery. Sometimes, the artery appears normal in a neutral position. The imaging study is then repeated with active, prolonged plantar flexion or passive dorsiflexion of the foot, which should provoke the compression (Fig. 6-58). Left untreated, the condition can lead to aneurysm formation, thrombosis, or distal embolization. The standard therapy is muscular or arterial release or bypass grafting.

Iliac Artery Endofibrosis

External iliac artery endofibrosis is an unusual disorder in which the intima is thickened by collagen, smooth muscle cells, and fibroblasts without any histologic evidence for atherosclerosis or inflammation. Endofibrosis is almost exclusively confined to the first few centimeters of the external iliac artery, and it is virtually seen only in high-performance athletes (particularly racing cyclists).[265,266] The etiology is unknown. Patients only complain of symptoms with vigorous activity. Screening is done with segmental blood pressure measurements during and after extreme exercise.

BOX 6-9   ■   Disorders Affecting the Popliteal Artery
Atherosclerosis
Embolism
Aneurysm
Trauma
Buerger's disease
Adventitial cystic disease
Entrapment
Extrinsic compression (e.g., Baker's cyst)

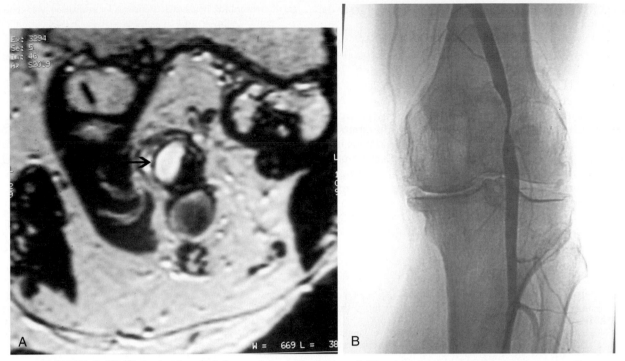

FIGURE 6-57 ■ Cystic adventitial disease of the popliteal artery. **A,** T2-weighted transverse MR image shows a cystic lesion *(arrow)* compressing the normal popliteal artery. **B,** Catheter angiogram reveals the classic hourglass appearance of the lesion. (Courtesy of Thomas Velling, MD, Newport Beach, Calif.)

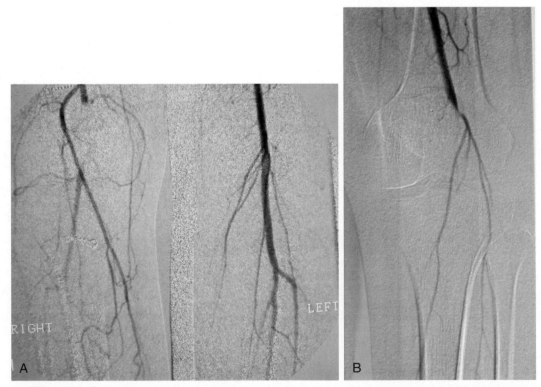

FIGURE 6-58 ■ Popliteal artery entrapment syndrome. **A,** Normal course of both popliteal arteries in neutral position. The right side is occluded. **B,** With active plantar flexion, the left popliteal artery becomes occluded. (Courtesy of John Kaufman, MD, Portland, Ore.)

Standard treatment is saphenous vein patch angioplasty or bypass graft placement.[267]

Neoplasms

Women with gynecologic tumors complicated by pelvic or vaginal bleeding may be treated with embolotherapy (see Chapter 11). Angiography has almost no role in the evaluation of neoplasms of the lower extremity. Occasionally, patients with highly vascular tumors undergo arteriography for preoperative planning or for embolotherapy to minimize bleeding during surgery.

REFERENCES

1. Caridi JG, Hawkins IF Jr, Klioze SD, et al: Carbon dioxide digital subtraction angiography: the practical approach. Tech Vasc Interv Radiol 2001;4:57.
2. Oliva VL, Denbow N, Therasse E, et al: Digital subtraction angiography of the abdominal aorta and lower extremities: carbon dioxide versus iodinated contrast material. J Vasc Interv Radiol 1999;10:723.
3. Diaz LP, Pabon IP, Garcia JS, et al: Assessment of CO_2 arteriography in arterial occlusive disease of the lower extremities. J Vasc Interv Radiol 2000;11:163.
4. Spinosa DJ, Kaufman JA, Hartwell GD, et al: Gadolinium chelates in angiography and interventional radiology: a useful alternative to iodinated contrast media for angiography. Radiology 2002;223:319.
5. Collins P, ed: Embryology and development. In: Williams PL, Bannister LH, Berry MM, et al, eds. Gray's Anatomy, 38th ed. New York, Churchill Livingstone, 1995:320.
6. Gabella G, ed: Cardiovascular system. In: Williams PL, Bannister LH, Berry MM, et al, eds. Gray's Anatomy, 38th ed. New York, Churchill Livingstone, 1995:1558.
7. Alson MD, Lang EV, Kaufman JA: Pedal arterial imaging. J Vasc Interv Radiol 1997;8:9.
8. Shinozaki T, Arita S, Watanabe H, et al: Aneurysm of a persistent sciatic artery. Arch Orthop Trauma Surg 1998;117:167.
9. Brantley SK, Rigdon EE, Raju S: Persistent sciatic artery: embryology, pathology, and treatment. J Vasc Surg 1993;18:242.
10. Kadir S, ed: Atlas of Normal and Variant Angiographic Anatomy. Philadelphia, WB Saunders, 1991:123.
11. Mauro MA, Jaques PF, Moore M: The popliteal artery and its branches: embryologic basis of normal and variant anatomy. AJR Am J Roentgenol 1988;150:435.
12. Piral T, Germain M, Princ G: Absence of the posterior tibial artery: implications for free transplants of the fibula. Surg Radiol Anat 1996;18:155.
13. Lutz BS, Wei FC, Ng SH, et al: Routine donor leg angiography before vascularized free fibula transplantation is not necessary: a prospective study in 120 clinical cases. Plast Reconstr Surg 1999;103:121.
14. Stoyioglou A, Jaff MR: Medical treatment of peripheral arterial disease: a comprehensive review. J Vasc Interv Radiol 2004;15:1197.
15. Murabito JM, D'Agostino RB, Silbershatz H, et al: Intermittent claudication. A risk profile from The Framingham Heart Study. Circulation 1997;96:44.
16. Criqui MH, Denenberg JO, Langer RD, et al: The epidemiology of peripheral arterial disease: importance of identifying the population at risk. Vasc Med 1997;2:221.
17. Blair JM, Glagov S, Zarins CK: Mechanism of superficial femoral artery adductor canal stenosis. Surg Forum 1990;41:359.
18. Mills JL, Porter JM: Basic data related to clinical decision making in acute limb ischemia. Ann Vasc Surg 1991;5:96.
19. Turnipseed WD: Clinical review of patients treated for atypical claudication: a 28-year experience. J Vasc Surg 2004;40:79.
20. Hertzer NR: The natural history of peripheral vascular disease: implications for its management. Circulation 1991;83(Suppl I):I-12.
21. Rutherford RB, Becker GJ: Standards for evaluating and reporting the results of surgical and percutaneous therapy for peripheral arterial disease. J Vasc Interv Radiol 1991;2:169.
22. Matchett WJ, McFarland DR, Eidt JF, et al: Blue toe syndrome: treatment with intra-arterial stents and review of therapies. J Vasc Interv Radiol 2000;11:585.
23. Rose SC: Noninvasive vascular laboratory for evaluation of peripheral arterial occlusive disease: Part II—clinical applications: chronic, usually atherosclerotic, lower extremity ischemia. J Vasc Interv Radiol 2000;11:1257.
24. Weitz JI, Byrne J, Clagett GP, et al: Diagnosis and treatment of chronic arterial insufficiency of the lower extremities: a critical review. Circulation 1996;94:3026.
25. Cambria RP, Kaufman JA, L'Italien GJ, et al: Magnetic resonance angiography in the management of lower extremity arterial occlusive disease: a prospective study. J Vasc Surg 1997;25:380.
26. Nelemans PJ, Leiner T, de Vet HC, et al: Peripheral arterial disease: meta-analysis of the diagnostic performance of MR angiography. Radiology 2000;217:105.
27. Quinn SF, Sheley RC, Semonsen KG, et al: Aortic and lower extremity arterial disease: evaluation with MR angiography versus conventional angiography. Radiology 1998;206:693.
28. Bertschinger K, Cassina PC, Debatin JF, et al: Surveillance of peripheral arterial bypass grafts with three-dimensional MR angiography: comparison with digital subtraction angiography. AJR Am J Roentgenol 2001;176:215.
29. Khilnani NM, Winchester PA, Prince MR, et al: Peripheral vascular disease: combined 3D bolus chase and dynamic 2D MR angiography compared with x-ray angiography for treatment planning. Radiology 2002;224:63.
30. Zhang HL, Khilnani NM, Prince MR, et al: Diagnostic accuracy of time-resolved 2D projection MR angiography for symptomatic infrapopliteal arterial occlusive disease. AJR Am J Roentgenol 2005;184:938.
31. Zhang HL, Ho BY, Chao M, et al: Decreased venous contamination on 3D gadolinium-enhanced bolus chase peripheral MR angiography using thigh compression. AJR Am J Roentgenol 2004;183:1041.
32. Kaufman JA, McCarter D, Geller SC, et al: Two-dimensional time-of-flight MR angiography of the lower extremities: artifacts and pitfalls. AJR Am J Roentgenol 1998;171:129.
33. Lee HM, Wang Y, Sostman HD, et al: Distal lower extremity arteries: evaluation with two-dimensional MR digital subtraction angiography. Radiology 1998;207:505.
34. Rubin GD, Shiau MC, Leung AN, et al: Aorta and iliac arteries: single versus multiple detector-row helical CT angiography. Radiology 2000;215:670.
35. Rubin GD, Schmidt AJ, Logan LJ, et al: Multi-detector row CT angiography of lower extremity arterial inflow and runoff: initial experience. Radiology 2001;221:146.
36. Duddalwar VA: Multislice CT angiography: a practical guide to CT angiography in vascular imaging and intervention. Br J Radiol 2004;77:S27.
37. Jakobs TF, Wintersperger BJ, Becker CR: MDCT-imaging of peripheral arterial disease. Semin Ultrasound CT MR 2004;25:145.
38. Rubin GD: MDCT imaging of the aorta and peripheral vessels. Eur J Radiol 2003;45(Suppl 1):S42.
39. Willmann JK, Mayer D, Banyai M, et al: Evaluation of peripheral arterial bypass grafts with multi-detector row CT angiography: comparison with duplex US and digital subtraction angiography. Radiology 2003;229:465.
40. Catalano C, Fraioli F, Laghi A, et al: Infrarenal aortic and lower-extremity arterial disease: diagnostic performance of multi-detector row CT angiography. Radiology 2004;231:555.
41. Kandarpa K, Becker GJ, Hunink MG, et al: Transcatheter interventions for the treatment of peripheral atherosclerotic lesions: part I. J Vasc Interv Radiol 2001;12:683.
42. de Vries SO, Visser K, de Vries JA, et al: Intermittent claudication: cost-effectiveness of revascularization versus exercise therapy. Radiology 2002;222:25.
43. Society of Interventional Radiology Standards of Practice Committee: Guidelines for percutaneous transluminal angioplasty. J Vasc Interv Radiol 2003;14(9 Pt 2):S209.
44. Dormandy JA, Rutherford RB: Management of peripheral arterial disease (PAD). TASC Working Group. TransAtlantic Inter-Society Consensus (TASC). J Vasc Surg 2000;31(1 Pt 2):S1.
45. Schillinger M, Exner M, Mlekusch W, et al: Vascular inflammation and percutaneous transluminal angioplasty of the femoropopliteal artery: association with restenosis. Radiology 2002;225:21.

46. Schillinger M, Exner M, Mlekusch W, et al: Endovascular revascularization below the knee: 6-month results and predictive value of C-reactive protein level. Radiology 2003;227:419.

47. Dibra A, Mehilli J, Braun S, et al: Association between C-reactive protein levels and subsequent cardiac events among patients with stable angina treated with coronary artery stenting. Am J Med 2003;114:715.

48. Walton BL, Dougherty K, Mortazavi A, et al: Percutaneous intervention for the treatment of hypoplastic aortoiliac syndrome. Catheter Cardiovasc Interv 2003;60:329.

49. Audet P, Therasse E, Oliva VL, et al: Infrarenal aortic stenosis: long-term clinical and hemodynamic results of percutaneous transluminal angioplasty. Radiology 1998;209:357.

50. Therasse E, Cote G, Oliva VL, et al: Infrarenal aortic stenosis: value of stent placement after percutaneous transluminal angioplasty failure. Radiology 2001;219:655.

51. Wescott MA, Bonn J: Comparison of conventional angioplasty with the Palmaz stent in the treatment of abdominal aortic stenoses from the STAR registry. J Vasc Intervent Radiol 1998;9:225.

52. Schedel H, Wissgott C, Rademaker J, et al: Primary stent placement for infrarenal aortic stenosis: immediate and midterm results. J Vasc Interv Radiol 2004;15:353.

53. Stoeckelhuber BM, Meissner O, Stoeckelhuber M, et al: Primary endovascular stent placement for focal infrarenal aortic stenosis: initial and midterm results. J Vasc Interv Radiol 2003;14:1443.

54. Sheeran SR, Hallisey MJ, Ferguson D: Percutaneous transluminal stent placement in the abdominal aorta. J Vasc Interv Radiol 1997;8:55.

55. Ligush J, Criado E, Burnham SJ, et al: Management and outcome of chronic atherosclerotic infrarenal aortic occlusion. J Vasc Surg 1996;24:394.

56. Cynamon J, Marin ML, Veith FJ, et al: Stent-graft repair of aortoiliac occlusive disease coexisting with common femoral artery disease. J Vasc Interv Radiol 1997;8:19.

57. Tetteroo E, van der Graaf Y, Bosch JL, et al: Randomised comparison of primary stent placement versus primary angioplasty followed by selective stent placement in patients with iliac-artery occlusive disease. Dutch Iliac Stent Trial Study Group. Lancet 1998;351:1153.

58. Bosch JL, Hunink MG: Meta-analysis of the results of percutaneous transluminal angioplasty and stent placement for aortoiliac occlusive disease. Radiology 1997;204:87.

59. Bosch JL, Haaring C, Meyerovitz MF, et al: Cost-effectiveness of percutaneous treatment of iliac artery occlusive disease in the United States. AJR Am J Roentgenol 2000;175:517.

60. Smith JC, Watkins GE, Taylor FC, et al: Angioplasty or stent placement in the proximal common iliac artery: is protection of the contralateral side necessary? J Vasc Interv Radiol 2001;12:1395.

61. Johnston KW: Iliac arteries: reanalysis of results of balloon angioplasty. Radiology 1993;186:207.

62. Tetteroo E, van Engelen AD, Spithoven JH, et al: Stent placement after iliac angioplasty: comparison of hemodynamic and angiographic criteria. Radiology 1996;201:155.

63. Henry M, Amor M, Ethevenot G, et al: Palmaz stent placement in iliac and femoropopliteal arteries: primary and secondary patency in 310 patients with 2-4 year follow-up. Radiology 1995;197:167.

64. Murphy KD, Encarnacion CE, Le VA, et al: Iliac artery stent placement with the Palmaz stent: follow-up study. J Vasc Interv Radiol 1995;6:321.

65. Sapoval MR, Chatellier G, Long AL, et al: Self-expandable stents for the treatment of iliac artery obstructive lesions: long-term success and prognostic factors. AJR Am J Roentgenol 1996;166:1173.

66. Murphy TP, Ariaratnam NS, Carney WI Jr, et al: Aortoiliac insufficiency: long-term experience with stent placement for treatment. Radiology 2004;231:243.

67. Schurmann K, Mahnken A, Meyer J, et al: Long-term results 10 years after iliac arterial stent placement. Radiology 2002;224:731.

68. Hamer OW, Borisch I, Finkenzeller T, et al: Iliac artery stent placement: clinical experience and short-term follow-up regarding a self-expanding nitinol stent. J Vasc Interv Radiol 2004;15:1231.

69. Sapoval MR, Long AL, Pagny J-V, et al: Outcome of percutaneous intervention in iliac artery stents. Radiology 1996;198:481.

70. Vorwerk D, Guenther RW, Schuermann K, et al: Late reobstruction in iliac arterial stents: percutaneous treatment. Radiology 1995;197:479.

71. Hausegger KA, Cragg AH, Lammer J, et al: Iliac artery stent placement: clinical experience with a nitinol stent. Radiology 1994;190:199.

72. Long AL, Page PE, Raynaud AC, et al: Percutaneous iliac artery stent: angiographic long-term follow-up. Radiology 1991;180:771.

73. Ponec D, Jaff MR, Swischuk J, et al: The Nitinol SMART stent vs Wallstent for suboptimal iliac artery angioplasty: CRISP-US trial results. J Vasc Interv Radiol 2004;15:911.

74. Leung DA, Spinosa DJ, Hagspiel KD, et al: Selection of stents for treating iliac arterial occlusive disease. J Vasc Interv Radiol 2003;14:137.

75. Strecker E-P, Boos IBL, Hagen B: Flexible tantalum stents for the treatment of iliac artery lesions: long-term patency, complications, and risk factors. Radiology 1996;199:641.

76. Long AL, Sapoval MR, Beyssen BM, et al: Strecker stent implantation in iliac arteries: patency and predictive factors for long-term success. Radiology 1995;194:739.

77. Laborde JC, Palmaz JC, Rivera FJ, et al: Influence of anatomic distribution of atherosclerosis on the outcome of revascularization with iliac stent placement. J Vasc Interv Radiol 1995;6:513.

78. Palmaz JC, Laborde JC, Rivera FJ, et al: Stenting of the iliac arteries with the Palmaz stent: experience from a multicenter trial. Cardiovasc Intervent Radiol 1992;15:291.

79. Timaran CH, Stevens SL, Freeman MB, et al: External iliac and common iliac artery angioplasty and stenting in men and women. J Vasc Surg 2001;34:440.

80. Park SI, Won JH, Kim BM, et al: The arterial folding point during flexion of the hip joint. Cardiovasc Intervent Radiol 2005;28:173.

81. Blum U, Gabelmann A, Redecker M, et al: Percutaneous recanalization of iliac artery occlusions: results of a prospective study. Radiology 1993;189:536.

82. Reyes R, Maynar M, Lopera J, et al: Treatment of chronic iliac artery occlusions with guide wire recanalization and primary stent placement. J Vasc Interv Radiol 1997;8:1049.

83. Vorwerk D, Guenther RW, Schuermann K, et al: Primary stent placement for chronic iliac artery occlusions: follow-up results in 103 patients. Radiology 1995;194:745.

84. Dyet JF, Gaines PA, Nicholson AA, et al: Treatment of chronic iliac artery occlusions by means of percutaneous endovascular stent placement. J Vasc Interv Radiol 1997;8:349.

85. Yedlicka JW Jr, Ferral H, Bjarnason H, et al: Chronic iliac artery occlusions: primary recanalization with endovascular stents. J Vasc Interv Radiol 1994;5:843.

86. Cragg AH, Dake MD: Treatment of peripheral vascular disease with stent-grafts. Radiology 1997;205:307.

87. Kofoed SC, Bismuth J, Just S, et al: Angioplasty for the treatment of buttock claudication caused by internal iliac artery stenoses. Ann Vasc Surg 2001;15:396.

88. Gruen B, Roth FJ: Percutaneous transluminal angioplasty of the deep femoral artery. Rofo Fortschr Geb Rontgenstr Neuen Bildgeb Verfahr 1995;163:163.

89. Hoffman U, Schneider E, Bollinger A: Percutaneous transluminal angioplasty of the deep femoral artery. Vasa 1992;21:69.

90. Silva JA, White CJ, Ramee SR, et al: Percutaneous profundaplasty in the treatment of lower extremity ischemia: results of long-term surveillance. J Endovasc Ther 2001;8:75.

91. Diehm N, Savolainen H, Mahler F, et al: Does deep femoral artery revascularization as an isolated procedure play a role in chronic critical limb ischemia? J Endovasc Ther 2004;11:119.

92. Hunink MG, Wong JB, Donaldson MC, et al: Revascularization for femoropopliteal disease. A decision and cost-effectiveness analysis. JAMA 1995;274:165.

93. Pentecost MJ, Criqui MH, Dorros G, et al: Guidelines for peripheral percutaneous transluminal angioplasty of the abdominal aorta and lower extremity vessels. Circulation 1994;89:511.

94. Capek P, McLean GK, Berkowitz HD: Femoropopliteal angioplasty. Factors influencing long-term success. Circulation 1991;83(Suppl I):I-70.

95. Taylor LM Jr, Porter JM: Clinical and anatomic considerations for surgery in femoropopliteal disease and the results of surgery. Circulation 1991;83(Suppl I):I-63.

96. Matsi PJ, Manninen HI, Vanninen RL, et al: Femoropopliteal angioplasty in patients with claudication: primary and secondary patency in 140 limbs with 1-3 year follow-up. Radiology 1994;191:727.

97. Johnston KW: Femoral and popliteal arteries: reanalysis of results of balloon angioplasty. Radiology 1992;183:767.

98. Matsi PJ, Manninen HI: Impact of different patency criteria on long-term results of femoropopliteal angioplasty: analysis of 106 consecutive patients with claudication. J Vasc Interv Radiol 1995;6:159.

99. Clark TW, Groffsky JL, Soulen MC: Predictors of long-term patency after femoropopliteal angioplasty: results from the STAR registry. J Vasc Interv Radiol 2001;12:923.

100. Jamsen TS, Manninen HI, Jaakkola PA, et al: Long-term outcome of patients with claudication after balloon angioplasty of the femoropopliteal arteries. Radiology 2002;225:345.

101. Jamsen T, Manninen H, Tulla H, et al: The final outcome of primary infrainguinal percutaneous transluminal angioplasty in 100 consecutive patients with chronic critical limb ischemia. J Vasc Interv Radiol 2002;13:455.

102. Rabbi JF, Kiran RP, Gersten G, et al: Early results with infrainguinal cutting balloon angioplasty limits distal dissection. Ann Vasc Surg 2004;18:640.

103. Laird J, Jaff MR, Biamino G, et al: Cryoplasty for the treatment of femoropopliteal arterial disease: results of a prospective, multicenter registry. J Vasc Interv Radiol 2005;16:1067.

104. Becquemin JP, Favre JP, Marzelle J, et al: Systematic versus selective stent placement after superficial femoral artery balloon angioplasty: a multicenter prospective randomized study. J Vasc Surg 2003;37:487.

105. Cejna M, Thurnher S, Illiasch H, et al: PTA versus Palmaz stent placement in femoropopliteal artery obstructions: a multicenter prospective randomized study. J Vasc Interv Radiol 2001;12:23.

106. Grimm J, Mueller-Huelsbeck S, Jahnke T, et al: Randomized study to compare PTA alone versus PTA with Palmaz stent placement for femoropopliteal lesions. J Vasc Interv Radiol 2001;12:935.

107. Muradin GS, Bosch JL, Stijnen T, et al: Balloon dilation and stent implantation for treatment of femoropopliteal arterial disease: meta-analysis. Radiology 2001;221:137.

108. Lugmayr HF, Holzer H, Kastner M, et al: Treatment of complex arteriosclerotic lesions with nitinol stents in the superficial femoral and popliteal arteries: a midterm follow-up. Radiology 2002;222:37.

109. Jahnke T, Voshage G, Mueller-Huelsbeck S, et al: Endovascular placement of self-expanding nitinol coil stents for the treatment of femoropopliteal obstructive disease. J Vasc Interv Radiol 2002;13:257.

110. Sabeti S, Schillinger M, Amighi J, et al: Primary patency of femoropopliteal arteries treated with nitinol versus stainless steel self-expanding stents: propensity score-adjusted analysis. Radiology 2004;232:516.

111. Vogel TR, Shindelman LE, Nackman GB, et al: Efficacious use of nitinol stents in the femoral and popliteal arteries. J Vasc Surg 2003;38:1178.

112. Ahmadi R, Schillinger M, Maca T, et al: Femoropopliteal arteries: immediate and long-term results with a Dacron-covered stent-graft. Radiology 2002;223:345.

113. Lammer J, Dake MD, Bleyn J, et al: Peripheral arterial obstruction: prospective study of treatment with a transluminally placed self-expanding stent-graft. International Trial Study Group. Radiology 2000;217:95.

114. Saxon RR, Coffman JM, Gooding JM, et al: Long-term results of ePTFE stent-graft versus angioplasty in the femoropopliteal artery: single center experience from a prospective, randomized trial. J Vasc Interv Radiol 2003;14:303.

115. Jahnke T, Andresen R, Mueller-Huelsbeck S, et al: Hemobahn stent-grafts for treatment of femoropopliteal arterial obstructions: midterm results of a prospective trial. J Vasc Interv Radiol 2003;14:41.

116. Deutschmann HA, Schedlbauer P, Berczi V, et al: Placement of Hemobahn stent-grafts in femoropopliteal arteries: early experience and midterm results in 18 patients. J Vasc Interv Radiol 2001;12:943.

117. Duda SH, Poerner TC, Wiesinger B, et al: Drug-eluting stents: potential applications for peripheral arterial occlusive disease. J Vasc Interv Radiol 2003;14:291.

118. Duda SH, Bosiers M, Lammer J, et al: Sirolimus-eluting versus bare nitinol stent for obstructive superficial femoral artery disease: The SIROCCO II trial. J Vasc Interv Radiol 2005;16:331.

119. Oliva VL, Soulez G: Sirolimus-eluting stents versus the superficial femoral artery: Second round. J Vasc Interv Radiol 2005;16:313.

120. Tielbeek AV, Vroegindeweij D, Buth J, et al: Comparison of balloon angioplasty and Simpson atherectomy for lesions in the femoropopliteal artery: angiographic and clinical results of a prospective randomized trial. J Vasc Interv Radiol 1996;7:837.

121. Maynar M, Reyes R, Cabrera V, et al: Percutaneous atherectomy as an alternative treatment for post-angioplasty obstructive intimal flaps. Radiology 1989;170:1029.

122. Zeller T, Rastan A, Schwarzwalder U, et al: Percutaneous peripheral atherectomy of femoropopliteal stenoses using a new-generation device: six-month results from a single center experience. J Endovasc Ther 2004;11:676.

123. Ruef J, Hofmann M, Haase J: Endovascular interventions in iliac and infrainguinal occlusive artery disease. J Interv Cardiol 2004;17:427.

124. Waksman R, Laird JR, Jurkovitz CT, et al: Intravascular radiation therapy after balloon angioplasty of narrowed femoropopliteal arteries to prevent restenosis: results of the PARIS feasibility clinical trial. J Vasc Interv Radiol 2001;12:915.

125. Krueger K, Zaehringer M, Bendel M, et al: De novo femoropopliteal stenoses: endovascular gamma irradiation following angioplasty—angiographic and clinical follow-up in a prospective randomized controlled trial. Radiology 2004;231:546.

126. Schillinger M, Minar E: Advances in vascular brachytherapy over the last 10 years: focus on femoropopliteal applications. J Endovasc Ther 2004;11(Suppl 2):II180.

127. Gordon IL, Conroy RM, Arefi M, et al: Three-year outcome of endovascular treatment of superficial femoral artery occlusion. Arch Surg 2001;136:221.

128. Rilinger N, Goerich J, Scharrer-Pamler R, et al: Short-term results with use of the Amplatz thrombectomy device in the treatment of acute lower limb occlusions. J Vasc Interv Radiol 1997;8:343.

129. Spinosa DJ, Leung DA, Matsumoto AH, et al: Percutaneous intentional extraluminal recanalization in patients with chronic critical limb ischemia. Radiology 2004;232:499.

130. Treiman GS, Whiting JH, Treiman RL, et al: Treatment of limb-threatening ischemia with percutaneous intentional extraluminal recanalization: a preliminary evaluation. J Vasc Surg 2003;38:29.

131. Spinosa DJ, Harthun NL, Bissonette EA, et al: Subintimal arterial flossing with antegrade-retrograde intervention (SAFARI) for subintimal recanalization to treat chronic critical limb ischemia. J Vasc Interv Radiol 2005;16:37.

132. Yilmaz S, Sindel T, Yegin A, et al: Subintimal angioplasty of long superficial femoral artery occlusions. J Vasc Interv Radiol 2003;14:997.

133. Lipsitz EC, Ohki T, Veith FJ, et al: Does subintimal angioplasty have a role in the treatment of severe lower extremity ischemia? J Vasc Surg 2003;37:386.

134. Bakal CW, Cynamon J, Sprayregen S: Infrapopliteal percutaneous transluminal angioplasty: what we know. Radiology 1996;200:36.

135. Bull PG, Mendel H, Hold M, et al: Distal popliteal and tibioperoneal transluminal angioplasty: long-term follow-up. J Vasc Interv Radiol 1992;3:45.

136. Brown KT, Moore ED, Getrajdman GI, et al: Infrapopliteal angioplasty: long-term follow-up. J Vasc Interv Radiol 1993;4:139.

137. Soder HK, Manninen HI, Jaakkola P, et al: Prospective trial of infrapopliteal artery balloon angioplasty for critical limb ischemia: angiographic and clinical results. J Vasc Interv Radiol 2000;11:1021.

138. Zeller T, Rastan A, Schwarzwaelder U, et al: Midterm results after atherectomy-assisted angioplasty of below-knee arteries with use of the Silverhawk device. J Vasc Interv Radiol 2004;15:1391.

139. Rutherford RB: Options in the surgical management of aorto-iliac occlusive disease: a changing perspective. Cardiovasc Surg 1999;7:5.

140. Abbott WM, Green RM, Matsumoto T, et al: Prosthetic above-knee femoropopliteal bypass grafting: results of a multicenter randomized prospective trial. Above-Knee Femoropopliteal Study Group. J Vasc Surg 1997;25:19.

141. Shah DM, Darling RC III, Chang BB, et al: Long-term results of in situ saphenous vein bypass: analysis of 2058 cases. Ann Surg 1995;222:438.

142. Johnson WC, Lee KK: A comparative evaluation of polytetrafluoroethylene, umbilical vein, and saphenous vein bypass grafts for femoral-popliteal above-knee revascularization: a prospective randomized Department of Veterans Affairs cooperative study. J Vasc Surg 2000;32:268.

143. Schneider JR, Walsh DB, McDaniel MD, et al: Pedal bypass versus tibial bypass with autogenous vein: a comparison of outcome and hemodynamic results. J Vasc Surg 1993;17:1029.

144. Darling RC 3rd, Chang BB, Paty PS, et al: Choice of peroneal or dorsalis pedis artery bypass for limb salvage. Am J Surg 1995;170:109.

145. Sharma PV, Babu SC, Shah PM, et al: Changing patterns of atheroembolism. Cardiovasc Surg 1996;4:573.

146. Karalis DG, Quinn V, Victor MF, et al: Risk of catheter-related emboli in patients with atherosclerotic debris in the thoracic aorta. Am Heart J 1996;131:1149.

147. Applebaum RM, Kronzon I: Evaluation and management of cholesterol embolization and blue toe syndrome. Curr Opin Cardiol 1996;11:533.

148. Bashore TM, Gehrig T: Cholesterol emboli after invasive cardiac procedures. J Am Coll Cardiol 2003;42:217.

149. Baumann DS, McGraw D, Rubin BG, et al: An institutional experience with arterial atheroembolism. Ann Vasc Surg 1994;8:258.

150. Keen RR, McCarthy WJ, Shireman PK, et al: Surgical management of atheroembolization. J Vasc Surg 1995;21:773.

151. Kumins NH, Owens EL, Oglevie SB, et al: Early experience using the Wallgraft in the management of distal microembolism from common iliac artery pathology. Ann Vasc Surg 2002;16:181.

152. Wagner H-J, Mueller-Huelsbeck S, Pitton MB, et al: Rapid thrombectomy with a hydrodynamic catheter: results from a prospective, multicenter trial. Radiology 1997;205:675.

153. Huettl EA, Soulen MC: Thrombolysis of lower extremity embolic occlusions: a study of the results of the STAR registry. Radiology 1995;197:141.

154. Spence LD, Hartnell GG, Reinking G, et al: Thrombolysis of infrapopliteal bypass grafts: efficacy and underlying angiographic pathology. AJR Am J Roentgenol 1997;169:717.

155. Rajan DK, Patel NH, Valji K, et al: Quality improvement guidelines for percutaneous management of acute limb ischemia. J Vasc Interv Radiol 2005;16:585.

156. Valji K: Evolving strategies for thrombolytic therapy of peripheral vascular occlusion. J Vasc Interv Radiol 2000;11:411.

157. Semba CP, Murphy TP, Bakal CW, et al: Thrombolytic therapy with use of alteplase (rt-PA) in peripheral arterial occlusive disease: review of the clinical literature. The Advisory Panel. J Vasc Interv Radiol 2000;11:149.

158. Benenati J, Shlansky-Goldberg R, Meglin A, et al: Thrombolytic and antiplatelet therapy in peripheral vascular disease with use of reteplase and/or abciximab. The SCVIR Consultants' Conference. J Vasc Interv Radiol 2001;12:795.

159. Razavi MK, Lee DS, Hofmann LV: Catheter-directed thrombolytic therapy for limb ischemia: current status and controversies. J Vasc Interv Radiol 2004;15:13.

160. Weaver FA, Comerota AJ, Youngblood M, et al: Surgical revascularization versus thrombolysis for nonembolic lower extremity native artery occlusions: results of a prospective randomized trial. The STILE Investigators. Surgery versus Thrombolysis for Ischemia of the Lower Extremity. J Vasc Surg 1996;24:513.

161. Ouriel K, Veith FJ, Sasahara AA: A comparison of recombinant urokinase with vascular surgery as initial treatment for acute arterial occlusion of the legs: Thrombolysis or Peripheral Arterial Surgery (TOPAS) Investigators. N Engl J Med 1998;338:1105.

162. Ouriel K, Shortell CK, Azodo MV, et al: Acute peripheral arterial occlusion: predictors of success in catheter-directed thrombolytic therapy. Radiology 1994;193:561.

163. Arepally A, Hofmann LV, Kim HS, et al: Weight-based rt-PA thrombolysis protocol for acute native arterial and bypass graft occlusions. J Vasc Interv Radiol 2002;13:45.

164. Swischuk JL, Fox PF, Young K, et al: Transcatheter intraarterial infusion of rt-PA for acute lower limb ischemia: results and complications. J Vasc Interv Radiol 2001;12:423.

165. Semba CP, Bakal CW, Calis KA, et al: Alteplase as an alternative to urokinase. Advisory Panel on Catheter-Directed Thrombolytic Therapy. J Vasc Interv Radiol 2000;11:279.

166. Davidian MM, Powell A, Benenati JF, et al: Initial results of reteplase in the treatment of acute lower extremity arterial occlusions. J Vasc Interv Radiol 2000;11:289.

167. Burkart DJ, Borsa JJ, Anthony JP, et al: Thrombolysis of occluded peripheral arteries and veins with tenecteplase: a pilot study. J Vasc Interv Radiol 2002;13:1099.

168. Ouriel K, Katzen B, Mewissen M, et al: Reteplase in the treatment of peripheral arterial and venous occlusions: a pilot study. J Vasc Interv Radiol 2000;11:849.

169. Castaneda F, Swischuk JL, Li R, et al: Declining-dose study of reteplase treatment for lower extremity arterial occlusions. J Vasc Interv Radiol 2002;13:1093.

170. Drescher P, McGuckin J, Rilling WS, et al: Catheter-directed thrombolytic therapy in peripheral artery occlusions: combining reteplase and abciximab. AJR Am J Roentgenol 2003;180:1385.

171. Ouriel K: Use of concomitant glycoprotein IIb/IIIa inhibitors with catheter-directed peripheral arterial thrombolysis. J Vasc Interv Radiol 2004;15:543.

172. Shlansky-Goldberg R: Platelet aggregation inhibitors for use in peripheral vascular interventions: what can we learn from the experience in the coronary arteries? J Vasc Interv Radiol 2002;13:229.

173. Ouriel K, Castaneda F, McNamara T, et al: Reteplase monotherapy and reteplase/abciximab combination therapy in peripheral arterial occlusive disease: results from the RELAX trial. J Vasc Interv Radiol 2004;15:229.

174. Duda SH, Tepe G, Luz O, et al: Peripheral artery occlusion: treatment with abciximab plus urokinase versus with urokinase alone—a randomized pilot trial (the PROMPT Study). Platelet Receptor Antibodies in Order to Manage Peripheral Artery Thrombosis. Radiology 2001; 221:689.

175. Kasirajan K, Gray B, Beavers FP, et al: Rheolytic thrombectomy in the management of acute and subacute limb-threatening ischemia. J Vasc Interv Radiol 2001;12:413.

176. Kasirajan K, Haskal ZJ, Ouriel K: The use of mechanical thrombectomy devices in the management of acute peripheral arterial occlusive disease. J Vasc Interv Radiol 2001;12:405.

177. Gorich J, Rilinger N, Sokiranski R, et al: Mechanical thrombolysis of acute occlusion of both the superficial and the deep femoral arteries using a thrombectomy device. AJR Am J Roentgenol 1998; 170:1177.

178. Fontaine AB, Borsa JJ, Hoffer EK, et al: Type III heart block with peripheral use of the Angiojet thrombectomy system. J Vasc Interv Radiol 2001;12:1223.

179. Wagner HJ, Starck EE: Acute embolic occlusions of the infrainguinal arteries: percutaneous aspiration embolectomy in 102 patients. Radiology 1992;182:403.

180. Ouriel K, Shortell CK, DeWeese JA, et al: A comparison of thrombolytic therapy with operative revascularization in the initial treatment of acute peripheral arterial ischemia. J Vasc Surg 1994;19:1021.

181. Diffin DC, Kandarpa K: Assessment of peripheral intraarterial thrombolysis versus surgical revascularization in acute lower-limb ischemia: a review of limb salvage and mortality statistics. J Vasc Interv Radiol 1996;7:57.

182. Vorwerk D, Guenther RW, Wendt G, et al: Ulcerated plaques and focal aneurysms of iliac arteries: treatment with noncovered, self-expanding stents. AJR Am J Roentgenol 1994;162:1421.

183. Mattos MA, van Bemmelen PS, Hodgson KJ, et al: Does correction of stenoses identified with color duplex scanning improve infrainguinal graft patency? J Vasc Surg 1993;17:54.

184. Beidle TR, Brom-Ferral R, Letourneau JG: Surveillance of infrainguinal vein grafts with duplex sonography. AJR Am J Roentgenol 1994;162:443.

185. Bergamini TM, George SM Jr, Massey HT, et al: Intensive surveillance of femoropopliteal-tibial autogenous vein bypasses improves long-term graft patency and limb salvage. Ann Surg 1995;221:507.

186. Idu MM, Blankenstein JD, deGier P, et al: Impact of a color-flow duplex surveillance program on infrainguinal vein graft patency: a five year experience. J Vasc Surg 1993;17:42.

187. Meissner OA, Verrel F, Tato F, et al: Magnetic resonance angiography in the follow-up of distal lower-extremity bypass surgery: comparison with duplex ultrasound and digital subtraction angiography. J Vasc Interv Radiol 2004;15:1269.

188. Loewe C, Cejna M, Schoder M, et al: Contrast material-enhanced, moving-table MR angiography versus digital subtraction angiography for surveillance of peripheral arterial bypass grafts. J Vasc Interv Radiol 2003;14:1129.

189. Whittemore AD, Donaldson MC, Polak JF, et al: Limitations of balloon angioplasty for vein graft stenosis. J Vasc Surg 1991;14:340.

190. Perler BA, Osterman FA, Mitchell SE, et al: Balloon dilatation versus surgical revision of infra-inguinal autogenous vein graft stenoses: long-term follow-up. J Cardiovasc Surg 1990;31:656.

191. Goh RH, Sniderman KW, Kalman PG: Long-term follow-up of management of failing in situ saphenous vein bypass grafts using endovascular intervention techniques. J Vasc Interv Radiol 2000; 11:705.

192. Engelke C, Morgan RA, Belli AM: Cutting balloon percutaneous transluminal angioplasty for salvage of lower limb arterial bypass grafts: feasibility. Radiology 2002;223:106.

193. Walker J, Chalmers N, Gillespie IN: A new use of the Simpson percutaneous atherectomy catheter: resection of retained valve cusps of an in situ vein graft. Cardiovasc Intervent Radiol 1995;18:50.

194. Hye RJ, Turner C, Valji K, et al: Is thrombolysis of occluded popliteal and tibial bypass grafts worthwhile? J Vasc Surg 1994;20:588.

195. Durham JD, Geller SC, Abbott WM, et al: Regional infusion of urokinase into occluded lower-extremity bypass grafts: long-term clinical results. Radiology 1989;172:83.

196. Sullivan KL, Gardiner GA Jr, Kandarpa K, et al: Efficacy of thrombolysis in infrainguinal bypass grafts. Circulation 1991;83(Suppl I):I-99.

197. Seabrook GR, Mewissen MW, Schmitt DD, et al: Percutaneous intra-arterial thrombolysis in the treatment of thrombosis of lower extremity arterial reconstructions. J Vasc Surg 1991;13:646.

198. Graor RA, Risius B, Young JR, et al: Thrombolysis of peripheral arterial bypass grafts: surgical thrombectomy compared with thrombolysis. J Vasc Surg 1988;7:347.

199. Richardson JW, Greenfield LJ: Natural history and management of iliac aneurysms. J Vasc Surg 1988;8:165.

200. Levi N, Schroeder TV: Arteriosclerotic femoral artery aneurysms: a short review. J Cardiovasc Surg 1997;38:335.

201. Vasquez G, Zamboni P, Buccoliero F, et al: Isolated true atherosclerotic aneurysms of the superficial femoral artery. Case report and literature review. J Cardiovasc Surg 1993;34:511.

202. Philpott JM, Parker FM, Benton CR, et al: Isolated internal iliac artery aneurysm resection and reconstruction: operative planning and technical considerations. Am Surg 2003;69:569.

203. Hsu RB, Tsay YG, Wang SS, et al: Surgical treatment for primary infected aneurysm of the descending thoracic aorta, abdominal aorta, and iliac arteries. J Vasc Surg 2002;36:746.

204. Sciannameo F, Ronca P, Caselli M, et al: The anastomotic aneurysms. J Cardiovasc Surg 1993;34:145.

205. Fahrni M, Lachat MM, Wildermuth S, et al: Endovascular therapeutic options for isolated iliac aneurysms with a working classification. Cardiovasc Intervent Radiol 2003;26:443.

206. Varga ZA, Locke-Edmunds JC, Baird RN, et al: A multicenter study of popliteal aneurysms. J Vasc Surg 1994;20:171.

207. Rubin GD: MDCT imaging of the aorta and peripheral vessels. Eur J Radiol 2003;45(Suppl 1):S42.

208. Pellerito JS: Current approach to peripheral arterial sonography. Radiol Clin North Am 2001;39:553.

209. Hollis HW Jr, Luethke JM, Yakes WF, et al: Percutaneous embolization of an internal iliac artery aneurysm: technical considerations and literature review. J Vasc Interv Radiol 1994;5:449.

210. Cynamon J, Marin ML, Veith FJ, et al: Endovascular repair of an internal iliac artery aneurysm with use of a stented graft and embolization coils. J Vasc Interv Radiol 1995;6:509.

211. Marin ML, Veith FJ, Lyon RT, et al: Transfemoral endovascular repair of iliac artery aneurysms. Am J Surg 1995;170:179.

212. Razavi MK, Dake MD, Semba CP, et al: Percutaneous endoluminal placement of stent-grafts for the treatment of isolated iliac artery aneurysms. Radiology 1995;197:801.

213. Tielliu IF, Verhoeven EL, Prins TR, et al: Treatment of popliteal artery aneurysms with the Hemobahn stent-graft. J Endovasc Ther 2003;10:111.

214. Paulson EK, Hertzberg BS, Paine SS, et al: Femoral artery pseudoaneurysms: value of color Doppler sonography in predicting which ones will thrombose without treatment. AJR Am J Roentgenol 1992;159:1077.

215. Morgan R, Belli A-M: Current treatment methods for postcatheterization pseudoaneurysms. J Vasc Interv Radiol 2003;14:697.

216. Krueger K, Zaehringer M, Soehngen F-D, et al: Femoral pseudoaneurysms: management with percutaneous thrombin injections—success rates and effects on systemic coagulation. Radiology 2003;226:452.

217. Heetveld MJ, Harris I, Schlaphoff G, Sugrue M: Guidelines for the management of haemodynamically unstable pelvic fracture patients. ANZ J Surg 2004;74:520.

218. Burgess AR, Eastridge BJ, Young JWR, et al: Pelvic ring disruptions: effective classification system and treatment protocols. J Trauma 1990;30:848.

219. Kimbrell BJ, Velmahos GC, Chan LS et al: Angiographic embolization for pelvic fractures in older patients. Arch Surg 2004;139:728.

220. Ben-Menachem Y, Coldwell DM, Young JWR, et al: Hemorrhage associated with pelvic fractures: causes, diagnosis, and emergent management. AJR Am J Roentgenol 1991;157:1005.

221. Shapiro M, McDonald AA, Knight D, et al: The role of repeat angiography in the management of pelvic fractures. J Trauma 2005;58:227.

222. Ramirez JI, Velmahos GC, Best CR, et al: Male sexual function after bilateral internal iliac artery embolization for pelvic fracture. J Trauma 2004;56:734.

223. Hafez HM, Woolgar J, Robbs JV: Lower extremity arterial injury: results of 550 cases and review of risk factors associated with limb loss. J Vasc Surg 2001;33:1212.

224. Frykberg ER: Advances in the diagnosis and treatment of extremity vascular trauma. Surg Clin North Am 1995;75:207.

225. Britt LD, Weireter LJ, Cole FJ: Newer diagnostic modalities for vascular injuries. Surg Clin North Am 2001;81:1263.

226. Smyth SH, Pond GD, Johnson PL, et al: Proximity injuries: correlation with results of extremity arteriography. J Vasc Interv Radiol 1991;2:451.

227. Kaufman JA, Parker JE, Gillespie DL, et al: Arteriography for proximity of injury in penetrating extremity trauma. J Vasc Interv Radiol 1992;3:719.

228. Dennis JW, Frykberg ER, Crump JM, et al: New perspectives on the management of penetrating trauma in proximity to major limb arteries. J Vasc Surg 1990;11:85.

229. Schwartz MR, Weaver FA, Bauer M, et al: Redefining the indications for arteriography in penetrating extremity trauma: a prospective analysis. J Vasc Surg 1993;17:116.

230. Knudson MM, Lewis FR, Atkinson K, et al: The role of duplex ultrasound arterial imaging in patients with penetrating extremity trauma. Arch Surg 1993;128:1033.

231. Gagne PJ, Cone JB, McFarland D, et al: Proximity penetrating extremity trauma: the role of duplex ultrasound in the detection of occult venous injuries. J Trauma 1995;39:1157.

232. Soto JA, Munera F, Morales C, et al: Focal arterial injuries of the proximal extremities: helical CT arteriography as the initial method of diagnosis. Radiology 2001;218:188.

233. Hoffer EK, Sclafani SJ, Herskowitz MM, et al: Natural history of arterial injuries diagnosed with arteriography. J Vasc Interv Radiol 1997;8:43.

234. Marin ML, Veith FJ, Panetta TF, et al: Transluminally placed endovascular stented graft repair for arterial trauma. J Vasc Surg 1994;20:466.

235. Olin JW: Thromboangiitis obliterans (Buerger's disease). N Engl J Med 2000;343:864.

236. Olin JW, Young JR, Graor RA, et al: The changing clinical spectrum of thromboangiitis obliterans (Buerger's disease). Circulation 1990;82(Suppl IV):IV-3.

237. Cutler DA, Runge MS: 86 years of Buerger's disease—what have we learned? Am J Med Sci 1995;309:74.

238. Hussein EA, Dorri A: Intra-arterial streptokinase as adjuvant therapy for complicated Buerger's disease: early trials. Int Surg 1993;78:54.

239. McKiernan TL, Bock K, Leya F, et al: Ergot induced peripheral vascular insufficiency, non-interventional treatment. Cathet Cardiovasc Diagn 1994;31:211.

240. Norton PT, Hagspiel K: Stationary arterial waves in magnetic resonance angiography. J Vasc Interv Radiol 2005;16:423.

241. Wing RJ, Waugh RC, Harris JP: Treatment of fibromuscular dysplasia of the external iliac artery by percutaneous transluminal angioplasty. Australas Radiol 1993;37:223.

242. Chuang VP: Radiation-induced arteritis. Semin Roentgenol 1994;29:64.

243. Enjolras O, Mulliken JB: Vascular tumors and malformations (new issues). Adv Dermatol 1997;13:375.

244. Konez O, Burrows PE: Magnetic resonance of vascular anomalies. Magn Reson Imaging Clin N Am 2002;10:363.

245. Laor T, Burrows PE, Hoffer FA: Magnetic resonance venography of congenital vascular malformations of the extremities. Pediatr Radiol 1996;26:371.

246. Dubois J, Garel L: Imaging and therapeutic approach of hemangiomas and vascular malformations in the pediatric age group. Pediatr Radiol 1999;19:879.

247. White RI Jr, Pollak J, Persing J, et al: Long-term outcome of embolotherapy and surgery for high-flow extremity arteriovenous malformations. J Vasc Interv Radiol 2000;11:1285.

248. Burrows PE, Mason KP: Percutaneous treatment of low flow vascular malformations. J Vasc Interv Radiol 2004;15:431.

249. Tan KT, Simons ME, Rajan DK, et al: Peripheral high-flow arteriovenous vascular malformations: a single-center experience. J Vasc Interv Radiol 2004;15:1071.

250. Pollak JS, White RI Jr: The use of cyanoacrylate adhesives in peripheral embolization. J Vasc Interv Radiol 2001;12:907.

251. Castaneda F, Goodwin SC, Swischuk JL, et al: Treatment of pelvic arteriovenous malformations with ethylene vinyl alcohol copolymer (Onyx). J Vasc Interv Radiol 2002;13:513.

252. Vogelzang RL, Nemcek AA Jr, Skrtic Z, et al: Uterine arteriovenous malformations: primary treatment with therapeutic embolization. J Vasc Interv Radiol 1991;2:517.

253. Vallance R, Quin RO, Forrest H: Arterio-venous shunting complicating occlusive atherosclerotic peripheral vascular disease. Clin Radiol 1986;37:389.
254. Dawson I, Sie RB, van Bockel JH: Atherosclerotic popliteal aneurysm. Br J Surg 1997;84:293.
255. Roggo A, Brunner U, Ottinger LW, et al: The continuing challenge of aneurysms of the popliteal artery. Surg Gynecol Obstet 1993;177:565.
256. Wright LB, Matchett WJ, Cruz CP, et al: Popliteal artery disease: diagnosis and treatment. Radiographics 2004;24:467.
257. Steffen CM, Ruddle A, Shaw JF: Adventitial cystic disease: multiple cysts causing common femoral artery occlusion. Eur J Vasc Endovasc Surg 1995;9:118.
258. Levien LJ, Benn CA: Adventitial cystic disease: a unifying hypothesis. J Vasc Surg 1998;28:193.
259. Elster EA, Hewlett S, DeRienzo DP, et al: Adventitial cystic disease of the axillary artery. Ann Vasc Surg 2002;16:134.
260. Peterson JJ, Kransdorf MJ, Bancroft LW, et al: Imaging characteristics of cystic adventitial disease of the peripheral arteries: presentation as soft-tissue masses. AJR Am J Roentgenol 2003;180:621.
261. Elias DA, White LM, Rubenstein JD, et al: Clinical evaluation and MR imaging features of popliteal artery entrapment and cystic adventitial disease. AJR Am J Roentgenol 2003;180:627.
262. Hoelting T, Schuermann G, Allenberg JR: Entrapment of the popliteal artery and its surgical management in a 20-year period. Br J Surg 1997;84:338.
263. Levien LJ: Popliteal artery entrapment syndrome. Semin Vasc Surg 2003;16:223.
264. Erdoes LS, Devine JJ, Bernhard VM, et al: Popliteal vascular compression in a normal population. J Vasc Surg 1994;20:978.
265. Abraham P, Bickert S, Vielle B, et al: Pressure measurements at rest and after heavy exercise to detect moderate arterial lesions in athletes. J Vasc Surg 2001;33:721.
266. Scavee V, Stainier L, Deltombe T, et al: External iliac artery endofibrosis: a new possible predisposing factor. J Vasc Surg 2003;38:180.
267. Abraham P, Bouye P, Quere I, et al: Past, present and future of arterial endofibrosis in athletes: a point of view. Sports Med 2004;34:419.

7

Upper Extremity Arteries

ARTERIOGRAPHY

The brachiocephalic, left carotid, and left subclavian arteries are typically catheterized from the aortic arch with a 5-French headhunter catheter (Fig. 7-1). In most patients, a guidewire can be advanced easily into the left subclavian artery directly from the descending thoracic aorta. If this is not possible, the catheter is advanced into the aortic arch, rotated, and withdrawn until the tip engages the vessel (see Fig. 7-1).

In older patients with ectasia of the aorta and arch vessels, a reverse-curve catheter may be useful (Fig. 7-2). During upper extremity arteriography, a high origin of the radial (or rarely the ulnar) artery from the brachial or axillary artery should be sought; if such origin is found, the catheter is placed proximal to its take-off. Extreme care should be

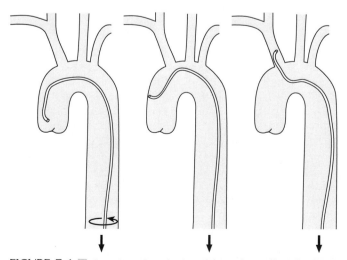

FIGURE 7-1 ■ Steps in catheterization of the arch vessels with a head-hunter catheter. The catheter can then be advanced into the right subclavian artery over a guidewire. Further withdrawal of the catheter *(third panel)* will cause it to jump into the left common carotid and then into the left sub-clavian artery. (Adapted from Kadir S: Diagnostic Angiography. Philadelphia, WB Saunders, 1986:177.)

taken when working in the aortic arch in patients with atherosclerotic disease to avoid atheroembolism to the brain or periphery.

Arteriography of the hand is performed with a catheter in the mid-brachial artery. The arteries of the hand and forearm are prone to vasospasm from many causes, including anxiety and pain.[1] Vasospasm is prevented or relieved by giving an intra-arterial vasodilator (e.g., 100 to 200 µg of nitroglycerin).

ANATOMY

Development

During early gestation, the upper limbs are nourished by the axial artery, which arises from the subclavian artery.[2] The axial artery evolves into the axillary, brachial, interosseous, and median arteries. The latter two vessels feed the arterial plexus of the hand in the fetus (Fig. 7-3). The ulnar artery is an outgrowth of the brachial artery at the elbow. The radial artery arises from a superficial branch of the proximal brachial artery, but its origin eventually migrates toward the elbow. In most cases, the distal interosseous and median arteries regress before birth.

Normal Anatomy

The *subclavian arteries* originate from the *brachiocephalic (innominate) artery* on the right and directly from the aortic arch on the left (Fig. 7-4).[3,4] The artery runs posterior to the subclavian vein and the anterior scalene muscle. It arches over the pulmonary apex surrounded by nerves of the brachial plexus. The subclavian artery has several major branches (Fig. 7-5; see also Fig. 7-4):

■ The *vertebral artery* arises from the superior aspect of the vessel and travels through the bony canal of the cervical transverse processes into the skull.

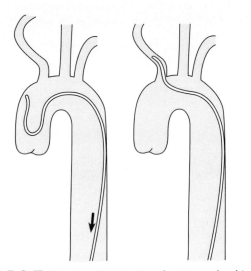

FIGURE 7-2 ■ Steps in catheterization of a tortuous brachiocephalic artery with a Simmons catheter. (Adapted from Kadir S: Diagnostic Angiography. Philadelphia, WB Saunders, 1986:178.)

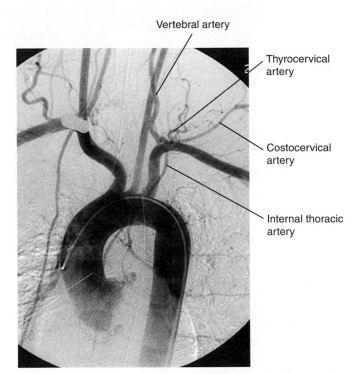

FIGURE 7-4 ■ Thoracic aorta and arch vessels in right posterior oblique projection.

■ The *internal thoracic (mammary) artery* arises from the undersurface of the subclavian artery opposite the vertebral artery and runs behind the costosternal junctions. The vessel divides into musculophrenic and superior epigastric branches. The internal thoracic artery and its musculophrenic branch give rise to the anterior intercostal arteries. The musculophrenic and superior epigastric branches have anastomoses with the inferior phrenic and inferior epigastric arteries, respectively, in the abdomen.

■ The *thyrocervical trunk* takes off beyond the vertebral artery origin and immediately divides into the inferior thyroid, suprascapular, and superficial cervical arteries.

■ The *costocervical trunk* gives rise to the superior intercostal artery (supplying the first, second, and, occasionally,

third posterior intercostal arteries) and the deep cervical artery. Small branches supply the anterior spinal artery.

■ The *dorsal scapular artery* is the final branch of the subclavian artery.

At the outer edge of the first rib, the subclavian artery becomes the *axillary artery* (see Fig. 7-5). The vessel runs behind the pectoralis major and minor muscles and lateral to the axillary vein. Its major branches include the superior thoracic, thoracoacromial, lateral thoracic, subscapular, and anterior and posterior humeral circumflex arteries. These branches supply muscles of the shoulder girdle, humerus, scapula, and chest wall.

At the lateral edge of the teres major muscle (approximately the lateral scapular border), the axillary artery becomes the *brachial artery* (Fig. 7-6; see also Fig. 7-5). In the upper arm, the artery lies in a fascial sheath along with the basilic vein, paired brachial veins, and the median nerve. Its major branches include the deep brachial and the superior and inferior ulnar collateral arteries (Fig. 7-7).

At about the level of the radial head, the brachial artery divides into the *radial* and *ulnar arteries* (Fig. 7-8). The radial recurrent artery and the posterior and anterior ulnar recurrent arteries arise immediately beyond the origins of their respective arteries to form anastomoses with branches of the brachial and deep brachial artery (see Fig. 7-7). The radial artery descends on the radial side of the forearm. The ulnar artery, which is larger than the radial artery in most cases, gives off the *common interosseous artery* and then descends on the ulnar side of the forearm. The interosseous artery divides into anterior and posterior branches that run on either side of the interosseous membrane. In less than 10% of cases, the anterior interosseous

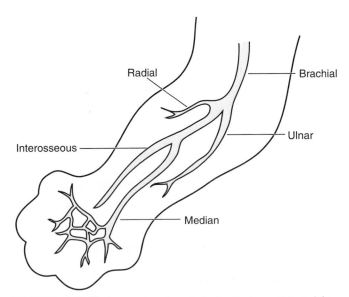

FIGURE 7-3 ■ Upper extremity arteries in the fetus. (Adapted from Williams PL, Bannister LH, Berry MM, et al, eds: Gray's Anatomy, 38th ed. New York, Churchill Livingstone, 1995:318.)

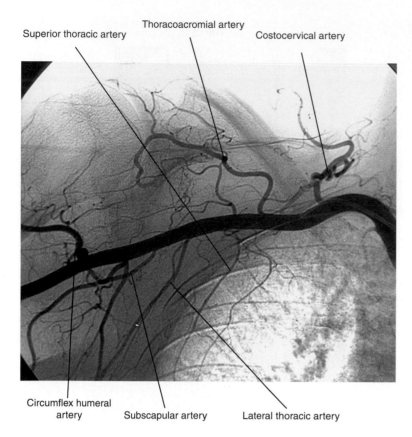

Superior thoracic artery

Thoracoacromial artery

Costocervical artery

Circumflex humeral artery

Subscapular artery

Lateral thoracic artery

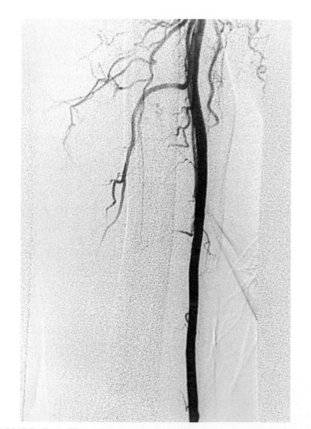

FIGURE 7-6 ■ Arteriogram of the right brachial artery. Note the proximal branches of the deep brachial artery.

or *median artery* persists and contributes to the palmar arch of the hand.[5]

The arterial anatomy of the hand is extremely variable, and deviations from the classic pattern described here are common.[5,6] The ulnar artery supplies the *superficial* palmar arch, and the radial artery supplies the *deep* palmar arch (Figs. 7-9 and 7-10). The arches often are in continuity with the opposing forearm artery through small branches at the wrist. The superficial arch is dominant and usually lies distal to the deep arch. The princeps pollicis and radialis indicis arteries arise from the radial artery and supply the thumb and index finger, respectively. The superficial palmar arch gives off three or four common palmar digital arteries, and the deep arch gives off the palmar metacarpal arteries. At the bases of the proximal phalanges, adjacent metacarpal vessels from each arch join and then immediately divide into proper digital arteries, which supply apposing surfaces of the fingers. A so-called *incomplete arch,* defined by a lack of continuity of the radial artery with the superficial arch and lack of supply of the thumb and medial index finger by the ulnar artery, is found in about 20% of the population in autopsy studies.[5] This pattern is found more frequently in angiographic series.[7]

Variant Anatomy

Anomalies of the subclavian artery origin are discussed in Chapter 4. In about one third of the population, the superficial

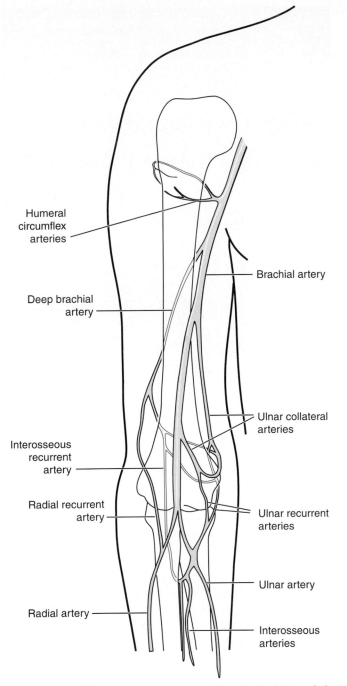

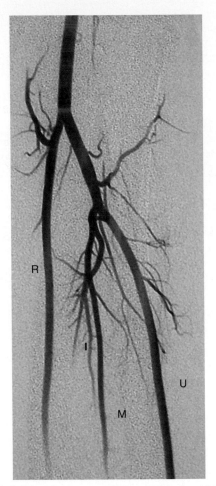

FIGURE 7-8 ■ Right forearm arteriogram. The brachial artery bifurcates into radial (R) and ulnar (U) arteries. The ulnar artery gives off anterior and posterior interosseous arteries (I). Also note an unusually prominent median artery (M).

FIGURE 7-7 ■ Arterial anatomy and collateral circulation of the upper arm and elbow.

cervical and dorsal scapular arteries have a common origin from the thyrocervical artery (i.e., *transverse cervical artery*). Variations in muscular branches of the axillary or brachial artery are common but do not have much clinical relevance.[8,9]

"High" origin of the radial artery from the axillary or upper brachial artery is an important variant (Fig. 7-11). This anomaly results when the radial artery origin in the fetus fails to migrate distally toward the elbow. It was found in 14% of cases in one autopsy series.[9] A high origin of the ulnar artery is much less common. Duplications of the brachial artery and

hypoplasia or aplasia of the radial and ulnar arteries are rare variants.

Persistent median artery results from lack of regression of the embryonic median branch arising from the common interosseous artery (Fig. 7-12). It is found in about 2% to 4% of the population.[4,10] This vessel may supply a palmar arch.

Collateral Circulation

With proximal subclavian artery obstruction, collateral blood flow from the contralateral vertebrobasilar system may run into the ipsilateral mid-subclavian artery (see below). When the obstruction is more distal, major collateral pathways are present across the thyroidal arterial system, between the internal thoracic and lateral thoracic arteries, and between the thyrocervical trunk and circumflex humeral arteries. With axillary artery obstruction, a rich network of muscular branches around the shoulder girdle provides collateral blood supply into the brachial artery.

In proximal brachial artery obstruction, the subscapular and posterior humeral circumflex arteries provide flow

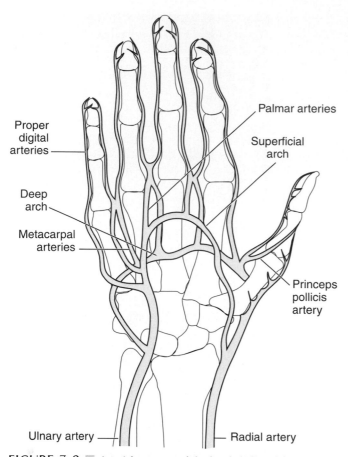

FIGURE 7-9 ■ Arterial anatomy of the hand. (Adapted from Loring LA, Hallisey MJ: Arteriography and interventional therapy for diseases of the hand. Radiographics 1995;15:1299.)

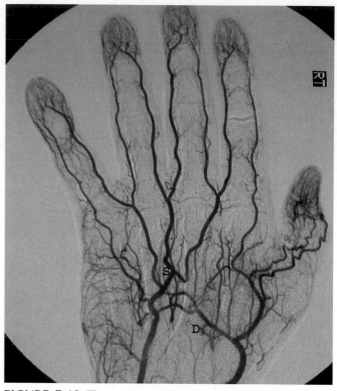

FIGURE 7-10 ■ Normal hand arteriogram. Note superficial (S) and deep (D) palmar arches.

through muscular branches into the distal brachial or forearm arteries (see Fig. 7-7).[3,11] In cases of mid-brachial artery occlusion, the deep brachial artery and superior ulnar collateral arteries supply the radial recurrent and ulnar recurrent arteries, respectively, above the elbow. The radial and ulnar recurrent arteries are the chief pathways across the elbow in patients with distal brachial artery occlusions.

When the radial or ulnar artery is obstructed, the opposing forearm artery, along with the anterior interosseous or median artery (if persistent into the wrist), supplies the hand. Collateral circulation with occlusion of the distal forearm or hand vessels depends on the individual anatomy and continuity of the palmar arches.

■ MAJOR DISORDERS

Acute Upper Extremity Ischemia

Etiology

Acute ischemia is far less common in the arm than in the leg.[12] This difference is partially explained by the extensive collateral network around the scapula and shoulder and by

the smaller muscle mass and metabolic needs of the arm. Emboli account for about 50% of cases of acute arterial occlusion, and most come from the heart.[13,14] Other potential sources of emboli include atherosclerotic plaque in the aorta or proximal upper extremity arteries, thrombus from subclavian artery aneurysms, endocarditis, and paradoxical emboli from the venous circulation.[15,16] About one fourth of cases result from iatrogenic or accidental trauma leading to arterial thrombosis.[14] In the remainder, acute thrombosis is caused by extension of a dissection or superimposed on underlying atherosclerotic plaque, injured artery (e.g., thoracic outlet syndrome [TOS]), aneurysm, or arteritis.

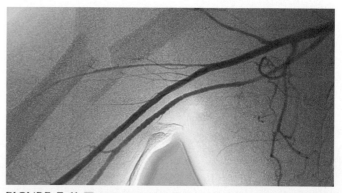

FIGURE 7-11 ■ High origin of the radial artery from the axillary artery. Note diffuse arterial spasm in the setting of acute fracture of the right humerus.

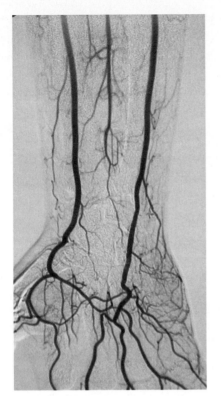

FIGURE 7-12 ■ Prominent persistent median artery.

Clinical Features

Most embolic occlusions occur in elderly patients with a history of cardiac dysrhythmias, myocardial infarction, or valvular heart disease. Embolization causes the sudden onset of arm pain, coolness, cyanosis, pallor, diminished or absent pulses, and, occasionally, sensorimotor deficits. Some patients are asymptomatic if the collateral circulation is adequate. The presence of arm swelling should raise the suspicion of severe venous thrombosis (see Chapter 15).

Imaging

Duplex sonography, CT angiography, or MR angiography is useful in the initial evaluation of patients who do not go directly for operation. However, catheter angiography is superior to these modalities for evaluation of distal vessels and is necessary if endovascular treatment is being considered. Regardless of the anatomic level of ischemia, the entire circulation from the aortic arch to the digital arteries of the hand should be evaluated to identify potential sources of emboli and to search for occult distal disease. An acute embolus produces a discrete filling defect with reconstitution of the distal vessels. However, it also may appear as a sharp cutoff point that mimics a thrombotic occlusion (Fig. 7-13). In greater than 50% of cases, emboli lodge in the brachial artery.[13,14,16] After the embolization has occurred, clot propagates proximally and distally to the next large collateral branches. Posttraumatic thrombosis results in an abrupt occlusion at or near the site of injury (Fig. 7-14).

Treatment

Blood flow to the arm must be restored promptly (within 4 to 6 hours after acute occlusion in the absence of preexisting obstructive disease) to avoid irreversible muscle necrosis and amputation. Delay in treatment can also lead to chronic ischemia or permanent neurologic deficits.

Surgical Therapy. Anticoagulation and embolectomy with a Fogarty catheter are standard treatment for embolic

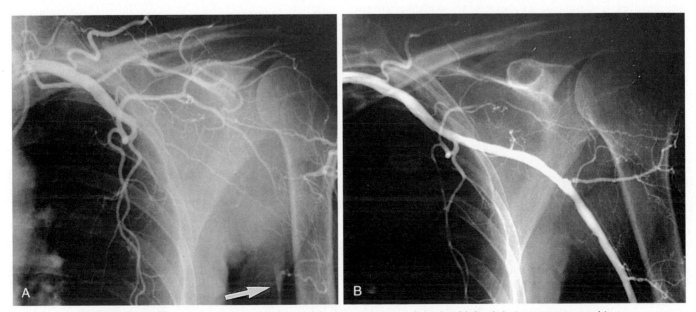

FIGURE 7-13 ■ Embolus to the brachial artery. **A,** Abrupt occlusion of the distal left subclavian artery occurred in a patient with atrial fibrillation and sudden onset of ischemic pain in the left arm. Notice the enlarged collaterals that reconstitute the mid-brachial artery *(arrow)*; the appearance mimics that of thrombotic occlusion. **B,** After infusion thrombolysis with urokinase, the occlusion completely resolves, with no evidence of underlying disease.

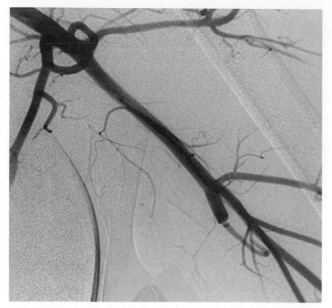

FIGURE 7-14 ■ Thrombosis of the left brachial artery after catheterization.

occlusions.[14,15] If the symptoms are mild and the clot burden is small, the patient can sometimes be managed with anticoagulation alone. Thrombotic occlusions are treated by direct thrombectomy, patch revision, or bypass grafting.[17]

Endovascular Therapy. Thrombolysis is an alternative to surgery for acute upper extremity arterial occlusions.[18-21] Acute embolic occlusions are very responsive to infusion thrombolysis, which achieves complete or near-complete clot lysis and limb salvage in many cases (see Fig. 7-13).[18,22-24] Liberal use of intra-arterial vasodilators is recommended to combat vasospasm, which occurs frequently with upper extremity artery manipulations. Because the collateral circulation in the arm and hand is so extensive, even partial lysis of an occlusion may avoid amputation or at least limit its extent. Occlusions less than 48 hours old respond better to thrombolysis than do older occlusions. An important advantage of lytic infusion over surgery is the ability to lyse clots in small vessels of the forearm and hand. Stroke from embolization of pericatheter clot has been reported with prolonged infusions, but it is a rare complication.

Chronic Upper Extremity Ischemia

Etiology

A variety of diseases may cause subacute or chronic upper extremity ischemia (Box 7-1).[25-27] Atherosclerosis usually affects the proximal segments of the subclavian artery and less often the brachiocephalic artery. Symptomatic disease is far more common in the left than in the right subclavian artery.[26] Significant atherosclerotic disease in the arm is uncommon. The various sources of thromboemboli were considered in the previous section.

Chronic occlusive disease of the upper extremity arteries is associated with several distinct clinical disorders:

- Stenosis or occlusion of the proximal subclavian artery may cause blood to flow from the contralateral vertebral artery through the basilar artery, in retrograde fashion in the ipsilateral vertebral artery, and into the post-stenotic subclavian artery. This pattern of flow may lead to cerebral ischemia during arm exercise *(subclavian steal syndrome)* (Fig. 7-15).[28]
- In patients with internal mammary artery bypass grafts to a coronary artery, a proximal subclavian artery stenosis may cause reversal of flow in the graft during arm exercise *(coronary-subclavian steal syndrome)*(Fig. 7-16).[29]
- Patients with hemodialysis access grafts in the arm may experience distal ischemia, usually from a combination of graft steal and underlying arterial disease.[30]
- In patients with extra-anatomic bypass grafts (e.g., axillofemoral grafts), subclavian artery stenosis may lead to ischemia in the leg or precipitate graft thrombosis.

Clinical Features

Chronic obstructions of the subclavian and axillary arteries may be entirely asymptomatic. Most patients with atherosclerosis-related thrombosis are older than 50 years of age. Arterial obstructions are manifested by ischemic symptoms such as exertional arm pain (claudication), rest pain, or tissue loss. Pulse deficits and blood pressure differences between the two arms (usually ≥20 mm Hg systolic) also may be found. Many patients have neurologic symptoms related to subclavian steal, including dizziness, syncope, visual disturbances, or ataxia. Patients with coronary-subclavian steal may develop angina during arm exercise. TOS is a common cause of arm ischemia in younger patients (see later).

Imaging

Cross-sectional Techniques. Duplex sonography[31-33] and MR imaging[34-36] often are used to evaluate patients with suspected proximal arterial obstruction, particularly when they have symptoms of subclavian steal (Fig. 7-17). Doppler ultrasound signs of obstructive disease include a parvus-et-tardus waveform (downstream lesion) and loss of normal diastolic

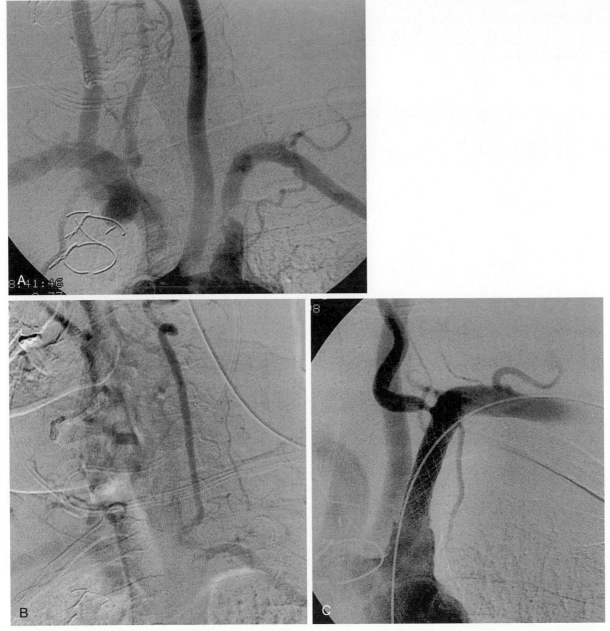

FIGURE 7-15 ■ Subclavian steal syndrome and subclavian artery stent placement. **A,** Arch aortogram shows an irregular stenosis of the proximal left subclavian artery. **B,** The late-phase arteriogram shows retrograde flow down the left vertebral artery into the subclavian artery beyond the stenosis. **C,** A stent was placed to relieve the obstruction. Note antegrade flow in the diseased vertebral artery.

flow reversal (upstream lesion).[33] Color flow imaging provides outstanding depiction of stenotic lesions and occlusions.

Angiography. Catheter arteriography is performed when noninvasive imaging studies are equivocal or endovascular therapy is contemplated. Atherosclerotic stenoses are typically found at the origins of the subclavian or brachiocephalic arteries (see Fig. 7-15). With proximal subclavian artery obstruction, flow in the ipsilateral vertebral artery may be reversed. Thrombotic occlusions produce an abrupt vessel cutoff. Arteriographic findings in TOS and rarer causes of chronic obstruction are considered in later sections.

Treatment

Medical Therapy. Many patients with chronic upper extremity ischemia can be initially treated conservatively with risk factor modification.

Surgical Therapy. The preferred method for treating subclavian artery occlusion is an extrathoracic bypass procedure, such as carotid-subclavian bypass, carotid-subclavian transposition, axilloaxillary bypass, or subclavian-subclavian bypass.[25,37] Brachial artery revascularization is done with autologous vein or synthetic graft material.[38]

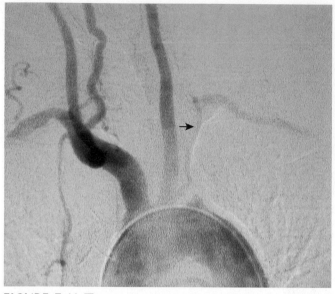

FIGURE 7-16 ▪ Coronary-subclavian steal in a patient with a left internal mammary artery (LIMA) coronary bypass graft. Early phase of arch aortogram shows occlusion at the origin of the left subclavian artery and retrograde flow up the LIMA *(arrow)* into the mid left subclavian artery.

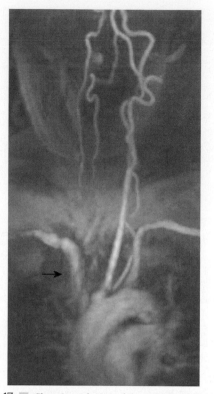

FIGURE 7-17 ▪ Chronic occlusion of the right brachiocephalic artery. Maximum intensity projection MR angiogram shows complete occlusion of the vessel with retrograde flow down the right vertebral and internal carotid arteries. The *arrow* denotes the right brachiocephalic vein.

Endovascular Therapy. In some cases, endovascular treatment (balloon angioplasty, primary stent placement, or selective stent placement) of subclavian and brachio-cephalic artery obstructions is a very attractive alternative to operative therapy.[39-40] Angioplasty is particularly effective in the treatment of subclavian steal syndrome[41,42] and coronary-subclavian steal syndrome (see Fig. 7-15).[43,44] Neurologic complications caused by angioplasty at or near the vertebral artery origin are rare, in part because of the delay ($\approx$20 seconds) in return of antegrade flow in the vessel after successful angioplasty.[45]

The overall technical success rate (with or without stent placement) is about 90% to 97%.[46-48] In the treatment of atherosclerotic stenoses, the results obtained have been fairly durable, with a 5-year patency of 72% in one large series.[47] However, results of balloon angioplasty for subclavian artery occlusions are less favorable.[49]

Thrombolytic therapy is effective in some patients with chronic upper extremity arterial occlusions.[20] Chronic occlusions are generally less responsive than are acute occlusions.

Thoracic Outlet Syndrome

Etiology

The various forms of TOS are a distinct set of clinical disorders of the upper extremity caused by extrinsic compression of the major nerves and blood vessels exiting or entering the thorax. In greater than 80% to 90% of cases, symptoms are caused by compression of the brachial plexus and related nerves; arterial compression is responsible for less than 5% of cases.[50-52]

Extrinsic arterial compression can be caused by a variety of musculoskeletal abnormalities, including cervical ribs, congenital fibromuscular bands, anomalies of the first rib, muscular hypertrophy, and clavicular fractures. The subclavian and axillary arteries are subject to compression at several sites; the most common are the costoclavicular space, scalene triangle, and subcoracoid (retropectal) space (Fig. 7-18).

Chronic arterial compression, which is made worse with certain arm positions, leads to intimal and medial injury from high-velocity flow and turbulence within the vessel. Over time, the result is post-stenotic dilation or frank aneurysm formation, premature atherosclerosis, embolization of platelet-fibrin deposits or thrombus from the diseased wall, or complete occlusion.

Clinical Features

TOS is typically seen in young or middle-aged adults. Women are affected more frequently than men. The arterial form of the disease causes arm pain, weakness, coolness, and pallor. Symptoms often are intermittent and usually provoked by certain arm positions or exercise. However, it may be difficult to distinguish neurogenic from vascular forms. A substantial number of patients has bilateral involvement. There may be evidence for distal embolization, such as digital ulcerations or cyanosis. Loss of the radial pulse with extreme abduction of the arm is normal in a minority of the population and is **not** diagnostic of the disease.[50] When symptoms are associated with arm swelling, the venous form of TOS should be considered (see Chapter 15).

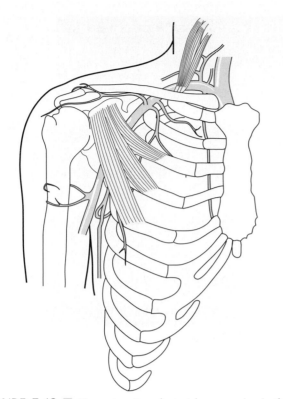

FIGURE 7-18 ■ The major sites of arterial compression in thoracic outlet syndrome are (medial to lateral) the scalene triangle, costoclavicular space, and subcoracoid (retropectal) space.

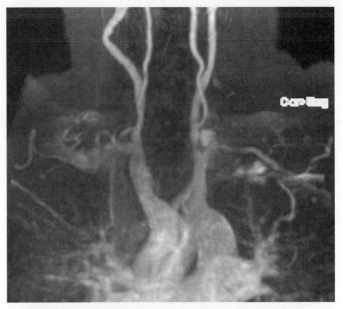

FIGURE 7-19 ■ Bilateral arterial thoracic outlet syndrome on maximum intensity projection MR angiogram in oblique sagittal plane. There is short-segment narrowing of the left subclavian artery beyond the vertebral artery origin. The right subclavian artery is occluded proximally.

Imaging

Cross-sectional Techniques. Duplex sonography,[33,53] MR angiography,[54-56] and helical CT angiography (with sagittal reformations)[57] are all useful in detecting arterial and venous abnormalities in patients with suspected TOS (Fig. 7-19). MR studies can be particularly helpful in characterizing fibromuscular abnormalities. However, asymptomatic compression of the subclavian artery has been identified in as many as 20% of normal volunteers by Doppler sonography.[53]

Studies should be performed in both neutral and stressed positions. A variety of arm positions can produce abnormal arterial impingement, including the Adson maneuver (i.e., depression of the shoulder with the head turned to the symptomatic side), military position (i.e., shoulders hyperflexed), hyperabduction of the arm, and the so-called "surrender" position (hands above the head).[50] As a practical matter, imaging should be performed in whatever position reproduces the patient's symptoms.

Angiography. The findings in patients with arterial TOS are varied.[58] Cervical ribs or elongated C7 transverse processes are present in many cases. With the arm in complete adduction, arteriographic findings may be normal or indicate only minimal compression or post-stenotic dilation (Fig. 7-20). In many patients, smooth, extrinsic narrowing of the artery is evident only with a provocative maneuver. Other possible angiographic findings include aneurysm formation with or without mural thrombus, distal embolization, and complete thrombosis (Fig. 7-21). The findings can be bilateral even when the symptoms are not.

Treatment

Surgical Therapy. For patients with mild symptoms and an imaging study showing normal subclavian and axillary arteries or only mild post-stenotic dilation in the neutral position, conservative therapy may be appropriate. For patients with disabling symptoms, florid imaging findings, or distal embolization, surgery usually is performed. The underlying musculoskeletal abnormality is corrected (e.g., removal of a cervical rib, release of fibrous bands) along with resection of the first rib.[50-52] Subclavian artery aneurysms are treated by resection and bypass.

Endovascular Therapy. Thrombolysis may be used to recanalize an acutely occluded artery from TOS (see Fig. 7-21). After flow is restored, anticoagulation is begun. Some time later, the underlying compressive abnormality is treated operatively. Stents should **not** be placed at the site of compression.

Digital Ischemia

Etiology

Ischemia of the digits may be caused by fixed obstructions of large or small arteries, intermittent vasospasm, or both. *Raynaud's disease* is a disorder of small arteries of the hand and less often of the feet in which vasoconstriction occurs with certain stimuli (e.g., cold, emotional stress) and leads to intermittent, reversible ischemia.[59] Although this condition is the most common cause of hand ischemia in some large referral populations,[60] functional vasospasm without fixed disease is unusual in angiographic series.[1,6]

Obstruction of large- or medium-sized arteries alone occasionally produces digital ischemia (see Box 7-1). More often,

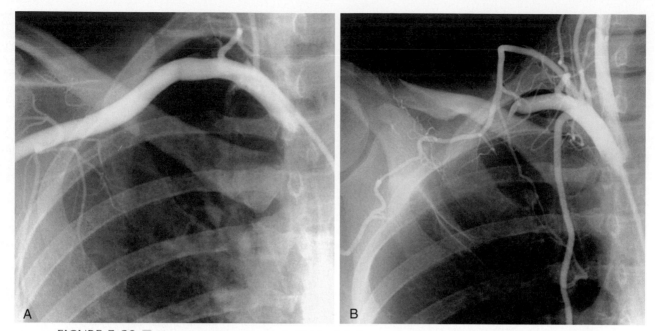

FIGURE 7-20 ■ Thoracic outlet syndrome. **A,** Right subclavian arteriogram in the neutral position is essentially normal. **B,** Repeat arteriogram with the arm abducted in a position that reproduced the patient's symptoms shows complete occlusion of the subclavian artery and enlarged collateral vessels.

the ischemia is caused by small vessel disease in the hand (Box 7-2).[6,60]

Emboli to the palmar and digital arteries may arise from many sources, including the heart, atherosclerotic plaque (usually in the subclavian artery), subclavian artery aneurysms (often related to TOS), arterial injury, endocarditis, and thrombosed hemodialysis grafts.[30,61] Buerger's disease is considered in a later section in this chapter.

Chronic, repetitive trauma to the hand, often from vibratory activity or repetitive pounding, can lead to intimal injury and eventual occlusion of palmar arteries. In patients with the *hypothenar hammer syndrome*, trauma to the distal ulnar artery as it runs across the hook of the hamate can result in aneurysm formation, occlusion, and distal embolization.[62] One study postulated that the entity occurs primarily in patients with underlying fibromuscular dysplasia of the ulnar artery. A similar disorder of the distal radial artery has also been described (*thenar hammer syndrome*).

Digital ischemia is relatively common in patients with certain collagen-vascular diseases. These heterogeneous disorders

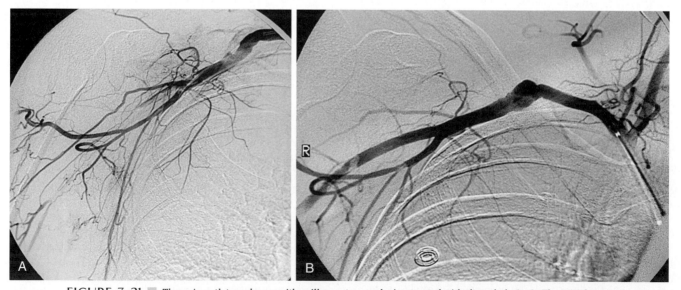

FIGURE 7-21 ■ Thoracic outlet syndrome with axillary artery occlusion treated with thrombolysis. **A,** The initial arteriogram shows complete occlusion of the right axillary and proximal brachial arteries. **B,** After pulse-spray and infusion thrombolysis with 750,000 IU of urokinase and balloon angioplasty, patency is restored, and an underlying subclavian artery aneurysm is revealed.

produce intimal thickening of small arteries of the wrist and hand that can lead to complete occlusion.[63]

Atherosclerosis of the small arteries of the arm and hand is commonly found in autopsy studies but rarely causes symptomatic digital ischemia. However, patients with chronic renal failure are prone to accelerated atherosclerotic disease of the digital arteries.[6]

The radial artery is sometimes harvested as a conduit for coronary artery bypass grafting.[64] Acute ischemia is rare, and numbness and paresthesias occur in less than 10% of cases.

Clinical Features

Patients with occlusions of the palmar or digital artery present with moderate to severe pain in the hand and fingers (which may be exacerbated by cold or stress), finger ulcerations, or even gangrene. Bluish discoloration of some of the fingers *(blue digit syndrome)* suggests microembolization of platelet-fibrin or cholesterol deposits from a proximal source. Many patients have a history of tobacco use, collagen-vascular disease, diabetes, chronic hand trauma (e.g., in karate enthusiasts or jackhammer users), or cardiac disease. Noninvasive studies, including finger and arm pressure measurements, Doppler flow studies, and plethysmography, are important in the diagnostic workup of these patients.[65]

Imaging

Although cross-sectional techniques such as MR angiography are sometimes used to evaluate the arteries of the hand, none of these methods yet approaches the diagnostic accuracy of catheter arteriography.[66,67] The purpose of arteriography is threefold:

- To identify emboli, which will require anticoagulant therapy and/or exclusion of the offending proximal source
- For specific diagnosis when prognosis is important (e.g., Buerger's disease)
- To localize treatable disease that may improve circulation to the hand

A complete study from the aortic arch to the digital arteries of the affected hand should be performed. Intra-arterial vasodilators often are given before arteriography to relieve functional vasospasm. Some radiologists do bilateral hand arteriography in selected cases even if the symptoms are unilateral. Most of the systemic disorders, including embolization from the heart or ascending aorta, produce angiographic abnormalities in both hands even if symptoms are confined to one side.

The angiographic findings depend on the underlying disorder.[1,6,68] When embolization is suspected, a careful search for a proximal source should be made (Fig. 7-22). The collagen-vascular diseases typically strike the proper digital arteries of

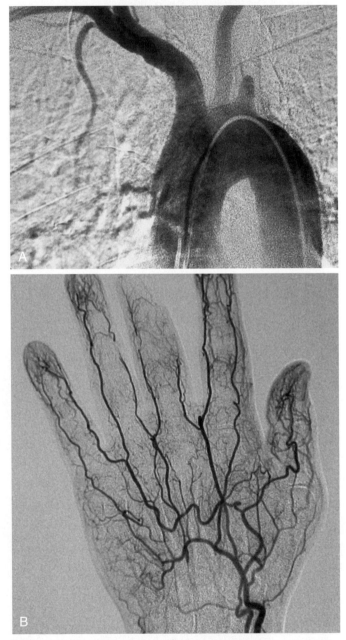

FIGURE 7-22 ▪ Hand ischemia from proximal atheroma embolization. **A,** Right posterior oblique arch aortogram shows a plaque on the inferior surface of the brachiocephalic artery. Also note occlusion of the proximal left subclavian artery. **B,** Hand angiogram shows occlusion of the distal ulnar artery and of multiple proper digital arteries.

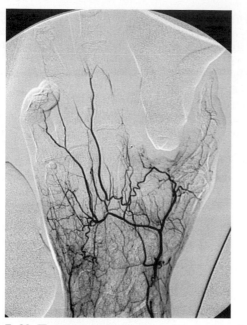

FIGURE 7-23 ▨ Scleroderma is characterized by abrupt occlusions of multiple proper digital arteries. The distal radial and ulnar arteries are occluded. Note prior second digit amputation.

the hand and the ulnar artery more frequently than the radial artery (Fig. 7-23).[6] The diagnosis of embolism can be made with confidence only if discrete intraluminal filling defects are found. Focal occlusion or an aneurysm of the ulnar artery near the hook of the hamate is diagnostic of hypothenar hammer syndrome (Fig. 7-24). The arteriographic findings in Buerger's disease are considered later (Fig. 7-25). Atherosclerosis produces stenoses and occlusions of the digital arteries with less severe disease in the palmar vessels. For patients who may have Raynaud's disease, angiography should be performed before and after injection of a vasodilator.

Treatment

Medical/Surgical Therapy. Many patients who present with chronic digital ischemia have little or no further progression of their symptoms.[60,63] For these patients, medical treatment with anticoagulants, antispasmodic agents, or both is appropriate. Vasodilators such as the prostacyclin analogue iloprost have been found to be beneficial in patients with some vasculitides such as systemic sclerosis.[69] Operative bypass procedures with autologous vein have been performed successfully for limb-threatening thrombotic or embolic disease involving the palmar and digital arteries.[70]

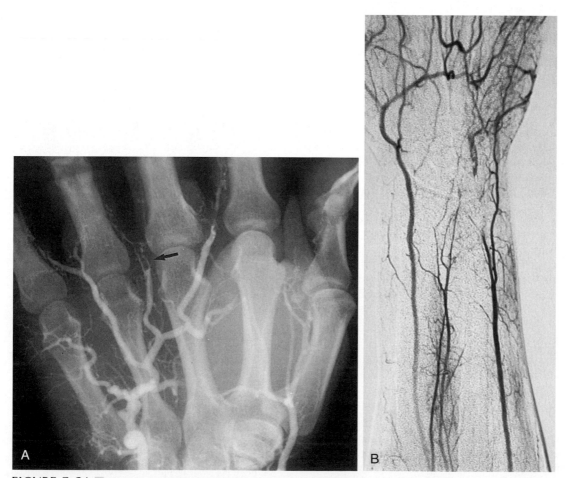

FIGURE 7-24 ▨ Hypothenar hammer syndrome. **A,** The patient has a pseudoaneurysm of the distal ulnar artery and an embolus in the palmar artery of the third web space *(arrow)*. **B,** Another patient has complete occlusion of the distal ulnar artery with reconstitution of a diseased vessel over the wrist.

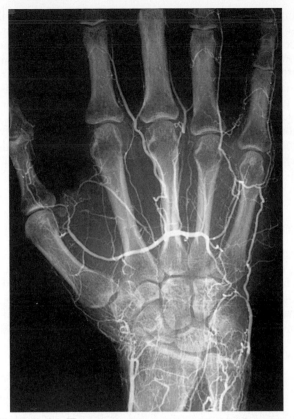

FIGURE 7-25 ■ Buerger's disease in this patient is characterized by abrupt occlusions of the distal radial and ulnar arteries and of multiple metacarpal and proper digital arteries. The intervening vessels are normal. Tortuous collaterals, which are most notable around the wrist, are characteristic of the disease.

Endovascular Therapy. Thrombolytic therapy has been used occasionally in some cases of acute or subacute arterial occlusion in the hand.[19,71,72]

Trauma

Etiology

The arteries of the upper extremity can be damaged in a variety of ways (Box 7-3).[73,74] Penetrating injury is far more common than blunt injury. Iatrogenic injuries may result from brachial or axillary artery catheterization, attempted vascular access placement in the chest or neck, or radial artery line insertion. The most common complications of axillary or brachial artery catheterization are local hematoma (occasionally with nerve compression) and arterial thrombosis; less commonly, pseudoaneurysms or arteriovenous fistulas may develop.[75,76] Skeletal injuries, especially humeral fractures, clavicular fractures, and anterior shoulder dislocations, can cause arterial damage. Chronic use of crutches may lead to axillary artery trauma.[77]

Clinical Features

The "hard signs" that strongly suggest a major arterial injury are listed in Box 7-4.[78-80] Significant arterial injuries are more common with shotgun blasts than with other forms of penetrating trauma. Because of the extensive collateral circulation in the arm, many patients with a significant proximal arterial injury have normal distal pulses.

Imaging

Over the last several decades, there has been a gradual evolution in the approach to suspected upper extremity arterial damage, from routine surgical exploration to routine arteriography for all "proximity" injuries to selected arteriography and observation.[78,81,82]

After clinical evaluation, some patients with hard signs of injury go directly to operation without imaging studies. In most cases, an ankle-brachial index (ABI) or Doppler arterial pressure index (API, ratio of distal pressure in affected versus unaffected arm) is determined. In the absence of hard signs of injury or with API or ABI greater than 0.90, patients may be observed or undergo color Doppler sonography.[78] Arteriography is reserved for patients with hard signs of injury or other accepted criteria (see Box 7-4), abnormal pressure measurements, or suspicious ultrasound studies.

Radiologic and surgical studies have found that the frequency of clinically silent arterial injuries distal to the axillary artery found by angiography that need repair is only 0 to 3%.[78,81-86] However, subclavian and axillary artery injuries are

---

BOX 7-3 ■ Causes of Trauma to Upper Extremity Arteries

Penetrating injury
  Accidental or criminal
  Iatrogenic (e.g., catheterization procedures)
Blunt injury
Bone fracture or joint dislocation
Chronic vibrational or pounding injury
Use of crutches
Thermal injury (e.g., frostbite, electrical injury)

BOX 7-4 ■ Indications for Arteriography in Cases of Trauma to the Upper Extremity

"Hard signs" of vascular injury
  Obvious arterial bleeding
  Expanding hematoma
  Absent or markedly diminished distal pulses
  Ischemic symptoms
  Bruit or thrill
Neurologic deficit
Shock in absence of other injuries
Shotgun blast
History of peripheral vascular disease
Thoracic outlet injury
Extensive bone or soft tissue injury
Delayed presentation

more difficult to detect on clinical grounds, and it is reasonable to obtain an arteriogram for proximity alone when these vessels are in jeopardy.

Sonography. In some centers, patients with suspected extremity arterial injuries are routinely evaluated with color Doppler sonography.[87-89] The accuracy and ability to exclude significant lesions in patients at low risk exceeds 95% in some studies. Pitfalls of the technique include limited evaluation of the thoracic outlet and confusion in the face of variant anatomy. Sonography is useful also for delayed diagnosis of posttraumatic pseudoaneurysms and arteriovenous fistulas, particularly in the subclavian and axillary arteries (Fig. 7-26).

Computed Tomography. CT angiography is quite accurate in assessing proximal upper extremity arterial injuries.[90] However, it is less useful for detecting injury to more distal vessels.

Angiography. Catheter arteriography is the most accurate technique for detecting traumatic injuries to upper extremity arteries.[91] Guidewires and catheters must be kept away from the area of injury so that catheterization-related vasospasm is not mistaken for vessel damage. Trauma can produce a wide spectrum of arterial abnormalities, including intimal tears, intraluminal thrombus, vasospasm, intramural hematoma, dissection, transection with or without thrombosis, vessel deviation, arteriovenous fistula formation, pseudoaneurysm formation, and compartment syndrome, which causes slow flow in proximal arteries (Figs. 7-27 through 7-29; see also Figs. 3-18, 7-11, 7-14, and 7-26).[73,74,91-93] Two projections often are needed to exclude subtle findings such as intimal tears. Arterial spasm may be difficult to differentiate from an intramural hematoma, but both entities usually are managed conservatively.

Treatment

Surgical Therapy. Injuries to small arterial branches are not repaired. Significant injuries to major arteries, such as occlusion, laceration, pseudoaneurysm, and flow-limiting dissection, require surgical treatment with resection or bypass grafting.[78-80] Time is of the essence in repairing occlusive injuries. Permanent ischemic injury can result if

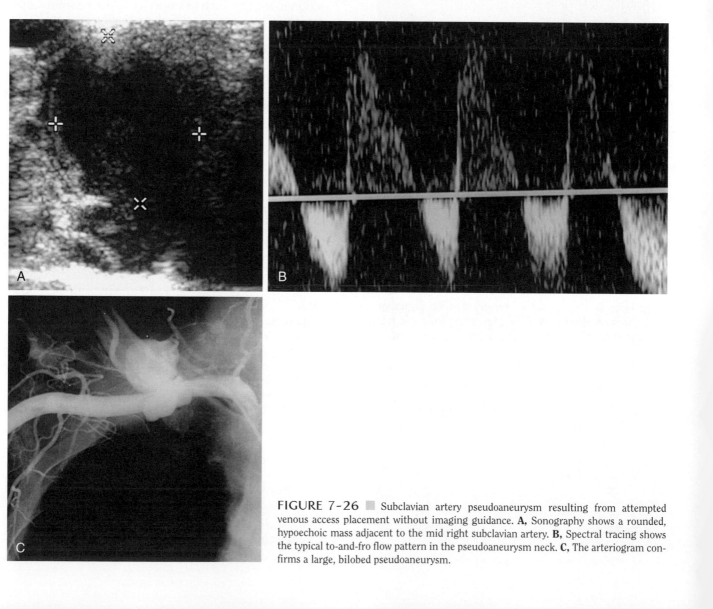

FIGURE 7-26 ■ Subclavian artery pseudoaneurysm resulting from attempted venous access placement without imaging guidance. **A,** Sonography shows a rounded, hypoechoic mass adjacent to the mid right subclavian artery. **B,** Spectral tracing shows the typical to-and-fro flow pattern in the pseudoaneurysm neck. **C,** The arteriogram confirms a large, bilobed pseudoaneurysm.

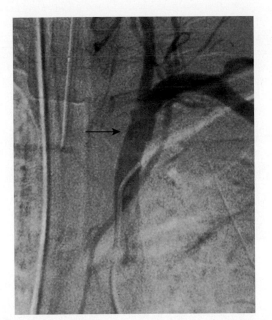

FIGURE 7-27 ■ Small pseudoaneurysm of the proximal left subclavian artery *(arrow)* after motor vehicle accident.

revascularization is not accomplished within about 4 to 6 hours of proximal injury (somewhat longer for more distal occlusions). The current trend is toward conservative management of minor vascular injuries such as nonocclusive intimal flaps, intramural hematomas, and small (<1 cm)

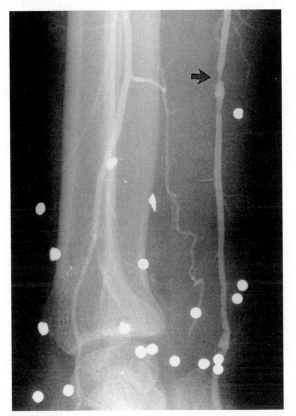

FIGURE 7-28 ■ Spasm or intramural hematoma *(arrow)* of the ulnar artery with possible distal intimal injury resulted from a gunshot blast.

pseudoaneurysms.[78,94] These lesions generally have a benign clinical course.

Endovascular Therapy. Large pseudoaneurysms or arteriovenous fistulas from a branch of a main upper extremity artery are best treated with embolotherapy.[93,95,96] Embolization usually is performed with Gelfoam pledgets or with coils (see Fig. 7-29). Pseudoaneurysms from brachial artery catheterization can sometimes be repaired by ultrasound-guided compression or percutaneous thrombin injection.[97,98] Traumatic pseudoaneurysms of the central arteries can be covered with stent-graft devices, although this technique is still investigational.[99,100] In cases with profound vasospasm, intra-arterial injection of a vasodilator (e.g., nitroglycerin 200 µg) can be useful. Finally, balloon catheters may be used to tamponade massive bleeding from a major arterial branch until the artery is repaired in the operating room.

Aneurysms

Etiology

A variety of diseases can produce true or false aneurysms of the upper extremity arteries (Box 7-5). Compared with the aorta and lower extremity arteries, degenerative aneurysms associated with atherosclerosis are uncommon in the upper extremity (see Chapter 3). They occur most frequently in the brachiocephalic and subclavian arteries.[101] Pseudoaneurysms often are the result of catheterization procedures such as brachial artery puncture, radial artery line placement, or attempted vascular access placement in the subclavian or jugular vein.[102] Aneurysms can develop near the site of extrinsic compression in patients with TOS. In the hand, aneurysms usually are caused by penetrating trauma or chronic blunt trauma (e.g., hypothenar hammer syndrome). Microaneurysms of small vessels of the hand are characteristic of a necrotizing vasculitis such as polyarteritis nodosa.[6]

Clinical Features

Subclavian artery aneurysms often are asymptomatic. Some patients present with chest pain, shoulder pain, or a pulsatile supraclavicular mass. Others have ischemia from distal embolization or aneurysmal thrombosis or have hypotension from rupture. Rarely, patients have massive hemoptysis from erosion into the lung.

Imaging

Cross-sectional Techniques. In patients with subclavian artery aneurysms, chest radiographs may show a right or left superior mediastinal mass. Duplex sonography, CT angiography, and MR angiography are used to diagnose central aneurysms (see Fig. 7-26).[103,104] Color Doppler sonography is used for detecting aneurysms of the brachial, forearm, and hand arteries.[105]

Angiography. Catheter angiography usually is reserved for cases in which the diagnosis cannot be made by cross-sectional

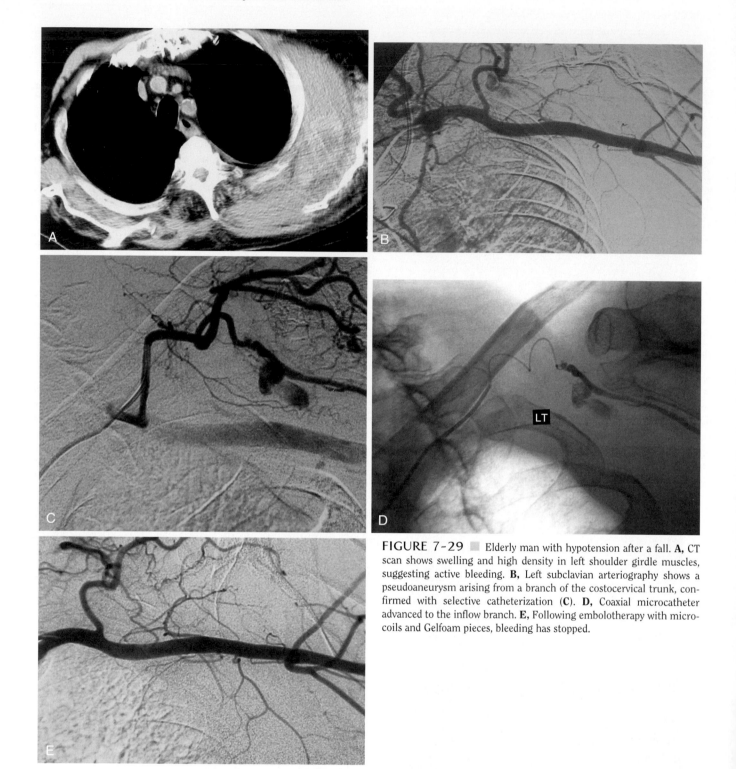

FIGURE 7-29 ■ Elderly man with hypotension after a fall. **A,** CT scan shows swelling and high density in left shoulder girdle muscles, suggesting active bleeding. **B,** Left subclavian arteriography shows a pseudoaneurysm arising from a branch of the costocervical trunk, confirmed with selective catheterization (**C**). **D,** Coaxial microcatheter advanced to the inflow branch. **E,** Following embolotherapy with microcoils and Gelfoam pieces, bleeding has stopped.

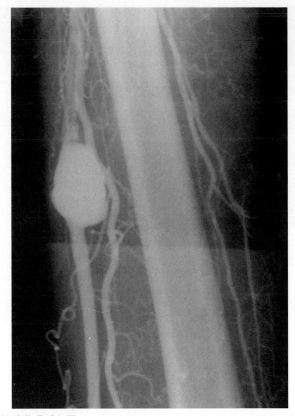

FIGURE 7-31 ■ Brachial artery aneurysm in a patient with Ehlers-Danlos syndrome.

methods, for preoperative planning, or when percutaneous therapy is being considered. Degenerative aneurysms, which are typically located in the brachiocephalic or subclavian arteries, usually are fusiform and calcified (Fig. 7-30; see also Fig. 3-18). Traumatic or infectious pseudoaneurysms are typically saccular, irregular, or multilobed (see Figs. 7-24 and 7-26). Aneurysms caused by connective tissue disorders may be fusiform or saccular (Fig. 7-31).

Treatment

Surgical Therapy. The standard treatment for upper extremity arterial aneurysms is surgical resection with end-to-end anastomosis or bypass grafting.[106]

Endovascular Therapy. Percutaneous therapy for posttraumatic aneurysms is described previously.

■ OTHER DISORDERS

Vasculitis

Several vasculitides affect the upper extremity arteries. Their pathogenesis is considered in more depth in Chapter 3.

Buerger's disease (thromboangiitis obliterans) is an occlusive panarteritis of medium-sized and small arteries and veins of the extremities.[107] The disease is classically seen in young to middle-aged men, all of whom are smokers. Buerger's disease almost always affects the lower extremities, and upper extremity involvement is seen in about 50% of cases. The occlusions usually are bilateral, although symptoms may be isolated to one arm. The proximal arteries (i.e., subclavian, axillary, and upper brachial) are unaffected. Abrupt, segmental occlusions begin in the arteries of the forearm.[6,108] A "corkscrew" appearance of the collateral vessels is said to be characteristic, but this often is not the case. Occlusions of palmar and digital arteries always occur (see Fig. 7-25). "Corrugation" of the arteries adjacent to obstructed segments has also been described. Subacute thromboses have been successfully treated with thrombolysis.[72]

Takayasu's arteritis is an inflammatory vasculitis affecting large- and medium-sized elastic arteries. The disease may

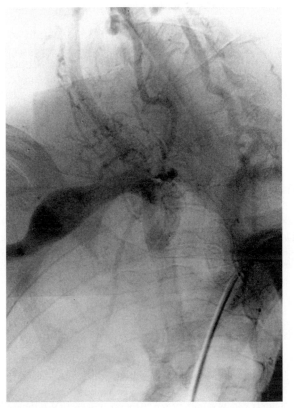

FIGURE 7-30 ■ Degenerative aneurysm of the right subclavian artery.

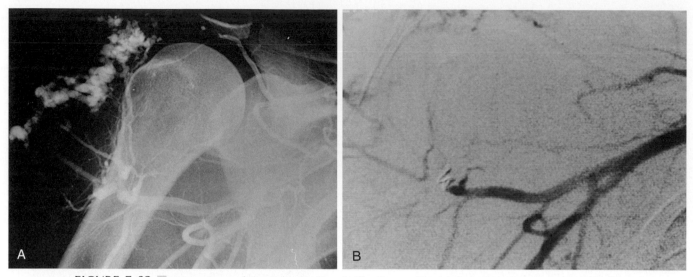

FIGURE 7-32 ■ Hemangioma of the right shoulder. **A,** The preoperative subclavian arteriogram shows markedly enlarged humeral circumflex arteries and puddling of contrast within the lesion. **B,** Embolization with coils reduces blood flow to the lesion before surgical resection.

cause long segmental stenoses or occlusions of branches of the aorta, especially the subclavian arteries (see Fig. 4-28).[109,110]

Giant cell (temporal) arteritis has many features that are similar to those of Takayasu's arteritis. However, it affects an older population, and the distribution of disease is different.[111] The neck and cranial vessels, particularly the carotid and temporal arteries, are most commonly affected. Occasionally, obstruction of the subclavian artery produces ischemic symptoms in the arm. Giant cell arteritis tends to cause long stenoses of the middle to distal segments of the subclavian artery, which may extend into the axillary artery.

Radiation arteritis is a rare complication of high-dose radiation therapy. Pathologic changes include intimal proliferation and fibrotic occlusion. These changes may only become apparent 5 years or more after treatment. Radiotherapy for breast carcinoma and lymphoma has caused obstructions of and, rarely, distal embolization from the subclavian and axillary arteries.[112,113]

Arteriovenous Communications

Vascular malformations and techniques for percutaneous treatment are discussed in Chapters 2 and 3. *Arteriovenous fistulas* are almost always acquired from accidental or iatrogenic trauma. Congenital *arteriovenous malformations* (AVMs) and *hemangiomas* are conditions that may affect the upper extremity.[114] Most patients with these lesions present as children or young adults with local hypertrophy, varices, pain, or a thrill or bruit over the site.

MR imaging has become the primary tool for diagnosis and staging of extremity AVMs. Angiography (arteriography or direct puncture) usually is reserved for embolotherapy or preoperative management. The angiographic findings vary with the type of AVM. With *arterial* malformations, markedly dilated inflow arteries, numerous feeding arterioles, pools of contrast within the AVM, and early filling of

draining veins may be seen (see Fig. 3-38). Hemangiomas may have a similar appearance (Fig. 7-32). Occasionally, vascular soft tissue or bony tumors can be confused with these congenital lesions.

Arteriovenous malformations are difficult to cure. None of the available treatments is likely to give permanent results, and recurrence is the rule. Therapy should be undertaken only when the patient has significant symptoms, such as bleeding, ulceration, pain, severe deformity, or high-output cardiac failure. When feasible, the treatment of choice is embolotherapy by an intra-arterial route or by direct percutaneous puncture.[115-118] Embolization is performed in stages to limit tissue loss. Ideally, the nidus of the AVM is obliterated. A permanent agent that can enter the substance of the AVM should be used, such as absolute alcohol or cyanoacrylate (glue). Proximal embolization must be strictly avoided. For venous malformations, direct injection with a sclerosing agent, such as absolute alcohol, can be extremely effective.

Neoplasms

Arteriography has virtually no role in the evaluation of patients with benign or malignant tumors of the shoulder or arm. Occasionally, patients with highly vascular tumors undergo arteriography for preoperative planning or for embolotherapy to reduce blood loss during surgery (see Fig. 7-32).

REFERENCES

1. Vogelzang RL: Arteriography of the hand and wrist. Hand Clin 1991;7:63.
2. Collins P, ed: Embryology and development. In: Williams PL, Bannister LH, Berry MM, et al, eds. Gray's Anatomy, 38th ed. New York, Churchill Livingstone, 1995:318.

3. Gabella G, ed: Cardiovascular system. In: Williams PL, Bannister LH, Berry MM, et al, eds. Gray's Anatomy, 38th ed. New York, Churchill Livingstone, 1995:1529.
4. Rose SC, Kadir S: Arterial anatomy of the upper extremities. In: Kadir S, ed. Atlas of Normal and Variant Angiographic Anatomy. Philadelphia, WB Saunders, 1991:55.
5. Coleman SS, Anson BJ: Arterial patterns in the hand based on a study of 650 specimens. Surg Gynecol Obstet 1961;113:409.
6. Bookstein JJ: Arteriography. In: Poznanski AK, ed. The Hand in Radiologic Diagnosis, 2nd ed. Philadelphia, WB Saunders, 1984:97.
7. Janevski BK: Anatomy of the arterial system of the upper extremities. In: Janevski BK, ed. Angiography of the Upper Extremities. The Hague, Martinus Nijhoff Publishers, 1982:41.
8. Keen JA: A study of the arterial variations in the limbs with special reference to symmetry of vascular patterns. Am J Anat 1961; 108:245.
9. McCormack LJ, Cauldwell EW, Anson BJ: Brachial and antebrachial arterial patterns: a study of 750 extremities. Surg Gynecol Obstet 1965;96:43.
10. Lindley SG, Kleinert JM: Prevalence of anatomic variations encountered in elective carpal tunnel release. J Hand Surg [Am] 2003; 28:849.
11. Yao JST, Bergan JJ, Neiman HL: Arteriography for upper-extremity and digital ischemia. In: Neiman HL, Yao JST, eds. Angiography of Vascular Disease. New York, Churchill Livingstone, 1985:353.
12. Eyers P, Earnshaw JJ: Acute non-traumatic arm ischemia. Br J Surg 1998;85:1340.
13. Wirsing P, Andriopoulous A, Bötticher R: Arterial embolectomies in the upper extremity after acute occlusion. Report on 79 cases. J Cardiovasc Surg 1983;24:40.
14. Ricotta JJ, Scudder PA, McAndrew JA, et al: Management of acute ischemia of the upper extremity. Am J Surg 1983;145:661.
15. Kaar G, Broe PJ, Bochier-Hayes DJ: Upper limb emboli. A review of 55 patients managed surgically. J Cardiovasc Surg 1989;30:165.
16. Kretz JG, Weiss E, Limuris A, et al: Arterial emboli of the upper extremity: a persisting problem. J Cardiovasc Surg 1984;25:233.
17. Katz SG, Kohl RD: Direct revascularization for the treatment of forearm and hand ischemia. Am J Surg 1993;165:312.
18. Widlus DM, Venbrux AC, Benenati JF, et al: Fibrinolytic therapy for upper extremity arterial occlusions. Radiology 1990;175:393.
19. Johnson SP, Durham JD, Subber SW: Acute arterial occlusions of the small vessels of the hand and forearm: treatment with regional urokinase therapy. J Vasc Interv Radiol 1999;10:869.
20. Michaels JA, Torrie EP, Galland RB: The treatment of upper limb vascular occlusions using intraarterial thrombolysis. Eur J Vasc Surg 1993; 7:744.
21. Browse DJ, Torrie EPH, Galland RB: Early results and 1-year follow-up after intra-arterial thrombolysis. Br J Surg 1993;80:194.
22. Coulon M, Goffette P, Dondelinger RF: Local thrombolytic infusion in arterial ischemia of the upper limb: mid-term results. Cardiovasc Intervent Radiol 1994;17:81.
23. Cejna M, Salomonowitz E, Wohlschlager: rt-PA thrombolysis in acute thromboembolic upper extremity occlusion. Cardiovasc Intervent Radiol 2001;24:218.
24. Sullivan KL, Minken SL, White RI Jr: Treatment of a case of thromboembolism resulting from thoracic outlet syndrome with intraarterial urokinase infusion. J Vasc Surg 1988;7:568.
25. Williams SJ II: Chronic upper extremity ischemia: current concepts in management. Surg Clinic North Am 1986;66:355.
26. Machleder HI: Arterial disorders. In: Machleder HI, ed. Vascular Disorders of the Upper Extremity, 2nd ed. Mount Kisco, NY, Futura Publishing, 1989:225.
27. Voyvodic F, Hayward M: Case report. Upper extremity ischaemia secondary to ergotamine poisoning. Clin Radiol 1996;51:589.
28. Webster MW, Downs L, Yonas H, et al: The effect of arm exercise on regional cerebral blood flow in the subclavian steal syndrome. Am J Surg 1994;168:91.
29. Westerband A, Rodriguez JA, Ramaiah VG, et al: Endovascular therapy in prevention and management of coronary-subclavian steal. J Vasc Surg 2003;38:699.
30. Valji K, Hye RJ, Roberts AC, et al: Hand ischemia in patients with hemodialysis access grafts: angiographic diagnosis and treatment. Radiology 1995;196:697.
31. Yip PK, Liu HM, Hwang BS, et al: Subclavian steal phenomenon: a correlation between duplex sonographic and angiographic findings. Neuroradiology 1992;34:279.
32. Walker DW, Acker JD, Cole CA: Subclavian steal syndrome detected with duplex pulsed Doppler sonography. Am J Neurorad 1982;3:615.
33. Rose SC: Noninvasive vascular laboratory for evaluation of peripheral arterial occlusive disease. Part III—clinical applications: nonatherosclerotic lower extremity arterial conditions and upper extremity arterial disease. J Vasc Interv Radiol 2001;12:11.
34. Krinsky G, Rofsky N, Flyer M, et al: Gadolinium-enhanced three-dimensional MR angiography of acquired arch vessel disease. AJR Am J Roentgenol 1996;167:981.
35. Carriero A, Salute L, Tartaro A, et al: The role of magnetic resonance angiography in the diagnosis of subclavian steal. Cardiovasc Intervent Radiol 1995;18:87.
36. Kumar S, Roy S, Radhakrishnan S, et al: Three-dimensional time of flight MR angiography of the arch of the aorta and its major branches: a comparative study with contrast angiography. Clin Radiol 1996; 51:18.
37. Salam TA, Lumsden AB, Smith RB III: Subclavian artery revascularization: a decade of experience with extrathoracic bypass procedures. J Surg Research 1994;56:387.
38. Roddy SP, Darling RC 3rd, Chang BB, et al: Brachial artery reconstruction for occlusive disease: a 12 year experience. J Vasc Surg 2001; 33:802.
39. Bogey WM, Demasi RJ, Tripp MD, et al: Percutaneous transluminal angioplasty for subclavian artery stenosis. Am Surg 1994;60:103.
40. Rodriguez-Lopez JA, Werner A, Martinez R, et al: Stenting for atherosclerotic occlusive disease of the subclavian artery. Ann Vasc Surg 1999;13:254.
41. Erbstein RA, Wholey MH, Smoot S: Subclavian artery steal syndrome: treatment by percutaneous transluminal angioplasty. AJR Am J Roentgenol 1988;151:291.
42. Motarjeme A, Keifer JW, Zuska AJ, et al: Percutaneous transluminal angioplasty for treatment of subclavian steal. Radiology 1985; 155:611.
43. Hallisey MJ, Rees JH, Meranze SG, et al: Use of angioplasty in the prevention and treatment of coronary-subclavian steal syndrome. J Vasc Interv Radiol 1995;6:125.
44. Westerbrand A, Rodriguez JA, Ramaiah VG, et al: Endovascular therapy in prevention and management of coronary-subclavian steal. J Vasc Surg 2003;38:699.
45. Vitek JJ: Subclavian artery angioplasty and the origin of the vertebral artery. Radiology 1989;170:407.
46. Selby JB Jr, Matsumoto AH, Tegtmeyer CJ, et al: Balloon angioplasty above the aortic arch: immediate and long-term results. AJR Am J Roentgenol 1993;160:631.
47. Bates MC, Broce M, Lavigne PS, et al: Subclavian artery stenting: factors influencing long-term outcome. Catheter Cardiovasc Interv 2004;61:5.
48. Millaire A, Trinca M, Marache P, et al: Subclavian angioplasty: immediate and late results in 50 patients. Cathet Cardiovasc Diag 1993;29:8.
49. Mathias KD, Lueth I, Haarmann P: Percutaneous transluminal angioplasty of proximal subclavian artery occlusions. Cardiovasc Intervent Radiol 1993;16:214.
49. Schmitter SP, Marx M, Bernstein R, et al: Angioplasty-induced subclavian artery dissection in a patient with internal mammary artery graft: treatment with endovascular stent and stent-graft. AJR Am J Roentgenol 1995;165:449.
50. Roos DB: Overview of thoracic outlet syndromes. In: Machleder HI, ed. Vascular Disorders of the Upper Extremity, 2nd ed. Mount Kisco, NY, Futura Publishing, 1989:155.
51. Maxey TS, Reece TB, Ellman PI, et al: Safety and efficacy of the supraclavicular approach to thoracic outlet decompression. Ann Thorac Surg 2003;76:396.
52. Balci AE, Balci TA, Cakir O, et al: Surgical treatment of thoracic outlet syndrome: effects and results of surgery. Ann Thorac Surg 2003;75:1091.
53. Longley DG, Yedlicka JW, Molina EJ, et al: Thoracic outlet syndrome: evaluation of the subclavian vessels by color duplex sonography. AJR Am J Roentgenol 1992;158:623.
54. Charon JP, Milne W, Sheppard DG, et al: Evaluation of MR angiographic technique in the assessment of thoracic outlet syndrome. Clin Radiol 2004;59:588.
55. Demondion X, Bacqueville E, Paul C, et al: Thoracic outlet: assessment with MR imaging in asymptomatic and symptomatic populations. Radiology 2003;227:461.
56. Krinsky G, Rofsky NM: MR angiography of the aortic arch vessels and upper extremity. MRI Clin North Am 1998;6:269.

57. Remy-Jardin M, Remy J, Masson P, et al: Helical CT angiography of thoracic outlet syndrome: functional anatomy. AJR Am J Roentgenol 2000;174:1667.

58. Adler J, Hooshmand I: The angiographic spectrum of the thoracic outlet syndrome: with emphasis on mural thrombosis and emboli and congenital vascular anomalies. Clin Radiol 1973;24:35.

59. Wigley FM: Clinical practice. Raynaud's phenomenon. N Engl J Med 2002;347:1001.

60. McLafferty RB, Edwards JM, Taylor LM Jr, et al: Diagnosis and long-term clinical outcome in patients diagnosed with hand ischemia. J Vasc Surg 1995;22:361.

61. Maiman MH, Bookstein JJ, Bernstein EF: Digital ischemia: angiographic differentiation of embolism from primary arterial disease. AJR Am J Roentgenol 1981;137:1183.

62. Ferris BL, Taylor LM Jr, Oyama K, et al: Hypothenar hammer syndrome: proposed etiology. J Vasc Surg 2000;31:104.

63. Hummers LK, Wigley FM: Management of Raynaud's phenomenon and digital ischemia in scleroderma. Rheum Dis Clin North Am 2003; 29:293.

64. Meharwal ZS, Trehan N: Functional status of the hand after radial artery harvesting: results in 3,977 cases. Ann Thorac Surg 2001; 72:1557.

65. Sumner DS: Noninvasive assessment of upper extremity and hand ischemia. J Vasc Surg 1986;3:560.

66. Rofsky NM: MR angiography of the hand and wrist. Magn Reson Imaging Clin North Am 1995;3:345.

67. Connell DA, Koulouris G, Thorn DA, et al: Contrast-enhanced MR angiography of the hand. Radiographics 2002;22:583.

68. Loring LA, Hallisey MJ: Arteriography and interventional therapy for diseases of the hand. Radiographics 1995;15:1299.

69. Bettoni L, Geri A, Airo P, et al: Systemic sclerosis therapy with iloprost: a prospective observational study of 30 patients treated for a median of 3 years. Clin Rheumatol 2002;21:244.

70. Nehler MR, Dalman RL, Harris EJ, et al: Upper extremity arterial bypass distal to the wrist. J Vasc Surg 1992;16:633.

71. Capek P, Holcroft J: Traumatic ischemia of the hand in a tennis player: successful treatment with urokinase. J Vasc Interv Radiol 1993; 4:279.

72. Lang EV, Bookstein JJ: Accelerated thrombolysis and angioplasty for hand ischemia in Buerger's disease. Cardiovasc Intervent Radiol 1989;12:95.

73. Pretre R, Hoffmeyer P, Bednarkiewicz M, et al: Blunt injury to the subclavian or axillary artery. J Am Coll Surg 1994;179:295.

74. Rose SC, Moore EE: Angiography in patients with arterial trauma: correlation between angiographic abnormalities, operative findings, and clinical outcome. AJR Am J Roentgenol 1987;149:613.

75. Scalea TM, Sclafani S: Interventional techniques in vascular trauma. Surg Clin North Am 2001;81:1281.

76. McCollum CH, Mavor E: Brachial artery injury after cardiac catheterization. J Vasc Surg 1986;4:355.

77. Feldman D, Vujic I, McKay D, et al: Crutch-induced axillary artery injury. Cardiovasc Intervent Radiol 1995;18:296.

78. Britt LD, Weireter LJ, Cole FJ: Newer diagnostic modalities for vascular injuries. Surg Clin North Am 2001;81:1263.

79. Fields CE, Latifi R, Ivatury RR: Brachial and forearm vessel injuries. Surg Clin North Am 2002;82:105.

80. Demetriades D, Asensio JA: Subclavian and axillary vascular injuries. Surg Clin North Am 2001;81:1357.

81. Weaver FA, Yellin AE, Bauer MA, et al: Is arterial proximity a valid indication for arteriography in penetrating extremity trauma? A prospective analysis. Arch Surg 1990;125:1256.

82. Francis H III, Thal ER, Weigelt JA, et al: Vascular proximity: is it a valid indication for arteriography in asymptomatic patients? J Trauma 1991;31:512.

83. Richardson JD, Vitale GC, Flint LM Jr: Penetrating arterial trauma. Analysis of missed vascular injuries. Arch Surg 1987;122:678.

84. Smyth SH, Pond GD, Johnson PL, et al: Proximity injuries: correlation with results of extremity arteriography. J Vasc Interv Radiol 1991;2:451.

85. Kaufman JA, Parker JE, Gillespie DL, et al: Arteriography for proximity of injury in penetrating extremity trauma. J Vasc Interv Radiol 1992; 3:719.

86. Schwartz MR, Weaver FA, Bauer M, et al: Refining the indications for arteriography in penetrating extremity trauma: a prospective analysis. J Vasc Surg 1993;17:116.

87. Fry WR, Smith RS, Sayers DV, et al: The success of duplex ultrasonographic scanning in diagnosis of extremity vascular proximity trauma. Arch Surg 1993;128:1368.

88. Knudson MM, Lewis FR, Atkinson K, et al: The role of duplex ultrasound arterial imaging in patients with penetrating extremity trauma. Arch Surg 1993;128:1033.

89. Edwards JW, Bergstein JB, Karp DL, et al: Penetrating proximity injuries—the role of duplex scanning: a prospective study. Journal of Vascular Technology 1993;17:257.

90. Soto JA, Munera F, Morales C, et al: Focal arterial injuries of the proximal extremities: helical CT arteriography as the initial method of diagnosis. Radiology 2001;218:188.

91. Reid JDS, Redman HC, Weigelt JA, et al: Wounds of the extremities in proximity to major arteries: value of angiography in the detection of arterial injury. AJR Am J Roentgenol 1988;151:1035.

92. Fisher RG, Ben-Menachem Y: Penetrating injuries of the thoracic aorta and brachiocephalic arteries: angiographic findings in 18 cases. AJR Am J Roentgenol 1987;149:607.

93. Sclafani SJA, Cooper R, Shaftan GW, et al: Arterial trauma: diagnostic and therapeutic angiography. Radiology 1986;161:165.

94. Frykberg ER, Crump JM, Dennis JW, et al: Nonoperative observation of clinically occult arterial injuries: a prospective evaluation. Surgery 1991;109:85.

95. Levey DS, Teitelbaum GP, Finck EJ, et al: Safety and efficacy of transcatheter embolization of axillary and shoulder arterial injuries. J Vasc Interv Radiol 1991;2:99.

96. Herbreteau D, Aymard A, Khayata MH, et al: Endovascular treatment of arteriovenous fistulas arising from branches of the subclavian artery. J Vasc Interv Radiol 1993;4:237.

97. Skibo L, Polak JF: Compression repair of a postcatheterization pseudoaneurysm of the brachial artery under sonographic guidance. AJR Am J Roentgenol 1993;160:383.

98. LaPerna L, Olin JW, Goines D, et al: Ultrasound-guided thrombin injection for the treatment of postcatheterization pseudoaneurysms. Circulation 2000;102:2391.

99. Hilfiker PR, Razavi MK, Kee ST, et al: Stent-graft therapy for subclavian artery aneurysms and fistulas: single center mid-term results. J Vasc Interv Radiol 2000;11:578.

100. Xenos ES, Freeman M, Stevens S, et al: Covered stents for injuries of subclavian and axillary arteries. J Vasc Surg 2003;38:451.

101. Dougherty MJ, Calligaro KD, Savarese RP, et al: Atherosclerotic aneurysm of the intrathoracic subclavian artery: a case report and review of the literature. J Vasc Surg 1995;21:521.

102. Johnson LW, Esente P, Giambartolomei A, et al: Peripheral vascular complications of coronary angioplasty by the femoral and brachial techniques. Cathet Cardiovasc Diagn 1994;31:165.

103. Cosottini M, Zampa V, Petruzzi P, et al: Contrast-enhanced three-dimensional MR angiography in the assessment of subclavian artery disease. Eur Radiol 2000;10:1737.

104. Meier RA, Marianacci EB, Costello P, et al: 3D image reconstruction of right subclavian artery aneurysms. J Comput Assist Tomogr 1993; 17:887.

105. Anderson SE, DeMonaco D, Buechler U, et al: Imaging features of pseudoaneurysms of the hand in children and adults. AJR Am J Roentgenol 2003;180:659.

106. Davidovic LB, Markovic DM, Pejkic SD, et al: Subclavian artery aneurysms. Asian J Surg 2003;26:7.

107. Olin JW: Thromboangiitis obliterans (Buerger's disease). N Engl J Med 2000;343:864.

108. Hagen B, Lohse S: Clinical and radiologic aspects of Buerger's disease. Cardiovasc Intervent Radiol 1984;7:283.

109. Tyagi S, Verma PK, Gambhir DS, et al: Early and long-term results of subclavian angioplasty in aortoarteritis (Takayasu disease): comparison with atherosclerosis. Cardiovasc Intervent Radiol 1998;21:219.

110. Sharma BK, Jain S, Bali HK, et al: A follow-up study of balloon angioplasty and de-novo stenting in Takayasu arteritis. Int J Cardiol 2000; 31(Suppl 1):S147.

111. Aburahma AF, Thaxton L: Temporal arteritis: diagnostic and therapeutic considerations. Am Surg 1996;62:449.

112. Rubin DI, Schomberg PJ, Shepherd RF, et al: Arteritis and brachial plexus neuropathy as delayed complications of radiation therapy. Mayo Clin Proc 2001;76:849.

113. Rhodes JM, Cherry KJ Jr, Clark RC, et al: Aortic-origin reconstruction of the great vessels: risk factors of early and late complications. J Vasc Surg 2000;31:260.

114. Carr MM, Mahoney JL, Bowen CVA: Extremity arteriovenous malformations: review of a series. Can J Surg 1994;37:293.

115. Yakes WF, Rossi P, Odink H: How I do it: arteriovenous malformations management. Cardiovasc Intervent Radiol 1996;19:65.

116. Gomes AS: Embolization therapy of congenital arteriovenous malformations: use of alternate approaches. Radiology 1994;190:191.

117. Yakes WF, Haas DK, Parker SH, et al: Symptomatic vascular malformations: ethanol embolotherapy. Radiology 1989;170:1059.

118. White RI Jr, Pollak J, Persing J, et al: Long-term outcome of embolotherapy and surgery for high-flow extremity arteriovenous malformations. J Vasc Interv Radiol 2000;11:1285.

8

Renal Arteries and Veins

◼ ARTERIOGRAPHY AND VENOGRAPHY

Evaluation of the renal arteries begins with abdominal aortography to detect aortic disease, renal artery ostial disease, and accessory arteries before selective catheterization is performed. A 4- or 5-French pigtail (or similar configuration) catheter is positioned with the side holes at the level of the main renal arteries (approximately the L1 or L2 vertebral body). Images are routinely obtained in an anteroposterior projection. With advancing age and aortic rotation, the origins of the right and left renal arteries often come to arise along the anterolateral and posterolateral aortic walls, respectively. Therefore, a shallow right posterior oblique view may place the ostia in profile.[1] Oblique projections or repeat injections with a lower catheter position are used to distinguish between accessory renal arteries and mesenteric branches.

Selective renal arteriography is performed with a 4- or 5-French cobra, visceral hook, or reverse curve (e.g., Simmons) catheter. Because the renal artery and its branches are prone to vasospasm and dissection, guidewires and catheters should be manipulated carefully. The average flow rate in the renal artery is 5 to 6 mL/second.

Renal venography is performed using a straight catheter (e.g., cobra shape) or an occlusion balloon (if evaluation of intrarenal veins is important). Valves at the origin of the veins may cause resistance to catheter passage. The valves can always be crossed with gentle guidewire probing. A guidewire is used to seat the catheter well within the vein. To partially overcome the rapid flow in a patent renal vein, a brisk, large-volume injection is required.

Several techniques have been described for renal vein renin sampling (see below). Blood specimens are taken from the main right renal vein, main left renal vein (beyond the orifice of the gonadal vein), and the infrarenal and suprarenal inferior vena cava (IVC). In patients with multiple renal veins, all main channels should be sampled. In patients with suspected renovascular hypertension and stenosis of intrarenal arterial branches, individual samples should be taken from the vein draining that renal segment.[2]

In patients with renal dysfunction (serum creatinine level greater than 1.2 to 1.5 mg/dL), carbon dioxide or gadolinium may be used instead of or to supplement iodinated contrast media to reduce the risk of contrast-induced renal failure (see Chapter 2).[3]

◼ ANATOMY

Development

In the fetus, the kidneys lie in the pelvis and receive their blood supply from neighboring vessels, including the median sacral and common iliac arteries.[4] With time, lateral splanchnic branches of the aorta begin to perfuse structures arising from the mesonephric ridge: adrenal glands, gonads, and kidneys. With the ascent of the kidneys to the mid-abdomen, they are ultimately supplied by the more caudal of these lateral splanchnic arteries. Anomalies in the origin and number of renal arteries can

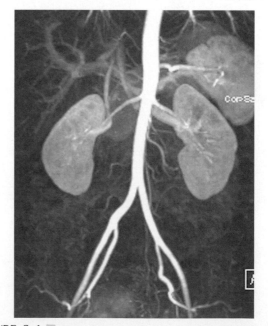

FIGURE 8-1 ◼ Normal renal arteries on gadolinium-enhanced MR angiography.

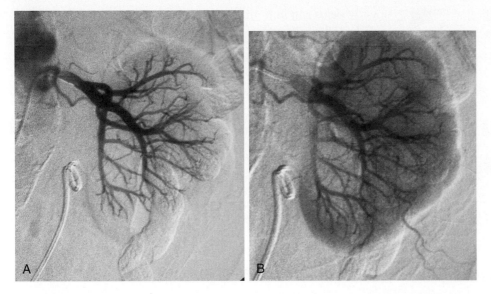

FIGURE 8-2 ■ Arteriogram of a normal left kidney. **A,** Early arterial phase. **B,** Late arterial phase.

be explained by incomplete regression of some of these primitive vessels.

Normal Anatomy

The *renal arteries* arise from the lateral surface of the aorta at about the L1-L2 vertebral level (Fig. 8-1).[5,6] The right renal artery runs posterior to the IVC and right renal vein to enter the renal hilum. The left renal artery passes behind the left renal vein. The proximal renal arteries have small *inferior adrenal, ureteric,* and *capsular branches,* which often are not seen on imaging studies.

At the renal hilum, the artery bifurcates into dorsal and ventral rami (Fig. 8-2). These trunks divide into segmental branches, which then further divide into lobar branches supplying the renal pyramids. The vessels successively branch into the *interlobar, arcuate,* and *interlobular arteries.* In the renal cortex, the interlobular arteries divide into afferent arterioles that supply the glomeruli. The intrarenal vessels are essentially end arteries; however, a collateral system exists between extrarenal arteries and segmental renal branches to maintain renal perfusion if the main renal artery becomes obstructed.

The renal venous system follows a branching pattern similar to that of the renal arteries. However, wide anastomoses exist among the intrarenal veins (Fig. 8-3). Both main renal

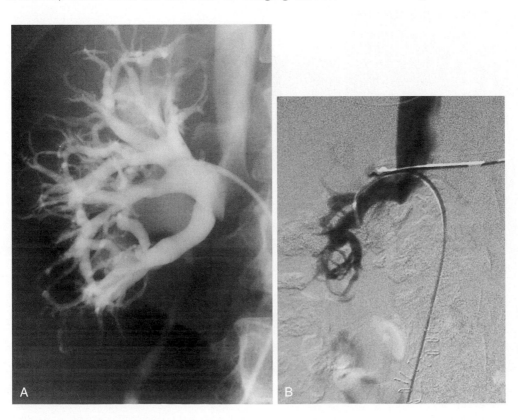

FIGURE 8-3 ■ **A,** Venogram of a normal right kidney after injection of 10 μg of epinephrine into the right renal artery with prominent filling of intrarenal veins. Notice the valve at the orifice to the inferior vena cava. **B,** Normal right renal venogram.

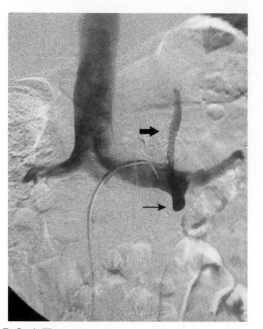

FIGURE 8-4 ▪ Normal left renal venogram with partial filling of the left phrenicoadrenal trunk *(thick arrow)* and gonadal vein to the level of the first valve *(thin arrow).*

veins run in front of their corresponding arteries. The *right renal vein* passes behind the duodenum and enters the right lateral surface of the IVC.[7] The *left renal vein*, which is about three times as long, runs between the aorta and superior mesenteric artery and then into the left lateral wall of the IVC. The *left gonadal vein* enters the left renal vein along its undersurface just to the left of the spine (Fig. 8-4). The *left adrenal vein* enters the left renal vein on its superior surface as a common trunk with the *left inferior phrenic vein*. The *right adrenal* and *gonadal veins* have separate entrances into the IVC at or near the origin of the right renal vein. In most patients, branches of the ascending lumbar and hemi-azygous venous systems enter the left renal and left gonadal veins. Some patients have valves in the renal veins between the hilum and the IVC.

Variant Anatomy

Accessory renal arteries are present in one or both kidneys in about 25% to 35% of the general population.[8-11] Most accessory renal arteries supply the lower pole of the kidney and may arise anywhere from the suprarenal aorta to the iliac artery (Figs. 8-5 and 8-6). Anomalies of position (i.e., ectopia), fusion, or rotation of the kidney are associated with variations in the origin and number of renal arteries (Fig. 8-7). The *horseshoe kidney* usually is supplied by three or more arteries arising from the aorta, iliac arteries, or both.

Several renal vein anomalies may be encountered (Table 8-1 and Figs. 8-8 through 8-10).[12-15] With the

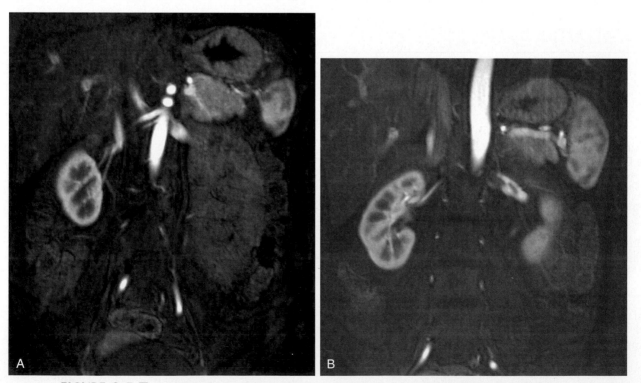

FIGURE 8-5 ▪ **A** and **B,** Accessory right renal artery documented on gadolinium-enhanced MR angiograms.

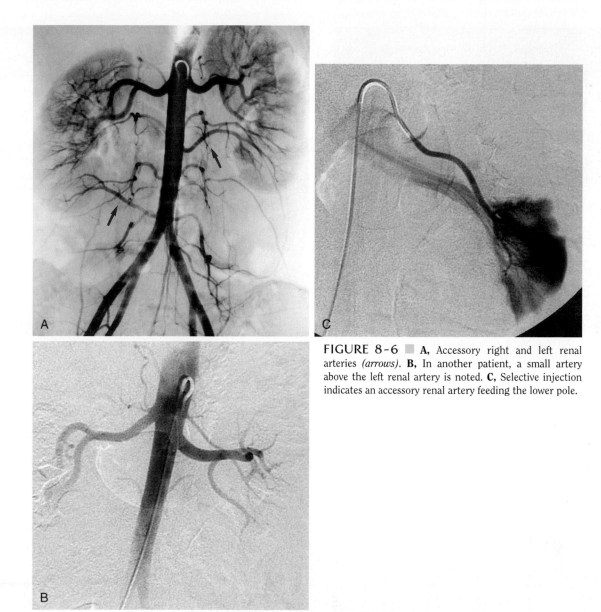

FIGURE 8-6 ■ **A,** Accessory right and left renal arteries *(arrows)*. **B,** In another patient, a small artery above the left renal artery is noted. **C,** Selective injection indicates an accessory renal artery feeding the lower pole.

circumaortic left renal vein, a "preaortic" segment enters the IVC in the usual location (see Fig. 8-9). A "retroaortic" segment arises from the renal hilum and drains into the low IVC. The two veins may or may not communicate in the renal hilum.

Collateral Circulation

With renal artery stenosis or occlusion, an extensive collateral circulation maintains blood flow to the kidney. Although renal arteries have been described as end arteries, communications between extrarenal arteries and segmental, interlobar, and arcuate vessels do exist. The classic description of collateral arterial flow in the kidney was made by Abrams and Cornell.[16] The intrarenal vessels are primarily supplied by three collateral networks: the capsular, peripelvic, and periureteric arteries. These three systems are ultimately fed by the lumbar arteries, aorta, internal iliac artery, inferior adrenal artery, and other vessels (Fig. 8-11).

In main renal vein obstruction, venous outflow occurs through ureteral, gonadal, adrenal, ascending lumbar, and capsular venous pathways (Fig. 8-12).

TABLE 8-1   RENAL VENOUS ANOMALIES

Type	Frequency (%)
Multiple right renal veins	8–15
Circumaortic left renal vein	2–10
Retroaortic left renal vein	2–7
Right gonadal vein enters right renal vein	<10

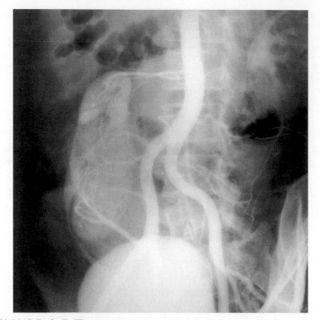

FIGURE 8-7 ■ The ptotic right kidney has multiple renal arteries arising from the abdominal aorta and the right iliac artery.

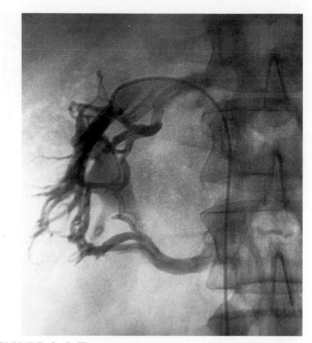

FIGURE 8-8 ■ Two right renal veins communicate in the renal hilum.

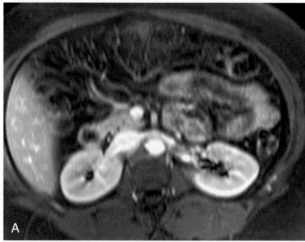

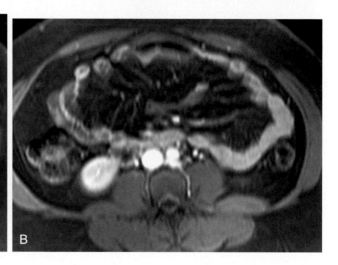

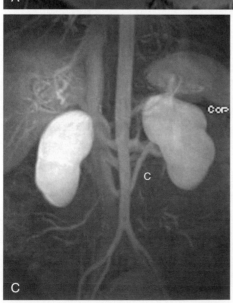

FIGURE 8-9 ■ Circumaortic left renal vein. **A,** Gadolinium-enhanced MR angiogram shows main left renal vein entering the inferior vena cava (IVC). **B,** Circumaortic component passes behind the aorta to join the IVC. **C,** Maximum intensity projection demonstrates the orthotopic and circumaortic (C) left renal veins.

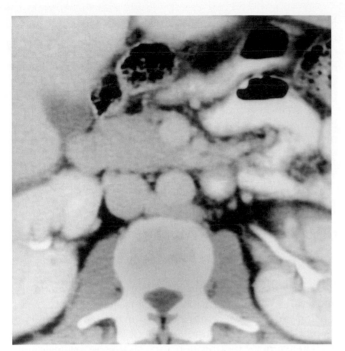

FIGURE 8-10 ■ Retroaortic left renal vein on CT scan.

■ MAJOR DISORDERS

Renal Transplant Living Donor Evaluation

Clinical Setting

Preoperative evaluation of potential kidney donors is done to prove their suitability for transplantation. The vascular components of imaging are needed to detect underlying renal vascular disease that might preclude organ donation and to guide selection of the kidney to be removed. In general, the left kidney is preferred over the right kidney because of the longer length of its vein.

Imaging

Certain information about the donor's anatomy is important to ascertain before a kidney is harvested:

- Presence and location of accessory renal arteries
- Early (prehilar) renal artery branching or proximal ureteral arteries (<2 cm from the aorta)
- Intrinsic renal artery disease (e.g., atherosclerosis, fibromuscular dysplasia, aneurysm, arteriovenous malformation [AVM])
- Aortic disease (e.g., abdominal aortic aneurysm)
- Renal vein and IVC variants (e.g., multiple renal veins)
- Ureteral anomalies
- Intrarenal masses

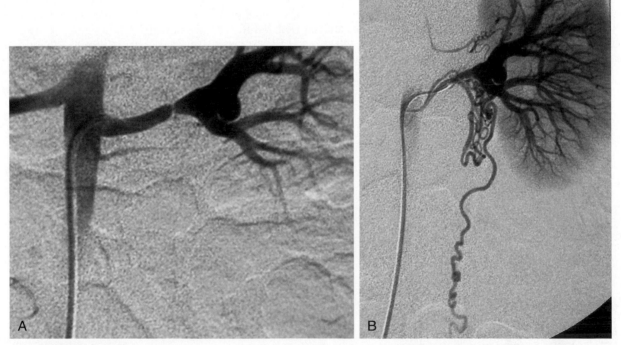

FIGURE 8-11 ■ Significant left renal artery stenosis from intimal or perimedial type fibromuscular dysplasia. **A,** Pretreatment arteriogram shows typical weblike appearance of lesion in the distal left renal artery. **B,** Following angioplasty, increased flow in the main artery causes antegrade flow in ureteric branches beyond the stenosis, which provided retrograde collateral circulation into the kidney before treatment.

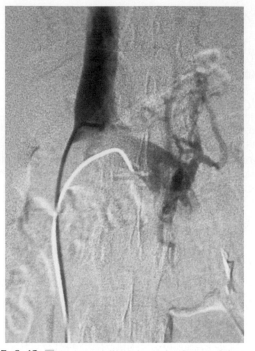

FIGURE 8-12 ■ Venous collaterals with chronic left renal vein stenosis caused by impingement between the superior mesenteric artery and aorta.

Highly accurate anatomic evaluation is particularly critical because laparoscopic donor nephrectomy (with its more limited view of anomalies) has become the standard of care in many centers.[17-19]

Computed Tomographic and Magnetic Resonance Angiography. These relatively noninvasive techniques provide thorough depiction of arterial, venous, ureteric, and parenchymal abnormalities that may influence kidney selection or suitability for donation.[11,17,20-22] Gadolinium-enhanced MR arteriography and venography is performed with maximum intensity projection images and multiplanar reconstructions for detection of vascular abnormalities (see Figs. 8-1 and 8-5). It avoids radiation exposure and the risks of iodinated contrast material. Multidetector CT angiography, on the other hand, provides somewhat better spatial resolution and may be more accurate in detecting accessory arteries or prehilar branching (Fig. 8-13). The sensitivity and specificity of the two methods is comparable (>90%). Small accessory arteries occasionally will be missed with both modalities.

Renovascular Hypertension and Ischemic Nephropathy

Etiology

Renovascular hypertension (RVH) is the most common secondary form of hypertension and refers specifically to hypertension caused by stenosis or occlusion of the renal artery or its branches. RVH accounts for about 3% to 5% of cases of hypertension.[23] The prevalence of significant renovascular disease (detected by duplex sonography) in the U.S. population of those older than 65 years of age is about 7%.[24]

Renal artery obstruction leads to a reduction in intrarenal arterial pressure that is sensed by the juxtaglomerular apparatus of the afferent arterioles. The renin-angiotensin-aldosterone system is triggered, leading to increased renin production, vasoconstriction of systemic arteries, sodium and water retention, and systemic hypertension. RVH may occur with disease in the main renal artery, accessory renal artery, or distal vessels. With time, untreated hypertension of any cause leads to thickening of the small arteries of the kidney (i.e., nephrosclerosis), which causes the distal intrarenal vessels to become irregular, tortuous, and pruned (Fig. 8-14).

Other *renal* causes of hypertension include trauma (e.g., Page kidney), cystic disease, renal cell carcinoma,

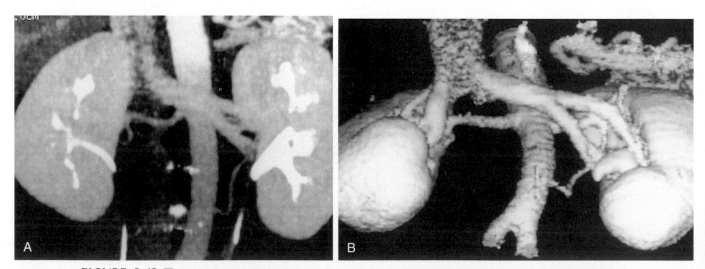

FIGURE 8-13 ■ Single detector CT angiogram of a renal donor. The maximum intensity projection (**A**) and three-dimensional reconstruction with surface shading in a caudocranial projection (**B**) show renal arterial and venous anatomy, with an accessory left renal artery arising low on the aorta. A catheter aortogram confirmed these findings.

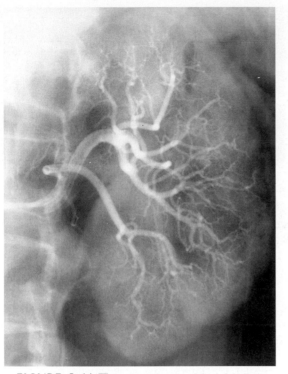

FIGURE 8-14 ■ Nephrosclerosis of the left kidney.

TABLE 8-2 CLASSIFICATION OF SUBTYPES OF RENAL ARTERY FIBROMUSCULAR DYSPLASIA

Type	Frequency (%)	Morphology
Medial fibroplasia	60–70	Alternating narrowing and aneurysms ("string of beads")
Perimedial fibroplasia	15–25	Irregular, beaded narrowing
Medial hyperplasia	5–15	Tubular, smooth narrowing
Medial dissection	5	False channel in media
Intimal fibroplasia	1–2	Focal, smooth narrowing
Periarterial fibroplasia	<1	Tubular, smooth narrowing

of the renal artery. In one study, atherosclerotic renal artery stenosis was found to be progressive in 44% of cases.[27]

Fibromuscular dysplasia (FMD) is a group of related disorders in which luminal narrowing results from overgrowth of fibrous or muscular tissue in one or more layers of the renal artery wall (see Chapter 3). Six types of FMD are described in one popular classification scheme; the most common type is medial fibroplasia (Table 8-2).[26,28]

Eventually, severe narrowing of the renal artery can lead to frank thrombosis and occlusion. Other causes of complete renal artery occlusion are listed in Box 8-2.

arteriovenous fistula, renal artery aneurysm, reninoma, and renal infarction.

Ischemic nephropathy, although variably defined, is essentially a loss of renal function related to hypoperfusion from main renal artery disease.[25] Atherosclerotic renal artery disease affecting both renal arteries or the artery to a solitary kidney is a common cause of ischemic nephropathy. Bilateral occlusions may eventually cause end-stage renal disease.

Renal artery stenoses have a variety of causes (Box 8-1). Atherosclerosis and fibromuscular dysplasia account for most cases. Uncommon causes for renal artery stenosis are considered later in this chapter.

Atherosclerosis is responsible for at least two thirds of cases of clinically significant renal artery stenosis.[26] Obstruction usually results from aortic plaque engulfing the renal artery ostium (i.e., within 5 to 10 mm of the aortic lumen). Less frequently, plaque develops independently in the truncal portion

Clinical Features

Most patients with RVH or ischemic nephropathy are middle aged or elderly and have one or more risk factors for atherosclerosis. Younger patients are more likely to suffer from one of the less common causes of RVH. FMD afflicts women more often than men. Although African Americans suffer from essential hypertension more frequently than do whites, RVH is relatively more common in the latter group.[29] Patients with thrombosis superimposed on underlying disease often are asymptomatic. However, worsening of hypertension or loss of renal function may occur if there is occlusion of the artery to a solitary functioning kidney.

Imaging

Because hypertension is common but RVH is not, screening should be reserved for patients at moderate to high risk

---

BOX 8-1 ■ Causes of Renal Artery Stenosis

Atherosclerosis
Fibromuscular dysplasia
Dissection
Vasculitis
Coarctation syndromes
  Neurofibromatosis
  Congenital rubella
  Williams syndrome
  Tuberous sclerosis
Extrinsic compression

BOX 8-2 ■ Causes of Renal Artery Occlusion

Thrombosis superimposed on underlying stenosis
Embolus (usually cardiac)
Trauma
  Accidental
  Iatrogenic (e.g., catheterization)
Aortic or renal artery aneurysm thrombosis
Dissection
Congenital (e.g., crossed fused ectopia)
Vasculitis
Hypercoagulable state
Nephrotic syndrome

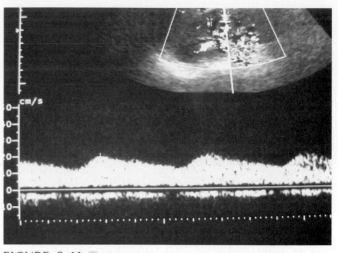

FIGURE 8-16 ■ Abnormal renal artery duplex ultrasound with damping and slowing of peak systole in intrarenal vessel distal to a significant stenosis.

for RVH. Criteria proposed by the Joint National Committee on Prevention, Detection, Evaluation, and Treatment of High Blood Pressure are listed in Box 8-3.[30]

Several metabolic screening tests are first performed to exclude rarer causes of RVH (e.g., pheochromocytoma, aldosteronoma). Noninvasive imaging procedures are then used to screen patients. Arteriography is employed only if results are equivocal or endovascular therapy is being considered. No single screening procedure has emerged as the ideal technique.

Color Doppler Sonography. Ultrasound is one of the principal tools for detecting RVH because it is quick, relatively inexpensive, and completely safe (Fig. 8-15). If the aorta and main renal artery can be imaged, criteria for significant renal artery stenosis include intrastenotic peak systolic velocity (PSV) of greater than 180 cm/second and PSV renal/aortic ratio of greater than 3.0–3.5.[31,32] If these structures cannot be seen due to technical factors, the intrarenal arteries are interrogated. With significant renal artery stenosis, damping and slowing of the time to peak systole ("parvus-et-tardus" waveform) is typical (Fig. 8-16).[33] In addition, the

acceleration is diminished and the acceleration time prolonged (<300 to 390 cm/second^2 and >0.06 to 0.07 seconds, respectively).[31,34] The resistive index usually is less than 0.45.[32] However, duplex sonography is highly operator dependent, and some studies have failed to confirm the accuracy of this technique.[35,36]

Magnetic Resonance Imaging. Many centers rely on gadolinium-enhanced MR angiography for screening all patients with suspected RVH. Several reports suggest that MR angiography is superior to color Doppler sonography in detection of disease in the main and accessory renal arteries.

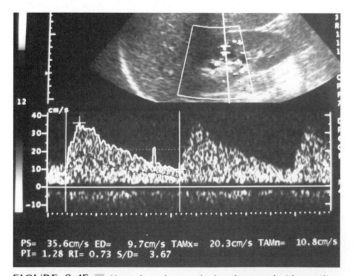

FIGURE 8-15 ■ Normal renal artery duplex ultrasound with sampling of intrarenal branches.

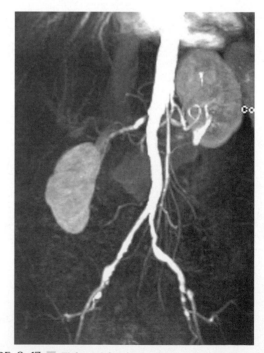

FIGURE 8-17 ■ Tight ostial right renal artery stenosis on gadolinium-enhanced MR angiography.

With current techniques, gadolinium-enhanced MR angiography can detect main renal artery stenoses with up to 90% to 100% sensitivity and 75% to 100% specificity (Figs. 8-17 and 8-18).[36-40] Weaknesses of the method include identification of disease in accessory and segmental renal arteries and artifacts related to metallic clips, intravascular stents, or patient motion. However, isolated significant stenoses of accessory arteries in this population are quite uncommon (<2%).[41]

Computed Tomography. Single detector CT angiography approaches the sensitivity and specificity of MR angiography in depicting renal artery stenosis (Fig 8-19).[36] Multidetector units should further improve on these results.[39,42] CT has better spatial resolution than MR imaging. In addition, CT is better for evaluation after renal artery stent placement. Its major disadvantage is the need for iodinated contrast in a population at increased risk for contrast nephropathy. Subtle lesions of FMD may be missed.[43]

Captopril Renal Scintigraphy. This technique provides functional rather than anatomic evidence of renal artery stenosis and overall kidney function. In a patient with a significant renal artery stenosis, the efferent arterioles of the glomeruli are constricted by angiotensin II to maintain glomerular filtration pressure in the face of diminished afferent arteriolar pressure. Administration of an angiotensin-converting enzyme (ACE) inhibitor decreases this angiotensin II–related constriction of the efferent arterioles, which reduces glomerular filtration.[44] This reduction can be quantified directly by using a glomerular filtered radionuclide agent such as ^{99m}Tc-diethylenetriamine-penta-acetic acid (^{99m}Tc-DTPA) or indirectly by changes in cortical renal activity using a tubular secreted agent such as ^{131}I-ortho-diodohippurate (IOH) or ^{99m}Tc-mercaptoacetyltriglycine (MAG3) (Fig. 8-20). A positive test result may be defined in several ways, including a significant decrease in kidney function by comparing renograms before and after captopril

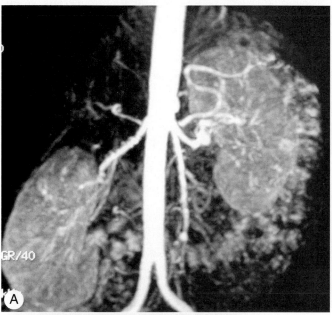

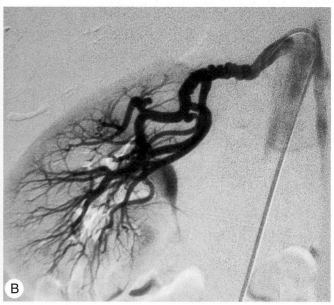

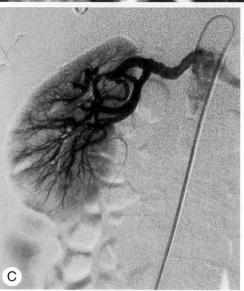

FIGURE 8-18 ■ Medial fibroplasia type of fibromuscular dysplasia of the right renal artery. **A,** MR angiogram shows classic "string of beads" appearance of distal portion of the artery. **B,** Catheter angiogram confirms these findings. Mild changes of fibromuscular dysplasia are noted beyond the main artery. A systolic pressure gradient of 50 mm Hg was found. **C,** Following angioplasty with a 6-mm balloon, the gradient was reduced to 5 mm Hg.

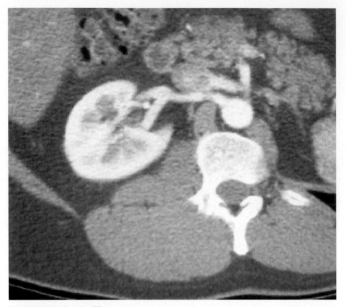

FIGURE 8-19 ▦ Transverse image from CT angiogram shows a mild to moderate stenosis of the proximal right renal artery.

administration or by asymmetry in excretion or uptake between the two kidneys.

The overall sensitivity and specificity of the test exceed 90% in some series.[45,46] However, some reports have called into question the accuracy of scintigraphy in clinical practice.[47] Many centers have abandoned this screening test in favor of cross-sectional imaging techniques. It may play a role in predicting response to intervention or in follow-up (see below).[48]

Renal Vein Renin Sampling. Normally, the ratio of renin activity in the renal vein to activity in the IVC is about 1.24.[49] In a patient with RVH, the affected kidney overproduces renin, and renin secretion from the contralateral kidney is suppressed. Several criteria have been used to diagnose RVH based on renal vein renin sampling, including a renal vein renin ratio between the involved and uninvolved kidney of greater than 1.5 and a ratio of (renal renin–IVC renin)/IVC renin of greater than 0.48 (Vaughan formula).[50] Analysis of numerous series shows an overall sensitivity of 80% and specificity of 62%.[51] Unfortunately, renin levels depend on several factors, including antihypertensive medications, body position, intravascular volume status, and

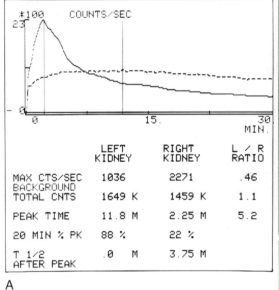

	LEFT KIDNEY	RIGHT KIDNEY	L / R RATIO
MAX CTS/SEC	1036	2271	.46
BACKGROUND TOTAL CNTS	1649 K	1459 K	1.1
PEAK TIME	11.8 M	2.25 M	5.2
20 MIN % PK	88 %	22 %	
T 1/2 AFTER PEAK	.0 M	3.75 M	

A

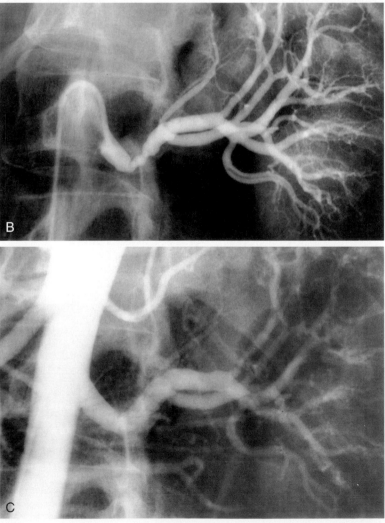

B

C

FIGURE 8-20 ▦ Renovascular hypertension from fibromuscular dysplasia in a young woman. **A,** Captopril renal scintigraphy shows a normal curve for the right kidney *(solid line)*. The curve for the left kidney *(dotted line)* shows slow uptake and a diminished peak. **B,** The left renal arteriogram shows an irregular, beaded appearance of the distal left renal artery of the medial fibroplasia type. Lucent area in the segmental branch to the lower pole is an inflow defect from unopacified collateral blood flow, a finding that confirms the hemodynamic significance of the stenosis. **C,** After balloon angioplasty, the artery is widely patent and the pressure gradient is abolished. The patient became normotensive without medication.

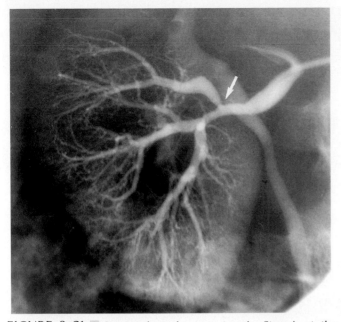

FIGURE 8-21 ■ Intrarenal renal artery stenosis. Stenosis at the origin of a segmental branch *(arrow)* produced renovascular hypertension in this child. The upper pole of the kidney is not filled because of injection into the dorsal ramus.

sampling technique.[52] This study is seldom used by most vascular radiologists.

Angiography. Catheter angiography is still the gold standard for the diagnosis of RVH. Angiographic evaluation includes abdominal aortography and bilateral selective renal arteriography. The initial aortogram is necessary to evaluate the renal artery ostia, identify accessory renal arteries, study the collateral circulation, and avoid mistaking guidewire-induced arterial spasm for fixed disease. Narrowing of accessory renal arteries or intrarenal branches can cause RVH and should be carefully sought; intrarenal stenoses are particularly common in children with RVH (Fig. 8-21).

Stenoses may go undetected for several reasons, including oblique origin of the renal artery from the aorta, overlap of renal and mesenteric vessels, and superimposition of intrarenal branches. Oblique views may be necessary to identify such hidden stenoses.

Atherosclerosis produces irregular narrowing of the renal ostium or proximal renal artery (Fig. 8-22). Bilateral disease is common, and infrarenal aortic atherosclerosis usually is present. FMD typically occurs in the middle to distal renal artery and less commonly in intrarenal branches. The aorta usually is disease free. Bilateral disease is seen in about two thirds of cases; the right kidney is affected more commonly than the left.[53] The classic appearance of the common medial fibroplasia type of FMD is a "string of beads" (see Fig. 8-18). The other forms of FMD have different morphologies (Figs. 8-23 and 8-24; see also Table 8-2). However, the pathologic subtype cannot always be predicted by the angiogram.[54] The angiographic features of rare causes of renal artery stenosis are illustrated later in this chapter.

After a stenosis has been identified, its hemodynamic significance **must** be proved by one of the following criteria:

■ Reduction in luminal diameter of greater than 75%
■ Systolic pressure gradient across stenosis greater than 10 to 20 mm Hg or greater than 20% of aortic systolic pressure

A stenosis with a 50% to 75% reduction in the luminal diameter may be hemodynamically significant, but in such cases, other signs should be sought. Pressure gradients are the most accurate indicator of hemodynamic significance.

Treatment

Selection of patients with RVH or ischemic nephropathy for endovascular or operative therapy is controversial (Box 8-4).[23] Many people with RVH and normal or mild renal insufficiency can be treated medically. The mere presence of a significant renal artery stenosis does not by itself warrant treatment, because not all such patients will have a positive clinical outcome from treatment. In addition, the procedure itself may worsen renal function by contrast nephropathy, atheroembolization, or, rarely, complete vessel occlusion.

In patients with hypertension, reopening the renal arteries is beneficial only if the obstruction is the sole cause of hypertension and long-standing hypertension has not produced significant nephrosclerosis of small renal vessels. In some situations, treatment may be of no clinical value:

■ Nonsignificant renal artery stenosis
■ Incidental finding of significant disease in the absence of hypertension or renal insufficiency
■ Significant renal artery stenosis with severe bilateral nephrosclerosis that may be responsible for hypertension

Revascularization for renal salvage is considered in patients with significant bilateral renal artery disease or disease in a solitary functioning kidney with some functional reserve. Even when the main renal artery is completely occluded, collateral circulation has often developed over time to keep the kidney viable, even up to 6 months or more after occlusion.[55] Renal salvageability is suggested by several criteria, including residual function documented on radionuclide studies, kidney size of 8 to 9 cm, renal biopsy showing preservation of glomeruli and tubules, and the presence of collateral circulation to the intrarenal arteries confirmed by arteriography.[56] There often is no benefit to revascularization of a kidney with minimal function. Improvement or stabilization of renal insufficiency is less likely when the serum creatinine exceeds 4.0 mg/dL.[57]

The primary indications for intervention in patients with suspected RVH or ischemic nephropathy are listed in Box 8-5.[58,59]

Renal Artery Angioplasty

Patient Selection

Angioplasty *alone* should be considered if renal artery stenosis is due to FMD, nonostial atherosclerosis, or Takayasu's arteritis.[60] There is common consent that angioplasty is

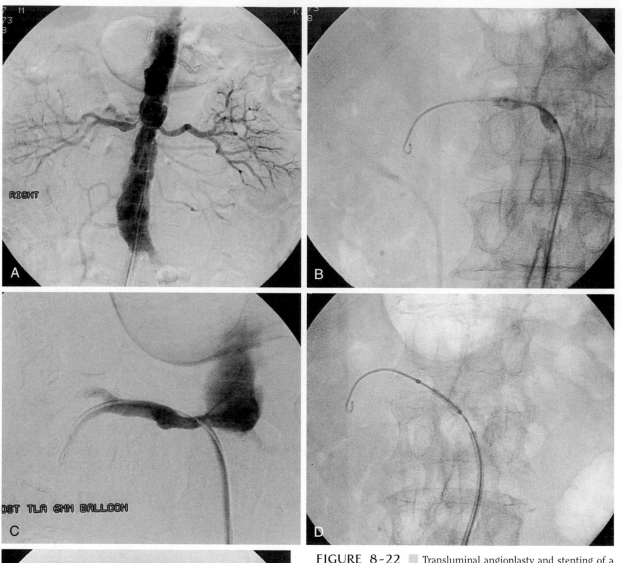

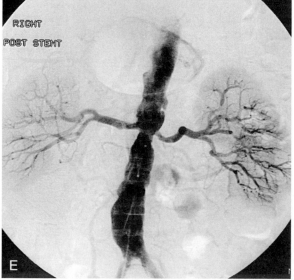

FIGURE 8-22   ■   Transluminal angioplasty and stenting of a renal artery stenosis in a patient with severe hypertension. **A,** The abdominal aortogram shows a right renal artery stenosis. The systolic gradient was 24 mm Hg. **B,** The stenosis was dilated with a 6-mm balloon. **C,** Although the lumen was widened, a systolic gradient of 20 mm Hg remained. **D,** A balloon-expandable stent mounted on a 6-mm angioplasty balloon is placed across the residual stenosis, with the end of the stent extending to the renal artery orifice. **E,** After stent deployment, the renal artery is widely patent. No residual gradient was detected.

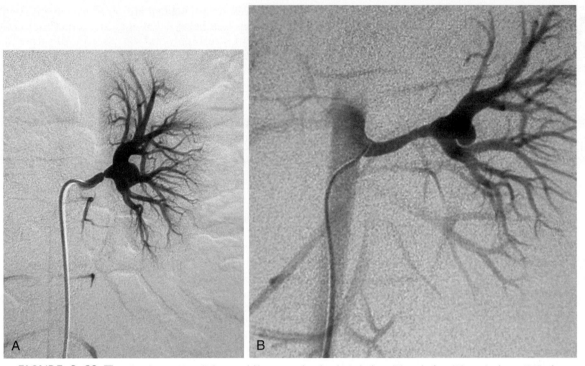

FIGURE 8-23 ■ Intimal or perimedial type of fibromuscular dysplasia before (**A**) and after (**B**) angioplasty. Note the intrarenal aneurysm.

the first-line treatment for FMD. The much more common atherosclerotic ostial stenoses require stent placement for optimal results (see below).[61]

In selecting patients for angioplasty, the interventionalist must remember that the risks increase when an abdominal aortic aneurysm or severe aortic atherosclerotic disease is present.

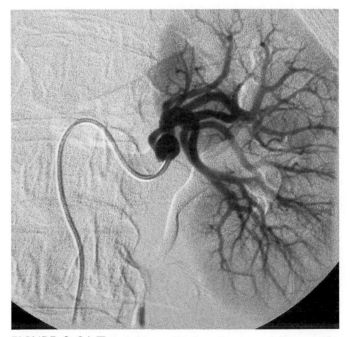

FIGURE 8-24 ■ Probable medial dissection type of fibromuscular dysplasia.

Technique

The classic description of renal artery angioplasty was formulated by Tegtmeyer and Sos.[62] Most interventionalists continue the patient's blood pressure medications until the procedure is completed. The dose of contrast material should be carefully monitored. Gadolinium- or CO_2-based arteriography should be used to supplement iodinated contrast.[3,63] Vigorous intravenous hydration and pharmacologic adjuncts to prevent contrast nephropathy should be administered (see Chapter 1).

Patients are pretreated with aspirin (325 mg PO). A reverse curve (e.g., Simmons or visceral hook) or straight catheter (e.g., cobra shape) is used to engage the stenosis; tight stenoses may be easier to cross with a reverse curve shape. Before traversing the stenosis, the patient is given heparin (5000 to 7000 units IV) and an intra-arterial vasodilator (100 to 200 µg of nitroglycerin).

BOX 8-4 ■ Indications for Endovascular Renal Artery Treatment

---

Likelihood of hypertension cure
Onset <30 or >60 years of age
Fibromuscular dysplasia
Refractory or accelerated hypertension
Malignant hypertension
Renal salvage (see Box 8-5)
Recurrent "flash" pulmonary edema

BOX 8-5 ■ Criteria for Revascularization in Ischemic Nephropathy

---

Unexplained decrease in kidney function
Decreased renal mass
Decreased renal function or acute renal failure from antihypertensive medications
Absence of nephrosclerosis at arteriography
Bilateral disease
Sudden onset of renal insufficiency
Doppler resistive index <80

The catheter is placed at the orifice of the renal artery, and the stenosis is crossed with a guidewire. A wide variety of guidewires may be used, although wires with a flexible tip (e.g., Bentson wire) or tapered floppy tip (e.g., TAD wire with 0.018-inch floppy tip and 0.035-inch stiff shaft) are generally preferred. Changes in the patient's respiration alter the angle of the renal artery, which may help the wire to negotiate the lesion.

The catheter is advanced over the guidewire across the stenosis, and its intraluminal location is confirmed with contrast injection. A heavy-duty exchange wire with a floppy tip (e.g., TAD or Rosen wire) is placed to provide support for the balloon catheter and avoid damage to the distal renal artery branches. However, great care must be taken because even a small-caliber floppy tipped nitinol wire can dissect the main vessel or perforate small renal artery branches, leading to occlusion or hemorrhage. The balloon diameter (usually 5 or 6 mm in adults) is chosen by measuring the lumen of the normal portion of the renal artery or contralateral artery on the diagnostic arteriogram. Placement of a guiding catheter may facilitate balloon/catheter exchanges and allow follow-up angiograms to be obtained while maintaining a guidewire across the stenosis.

The balloon is inserted, advanced and centered across the stenosis, and inflated with an inflation device. The distal portion of the balloon must be kept away from smaller branch vessels when it is expanded. FMD lesions may require pressures in excess of the 4 to 12 mm Hg needed to crack atherosclerotic plaques. After two or three 30- to 60-second inflations, the balloon is withdrawn. If the patient complains of severe pain, the vessel may be overstretched, and the balloon should be immediately deflated. Renal artery perforation is rare but should be temporized by repeat inflation of the balloon to control bleeding while a vascular surgeon is contacted. In this rare situation, the problem may be remedied by prolonged balloon inflation or placement of a covered stent.

If a small-caliber wire is kept across the dilated segment, an angiogram may be performed by injecting the balloon or a diagnostic catheter around a hemostatic valve, avoiding the need to cross the lesion again if larger balloons or stents are needed to achieve a good result. Angioplasty is considered successful when the residual stenosis is less than 30% and the systolic pressure gradient is less than 10 mm Hg. An irregular, "ratty" luminal surface alone is not an indication for stent placement as these vessels often remodel over time.

If results are inadequate, stent placement should be considered (see below). Patients are sometimes continued on heparin overnight and on aspirin or other antiplatelet agents for life. Blood pressure should be monitored carefully in the immediate period after treatment, as precipitous drops in pressure can occur.

Results

Success in renal artery revascularization for RVH is judged by blood pressure response, with clinical benefit defined as *cure* (i.e., blood pressure lower than 140/90 mm Hg without medication) or *improvement* (i.e., reduced number of medications required to maintain blood pressure below 140/90 mm Hg or a 15-mm Hg reduction in blood pressure on the same or reduced number of medications).[23] In patients treated for renal salvage, a reduction in the serum creatinine level of greater than 20% may be considered a successful treatment.

The outcome of renal artery angioplasty depends on the type of lesion, indication for treatment, and factors such as age, coexistent essential hypertension, and nephrosclerosis. For **atherosclerotic** lesions, technical success is achieved in about 75% to 95% of cases.[64-67] With angioplasty alone, long-term cure or improvement can be expected only in about 50% to 60% of patients.[68]

For **FMD**, technical success occurs in greater than 90% of cases.[69,70] Clinical benefit is noted in 90% of cases, and results usually are long lasting. However, these figures primarily apply to the common medial fibroplasia type of disease, as large series studying the less common subtypes are unavailable. For patients with Takayasu's arteritis treated in the chronic phase, the technical and long-term results are excellent.

For renal salvage, the results are less favorable. Improvement in renal function occurs in 40% to 60% of cases.[71-73] Patients with baseline serum creatinine levels greater than 4.0 mg/dL are unlikely to improve. Results are better in patients who undergo bilateral renal artery revascularization.

Complications

Complications are reported in 5% to 10% of cases and include renal artery dissection, thrombosis, rupture, distal renal or aortic embolization of clot, cholesterol embolization, and access site complications (e.g., groin hematoma). Many complications are related to injury of the renal artery or its branches by guidewires. Renal failure, which usually is transient, affects about 2% of patients.[74]

Renal Artery Stent Placement

Patient Selection

The primary indications for stent placement are outlined in Box 8-6. Stents significantly improve the technical success of renal artery angioplasty for atherosclerotic disease, particularly for ostial lesions (from 55% to 70% to more than 95%).[75] This improvement alone may largely explain the better long-term patency rates associated with stent placement. It is not clear that routine placement of stents in truncal lesions is beneficial.[76] Use of stents in renal arteries with nominal diameter of less than 5 mm usually is avoided due to the relatively higher rates of clinically significant restenosis in this setting.[77] Stents are generally not useful or necessary for FMD lesions.

Technique

Off-label use of a variety of stainless steel and nitinol devices is standard practice. Some interventionalists prefer to predilate lesions with a balloon catheter before stent placement. This approach ensures that the lesion will fully respond to dilation and that the lesion can be traversed with the device. In addition, proper stent and balloon size can be chosen to avoid poor wall apposition from undersizing or dissection or rupture from oversizing. Other practitioners choose primary stent placement to avoid distal embolization with initial balloon dilation; difficulty with lesion traversal is avoided by using low-profile monorail systems.

The stent device is operator- or factory-mounted on an appropriately sized angioplasty balloon (typically 6 to 7 mm) and preloaded in a preformed 5- to 8-French guiding catheter. The antiplatelet, anticoagulant, and antispasmodic drug regimen is identical to that used for angioplasty (see above). The system is advanced though a vascular sheath at the groin into the renal artery over an 0.035-inch heavy-duty guidewire (see Fig. 8-22). The stent is exposed by withdrawing the guiding catheter from the renal artery. Alternatively, a steerable 0.014-inch wire is placed and a low-profile monorail stent-balloon catheter is advanced directly into the artery.

For ostial lesions, the stent is positioned with the proximal end about 1 mm inside the aortic lumen to completely cover the overhanging plaque. Multiple angiograms are obtained through the guiding catheter to ensure precise positioning. The stent is deployed by expansion of the balloon with an inflation device. Additional stents are placed as needed. Care should be taken to avoid placing stents into the distal renal artery, which could preclude later surgical revascularization or damage branch vessels.

If difficulty is encountered traversing the lesion with the stent, several maneuvers should be tried. Changes in the patient's respiration can dramatically alter the aortic-renal artery angle. Stiffer (or sometimes less stiff) guidewires may be used. If all attempts fail, placement through a high brachial puncture should be considered.

Results

A widely patent artery can be created with a metallic stent in greater than 95% of cases.[23,78-81] In *atherosclerotic RVH*, actual cure of hypertension is achieved in less than 10% to 20% of cases whether stents are used or not.[23,81,82] Improvement can be expected in about 50% to 80% of patients. In *medial fibroplasia FMD–related RVH*, cure of hypertension is seen in about 40% to 50% of patients.

The angiographic restenosis rate is about 20%.[77-80] Luminal compromise seems to increase slowly over time. The predictive factor in restenosis is small initial vessel diameter (<4 to 5 mm). Restenosis is treated by repeated balloon angioplasty usually *without* additional stent placement (Fig. 8-25).[83]

In *ischemic nephropathy*, clinical benefit from revascularization is defined as reduction or stabilization in serum creatinine or flattening of the progression of renal dysfunction (1/creatinine versus time). Angioplasty and stent placement leads to improvement or stabilization of renal insufficiency in about 70% of cases, although the benefit diminishes over time.[77,81,82,84]

Major complications occur in about 8% to 15% of procedures.[23,85] Permanent decline in renal function is noted in about 6% of cases and usually is caused by contrast nephropathy or microembolization. Distal protective devices (occlusion balloons or permeable filters) have been shown to collect significant amounts of debris (small atheroma, cholesterol crystals, acute or chronic clots) in at least two thirds of cases.[86,87] There is growing evidence that use of such devices may prevent microembolic injury to the treated kidney.

Surgical Therapy

In patients with RVH or ischemic nephropathy, surgery is preferred for patients with obstructions and associated aortic disease that require open operation and for most renal artery occlusions.[88] If minimal aortic disease is present, the standard procedure is aortorenal bypass grafting with autologous vein. In patients with severe aortic atherosclerosis or an aortic aneurysm, the hepatic or splenic artery may be used as a bypass conduit for the right or left renal artery, respectively.[89,90] If the main renal artery is occluded but the distal artery reconstitutes through collaterals, bypass is sometimes done to improve function or treat RVH.[90] Otherwise, hypertension may be treated with nephrectomy.

Acute Renal Artery Obstruction

Etiology

The major causes of renal artery occlusion are listed in Box 8-2.[91,92] The most common reason for acute occlusion is embolism, which originates from the heart in about 90% of cases.[93] Bilateral renal artery embolization occurs in about 30% of cases. Blunt or penetrating abdominal trauma can produce an intimal tear, dissection, or complete avulsion of the renal artery, any of which can lead to acute thrombosis. Renal artery dissection may result from underlying atherosclerosis, FMD, trauma, or extension of an aortic dissection.

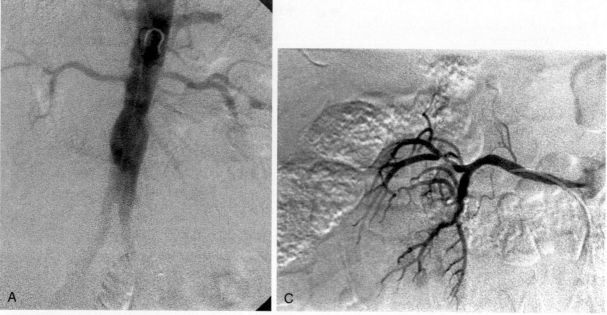

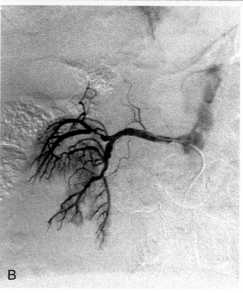

FIGURE 8-25   ■   Restenosis 5 years after renal artery stent placement. Patient presented with stable renal insufficiency and difficult to control hypertension. **A,** Gadolinium catheter angiogram suggests normal renal arteries bilaterally. **B,** Iodine-based selective angiogram shows intrastent narrowing. Transstent systolic pressure gradient was 33 mm Hg. **C,** Following dilation with a 6-mm balloon, luminal patency is improved. Residual pressure gradient was 5 mm Hg. Occlusion of segmental arteries has caused some renal parenchymal loss.

Clinical Features

Most patients are elderly and have a history of heart disease, particularly atrial fibrillation or coronary artery disease. Patients with acute occlusion of a previously patent renal artery may complain of sudden flank pain and hematuria. However, embolic occlusions often are silent and may be missed for some time.

Imaging

Ultrasound, Computed Tomographic, and Magnetic Resonance Angiography. Color Doppler sonography is the simplest method for detecting renal artery occlusion.[94] If results are equivocal, CT or MR angiography should be performed (Fig. 8-26).

Angiography. Catheter arteriography is performed only if endovascular therapy is being considered. An embolus appears as a filling defect or complete occlusion with concave margin (Fig. 8-27). Emboli tend to lodge in the proximal renal artery or at a branch point.[95] When embolization occurs to a previously normal artery, the collateral circulation may be inadequate to perfuse the kidney. Embolization of intrarenal vessels produces segmental infarction. Traumatic occlusions usually produce an abrupt cutoff of the vessel at the site of injury (Fig. 8-28).

Treatment

Although the viability of the native human kidney suddenly deprived of blood flow may be a matter of hours, revascularization of kidneys suffering acute occlusion has been successful after much longer intervals.[92,96,97] This is because collateral circulation can maintain kidney function for weeks or even months after occlusion of a previously normal renal artery. Therefore, treatment should not be withheld

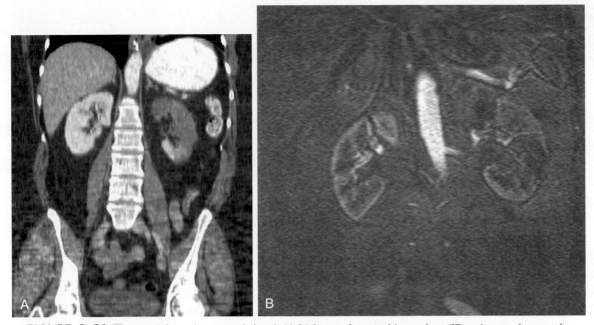

FIGURE 8-26 ■ Acute left renal artery embolus. **A,** Multiplanar reformatted image from CT angiogram shows perfusion defect occupying most of the left kidney. **B,** Coronal gadolinium-enhanced MR angiogram shows filling defect in the mid to distal left renal artery.

based solely on estimated time from occlusion. Scintigraphy and sonography should be used to determine viability and residual mass.

Surgical Therapy. Renal artery embolus is easily removed by surgical embolectomy. However, there is substantial morbidity and mortality associated with this procedure, mostly related to patients' underlying cardiac disease. Return of renal function can be anticipated in many cases after conservative treatment with anticoagulation and temporary dialysis, as needed.[98] Embolectomy is therefore often reserved for cases of bilateral embolism or embolism to a solitary kidney.

Endovascular Therapy. Although catheter-directed thrombolytic therapy can reopen most acute embolic occlusions, long-term kidney salvage is uncommon unless flow is restored within about 3 hours of occlusion (see Fig. 8-27).[99]

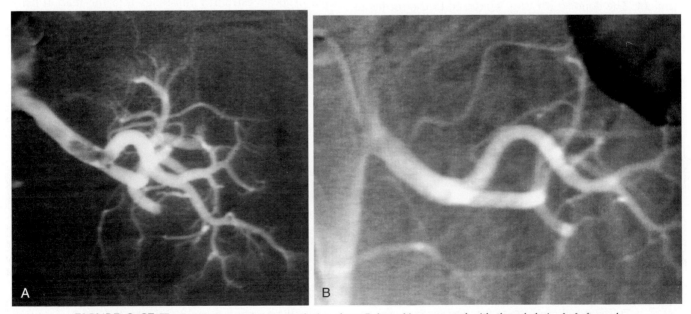

FIGURE 8-27 ■ An embolic renal artery occlusion about 5 days old was treated with thrombolysis. **A,** Left renal angiogram shows a filling defect in the distal artery. **B,** After intra-arterial infusion of urokinase, complete lysis has occurred. The renal function of the patient returned.

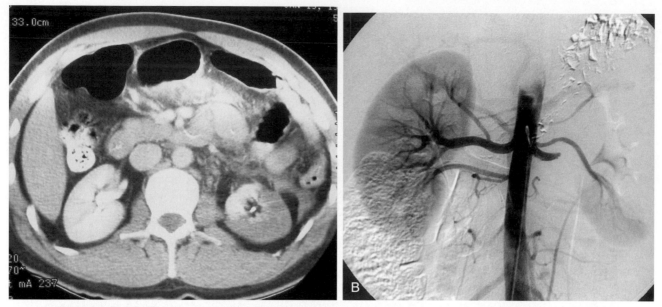

FIGURE 8-28 ■ Traumatic renal artery occlusion after a motor vehicle accident. **A,** The CT scan shows almost complete lack of enhancement of the left kidney. **B,** The arteriogram shows traumatic occlusion of the main left renal artery and preservation of the accessory artery to the lower pole.

Angioplasty and stent placement have successfully reestablished function in some cases with proven viability.[100]

Vascular Complications after Renal Transplantation

Etiology

The harvested kidney is placed into either iliac fossa of the recipient. The donor renal vein is sutured to the recipient external iliac vein in an end-to-side fashion or internal iliac vein in an end-to-end fashion. The donor artery is connected in one of two ways. The surgeon may construct an end-to-side anastomosis to the recipient external (or common) iliac artery (Fig. 8-29). In cadaveric transplants, an oval patch of aorta surrounding the donor artery *(Carrell patch)* may be incorporated. Otherwise, an end-to-end anastomosis to the recipient's ligated internal iliac artery is made. If the donor kidney has multiple arteries, the accessory branches may be tied individually into the main vessel. In cadaveric transplants, a large aortic patch incorporating both vessels may be inserted onto the recipient external iliac artery.

Vascular complications develop in up to 25% of patients after kidney transplantation.[101] *Arterial stenosis* is the most common vascular problem, encountered in about 5% to 10% of transplant recipients.[101-103] Most lesions develop between 3 months and 2 years after placement. The stenosis occurs most frequently at the anastomosis and less often in the recipient or graft artery. Inflow iliac artery lesions also may contribute to declining allograft function. Stenoses are more common in cadaveric transplants than in organs from living-related donors. Immune-related proliferative narrowing

has been postulated as the cause of some cases of graft arterial stenosis.[104]

Arterial thrombosis usually is the result of operative injury of the donor or recipient artery, kinking of the arterial connection, underlying atherosclerosis, acute rejection, hypercoagulable states, or hypotension. While the frequency of complete main renal artery thrombosis is less than 1%, thrombosis of accessory branches or segmental infarcts are more common.[105] *Venous thrombosis* may be caused by intraoperative damage to the vein, hypotension, renal vein compression by an extrinsic mass (e.g., lymphocele), extension of lower extremity thrombus into the iliac veins, or graft infection.

Aneurysm or *pseudoaneurysm* may develop after graft infection, loss of integrity of the arterial anastomosis, or transplant biopsy. *Intrarenal arteriovenous fistula* is relatively common after graft biopsy, but most of these communications close spontaneously.

Clinical Features

The most common signs of transplant renal artery obstruction are hypertension, worsening renal function, and a bruit heard over the allograft. Because elevated blood pressure is common after transplantation, only patients with severe or refractory hypertension are evaluated for treatable causes. In addition to arterial stenosis or occlusion, a decline in renal function after transplantation may be caused by acute or chronic rejection, acute tubular necrosis, drug reaction from immunosuppressive agents, or the development of intrinsic disease in the transplant.

The classic signs of transplant renal vein thrombosis (RVT) are swelling and tenderness of the graft and impaired renal function. Patients with renal artery aneurysms may develop a pulsatile mass over the graft. Although hematuria is common

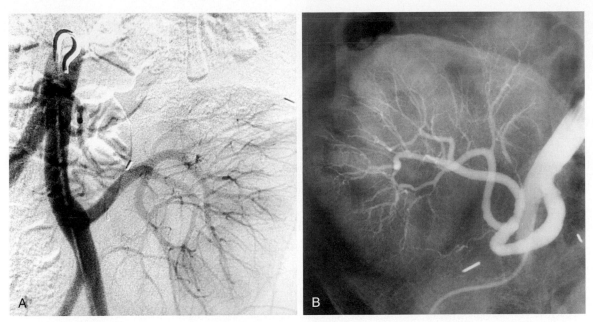

FIGURE 8-29 ■ Kidney transplant arterial connections. **A,** End-to-side anastomosis to the left common iliac artery. **B,** End-to-end anastomosis to the right internal iliac artery. Irregular stenoses and occlusions of distal renal arterial branches are consistent with the clinical diagnosis of chronic rejection.

after percutaneous renal transplant biopsy, an angiogram should be performed to look for an arteriovenous fistula or pseudoaneurysm if bleeding is persistent or massive.

Imaging

Imaging is used to distinguish vascular, medical, and urinary tract complications as the cause of allograft dysfunction.

Sonography. Color or power Doppler sonography has become the standard tool for screening patients with suspected vascular complications after renal transplantation.[105-108] The criteria for significant arterial stenosis include a PSV ratio of 2:1 or more (stenosis versus adjacent normal segment), color aliasing, and a PSV of greater than 2 m/second. Spectral analysis of intrarenal vessels may show a marked prolongation of acceleration time as an indirect indicator of a proximal stenosis. Segmental infarcts appear as sharply defined regions of absent flow in small parenchymal vessels. Sonography is useful also in detecting renal artery thrombosis, RVT, renal vein kinks, arteriovenous fistulas, and pseudoaneurysms (Fig. 8-30).

Magnetic Resonance Angiography. This technique is an alternative to ultrasound evaluation.[109-111] MR is superior to sonography in detecting associated iliac artery stenoses. Causes for nondiagnostic or inaccurate studies include motion or surgical clip artifact or venous contamination.

Angiography. Although catheter arteriography and venography remain the gold standards for diagnosis, they are employed only if noninvasive studies are equivocal or endovascular therapy is being considered. Grafts with end-to-side anastomoses to the external iliac artery are best approached with a hockey stick–shaped catheter from the

ipsilateral femoral artery. Grafts with end-to-end anastomoses to the internal iliac artery usually are studied with a cobra or long reverse-curve catheter from the contralateral groin. The renal vein may be approached from the ipsilateral groin. Care must be taken to strictly limit the volume of iodinated contrast material. The risk of contrast nephropathy is almost completely eliminated if carbon dioxide or gadolinium is used as the contrast agent.[112,113] Steep oblique projections often are required to lay out the arterial anastomosis. However, a single pressure gradient across the anastomosis is far more accurate than multiple images for excluding a hemodynamically significant stenosis.

Arterial stenoses usually occur directly at the anastomosis and produce little change in renal blood flow (Fig. 8-31). Other possible findings include iliac artery stenosis, segmental artery occlusion, main transplant artery stenosis, and vessel kink. Acute or chronic rejection causes markedly diminished flow (<5 to 6 mL/second), severe pruning of distal intrarenal branches, and a faint or absent nephrogram (Fig. 8-32). Renal artery or vein thrombosis appears as complete or near-complete occlusion of the vessel. Venous kinks also have been described (see Fig. 8-30). Arteriovenous fistulas and pseudoaneurysms have a characteristic appearance and are virtually always intrarenal (see later).

Treatment

Endovascular Therapy. Transcatheter techniques are effective in treating most vascular complications of renal transplantation. Balloon angioplasty has been used with great success in treating arterial stenoses (see Fig. 8-31).[103,104,114] Angioplasty is performed in a fashion similar to that for

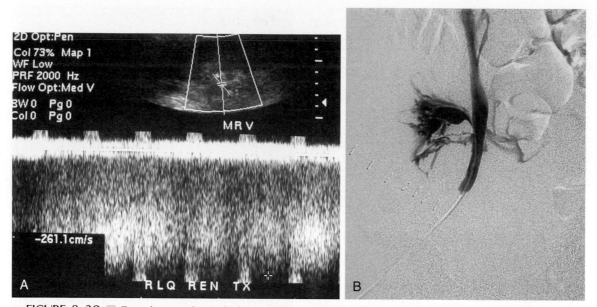

FIGURE 8-30 ■ Transplant renal vein kink. **A,** Duplex sonography demonstrates markedly increased velocity and turbulence at the renal vein anastomosis. **B,** Selective catheter venogram confirms tight narrowing due to a kink in the vessel.

treatment of native renal arterial stenoses. About 80% to 90% of procedures show initial clinical success (reduction in serum creatinine, cure or improvement in hypertension); long-term renal salvage is achieved in about two thirds of cases. Even investigators reporting less encouraging results often support a trial of angioplasty in most patients.[114] The use of intravascular stents should further improve the durability of this technique.[115] Complications, which are uncommon, include arterial dissection, perforation, and rupture; however, loss of the allograft is rare (Fig. 8-33).

Thrombolytic therapy has been used to treat arterial and venous thromboses of renal transplants. Renal vein clot is lysed with selective intravenous and intra-arterial fibrinolytic infusion, alone or in combination.[116,117]

Percutaneous treatment of postbiopsy arteriovenous fistulas and pseudoaneurysms is preferred over surgery (see below).[118-120] Tissue loss is minimized by superselective embolization with microcoils deposited through coaxial microcatheters directly at the site of abnormality.

Surgical Therapy. Operative treatment of arterial stenoses usually is reserved for patients with a poor response to balloon angioplasty. Surgical thrombectomy and revision may be performed for cases of acute arterial or venous thrombosis, although long-term salvage is uncommon.

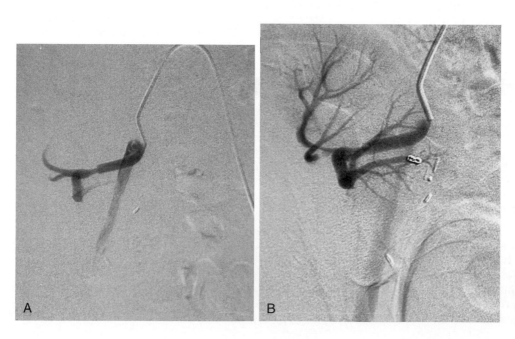

FIGURE 8-31 ■ Transplant renal artery anastomotic stenosis on catheter arteriogram before (**A**) and after (**B**) angioplasty.

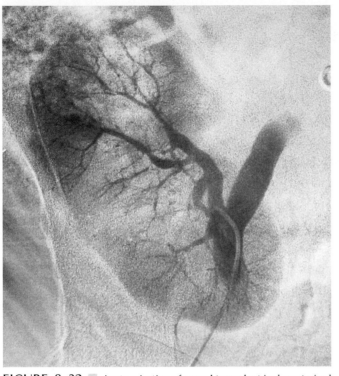

FIGURE 8-32 ■ Acute rejection of a renal transplant is characterized by severe pruning of the intrarenal branches.

Trauma

Etiology

Injury to the renal artery can occur from blunt trauma (e.g., motor vehicle accidents), penetrating trauma (e.g., criminal assault), or medical procedures (e.g., percutaneous biopsy, percutaneous nephrostomy, nephrolithotomy, or open surgery). Blunt trauma can produce a spectrum of renal injuries. The most severe injuries affect the renal pedicle and include intimal damage, dissection, thrombotic occlusion, or complete avulsion of the artery.[121] A subcapsular hematoma can ultimately produce RVH by a compressive effect *(Page kidney)*. Other traumatic lesions include pseudoaneurysms, arteriovenous fistulas, and frank extravasation.

Penetrating injuries may cause perirenal hematomas, arteriovenous fistulas, pseudoaneurysms, arteriocaliceal fistulas, or complete arterial occlusion.[122] Arteriovenous fistulas may occur after percutaneous renal biopsy, although most of these lesions close spontaneously.[118] Percutaneous nephrostomy is complicated by a significant vascular injury in about 1% of cases.[123] A retroperitoneal hematoma may develop from acute laceration of an artery or delayed rupture of a pseudoaneurysm.

Clinical Features

Minor bleeding is common immediately after percutaneous renal interventions. Most lesions resolve spontaneously within days to weeks. Patients with persistent or recurrent gross hematuria may have an injury that requires treatment.

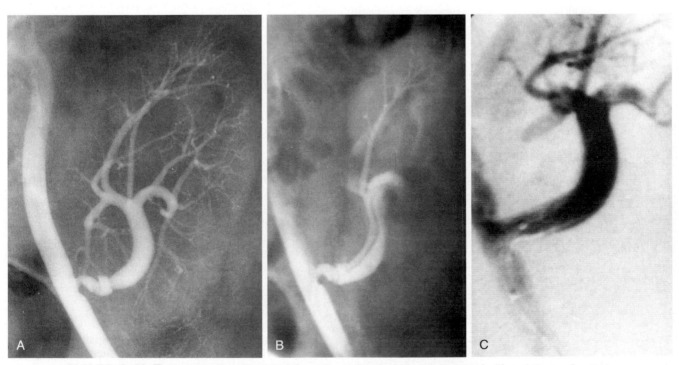

FIGURE 8-33 ■ Postangioplasty dissection of a renal artery transplant stenosis treated with an intravascular stent. **A,** The iliac arteriogram shows a tight anastomotic stenosis. **B,** After angioplasty, a large flow-limiting dissection extends into the distal artery. **C,** After stent placement, the stenosis and dissection have been abolished.

In some patients, symptoms occur days to weeks after the injury, particularly in the case of arteriovenous fistulas or pseudoaneurysms that expand and eventually rupture into the kidney parenchyma or collecting system. Left untreated, some of these abnormalities may result in RVH or renal ischemia, leading to renal failure if the kidney is solitary.

Imaging[124]

Computed Tomography and Magnetic Resonance Imaging. Patients with blunt abdominal injury are initially evaluated and staged with CT. Findings of vascular injury include main renal artery occlusion, segmental infarcts, active bleeding, perinephric hematoma, lacerations, arteriovenous fistulas, and pseudoaneurysms (Fig. 8-34; see also Fig. 8-28).

Arteriography. Catheter angiography is reserved for confirmation of CT findings, endovascular treatment, or the following situations:

▪ Hematuria with hypotension or falling hematocrit
▪ Persistent or recurrent hematuria
▪ Hypotension or hypertension after documented renal injury
▪ Retroperitoneal hematoma detected by CT or during surgery

Evaluation should begin with an abdominal aortogram to identify accessory renal arteries, determine the status of the renal artery origins, and identify other pathology (e.g., bleeding from a lumbar artery). Angiographic findings vary widely and may include perirenal hematoma, arteriovenous fistula, pseudoaneurysm, frank extravasation, evidence for retroperitoneal hematoma, intimal injury, or complete renal artery occlusion (Figs. 8-35 and 8-36; see also Fig. 8-28).

Treatment

Endovascular Therapy. Transcatheter embolization is the primary treatment for bleeding traumatic lesions of the kidney.[120,125,126] Surgery, which almost always leads to greater parenchymal damage, is reserved only for cases that cannot be treated by endovascular means. To minimize tissue loss, the embolic agent should be placed as close to the lesion as possible (see Figs. 8-35 and 8-36). Gelfoam pieces and microcoils placed through coaxial microcatheters are favored for embolization of both large and small arterial branches. In patients with arteriovenous fistulas, the coil should be large enough to avoid escape through the fistula into the venous system. Stents have been used to tack down posttraumatic renal artery intimal flaps and avoid thrombosis or distal embolization.[127]

Postembolization syndrome (fever, flank pain) is seen in a few patients. Nontarget embolization (usually of uninvolved renal vessels) is a rare complication of the procedure. Postembolization hypertension is unusual and usually transient.

Neoplasms

Etiology

The major benign and malignant neoplasms of the kidney are outlined in Box 8-7. *Renal cell carcinoma* (RCC) is the most common malignant neoplasm of the kidney. This tumor is largely composed of clear cells, often encapsulated, and usually quite vascular. Tumor growth from the renal vein into the IVC is relatively uncommon (5% to 10%).[128] Multiple, bilateral tumors may be seen in patients with von Hippel-Lindau disease.[129] For unknown reasons, the incidence of RCC has been rising, only partly explained by more frequent detection of asymptomatic patients with cross-sectional imaging.

Wilms' tumor is composed of a variety of cellular elements and frequently produces areas of hemorrhage and necrosis.[130] *Angiomyolipoma* is a renal hamartoma made up of blood vessels, smooth muscle cells, lipid, and connective tissue.[131] Angiomyolipomas may be solitary or may be multiple and bilateral, as in patients with tuberous sclerosis. *Adenoma* is a benign tumor of epithelial cell origin. *Oncocytoma* is one form of adenoma composed partly of cells with eosinophilic cytoplasm. The lesion usually is solitary and encapsulated and has a central scar.

Clinical Features

With widespread use of cross-sectional imaging, renal neoplasms often are discovered as an incidental finding. Most patients with malignant neoplasms are older than 50 years of age. RCC affects men more frequently than women. Angiomyolipomas are commonly seen in middle-aged women.

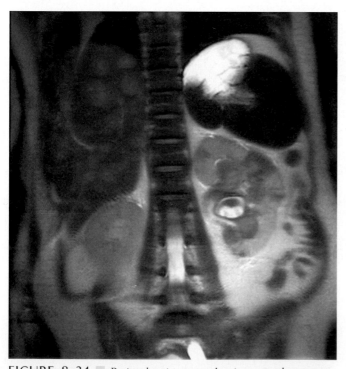

FIGURE 8-34 ▪ Postnephrostomy renal artery pseudoaneurysm. Coronal T2-weighted MR image shows a round mass in the left renal pelvis with swirling flow, indicating an aneurysm.

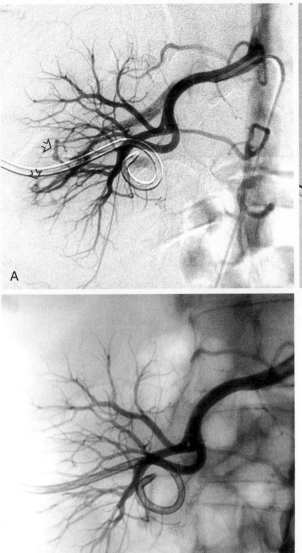

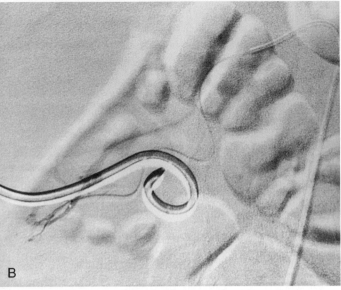

FIGURE 8-35 ■ Arteriovenous fistula in a patient with persistent bleeding after right nephrostomy placement. **A,** The initial arteriogram shows two lower pole fistulas with early venous drainage *(arrows)*. **B,** A coaxial microcatheter was advanced to the branch feeding both fistulas. **C,** After placement of two microcoils, the fistulas are closed.

Tumors associated with tuberous sclerosis tend to be more aggressive. Larger tumors are more likely to bleed. Most patients with Wilms' tumor are less than 5 years old. The most common symptoms of malignant tumors are hematuria, flank pain, and a palpable abdominal mass.[132] Rarely, patients may have hypertension directly related to the tumor. Male patients with neoplastic invasion of the left renal vein may present with a left-sided varicocele.

Imaging

Computed Tomography and Magnetic Resonance Imaging.
Diagnosis and staging of benign and malignant renal neoplasms is accomplished with CT or MR imaging (Figs. 8-37 and 8-38). Assessing the extent of IVC thrombosis with RCC is crucial to operative planning: less than 2 cm above the renal veins (level 1), below the most inferior hepatic vein (level 2), below the diaphragm (level 3), or supradiaphragmatic (level 4).[128]

Angiography.
Arteriography is indicated as a preoperative procedure before partial (kidney-sparing) nephrectomy to determine vascular supply and the presence of parasitized vessels, for preoperative embolization of malignant tumors, as definitive embolotherapy in selected cases, and for treatment (or prevention) of spontaneous tumor-related bleeding.

In RCC, the typical angiographic features are neovascularity, hypervascularity, dilation of the main renal artery, tumor stain, contrast puddling, displacement of normal renal vessels, and arteriovenous shunts with early venous drainage (Fig. 8-39).[133] Parasitization of neighboring vessels (e.g., inferior mesenteric or lumbar arteries) is relatively common. About 6% of tumors are hypovascular, and most of these are of the papillary type (Fig. 8-40). A cystic renal cell carcinoma may be impossible to differentiate from a benign cyst and is fortunately rare. Extension of tumor into the renal vein occurs in 15% to 30% of cases; IVC invasion is less common.[134]

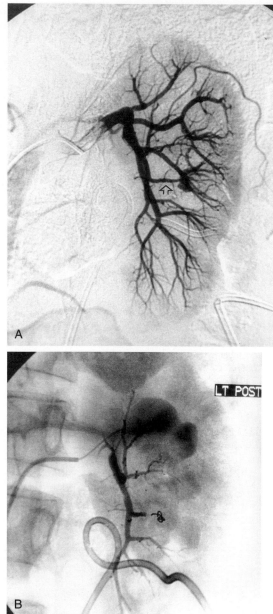

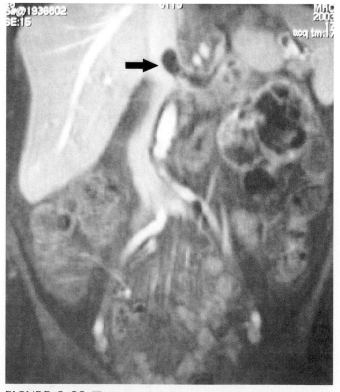

FIGURE 8-37 ■ CT image shows a renal cell carcinoma invading the left renal vein.

FIGURE 8-36 ■ Iatrogenic pseudoaneurysm of the left kidney after percutaneous nephrostomy. **A,** Pseudoaneurysm of a midpolar branch *(arrow).* **B,** A 3-French microcatheter was used to deposit two microcoils in the feeding branch to obliterate the pseudoaneurysm.

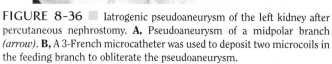

BOX 8-7 ■ Major Renal Neoplasms

Benign Tumors
Adenoma (including oncocytoma)
Angiomyolipoma (hamartoma)

Malignant Tumors
Renal cell carcinoma (hypernephroma)
Transitional cell carcinoma
Wilms' tumor
Metastases (including lymphoma)

FIGURE 8-38 ■ MR angiogram shows renal cell carcinoma invading the left renal vein and inferior vena cava *(arrow).*

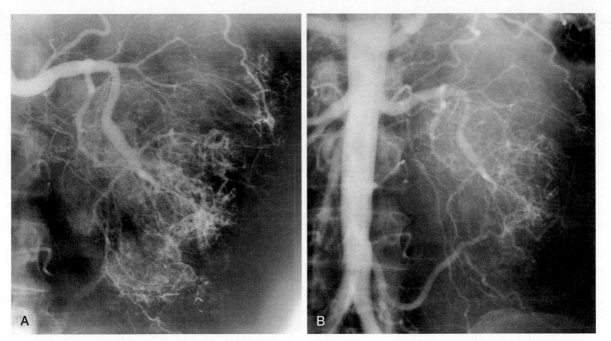

FIGURE 8-39 ■ Renal cell carcinoma. **A,** Markedly hypervascular left renal mass with bizarre neovascularity. **B,** Parasitization of the inferior mesenteric artery branches by the tumor.

In contrast, Wilms' tumor usually is moderately vascular.[130] Arteriography shows displacement of normal renal vessels around the tumor mass with encasement or occlusion of vessels. Transitional cell carcinoma is typically hypovascular with encasement of vessels, presence of tumor stain, and fine neovascularity.[135] Lymphoma may be hypovascular or hypervascular.

Renal oncocytoma, a subtype of benign adenoma, has a characteristic angiographic appearance with a dense, homogeneous stain and "spoke-wheel" arrangement of vessels corresponding to the central scar (Fig. 8-41).[136] Angiomyolipomas, which may be solitary or multiple, are hypervascular, with bizarre vascularity and multiple small aneurysms.[131]

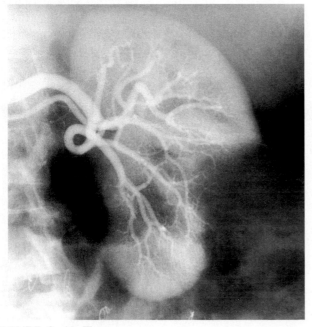

FIGURE 8-40 ■ Hypovascular, papillary-type renal cell carcinoma.

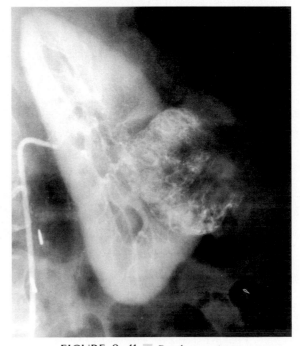

FIGURE 8-41 ■ Renal oncocytoma.

Treatment

Percutaneous Therapy. Transcatheter embolization is used in patients with renal neoplasms for several reasons[137-139]:

- Preoperative devascularization to ease resection, minimize blood loss, and possibly heighten the immune response against the tumor
- Palliative treatment in patients with unresectable disease
- Treatment or prevention of hemorrhagic complications

For RCC, the preoperative procedure usually is performed within 24 hours of nephrectomy. The most popular embolic agent is ethanol. An occlusion balloon is placed in the distal renal artery beyond adrenal and ureteral branches to avoid reflux of alcohol into the aorta, which may have disastrous consequences. The volume of alcohol can be estimated by measuring the volume of contrast required to fill the renal artery and branches with the occlusion balloon inflated. Alcohol is slowly injected in small aliquots (1 to 5 mL) into the main renal artery (Fig. 8-42). The balloon is kept inflated for several minutes after injection and is then slowly deflated. Accessory or parasitized arteries may be treated in a similar fashion if there is virtually no chance of nontarget embolization. Patients commonly experience a florid postembolization syndrome, characterized by fever, severe flank pain, and nausea.

Recently, radiofrequency ablative techniques have been employed to treat small renal cell carcinomas up to 5 cm in size.[140-143] Exophytic tumors are the best candidates; treatment of central lesions near the renal sinus is more difficult, owing to the presence of the collecting system and vessels. Midterm results are promising.

For patients with angiomyolipomas, embolization has emerged as a useful alternative to surgery, particularly for symptomatic lesions and silent tumors larger than 4 cm (which have a propensity to growth and hemorrhage).[131,139,144,145] Tumor shrinkage and pain relief occur in most cases. Smaller tumors should be followed with annual imaging.

Surgical Therapy. The standard treatment for RCC is radical nephrectomy with removal of Gerota's fascia.[134] The adrenal gland may be spared if there is no involvement of the gland or upper pole of the kidney. Renal vein or IVC invasion does not preclude surgical resection. Kidney-sparing procedures are indicated in patients with bilateral tumors, malignancy in a solitary kidney and angiomyolipomas.

Miscellaneous Conditions

Several common renal diseases may appear as incidental findings at abdominal aortography or renal arteriography.

Renal cysts appear as rounded, avascular filling defects in the renal parenchyma, with draping of vessels around the cyst (Fig. 8-43). Hypovascular neoplasms rarely mimic benign cysts; sonography or CT is recommended to exclude a hypovascular or cystic tumor.

Hydronephrosis typically has a "soap bubble" appearance, with displacement of intrarenal branches around the dilated collecting system (Fig. 8-44). *End-stage renal disease* causes the kidneys to shrink. Flow into the renal arteries is markedly diminished, but the central vessels usually remain patent.

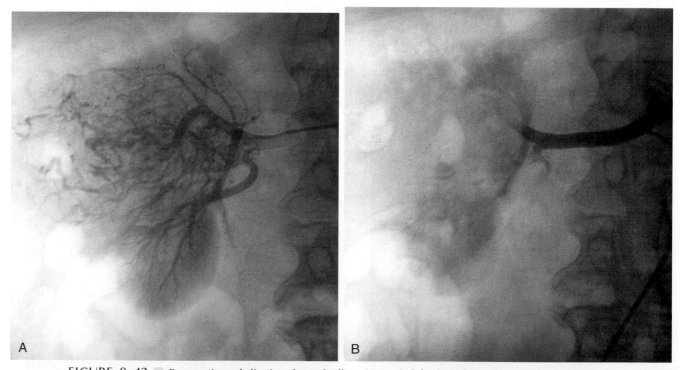

A

B

FIGURE 8-42 ■ Preoperative embolization of a renal cell carcinoma. **A,** Selective right renal arteriogram shows a large mass with bizarre vascularity occupying most of the upper pole. **B,** Following ethanol injection, the kidney has been entirely devascularized.

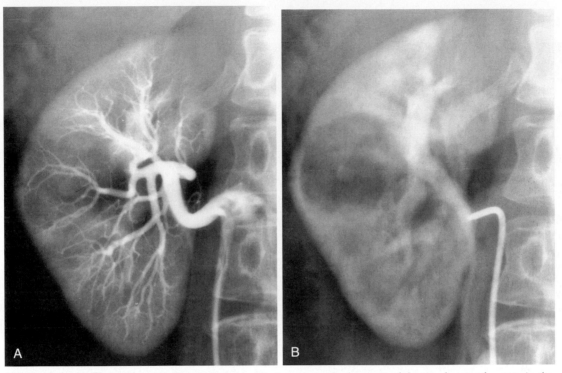

FIGURE 8-43 ■ Renal cyst. **A,** The early-phase angiogram shows displacement of the vessels around a mass in the middle pole of the kidney. An accessory renal artery feeds the most superior portion of the kidney, leading to an apparent filling defect in this region. **B,** The midpole nephrographic defect corresponds to a renal cyst.

■ OTHER DISORDERS

Aneurysms

Extrarenal artery aneurysms are most commonly caused by degeneration, FMD, arteritis, trauma, infection, or congenital abnormality. Degenerative aneurysms are the most common, and atherosclerotic changes, including calcification,

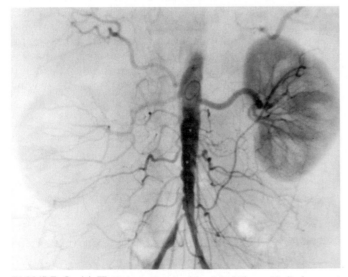

FIGURE 8-44 ■ Hydronephrosis of the right kidney with displacement of intrarenal branches around a dilated collecting system.

are probably a secondary effect rather than causative. Pseudoaneurysms usually are caused by trauma or infection.[146] *Intrarenal* aneurysms, which usually are multiple, are most commonly caused by a necrotizing arteritis (e.g., polyarteritis nodosa) or illicit drug use (e.g., cocaine, methamphetamines).

Renal artery aneurysms are more common on the right side and at arterial bifurcations; they may be multiple or bilateral. Most aneurysms are asymptomatic. Some patients present with hypertension, which may be essential or aneurysm-related (segmental ischemia from distal embolization of mural thrombus, stenotic disease adjacent to the aneurysm, or, rarely, extrinsic compression of an arterial branch).[147] The major complications of renal artery aneurysm are rupture and thrombosis. Although the overall likelihood of rupture is low, this risk is apparently heightened in pregnant women.[148]

The typical appearance of large- or medium-vessel aneurysms is saccular or fusiform dilation of the renal artery (often near a branch point), sometimes with mural calcification (Fig. 8-45; see also Figs. 8-34 and 8-36). Polyarteritis nodosa produces multiple aneurysms of small intrarenal vessels (Fig. 8-46).

Indications for treatment (operative aneurysmectomy, bypass, or endovascular covered stent placement) include rupture, symptoms from aneurysm expansion, distal embolization, renal artery stenoses causing hypertension, and women of child-bearing age. Asymptomatic lesions are treated when they exceed about 2 cm. Case reports have described treatment of a bleeding aneurysm with percutaneous thrombosis and of degenerative and fibromuscular dysplastic aneurysms with stent-grafts.[149-152]

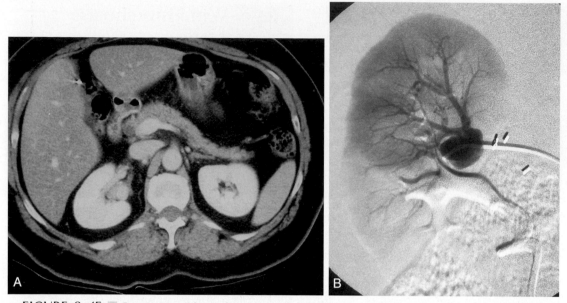

FIGURE 8-45 ■ Degenerative right renal artery aneurysm. **A,** CT scan reveals a round vascular mass with rim calcification in the renal pelvis. **B,** Catheter angiogram displays the aneurysm.

Dissection

Renal artery dissection may result from a variety of causes (Box 8-8). Dissections are seen more commonly in men than in women. Patients with acute dissection often present with flank pain, hematuria, or hypertension. Patients with chronic dissection usually are hypertensive. Imaging findings include an intimal flap, an irregularly dilated vessel from filling of a false lumen (especially in dissections from FMD), or complete vessel occlusion (see Fig. 8-33). Branch vessels often are involved. Surgical treatment consists of aortorenal bypass (when feasible) or nephrectomy to treat severe hypertension. Intravascular stents have been used to repair spontaneous renal artery dissections and those extending from an aortic dissection.[153-155]

Arteriovenous Fistulas and Malformations

Acquired arteriovenous fistulas in the kidney usually are the result of trauma, especially percutaneous biopsy. Massive renal arteriovenous fistulas can cause high-output heart failure.[156] Congenital AVMs of the kidney are exceedingly rare.[157] These lesions consist of numerous dilated, tortuous vessels within the subepithelium of the collecting system. When symptomatic, they usually present with gross hematuria and less commonly are associated with hypertension or an abdominal bruit. Color Doppler sonography, CT, and MR imaging are useful in detecting some of these lesions.[157,158]

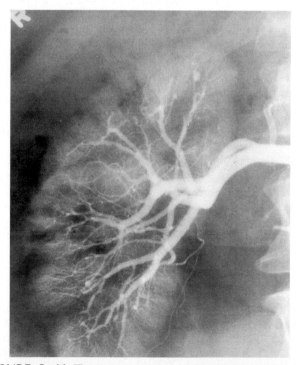

FIGURE 8-46 ■ Polyarteritis nodosa with multiple distal renal artery branch aneurysms.

BOX 8-8 ■ Causes of Renal Artery Dissection
Extension of aortic dissection
Iatrogenic (e.g., catheterization)
Blunt or penetrating trauma
Degeneration (atherosclerosis)
Fibromuscular dysplasia
Segmental arterial mediolysis
Spontaneous

At angiography, an arteriovenous fistula produces dilation of the feeding branch and early filling of the draining renal vein (Fig. 8-47; see also Fig. 8-35). Numerous segmental or interlobar arteries feed the renal AVM, which is composed of dilated, tortuous channels with rapid shunting into the renal vein and IVC (Fig. 8-48).

Transcatheter embolization is the first-line treatment for most of these lesions.[123,156,159,160] Coils are effective for treatment of fistulas. In AVMs, the nidus should be obliterated using a liquid agent such as cyanoacrylate (glue).

Renal Vein Thrombosis

The causes of RVT are outlined in Box 8-9.[161] The most common cause in adults is the *nephrotic syndrome*, resulting from a variety of renal or systemic disorders, particularly membranous glomerulonephritis. The combination of intravascular volume depletion and a thrombophilic state makes these patients especially prone to RVT. The most common cause in children is dehydration.

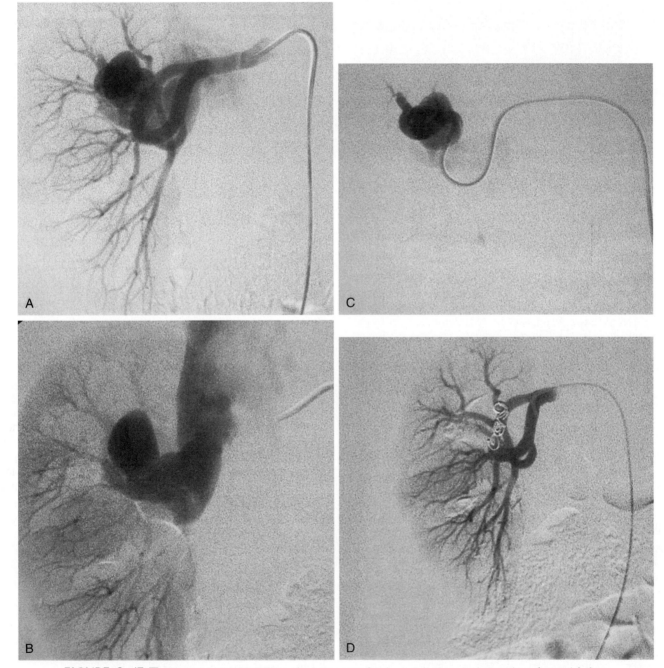

FIGURE 8-47 ■ Massive congenital right renal arteriovenous fistula. **A,** Selective arteriogram in early arterial phase shows early filling of large venous structures. **B,** Late arterial phase shows rapid washout through engorged venous channels into the inferior vena cava. **C,** Selective catheterization to the center of the connection. **D,** Following coil embolization, the connection is obliterated. Overall perfusion to the kidney is improved.

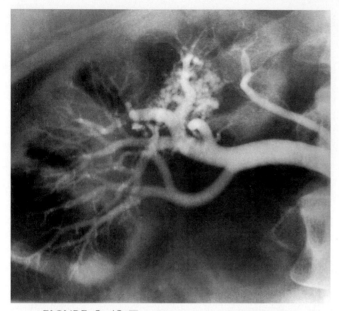

FIGURE 8-48 ■ Renal arteriovenous malformation.

Many of these patients have bilateral RVT. IVC or iliofemoral vein thrombosis and pulmonary embolism are relatively common.[162] Acute occlusion leads to kidney swelling, flank pain, hematuria, and, ultimately, hemorrhagic infarction. More commonly, the disease is progressive, collateral channels have time to develop, and kidney loss can be avoided. Many of these patients are asymptomatic.

The diagnosis of RVT is made by color Doppler sonography, CT, or MR venography.[163,164] A filling defect or flow void is noted in the main renal vein (see Figs. 8-37 and 8-38). Distension of the vein suggests acute thrombus. Vein retraction and abundant collaterals indicate chronic occlusion. The appearance at renal venography is varied. Clot may extend to the IVC and preclude catheterization. Nonocclusive thrombus may fill part of the main renal vein or intrarenal branches. In patients with chronic RVT, the venous branches may be small and irregular, and collateral vessels or varices may exist.

The standard treatment for RVT is anticoagulation and, in selected cases with acute thrombosis, surgical thrombectomy

or endovascular therapy. Several reports have described successful treatment of acute native RVT with thrombolytic infusion into the renal vein, renal artery, or both.[165,166] Intra-arterial injection may assist in lysis of thrombi within small intrarenal veins. IVC filter placement should be considered in patients who have a contraindication to anticoagulation or history of recurrent pulmonary embolism.

Renal Vein Varices

Renal vein varices may develop for several reasons (Box 8-10). They are an incidental finding in about 6% of the population.[167] Varices virtually always occur on the left side. It has been postulated that compression of the left renal vein between the superior mesenteric artery and the aorta (nutcracker phenomenon) may be responsible for renal vein hypertension and development of varices in some cases (see Fig. 8-12).[168]

Although renal vein varices may be asymptomatic, some patients develop intermittent or persistent hematuria and flank pain, which can be localized to the left kidney. Varices are among several possible causes of unexplained bleeding from the kidney (Box 8-11). Women also may suffer from pelvic congestion syndrome (pelvic pain, dyspareunia, dysmenorrhea) due to impeded outflow from the left ovarian vein.[168] The diagnosis is initially made by noninvasive vascular imaging.[169] Angiographic features include a pressure gradient across the left renal vein of 4 mm Hg or greater and dilated intrarenal veins and venous collaterals (Fig. 8-49). The treatment is either surgical (bypass or stent placement) or endovascular stent placement.[168,170,171]

Vasculitis and Coarctation Syndromes

Several types of vasculitis may affect the renal arteries, including Takayasu's arteritis, radiation-induced arteritis, and polyarteritis nodosa.[60,172,173] The rare congenital abdominal coarctation syndromes may cause narrowing of the renal arteries with RVH in children and young adults (Fig. 8-50).[174,175] Endovascular treatment with angioplasty and stent placement is appropriate in selected cases.[176] These disorders are considered further in Chapters 3 and 5.

Polyarteritis nodosa produces multiple microaneurysms in the kidney and many other vascular beds (see Fig. 8-46).

BOX 8-9 ■ **Causes of Renal Vein Thrombosis**

Nephrotic syndrome
Glomerulonephritis (membranous)
Renal cell carcinoma
Extension of clot or tumor from the inferior vena cava
Dehydration (in children)
Thrombophilic states
Lupus nephropathy
Diabetic nephropathy
Amyloidosis
Extrinsic renal vein compression
Trauma (e.g., postoperative)
Idiopathic causes

BOX 8-10 ■ **Causes of Renal Vein Varices**

Chronic renal vein thrombosis
Renal vein hypertension (nutcracker syndrome)
Portal hypertension with development of splenorenal or other
    shunts
Compressed retroaortic left renal vein
Congenital anomalies
Idiopathic causes

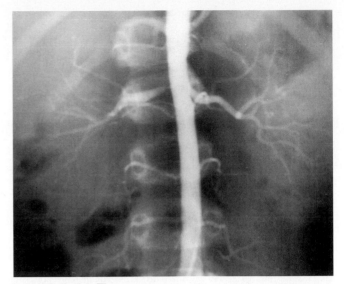

FIGURE 8-50 ■ Renal artery stenosis caused by neurofibromatosis.

BOX 8-11 ■ Causes of Occult Renal Bleeding

Neoplasm (e.g., renal cell carcinoma, angiomyolipoma)
Arteriovenous malformation
Arteriovenous fistula
Renal artery aneurysm
Renal vein varices
Arteritis (e.g., polyarteritis nodosa)
Idiopathic causes

Large- and medium-vessel aneurysms are seen less frequently.[177] Patients may present with spontaneous perinephric bleeding.[178,179] Catheter angiography usually is required for definitive diagnosis.

Segmental Arterial Mediolysis

This extremely rare disorder (which may be related to fibromuscular dysplasia) primarily attacks the coronary, splanchnic, and renal arteries.[180,181] The disease begins with destruction of medial smooth muscle and replacement by fibrin and granulation tissue. Extension to other layers of the arterial wall can lead to spontaneous dissection or aneurysm formation. The cause of the disorder is unknown.

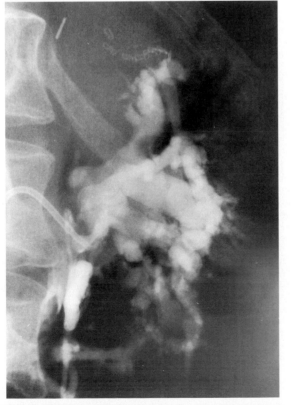

FIGURE 8-49 ■ Renal vein varices with a 5-mm Hg gradient across the left renal vein. The patient had intermittent hematuria localized to the left kidney.

REFERENCES

1. Verschuyl E-J, Kaatee R, Beek FJA, et al: Renal artery origins: best angiographic projection angles. Radiology 1997;205:115.
2. Harrington DP, Whelton PK, Mackenzie EJ, et al: Renal venous renin sampling: prospective study of technique and methods. Radiology 1981;138:571.
3. Caridi JG, Stavropoulos SW, Hawkins IF Jr: CO_2 digital subtraction angiography for renal artery angioplasty in high-risk patients. AJR Am J Roentgenol 1999;173:1551.
4. Collins P, ed: Embryology and development. In: Williams PL, Bannister LH, Berry MM, et al, eds. Gray's Anatomy, 38th ed. New York, Churchill Livingstone, 1995:204, 318.
5. Gabella G, ed: Cardiovascular system. In: Williams PL, Bannister LH, Berry MM, et al, eds. Gray's Anatomy, 38th ed. New York, Churchill Livingstone, 1995:1557.
6. Dyson M, ed: Urinary system. In: Williams PL, Bannister LH, Berry MM, et al, eds. Gray's Anatomy, 38th ed. New York, Churchill Livingstone, 1995:1826.
7. Gabella G, ed: Cardiovascular system. In: Williams PL, Bannister LH, Berry MM, et al, eds. Gray's Anatomy, 38th ed. New York, Churchill Livingstone, 1995:1601.
8. Shokeir AA, el-Diasty TA, Nabeeh A, et al: Digital subtraction angiography in potential live-kidney donors: a study of 1000 cases. Abdom Imaging 1994;19:461.
9. Gupta A, Tello R: Accessory renal arteries are not related to hypertension risk: a review of MR angiography data. AJR Am J Roentgenol 2004; 182:1521.
10. Platt JF, Ellis JH, Korobkin M, et al: Helical CT evaluation of potential kidney donors: findings in 154 subjects. AJR Am J Roentgenol 1997;169:1325.
11. Rankin SC, Jan W, Koffman CG: Noninvasive imaging of living related kidney donors: evaluation of CT angiography and gadolinium enhanced MR angiography. AJR Am J Roentgenol 2001;177:349.
12. Kaufman JA, Waltman AC, Rivitz SM, et al: Anatomical observations on the renal veins and inferior vena cava at magnetic resonance angiography. Cardiovasc Intervent Radiol 1995;18:153.
13. Hicks ME, Malden ES, Vesely TM, et al: Prospective anatomic study of the inferior vena cava and renal veins: comparison of selective renal venography with cavography and relevance in filter placement. J Vasc Interv Radiol 1995;6:721.

14. Trigaux JP, Vandroogenbroek S, deWispelaere JF, et al: Congenital anomalies of the inferior vena cava and left renal vein: evaluation with spiral CT. J Vasc Interv Radiol 1998;9:339.
15. Aljabri B, MacDonald PS, Satin R, et al: Incidence of major venous and renal anomalies relevant to aortoiliac surgery as demonstrated by computed tomography. Ann Vasc Surg 2001;15:615.
16. Abrams HL, Cornell SH: Patterns of collateral flow in renal ischemia. Radiology 1965;84:1001.
17. Jha RC, Korangy SJ, Ascher SM, et al: MR angiography and preoperative evaluation for laparoscopic donor nephrectomy. AJR Am J Roentgenol 2002;178:1489.
18. Sasaki TM, Finelli F, Bugarin E, et al: Is laparoscopic donor nephrectomy the new criterion standard? Arch Surg 2000;135:943.
19. Matas AJ, Bartlett ST, Leichtman AB, et al: Morbidity and mortality after living kidney donation, 1999-2001: survey of United States transplant centers. Am J Transplant 2003;3:830.
20. Liem YS, Kock MCJM, Ijzermans JNM, et al: Living renal donors: optimizing the imaging strategy: decision and cost-effectiveness analysis. Radiology 2003;226:53.
21. Halpern EJ, Mitchell DG, Wechsler RJ, et al: Preoperative evaluation of living renal donors: comparison of CT angiography and MR angiography. Radiology 2000;216:433.
22. Hussain SM, Kock MC, Ijzermans JN, et al: MR imaging: "one-stop shop" modality for preoperative evaluation of potential living kidney donors. Radiographics 2003;23:505.
23. Martin LG, Rundback JH, Sacks D, et al: Quality improvement guidelines for angiography, angioplasty, and stent placement in the diagnosis and treatment of renal artery stenosis in adults. J Vasc Interv Radiol 2003; 4:S297.
24. Hansen KJ, Edwards MS, Craven TE, et al: Prevalence of renovascular disease in the elderly: a population-based study. J Vasc Surg 2002; 36:443.
25. Rundback JH, Murphy TP, Cooper C, et al: Chronic renal ischemia: pathophysiologic mechanisms of cardiovascular and renal disease. J Vasc Interv Radiol 2002;13:1085.
26. Harrison EG Jr, McCormack LJ: Pathologic classification of renal arterial disease in renovascular hypertension. Mayo Clin Proc 1971; 46:161.
27. Schreiber MJU, Pohl MA, Novick AC: The natural history of atherosclerotic and fibrous renal artery disease. Urol Clin North Am 1984; 11:383.
28. Luescher TF, Lie JT, Stanson AW, et al: Arterial fibromuscular dysplasia. Mayo Clin Proc 1987;62:931.
29. Ram CV, Clagett GP, Radford LR: Renovascular hypertension. Semin Nephrol 1995;15:152.
30. Chobanian AV, Bakris GL, Black HR, et al: Seventh report of the Joint National Committee on Prevention, Detection, Evaluation, and Treatment of High Blood Pressure. Hypertension 2003;42:1206.
31. House MK, Dowling RJ, King P, et al: Using Doppler sonography to reveal renal artery stenosis: an evaluation of optimal imaging parameters. AJR Am J Roentgenol 1999;173:761.
32. Zucchelli PC: Hypertension and atherosclerotic renal artery stenosis: diagnostic approach. J Am Soc Nephrol 2002;13:S184.
33. Patriquin HB, Lafortune M, Jequier J-C, et al: Stenosis of the renal artery: assessment of slowed systole in the downstream circulation with Doppler sonography. Radiology 1992;184:479.
34. Qanadli SD, Soulez G, Therasse E, et al: Detection of renal artery stenosis: prospective comparison of captopril-enhanced Doppler sonography, captopril-enhanced scintigraphy, and MR angiography. AJR Am J Roentgenol 2001;177:1123.
35. Stavros AT, Parker SH, Yakes WF, et al: Segmental stenosis of the renal artery: pattern recognition of tardus and parvus abnormalities with duplex sonography. Radiology 1992;184:487.
36. Vasbinder GB, Nelemans PJ, Kessels AG, et al: Diagnostic tests for renal artery stenosis in patients suspected of having renovascular hypertension: meta-analysis. Ann Intern Med 2001;135:401.
37. Fain SB, King BF, Breen JF, et al: High-spatial resolution contrast-enhanced MR angiography of the renal arteries: a prospective comparison with digital subtraction angiography. Radiology 2001;218:481.
38. DeCobelli F, Venturini M, Vanzulli A, et al: Renal arterial stenosis: prospective comparison of color Doppler US and breath-hold, three dimensional dynamic, gadolinium-enhanced MR angiography. Radiology 2000;214:373.
39. Willmann JK, Wildermuth S, Pfammatter T, et al: Aortoiliac and renal arteries: prospective intraindividual comparison of contrast-enhanced three-dimensional MR angiography and multi-detector row CT angiography. Radiology 2003;226:798.
40. Bakker J, Beek FJA, Beutler JJ, et al: Renal artery stenosis and accessory renal arteries: accuracy of detection and visualization with gadolinium-enhanced breath-hold MR angiography. Radiology 1998;207:497.
41. Bude RO, Forauer AR, Caoili EM, et al: Is it necessary to study accessory arteries when screening the renal arteries for renovascular hypertension? Radiology 2003;226:411.
42. Pannu HK, Fishman EK: Multidetector computed tomographic evaluation of the renal artery. Abdom Imaging 2002;27:611.
43. Beregi J-P, Louvegny S, Gautier C, et al: Fibromuscular dysplasia of the renal arteries: comparison of helical CT angiography and arteriography. AJR Am J Roentgenol 1999;172:27.
44. Taylor A Jr, Nally JV: Clinical applications of renal scintigraphy. AJR Am J Roentgenol 1995;164:31.
45. Setaro JF, Saddler MC, Chen CC, et al: Simplified captopril renography in diagnosis and treatment of renal artery stenosis. Hypertension 1991;18:289.
46. Dondi M, Monetti N, Fanti S, et al: Use of technetium-99m-MAG$_3$ for renal scintigraphy after angiotensin-converting enzyme inhibition. J Nucl Med 1991;32:424.
47. Huot SJ, Hansson JH, Dey H, et al: Utility of captopril renal scans for detecting renal artery stenosis. Arch Intern Med 2002;162:1981.
48. Soulez G, Therasse E, Qanadli SD, et al: Prediction of clinical response after renal angioplasty: respective value of renal Doppler sonography and scintigraphy. AJR Am J Roentgenol 2003;181:1029.
49. Vaughan ED Jr, Buehler FR, Laragh JH, et al: Renovascular hypertension: renin measurements to indicate hypersecretion and contralateral suppression, estimate renal plasma flow, and score for surgical curability. Am J Med 1973;55:402.
50. Vaughan ED Jr: Renin sampling: collection and interpretation. N Engl J Med 1974;290:1195.
51. Rudnick MR, Maxwell MH: Diagnosis of renovascular hypertension: limitations of renin assays. In: Narins R, ed. Controversies in Nephrology and Hypertension. New York, Churchill Livingstone, 1984:123.
52. Roubidoux MA, Dunnick NR, Klotman PE, et al: Renal vein renins: inability to predict response to revascularization in patients with hypertension. Radiology 1991;178:819.
53. Stanley JC, Fry WJ: Renovascular hypertension secondary to arterial fibrodysplasia in adults. Criteria for operation and results of surgical therapy. Arch Surg 1975;110:922.
54. Scott JA, Rabe FE, Becker GJ, et al: Angiographic assessment of renal artery pathology: how reliable? AJR Am J Roentgenol 1983; 141:1299.
55. Mercier C, Piquet P, Alimi Y, et al: Occlusive disease of the renal arteries and chronic renal failure: the limits of reconstructive surgery. Ann Vasc Surg 1990;4:166.
56. Middleton JP: Ischemic disease of the kidney: how and why to consider revascularization. J Nephrol 1998;11:123.
57. Novick AC: Current concepts in the management of renovascular hypertension and ischemic renal failure. Am J Kidney Dis 1989; 13(Suppl 1):33.
58. Radermacher J, Haller H: The right diagnostic work-up: investigating renal and renovascular disorders. J Hypertens Suppl 2003;21:S19.
59. Radermacher J, Chavan A, Bleck J, et al: Use of Doppler ultrasonography to predict the outcome of therapy for renal artery stenosis. N Engl J Med 2001;344:410.
60. Sharma S, Thatai D, Saxena A, et al: Renovascular hypertension resulting from nonspecific aortoarteritis in children: midterm results of percutaneous transluminal renal angioplasty and predictors of restenosis. AJR Am J Roentgenol 1996;166:157.
61. van Jaarsveld BC, Krijnen P, Pieterman H, et al: The effect of balloon angioplasty on hypertension in atherosclerotic renal artery stenosis. Dutch Renal Artery Stenosis Intervention Cooperative Study Group. N Engl J Med 2000;342:1007.
62. Tegtmeyer CJ, Sos TA: Techniques of renal angioplasty. Radiology 1986;161:577.
63. Spinosa DJ, Matsumoto AH, Angle JF, et al: Safety of CO_2- and gadodiamide-enhanced angiography for the evaluation and percutaneous treatment of renal artery stenosis in patients with chronic renal insufficiency. AJR Am J Roentgenol 2001;176:1305.
64. Martin LG, Price RB, Casarella WJ, et al: Percutaneous angioplasty in clinical management of renovascular hypertension: initial and long-term results. Radiology 1985;155:629.

65. Klinge J, Mali WPTM, Puijlaert CBAJ, et al: Percutaneous transluminal renal angioplasty: initial and long-term results. Radiology 1989; 171:501.

66. Tegtmeyer CJ, Kellum CD, Ayers C: Percutaneous transluminal angioplasty of the renal artery: results and long-term follow-up. Radiology 1984;153:77.

67. Canzanello VJ, Millan VG, Spiegel JE, et al: Percutaneous transluminal renal angioplasty in management of atherosclerotic renovascular hypertension: results in 100 patients. Hypertension 1989; 13:163.

68. Giroux M-F, Soulez G, Therasse E, et al: Percutaneous revascularization of the renal arteries: predictors of outcome. J Vasc Interv Radiol 2000;11:713.

69. Tegtmeyer CJ, Selby JB, Hartwell GD, et al: Results and complications of angioplasty in fibromuscular disease. Circulation 1991;83(Suppl I):I155.

70. Sos TA, Pickering TG, Sniderman K, et al: Percutaneous transluminal renal angioplasty in renovascular hypertension due to atheroma or fibromuscular dysplasia. N Engl J Med 1983;309:274.

71. Martin LG, Casarella WJ, Gaylord GM: Azotemia caused by renal artery stenosis: treatment by percutaneous angioplasty. AJR Am J Roentgenol 1988;150:839.

72. Pattynama PM, Becker GJ, Brown J, et al: Percutaneous angioplasty for atherosclerotic renal artery disease: effect on renal function in azotemic patients. Cardiovasc Intervent Radiol 1994;17:143.

73. Pickering TG, Sos TA, Saddekni S, et al: Renal angioplasty in patients with azotaemia and renovascular hypertension. J Hypertens 1986; 4(Suppl 6):S667.

74. Martin LG, Casarella WJ, Alspaugh JP, et al: Renal artery angioplasty: increased technical success and decreased complications in the second 100 patients. Radiology 1986;159:631.

75. Rees CR: Stents for atherosclerotic renovascular disease. J Vasc Interv Radiol 1999;10:689.

76. Baumgartner I, von Aesch K, Do DD, et al: Stent placement in ostial and nonstial atherosclerotic renal arterial stenoses: a prospective follow-up study. Radiology 2000;216:498.

77. Lederman RJ, Mendelsohn FO, Santos R, et al: Primary renal artery stenting: characteristics and outcomes after 363 procedures. Am Heart J 2001;142:314.

78. Bakker J, Goffette PP, Henry M, et al: The Erasme study: a multicenter study on the safety and technical results of the Palmaz stent used for the treatment of atherosclerotic ostial renal artery stenosis. Cardiovasc Intervent Radiol 1999;22:468.

79. Blum U, Krumme B, Fluegel P, et al: Treatment of ostial renal-artery stenoses with vascular endoprostheses after unsuccessful balloon angioplasty. N Engl J Med 1997;336:459.

80. Henry M, Amor M, Henry I, et al: Stent placement in the renal artery: three-year experience with the Palmaz stent. J Vasc Interv Radiol 1996;7:343.

81. Gill KS, Fowler RC: Atherosclerotic renal arterial stenosis: clinical outcomes of stent placement for hypertension and renal failure. Radiology 2003;226:821.

82. Leertouwer TC, Gussenhoven EJ, Bosch JL, et al: Stent placement for renal arterial stenosis: where do we stand? A meta-analysis. Radiology 2000;216:78.

83. Bax L, Mali WP, Van De Ven PJ, et al: Repeated intervention for in-stent restenosis of the renal arteries. J Vasc Interv Radiol 2002; 13:1219.

84. Rundback JH, Gray RJ, Rozenblit G, et al: Renal artery stent placement for the management of ischemic nephropathy. J Vasc Interv Radiol 1998;9:413.

85. Ivanovic V, McKusick MA, Johnson CM III, et al: Renal artery stent placement: complications at a single tertiary care center. J Vasc Interv Radiol 2003;14:217.

86. Holden A, Hill A: Renal angioplasty and stenting with distal protection of the main renal artery in ischemic nephropathy: early experience. J Vasc Surg 2003;38:962.

87. Henry M, Henry I, Klonaris C, et al: Renal angioplasty and stenting under protection: the way for the future? Catheter Cardiovasc Interv 2003;60:299.

88. Hassen-Khodja R, Sala F, Declemy S, et al: Renal artery revascularization in combination with infrarenal aortic reconstruction. Ann Vasc Surg 2000;14:577.

89. Rigdon EE, Durham JR, Massop DW, et al: Hepatorenal and splenorenal artery bypass for salvage of renal function. Ann Vasc Surg 1991;5:133.

90. Geroulakos G, Wright IG, Tober JC, et al: Use of the splenic and hepatic artery for renal revascularization in patients with atherosclerotic renal artery disease. Ann Vasc Surg 1997;11:85.

91. van der Wal MA, Wisselink W, Rauwerda JA, et al: Traumatic bilateral renal artery thrombosis: case report and review of the literature. Cardiovasc Surg 2003;11:527.

92. Wright MPJ, Persad RA, Cranston DW: Renal artery occlusion. BJU Int 2001;87:9.

93. Lessman RK, Johnson SF, Coburn JW, et al: Renal artery embolism: clinical features and long-term follow-up of 17 cases. Ann Intern Med 1978;89:477.

94. Carman TL, Olin JW, Czum J: Noninvasive imaging of the renal arteries. Urol Clin North Am 2001;28:815.

95. Ouriel K, Andrus CH, Ricotta JJ, et al: Acute renal artery occlusion: when is revascularization justified? J Vasc Surg 1987;5:348.

96. Towne JB, Bernhard VM: Revascularization of the ischemic kidney. Arch Surg 1978;113:216.

97. Morris D, Kisly A, Stoyka CG, et al: Spontaneous bilateral renal artery occlusion associated with chronic atrial fibrillation. Clin Nephrol 1993;39:257.

98. Nicholas GG, DeMuth WE Jr: Treatment of renal artery embolism. Arch Surg 1984;119:278.

99. Blum U, Billmann P, Krause T, et al: Effect of local low-dose thrombolysis on clinical outcome in acute embolic renal artery occlusion. Radiology 1993;189:549.

100. Dwyer KM, Vrazas JI, Lodge RS, et al: Treatment of acute renal failure caused by renal artery occlusion with renal artery angioplasty. Am J Kidney Dis 2002;40:189.

101. Orons PD, Zajko AB: Angiography and interventional aspects of renal transplantation. Radiol Clin North Am 1995;33:461.

102. Bruno S, Remuzzi G, Ruggenenti P: Transplant renal artery stenosis. J Am Soc Nephrol 2004;15:134.

103. Patel NH, Jindal RM, Wilkin T, et al: Renal arterial stenosis in renal allografts: retrospective study of predisposing factors and outcome after percutaneous transluminal angioplasty. Radiology 2001; 219:663.

104. Matalon TAS, Thompson MJ, Patel SK, et al: Percutaneous transluminal angioplasty for transplant renal artery stenosis. J Vasc Interv Radiol 1992;3:55.

105. Claudon M, Lefevre F, Hestin D, et al: Power Doppler imaging: evaluation of vascular complications after renal transplantation. AJR Am J Roentgenol 1999;173:41.

106. Tublin ME, Dodd GD III: Sonography of renal transplantation. Radiol Clin North Am 1995;33:447.

107. Finlay DE, Letourneau JG, Longley DG: Assessment of vascular complications of renal, hepatic, and pancreatic transplantation. Radiographics 1992;12:981.

108. Baxter GM: Imaging in renal transplantation. Ultrasound Q 2003; 19:123.

109. Huber A, Heuck A, Scheidler J, et al: Contrast-enhanced MR angiography in patients after kidney transplantation. Eur Radiol 2001;11:2488.

110. Ferreiros J, Mendez R, Jorquera M, et al: Using gadolinium-enhanced three-dimensional MR angiography to assess arterial inflow stenosis after kidney transplantation. AJR Am J Roentgenol 1999;172:751.

111. Fany YC, Siegelman ES: Complications of renal transplantation: MR findings. J Comput Assist Tomogr 2001;25:836.

112. Kuo PC, Petersen J, Semba C, et al: CO_2 angiography—a technique for vascular imaging in renal allograft dysfunction. Transplantation 1996;61:652.

113. Spinosa DJ, Matsumoto AH, Angle JF, et al: Gadolinium-based contrast and carbon dioxide angiography to evaluate renal transplants for vascular causes of renal insufficiency and accelerated hypertension. J Vasc Interv Radiol 1998;9:909.

114. Benoit G, Moukarzel M, Hiesse C, et al: Transplant renal artery stenosis: experience and comparative results between surgery and angioplasty. Transplant Int 1990;3:137.

115. Newman-Sanders APG, Gedroyc WG, Al-Kutoubi MA, et al: The use of expandable metal stents in transplant renal artery stenosis. Clin Radiol 1995;50:245.

116. Modrall JG, Teitelbaum GP, Diaz-Luna H, et al: Local thrombolysis in a renal allograft threatened by renal vein thrombosis. Transplantation 1993;56:1011.

117. Robinson JM, Cockrell CH, Tisnado J, et al: Selective low-dose streptokinase infusion in the treatment of acute transplant renal vein thrombosis. Cardiovasc Intervent Radiol 1986;9:86.

118. deSouza NM, Reidy JF, Koffman CG: Arteriovenous fistulas complicating biopsy of renal allografts: treatment of bleeding with superselective embolization. AJR Am J Roentgenol 1991;156:507.

119. Perini S, Gordon RL, LaBerge JM, et al: Transcatheter embolization of biopsy-related vascular injury in the transplant kidney: immediate and long-term outcome. J Vasc Interv Radiol 1998;9:1011.

120. Maleux G, Messiaen T, Stockx L, et al: Transcatheter embolization of biopsy-related vascular injuries in renal allografts. Long-term technical, clinical, and biochemical results. Acta Radiol 2003;44:13.

121. Smith JK, Kenney PJ: Imaging of renal trauma. Radiol Clin North Am 2003;41:1019.

122. Fisher RG, Ben-Menachem Y, Whigham C: Stab wounds of the renal artery branches: angiographic diagnosis and treatment by embolization. AJR Am J Roentgenol 1989;152:1231.

123. Beaujeux R, Saussine C, Al-Fakir A, et al: Superselective endo-vascular treatment of renal vascular lesions. J Urol 1995;153:14.

124. Kawashima A, Sandler CM, Corl FM, et al: Imaging of renal trauma: a comprehensive review. Radiographics 2001;21:557.

125. Eastham JA, Wilson TG, Larsen DW, et al: Angiographic embolization of renal stab wounds. J Urol 1992;148:268.

126. Uflacker R, Paolini RM, Lima S: Management of traumatic hematuria by selective renal artery embolization. J Urol 1984;132:662.

127. Whigham CJ Jr, Bodenhamer JR, Miller JK: Use of the Palmaz stent in primary treatment of renal artery intimal injury secondary to blunt trauma. J Vasc Interv Radiol 1995;6:175.

128. Oto A, Herts BR, Remer EM, et al: Inferior vena cava tumor thrombus in renal cell carcinoma: staging by MR imaging and impact on surgical treatment. AJR Am J Roentgenol 1998;171:1619.

129. Miller DL, Choyke PL, Walther MM, et al: von Hippel-Lindau disease: inadequacy of angiography for identification of renal cancers. Radiology 1991;179:833.

130. Clark RE, Moss AA, DeLorimier AA, et al: Arteriography of Wilms' tumor. AJR Am J Roentgenol 1971;113:476.

131. Han Y-M, Kim J-K, Roh B-S, et al: Renal angiomyolipoma: selective arterial embolization-effectiveness and changes in angiomyogenic components in long-term follow-up. Radiology 1997;204:70.

132. McClennan BL, Deyoe LA: The imaging evaluation of renal cell carcinoma: diagnosis and staging. Radiol Clin North Am 1994;32:55.

133. Watson RC, Fleming RJ, Evans JA: Arteriography in the diagnosis of renal carcinoma. Review of 100 cases. Radiology 1968;91:888.

134. Couillard DR, deVere White RW: Surgery of renal cell carcinoma. Urol Clin North Am 1993;20:263.

135. Rabinowitz JG, Kinkhabwala M, Himmelfarb E, et al: Renal pelvic carcinoma: an angiographic re-evaluation. Radiology 1972;102:551.

136. Quinn MJ, Hartman DS, Friedman AC, et al: Renal oncocytoma: new observations. Radiology 1984;153:49.

137. Bakal CW, Cynamon J, Lakritz PS, et al: Value of preoperative renal artery embolization in reducing blood transfusion requirements during nephrectomy for renal cell carcinoma. J Vasc Interv Radiol 1993;4:727.

138. Park JH, Kim SH, Han JK, et al: Transcatheter arterial embolization of unresectable renal cell carcinoma with a mixture of ethanol and iodized oil. Cardiovasc Intervent Radiol 1994;17:323.

139. Harabayashi T, Shinohara N, Katano H, et al: Management of renal angiomyolipomas associated with tuberous sclerosis complex. J Urol 2004;171:102.

140. Gervais DA, McGovern FJ, Arellano RS, et al: Renal cell carcinoma: clinical experience and technical success with radio-frequency ablation of 42 tumors. Radiology 2003;226:417.

141. Matlaga BR, Zagoria RJ, Clark PE, et al: Radiofrequency ablation of renal tumors. Curr Urol Rep 2004;5:39.

142. Farrell MA, Charboneau WJ, DiMarco DS, et al: Imaging-guided radiofrequency ablation of solid renal tumors. AJR Am J Roentgenol 2003;180:1509.

143. Mayo-Smith WW, Dupuy DE, Parikh PM, et al: Imaging-guided percutaneous radiofrequency ablation of solid renal masses: technique and outcomes of 38 treatment sessions in 32 consecutive patients. AJR Am J Roentgenol 2003;180:1503.

144. Soulen MC, Faykus MH Jr, Shlansky-Goldberg RD, et al: Elective embolization for prevention of hemorrhage from renal angiomyolipomas. J Vasc Interv Radiol 1994;5:587.

145. Nelson CP, Sanda MG: Contemporary diagnosis and management of renal angiomyolipoma. J Urol 2002;168:1315.

146. Lee RS, Porter JR: Traumatic renal artery pseudoaneurysm: diagnosis and management techniques. J Trauma 2003;55:972.

147. Henke PK, Stanley JC: Renal artery aneurysms: diagnosis, management, and outcomes. Minerva Chir 2003;58:305.

148. Cohen JR, Shamash FS: Ruptured renal artery aneurysms during pregnancy. J Vasc Surg 1987;6:51.

149. Bui BT, Oliva VL, Leclerc G, et al: Renal artery aneurysm: treatment with percutaneous placement of a stent-graft. Radiology 1995;195:181.

150. Routh WD, Keller FS, Gross GM: Transcatheter thrombosis of a leaking saccular aneurysm of the main renal artery with preservation of renal blood flow. AJR Am J Roentgenol 1990;154:1097.

151. Rundback JH, Rizvi A, Rozenblit GN, et al: Percutaneous stent-graft management of renal artery aneurysms. J Vasc Interv Radiol 2000;11:1189.

152. Bisschops RHC, Popma JJ, Meyerovitz MF: Treatment of fibromuscular dysplasia and renal artery aneurysm with use of a stent-graft. J Vasc Interv Radiol 2001;12:757.

153. Lacombe P, Mulot R, Labedan F, et al: Percutaneous recanalization of a renal artery in aortic dissection. Radiology 1992;185:829.

154. Starnes BW, O'Donnell SD, Gillespie DL, et al: Endovascular management of renal ischemia in a patient with acute aortic dissection and renovascular hypertension. Ann Vasc Surg 2002;16:368.

155. Lee SH, Lee HC, Oh SJ, et al: Percutaneous intervention of spontaneous renal artery dissection complicated with renal infarction: a case report and literature review. Catheter Cardiovasc Interv 2003;60:335.

156. Khawaja AT, McLean GK, Srinivasa V: Successful intervention for high-output cardiac failure caused by massive renal arteriovenous fistula—a case report. Angiology 2004;55:205.

157. Crotty KL, Orihuela E, Warren MM: Recent advances in the diagnosis and treatment of renal arteriovenous malformations and fistulas. J Urol 1993;150:1355.

158. Takebayashi S, Aida N, Matsui K: Arteriovenous malformations of the kidneys: diagnosis and follow-up with color Doppler sonography in six patients. AJR Am J Roentgenol 1991;157:991.

159. Allione A, Pomero F, Valpreda S, et al: Worsening of hypertension in a pregnant women with renal arteriovenous malformation: a successful superselective embolization after delivery. Clin Nephrol 2003;60:211.

160. Takebayashi S, Hosaka M, Ishizuka E, et al: Arteriovenous malformations of the kidneys: ablation with alcohol. AJR Am J Roentgenol 1988;150:587.

161. Witz M, Kantarovsky A, Morag B, et al: Renal vein occlusion: a review. J Urol 1996;155:1173.

162. Llach F, Arieff AI, Massry SG: Renal vein thrombosis and nephrotic syndrome: a prospective study of 36 adult patients. Ann Intern Med 1975;83:8.

163. Kawashima A, Sandler CM, Ernst RD, et al: CT evaluation of renovascular disease. Radiographics 2000;20:1321.

164. Butty S, Hagspiel KD, Leung DA, et al: Body MR venography. Radiol Clin North Am 2002;40:899.

165. Huang AB, Glanz S, Hon M, et al: Renal vein thrombolysis with selective simultaneous renal artery and renal vein infusions. J Vasc Interv Radiol 1995;6:581.

166. Vogelzang RL, Moel DI, Cohn RA, et al: Acute renal vein thrombosis: successful treatment with intraarterial urokinase. Radiology 1988;169:681.

167. Beckmann CF, Abrams HL: Idiopathic renal vein varices: incidence and significance. Radiology 1982;143:649.

168. Scultetus AH, Villavicencio JL, Gillespie DL: The nutcracker syndrome: its role in the pelvic venous disorders. J Vasc Surg 2001;34:812.

169. Takebayashi S, Ueki T, Ikeda N, et al: Diagnosis of the nutcracker syndrome with color Doppler sonography: correlation with flow patterns on retrograde left renal venography. AJR Am J Roentgenol 1999;172:39.

170. Chiesa R, Anzuini A, Marone EM, et al: Endovascular stenting for the nutcracker phenomenon. J Endovasc Ther 2001;8:652.

171. Wei SM, Chen ZD, Zhou M: Intravenous stent placement for treatment of the nutcracker syndrome. J Urol 2003;170:1934.

172. Chuang VP: Radiation-induced arteritis. Semin Roentgenol 1994;29:64.

173. Kissin EY, Merkel PA: Diagnostic imaging in Takayasu arteritis. Curr Opin Rheumatol 2004;16:31.

174. Itzchak Y, Katznelson D, Boichis H, et al: Angiographic features of arterial lesions in neurofibromatosis. AJR Am J Roentgenol 1974;122:643.

175. Sumboonnanonda A, Robinson BL, Gedroyc WMW, et al: Middle aortic syndrome: clinical and radiological findings. Arch Dis Child 1992;67:501.

176. Both M, Jahnke T, Reinhold-Keller E, et al: Percutaneous management of occlusive arterial disease associated with vasculitis: a single center experience. Cardiovasc Intervent Radiol 2003;26:19.

177. Brogan PA, Davies R, Gordon I, et al: Renal angiography in children with polyarteritis nodosa. Pediatr Nephrol 2002;17:277.

178. Nguan C, Leone E: A case of spontaneous perirenal hemorrhage secondary to polyarteritis nodosa. Can J Urol 2002;9:1704.
179. Allen AW, Waybill PN, Singh H, et al: Polyarteritis nodosa presenting as spontaneous perirenal hemorrhage: angiographic diagnosis and treatment with microcoil embolization. J Vasc Interv Radiol 1999;10:1361.
180. Slavin RE, Saeki K, Bhagavan B, et al: Segmental arterial mediolysis: a precursor to fibromuscular dysplasia? Mod Pathol 1995; 8:287.
181. Soulen MC, Cohen DL, Itkin M, et al: Segmental arterial mediolysis: angioplasty of bilateral renal artery stenoses with 2-year imaging follow-up. J Vasc Interv Radiol 2004;15:763.

9

Mesenteric Arteries

■ ARTERIOGRAPHY

A wide variety of catheters is available for celiac and superior mesenteric arteriography, including visceral hook, side-winder, and cobra shapes (see Figs. 2-20 and 2-21). These vessels are engaged by searching the anterior aortic wall at about the T12 and L1-L2 levels, respectively. Typical contrast injection rates are 6 mL/second for 8 seconds for the celiac artery and 7 mL/second for 7 seconds for the superior mesenteric artery (SMA). Inferior mesenteric arteriography is done with a visceral hook or reverse-curve catheter. The artery originates from the left anterolateral surface of the aorta at about the L3-L4 level. Typical injection rate is 2 mL/second for 5 seconds. If the desired vessel is not easily found, a steeply oblique aortogram often shows an obstructed origin or anomalous location.

For selective catheterization of large caliber celiac artery branches (e.g., hepatic, splenic, or gastroduodenal artery), the catheter often can be advanced using steerable, hydrophilic guidewires. Otherwise, an exchange is done with a more suitably shaped catheter (Fig. 9-1). There are several methods for engaging the left gastric artery; one technique is outlined in Figure 9-2. Superselective catheterization for intervention is usually accomplished with coaxial microcatheters.

■ ANATOMY

Development

In the fetus, a series of vitelline arteries arising from the fused dorsal aortae supply the abdominal viscera.[1] These branches are initially connected by a ventral anastomotic channel (Fig. 9-3). The *celiac artery, SMA,* and *inferior mesenteric artery* (IMA) originate from three of these vitelline segments; the remaining segments regress before birth. Common variants in mesenteric artery anatomy can

be explained by abnormal persistence of vitelline segments or portions of the ventral anastomosis.

Normal Anatomy

The celiac artery originates from the anterior surface of the aorta at about the T12 level (Fig. 9-4).[2-4] The main trunk can take an upward, downward, or forward course. Within 1 to 2 cm of its origin, it gives off the *left gastric artery* and then divides into the common hepatic and splenic arteries. Sometimes, the *inferior phrenic* or *dorsal pancreatic artery* arises directly from the celiac trunk.

The *common hepatic artery* runs toward the liver. After giving off the *gastroduodenal artery*, it becomes the *proper hepatic artery* and then divides into *right* and *left* (and occasionally *middle*) *hepatic arteries*. The *middle hepatic artery* supplies the quadrate lobe. Hepatic arterial anatomy is detailed in Chapter 10. The *right gastric artery* usually takes off from the common or left hepatic artery but often is not visualized at angiography. It supplies the pylorus and the lesser curvature of the stomach and communicates with distal branches of the left gastric artery. The *cystic artery* usually originates from the right hepatic artery, although it may arise more proximally.

The gastroduodenal artery runs between the neck of the pancreas and the duodenum. Its first major branch is the *posterior superior pancreaticoduodenal artery*. This vessel gives off branches to the pancreas on the left and to the duodenum on the right. The gastroduodenal artery then divides into its terminal branches, the *anterior superior pancreaticoduodenal artery* and the *right gastroepiploic artery*. The **superior** pancreaticoduodenal arteries lead into an arterial network that supplies the head of the pancreas. These vessels have rich anastomoses with the corresponding branches of the *inferior pancreaticoduodenal artery*, which originates from the SMA (see below). The right gastroepiploic artery runs along the greater curvature of the stomach and

240

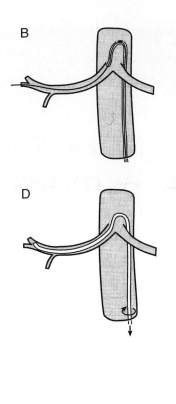

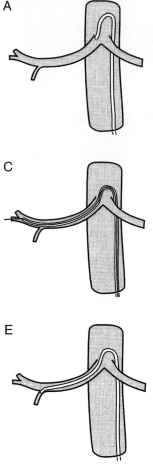

E

FIGURE 9-1 ▮ Selective catheterization of the hepatic and gastroduodenal arteries. The visceral hook catheter is exchanged for a headhunter catheter. (Adapted from Reuter SR, Redman HC, Cho KJ: Gastrointestinal Angiography, 3rd ed. Philadelphia, WB Saunders, 1986:21.)

communicates with the left gastroepiploic branch of the splenic artery.

The *splenic artery* supplies the spleen, pancreas, and stomach (see Chapter 10). It runs along the upper border of the pancreas along with the splenic vein. Its branches include the dorsal pancreatic, pancreatica magna, short gastric, and

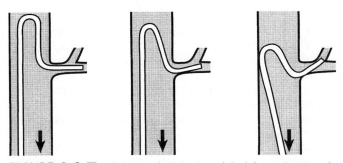

FIGURE 9-2 ▮ Selective catheterization of the left gastric artery. As the sidewinder-shaped catheter with its tip well into the celiac artery is withdrawn at the groin, the tip begins to point upward and eventually engages the left gastric artery.

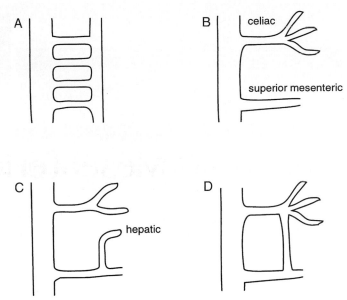

FIGURE 9-3 ▮ Embryologic development of the mesenteric arteries (right lateral view). **A,** In the fetus, the dorsal aorta on the left and the ventral anastomotic channel on the right are connected by a series of vitelline arteries. **B,** Normal anatomy at birth. **C,** Failure of a portion of the ventral anastomosis to regress causes the hepatic artery to be "replaced" to the superior mesenteric artery. **D,** Failed regression of a segment of the ventral anastomosis between the celiac and superior mesenteric arteries leaves a direct collateral pathway (i.e., *arc of Buehler*). (Adapted from Reuter SR, Redman HC, Cho KJ: Gastrointestinal Angiography, 3rd ed. Philadelphia, WB Saunders, 1986:34.)

polar arteries. The splenic artery divides into superior and inferior branches near the splenic hilum. The inferior polar artery gives rise to the left gastroepiploic artery, which courses along the greater curvature of the stomach.

The left gastric artery originates from the upper surface of the celiac artery and runs toward the cardia of the stomach (Fig. 9-5). At this point, it divides into several branches that supply the distal esophagus and fundus of the stomach. These vessels communicate with short gastric branches of the splenic artery, the right gastric artery, and the left inferior phrenic artery.

The SMA supplies the bowel from the distal duodenum to the mid-transverse colon (Fig. 9-6). It originates from the anterior surface of the aorta at about the L1-L2 level, approximately 1 to 2 cm below the celiac trunk. The SMA runs behind the body of the pancreas and then enters the root of the mesentery. The *superior mesenteric vein* lies along the right side of the artery. The inferior pancreaticoduodenal artery is the first branch of the SMA, although it may arise in a common trunk with the first jejunal artery. It runs to the right and superiorly into the head of the pancreas, where it communicates with the superior pancreaticoduodenal branches of the gastroduodenal artery. A series of jejunal and ileal branches occupy most of the main trunk of the SMA. Usually, these vessels fan out from the left upper quadrant to the right lower quadrant. A system of arcades between these branches feed the *vasa recta* that directly supply the wall of the bowel. The *ileocolic artery* is the terminal continuation of the SMA. It gives off branches to the ileum, appendix, cecum, and right colon. The *right* and

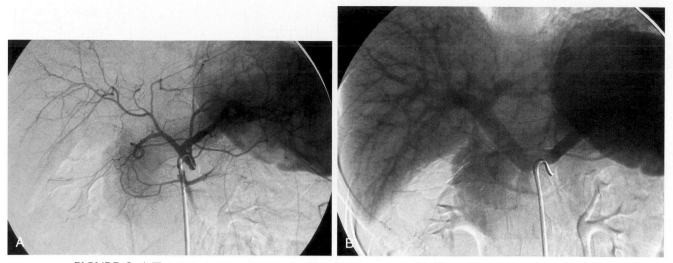

FIGURE 9-4 ■ Celiac arteriogram. **A,** Arterial phase. **B,** Venous phase with filling of the splenic and portal veins.

middle colic arteries arise separately or as a common trunk on the right side of the SMA. These vessels supply the ascending and transverse colon. Small bowel branches of the SMA can be differentiated from colonic branches by their more extensive arcade system and longer vasa recta (see Fig. 9-6).

The IMA supplies the colon from its mid-transverse segment to the rectum (Fig. 9-7). It originates from the left anterolateral surface of the aorta at about the L3-L4 level. The vessel runs inferiorly for several centimeters and then gives off the left colic artery. An ascending branch of this artery joins the middle colic branch of the SMA. Descending colic (sigmoid) branches take off from the *left colic artery* and distal IMA to supply the lower descending and sigmoid colon. The terminal branch of the IMA is the *superior rectal (hemorrhoidal) artery*, which divides into right and left branches that supply blood to the rectum.

Variant Anatomy

Anomalies in the origins of the central mesenteric arteries are rare. Anomalies in the branching patterns of the mesenteric arteries are common. It is vital to be alert to potential variants when performing angiographic procedures. The important variants formulated by the classic anatomic studies of Michel and coworkers are outlined in Table 9-1 (Figs. 9-8 and 9-9; see also Figs. 5-4 and 5-5).[5] The reported frequencies vary somewhat in postmortem and angiographic studies.

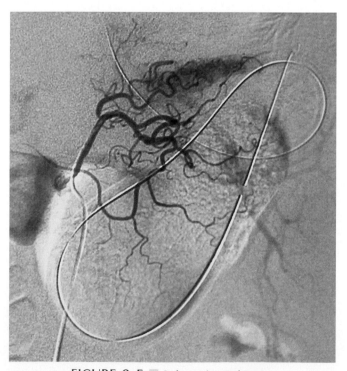

FIGURE 9-5 ■ Left gastric arteriogram.

TABLE 9-1   IMPORTANT ANOMALIES OF THE MESENTERIC ARTERIES

Artery	Anomalous Origin	Frequency (%)
Replaced common hepatic	Superior mesenteric	2.5
Replaced right hepatic	Superior mesenteric	10
Accessory right hepatic	Superior mesenteric	6
Replaced left hepatic	Left gastric	10–12
Accessory left hepatic	Left gastric	8–13
Inferior phrenic	Celiac	35
Dorsal pancreatic	Celiac	22
Gastroduodenal	Right or left hepatic	18
Left gastric, splenic, or hepatic	Aorta	<1
Celiomesenteric trunk	Aorta	<1
Middle colic	Dorsal pancreatic, splenic, hepatic	<1

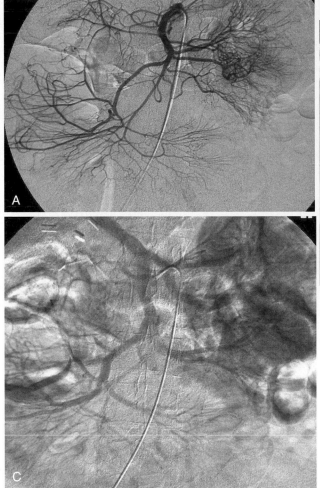

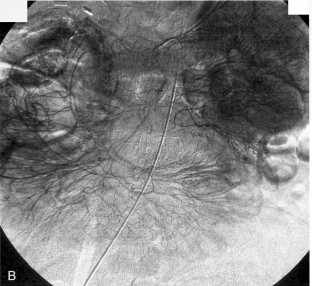

FIGURE 9-6 ■ Superior mesenteric arteriogram. **A,** Arterial phase. There is variable enhancement of bowel wall. **B,** Capillary phase. **C,** Venous phase.

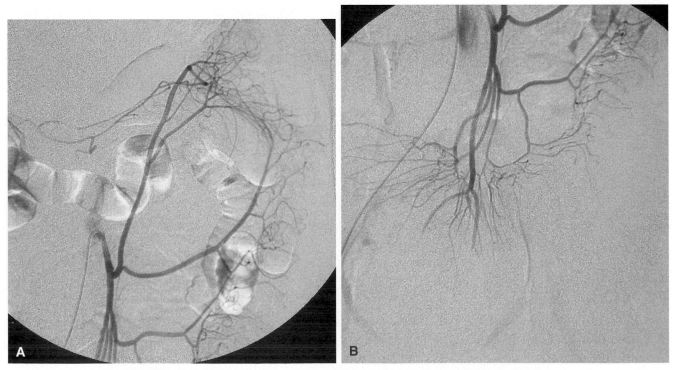

FIGURE 9-7 ■ Inferior mesenteric arteriogram. **A,** Superior imaging. **B,** Inferior imaging.

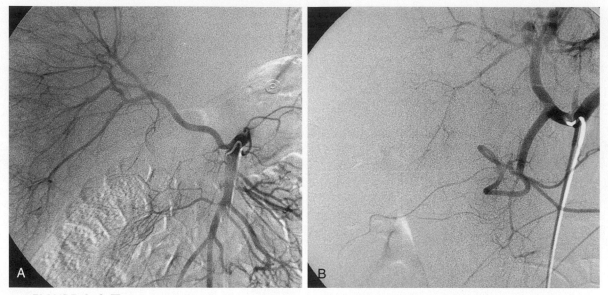

FIGURE 9-8   ■   **A,** Replaced right hepatic artery to the superior mesenteric artery. **B,** No filling of the right hepatic branches is seen on the celiac arteriogram.

A *replaced* hepatic artery exists when an *entire* hepatic lobe is supplied by a vessel with an aberrant origin (see Fig. 9-8). An *accessory* hepatic artery exists when a *portion* of the affected lobe is supplied by a vessel with an aberrant origin (Fig. 9-10). Accessory hepatic arteries supply isolated hepatic segments and are not redundant arteries. As a rule of thumb,

a replaced or accessory hepatic artery arises from the left gastric artery in 20% of patients and from the SMA in 20%.

Other rare variants include common origin of the celiac artery and SMA *(celiomesenteric trunk)*, separate origin of one or more major celiac branches from the aorta, and splenic artery arising from the SMA (Fig. 9-11; see also Fig. 5-4).

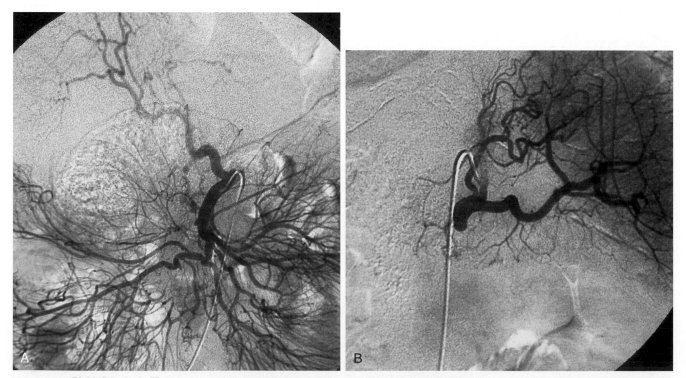

FIGURE 9-9   ■   Replaced common hepatic artery. **A,** The common hepatic artery originates from the superior mesenteric artery. **B,** At celiac angiography, only the left gastric and splenic arteries are seen.

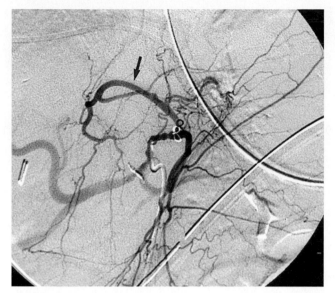

FIGURE 9-10 ■ Left gastric arteriogram. Note the accessory left hepatic artery *(arrow)*.

TABLE 9-2	MAJOR MESENTERIC ARTERIAL COLLATERAL PATHWAYS
Pathway	**Communication**
Intraceliac Branches (see Fig. 9-13)	
Gastric arcade	Left and right gastric arteries
Gastroepiploic arcade	Left and right gastroepiploic arteries
Arc of Barkow	Left and right epiploic arteries (within omentum)
Celiac and Superior Mesenteric Arteries (see Figs. 9-3 and 9-12)	
Pancreatic arcade	Gastroduodenal and inferior pancreatico-duodenal arteries
Arc of Buehler	Direct embryologic pathway
Superior and Inferior Mesenteric Arteries (see Figs. 9-14 and 9-15)	
Marginal artery (of Drummond)	Branches of middle and left colic arteries
Arc of Riolan	Central vessel from middle to left colic artery
Inferior Mesenteric and Iliac Arteries	
Rectal (hemorrhoidal) arcade	Superior and middle/inferior rectal arteries

Collateral Circulation

The intestinal tract has an extensive collateral network that prevents or limits bowel ischemia when central arteries become obstructed. The more important pathways are outlined in Table 9-2 and shown in Figures 9-12 through 9-15.[5] The different collateral routes between the SMA and IMA are often confused. The *marginal artery (of Drummond)* is a longitudinal vessel formed by trunks or distal branches of the right, middle, and left colic arteries. It runs along the entire mesenteric border of the colon. The *arc of Riolan* is a central vessel running in the mesentery that directly connects the middle colic artery with the left colic artery.

■ MAJOR DISORDERS

Acute Mesenteric Ischemia

Etiology

Several vascular diseases that reduce blood flow to or from the intestinal arteries or veins can lead to acute mesenteric ischemia (Box 9-1).[6-9] *SMA embolism* is the one of the most common causes of acute mesenteric vascular obstruction. Most emboli come from the heart. The embolus typically lodges in the SMA just **below** the origin of the middle colic artery, although single or multiple emboli may pass into the

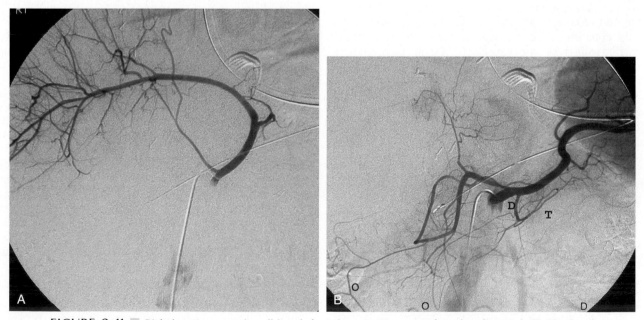

FIGURE 9-11 ■ Right hepatic artery takes off directly from the aorta (**A**), separate from the celiac trunk (**B**). The dorsal pancreatic artery (D), transverse pancreatic artery (T), and omental branches (O) are seen.

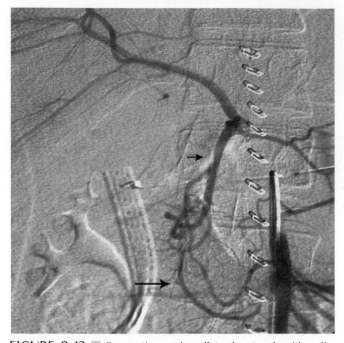

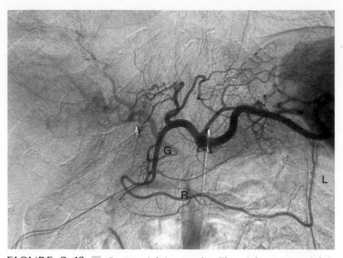

FIGURE 9-13 ■ Gastroepiploic arcade. The right gastroepiploic artery (R), the terminal branch of the gastroduodenal artery (G), continues to the left gastroepiploic artery (L) in the splenic hilum. This pathway provides collateral circulation with splenic artery obstruction. Also note the replaced right hepatic artery.

FIGURE 9-12 ■ Pancreatic arcade collateral network with celiac artery occlusion. Superior mesenteric arterial injection fills dilated inferior pancreaticoduodenal arteries *(long arrow)* and pancreatic arcades. Retrograde flow in the gastroduodenal artery *(short arrow)* then backfills the hepatic artery.

distal SMA trunk or its branches. The arteries beyond the obstruction undergo reflex vasoconstriction, which further worsens bowel ischemia.

SMA thrombosis is another common cause for acute intestinal ischemia. Thrombosis is usually superimposed on severe atherosclerotic disease near the origin of the SMA.

Nonocclusive mesenteric ischemia is responsible for a substantial number of cases of bowel ischemia.[10,11] The disorder is caused by hypotension or hypovolemia in the setting of acute cardiac disease, sepsis, or liver or kidney disease and after recent surgery. Certain drugs (including digitalis, dopamine, and vasopressin) have also been implicated. Regardless of the cause, the result is persistent vasoconstriction of the SMA and its branches leading to intestinal hypoxia.

Superior mesenteric vein thrombosis may be spontaneous or secondary to portal hypertension, hypercoagulable states, trauma, abdominal surgery, inflammatory bowel disease, sepsis, neoplasm, or pancreatitis.[12] If the venous collateral circulation is inadequate, the bowel wall becomes edematous, and arterial inflow is diminished.

Reflex vasospasm in the distal mesenteric branches (which may persist even after the proximal obstruction is relieved) often limits the effectiveness of collateral pathways and worsens the ischemic symptoms. Acute obstruction of the celiac artery or IMA rarely causes symptomatic mesenteric ischemia, provided that adequate collaterals exist.

Clinical Features

Most patients with acute mesenteric ischemia are elderly. Many have associated conditions such as congestive heart failure, coronary artery disease, valvular heart disease, dysrhythmias, or hypotension. Patients usually present with acute onset of moderate to severe abdominal pain, sometimes with nausea and vomiting or gastrointestinal bleeding. Classically, the symptoms are out of proportion to the relatively benign findings on physical examination. Often, a leukocytosis and metabolic acidosis are present. If bowel infarction occurs, signs of an acute abdomen will develop. Prompt diagnosis is important to avoid irreversible bowel damage, perforation, and sepsis, which usually occurs within 12 to 24 hours of occlusion unless the collateral circulation is already well developed. The mortality rate can be as high at 60% to 100%.[13]

Imaging

Patients with a high likelihood of acute ischemia and evidence of peritonitis or shock often undergo immediate operation without a complex imaging workup.

Cross-sectional Techniques. Duplex ultrasound, CT, and MR imaging can play an important role in the diagnosis and are particularly useful for excluding other sources of abdominal pain.[13-16] Sonography is used primarily to assess the patency of the central mesenteric vessels. Findings on CT (or MR) include bowel distension, bowel wall thickening, edema of the mesentery, intramural gas, and, sometimes, diminished bowel wall enhancement.[17,18] Nonopacification of the major mesenteric arteries and veins should be carefully assessed (Figs. 9-16 and 9-17). However, these methods cannot diagnose nonocclusive mesenteric ischemia or accurately assess the extent of distal embolization and status of any collateral circulation.

Angiography. Arteriography is performed emergently when there is a high index of suspicion without peritoneal signs or when noninvasive imaging suggests arterial occlusion. The study includes frontal and lateral (or steep

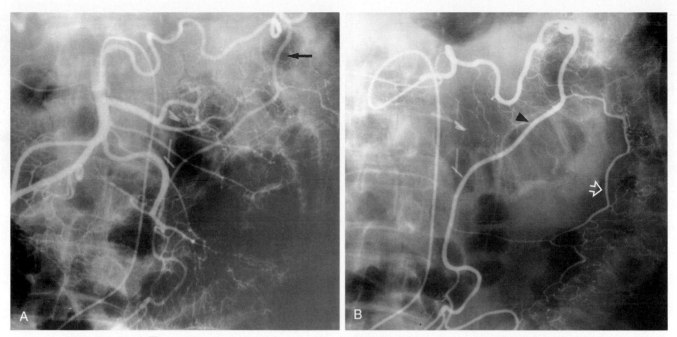

FIGURE 9-14 ■ Marginal artery of Drummond and arc of Riolan with inferior mesenteric artery (IMA) occlusion. **A,** Superior mesenteric arteriogram shows dilation of the middle colic artery with flow into the IMA distribution *(arrow)*. **B,** Selective middle colic artery injection shows filling of the arc of Riolan *(arrowhead)* and the marginal artery *(open arrow)*.

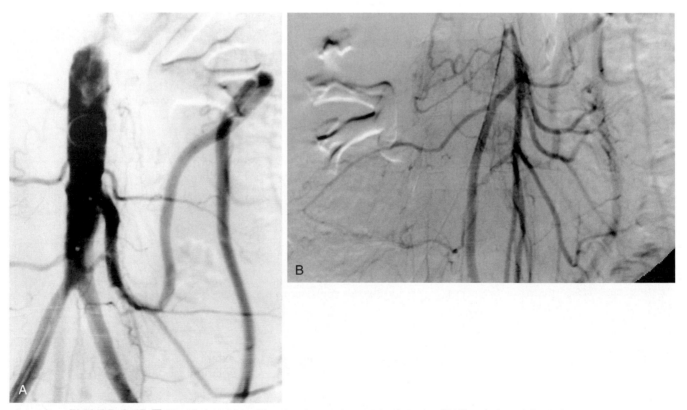

FIGURE 9-15 ■ Meandering mesenteric artery in superior mesenteric artery (SMA) occlusion. Abdominal aortogram shows markedly enlarged inferior mesenteric and left colic arteries (**A**), with retrograde filling of the main trunk of the superior mesenteric artery on later images (**B**). The SMA origin has a tapered occlusion.

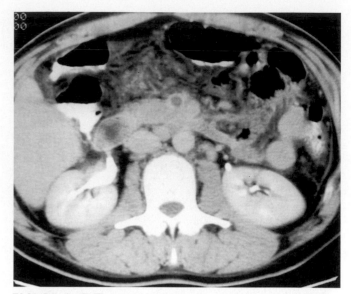

FIGURE 9-17 ■ Superior mesenteric vein thrombosis. The CT scan shows a clot in the superior mesenteric vein and dilated, thickened small bowel loops.

oblique) abdominal aortography and selective SMA and IMA arteriography if the vessel origins are not occluded. Blood flow in the SMA (normally about 6 to 7 mL/second) can be estimated based on the contrast injection rate and the degree of contrast spillover into the aorta.

Arteriographic findings depend on the cause of occlusive disease.[19] A fresh embolus produces a discrete filling defect (Fig. 9-18). In some cases, residual flow is seen around the clot. Reconstitution of the distal SMA is usually poor or non-existent. Occasionally, small clots are seen in distal SMA branches or other abdominal and pelvic arteries.

Thrombotic occlusion produces complete obstruction in the most proximal portion of the SMA trunk (see Fig. 9-15). It may be impossible to distinguish thrombotic and embolic occlusions by angiography. Because thrombosis occurs at a site of previous narrowing, the collateral circulation is often well developed.

Nonocclusive mesenteric ischemia is characterized by slow flow in the SMA, diffuse narrowing of SMA branches and arcades, segments of alternating spasm and dilation of these branches, and poor filling of the vasa recta (Fig. 9-19).[10,13,20] Contrast persists in intestinal branches for greater than 2 seconds after the injection has ended. Profound systemic hypotension (shock bowel) and certain vasoconstricting drugs can produce similar findings (see below).

Superior mesenteric vein thrombosis is diagnosed by the presence of numerous collateral channels in place of the

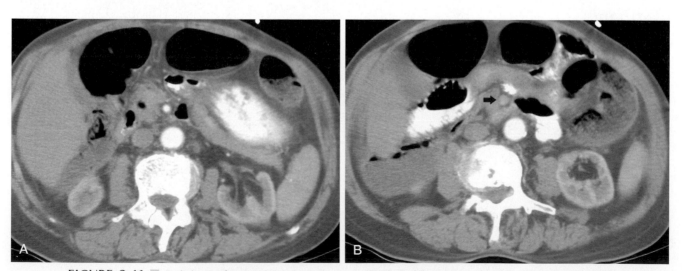

FIGURE 9-16 ■ Embolus to the superior mesenteric artery (SMA). **A,** CT scan near the SMA origin shows normal opacification. **B,** CT scan just caudal shows no opacification in the vessel *(arrow)*. There is no evidence of preexisting disease.

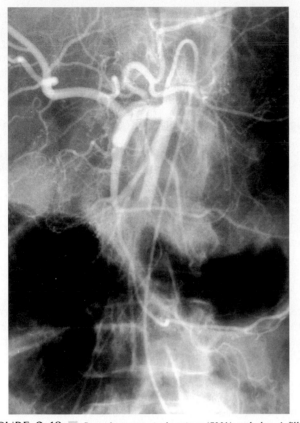

FIGURE 9-18 ■ Superior mesenteric artery (SMA) embolus. A filling defect is present in the SMA beyond the origin of the middle colic artery. The common hepatic artery is replaced to the SMA.

superior mesenteric vein during the late-phase SMA arteriogram. Sometimes, a filling defect in the main trunk of the vein is seen. Venous obstruction is usually associated with slow flow in the SMA and slow washout of mesenteric branches. Chronic mesenteric artery or vein occlusion may be an incidental finding in patients with acute abdominal pain from other causes.

Treatment

Surgical Therapy. Patients are sent for laparotomy based on the presence of peritoneal signs and the extent of collateral circulation seen at angiography. Acute SMA occlusion is treated by embolectomy, thromboendarterectomy, or bypass grafting along with removal of infarcted bowel. With severe aortic disease, an iliac artery may be used as an inflow vessel for a bypass graft. Multiple, small, distal SMA emboli are often treated conservatively with anticoagulation and vasodilators.

Endovascular Therapy. Infusion of the vasodilator *papaverine* directly into the SMA (60-mg bolus followed by an infusion at 30 to 60 mg/hour) is effective as primary treatment for nonocclusive mesenteric ischemia or as a preoperative maneuver for other forms of acute mesenteric ischemia.[6,20] Thrombolysis has also been used effectively for acute SMA embolism and acute superior mesenteric venous thrombosis.[21,22] It may be particularly appropriate in

patients without evidence of frank bowel necrosis. Balloon angioplasty with stent placement is also an attractive alternative to surgery in very high-risk patients with critical stenoses or extensions of dissection.[23,24] Immediate clinical benefit is the rule, but long-term durability has not been established.

Chronic Mesenteric Ischemia

Etiology

Symptomatic chronic obstruction of the mesenteric vessels is less common than acute intestinal ischemia. The primary cause of chronic obstruction is atherosclerotic disease (Box 9-2).[7,13,25] The stenoses are often caused by plaques on the abdominal aortic wall that engulf the ostia of the mesenteric arteries. Subacute or chronic superior mesenteric vein thrombosis can mimic chronic arterial obstruction.

Clinical Features

Most patients are elderly women with one or more risk factors for atherosclerosis. The classic symptom complex is a long history of abdominal pain after eating (intestinal angina), fear of food, and weight loss. Some patients have diarrhea, nausea, or intermittent vomiting. The abdominal

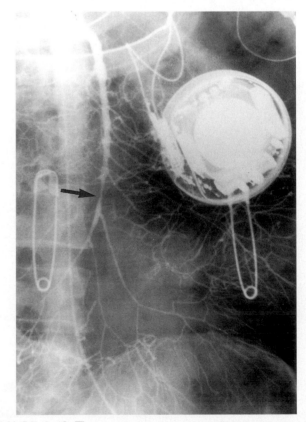

FIGURE 9-19 ■ Nonocclusive mesenteric ischemia. There is slow flow in the superior mesenteric artery (SMA), constriction of intestinal branches, and alternating segments of dilation and narrowing in the distal SMA *(arrow)*.

angiography can also identify mesenteric vascular stenoses and occlusions (Fig. 9-21).[14,29,30] It is commonly accepted that at least two of the three mesenteric arteries must have significant stenoses or occlusions to make the diagnosis of chronic mesenteric ischemia. On the other hand, the mere presence of severe multivessel mesenteric artery disease can be an incidental finding in a patient with other causes for abdominal pain.

Angiography. Arteriography is often obtained to confirm the diagnosis before surgery or for endovascular therapy. The approach is identical to the workup for acute mesenteric ischemia. Several entities should be considered in the differential diagnosis of mesenteric artery narrowing (see Box 9-2). Because of the chronic nature of the disease, the collateral circulation is usually extensive. Obstruction of the IMA is suggested by enlargement of the marginal artery (or arc of Riolan) with retrograde flow into the IMA trunk (see Fig. 9-14).

examination findings are usually benign, although an epigastric bruit may be heard.

Imaging

Cross-sectional Techniques. Because the symptoms of chronic mesenteric ischemia are often vague and intermittent, the diagnosis is often delayed. Duplex sonography is the primary imaging tool for screening suspected patients. Criteria include major vessel occlusion, high-grade stenosis, and peak systolic velocities in the celiac and SMA arteries of greater than 200 cm/second and greater than 275 cm/second in the fasting state, respectively (Fig. 9-20).[26-28] CT or MR

Treatment

Revascularization is performed to relieve chronic ischemic symptoms, prevent the development of life-threatening acute mesenteric ischemia, or avoid postoperative ischemia if the IMA is to be ligated during an aortic operation.

Surgical Therapy. The most common procedures for mesenteric revascularization are transaortic thromboendarterectomy, aortovisceral bypass, and arterial reimplantation.[31]

Endovascular Therapy. Balloon angioplasty (usually with stent placement) of the celiac artery and SMA is an acceptable alternative to surgery in some cases, particularly

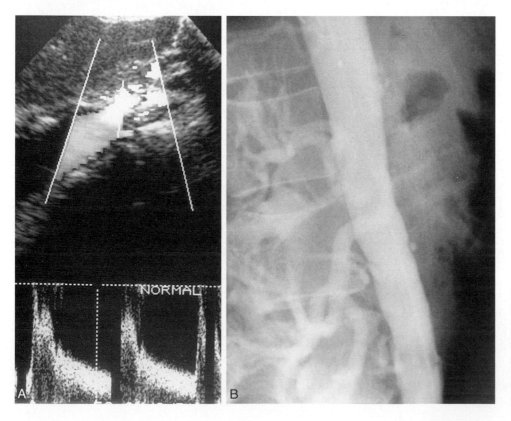

FIGURE 9-20 ■ Chronic mesenteric ischemia. **A,** Duplex sonography shows a stenosis at the origin of the superior mesenteric artery (SMA) with a peak systolic velocity of 302 cm/second. **B,** The lateral aortogram 3 weeks later showed complete occlusion of the celiac artery and SMA. The inferior mesenteric artery supplied the entire bowel.

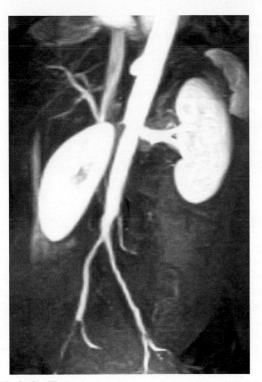

FIGURE 9-21 ■ Recurrent symptoms of chronic mesenteric ischemia after celiac/superior mesenteric artery bypass. Gadolinium-enhanced MR angiogram in sagittal projection shows stump of bypass with no filling of central mesenteric arteries.

when the patient is at high risk for operative complications (Fig. 9-22).[32-37] Technical success is reported in 30% to 90% of cases; long-term relief of symptoms occurs in more than two thirds of patients with atherosclerotic obstructions. However, major complications occur frequently (16% to 33%)

in some series. Surgery is more effective than balloon angioplasty and yields more durable results. Angioplasty is **not** useful in patients with celiac artery compression syndrome or extrinsic narrowing from tumor.

Acute Gastrointestinal Bleeding

The diagnosis and treatment of acute gastrointestinal bleeding have undergone a revolution over the last several decades. The widespread use of H_2 blockers and "proton pump" inhibitors has markedly reduced the incidence of peptic ulcer disease and associated bleeding. Fiberoptic endoscopy has largely supplanted angiography in the management of upper gastrointestinal hemorrhage. Endoscopy has also assumed a larger role in the evaluation and treatment of lower intestinal tract bleeding. Despite these advances, angiography is still required in many patients with this difficult clinical problem.

Etiology

For several reasons, acute gastrointestinal bleeding is typically categorized as being from an upper gastrointestinal source (from the esophagus to the ligament of Treitz) or a lower gastrointestinal source (from the small bowel, colon, or rectum). The major causes of upper gastrointestinal bleeding are outlined in Box 9-3. The most common are duodenal or gastric ulcer disease, gastritis, Mallory-Weiss tear, and gastroesophageal varices.

Gastroesophageal varices are a common source of upper gastrointestinal bleeding in patients with portal hypertension. However, patients with varices may bleed from other lesions. Variceal bleeding is usually detected by endoscopy. Angiography may show the varices but rarely shows active bleeding.

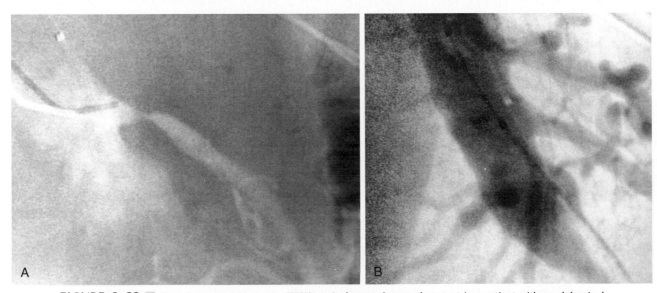

FIGURE 9-22 ■ Superior mesenteric artery (SMA) angioplasty and stent placement in a patient with an abdominal aortic aneurysm and occlusion of the inferior mesenteric artery. **A,** The lateral aortogram shows a tight proximal SMA stenosis. **B,** After placement of a stent mounted on a 6-mm angioplasty balloon using a high brachial approach, the stenosis is relieved. The residual systolic pressure gradient was 7 to 8 mm Hg.

Mallory-Weiss tear is a laceration at the gastroesophageal junction, often seen in alcoholics after repeated episodes of vomiting.[38] *Pseudoaneurysms* of the gastroduodenal, pancreaticoduodenal, and splenic arteries may develop in patients with pancreatitis or trauma.[39]

Medical interventions such as endoscopic biliary procedures and surgery can cause bleeding from direct injury to the bowel. *Hemobilia* can manifest as acute gastrointestinal hemorrhage, usually after percutaneous liver biopsy, biliary drainage procedures, hepatic surgery, or trauma. Bleeding can be immediate or delayed.

Aortoenteric fistula occurs in less than 1% of patients after aortic graft replacement. The fistula develops between the bowel (usually the transverse duodenum) and the graft as a consequence of graft infection.[40]

Marginal ulcers occasionally develop after gastrojejunostomy.[41,42] Ulcers are located on the jejunal side of the anastomosis; however, bleeding may occur from branches of the celiac artery or SMA.

Dieulafoy's disease is a noninflammatory disorder in which a small superficial gastric mucosal erosion covers a submucosal artery and may result in bleeding.[43] The lesion is usually found in the cardia or fundus of the stomach.

Hemosuccus pancreaticus can result when a pseudoaneurysm develops in the setting of acute or chronic pancreatitis and causes bleeding into the pancreatic duct and then the duodenum.[44]

The major causes of lower gastrointestinal bleeding are outlined in Box 9-4. The most common sources are angiodysplasia (or arteriovenous malformation), diverticulosis, and bleeding after endoscopic biopsy. At least two thirds of cases are localized to the large bowel.[45]

Diverticular disease is sometimes complicated by hemorrhage. Bleeding is minor and self-limited in most cases. Massive or recurrent bleeding is an indication for angiography. Hemorrhage occurs from a branch of the vasa recta in continuity with the body of the diverticulum.[46] Although diverticula are most common in the sigmoid and left colon, massive bleeding occurs in the right colon in greater than 50% of cases.[45-47]

Angiodysplasia (vascular ectasia) is a developmental vascular anomaly consisting of clusters of dilated submucosal veins and capillaries in the bowel wall, most frequently in the ascending colon.[48] The cause is unknown. There is speculation that intermittent elevation in intraluminal pressure causes venous obstruction, which over time leads to venous engorgement and bleeding. Lesions are often multiple. Angiodysplasia is relatively common in the elderly and may be an incidental finding in patients with other sources for gastrointestinal bleeding.

Acquired immunodeficiency syndrome can cause lower or upper gastrointestinal hemorrhage. A wide variety of lesions may bleed, including Kaposi's sarcoma, lymphoma, and a host of opportunistic infections.[49]

Clinical Features

Patients with significant upper gastrointestinal bleeding have bright red or coffee-ground hematemesis or melena. Patients with lower gastrointestinal bleeding present with hematochezia or melena. However, about 10% of patients with major upper gastrointestinal hemorrhage have bright red rectal bleeding that suggests a lower tract source. About 75% of patients with acute gastrointestinal bleeding respond to supportive measures and minor blood transfusions. The remainder require direct intervention.

Imaging

After the patient is resuscitated and a nasogastric tube is placed, endoscopy or anoscopy is usually performed to identify and possibly treat a culprit lesion. Imaging is needed only when the bleeding site cannot be identified or transcatheter treatment is contemplated. Radionuclide scans are useful for assessing hemodynamically stable patients with mild to moderate bleeding or intermittent bleeding. The scan may localize the hemorrhage and determine whether it is brisk enough that its origin can be detected by angiography. Continuous rapid bleeding is signaled by persistent passage or aspiration of large volumes of blood, transfusion of more than 4 to 6 units of packed red blood cells over 24 hours, or hemodynamic instability. These patients should undergo angiography without delay.

Radionuclide Scanning. Scintigraphy is done with ^{99m}Tc-sulfur colloid or ^{99m}Tc-labeled red blood cells.[50,51] The threshold for detection of gastrointestinal bleeding is quoted as ranging from 0.05 to 0.4 mL/minute, compared with a rate of about 0.5 mL/minute with angiography.[52-54] However, these figures are based on animal models, phantom studies, and estimated transfusion requirements and are only approximations.

Most centers prefer red blood cell scanning over sulfur colloid scanning. Red blood cell scans are more sensitive, avoid significant background activity over the liver and spleen, and can show intermittent bleeding through delayed imaging (Fig. 9-23A).[55-57] Both methods can localize the bleeding site. However, forward or backward movement of tracer in the bowel can mislead the reader.[58] Patients with negative scan results are observed. Patients with positive scan results should undergo immediate angiography.

Angiography. Nusbaum and Baum pioneered the angiographic technique for evaluating gastrointestinal hemorrhage.[54,59]

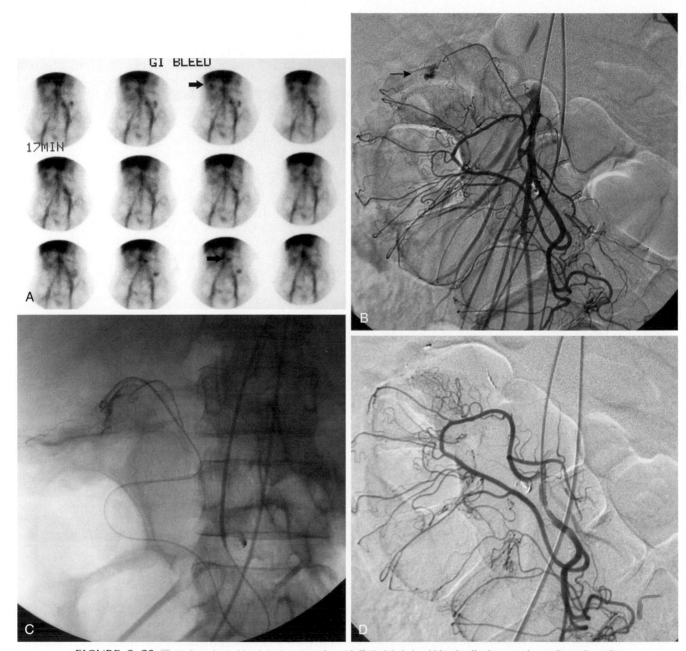

FIGURE 9-23 ■ Right colonic bleed. **A,** Scintigraphy with ^{99m}Tc-labeled red blood cells shows early uptake in the right upper quadrant, which is consistent with hepatic flexure bleed *(arrow)*. **B,** The superior mesenteric arteriogram shows extravasation from a branch of the right colic artery *(arrow)*. **C,** Coaxial microcatheter is advanced to the site of bleeding. **D,** After placement of several microcoils and small Gelfoam pieces, bleeding has stopped.

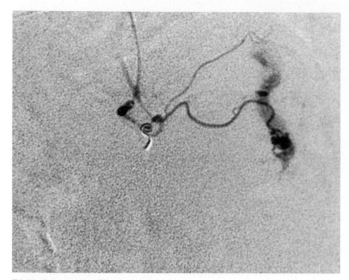

FIGURE 9-24 ■ "Pseudovein" sign of gastrointestinal hemorrhage. The curvilinear, wormlike density in the middle descending colon persisted through the venous phase.

The vessel most likely to supply the bleeding site (based on clinical scenario and results of endoscopy or scintigraphy) is studied first. Upper gastrointestinal bleeding is evaluated by celiac arteriography, followed by superior mesenteric arteriography. If no bleeding site is found, selective left gastric or gastroduodenal arteriography may detect a subtle bleed. If results of all these studies are negative, inferior mesenteric arteriography should be considered. Presumed lower gastrointestinal bleeding is evaluated by superior mesenteric arteriography, followed by inferior mesenteric arteriography. If results of both studies are negative, celiac arteriography should be performed. Aortography is needed only when ostial disease or variant anatomy makes catheterization difficult or when the examiner is trying to find other aortic branches that may be the source of bleeding (e.g., inferior phrenic artery). The entire length of bowel supplied by the injected artery must be visualized by using careful patient positioning and multiple angiographic runs. Selective injections are used to confirm suspicious findings on nonselective angiograms. Patients with suspected aortoenteric fistulas are studied by CT rather than angiography.

The hallmark of gastrointestinal hemorrhage is extravasation of contrast material into the bowel (see Fig. 9-23).[60] Occasionally, extravasated contrast has a curvilinear shape that mimics a vascular structure (pseudovein sign) (Fig. 9-24). Several entities can be confused with extravasation, including hypervascular mucosa and adrenal gland opacification.

The angiogram often can identify the bleeding site but provide no clue to the underlying condition. At other times, a pathologic diagnosis is suggested.

Peptic ulcer disease produces puddles of contrast outlining the gastric or duodenal mucosa. With gastric ulcers, the bleeding source may be the left or right gastric artery, left or right gastroepiploic artery, or short gastric branches of the splenic artery. With pyloric and duodenal ulcers, bleeding usually comes from duodenal branches of the gastroduodenal artery or the right gastroepiploic artery (Fig. 9-25).

Gastritis causes hypervascularity and dense staining of the gastric mucosa. The disease may be localized or diffuse. A *Mallory-Weiss tear* causes extravasation in the region of the gastroesophageal junction with retrograde flow of contrast into the esophagus in some cases (Fig. 9-26).

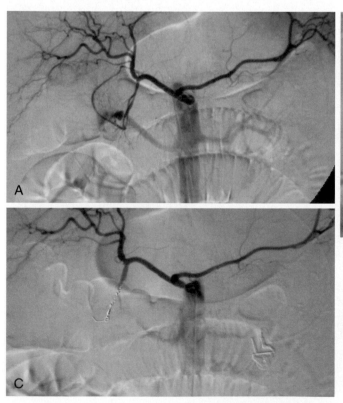

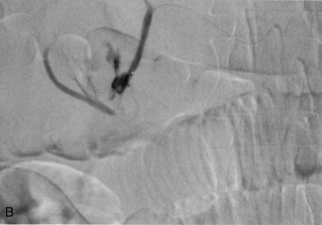

FIGURE 9-25 ■ Duodenal ulcer hemorrhage. **A,** Extravasation has occurred from duodenal branches of the gastroduodenal artery. **B,** Coils are placed across the gastroduodenal artery to isolate the bleeding vessels and prevent backflow from the superior mesenteric artery. **C,** Bleeding has ceased.

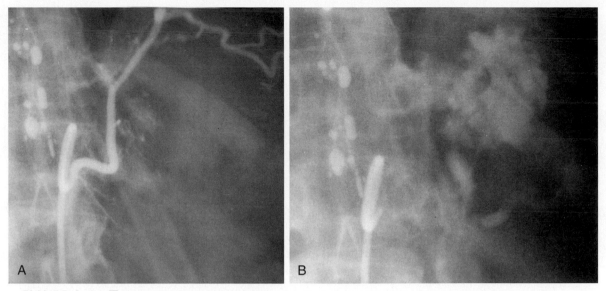

FIGURE 9-26 ■ Mallory-Weiss tear. The left inferior phrenic arteriogram (**A**) shows massive extravasation on late-phase images (**B**).

Diverticular bleeding does not have a characteristic appearance unless contrast fills the diverticulum itself (Fig. 9-27). *Angiodysplasia* is diagnosed by early and then persistent filling of a draining vein and by an abnormal cluster of vessels in the bowel wall (Fig. 9-28).[61] Lesions can be multiple. The abnormality is identified by early venous drainage from one portion of the bowel or a "tram track" sign from simultaneous opacification of the feeding artery and draining vein. Contrast extravasation usually is not seen. Because angiodysplasia is relatively common in elderly patients and may be an incidental finding, other sources of bleeding should be considered. Congenital *arteriovenous malformations* can look identical (Fig. 9-29).

Pseudoaneurysms are classically seen in patients with chronic pancreatitis and inflammatory erosion into the gastroduodenal, pancreatic, or splenic artery. *Variceal bleeding* itself is rarely detected by angiography. However, filling of varices at unsuspected sites (e.g., duodenum, cecum) may suggest a possible source for hemorrhage (Fig. 9-30).[62]

Angiography identifies a bleeding source in 50% to 90% of cases.[63-67] Extravasation is almost always seen if the hemorrhage is active and brisk at the time of angiography. The study may be normal if bleeding has stopped, is intermittent, or is below the threshold for angiography.[68] Other reasons for a negative angiographic result include venous

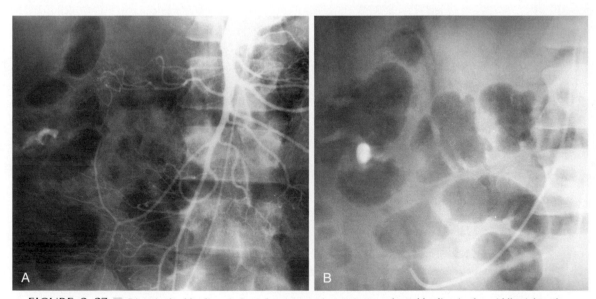

FIGURE 9-27 ■ Diverticular bleeding. **A,** Superior mesenteric arteriogram shows bleeding in the middle right colon. **B,** A scout film before a selective right colic arteriogram shows a rounded contrast collection within a bleeding diverticulum from prior contrast injection.

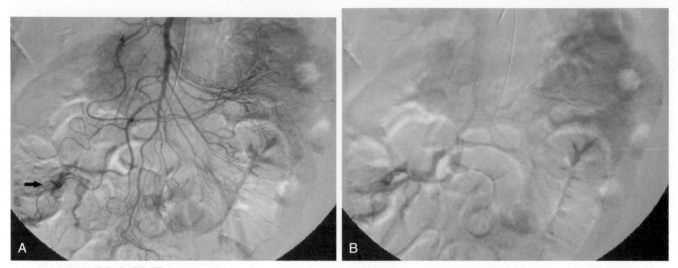

FIGURE 9-28 ■ Angiodysplasia of the cecum. **A,** Early phase of superior mesenteric arteriogram shows a tangle of vessels in the cecum *(arrow)*. **B,** Capillary phase exhibits early opacification of draining vein. Note that no venous drainage is seen from other portions of the bowel.

bleeding, failure to inject the correct artery, or bleeding outside the field of imaging.

Treatment
Vasopressin Infusion Therapy

Among other effects, the natural hormone vasopressin (Pitressin) causes constriction of smooth muscle of the bowel wall and splanchnic blood vessels. Infusion of the drug proximal to a bleeding mesenteric artery reduces blood flow, lowers the pulse pressure, and allows a clot to form.[69]

Intra-arterial infusion is more effective and safer than systemic infusion for mesenteric arterial bleeding.[70]

Indications. While some interventionalists continue to use vasopressin infusion as a first-line treatment for certain types of gastrointestinal hemorrhage, most practitioners favor embolotherapy when feasible (see below). Vasopressin is not used in the following situations:

- Bleeding directly from a large artery (e.g., gastroduodenal bleed, splenic artery pseudoaneurysm)
- Bleeding at sites with dual blood supply (e.g., pyloroduodenal bleeding)

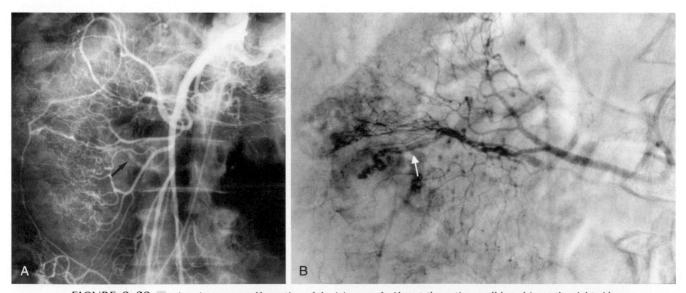

FIGURE 9-29 ■ Arteriovenous malformation of the jejunum. **A,** Almost the entire small bowel is on the right side of the abdomen on the superior mesenteric arteriogram. Early filling of a jejunal vein *(arrow)* can be seen. **B,** Selective injection of the second jejunal branch shows an abnormal tuft of vessels in the bowel wall and early filling of a draining vein *(arrow)*.

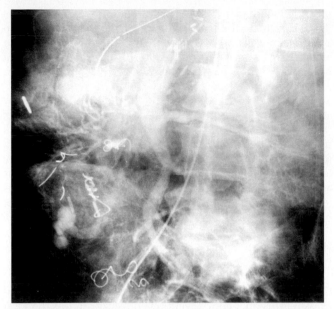

FIGURE 9-30 ■ Cecal varices are demonstrated on the late-phase superior mesenteric arteriogram of a patient with lower gastrointestinal bleeding. The patient had undergone a transjugular intrahepatic portosystemic shunt procedure for portal hypertension and prior embolization of bleeding intestinal varices.

■ Patients with a contraindication to vasopressin therapy (e.g., severe coronary artery disease, dysrhythmias, severe hypertension)
■ After embolotherapy, because of the significant risk of bowel infarction

Technique. The catheter is placed in the central vessel feeding the bleeding site (celiac artery, left gastric artery, SMA, or IMA).[71-75] Vasopressin is infused at 0.2 units per minute. After 20 to 30 minutes, arteriography is repeated to look for residual bleeding and the presence of some direct or collateral blood flow to the viscera (see Fig. 3-4). If bleeding has stopped, the infusion is continued while the patient is monitored in an intensive care unit. If bleeding persists, the infusion rate is increased to 0.3 or 0.4 units per minute, and arteriography is repeated 20 to 30 minutes later. If the lesion is still bleeding, alternate forms of therapy should be pursued. Higher doses of vasopressin are generally not recommended. Vasopressin therapy is continued for 6 to 24 hours. The rate is then gradually tapered over 12 to 48 hours. After the infusion has been stopped, the catheter is kept in place for 12 to 24 hours in case rebleeding occurs.

Results. Vasopressin therapy is initially very effective for certain types of gastrointestinal hemorrhage, particularly colonic diverticular and gastric mucosal hemorrhage. Initial success rates range from 60% to 90%.[47,64,65,76-79] However, rebleeding has been reported in up to 50% of cases.

Complications. Patients often have mild abdominal pain at the onset of infusion. Persistent pain can be a sign of bowel ischemia, in which case the infusion rate should be slowed. Possible side effects of vasopressin treatment include angina, dysrhythmias, hypertension, bradycardia, cardiac arrest,

bowel ischemia or infarction, fluid retention (a consequence of its antidiuretic effect), allergic reactions, and complications from prolonged femoral artery catheterization.[80,81] Major adverse events are reported in up to 20% of cases.

Embolization

The goal of embolotherapy is to stop blood flow to the bleeding artery while maintaining viability of the bowel. For many years, embolization, particularly in the small intestine and colon, was avoided by angiographers because of the fear of bowel infarction. However, with the development of coaxial microcatheters (which can be negotiated directly to the site of bleeding) and newer embolic agents (e.g., microcoils, polyvinyl alcohol [PVA] particles), the risk of significant bowel ischemia is minimal. Embolotherapy has the advantage of immediate and theoretically permanent cessation of bleeding without the risks of vasopressin infusion or prolonged catheterization (Table 9-3). For these reasons, the procedure has become widely popular as first-line therapy for acute gastrointestinal hemorrhage.[45,71,82] Even in the absence of extravasation, empiric embolization of the left gastric artery often is done to prevent recurrent bleeding in patients with massive upper gastrointestinal bleeding but negative angiograms.[83-85]

Angiodysplasia and arteriovenous malformations may respond to embolotherapy alone.[86,87] However, recurrent bleeding can occur, and those lesions must be removed operatively. In the case of right-sided angiodysplasia, a right hemicolectomy is performed to eliminate the bleeding lesion and any other occult lesions. Small bowel arteriovenous malformations, however, are often exceedingly difficult to find at surgery. The involved segment of bowel is much easier to locate if a coil is deposited in a distal feeding branch or a coaxial microcatheter is left in place for methylene blue injection during the operation.[88,89]

Embolotherapy is feasible because of the extensive intestinal collateral circulation (particularly in the upper tract) through arterial arcades, communications between vasa recta, and submucosal interconnections. However, embolization is risky in the setting of previous gastric or bowel surgery or radiation therapy or when the collateral circulation is otherwise inadequate.[90]

Technique. Embolotherapy has become much safer and simpler with the availability of coaxial catheter systems

TABLE 9-3   ADVANTAGES OF VASOPRESSIN VS. EMBOLOTHERAPY

	Vasopressin	Embolotherapy
Limited catheter manipulation	×	
Shorter overall procedure time		×
Immediate result		×
Better long-term success		×
Decreased complication rate		×
Access-related (catheter duration)		
Injury parent artery		
Non-target infusion		
Cardiac		
Systemic		

and microcoils. These devices allow precise placement of agents even through small or tortuous intestinal branches. A coaxial microcatheter is directed through the diagnostic catheter placed in the main trunk of the feeding artery. Care must be taken to minimize vasospasm. Since it is difficult to determine precisely which branches are supporting the bleeding site, sequential injection into multiple likely candidates often is necessary. The optimal location for placing embolic material is controversial. Early teaching favored proximal occlusion. Experts now recommend more distal embolization at the level of the vasa recta feeding the bleeding site (or just proximal to the vasa recta) to minimize the length of bowel at risk for ischemia (see Fig. 2-38).[82,91,92]

The most commonly used embolic agents are microcoils, Gelfoam pieces, and PVA particles. Recanalization seems to be more frequent when microcoils are used alone.[85] Large PVA particles have been used safely by some groups.[93] Smaller PVA particles or microspheres (less than 300 μm) should generally be avoided. Coils can be delivered with more precision and are permanent. Contrast is injected after each delivery. Embolization is continued until bleeding has stopped. The proximal mesenteric artery is restudied to be certain there is no extravasation through collateral vessels.

If a lesion is situated within an arcade fed by two mesenteric arteries, angiography is performed at both levels. For example, after embolizing the gastroduodenal artery for a duodenal ulcer hemorrhage, a superior mesenteric arteriogram is done to evaluate the inferior pancreaticoduodenal supply to the duodenum. Embolization of the other entrance to the arcade may be necessary, although this increases the risk of ischemia.[94,95]

Results. In recent series, embolotherapy successfully stopped gastrointestinal bleeding in about 80% of patients (Figs. 9-31 to 9-33).[45,71,87,93,96-101] Recurrent hemorrhage is uncommon (less than 20% in most series) (Box 9-5).[45,101] Rebleeding may be more frequent with inflammatory lesions and arteriovenous malformations. If it occurs, repeat angiography (and embolization) may improve success rates by identification of recanalized sites and new sources of bleeding (Fig. 9-34). In general, clinical success is more likely with embolization than with vasopressin therapy. However, angiodysplasias and arteriovenous malformations typically rebleed and require surgical removal.

Complications. Overall, embolotherapy is safer than vasopressin infusion. Major adverse events occur in less than 2% of patients. Self-limited subclinical bowel ischemia can be identified in a substantial number of patients by endoscopy or pathology.[99] Patients should be monitored closely for clinical signs of ischemia (e.g., abdominal pain, elevated serum lactate), which occurs in less than 20% of cases.[45,93,102,103] In many patients, small areas of infarction are well tolerated

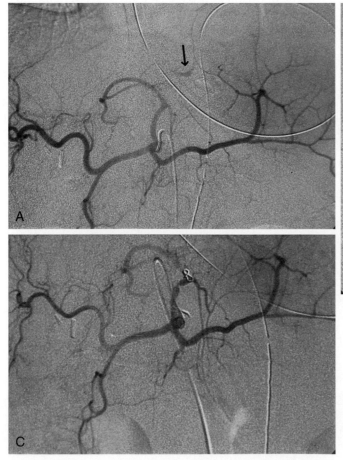

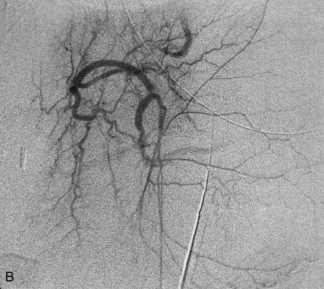

FIGURE 9-31 ■ Gastric fundus bleeding. **A,** Celiac arteriogram shows extravasation from a branch of the left gastric artery *(arrow).* **B,** Left gastric arteriogram confirms bleeding. Also note replaced left hepatic artery. **C,** After Gelfoam and microcoil embolization, bleeding has stopped.

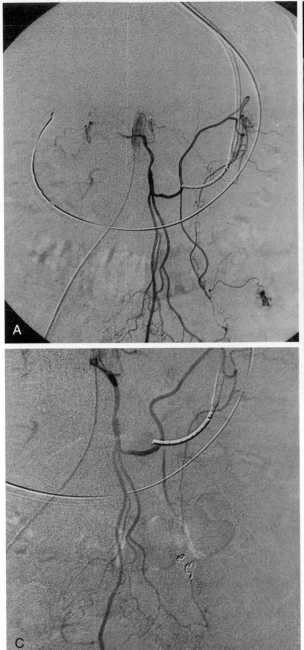

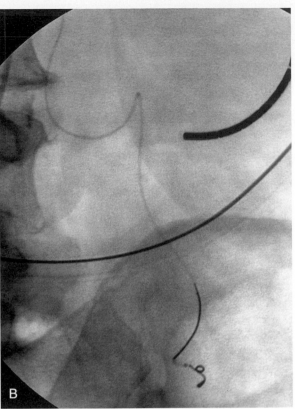

FIGURE 9-32 ■ Massive lower gastrointestinal hemorrhage was treated with microcoil embolization. **A,** The inferior mesenteric arteriogram shows extravasation in the distal left colon. **B,** A coaxial microcatheter has been advanced to a site proximal to the vasa recta supplying the bleed. A second microcoil is being deployed. **C,** Extravasation has stopped on repeat injection of the inferior mesenteric artery, with preservation of flow to the remainder of the bowel.

and do not require surgery. Most recent series report no cases of clinically significant bowel ischemia or infarction.

Surgical Therapy

Emergency operation for acute gastrointestinal bleeding has a mortality of up to 50%.[104,105] Surgery is necessary when the disease cannot be treated definitively by transcatheter means, as with arteriovenous malformations, or when the lesion is malignant. Even in these cases, transcatheter therapy may be used to stop or reduce bleeding and allow the operation to be postponed until the patient is stabilized and the bowel is cleansed.

Chronic and Occult Gastrointestinal Bleeding

Etiology

Almost every patient with gastrointestinal hemorrhage stops bleeding spontaneously or has a bleeding source identified and treated. However, about 5% of patients suffer from persistent, intermittent bleeding that may be difficult to localize (so-called "obscure" bleeding).[106] Arteriovenous malformations and neoplasms account for most of these cases (Box 9-6).[107,108] Most lesions are

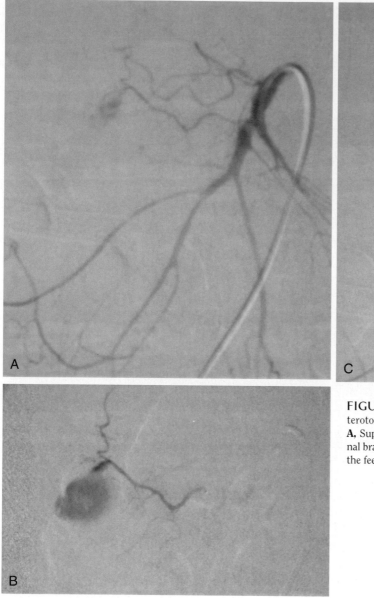

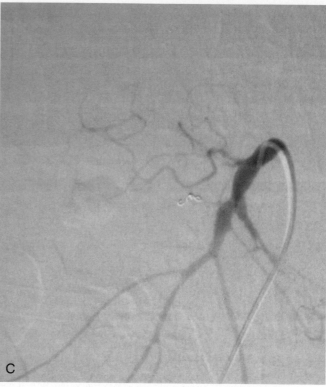

FIGURE 9-33 ◼ Duodenal hemorrhage after endoscopic sphincterotomy during endoscopic retrograde cholangiopancreatography. **A,** Superior mesenteric arteriogram shows extravasation from a duodenal branch of the first jejunal artery. **B,** A microcatheter is advanced into the feeding vessel. **C,** After embolization, hemorrhage has stopped.

BOX 9-5 ◼ Causes of Failure of Embolotherapy/
Vasopressin Therapy

Initial
Unable to catheterize main mesenteric artery (e.g., inferior mesenteric artery stenosis)
Unable to select branch vessel (spasm, tortuosity)
Uncorrectable coagulopathy
Catheter dislodgement (vasopressin infusion)

Delayed
Recanalization of embolized site or vasopressin-induced clot
Collateral flow
New bleeding site
Persistent coagulopathy
Multiorgan failure
Sepsis
Steroid therapy

---

found in the small bowel or ascending colon, which are the most difficult sites to inspect with fiberoptic endoscopy. However, video capsule endoscopy is showing promise as a method to detect bleeding lesions at these remote sites.[109]

Clinical Features

Patients typically have recurrent episodes of (usually lower) gastrointestinal bleeding that persist for months or years. Anemia is common. Some patients have undergone one or more operations to locate the bleeding source. Bleeding is typically not active at the time angiography is requested.

Imaging

Angiography. Most patients have been through an exhaustive workup before an angiogram is requested.

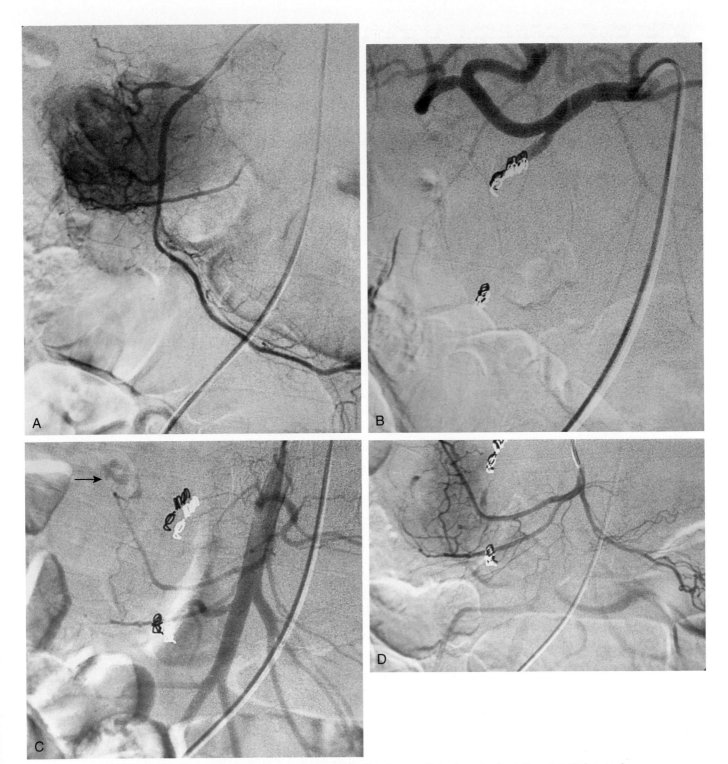

FIGURE 9-34 ■ Recurrent upper gastrointestinal bleeding due to collateral arcade circulation. **A,** Initial gastroduodenal arteriogram shows marked hypervascularity without frank extravasation. The feeding branches could not be selectively catheterized. **B,** Embolization was performed across the gastroduodenal artery. **C,** Patient developed recurrent bleeding. Repeat gastroduodenal arteriography confirmed persistent occlusion (not shown). Superior mesenteric arteriography is suspicious for bleeding from the inferior pancreaticoduodenal artery *(arrow)*. **D,** Selective catheterization confirms the bleeding. *Continued*

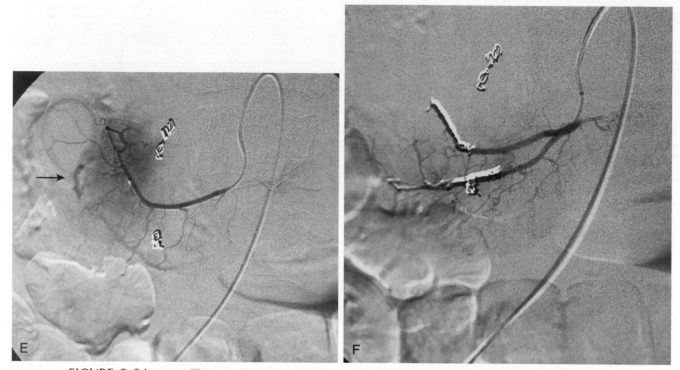

FIGURE 9-34 *Cont'd* ■ **E,** The first of two feeding vessels is selected up to the site of bleeding *(arrow).* **F,** After embolization of both distal vessels, bleeding has stopped.

The approach to patients with chronic, intermittent bleeding is similar to the study of acute gastrointestinal hemorrhage. A bleeding source (i.e., pathologic finding or extravasation) is found in about half of studies (see Fig. 9-29).[107-108] Provocative maneuvers can be used to induce hemorrhage, including heparinization, intra-arterial injection of vasodilators, and intra-arterial fibrinolytic infusion.[110-114] This heroic approach will undercover a bleeding site in more than one half of cases. Before attempting to induce bleeding, blood products and surgical backup should be available. It is worthwhile to repeat the angiogram if the result of the first study is negative for patients with this difficult problem.

BOX 9-6 ■ Causes of Chronic Gastrointestinal Bleeding

Arteriovenous malformation
Angiodysplasia (vascular ectasia)
Neoplasm
Visceral artery aneurysm
Polyp
Diverticulum (e.g., Meckel's)
Gastritis
Inflammatory bowel disease
Ulcer
Radiation enteritis

Treatment

Most lesions that cause chronic gastrointestinal hemorrhage of obscure origin require operative removal.

Inflammatory Diseases

Angiography is not used for the diagnosis of inflammatory disorders of the bowel unless certain complications occur, such as gastrointestinal bleeding or pseudoaneurysm formation. However, these conditions may be incidental findings with arteriography. For the most part, the acute inflammatory diseases show hypervascularity, increased parenchymal staining, and early, dense venous filling. In the chronic phase, narrowing and encasement of large and small arteries and veins may be found.

Neoplasms

Angiography plays no role in the evaluation of patients with suspected mesenteric neoplasms unless gastrointestinal bleeding occurs. Hypervascular intestinal tumors include leiomyomas, leiomyosarcomas, adenomas, adenocarcinomas with inflammatory reaction, and hypervascular metastases (e.g., choriocarcinoma, melanoma) (Fig. 9-35).[115] Adenocarcinomas and most metastatic lesions are hypovascular. *Carcinoid* of the small intestine has a characteristic appearance (Fig. 9-36). Because the tumor liberates hormones that incite an infiltrating, desmoplastic reaction in the mesentery, the arteries

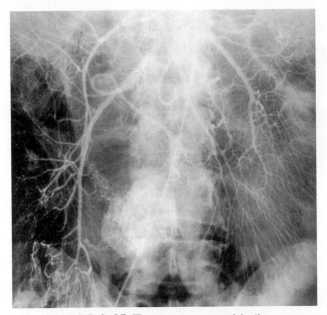

FIGURE 9-35 ■ Leiomyosarcoma of the ileum.

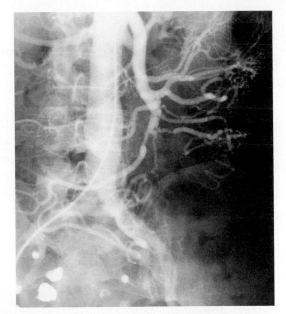

FIGURE 9-36 ■ Carcinoid of the small bowel. There is narrowing, encasement, and retraction of mesenteric branches within and around the tumor.

are retracted, narrowed, irregular, or obstructed.[116] Tumors outside the intestinal tract can invade mesenteric vessels (Fig. 9-37).

■ OTHER DISORDERS

Celiac Artery Compression (Median Arcuate Ligament) Syndrome

The root of the celiac artery is close to the median arcuate ligament, which connects the crura of the diaphragm. Mild to moderate compression of the superior aspect of the artery by this ligament is seen frequently on conventional, CT, or MR angiograms in patients without intestinal symptoms (Fig. 9-38).[117-121] A few patients with severe compression or occlusion of the artery also complain of abdominal pain, weight loss, and nausea. The syndrome is classically seen in young, asthenic women. Compression is exaggerated during expiration.

The relationship between celiac artery compression and the associated clinical syndrome is controversial. The other mesenteric arteries are usually patent in these patients, and the existing collateral circulation should be adequate to prevent intestinal ischemia. Nonetheless, symptoms have been attributed to visceral ischemia or to compression of the celiac neural plexus. Surgical treatment, which may include division of the crus, release of sympathetic nerve fibers, and revascularization, is often curative, although the results may not be durable.[122]

Aneurysms

Aneurysms of the mesenteric arteries are rare. Splenic and hepatic artery aneurysms, which are the most common

splanchnic aneurysms, are considered in Chapter 10.[123] *SMA* and *celiac artery aneurysms* are usually caused by atherosclerosis, infection, degenerative diseases, or trauma.[124] Some patients present with abdominal pain, although others are diagnosed by incidental findings on imaging studies. The natural history of these aneurysms is that of expansion, rupture, or thrombosis. Rupture is almost always associated with lack of calcification.[125] Surgery is recommended in most cases. However, stent-graft placement has been reported.[126]

Gastric, duodenal, or *pancreaticoduodenal artery pseudoaneurysm* is a rare complication of an adjacent inflammatory process (e.g., pancreatitis, peptic ulcer disease) or trauma.[127] Many of these patients present with gastrointestinal tract or

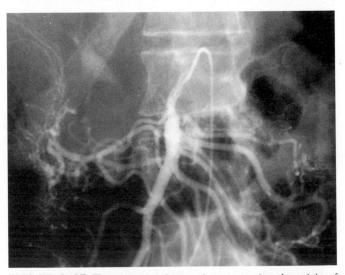

FIGURE 9-37 ■ Pancreatic adenocarcinoma encasing the origin of the superior mesenteric artery.

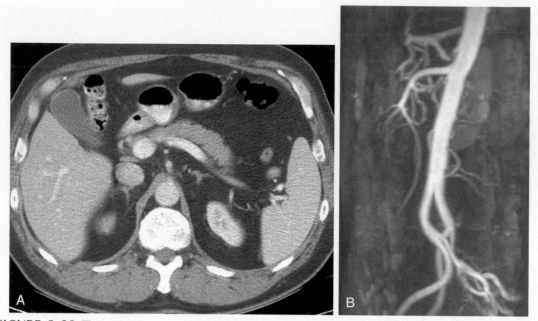

FIGURE 9-38 ■ Celiac artery compression in an asymptomatic patient. **A,** Transverse CT image reveals impingement of diaphragmatic crus on the superior aspect of the celiac artery origin. **B,** Gadolinium-enhanced MR angiogram in sagittal projection depicts proximal celiac artery stenosis.

intra-abdominal bleeding and abdominal pain (see Fig. 11-7). These aneurysms are sometimes lethal without treatment. The preferred therapy is transcatheter embolization.[128,129]

Vasculitis

Mesenteric arteritis is rare. A wide variety of small vessel vasculitides may cause nonspecific findings on CT and MR (segments of bowel wall thickening and enhancement, bowel distension, venous thrombosis) related to inflammation, ulcerations, ischemia, and perforation.[130] These include Wegener's granulomatosis, microscopic polyangiitis, Henoch-Schönlein purpura, collagen vascular diseases, and Behçet's syndrome.

Takayasu's arteritis is an inflammatory vasculitis of large- and medium-sized arteries (see Chapter 3).[131,132] Stenosis or, rarely, complete occlusion of the mesenteric arteries associated with abdominal aortic narrowing occurs in about 20% to 25% of cases.

Polyarteritis nodosa is a necrotizing vasculitis that can affect distal branches of the mesenteric arteries, producing multiple small saccular aneurysms (Fig. 9-39).[133] Some of these patients present with abdominal pain, gastrointestinal hemorrhage, or ischemia. Branches of the renal, hepatic, splenic, and pancreatic arteries often are involved.

Radiation arteritis can develop after high-dose radiation therapy for abdominal malignancies. The condition may lead to irregular narrowing and occlusion of mesenteric arteries and veins.[134]

Buerger's disease (i.e., *thromboangiitis obliterans*) is an occlusive vasculitis that primarily affects small vessels of the extremities (see Chapter 3). However, mesenteric artery involvement also has been described.[135]

Arteriovenous Malformations

Four types of abnormal arteriovenous communications can be seen in the mesenteric vessels: arteriovenous malformations, angiodysplasia, telangiectasias and angiomas, and arteriovenous fistulas.

Arteriovenous malformations are **congenital** lesions that can occur at any site in the intestinal tract. They may cause chronic, intermittent gastrointestinal hemorrhage (see Fig. 9-29). *Angiodysplasia* (i.e., vascular ectasia) is an **acquired**

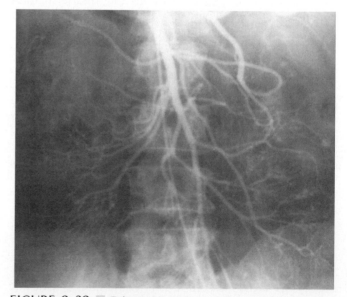

FIGURE 9-39 ■ Polyarteritis nodosa of the superior mesenteric artery branches with numerous microaneurysms.

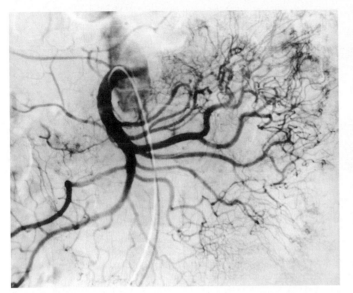

FIGURE 9-40 ■ Multiple telangiectasias of the jejunum in a patient with hereditary hemorrhagic telangiectasia.

anomaly of submucosal veins found primarily in the ascending colon (see Fig. 9-28). *Telangiectasias* and *angiomas* are usually associated with congenital or hereditary syndromes, including hereditary hemorrhagic telangiectasia, Klippel-Trenaunay syndrome, and blue rubber nevus syndrome.[136-138] In these disorders, multiple, punctate hypervascular lesions are typically scattered throughout the bowel (Fig. 9-40). In advanced cases, vascular tangles and arteriovenous shunting may be seen. *Arteriovenous fistulas* are acquired lesions that usually result from penetrating trauma.[139]

Trauma

Most injuries are caused by penetrating trauma, although SMA or superior mesenteric vein damage can occur with blunt or decelerating trauma or catheterization procedures.[140,141] Patients with penetrating trauma to the central mesenteric arteries usually die before reaching medical care. Those who survive present with massive hemoperitoneum or mesenteric hematoma and usually undergo emergency laparotomy without imaging evaluation. Trauma may also lead to vascular occlusion, arteriovenous fistula, or pseudoaneurysm. Isolated mesenteric artery injuries have been successfully treated with embolotherapy.[139,142]

Drug-Induced Vasospasm

Chronic ingestion of ergot derivatives can cause functional spasm at a variety of sites, including the extremities and mesenteric vessels (Fig. 9-41).[143] Typically, the patient has diffuse irregular narrowing of the proximal portions of the mesenteric branches. These findings resolve after the drug is stopped. Vasopressin therapy and nonocclusive mesenteric ischemia cause similar changes in intestinal vessels.

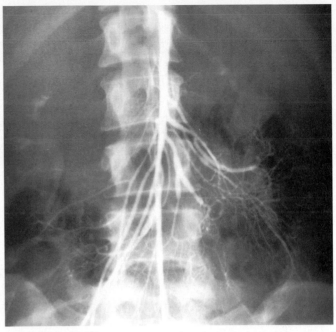

FIGURE 9-41 ■ Ergot arteritis. There is narrowing and beading of multiple branches of the superior mesenteric artery.

Segmental Arterial Mediolysis

This extremely rare noninflammatory condition, which may be related to fibromuscular dysplasia, results in patchy destruction of medial smooth muscles cells that are replaced by fibrin, collagen, and granulation tissue.[144-147] The weakened arterial wall is predisposed to aneurysms and spontaneous dissection (Fig. 9-42). The etiology is unknown. Unlike fibromuscular

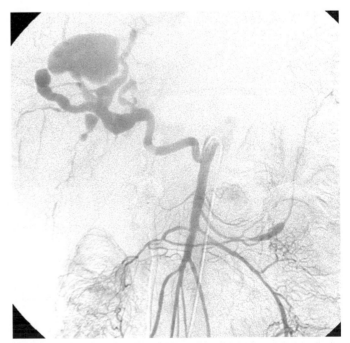

FIGURE 9-42 ■ Probable segmental arterial mediolysis. A fusiform aneurysm of the middle colic artery is identified. Also seen are multiple saccular aneurysms of branches of the hepatic artery.

dysplasia, this disorder primarily affects the visceral and coronary arteries. In the abdomen, patients present with vessel rupture and massive bleeding. Celiac artery branches are most commonly affected. Multiple lesions may be present.

Fibromuscular dysplasia can affect the mesenteric arteries, although this is extremely unusual.[148]

Coarctation Syndromes

The abdominal coarctation syndromes are rare congenital disorders that can narrow the abdominal aorta and its major branches (see Chapter 3). Abdominal coarctation is seen in patients with neurofibromatosis, congenital rubella, Williams syndrome, and tuberous sclerosis. Although renovascular hypertension from renal artery stenoses is common, mesenteric ischemia is rare.

REFERENCES

1. Collins P, ed: Embryology and development. In: Williams PL, Bannister LH, Berry MM, et al, eds. Gray's Anatomy, 38th ed. New York, Churchill Livingstone, 1995:318.
2. Gabella G, ed: Cardiovascular system. In: Williams PL, Bannister LH, Berry MM, et al, eds. Gray's Anatomy, 38th ed. New York, Churchill Livingstone, 1995:1548.
3. Kornblith PL, Boley SJ, Whitehouse BS: Anatomy of the splanchnic circulation. Surg Clin North Am 1992;72:1.
4. Nesebar RA, Kornblith PL, Pollard JJ, et al: Celiac and Superior Mesenteric Arteries: A Correlation of Angiograms and Dissections. Boston, Little, Brown, 1969.
5. Michels NA, Siddharth P, Kornblith PL, et al: Routes of collateral circulation of the gastrointestinal tract as ascertained in a dissection of 500 bodies. Int Surg 1968;49:8.
6. Park WM, Gloviczki P, Cherry KJ, et al: Contemporary management of acute mesenteric ischemia: factors associated with survival. J Vasc Surg 2002;35:445.
7. Kim AY, Ha HK: Evaluation of suspected mesenteric ischemia: efficacy of radiologic studies. Radiol Clin North Am 2003;41:327.
8. Hassoun Z, Lacrosse M, DeRonde T: Intestinal involvement in Buerger's disease. J Clin Gastroenterol 2001;32:85.
9. Osorio J, Farreras N, Ortiz De Zarate L, et al: Cocaine-induced mesenteric ischemia. Dig Surg 2000;17:648.
10. Bassiouny HS: Non-occlusive mesenteric ischemia. Surg Clin North Am 1997;77:319.
11. Kolkman JJ, Mensink PB: Non-occlusive mesenteric ischemia: a common disorder in gastroenterology and intensive care. Best Pract Res Clin Gastroenterol 2003;17:457.
12. Warshauer DM, Lee JKT, Maura MA et al: Superior mesenteric vein thrombosis with radiologically occult cause: a retrospective study of 43 cases. AJR Am J Roentgenol 2001;177:837.
13. Chang JB, Stein TA: Mesenteric ischemia: acute and chronic. Ann Vasc Surg 2003;17:323.
14. Kim JK, Ha HK, Byun JY, et al: CT differentiation of mesenteric ischemia due to vasculitis and thromboembolic disease. J Comput Assist Tomogr 2001;25:604.
15. Klein H-M, Lensing R, Klosterhalfen B, et al: Diagnostic imaging of mesenteric infarction. Radiology 1995;197:79.
16. Shirkhoda A, Konez O, Shetty AN, et al: Mesenteric circulation: three-dimensional MR angiography with a gadolinium-enhanced multiecho gradient-echo technique. Radiology 1997;202:257.
17. Taourel PG, Deneuville M, Pradel JA, et al: Acute mesenteric ischemia: diagnosis with contrast-enhanced CT. Radiology 1996;199:632.
18. Bradbury MS, Kavanagh PV, Bechtold RE, et al: Mesenteric venous thrombosis: diagnosis and non-invasive imaging. Radiographics 2002;22:527.
19. Bakal CW, Sprayregen S, Wolf EL: Radiology in intestinal ischemia: angiographic diagnosis and management. Surg Clin North Am 1992; 72:125.
20. Lock G, Schoelmerich J: Non-occlusive mesenteric ischemia. Hepatogastroenterology 1995;42:234.
21. Badiola CM, Scoppetta DJ: Rapid revascularization of an embolic superior mesenteric artery occlusion using pulse-spray pharmacomechanical thrombolysis with urokinase. AJR Am J Roentgenol 1997;169:55.
22. Rivitz SM, Geller SC, Hahn C, et al: Treatment of acute mesenteric venous thrombosis with transjugular intramesenteric urokinase infusion. J Vasc Interv Radiol 1995;6:219.
23. Vedantham S, Picus D, Sanchez LA, et al: Percutaneous management of ischemic complications in patients with type B aortic dissection. J Vasc Interv Radiol 2002;14:181.
24. Loomer DC, Johnson SP, Diffin DC, et al: Superior mesenteric artery stent placement in a patient with acute mesenteric ischemia. J Vasc Interv Radiol 1999;10:29.
25. Cunningham CG, Reilly LM, Stoney R: Chronic visceral ischemia. Surg Clin North Am 1992;72:231.
26. Moneta GL, Lee RW, Yeager RA, et al: Mesenteric duplex scanning: a blinded, prospective study. J Vasc Surg 1993;17:79.
27. Lim HK, Lee WJ, Kim SH, et al: Splanchnic arterial stenosis or occlusion: diagnosis at Doppler US. Radiology 1999;211:405.
28. Moneta GL: Screening for mesenteric vascular insufficiency and follow-up of mesenteric artery bypass procedures. Semin Vasc Surg 2001;14:186.
29. Li KC: MR angiography of abdominal ischemia. Semin Ultrasound CT MR 1996;17:352.
30. Burkart DJ, Johnson CD, Reading CC, et al: MR measurements of mesenteric venous flow: prospective evaluation in healthy volunteers and patients with suspected chronic mesenteric ischemia. Radiology 1995;194:801.
31. Calderon M, Reul GJ, Gregoric ID, et al: Long-term results of the surgical management of symptomatic chronic intestinal ischemia. J Cardiovasc Surg 1992;33:723.
32. Rose SC, Quigley TM, Raker EJ: Revascularization for chronic mesenteric ischemia: comparison of operative arterial bypass grafting and percutaneous transluminal angioplasty. J Vasc Interv Radiol 1995;6:339.
33. Hallisey MJ, Deschaine J, Illescas FF, et al: Angioplasty for the treatment of visceral ischemia. J Vasc Interv Radiol 1995;6:785.
34. Matsumoto AH, Tegtmeyer CJ, Fitzcharles EK, et al: Percutaneous transluminal angioplasty of visceral arterial stenoses: results and long-term clinical follow-up. J Vasc Interv Radiol 1995;6:165.
35. Sharafuddin MJ, Olson CH, Sun S, et al: Endovascular treatment of celiac and mesenteric arteries stenoses: applications and results. J Vasc Surg 2003;38:692.
36. Peene P, Vanrusselt J, Coenegrachts JL, et al: Strecker stent placement in the superior mesenteric artery for recurrent ischemic colitis. J Belge Radiol 1996;79:168.
37. Sheeran SR, Murphy TP, Khwaja A, et al: Stent placement for treatment of mesenteric artery stenoses or occlusions. J Vasc Interv Radiol 1999;10:861.
38. Knauer CM: Mallory-Weiss syndrome. Characteristics of 75 Mallory-Weiss lacerations in 528 patients with upper gastrointestinal hemorrhage. Gastroenterology 1976;71:5.
39. Sawlani V, Phadke RV, Baijal SS, et al: Arterial complications of pancreatitis and their radiologic management. Australas Radiol 1996;40:381.
40. Goldstone J: The infected infra-renal aortic graft. Acta Chir Scand 1987;538:72.
41. Rosenbaum A, Siegelman SS, Sprayregen S: The bleeding marginal ulcer. Catheterization diagnosis and therapy. AJR Am J Roentgenol 1975;125:812.
42. Oglevie SB, Smith DC, Mera SS: Bleeding marginal ulcers: angiographic evaluation. Radiology 1990;174:943.
43. Durham JD, Kumpe DA, Rothbarth LJ, et al: Dieulafoy disease: arteriographic findings and treatment. Radiology 1990;174:937.
44. Dasgupta R, Davies NJ, Williamson RC, et al: Haemosuccus pancreaticus: treatment by arterial embolization. Clin Radiol 2002;57:1021.
45. Sebrechts C, Bookstein JJ: Embolization in the management of lower gastrointestinal hemorrhage. Semin Intervent Radiol 1988;5:39.
46. Meyers MA, Alonso DR, Baer JW: Pathogenesis of massively bleeding colonic diverticulosis: new observations. AJR Am J Roentgenol 1976; 127:901.
47. Athanasoulis CA, Baum S, Roesch J, et al: Mesenteric arterial infusions of vasopressin for hemorrhage from colonic diverticulosis. Am J Surg 1975;129:212.

48. Boley SJ, Brandt LJ: Vascular ecstasias of the colon—1986. Dig Dis Sci 1986;31(9 Suppl):26S.
49. Sharma VS, Valji K, Bookstein JJ: Gastrointestinal hemorrhage in AIDS: arteriographic diagnosis and transcatheter treatment. Radiology 1992;185:447.
50. Alavi A: Detection of gastrointestinal bleeding with ^{99m}Tc-sulfur colloid. Semin Nucl Med 1982;12:126.
51. Srivastava SC, Chervu LR: Radionuclide-labeled red blood cells: current status and future prospects. Semin Nucl Med 1984;14:68.
52. Smith R, Copely DJ, Bolen FH: ^{99m}Tc RBC scintigraphy: correlation of gastrointestinal bleeding rates with scintigraphic findings. AJR Am J Roentgenol 1987;148:869.
53. Chandeysson PL, Hanson RJ, Watson CE, et al: Minimum gastrointestinal bleeding rate detectable by abdominal scintigraphy (abstract). J Nucl Med 1983;24:P97.
54. Nusbaum M, Baum S: Radiographic demonstration of unknown sites of gastrointestinal bleeding. Surg Forum 1963;14:374.
55. Zuckerman DA, Bocchini TP, Birnbaum EH: Massive hemorrhage in the lower gastrointestinal tract in adults: diagnostic imaging and intervention. AJR Am J Roentgenol 1993;161:703.
56. Bunker SR, Lull RJ, Tanasescu DE, et al: Scintigraphy of gastrointestinal hemorrhage: superiority of ^{99m}Tc red blood cells over ^{99m}Tc sulfur colloid. AJR Am J Roentgenol 1984;143:543.
57. Maurer AH, Rodman MS, Vitti RA, et al: Gastrointestinal bleeding: improved localization with cine scintigraphy. Radiology 1992;185:187.
58. Hunter JM, Pezim ME: Limited value of technetium 99m-labeled red cell scintigraphy in localization of lower gastrointestinal bleeding. Am J Surg 1990;159:504.
59. Nusbaum M, Baum S, Blakemore W, et al: Demonstration of intraabdominal bleeding by selective arteriography. JAMA 1965;191:117.
60. Rosen RJ, Sanchez G: Angiographic diagnosis and management of gastrointestinal hemorrhage. Current concepts. Radiol Clin North Am 1994;32:951.
61. Baum S, Athanasoulis CA, Waltman AC, et al: Angiodysplasia of the right colon: a cause of gastrointestinal bleeding. AJR Am J Roentgenol 1977;129:789.
62. Martin EC, Laffey KJ, Bixon R: Recanalization of the superior mesenteric vein for massive bleeding in Crohn disease. J Vasc Interv Radiol 1995;6:703.
63. Whitaker SC, Gregson RHS: The role of angiography in the investigation of acute or chronic gastrointestinal haemorrhage. Clin Radiol 1993;47:382.
64. Browder W, Cerise EJ, Litwin MS: Impact of emergency angiography in massive lower gastrointestinal bleeding. Ann Surg 1986;204:530.
65. Rahn NH III, Tishler JM, Han SY, et al: Diagnostic and interventional angiography in acute gastrointestinal hemorrhage. Radiology 1982;143:361.
66. Allison DJ, Hemingway AP, Cunningham DA: Angiography in gastrointestinal bleeding. Lancet 1982;2:30.
67. Wagner HE, Stain SC, Gilg M, et al: Systematic assessment of massive bleeding of the lower part of the gastrointestinal tract. Surg Gynecol Obstet 1992;175:445.
68. Sos TA, Lee JG, Wixson D, et al: Intermittent bleeding from minute to minute in acute massive gastrointestinal hemorrhage: arteriographic demonstration. AJR Am J Roentgenol 1978;131:1015.
69. Baum S, Athanasoulis CA, Waltman AC: Angiographic diagnosis and control of large-bowel bleeding. Dis Colon Rectum 1974;17:447.
70. Davis GB, Bookstein JJ, Coel MN: Advantage of intraarterial over intravenous vasopressin infusion in gastrointestinal hemorrhage. AJR Am J Roentgenol 1977;128:733.
71. Gomes AS, Lois JF, McCoy RD: Angiographic treatment of gastrointestinal hemorrhage: comparison of vasopressin infusion and embolization. AJR Am J Roentgenol 1986;146:1031.
72. Waltman AC, Greenfield AJ, Novelline RA, et al: Pyloroduodenal bleeding and intraarterial vasopressin: clinical results. AJR Am J Roentgenol 1979;133:643.
73. Ledermann HP, Schoch E, Jost R: Superselective coil embolization in acute gastrointestinal hemorrhage: personal experience in 10 patients and review of the literature. J Vasc Interv Radiol 1998;9:753.
74. Prochaska JM, Flye MW, Johnsrude IS: Left gastric artery embolization for control of gastric bleeding: a complication. Radiology 1973;107:521.
75. Baum S, Nusbaum M: The control of gastrointestinal hemorrhage by selective mesenteric arterial infusion of vasopressin. Radiology 1971;98:497.
76. Clark RA, Colley DP, Eggers FM: Acute arterial gastrointestinal hemorrhage: efficacy of transcatheter control. AJR Am J Roentgenol 1981;136:1185.
77. Eckstein MR, Kelemouridis V, Athanasoulis CA, et al: Gastric bleeding: therapy with intraarterial vasopressin and transcatheter embolization. Radiology 1984;152:643.
78. Roesch J, Dotter CT, Antonovic R: Selective vasoconstrictor infusion in the management of arterio-capillary gastrointestinal hemorrhage. AJR Am J Roentgenol 1972;116:279.
79. Baum S, Roesch J, Dotter CT, et al: Selective mesenteric arterial infusions in the management of massive diverticular hemorrhage. N Engl J Med 1973;288:1269.
80. Conn HO, Ramsby GR, Storer EH: Selective intra-arterial vasopressin in the treatment of upper gastrointestinal hemorrhage. Gastroenterology 1972;63:634.
81. Roberts C, Maddison FE: Partial mesenteric arterial occlusion with subsequent ischemic bowel damage due to pitressin infusion. AJR Am J Roentgenol 1976;126:829.
82. Darcy M: Treatment of lower gastrointestinal bleeding: vasopressin infusion versus embolization. J Vasc Interv Radiol 2003;14:535.
83. Lang EV, Picus D, Marx MV, et al: Massive upper gastrointestinal hemorrhage with normal findings at arteriography: value of prophylactic embolization of the left gastric artery. AJR Am J Roentgenol 1992;158:547.
84. Morris DC, Nichols DM, Connell DG, et al: Embolization of the left gastric artery in the absence of angiographic extravasation. Cardiovasc Intervent Radiol 1986;9:195.
85. Aina R, Oliva VL, Therasse E, et al: Arterial embolotherapy for upper gastrointestinal hemorrhage: outcome assessment. J Vasc Interv Radiol 2001;12:195.
86. Defreyne L, Vanlangenhove P, DeVos M, et al: Embolization as a first approach with endoscopically unmanageable acute nonvariceal gastrointestinal hemorrhage. Radiology 2001;218:739.
87. Funaki B, Kostelic JK, Lorenz J, et al: Superselective microcoil embolization of colonic hemorrhage. AJR Am J Roentgenol 2001;177:829.
88. Athanasoulis CA, Moncure AC, Greenfield AJ, et al: Intraoperative localization of small bowel bleeding sites with combined use of angiographic methods and methylene blue injection. Surgery 1980;87:77.
89. Schmidt SP, Boskind JF, Smith DC, et al: Angiographic localization of small bowel angiodysplasia with use of platinum coils. J Vasc Interv Radiol 1993;4:737.
90. Roesch J, Keller FS, Kozak B, et al: Gelfoam powder embolization of the left gastric artery in treatment of massive small-vessel gastric bleeding. Radiology 1984;151:365.
91. Palmaz JC, Walter JF, Cho KJ: Therapeutic embolization of the small-bowel arteries. Radiology 1984;152:377.
92. Okazaki M, Furui S, Higashihara H, et al: Emergent embolotherapy of small intestinal hemorrhage. Gastrointest Radiol 1992;17:223.
93. Guy GE, Shetty PC, Sharma RP, et al: Acute lower gastrointestinal hemorrhage: treatment by superselective embolization with polyvinyl alcohol particles. AJR Am J Roentgenol 1992;159:521.
94. Bell SD, Lau KY, Sniderman KW: Synchronous embolization of the gastroduodenal artery and the inferior pancreaticoduodenal artery in patients with massive duodenal hemorrhage. J Vasc Interv Radiol 1995;6:531.
95. Okazaki M, Higashihara H, Ono H, et al: Embolotherapy of massive duodenal hemorrhage. Gastrointest Radiol 1992;17:319.
96. Uflacker R: Transcatheter embolization for treatment of acute lower gastrointestinal bleeding. Acta Radiol 1987;28:425.
97. Encarnacion CE, Kadir S, Beam CA, et al: Gastrointestinal bleeding: treatment with gastrointestinal arterial embolization. Radiology 1992;183:505.
98. Patel TH, Cordts PR, Abcarian P, et al: Will transcatheter embolotherapy replace surgery in the treatment of gastrointestinal bleeding? Curr Surg 2001;58:323.
99. Bandi R, Shetty PC, Sharma RP, et al: Superselective arterial embolization for the treatment of lower gastrointestinal hemorrhage. J Vasc Interv Radiol 2001;12:1399.
100. Kuo WT, Lee DE, Saad WE, et al: Superselective microcoil embolization for the treatment of lower gastrointestinal hemorrhage. J Vasc Interv Radiol 2003;14:1503.
101. Schenker MP, Duszak R, Soulen MC, et al: Upper gastrointestinal hemorrhage and transcatheter embolotherapy: clinical and technical

factors impacting success and survival. J Vasc Interv Radiol 2001; 12:1263.

102. Peck DJ, McLoughlin RF, Hughson MN: Percutaneous embolotherapy of lower gastrointestinal hemorrhage. J Vasc Interv Radiol 1998;9:747.

103. Rosenkrantz H, Bookstein JJ, Rosen RJ, et al: Postembolic colonic infarction. Radiology 1982;142:47.

104. Boley SJ, DiBiase A, Brandt LJ, et al: Lower intestinal bleeding in the elderly. Am J Surg 1979;137:57.

105. Giacchino JL, Geis WP, Pickleman JR, et al: Changing perspectives in massive lower intestinal hemorrhage. Surgery 1979;86:368.

106. Steger AC, Spencer J: Obscure gastrointestinal bleeding. Br Med J 1988;296:3.

107. Rollins ES, Picus D, Hicks ME, et al: Angiography is useful in detecting the source of chronic gastrointestinal bleeding of obscure origin. AJR Am J Roentgenol 1991;156:385.

108. Lau WY, Ngan H, Chu KW, et al: Repeat selective visceral angiography in patients with gastrointestinal bleeding of obscure origin. Br J Surg 1989;76:226.

109. Costamagna G, Shah SK, Riccioni ME, et al: A prospective trial comparing small bowel radiographs and video capsule endoscopy for suspected small bowel disease. Gastroenterology 2002;123:999.

110. Koval G, Benner KG, Roesch J, et al: Aggressive angiographic diagnosis in acute lower gastrointestinal hemorrhage. Dig Dis Sci 1987;32:248.

111. Roesch J, Keller FS, Wawrukiewicz AS, et al: Pharmacoangiography in the diagnosis of recurrent massive lower gastrointestinal bleeding. Radiology 1982;145:615.

112. Glickerman DJ, Kowdley KV, Rosch J: Urokinase in gastrointestinal tract bleeding. Radiology 1988;168:375.

113. Reeves TQ, Osborne TM, List AR, et al: Dieulafoy disease: localization with thrombolysis-assisted angiography. J Vasc Interv Radiol 1993;4:119.

114. Ryan JM, Key SM, Dumbleton SA, et al: Nonlocalized lower gastrointestinal bleeding: provocative bleeding studies with intraarterial tPA, heparin, and tolazoline. J Vasc Interv Radiol 2001;12:1273.

115. Ramer M, Mitty HA, Baron MG: Angiography in leiomyomatous neoplasms of the small bowel. AJR Am J Roentgenol 1971;113:263.

116. Boijsen E, Kaude J, Tylen U: Radiologic diagnosis of ileal carcinoid tumors. Acta Radiol 1974;15:65.

117. Lee VS, Morgan JN, Tan AG, et al: Celiac artery compression by the median arcuate ligament: a pitfall of end-expiratory MR imaging. Radiology 2003;228:437.

118. Bech FR: Celiac artery compression syndromes. Surg Clin North Am 1997;77:409.

119. Taylor DC, Moneta GL, Crammer MM, et al: Extrinsic compression of the celiac artery by the median arcuate ligament of the diaphragm: diagnosis by duplex ultrasound. J Vasc Technol 1987;11:236.

120. Takach TJ, Livesay JJ, Reul GJ Jr, et al: Celiac compression syndrome: tailored therapy based on intraoperative findings. J Am Coll Surg 1996;183:606.

121. Holland AJ, Ibach EG: Long-term review of coeliac axis compression syndrome. Ann R Coll Surg Engl 1996;78:470.

122. Geelkerken RH, vanBockel JH, deRoos WK, et al: Coeliac artery compression syndrome: the effect of decompression. Br J Surg 1990;77:807.

123. Graham JM, McCollum CH, DeBakey ME: Aneurysms of the splanchnic arteries. Am J Surg 1980;140:797.

124. Stanley JC, Wakefield TW, Graham LM, et al: Clinical importance and management of splanchnic artery aneurysms. J Vasc Surg 1986;3:836.

125. Stone WM, Abbas M, Cherry KJ, et al: Superior mesenteric artery aneurysms: is presence an indication for intervention? J Vasc Surg 2002;36:234.

126. Appel N, Duncan JR, Schuerer DJ: Percutaneous stent-graft treatment of superior mesenteric and internal iliac artery pseudoaneurysms. J Vasc Interv Radiol 2003;14:917.

127. Eckhauser FE, Stanley JC, Zelenock GB, et al: Gastroduodenal and pancreaticoduodenal artery aneurysms: a complication of pancreatitis causing spontaneous gastrointestinal hemorrhage. Surgery 1980; 88:335.

128. Guijt M, Delden OM, Koedam NA, et al: Rupture of true aneurysms of the pancreaticoduodenal arcade: treatment with transcatheter arterial embolization. Cardiovasc Intervent Radiol 2003;26:166.

129. Boudghene F, L'Hermine C, Bigot J-M: Arterial complications of pancreatitis: diagnostic and therapeutic aspects in 104 cases. J Vasc Interv Radiol 1993;4:551.

130. Ha HK, Lee SH, Rha SE, et al: Radiologic features of vasculitis involving the gastrointestinal tract. Radiographics 2000;20:779.

131. Yamato M, Lecky JW, Hiramatsu K, et al: Takayasu arteritis: radiographic and angiographic findings in 59 patients. Radiology 1986; 161:329.

132. Park JH, Han MC, Kim SH, et al: Takayasu arteritis: angiographic findings and results of angioplasty. AJR Am J Roentgenol 1989;153:1069.

133. Chudacek Z: Angiographic diagnosis of polyarteritis nodosa of the liver, kidney, and mesentery. Br J Radiol 1967;40:864.

134. Dencker H, Holmdahl KH, Lunderquist A, et al: Mesenteric angiography in patients with radiation injury of the bowel after pelvic irradiation. AJR Am J Roentgenol 1972;114:476.

135. Broide E, Scapa E, Peer A, et al: Buerger's disease presenting as acute small bowel ischemia. Gastroenterology 1993;104:1192.

136. Ghahremani GG, Kangarloo H, Volberg F, et al: Diffuse cavernous hemangioma of the colon in the Klippel-Trenaunay syndrome. Radiology 1976;118:673.

137. Nyman U, Boijsen E, Lindstrom C, et al: Angiography in angiomatous lesions of the gastrointestinal tract. Acta Radiol 1980;21:21.

138. Baker AL, Kahn PC, Binder SC, et al: Gastrointestinal bleeding due to blue rubber bleb nevus syndrome: a case diagnosed by angiography. Gastroenterology 1971;61:530.

139. Repasky RG, Tisnado J, Freedman AM: Transcatheter embolization of a superior mesenteric artery pseudoaneurysm and arteriovenous fistula. J Vasc Interv Radiol 1993;4:241.

140. Mullins RJ, Huckfeldt R, Trunkey DD: Abdominal vascular injuries. Surg Clin North Am 1996;76:813.

141. Bourland WA, Kispert JF, Hyde GL, et al: Trauma to the proximal superior mesenteric artery: a case report and review of the literature. J Vasc Surg 1992;15:669.

142. Gabata T, Matsui O, Nakamura Y, et al: Transcatheter embolization of traumatic mesenteric hemorrhage. J Vasc Interv Radiol 1994;5:891.

143. Greene FL, Ariyan S, Stansel HC Jr: Mesenteric and peripheral vascular ischemia secondary to ergotism. Surgery 1977;81:176.

144. LaBerge JM, Kerlan RK Jr: Segmental arterial mediolysis (SAM) resulting in spontaneous dissections of the middle colic and left renal arteries and occlusion of the SMA. J Vasc Interv Radiol 1999;10:509.

145. Slavin RE, Saeki K, Bhagavan B, et al: Segmental arterial mediolysis: a precursor to fibromuscular dysplasia? Mod Pathol 1995;8:287.

146. Lee SI, Chew FS: Splanchnic segmental arterial mediolysis. AJR Am J Roentgenol 1998;170:122.

147. Chan RJ, Goodman TA, Aretz TH, et al: Segmental mediolytic arteriopathy of the splenic and hepatic arteries mimicking systemic necrotizing vasculitis. Arthritis Rheum 1998;41:935.

148. Sandmann W, Schulte KM: Multivisceral fibromuscular dysplasia in childhood: case report and review of the literature. Ann Vasc Surg 2000;14:496.

10

Hepatic, Splenic, and Portal Vascular Systems

■ ARTERIOGRAPHY AND VENOGRAPHY

Techniques for celiac and superior mesenteric arteriography are described in Chapter 9. Splenic or common hepatic arteriography is performed with a variety of catheters, including cobra and sidewinder shapes. Steerable, hydrophilic guide-wires simplify catheter placement. Alternatively, high-flow coaxial microcatheters are used to select the main splenic or hepatic arteries and their branches.

The hepatic veins are studied from an internal jugular vein approach using a cobra or headhunter catheter. When the femoral route is required, a straight catheter and tip-deflecting wire or a cobra catheter is used. Wedged hepatic manometry and venography are done by inflating a balloon occlusion catheter within an hepatic vein branch. Pressure measurements should be obtained before contrast injection, which may spuriously elevate the sinusoidal pressure. A flat waveform indicates a wedged position. Overinjection can produce subcapsular extravasation and liver perforation. Retrograde filling of the portal vein is enhanced when CO_2 is used as the contrast agent (30 to 60 mL of gas injected rapidly).

The splenic, superior mesenteric, and portal veins are visualized on the late phases of celiac or superior mesenteric arteriography ("indirect portography"). Direct splenoportography and transhepatic portography are occasionally required for the evaluation of patients with portal hypertension. The original description of splenoportography involved placement of a large caliber needle or Teflon sheath into the substance of the spleen from a mid-axillary subcostal approach. Iodinated contrast is injected during image acquisition, and the tract is embolized with Gelfoam during catheter withdrawal. Many practitioners now prefer to use CO_2 (15 to 20 mL injected over 2 to 3 seconds). Because of the low viscosity of the gas, very-small-caliber needles (25 to 27 gauge, placed with ultrasound guidance) can be used to minimize the risk of hemorrhage occasionally noted with larger catheters.[1-3]

■ ANATOMY

Development

The liver bud develops between the pericardial cavity and the stalk of the primitive yolk sac.[4] Liver cords insinuate between tributaries of the *vitelline* and *umbilical veins* to form the hepatic sinusoids. Branches of the right vitelline veins around the duodenum develop into the central portal veins.[5] The right umbilical vein involutes, and the left umbilical vein becomes the primary inflow vessel to the liver. The hepatic venous outflow is directed toward the upper portion of the right vitelline vein, which ultimately forms the hepatic veins and the intrahepatic portion of the inferior vena cava (IVC). The *ductus venosus* connects the left umbilical vein (portal venous inflow) to the right vitelline vein (hepatic outflow). Shortly after birth, the ductus venosus and left umbilical vein close and form the *ligamentum venosum* and *ligamentum teres*, respectively.

Normal Anatomy

Liver

With the advent of living-related split-liver donor transplants, more ambitious surgical techniques for segmental hepatic resection, transcatheter methods for treatment of liver tumors, a detailed understanding of the normal, variant, and collateral hepatic circulations is critical for the vascular interventionalist. For preoperative planning, high-quality CT or MR arteriography and venography are highly accurate.[6-9] For transarterial therapy, selective digital angiography is required, including celiac and superior mesenteric arteriography, right and left hepatic arteriography, and (occasionally) gastroduodenal arteriography.[10]

The liver is divided into *right* and *left lobes* separated by the major fissure. The right lobe has anterior and posterior segments; the left lobe has medial and lateral segments.

The *caudate lobe* is anatomically distinct from the right and left lobes. By convention, segmental anatomy is based on the original system of Couinaud demarcated by the three main hepatic veins and a transverse plane at the level of the portal vein bifurcation (Fig. 10-1).[11,12] However, the relationship between these landmarks identified on cross-sectional imaging and the true anatomic segmental anatomy is only approximate.[13]

The liver is supplied by the common hepatic artery and portal vein. Normally, about three fourths of the blood supply to the liver comes from the portal vein. Any reduction in hepatic arterial or portal venous blood flow leads to a compensatory increase in flow through the companion system. The biliary tree is nourished by branches of the hepatic arteries.

The *common hepatic artery* arises from the *celiac artery* (Fig. 10-2). After giving off the *gastroduodenal artery*, it

becomes the *proper hepatic artery*. This vessel enters the porta hepatis and divides into the *right hepatic artery* (RHA) and *left hepatic artery* (LHA), which feed their respective lobes. The RHA supplies segments V to VIII (and sometimes segment I, caudate lobe). The LHA supplies segments II, III, IVa, and IVb. The inconsistent *middle hepatic artery* (which, if present, feeds segments IVa and IVb) usually originates from the right hepatic artery or forms a true trifurcation. Variations in hepatic arterial anatomy are common (see below). Although the hepatic arteries are considered end-arteries, intrahepatic and extrahepatic anastomoses do exist. The origins of important branches are outlined in Table 10-1.

The *portal vein* (PV) is formed by the confluence of the *superior mesenteric vein* (SMV) and *splenic vein* (Fig. 10-3).[14] It is valveless. Normal main portal vein pressure is about 3 to 5 mm Hg. The SMV has numerous jejunal, ileal, and colonic tributaries. The *inferior mesenteric vein* (IMV) joins the splenic

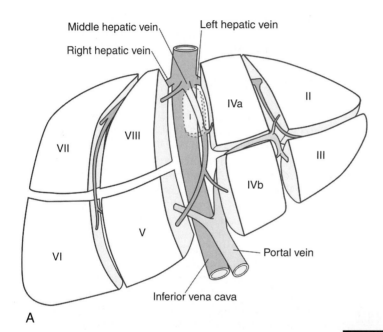

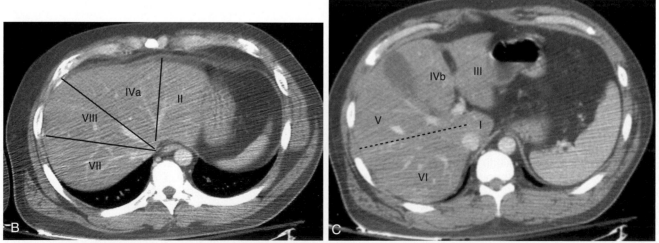

FIGURE 10-1 ▪ Segmental anatomy of the liver. **A,** Schematic drawing shows segmental divisions along with portal vein inflow and hepatic vein outflow. Segment I (caudate lobe) lies posterior to segments III and IV and in front of the inferior vena cava. CT scans through the upper (**B**) and lower (**C**) aspects of the liver, with segments noted. (**A,** Adapted with permission from the website of the American Hepato-Pancreato-Biliary Association, www.ahpba.org.)

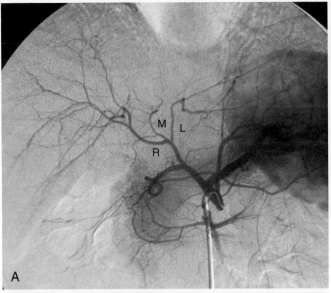

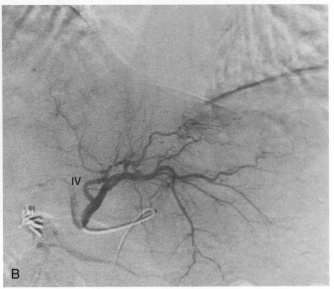

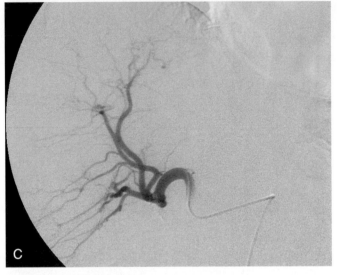

FIGURE 10-2 ■ Normal hepatic arterial anatomy. **A,** Celiac arteriography shows right (R), middle (M), and left (L) hepatic arteries. Normal left (**B**) and right (**C**) hepatic arteriograms.

vein or the SMV.[15] The right gastroepiploic, pancreaticoduodenal, and right colonic veins often merge into a common *gastrocolic trunk* that drains into the right side of the SMV near its confluence with the PV. The *right* and *left gastric (coronary) veins* enter the superior surface of the main portal or central splenic vein. Multiple coronary veins often exist.

The portal vein runs in front of the IVC and behind the head of the pancreas before entering the liver. The PV bifurcation is outside the liver capsule in about half of the population.[16] The right and left PVs and their branches follow the hepatic artery into the liver. The left PV supplies segments I to IV.[17] The right anterior PV supplies segments V and VIII; the right posterior PV supplies segments VI and VII. The caudate lobe is usually fed by branches of the left PV. The remnant of the umbilical vein (ligamentum teres) is connected to the left PV. A patent paraumbilical vein arising from the **left** PV is sometimes seen in patients with portal hypertension.

TABLE 10-1	IMPORTANT BRANCHES OF THE HEPATIC ARTERIES

Vessel	Typical and Atypical Origins
Right gastric artery	PHA
	LHA
	CHA, GDA, RHA, MHA
Cystic artery	RHA
	Replaced/accessory RHA
	LHA or CHA
	GDA
Supraduodenal artery	GDA, CHA, LHA, RHA, cystic
Dorsal pancreatic artery	SA
	Celiac artery, RHA, SMA
Falciform artery	MHA, LHA

CHA, common hepatic artery; GDA, gastroduodenal artery; LGA, left gastric artery; LHA, left hepatic artery; MHA, middle hepatic artery; PHA, proper hepatic artery; RHA, right hepatic artery; SA, splenic artery; SMA, superior mesenteric artery.

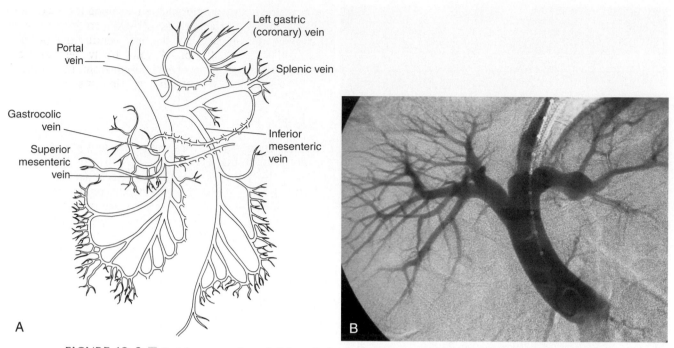

FIGURE 10-3 ▪ Portal venous anatomy. **A,** Schematic drawing. **B,** Direct transhepatic portogram through an obstructed transjugular intrahepatic portosystemic shunt. (**A,** From Lundell C, Kadir S: The portal venous system and hepatic vein. In: Kadir S, ed. Atlas of Normal and Variant Angiographic Anatomy. Philadelphia, WB Saunders, 1991:370.)

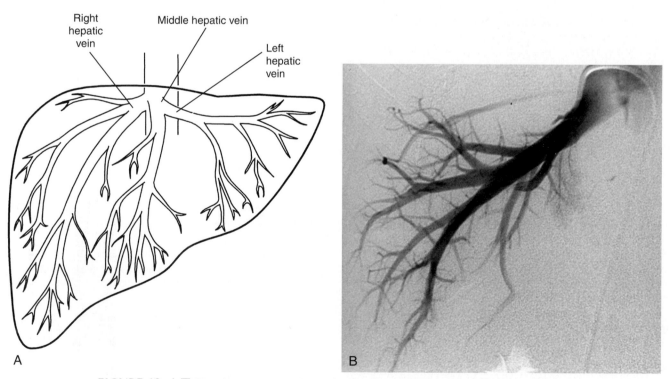

FIGURE 10-4 ▪ Hepatic venous anatomy. **A,** Schematic drawing. **B,** Normal right hepatic venogram.

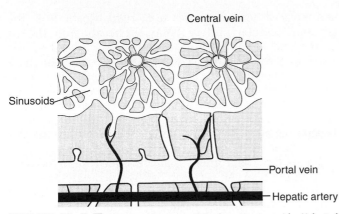

FIGURE 10-5 ■ Microarchitecture of the hepatic sinusoids. (Adapted from Cho KJ, Lunderquist A: The peribiliary vascular plexus: the microvascular architecture of the bile duct in the rabbit and in clinical cases. Radiology 1983;147:357.)

The liver is drained by the hepatic veins. The *right* and *left hepatic veins* run between the segments of the right and left lobes of the liver, and the *middle hepatic vein* lies in the main lobar fissure (Fig. 10-4). These vessels enter the IVC within several centimeters of the diaphragm. The right hepatic vein (draining segments VI and VII) joins the right posterolateral surface of the IVC. The middle hepatic vein (draining segments V and VIII) and left hepatic vein (draining segments II and III) confluence enters the anteromedial surface of the IVC. Segments IVa and IVb are drained by the left or middle hepatic vein. The caudate lobe empties separately into the intrahepatic IVC.

The liver parenchyma is composed of hepatic *lobules*, which contain the hepatocytes and sinusoidal spaces that form the functional units of the liver (Fig. 10-5).[18] Neighboring lobules are organized into *acini*. Hepatic arterial, portal venous, and biliary duct branches run along the edges of the lobules. Hepatic arterioles feed the sinusoids directly and through communications with portal venules that perforate the lobules. Normally, blood flows freely between acini. Central veins at the core of each lobule drain the sinusoids. These venules coalesce into the hepatic veins.

Spleen

The *splenic artery* supplies the spleen and portions of the pancreas and stomach (Fig. 10-6).[19] It runs along the superior edge of the pancreas along with the splenic vein. With advancing age, the splenic artery can become extremely tortuous. Near the splenic hilum, the artery usually divides into superior and inferior branches. *Superior* and *inferior polar arteries* often arise from the mid-splenic artery and supply their respective splenic segments. The *left gastroepiploic artery* originates from the distal inferior polar artery and then courses along the greater curvature of the stomach. Numerous *short gastric branches* feed the fundus of the stomach. The splenic artery also has numerous branches to the body and tail of the pancreas. The largest of these vessels are the *dorsal pancreatic artery* (which may originate on the celiac trunk) and the *pancreatica magna artery* (see Fig. 10-6).

The *splenic vein* lies behind the upper border of the pancreas below the splenic artery (see Fig. 10-6B). Its tributaries include the short gastric, left gastroepiploic, pancreatic, and inferior mesenteric veins (see Fig. 10-3).

Variant Anatomy

Anomalies of hepatic artery origin and number are common (Table 10-2).[10,20-23] The most frequent variants are accessory

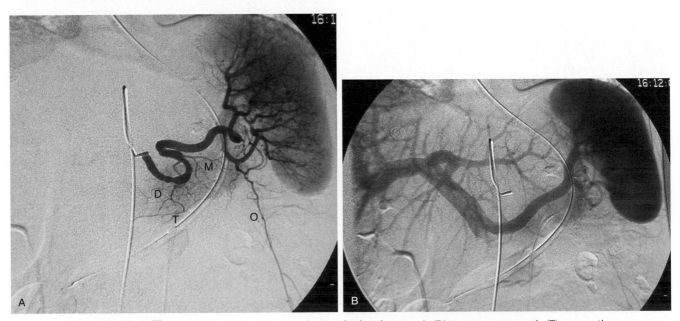

FIGURE 10-6 ■ **A,** Normal splenic arteriogram showing the dorsal pancreatic (D), transverse pancreatic (T), pancreatica magna (M), and omental (O) branches. Proximal irregularity is guidewire-related spasm. **B,** Late-phase indirect splenoportogram. Diminished density in the main portal vein is due to unopacified inflow from the superior mesenteric vein.

TABLE 10-2   VARIANT HEPATIC ARTERIAL ANATOMY

Type	Michels (%)	Recent Series (%)
I: Classic Anatomy	55	58–79
II: Replaced LHA	10	3–12
III: Replaced RHA	11	6–15
IV: Replaced RHA and LHA	1	1–2
V: Accessory LHA from LGA	8	3–11
VI: Accessory RHA from SMA	7	3–12
VII: Accessory RHA and LHA	1	0–1
VIII: Accessory RHA/LHA + replaced LHA or RHA	2	1–3
IX: Replaced CHA to SMA	4.5	1–2
X: Replaced CHA to LGA	0.5	0
Double hepatic artery		1–4
Triple hepatic artery		0–7
Separate CHA origin from aorta		0.4–2
Replaced PHA to SMA, GDA origin from aorta		0.3
Other		1.5–4

CHA, common hepatic artery; GDA, gastroduodenal artery; LGA, left gastric artery; LHA, left hepatic artery; PHA, proper hepatic artery; RHA, right hepatic artery; SMA, superior mesenteric artery.

and replaced hepatic arteries (e.g., right hepatic from the superior mesenteric artery [SMA], left hepatic from the left gastric, and common hepatic from the SMA) (Fig. 10-7; see also Figs. 9-8 and 9-10). *Accessory hepatic arteries* are those in which a **portion** of the affected lobe is supplied by a vessel with an aberrant origin. *Replaced hepatic arteries* are those in which the **entire** lobe is supplied by a vessel with an aberrant origin. Accessory hepatic arteries supply isolated hepatic segments and are believed by most authorities not to be redundant arteries.[24]

Rarely, the splenic artery originates directly from the aorta or from the SMA. An accessory left gastric artery may arise from the proximal splenic artery. Splenic anomalies include an accessory spleen (usually located in the tail of the pancreas), asplenia, polysplenia, and the ectopic or "wandering" spleen.[25]

Classic PV anatomy is found in 65% to 75% of the population. Surgically significant variants of the portal venous system include trifurcation of the main PV (type 2, 9% to 16%), origin of the right posterior branch from the main PV (type 3 or "Z type," 8% to 13%), and separate segment VI or VII branches from the right portal vein (types 4 and 5, 7%).[16,17,26]

Accessory right hepatic veins are found in 25% or more of the population (Fig. 10-8). An *inferior right hepatic vein* (entering the IVC well below the diaphragm) is the dominant venous drainage for the right lobe in about 3% of patients.[16]

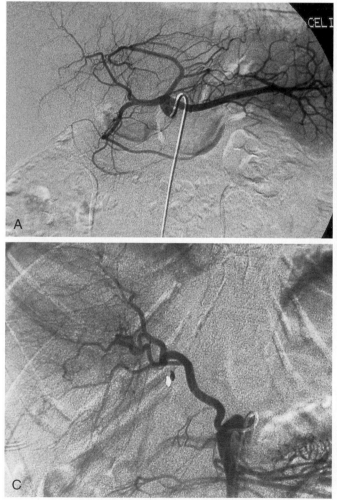

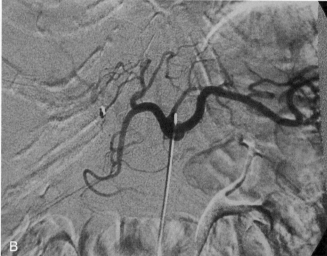

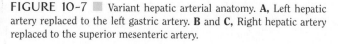

FIGURE 10-7 ■ Variant hepatic arterial anatomy. **A,** Left hepatic artery replaced to the left gastric artery. **B** and **C,** Right hepatic artery replaced to the superior mesenteric artery.

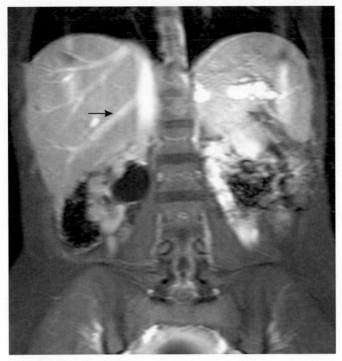

FIGURE 10-8 ■ Accessory inferior right hepatic vein *(arrow)* on coronal maximum intensity projection MR venogram.

Collateral Circulation

With extrahepatic arterial obstruction, the major collateral pathways are

- SMA to pancreaticoduodenal arcades and choledochal arteries (Fig. 10-9)
- Diaphragmatic inferior phrenic branches to intrahepatic arteries (see Fig. 10-9)
- Splenic artery to pancreatic, gastric, and gastroepiploic branches

In the presence of intrahepatic arterial obstruction, the liver is primarily supplied by accessory hepatic arteries (if present) and extracapsular branches.

With splenic artery obstruction, several collateral routes are available:

- Left gastric to short gastric arteries
- Right gastroepiploic to left gastroepiploic artery
- Pancreatic arcades or dorsal pancreatic artery to distal pancreatic arteries

Patterns of collateral flow in the portal and hepatic venous systems are discussed subsequently.

■ MAJOR DISORDERS

Cirrhosis and Portal Hypertension

Etiology

Liver cirrhosis is a progressive disease characterized by generalized necrosis, regeneration, and widespread fibrosis.[27] Initially, inflammation or steatosis predominates. Fibrotic tissue then infiltrates the sinusoidal spaces and obstructs central veins while preserving portal venules. Masses (either micronodular or macronodular) begin to develop, including regenerative, dysplastic, and malignant lesions. As the vascular resistance in the liver increases, PV pressure rises, but flow is still directed into the liver *(hepatopetal)*. An imbalance between nitric oxide (a vasodilator) and endothelin-1 (a vasoconstrictor) is implicated in these important alterations in hepatic, splanchnic, and peripheral hemodynamics that follow.[28,29] With progression of cirrhosis, systemic and splanchnic vasodilation occurs, leading to increased cardiac output (a hyperdynamic circulatory state) and humorally mediated renal and hepatic vasoconstriction, thus further decreasing liver blood flow.[30,31] Extrahepatic portal flow

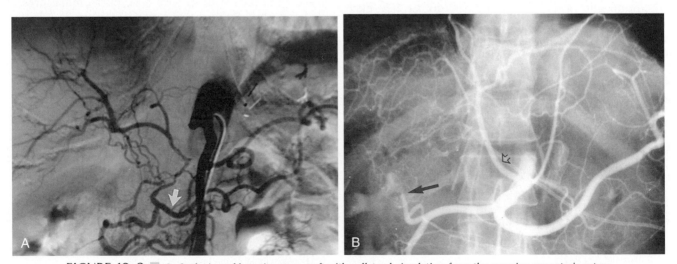

FIGURE 10-9 ■ **A,** Occlusion of hepatic artery graft with collateral circulation from the superior mesenteric artery through the pancreatic arcades *(arrow)*. **B,** Occlusion of the proper hepatic artery *(arrow)* with collateral circulation into the liver from an enlarged right inferior phrenic artery *(open arrow)*.

BOX 10-1 ■ Forms of Portal Hypertension

Extrahepatic portal vein obstruction (see Box 10-2)
Presinusoidal intrahepatic obstruction (see Box 10-3)
Sinusoidal intrahepatic obstruction (see Box 10-4)
Postsinusoidal obstruction (see Box 10-5)
Hyperdynamic portal hypertension

BOX 10-3 ■ Causes of Presinusoidal Intrahepatic Obstruction

Hepatitis
Schistosomiasis
Biliary cirrhosis
    Primary form
    Chronic obstruction
Toxic agents (e.g., vinyl chloride, cytotoxic drugs)
Metabolic disorders (e.g., hemochromatosis)
Malignancies
    Myeloproliferative disorders
    Reticuloendothelial tumors
Sarcoidosis
Congenital hepatic fibrosis
Idiopathic portal hypertension

---

increases while intrahepatic portal flow decreases; in a compensatory fashion, hepatic arterial flow is augmented.

With end-stage cirrhosis, the liver shrinks, and portal venules and hepatic arterial branches are severely compressed by fibrotic infiltration and regenerating nodules. Hepatic vein outflow is markedly diminished. Intrahepatic pressure becomes so great that the portal system is decompressed through portosystemic collateral channels (see below). Finally, flow in the PV is completely reversed *(hepatofugal)*.

Although cirrhosis is by far the most frequent cause of portal hypertension, many other diseases can produce similar physiologic effects. Portal hypertension is traditionally classified by the site of obstruction relative to the hepatic sinusoids (Boxes 10-1 through 10-5).[30-32] Some diseases may first cause obstruction at one level and then extend to others.

Alcoholic cirrhosis is the most common form of the disease in the United States. It evolves from the initial stage of fatty liver to sinusoidal scarring, formation of regenerative nodules (i.e., micronodular cirrhosis), and finally widespread fibrosis with liver shrinkage. *Viral hepatitis,* including hepatitis B and particularly hepatitis C, may progress to chronic liver disease.[33] Hepatitis C is rapidly becoming a dominant cause of cirrhosis in Western countries, as it is in many parts of Asia. *Hepatic schistosomiasis,* which is endemic in Africa and parts of Asia, causes infiltration of portal venules and periportal spaces, leading to presinusoidal obstruction.[34]

Primary biliary cirrhosis is a cholestatic liver disease of immunologic origin that results in diffuse bile duct obstruction.[35] It is typically seen in middle-aged women. In patients with *chronic bile duct obstruction,* portal fibrosis rather than diffuse cirrhosis is the cause for portal hypertension. *Congenital hepatic fibrosis* presents in late childhood with evidence of portal hypertension but normal liver function. *Idiopathic portal hypertension (non-cirrhotic portal fibrosis)* is a rare condition in which PV pressure is elevated without underlying liver disease.[36] Destruction of intrahepatic portal radicles, portal fibrosis, and liver atrophy are characteristic.

Hyperdynamic portal hypertension, defined as increased flow through the portal venous system in the absence of resistive changes, is a rare cause of elevated portal pressures. The most common etiology is an arterioportal fistula (which is often the result of penetrating trauma) or rupture of a hepatic artery aneurysm.[37] In such cases, embolization of the fistula may be curative. PV thrombosis and hepatic venous outflow obstruction are considered later in the chapter.

Clinical Features

The most frequent clinical sequela of portal hypertension is bleeding from ruptured gastroesophageal varices that form portosystemic collaterals to decompress the fibrotic liver. Varices develop in about one half of patients with cirrhosis, but only about one third of those will bleed.[29] The risk of bleeding is related to variceal size, intraluminal pressure, and the Child-Pugh classification (Table 10-3).[38] Between 40% and 70% of patients die from the first episode of variceal hemorrhage. Bleeding is unlikely when the portosystemic pressure gradient is less than 12 mm Hg.[39]

BOX 10-2 ■ Causes of Portal Vein Obstruction

Thrombosis (bland or neoplastic invasion)
Extrinsic compression
    Tumor
    Inflammatory mass
Postoperative
Congenital

BOX 10-4 ■ Causes of Sinusoidal Intrahepatic Obstruction

Cirrhosis
    Alcoholic (i.e., Laënnec's)
    Cryptogenic
    Congestive
    Postnecrotic
Hepatitis
Hepatocellular carcinoma
Sclerosing cholangitis
Felty's syndrome

BOX 10-5 ■ Causes of Postsinusoidal Hepatic

BOX 10-5 ■ Causes of Postsinusoidal Hepatic
Obstruction

Hepatic vein thrombosis (classic Budd-Chiari disease)
Hepatic veno-occlusive disease
Inferior vena cava or hepatic vein outflow obstruction
Hepatic vein or inferior vena cava tumor
Constrictive pericarditis
Right atrial tumor

Fiberoptic endoscopy is performed routinely in all patients with suspected variceal bleeding to document variceal size and stigmata of recent rupture (e.g., red wales, cherry spots). However, these patients may have other causes for acute gastrointestinal bleeding.

Ascites is another important complication of portal hypertension. The cause of ascites in this condition is manifold. Increased splanchnic blood flow produces elevated microcirculatory pressures and increased production of lymph, which leaks from the liver and intestines.[40] In addition, peripheral arterial dilation (a response to vasoactive factors liberated from the gastrointestinal tract) causes a reduction in effective plasma volume and retention of salt and water by the kidneys. The hepatic lymphatic system becomes overwhelmed, leading to peritoneal leakage and a vicious cycle of further reduction in the plasma volume and worsening ascites.

These patients also are at risk for hepatic encephalopathy, spontaneous bacterial peritonitis, splenomegaly and pancytopenia, hepatocellular carcinoma, and fulminant hepatic failure.

Finally, less common complications include hepatorenal syndrome, hepatopulmonary syndrome, portopulmonary hypertension, and hepatohydrothorax.[41] Some of these conditions are related to the misregulation of vasodilating and vasoconstricting factors.[42] *Hepatorenal syndrome* is characterized by diffuse splanchnic and peripheral vasodilation and decreased effective plasma volume, leading to reflex renal vasoconstriction.[43] While the chronic form is treatable, the acute type is almost universally fatal.

TABLE 10-3 MODIFIED CHILD-PUGH CLASSIFICATION FOR HEPATIC FAILURE

Determinant	Threshold*
Ascites	Moderate
Encephalopathy	Moderate
Prothrombin time	15–17 sec
Bilirubin	2–3 mg/dL
Albumin	2.8–3.4 mg/dL

Classification	Points
Class A	5–6
Class B	7–9
Class C	10–15

*Score 2 points if within threshold, score 1 point if better than threshold, and score 3 points if worse than threshold.

Imaging and Tissue Diagnosis

Virtually all patients with suspected cirrhosis or portal hypertension undergo radiologic tests to confirm the existence and assess the extent of liver disease and to detect occult hepatic malignancies. The primary indications for **diagnostic** invasive vascular procedures in these patients are confirmation or quantitation of portal hypertension and transvenous liver biopsy.

Hepatic Vein Manometry. Direct measurement of PV pressure rarely is needed for diagnosing portal hypertension. Clinical studies have shown that the *hepatic vein wedged (HVW) pressure* is equal to PV pressure in most patients. The difference between HVW and IVC pressure is the *corrected sinusoidal pressure*, which reflects the portosystemic gradient. However, the measurements are valid only when the PVs and hepatic sinusoids are in continuity. In patients with extrahepatic PV obstruction, splenic vein obstruction ("segmental" portal hypertension), or presinusoidal portal hypertension, this disconnection leads to a spuriously low HVW pressure. Normally, the portosystemic gradient is less than 5 mm Hg. Portal hypertension is defined as a gradient of greater than 6 mm Hg. The risk of bleeding from gastroesophageal varices becomes significant when the gradient is greater than 12 mm Hg (Fig. 10-10).[39]

Hepatic Venography. Free hepatic venography is done during the transjugular intrahepatic portosystemic shunt (TIPS) procedure and transvenous liver biopsy. Balloon-occluded or catheter-wedged hepatic venography with CO_2 is routinely performed with TIPS creation to provide a target for the PV puncture. Hepatic veins have a pinnate (featherlike) branching pattern; PVs branch dichotomously.

Arteriography and Indirect Portography. With advanced cirrhosis, the hepatic arteries take on a corkscrew appearance because of increased arterial flow and liver shrinkage, and the spleen and splenic artery are enlarged (Fig. 10-11). The demand for hepatic artery flow can become so great that flow in the gastroduodenal artery is reversed. In some cases, arterioportal shunting is seen (see Fig. 3-43).

In the early stages of cirrhosis, PV flow is relatively normal. As the disease advances and portal hypertension becomes significant, several changes occur. The most important is the appearance of *portosystemic collateral pathways*, which include the following principal channels (Fig. 10-12):

- Left gastric (coronary) and short gastric veins through gastroesophageal veins to the azygous vein
- Left PV through a paraumbilical vein to systemic abdominal wall veins around the umbilicus ("caput medusae")
- IMV through rectal (hemorrhoidal) vein to the internal iliac vein
- Splenic or short gastric veins through retroperitoneal branches to the left adrenal/inferior phrenic veins and then to the left renal vein (*spontaneous splenorenal shunt*)

Less common routes of decompression are gastric veins to pulmonary or intercostal veins, duodenal varices ultimately draining into the right gonadal vein (Fig. 10-13), left

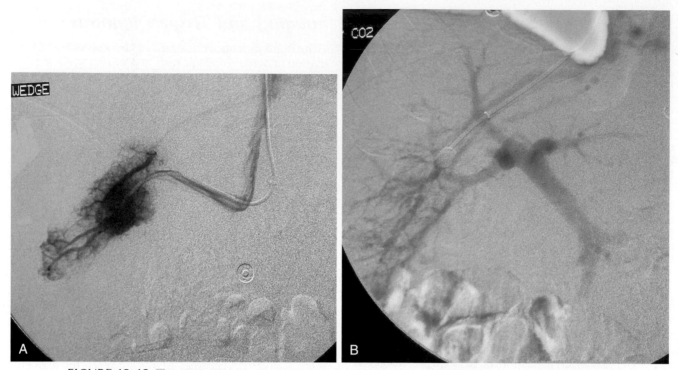

FIGURE 10-10 ■ **A,** Wedged hepatic venography shows homogeneous parenchymal stain and filling of adjacent hepatic venules and veins. **B,** Balloon-occluded hepatic venography with CO_2 in a patient with cirrhosis and portal hypertension prior to transjugular intrahepatic portosystemic shunt procedure. Note excellent opacification of the portal vein.

colic vein to left renal vein through the left gonadal vein, ileocolic vein to the IVC through hemorrhoidal veins, and intrahepatic portal venous branches to diaphragmatic veins. Gastroesophageal varices may be present but not seen on indirect portography.

The direction of flow in the PV also changes as portal hypertension worsens. With mild cirrhosis, PV flow is

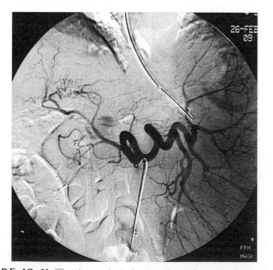

FIGURE 10-11 ■ Advanced cirrhosis. The celiac arteriogram shows "corkscrew" intrahepatic arteries, liver shrinkage, splenic artery enlargement, and massive splenomegaly.

hepatopetal (see Fig. 10-3). As resistance increases, bidirectional flow in the PV may develop and the PV may not fill at all. With severe portal hypertension, the PV becomes an outflow conduit for the liver, and flow is hepatofugal (Fig. 10-14).

Splenoportography. This procedure is indicated only in rare cases in which noninvasive imaging or indirect arterial portography fails to adequately document patency of the portal or splenic vein (Fig. 10-15). This situation is most common in patients with massive splenomegaly in whom the splenic vein does not opacify despite selective splenic artery injection.

Transjugular Liver Biopsy

Patient Selection. Tissue samples for histologic diagnosis of diffuse liver disease are usually obtained by percutaneous liver biopsy. For patients with one of the following conditions, transhepatic biopsy may be relatively unsafe:

- Uncorrectable coagulopathy
- Massive ascites
- Morbid obesity
- Grossly shrunken liver

In such cases, transvenous liver biopsy is preferred. This approach is used also in patients already undergoing hepatic vein catheterization (e.g., for the diagnosis of portal hypertension, during the TIPS procedure).

Technique. From the right (or left) internal jugular vein, a 10-French sheath is advanced into the right or middle

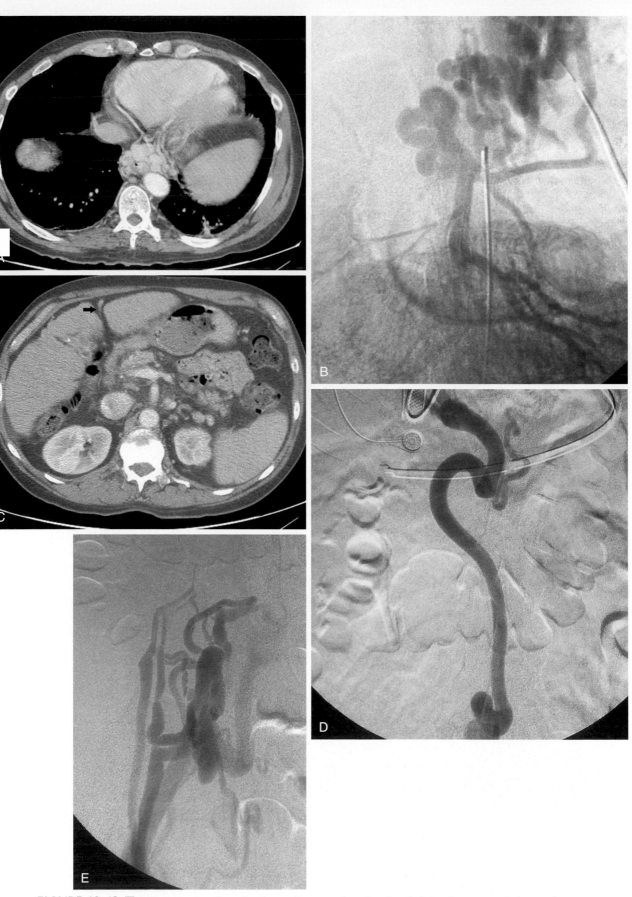

FIGURE 10-12 ■ Portosystemic collateral pathways. Gastroesophageal varices draining the coronary (left gastric) vein into the azygous system on CT scan (**A**) and late phase of superior mesenteric arteriography (**B**). Paraumbilical vein drains the left portal vein through internal iliac venous channels into the inferior vena cava seen on CT scan (**C,** *arrow*) and early and late phases of a direct portogram (**D** and **E**).

Continued

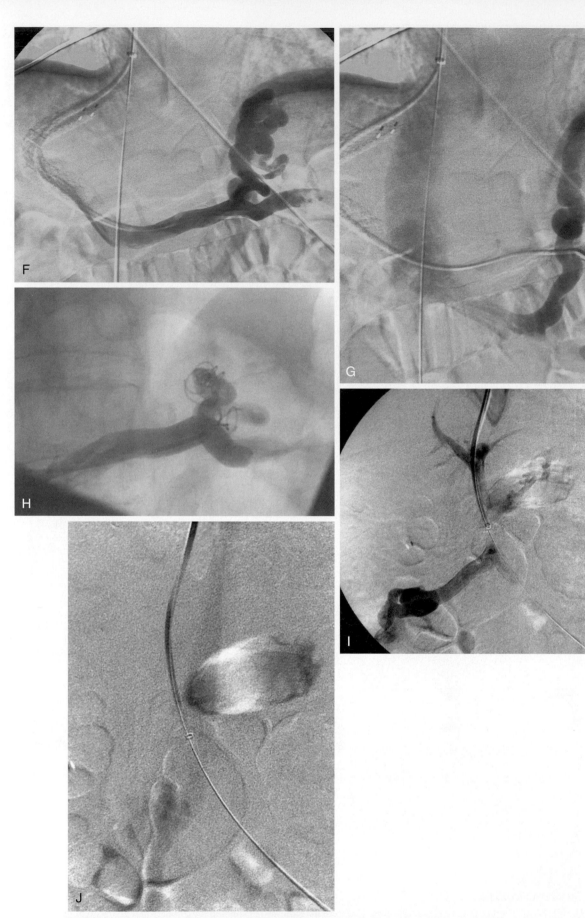

FIGURE 10-12 *Cont'd* ▮ Splenorenal shunt drains short gastric varices from the splenic hilum into the left renal vein and then the inferior vena cava on early (**F**) and late (**G**) phases of a direct splenic venogram through a transjugular intrahepatic portosystemic shunt. Such shunts are occasionally embolized to prevent bleeding, relieve hepatic encephalopathy, or improve overall liver perfusion (**H**). Cecal varices fill by direct portal vein injection (**I**) and then drain through systemic pelvic collaterals into the inferior vena cava (**J**).

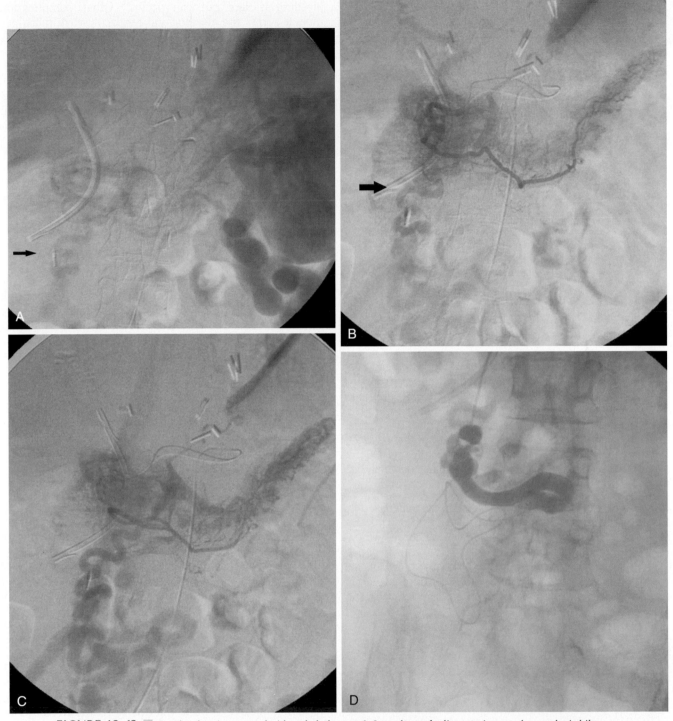

FIGURE 10-13 ■ Duodenal varices treated with embolotherapy. **A,** Late phase of celiac arteriogram shows splenic hilar varices and duodenal varices *(arrow)*. **B,** The duodenal varices are better seen with selective gastroduodenal arteriography through a coaxial microcatheter. **C,** Pelvic collaterals were found to drain into the right ovarian vein and then into the inferior vena cava. **D,** The ovarian vein is catheterized, a microcatheter is negotiated to the site of the varices, and ethanolamine oleate was injected to induce sclerosis.

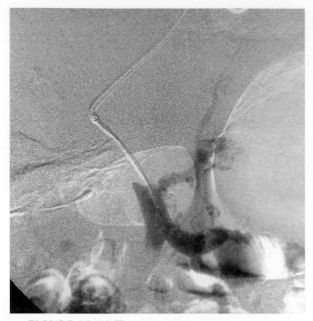

FIGURE 10-14 ■ Hepatofugal flow in the portal vein.

hepatic vein (Fig. 10-16). A stainless steel stiffening cannula is placed through the sheath. A flexible biopsy forceps or biopsy needle (e.g., Quick-Core, Cook Inc., Bloomington, Ind.) is then inserted through the cannula and torqued within the hepatic vein until resistance is met.[44] The device is buried in the parenchyma and triggered, and a piece of tissue is removed. Several specimens may be needed to ensure that adequate material is obtained for analysis. Sampling from different areas of the liver is advisable.

Results and Complications. Biopsy samples adequate for pathologic diagnosis are obtained in greater than 90% of cases.[45-48] In series using the Quick-Core biopsy needle (which provides better results than simple aspiration), the diagnostic accuracy has approached 100%.[44,49] The major risk of the procedure is liver capsule perforation. Abdominal bleeding occurs in less than 6% of cases.[44,46-48] Fatal intraperitoneal

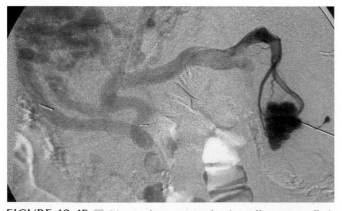

FIGURE 10-15 ■ Direct splenoportography. A small-gauge needle is inserted into the splenic pulp. Contrast injection fills the peripheral splenic vein, but the central vein is occluded. Collateral channels drain into the liver hilum, where bizarre periportal collaterals indicate portal vein occlusion (cavernous transformation).

bleeding is rare but can occur.[49] Other complications include access site bleeding and cardiac dysrhythmias.

Treatment

Pharmacologic Therapy. Prophylactic treatment with beta-adrenergic blocking agents (alone or in combination with isosorbide nitrate) is routinely prescribed in patients with documented gastroesophageal varices to prevent initial or recurrent bleeding by reducing portal venous pressure.[50] If bleeding occurs, emergent management begins with resuscitation and pharmacologic therapy: the somatostatin analogue *octreotide,* or infusion of *vasopressin* or synthetic *terlipressin* (which constrict mesenteric arteries and thereby reduce portal venous pressure and flow).[29]

Endoscopic Treatment. Sclerotherapy or band ligation is highly effective for the initial management and primary or secondary prevention of variceal hemorrhage.[29,51-54] A sclerosing agent such as ethanolamine oleate or polidocanol injected into or around varices causes variceal thrombosis. Variceal banding is just as effective and is associated with fewer complications. About 70% to 90% of patients stop bleeding after one or two sessions. However, sclerotherapy does not remedy the underlying hemodynamics of portal hypertension. Rebleeding is observed in about one half of patients. Serious complications are encountered in about 10% of cases.

Transcatheter Variceal Embolization. Embolization of the coronary vein was quite popular before the widespread use of endoscopic sclerotherapy.[55] Coils, with or without a sclerosing agent, are placed to obstruct the inflow vein. Although immediate results are excellent, rebleeding occurs in greater than 50% of cases as new collateral channels develop.[56] This procedure has limited use as an adjunct to TIPS placement (see below).

Balloon-occluded Retrograde Transvenous Obliteration of Gastric and Duodenal Varices. In Japan and other parts of Asia, balloon-occluded retrograde transvenous obliteration (BRTO) has become a popular alternative to prevent or control bleeding from these isolated variceal clusters.[57-60] In some cases, these massive shunts can cause intractable hepatic encephalopathy. Gastric and duodenal varices are notoriously difficult to treat with endoscopy because of their location and size.

Prior to BRTO, indirect portography via celiac and SMA arteriography is done to establish the portal venous anatomy and hemodynamics. The outflow vein for the varices (typically the left inferior phrenic/adrenal to left renal vein for gastric varices, right gonadal vein for duodenal varices) is selectively engaged with a diagnostic catheter. A 6-French balloon occlusion catheter (e.g., 11 or 20 mm diameter) is advanced into the main trunk and inflated, and venography is performed to classify the varices and collateral veins.

For simple types of varices, 10 mL of ethanolamine oleate 10% mixed with 10 mL of contrast material is slowly injected with the balloon inflated until the varices are completely filled to induce thrombosis. The agent is left in place from 1 to 24 hours, aspirated, and the balloon removed. More complex types of variceal communications may require use of a microcatheter or initial partial splenic embolization

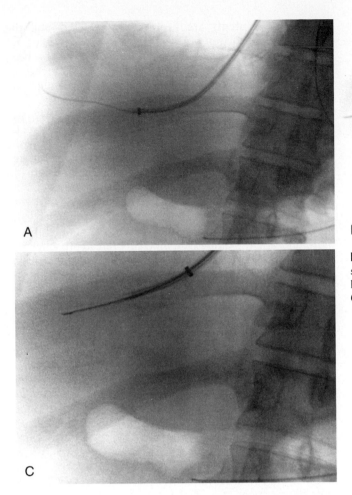

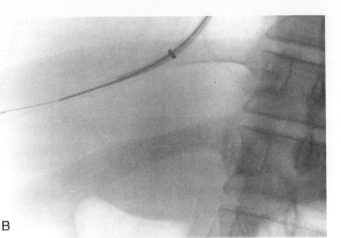

FIGURE 10-16 ■ Transjugular liver biopsy. **A,** A sheath and inner stiffening cannula are directed from the right jugular vein into the right hepatic vein. **B,** The biopsy device is advanced into the liver parenchyma. **C,** The gun is triggered to obtain liver tissue.

to reduce flow through the shunts.[57,58] Obliteration of varices is documented with contrast CT. In experienced hands, BRTO is effective in preventing further bleeding and improving encephalopathy in greater than 80% of attempts (see Fig. 10-13).[61]

There are some risks to using ethanolamine oleate, including renal failure, pulmonary edema, and anaphylaxis. In Asia, it is routine to administer IV *haptoglobin* (which binds free hemoglobin) to prevent hemolysis-induced kidney damage.

Transjugular Intrahepatic Portosystemic Shunts. The therapeutic applications of TIPS are discussed later in a separate section.

Surgical Therapy. Varices can be obliterated by operative ligation or transsection. However, such procedures fail to treat the underlying cause of variceal formation.

In the past, surgical portocaval shunts were commonly recommended for management of these difficult patients.[62,63] Side-to-side portacaval and mesocaval shunts are nonselective conduits that direct all portal blood flow away from the liver and reduce PV pressure to normal levels. The distal splenorenal (Warren) shunt is a selective communication that diverts flow from gastroesophageal varices but maintains intestinal portal flow to the liver. In this procedure, the splenic vein is divided, and the left gastric, right gastric, and gastroepiploic veins are ligated. Surgical mortality rates for all operative shunts are similar (10% to 20%). Rebleeding from

varices occurs in about 5% to 15% of cases and is more frequent with selective shunts. In most centers, operative shunts are rarely performed anymore.

Liver Transplantation. Liver transplantation is the definitive treatment for relieving portal hypertension from chronic liver disease and provides the best long-term outcome compared with all other methods. Current 5-year survival rates for non–hepatitis C virus-related cirrhosis range from 75% to 85%. Unfortunately, not all patients are candidates for transplantation, and donor organs are in short supply.

Transjugular Intrahepatic Portosystemic Shunts

The TIPS procedure has been in widespread practice for more than 15 years and has revolutionized the management of patients with complications related to portal hypertension.

Patient Selection

The indications for TIPS are still controversial despite well-supported recommendations by several expert groups, including the National Digestive Diseases Advisory Board and, more recently, the American Association for the Study of Liver Diseases (Box 10-6).[64-66] TIPS is most commonly performed for prevention of recurrent gastroesophageal variceal hemorrhage and management of refractory ascites. Given the inherent risks of the procedure, that many patients with varices will never bleed, and that only about half of those who do will rebleed, TIPS should be reserved for patients who suffer one or more bleeding episodes that have not been managed successfully with endoscopic methods. Refractory ascites implies that sodium restriction and maximum diuretic therapy are unsuccessful. TIPS may afford better quality of life than repeated large-volume paracentesis, but encephalopathy may get worse and survival is not clearly improved.

There are differing opinions about the value of TIPS as a bridge to liver transplantation.[67] Unlike surgical shunts, a TIPS does not interfere with subsequent liver transplantation

(provided that stents are kept out of the IVC and the retropancreatic portion of the portal vein). In some but not all series, pretransplantation TIPS procedure has been shown to improve the general condition and nutritional status of the patient, reduce operative blood loss and procedure time, and decrease hospital stay.[68]

TIPS is effective in some patients with portal hypertensive bleeding at atypical sites (e.g., colonic, stomal, anorectal varices), and for portal hypertensive gastropathy.[69,70] While polycystic liver disease and hepatic neoplasm are considered absolute or relative contraindications, the TIPS procedure has been performed successfully and safely in these situations.[71,72]

The decision to insert a TIPS demands thoughtful consideration by the patient, family, referring physician, and interventionalist. The procedure has a small but significant morbidity, and the immediate mortality rate approaches 2%. In addition, a substantial number of patients dies soon afterward, largely from underlying liver disease but partly as a consequence of diversion of portal venous flow (which can precipitate fulminant hepatic failure).

It is useful in counseling patients and referring physicians to provide guidance regarding the likelihood of survival following shunt creation. The severity of liver failure often is graded by the Child-Pugh classification (see Table 10-3). A second model is the EMORY score, which assigns points based on elevated alanine transaminase (ALT) and bilirubin, presence of encephalopathy, and need for emergent TIPS. Recently, the MELD (Mayo Endstage Liver Disease) score has been adopted by many centers to estimate prognosis in patients being considered for liver transplantation or TIPS. This score is based on the serum bilirubin, creatinine, international normalized ratio, and recent need for dialysis (for calculation, go to http://www.mayoclinic.org/gi-rst/mayomodel6.html).

Early mortality after TIPS procedure is especially high in patients with a MELD score greater than 18 to 25, Child-Pugh score greater than 12 (class C), Emory score greater than 4 to 5, APACHE severity of illness score greater than 18 to 20, or bilirubin greater than 3 mg/dL.[64,73-76] Changes in liver hemodynamics assessed with dynamic imaging studies have also been employed to predict survival.[77-79] For example, reduced total hepatic perfusion and delayed arterial hepatic enhancement may portend a poor outcome.

Technique

Acute bleeding is controlled with variceal sclerotherapy or banding, systemic vasopressin or octreotide infusion, placement of an esophageal tamponade balloon, or some combination of these measures. Coagulation defects should be corrected and broad-spectrum antibiotics given before the procedure. Color Doppler sonography (or occasionally MR imaging) is obtained to establish PV patency and flow direction, the status of the hepatic veins, degree of ascites, liver size, and to exclude a liver tumor or polycystic liver disease.

The TIPS procedure is often performed with moderate sedation under the direction of the interventionalist. However, unstable or uncooperative patients are best managed by an anesthesiologist who can induce deep sedation or general anesthesia if needed.

Access is gained through the right internal jugular vein (Fig. 10-17).[80,81] The procedure can also be done through the

---

BOX 10-6 ■ Indications and Contraindications for the Transjugular Intrahepatic Portosystemic Shunt Procedure

Accepted Indications
Acute variceal bleeding unresponsive to medical therapy (including sclerotherapy/banding)
Prevention of recurrent gastroesophageal variceal bleeding unresponsive to medical therapy (including repeated sclerotherapy/banding)
Refractory ascites
Refractory hepatic hydrothorax
Prevention of rebleeding with gastric and ectopic varices (colonic, stomal, anorectal)
Prevention of recurrent bleeding with portal hypertensive gastropathy on beta-blocker medication

Debated Indications
Budd-Chiari syndrome
Bridge to liver transplantation
Prevention of variceal bleeding after a single episode

Generally Not Acceptable
Primary prevention of variceal bleeding
Bleeding from gastric antral vascular ectasia
Hepatorenal syndrome
Hepatopulmonary syndrome

Absolute Contraindications
Polycystic liver disease
Severe hepatic failure
Severe right-sided heart failure (right atrial pressure >20 mm Hg)
Severe pulmonary hypertension (mean >45 mm Hg)
Uncontrolled systemic infection or sepsis
Unrelieved biliary obstruction

Relative Contraindications
Severe or uncontrollable hepatic encephalopathy
Hypervascular liver tumor
Portal vein thrombosis
Severe active infection
Complete hepatic vein obstruction
Uncorrectable severe coagulopathy
Moderate pulmonary hypertension

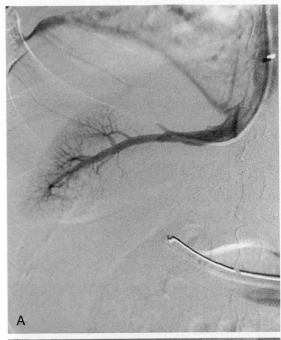

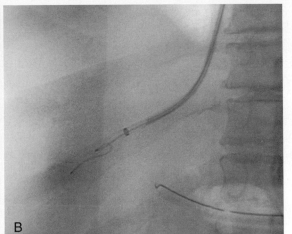

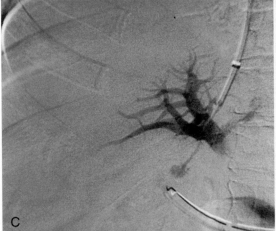

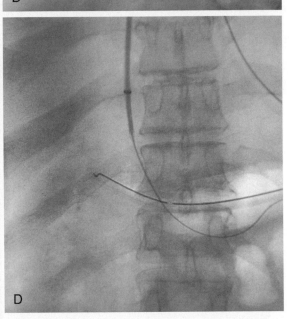

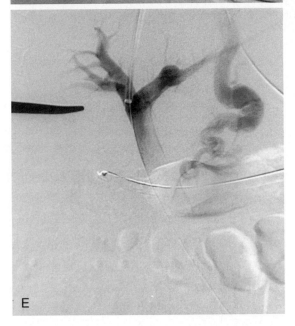

FIGURE 10-17 Transjugular intrahepatic portosystemic shunt procedure with uncovered stent. **A,** Right hepatic vein catheterization. Note that massive ascites has displaced the liver. **B,** Outer sheath and stiffening cannula placement. **C,** Entry of inner 5-French catheter into the portal system after transhepatic needle passage. **D,** Guidewire placement into the splenic vein. **E,** Portal venogram shows the entry site into the proximal right portal vein and large gastroesophageal varices. *Continued*

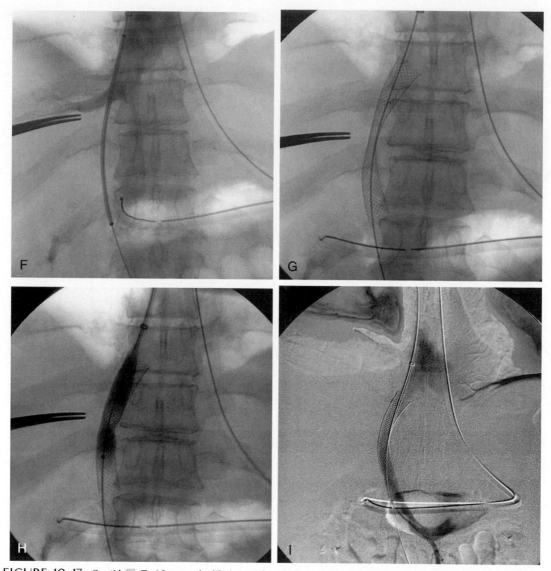

FIGURE 10-17 *Cont'd* ■ **F,** After track dilation with a balloon catheter, a 12 × 90-mm Wallstent is positioned. **G,** Complete stent deployment with residual narrowing along the intraparenchymal track. **H,** Balloon angioplasty of the stent and outflow vein. **I,** Completion portal venogram shows a widely patent shunt and no filling of varices or intrahepatic portal venous branches.

right external jugular vein or even the left internal jugular vein if necessary. A long, 10-French sheath (Cook Inc., Bloomington, Ind.) is advanced into the right atrium. Right atrial and IVC pressures are measured.

The right hepatic vein is engaged with a curved catheter and steerable guidewire. If the right hepatic vein is small, has a very acute angle with the IVC, or is difficult to cannulate, TIPS can be created from the middle or left hepatic vein. It is important to establish which vein is being used so that the intrahepatic puncture toward the PV is made in the appropriate direction. This can be accomplished in several ways, including steep oblique/lateral fluoroscopy or with ultrasound interrogation. About 3% of the population has a dominant inferior right hepatic vein. In this situation, TIPS can be formed from the right common femoral vein (Fig. 10-18; see also Fig. 10-8).

Several methods are used to select a site for puncture from the hepatic vein toward the PV (Fig. 10-19). The most popular techniques are reliance on bony landmarks and

injection of CO_2 through a balloon occlusion catheter to fill the central portal venous system (see Fig. 10-10).[82,83] The right PV trunk typically runs at the level of the 11th rib, about 0.5 to 1.5 vertebral widths from the lateral border of the spine. Three-dimensional ultrasound also may minimize the number of needle passes required to gain entry.[84] The site of venous puncture is critical. Because the portal vein bifurcation is extrahepatic in about one half of patients, entry must be peripheral to this point to avoid extrahepatic puncture and the possibility of exsanguinating hemorrhage.[85]

After the outer sheath is inserted well into the vein, the stiffening cannula and catheter-needle system are inserted (e.g., 16-gauge Rosch-Uchida catheter-trocar set, Cook Inc., Bloomington, Ind.). The catheter-trocar is advanced within the protective outer sheath until they are tip to tip.

When the right hepatic vein is used, the needle is turned anteromedially toward the right PV, and the puncture is made. From the middle hepatic vein, an anterior or posterior

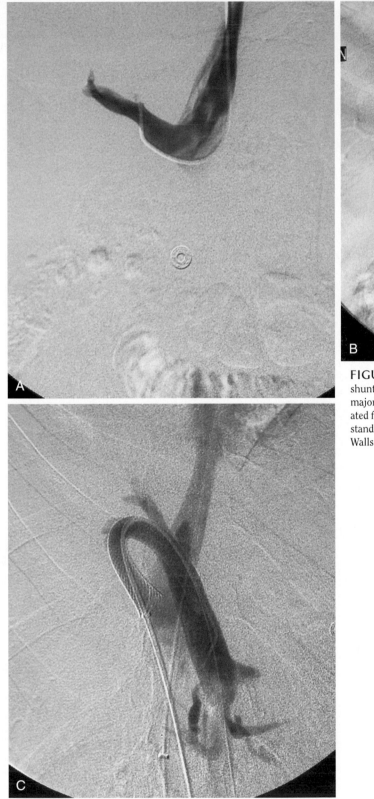

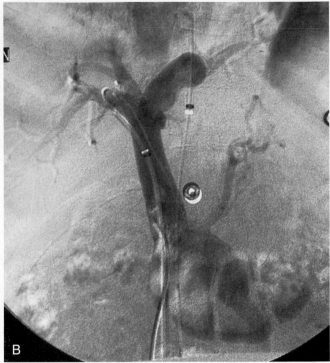

FIGURE 10-18 ■ Femoral transjugular intrahepatic portosystemic shunt (TIPS) procedure. **A,** From right internal jugular vein access, the major draining vein is an inferior right hepatic vein. TIPS cannot be created from above. **B,** Through a right common femoral vein approach, the standard TIPS set is used to enter the right portal vein. **C,** An uncovered Wallstent is placed to create the shunt.

puncture (toward the left or right portal vein, respectively) is chosen. The catheter is gradually withdrawn, and contrast is injected when blood is aspirated. It is common to obtain ascitic fluid or to opacify biliary ducts, hepatic arterial branches, or even lymphatic channels. It is important not to mistake them for the portal venous system and inadvertently create a shunt into these structures. When a PV branch fills and the vessel appears suitable, a guidewire (e.g., angled hydrophilic steerable wire) is advanced into the PV and negotiated into the splenic vein or SMV.

An endhole catheter is placed for PV pressure measurements to determine the initial portosystemic gradient.

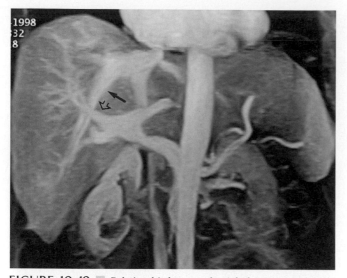

FIGURE 10-19 ■ Relationship between the right hepatic vein *(arrow)* and the right portal vein *(open arrow)* on coronal gadolinium-enhanced MR angiogram.

Then, a marking pigtail catheter is advanced into the main portal vein for venography. The suitability of the portal puncture site is confirmed. The parenchymal track is then dilated with an 8- or 10-mm angioplasty balloon.

Most interventionalists use the Viatorr PTFE-covered stent graft (W. L. Gore and Associates, Flagstaff, Ariz) because of its superior long-term results. In the past, bare stents were used (e.g., Wallstent [Boston Scientific, Natick, Mass.]). A stent is chosen based on the magnitude of the portosystemic gradient and the measured length of the track (with 2 cm added to account for projection artifact). Ideally, the uncovered portion of the stent (always 2 cm in length) should be entirely within the portal vein. The remaining polytetrafluoroethylene (PTFE)-covered segment should encompass the parenchymal track and outflow hepatic vein but *not* extend into the IVC. Future liver transplantation is made more difficult or impossible if the stent protrudes into the IVC or the retropancreatic portion of the main PV. Optimal stent diameter is controversial. With the bare Wallstent, 10 or 12 mm sizes were customary. With the Viatorr stent, some practitioners believe smaller diameters will limit postprocedure encephalopathy.

The Viatorr stent-graft is loaded into the outer sheath, which has been advanced into the portal vein. The sheath is withdrawn to expose the uncovered segment. The entire unit is pulled back to snug the covered portion against the parenchymal track. The sheath is withdrawn into the right atrium and the release cord is pulled, deploying the remainder of the device. The track is then dilated with an 8-, 10-, or 12-mm balloon.

In patients treated for variceal hemorrhage, the conventional endpoint is a portosystemic gradient of less than 12 mm Hg. However, there is some evidence that relative reduction of the gradient (e.g., by 50% of baseline) may be sufficient to prevent variceal rebleeding. The threshold for patients with refractory ascites is more controversial.[64] Some experts believe gradients less than 8 mm Hg are necessary; others argue that it is prudent to accept a larger gradient (and thus reduce the risk of encephalopathy and hepatic insufficiency).

At the end of the procedure, a portal venogram is done to document shunt patency, lack of filling of intrahepatic PV branches, and nonvisualization of gastroesophageal varices. If the portosystemic gradient remains elevated despite use of a 12-mm balloon or if varices continue to fill, embolization of varices should be considered (Fig. 10-20).[86,87]

Postprocedure care includes observation for signs of abdominal bleeding, evaluation of hepatic and renal function, treatment of encephalopathy, and follow-up duplex sonography of the shunt. Because of air trapped in the graft fabric, Viatorr stent visualization is possible only days to weeks after deployment.

Early Results

A shunt can be created successfully in greater than 90% to 95% of attempts, leaving a portosystemic gradient below 12 mm Hg or reduced by greater than 50% in most cases.[64,81,88,89] In patients treated for variceal hemorrhage, early rebleeding (before 6 months) occurs in up to 15% of patients. TIPS is more effective than sclerotherapy or banding in preventing rebleeding, although survival may not be prolonged.[90] About 50% to 75% of patients treated for refractory ascites have partial or complete resolution within about 1 month of placement.[91-93] Early (30-day) mortality after TIPS can be substantial, but this is largely due to the underlying liver disease rather than direct complications of the procedure.[64] There is equivocal evidence that mortality is greater in patients treated for refractory ascites than variceal bleeding prevention.

Complications

Major procedure-related complications develop in about 3% of patients. Adverse events from the TIPS procedure are listed in Table 10-4.[64,81,87,89,94] Other complications include

TABLE 10-4	MAJOR COMPLICATIONS OF THE TRANSJUGULAR INTRAHEPATIC PORTOSYSTEMIC SHUNT (TIPS) PROCEDURE

Complication	Frequency (%)
Transcapsular puncture	33
Bleeding	
Intraperitoneal	1–13
Hemobilia	1–4
Liver dysfunction	
Transient worsening	10–20
Fulminant hepatic failure or infarction	3–7
Hepatic encephalopathy	
New onset or worsened	10–44
Uncontrollable	5–10
Sepsis	2–10
Stent malposition or migration	1–3
Other	
Hemolysis	10–15
Fistula	<1
Infection of TIPS	<1

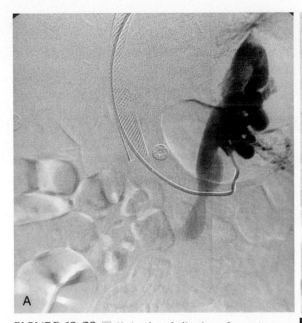
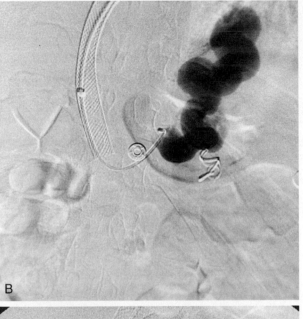
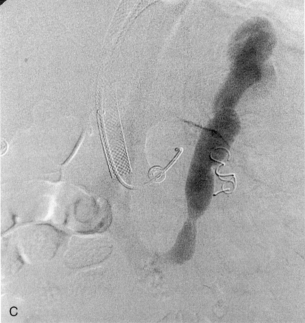

FIGURE 10-20 ■ Variceal embolization after a transjugular intrahepatic portosystemic shunt procedure. **A,** Varices continue to fill despite pressure gradient reduction from 13 to 7 mm Hg because of a low-resistance shunt to the renal vein. **B,** A second channel of varices is found after initial embolization. **C,** Rapid drainage into the inferior vena cava is noted.

acute renal failure, access site bleeding, cardiac dysrhythmias, and reactions to contrast material.

The riskiest step in the TIPS procedure is the transhepatic needle puncture. Liver capsule perforation and injury to small hepatic artery or bile duct branches are common and usually inconsequential. Rarely, needle passes cause gallbladder perforation, hepatic artery pseudoaneurysms, or arteriovenous fistula formation. Massive hemorrhage from extracapsular, IVC, or PV perforation is rare.

Acute shunt thrombosis is reported in about 3% to 4% of cases and may be caused by a residual stenosis or incomplete coverage of the track. Thrombosed shunts are salvaged by mechanical or enzymatic thrombolysis and placement of additional stents as needed (Fig. 10-21).[95,96]

Hepatic encephalopathy is a major concern after any side-to-side portosystemic shunt. With diversion of mesenteric venous blood into the shunt, nitrogen-containing compounds (among several other substances) produced by bacterial action in the gut are not metabolized by the liver before entering the circulation. Blood ammonia levels can rise sharply and result in encephalopathy. In this population, encephalopathy also may be related to increased protein intake, gastrointestinal bleeding, sepsis, dehydration, or acute hepatitis. This complication is more likely when the residual portosystemic gradient is less than 10 mm Hg.[97,98] Although about 25% of patients develop new or worsened encephalopathy, less than 5% to 10% are unresponsive to medical therapy (e.g., low-protein diet, daily lactulose, neomycin).

A transient elevation in liver enzymes is common after TIPS. However, isolated persistent hyperbilirubinemia may be related to hemolysis. Fulminant hepatic failure is seen in less than 7% of cases.

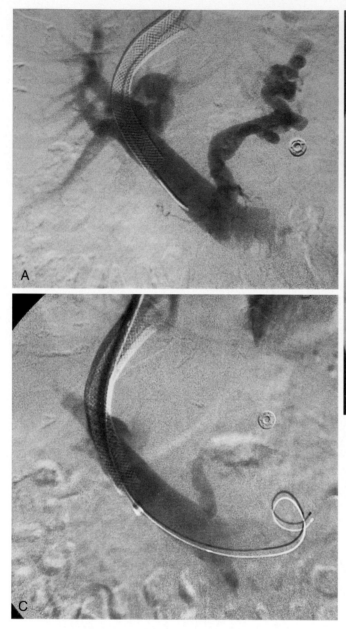

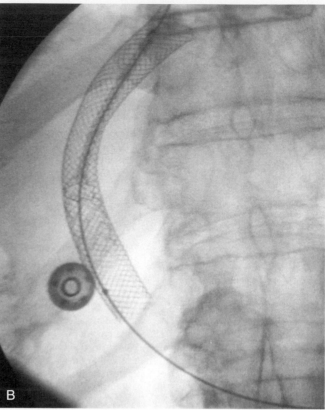

FIGURE 10-21 ■ Acute transjugular intrahepatic portosystemic shunt (TIPS) thrombosis. **A,** Complete shunt occlusion was suspected on the basis of post-TIPS ultrasound findings and confirmed by direct cannulation of the shunt. **B,** A covered Viatorr stent was deployed within the track. **C,** The shunt is recanalized, and portal flow is now hepatofugal.

The immediate mortality rate is 0 to 2%, although this figure may be higher for less-experienced operators. Early procedure-related death is usually the result of extracapsular perforation with intraperitoneal bleeding, hepatic artery thrombosis with fulminant hepatic failure, or acute right heart failure. The reported 30-day mortality rate varies from 3% to 45%.[94]

Late Results

Despite the excellent short-term results of the TIPS procedure using **uncovered** stents, most shunts do not remain patent without repeated intervention. The reported primary patency rate for TIPS with these devices is 25% to 66% (average, 50%) at 1 year and 26% to 32% at 2 years.[89,99-101]

After a TIPS is created with a bare stent, a layer of pseudointima begins to cover the stented segment, which protects it from late thrombosis.[102] Neointimal hyperplasia progresses within the track and in the denuded outflow veins. An inflammatory reaction to injured bile ducts may be an important cause of this process (Fig. 10-22).[103,104] Significant stenoses develop within the body of the stent and the outflow vein; however, PV stenoses are exceedingly uncommon.[101]

There is incontrovertible evidence that **PTFE-covered** stent-grafts dramatically improve long-term durability, with 1- and 2-year primary patency rates of about 81% to 86% and 80%, respectively.[105-108]

Surveillance and Shunt Management

Recurrent variceal hemorrhage or refractory ascites after TIPS procedure is usually a sign of shunt stenosis or occlusion. However, shunt closure is usually silent until rebleeding occurs. Vigorous surveillance programs have become routine, although this approach may change with widespread use of

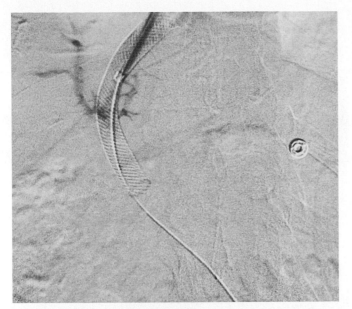

FIGURE 10-22 ■ Biliary fistula is noted upon injection of a thrombosed transjugular intrahepatic portosystemic shunt track.

covered stents. CT angiography is helpful in detecting impending TIPS failure, but color Doppler sonography is the best tool for long-term screening because of its simplicity and low cost.[109] Sonography is routinely performed following and 1 month after the TIPS procedure, at 3-month intervals for the first year and at 6- to 12-month intervals thereafter. Several criteria signal shunt dysfunction[110-114]:

■ Absent flow
■ Significant rise or fall in shunt velocity (>50 cm/second) compared with the first post-TIPS study
■ Low-peak shunt velocity (<50 to 90 cm/second)
■ High-peak shunt velocity (greater than 190 cm/second)
■ Low main PV velocity (<30 cm/second)
■ Return of antegrade flow in intrahepatic PVs
■ Reversed flow in the peripheral segment of the hepatic vein draining the shunt

However, recently it has become apparent that color Doppler sonography is **not** as accurate in detecting shunt dysfunction as was once thought. While quite specific in identifying abnormalities (about 90%), color Doppler sonography is not particularly sensitive in this regard (about 50%).[64] Therefore, shunt angiography is required if varices reappear at endoscopy.

When shunt dysfunction is suspected, a direct portal venogram is performed from a right internal jugular vein approach. A patent shunt almost always can be cannulated with an angiographic catheter (e.g., headhunter or cobra shape) and an angled hydrophilic guidewire. The presence of shunt occlusion, stenosis of greater than 50%, portosystemic gradient of greater than 12 mm Hg, and filling of gastroesophageal varices are indications for intervention. If a bare stent was placed originally, insertion of a covered device usually is appropriate (Fig. 10-23). With covered stents, in-stent stenosis is rare. In most cases, lesions

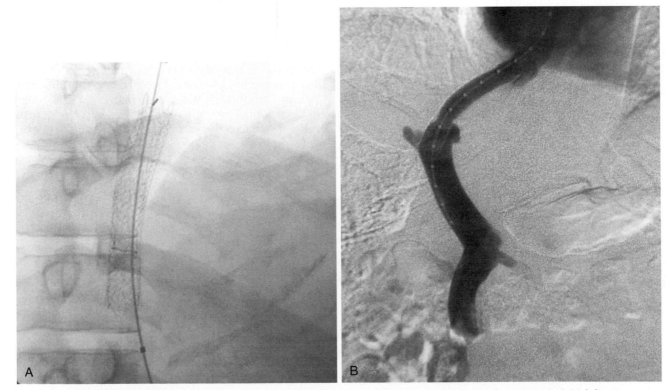

FIGURE 10-23 ■ Covered stent placement for transjugular intrahepatic portosystemic shunt stenosis. Initial direct portogram revealed in-stent neointimal hyperplasia and hepatopetal flow (see Fig. 10-3B). **A,** A covered stent is placed across the shunt, taking care to keep the covered portion (above the lower stent markers) within the liver track and hepatic outflow vein. **B,** Widely patent shunt after deployment.

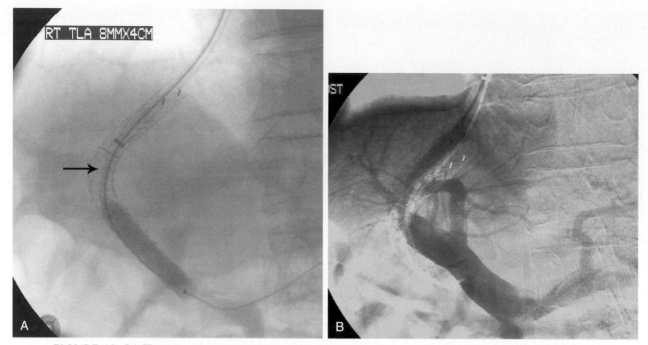

FIGURE 10-24 ■ Shunt reduction in a patient with liver failure following transjugular intrahepatic portosystemic shunt procedure. Initial portogram showed a widely patent shunt. A suture was used to make a waist around the middle of a covered Viatorr stent, which was then inserted into the existing shunt (**A**). **B,** Follow-up portogram demonstrates flow both in the shunt and the intrahepatic portal vein.

develop in unstented portions of the outflow veins, which then require placement of additional covered stents. However, care must be taken to avoid stent extension into the IVC, which can precipitate thrombosis.[115]

Occasionally, patients develop uncontrollable hepatic encephalopathy or progressive liver failure. In these cases, portal venous flow can be augmented in several ways (Fig. 10-24)[116-118]:

■ *Shunt occlusion* is accomplished by embolization with coils or prolonged inflation (24 to 48 hours) of an occlusion balloon in the tract. Obviously, the patient will then be at risk for the symptoms of portal hypertension for which he or she was first treated. More importantly, cases of life-threatening or fatal hemodynamic changes have been reported.[116,119]

■ *Shunt reduction* is accomplished by several means, most of which involve placement of a covered, partially constrained stent within the existing shunt. Some of these devices, fashioned sterilely on the interventional table, can later be adjusted using balloons to achieve controlled reduction in shunt flow.

■ *Splenorenal shunt embolization* using the BRTO methods (see above) can be effective in appropriate patients with intractable encephalopathy.

Portal and Splenic Vein Thrombosis

Etiology

Portal vein thrombosis has many causes (Box 10-7).[120,121] It was once thought that most cases were idiopathic. In fact, a precipitating condition can be identified in up to 80% of affected patients.[121] The etiology is often multifactorial. In children, sepsis is frequently implicated.

PV thrombosis can be confined to the PV itself, include the SMV but spare mesenteric vessels, or reflect widespread involvement (with or without an adequate collateral circulation).

Splenic vein thrombosis is usually the result of pancreatitis, pancreatic neoplasms, splenectomy, thrombophilic states, or trauma.[122] With obstruction of the splenic vein, "segmental" or "left-sided" portal hypertension may develop. The spleen then drains through several portoportal collateral routes (see below).

BOX 10-7 ■ **Causes of Portal Vein Thrombosis**

Inflammatory
    Infection/sepsis
    Pancreatitis
    Appendicitis or diverticulitis
    Schistosomiasis
Thrombophilic state
    Oral contraceptives/pregnancy
Neoplasms (hepatic or pancreatic)
Cirrhosis
Posttraumatic
    After transplantation
    After shunt placement
    After neonatal umbilical vein catheter placement
Dehydration
Idiopathic

some patients do have coexisting esophageal varices if the left gastric vein drains into the occluded portion of the splenic vein.[122]

Imaging

Cross-sectional Techniques. Portal and splenic vein thrombosis is detected with color Doppler sonography or CT or MR angiography.[123,124] In the acute phase, signs of the underlying causes (e.g., cirrhosis, pancreatitis, recent splenectomy) may be evident along with thrombus in the portal, splenic, superior mesenteric and/or branch mesenteric veins, bowel wall edema, varices, and ascites.

In the chronic phase, numerous collateral venous channels in the porta hepatis and gallbladder fossa often bypass the occlusion and fill intrahepatic PVs. This appearance is inappropriately referred to as *cavernous transformation* of the PV, even though the PV itself remains occluded. Other portoportal and portosystemic collaterals may bypass the occlusion. Calcification of the PV, liver atrophy, and splenomegaly also are characteristic.

Angiography. Because the obstruction in portal and splenic vein thrombosis is proximal to the hepatic sinusoids, the normal pressures obtained at HVW manometry do not reflect true portal hemodynamics. In acute or partial PV thrombosis, a filling defect may be seen on the late-phase celiac or SMA arteriogram. However, a patent PV may not opacify if flow is hepatofugal. In cases of subacute or chronic PV thrombosis, changes of cavernous transformation are found (Fig. 10-25).

With splenic vein occlusion, the spleen drains through portoportal collateral pathways such as short gastric veins to the left gastric vein, left gastroepiploic vein to the SMV, the venous arc of Barkow running in the greater omentum, IMV to rectal veins (with central splenic vein occlusion), and splenorenal and splenoretroperitoneal shunts (Fig. 10-26). Even with a large-volume contrast injected directly into the

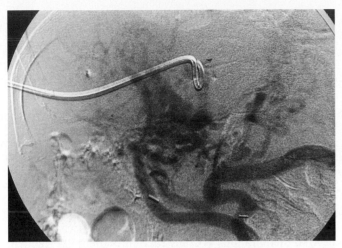

FIGURE 10-25 ■ Cavernous transformation of the portal vein with numerous collateral channels in the gallbladder fossa is seen on the late-phase splenic arteriogram. Gastroesophageal varices also are evident.

Clinical Features

Classically, patients with **acute** PV thrombosis complain of fever, abdominal pain, nausea, and (sometimes) new-onset ascites. Some of these cases resolve spontaneously. Patients with **chronic** PV thrombosis usually present with symptoms related to resulting portal hypertension. Sometimes, the liver size is normal, signs of liver failure are absent, and the liver biopsy is unremarkable. The most feared outcome is bowel infarction. Biliary complications related to mass effect by collateral veins on the extrahepatic bile ducts also can occur.

Patients with isolated splenic vein thrombosis may be asymptomatic or can develop variceal bleeding or abdominal pain. At endoscopy, bleeding gastric varices without associated esophageal varices are characteristic. However,

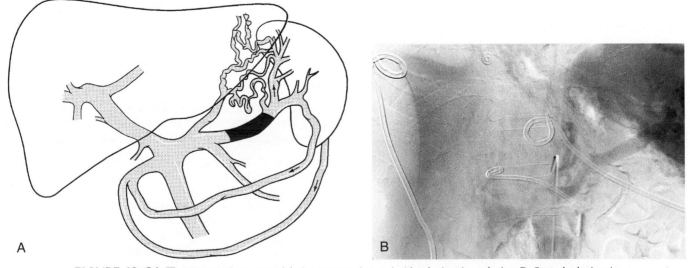

FIGURE 10-26 ■ **A,** Potential portoportal drainage routes *(arrows)* with splenic vein occlusion. **B,** Central splenic vein occlusion with filling of short gastric varices on the late phase of a splenic arteriogram. (**A,** Adapted from Reuter SR, Redman HC, Cho KJ: Gastrointestinal Angiography, 3rd ed. Philadelphia, WB Saunders, 1986:389.)

splenic artery, a patent splenic vein may not be identified in some patients with massive splenomegaly, hepatofugal flow in the splenic vein, or gastroesophageal varices. In such cases, direct splenoportography is helpful.

Treatment

Medical Therapy. In patients with acute PV or splenic vein thrombosis, the standard treatment is anticoagulation. Many of the former group exhibit endogenous lysis.

Endovascular Therapy. Thrombolysis should strongly be considered when acute PV thrombosis is found.[121,125] If thrombus is truly acute (<2 to 4 weeks old), lysis and improvement in symptoms are the rule.[126-129] Although acute PV thrombosis makes the TIPS procedure quite challenging, shunt placement can be accomplished in some cases.[130,131] Chronic thrombosis rarely responds to thrombolytic therapy or allows a TIPS insertion.

Endoscopic banding of isolated gastric varices from splenic vein thrombosis is difficult because of large variceal size and the sharp angles required to access the dilated veins. In an effort to reduce flow through the varices, proximal splenic artery embolization with coils may be attempted.[132]

Surgical Therapy. Operative treatment of PV thrombosis involves thrombectomy or bowel resection (for acute disease), portomesenteric shunt placement, or liver transplantation.[133] In patients with splenic vein thrombosis, splenectomy may be performed to eliminate variceal flow.[122]

Hepatic Vein Outflow Obstruction

Etiology

Obstruction to venous drainage of the liver *(Budd-Chiari syndrome)* can occur at several levels[134]:

■ *Hepatic venules (hepatic veno-occlusive disease).* This form of hepatic venous obstruction usually follows ingestion of certain toxic substances (e.g., pyrrolizidine alkaloids) or chemotherapy and irradiation for bone marrow transplantation.[135]
■ *Hepatic vein thrombosis.* The classic form of Budd-Chiari disease results from clotting of the main hepatic veins and is often associated with a thrombophilic state such as polycythemia vera, oral contraceptive use, sickle cell anemia, or malignancy.
■ *Hepatic vein confluence, IVC, or right atrium.* Obstruction of the IVC or entrance of the hepatic veins is caused by congenital membranes, bland thrombus, tumor, or extrinsic compression.[136] Constrictive pericarditis, right heart failure, and right atrial tumors also may cause Budd-Chiari syndrome.

The unifying features of these disparate conditions are venous hypertension, hypoxic and oxidative hepatocyte injury, and, ultimately, centrilobular necrosis and fibrosis. Early on, symptoms reflect hepatic congestion, but liver function is maintained. With advanced disease, cirrhosis, postsinusoidal portal hypertension, and fulminant hepatic failure may develop.

Most patients have an identifiable thrombophilic state, most notably a hematologic disorder (see Box 3-5).[134] Less common causes include neoplastic invasion (especially hepatocellular, adrenal, and renal cell carcinoma), aspergillosis, Behçet's syndrome, trauma, and inflammatory bowel disease.

Clinical Features

Fulminant, acute, subacute, and chronic forms of the disease exist. The classic triad of symptoms is hepatomegaly, abdominal pain, and ascites. Some patients are jaundiced and may suffer from variceal bleeding. Others are entirely asymptomatic. In Western countries, central hepatic vein thrombosis is the most common form of the disease and typically is seen in young women. In South Africa and parts of Asia, membranous IVC obstruction is the most frequent cause of Budd-Chiari syndrome.[136]

Imaging

Cross-sectional Techniques. Usually the diagnosis is made by color Doppler sonography, CT, or MR imaging; each study has its own particular advantages.[137,138] Hepatic vein wall thickening, stenoses, or occlusions and intrahepatic collateral channels are characteristic. Secondary findings of ascites, hepatomegaly, areas of necrosis, right lobe atrophy and caudate lobe enlargement (a consequence of its separate and intact venous drainage into the IVC), cirrhosis, and malignancy are well depicted by all modalities (Fig. 10-27).

Angiography. Venography and hepatic vein manometry are required when cross-sectional studies are equivocal, when transcatheter therapy is contemplated, and in some patients before shunt procedures. Bone marrow transplantation patients with suspected veno-occlusive disease can go directly to percutaneous or transvenous liver biopsy (with hepatic venography and manometry).[139] With contrast injection in the hepatic vein orifice, the "spider-web" pattern of intrahepatic venous collaterals is pathognomonic of central Budd-Chiari disease (Fig. 10-28). The intrahepatic IVC often is narrowed by ascites or an enlarged caudate lobe. Membranes, webs, and thrombus (bland or neoplastic) also may be identified. In the advanced stages of the disease, patients may have features of portal hypertension.

Treatment

The goals of treatment are prevention of fulminant hepatic failure and management of complications related to portal hypertension, including variceal bleeding and ascites.

Endovascular Therapy. For central hepatic vein or IVC obstruction, catheter-directed thrombolysis (in the acute setting), angioplasty, and stent placement have been used effectively in selected patients with acute or chronic disease.[140-143]

The TIPS procedure is beneficial in some patients with Budd-Chiari syndrome, often as a bridge to transplantation.[135,144-146] A shunt improves venous drainage from the liver.

Surgical Therapy. Operative procedures include mesenteric-systemic shunts (e.g., mesoatrial shunt) and liver transplantation.[147]

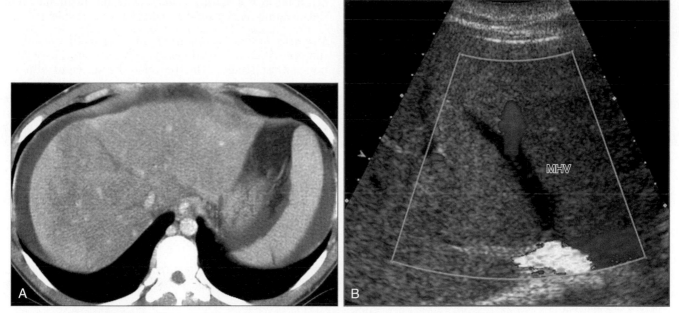

FIGURE 10-27 ■ Budd-Chiari syndrome. **A,** Contrast CT scan shows a mottled parenchymal pattern and lack of filling of central hepatic veins. **B,** Color Doppler ultrasound fails to identify flow in the middle hepatic vein.

Hepatocellular Carcinoma and Metastatic Liver Neoplasms

Pathology and Etiology

Hepatocellular carcinoma (HCC) is the most common primary neoplasm of the liver.[148,149] It is a leading malignancy in many parts of Asia and sub-Saharan Africa, and the incidence is rapidly increasing in many Western countries due to the epidemic of hepatitis C virus (HCV) infection. HCC takes several forms, including solitary lesions, multiple nodules, or diffuse infiltration of the liver. A fibrous capsule usually surrounds mature focal lesions. Hemorrhage or necrosis is common within larger nodules. Neoplastic extension into the portal or hepatic veins is a hallmark of the disease. Pathologically, HCC ranges from highly to poorly differentiated. Metastases occur to lymph nodes, lung, bone, and the adrenal glands. Tumor nodules receive almost their entire blood supply from the hepatic artery and usually are quite vascular. *Alpha-fetoprotein* (AFP), along with several other enzymes such as des-gamma-carboxy prothrombin (protein induced by vitamin K absence [*PIVKA*]), is used as a marker for disease diagnosis and treatment effect.[150]

Most patients with HCC have long-standing liver disease, particularly cirrhosis (from any cause) or chronic viral hepatitis.[148,149] Almost all cases of HCV-associated HCC occur in patients with cirrhosis; this is not true with chronic hepatitis B virus (HBV) infection. In the United States, hepatitis C infection is the most common cause for the malignancy.

A wide variety of metastatic lesions affects the liver (Box 10-8). Patients suffering from these diseases are often referred to the interventionalist for palliative treatment.

Clinical Features

Most patients with HCC are middle-aged or elderly. They may present with hepatomegaly, abdominal pain, weight loss, ascites, fever, or jaundice. Increasingly, however, HCC is being detected through routine screening of high-risk populations and as an incidental finding on abdominal imaging studies. The AFP level is elevated in about 70% of cases.[151]

Diagnosis and Imaging

Patients with suspected metastatic lesions from a known primary tumor usually undergo percutaneous biopsy to

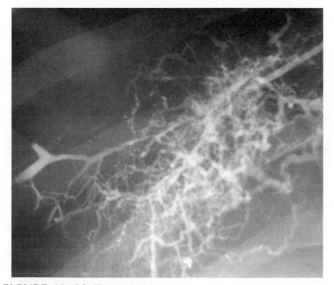

FIGURE 10-28 ■ Budd-Chiari syndrome from central hepatic vein thrombosis. The classic spider-web pattern with injection of the right hepatic vein is caused by innumerable intrahepatic venous collaterals.

BOX 10-8   ■   Liver Neoplasms

Benign
Hemangioma
Adenoma
Focal nodular hyperplasia (hamartoma)
Regenerating nodule
Biliary cystadenoma

Malignant
Hepatocellular carcinoma
Cholangiocarcinoma
Angiosarcoma
Biliary carcinoma
Lymphoma

Metastatic
Gastrointestinal tract
Breast
Pancreas
Lung
Kidney
Islet cell (i.e., pancreas)
Carcinoid

Pediatric
Metastases (e.g., neuroblastoma, Wilms' tumor)
Hepatoblastoma
Hemangioendothelioma
Hemangioma
Hepatocellular carcinoma

---

guide management. However, tissue diagnosis of HCC is not necessary when contrast-enhanced CT or MR imaging findings are diagnostic **in the setting of cirrhosis** or the AFP (or other tumor marker) is greatly elevated (>400 to 500 ng/mL).[149]

Color Doppler Sonography. The primary role of color Doppler sonography is **detection** of liver masses in high-risk populations for HCC. The overall sensitivity and specificity exceed 60% and 90%, respectively.[152] The common findings include hypervascularity, solitary or multiple hypo- (or hyper-) echoic lesions, or diffuse heterogeneity (mosaic pattern), often along with the usual features of cirrhosis. Portal or hepatic vein invasion may be evident. Differentiation between multifocal HCC and cirrhosis can be difficult. Characterization of liver masses is improved with microbubble contrast agents.[153] HCC typically shows dysmorphic hypervascularity, increased enhancement in the arterial phase, decreased enhancement in the portal venous phase, and overall washout with time.

Computed Tomography. Triple-phase contrast CT is necessary to optimize detection of HCC. The tumor appears as solitary or multiple discrete masses with prominent arterial enhancement, hypervascularity, and rapid washout in the portal venous and equilibrium phases (Fig. 10-29).[154,155] A capsule or septations may be identified. Occasionally, one may identify arterioportal shunts, tumor necrosis, calcification, or hemorrhage. Portal (and, less frequently, hepatic) vein invasion also is characteristic (Fig. 10-30). However,

detection in the setting of cirrhosis and distinction from regenerating and dysplastic nodules can be problematic.

Magnetic Resonance Imaging. Like many other malignant tumors, HCC is sometimes hypointense on T1-weighted noncontrast studies. On the other hand, about 50% are actually iso- or hyperintense. Some but not all HCCs are hyperintense on T2-weighted images.[156] Dramatic enhancement is seen in the arterial phase after gadolinium infusion, with rapid washout observed through the portal venous phase. Because HCC typically does not lose signal after administration of superparamagnetic iron oxide reticuloendothelial contrast agent such as Feridex, subtle enhancement of the tumor can be detected.

Hepatocellular carcinoma may be distinguished from metastases by the presence of heterogenous enhancement, irregular tumor vessels, portal or hepatic vein invasion, and arterioportal shunting.

Angiography. Certain features of focal or multinodular HCC are typical (see Fig. 10-29):

- Enlargement of the hepatic artery
- Hypervascularity and neovascularity
- Tumor stain, sometimes with contrast puddles
- Arterioportal shunting, which is almost pathognomonic
- PV invasion with vascularized tumor thrombus (i.e., "threads and streaks" sign)
- Hepatic vein invasion

Lesions from gastrointestinal tract adenocarcinoma, pancreatic adenocarcinoma, bronchogenic carcinoma, and breast carcinoma are typically **hypovascular** and show displacement of vessels and parenchymal defects. Lesions from renal cell carcinoma, pancreatic islet cell tumors, and gastrointestinal carcinoid are typically **hypervascular** with increased number of vessels, neovascularity, and variable tumor stain.

Treatment

Hepatocellular carcinoma is a lethal disease. The median survival in patients with cirrhosis is 13 months, and only one third of patients are alive at 2 years.[154] Prognosis is in large part a function of underlying hepatic reserve, categorized by the Okuda stage (I to III). Generally, metastatic disease to the liver portends a poor outcome from most primary sites.

The choice of treatment depends largely on the tumor stage and the severity of cirrhosis or other underlying chronic liver disease. Earlier interest in systemic chemotherapy and direct intra-arterial chemotherapy for HCC has waned because of the poor survival rates with the former and substantial complication rates with the latter.

Surgical Resection

Partial hepatectomy for primary or metastatic liver tumors is a favored treatment, but unfortunately only a small percentage of patients are candidates due to the extent of tumor involvement, underlying liver disease, or other contraindications. For HCC, 5-year survival rates are about 20% to 70%, but more than 50% of patients develop recurrence after this time.[149,154]

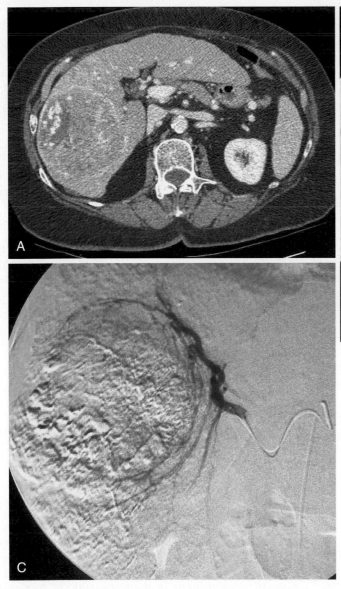

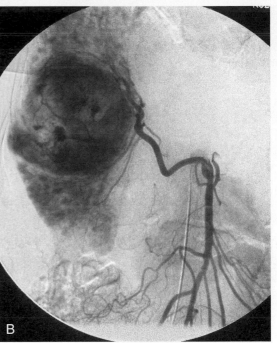

FIGURE 10-29 ■ Hepatocellular carcinoma. **A,** Contrast CT scan in the arterial phase reveals a large hypervascular mass in the right lobe of the liver with central puddling of contrast. **B,** Superior mesenteric arteriography with replaced right hepatic artery confirms a large vascular mass with displacement of vessels. **C,** Following chemoembolization, flow has been abolished and lipidol has accumulated within the tumor.

As a rule, 25% to 40% of total hepatic volume must remain following resection in patients with normal or chronically diseased livers, respectively. Preoperative *portal vein embolization* is a technique designed to cause hypertrophy of the "future liver remnant" and thus increase the number of candidates for potential cure.[157-160] The procedure usually is avoided in patients with total portal vein occlusion.

Sonographic guidance is used to access a right (or left) portal venous branch. After placement of a vascular sheath, main and selective right and left portograms are obtained to outline the venous anatomy (Fig. 10-31). Prior to right hepatectomy, segments V to VIII are selectively embolized. A variety of agents has been used, but many experts prefer polyvinyl alcohol particles or microspheres for occlusion of distal and then proximal branches, followed by microcoils to complete the procedure. Embolization of segments IVa and IVb is required before extended right hepatectomy (right trisegmentectomy). The access tract is then coiled during sheath removal. Complications include pseudoaneurysm

formation, pneumothorax, hemobilia, subcapsular hematoma, and portal vein thrombosis.[161] The procedure invokes adequate hypertrophy to allow operation in the majority of patients. Regeneration usually is maximal at about 2 weeks.

Liver Transplantation

In appropriate candidates, orthotopic or living-donor–related split-liver transplantation offers the best hope for survival and cure. The strategies for organ allocation and operative technique are beyond the scope of this chapter. Median survival may be prolonged to almost 5 years. All patients treated with percutaneous palliative techniques should be considered as possible candidates for transplantation.

Percutaneous Ethanol Ablation

Absolute alcohol causes instant dehydration and death of tumor and normal cells, followed by vascular thrombosis

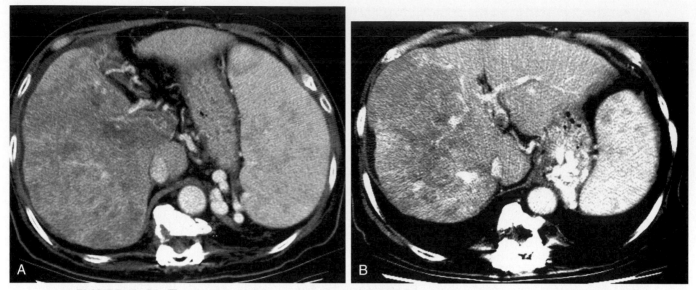

FIGURE 10-30 ■ Portal vein infiltration by hepatocellular carcinoma (HCC). **A,** Contrast-enhanced CT scans show vascularized thrombus in the main portal vein due to a large HCC. **B,** Also note gastroesophageal and splenic hilar varices due to portal hypertension.

and tissue ischemia. Direct ethanol injection has been used to treat patients with focal HCCs. The technique is most effective when the patient has three or fewer lesions less than 4 cm in diameter. Although survival rates are encouraging, local radiofrequency ablation has largely supplanted this procedure.[162,163]

Radiofrequency Ablation

Radiofrequency ablation (RFA) is one of several emerging technologies for thermal destruction of solid organ tumors, which also include high-intensity focused ultrasound, microwaves, laser, and cryotherapy.[162,163] A generator creates an electric field between a probe placed into the tumor and a second electrode, which is usually a cutaneous grounding pad fixed to the patient's thigh. Frictional heat is produced. Coagulation necrosis develops in a small region surrounding the probe when temperatures climb into the 50° to 100°C range.

The destruction of an entire tumor of irregular shape that also encompasses 5 to 10 mm of surrounding normal tissue is limited by device configuration and tissue effects. Some novel alterations in design have partially addressed this issue. Umbrella-shaped or cluster electrodes with multiple tines or probes allow coagulation of moderate-sized (3 to 5 cm) tumors (Fig. 10-32).

Internally cooled electrodes perfused with cold fluid create a "heat sink" that lowers probe tip temperature, allows more gradual tissue heating, and therefore avoids central charring or rapid surges in tissue impedance that can limit heat conductance to the periphery of the tumor.

Animal and human studies suggest that saline injection into tissue may further enhance energy conduction and the volume of ablated tissue.[164]

Arterial or venous blood flowing through the site of treatment also produces a heat sink that limits coagulation necrosis in the region. Routine temporary proximal vascular occlusion may someday become an important step to increase the ablation volume.[165]

Patient Selection. RFA is an alternative to but not a replacement for surgical resection. It may serve as a first-line treatment, adjunct to chemoembolization, palliative measure to control symptoms, a "bridge" to transplantation, or salvage for failures of other modalities.[166] There is mounting evidence that the combination of RFA and chemoembolization is the most effective strategy in many patients. In most centers, RFA has replaced percutaneous ethanol ablation as a primary treatment for limited disease because of apparently better outcomes.[149,163]

RFA is used primarily to treat HCC and colorectal metastatic disease, but it also has shown promising results with other metastatic lesions (e.g., breast, gastrointestinal tract, neuroendocrine neoplasms, sarcomas).[167] Although guidelines are continuously evolving, the ideal candidates have 3 to 4 or fewer lesions, all of which are less than 5.0 cm in diameter. The major contraindication for the percutaneous approach is location of the lesion contiguous with a sensitive organ (e.g., colon, gallbladder, stomach).

Technique.[168] RFA is performed either by open or laparoscopic surgery or percutaneously with imaging guidance.[169] The choice between moderate sedation and general anesthesia depends on many factors, including lesion size, number, and location; the patient's condition; and operator preference and experience. Broad-spectrum antibiotics usually are given beforehand.

Currently, the most popular devices are the *RITA* and *Radiotherapeutics* hooked electrode devices (Mountain View,

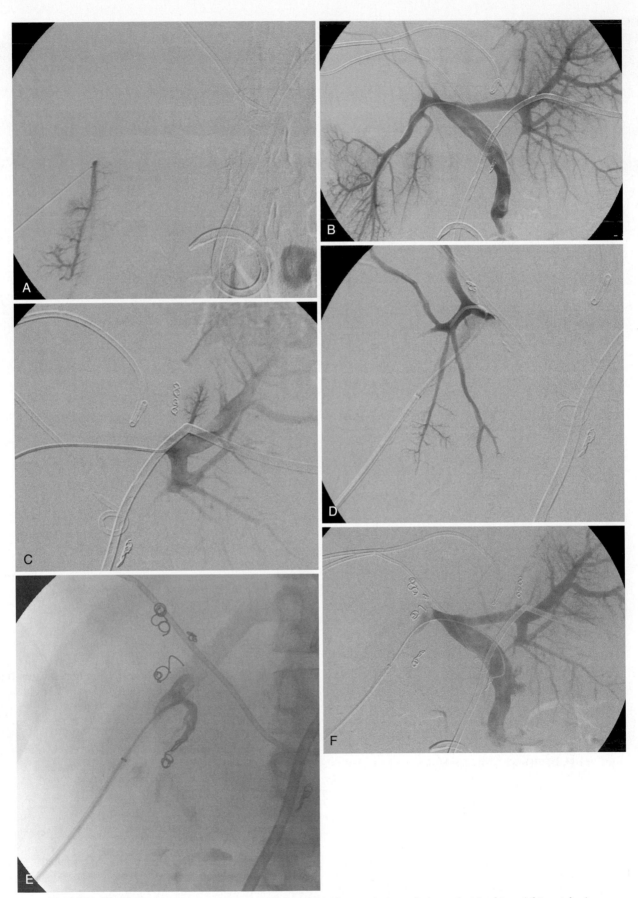

FIGURE 10-31 ■ Portal vein embolization prior to right trisegmentectomy. **A,** Access is gained to a right portal vein branch with sonographic guidance. **B,** A vascular sheath has been placed, followed by portography, which shows distortion of right portal branches by tumor. **C,** Portal branches to segment IV have been embolized. **D** and **E,** Right portal venous branches are engaged and then occluded. **F,** Final portogram shows complete obstruction of branches to segments IV–VIII.

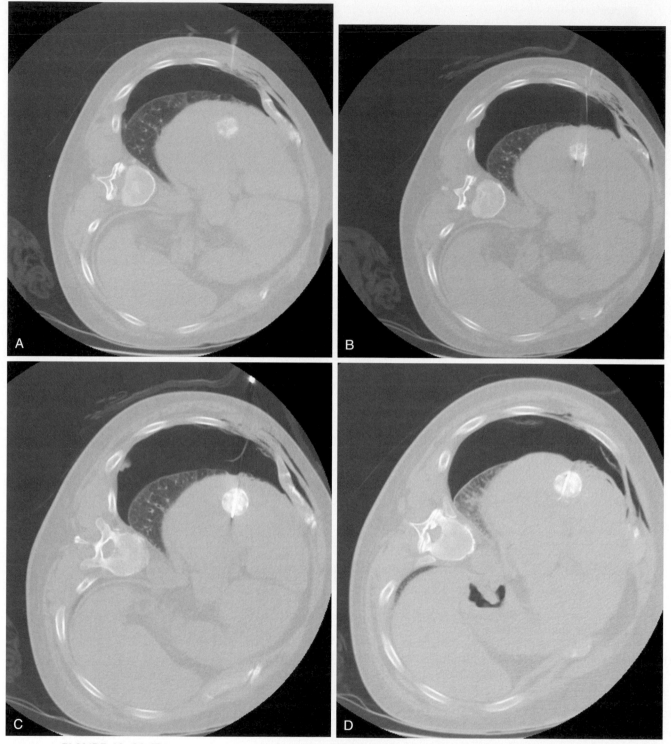

FIGURE 10-32 ■ Radiofrequency ablation for hepatocellular carcinoma. **A,** A pneumothorax has been induced to allow transthoracic entry into the lesion in the dome of the liver. Ethiodol from previous chemoembolization demarcates the tumor. **B,** A second pass is required for central needle placement. **C,** The radiofrequency probe is advanced to the far end of the lesion. **D,** The tines are deployed, and ablation is begun.

Calif.) and the *Radionics* internally cooled probes (Burlington, Mass.). Each device has its own performance characteristics. Probes (typically 14 to 16 gauge) are advanced into the lesion with imaging guidance (CT fluoroscopy or ultrasound). Occasionally, transthoracic entry into the dome of the liver is necessary.[170] Tines are first deployed usually on the far end

of the tumor and repositioned as needed to encompass the entire lesion. The endpoints for completion are based on measurement of adjacent tissue temperatures and imaging assessment. With ultrasound guidance, an intensely hyperechoic band caused by heat-produced microbubbles eventually obscures the lesion. Contrast-enhanced CT can be obtained immediately afterward to ensure that adequate ablation has been achieved. Patients with multiple lesions may require several sessions of therapy.

Results and Complications. The likelihood of eradication of a tumor less than 2.5 cm in diameter is about 90% and of a tumor between 2.5 and 3.5 cm greater than 70%.[171] Results are better with HCC than with colorectal metastases. Estimated 3-year survival with colorectal metastases was 46% in one study.[172] However, about 40% of lesions showed some recurrence after treatment. Tumor size is the most important factor in predicting success. Periodic imaging follow-up and assessment of tumor markers is required to document complete destruction and absence of new disease.

The major complication rate is about 2%.[173] Adverse events include pleural effusion, bleeding, abscess formation, track seeding, and intestinal perforation.

Intra-arterial Hepatic Infusion Chemotherapy

Although this technique continues to be popular in some countries, it has not been generally embraced.

Hepatic Transarterial Embolization and Chemoembolization

The concept behind hepatic artery chemoembolization is twofold. First, chemotherapeutic agents are infused directly into the liver using iodized poppyseed oil (e.g., Ethiodol) as a carrier to maximize their concentration and exposure time in the tumor. At the same time, hepatic arterial branches supplying the tumor are embolized to induce tumor necrosis. Poppyseed oil droplets also assist with vascular occlusion at the level of arterioportal shunts.

Patient Selection. Transarterial chemoembolization (TACE) is suitable for patients with large HCC burden not amenable to thermal ablative techniques. It is used also as an adjunct to RFA to improve overall results. There is now substantial evidence that TACE prolongs survival for HCC compared with conservative therapy, but it is clear that some patients benefit more than others. Variables that predict diminished survival included high MELD score, Child-Pugh class C, large tumor volume (>5 cm), less than 50% residual functional liver volume, and elevated bilirubin.[149,174,175] Patients may be excluded on the basis of extrahepatic metastases, unresolved biliary obstruction, or malignant ascites. Portal vein thrombosis is no longer considered an absolute contraindication to the procedure.[176]

TACE has been used also in patients with inoperable liver metastases. Results generally are not as encouraging as with HCC, although hypervascular tumors seem to respond more favorably than hypovascular ones.[177-185]

Technique. A Foley catheter is placed, and vigorous hydration is begun (normal saline at 200 mL/hour). A standard protocol is outlined in Box 10-9. Diagnostic celiac, SMA, and hepatic arteriography is performed using 5-French catheters to lay out the anatomy and identify anatomic variants. A coaxial microcatheter is then used to superselect the individual branches feeding all tumors in the lobe with dominant disease.[178] Superselective embolotherapy appears

---

> **BOX 10-9** ■ **Hepatic Transarterial Chemoembolization Protocol**
>
> ***Preprocedure Regimen***
> Cephazolin 1 g IV
> Benadryl 25 mg IV
> Metronidazole 1 g IV
> Granisetron 3 mg IV over 15 min starting 30 min before chemoinfusion
> Dexamethasone 8 mg IV and 4 mg PO immediately before chemoinfusion
>
> ***Chemoembolization Regimen***
> Adriamycin 50 mg
> Mitomycin C 10 mg
> Cis-platin 100 mg
> Contrast material 10 mL
> Ethiodol 10 mL
> Polyvinyl alcohol particles or microspheres
> Gelfoam pledgets
>
> ***Postprocedure Regimen***
> Saline hydration × 24 hr
> Cefazolin 1 g IV q8hr
> Dexamethasone 4 mg PO q6hr × 24 hr
> Metronidazole 500 mg PO q8hr
> Patient-controlled analgesia pump
> Antiemetics (prochlorperazine or droperidol)

---

safer than nonselective injection.[176] Infusion of the viscera, including the gallbladder, should be avoided if possible.[186] Either bland embolization or chemoembolization is used (Fig. 10-33; see also Box 10-9). The sterile chemoembolic mixture is partitioned roughly based on the gross volume of disease within various segments of the liver. Only syringes and stopcocks compatible with the iodized oil should be used. A three-way stopcock is used to allow emulsification between the reservoir syringe and a 3-mL delivery syringe, which ensures adequate admixing. Sometimes, central embolization of the right or left hepatic artery follows.

Most patients experience a moderate to severe *postembolization syndrome* (i.e., fever, abdominal pain, nausea) for several days after the procedure. Lesions in the right and left lobes usually are treated in separate sessions, but the timing must be tailored to the individual patient.

Recurrent or unresponsive disease may be the result of collateral circulation to the tumor from the internal thoracic (mammary), inferior phrenic, cystic, or omental arteries (Fig. 10-34).[187-190] When follow-up imaging suggests incomplete treatment of a lesion, these potential sources should be sought and embolized to eradicate residual tumor.

Results and Complications. For years, the benefit of TACE for HCC with respect to improved survival or quality of life was questioned.[191] However, two randomized controlled trials and a rigorous meta-analysis of recent clinical reports have established the value of TACE compared with medical therapy, with 2-year survival rates of up to 63%.[192-194] Major complications, including nontarget embolization (e.g., surgical cholecystitis), liver failure or infarction, hepatic abscess, and gastrointestinal bleeding, occur in about 4% to 6% of cases.[175,176]

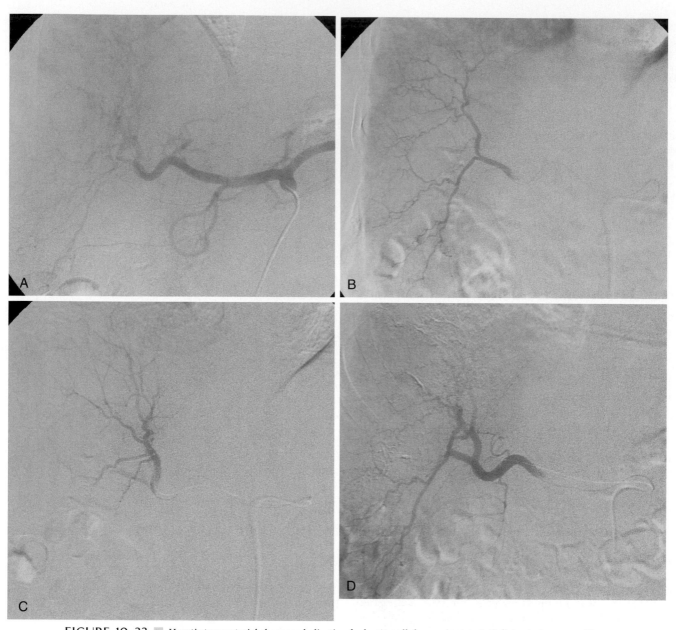

FIGURE 10-33 ■ Hepatic transarterial chemoembolization for hepatocellular carcinoma. **A,** Celiac arteriogram outlines hepatic arterial anatomy. **B** and **C,** Superselective right hepatic arteriography prior to chemoembolization infusion. Hypervascular tumor is evident. **D,** Final right hepatic arteriogram shows marked diminution in vascularity to the region of the tumor.

Liver abscess is seen most often in patients with prior bilioenteric anastomoses.[195]

Although lesion shrinkage is common after TACE for metastatic disease, improvements in quality of life and survival compared with medical therapy have not been studied as rigorously (Fig. 10-35). Most of the experience to date is with colorectal metastases.

Radiotherapy

Yttrium-90 (^{90}Y) is a beta-emitter with a physical half-life of 64.2 hours.[196] Radiation effects in tissue average 2.5 mm. Intra-arterial radiotherapy with ^{90}Y bonded to microspheres made of glass (*TheraSpheres*, MDS Nordion, Ottawa, Canada)

or resin (*SIR Spheres*, Sirtex, Lake Forest, Ill.) causes local tumor destruction with minimal effect on normal liver tissue.

Patient Selection and Pretreatment Management. Radiotherapy is applied to patients with both HCC and metastatic liver lesions, principally colorectal carcinoma. Response to this therapy is based largely on functional status and liver reserve as determined by the Okuda stage, Eastern Cooperative Oncology Group classification, Karnovsky scale, or Cancer of the Liver Italian Program (CLIP) scale.[196] The specific contraindication to radiotherapy is the presence of significant hepatopulmonary shunting. Potentially life-threatening radiation pneumonitis may occur in such cases.

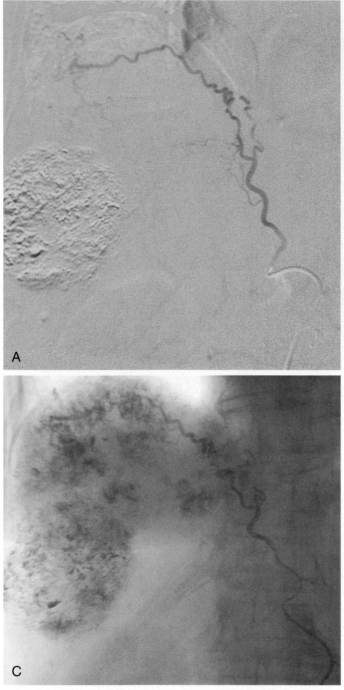

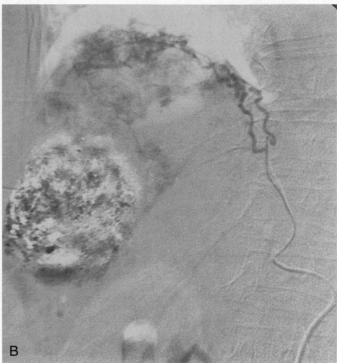

FIGURE 10-34 ■ Chemoembolization (TACE) of collateral circulation to hepatocellular carcinoma. Residual tumor was evident on contrast CT scan following initial right hepatic TACE. Proximal (**A**) and distal (**B**) injection of the right inferior phrenic artery reveals tumor vessels feeding the superior portion of the lesion. Note Ethiodol residing in tumor from prior TACE. **C,** Following chemoembolic infusion, there is stasis in the inferior phrenic artery and more Ethiodol accumulation in the tumor.

Angiography is performed in advance of the procedure (Fig. 10-36). ^{99m}Tc-labeled macroaggregated albumin is injected into the hepatic artery with dominant disease. Scanning is then performed; if the shunt ratio exceeds a certain threshold, the patient is not a candidate. Because the gastrointestinal tract is highly sensitive to these radiopharmaceuticals, proximal embolization of all potential targets are done at this time, including the right and left gastric arteries and the cystic artery.[10,196] Finally, CT or MR scans are used to calculate the volume of each hepatic lobe to calculate the appropriate radiotherapeutic dose. In general, a dose of 100 to 150 Gy is ideal for each lobe.

Technique. Strict radiation safety measures must be taken during the entire procedure. The operator should have thorough training and proctoring before performing radiotherapy independently. The case should be done with advice and supervision of the institution's radiation safety officer. However, no special precautions are necessary for the patient or contacts afterward.

The material is delivered into the right or left hepatic lobe, usually with a coaxial high-flow microcatheter placed through a standard angiographic catheter. Afterward, patients are routinely given antacids and proton pump inhibitors for several weeks, although the likelihood of

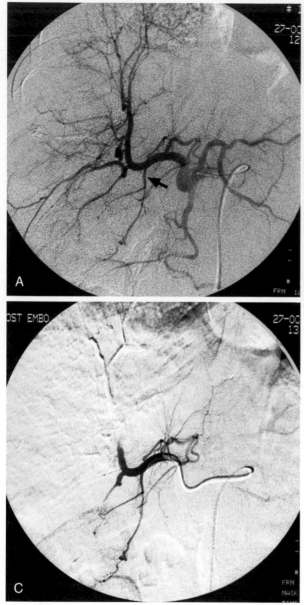

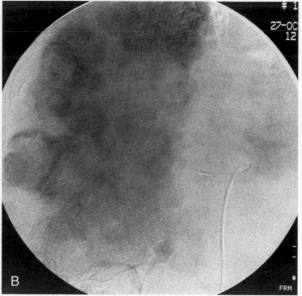

FIGURE 10-35 ■ Hepatic artery chemoembolization for carcinoid metastases. **A** and **B,** The common hepatic arteriogram shows multiple hypervascular masses. The cystic artery (**A,** *arrow*) is easily identified. **C,** After embolization, the right hepatic artery is occluded.

gastric ulceration is small when the above measures are followed.

Results and Complications. Evidence for radiation-induced liver toxicity is not uncommon and is particularly associated with preprocedure bilirubin level and radiation dose. Although this technology is evolving, preliminary results with both HCC and colorectal metastatic disease is encourgaging.[197-200]

Other Liver Neoplasms

The liver is affected by a wide variety of other benign and malignant tumors (see Box 10-8).

Hemangioma is the most common benign mass found in the liver. The lesion is a type of arteriovenous malformation characterized by collections of blood spaces lined with an endothelium (see Chapter 3).[201] They are usually small (<3 cm in diameter), may be multiple, and are more common in women than men. Patients often are asymptomatic, although the tumor can cause abdominal pain or hemorrhage. On CT, hemangiomas show peripheral enhancement in the arterial phase of contrast injection, with gradual fill-in through the portal and equilibrium phases. On MR, they show a similar pattern and are intensely bright on T2-weighted and gadolinium-enhanced images. The angiographic appearance is quite characteristic, with a normal-caliber hepatic artery, absence of neovascularity, and pooling of contrast in amorphous spaces (Fig. 10-37). Contrast puddles linger well into the venous phase of the arteriogram because of slow flow in the lesion. These features differentiate hemangioma from HCC. Although surgery is rarely indicated, transcatheter embolization has been performed preoperatively for large, symptomatic masses.[202,203]

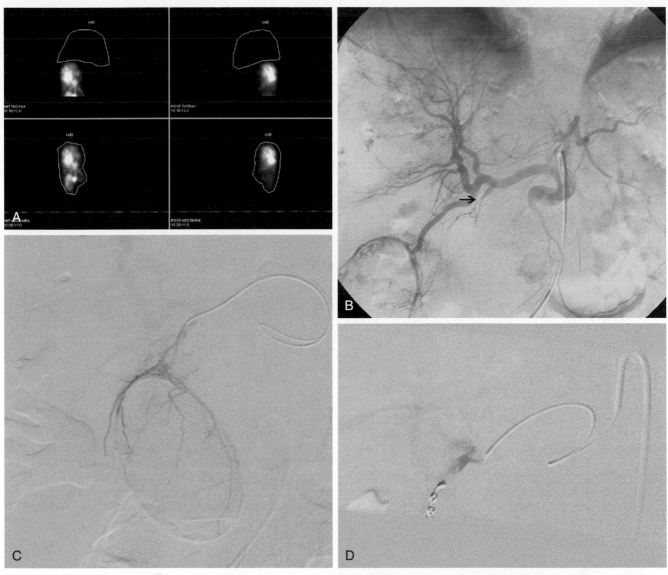

FIGURE 10-36 ■ Yttrium-90 (^{90}Y) radiotherapy for colorectal liver metastases. **A,** Radionuclide scanning following intra-arterial injection of ^{99m}Tc macroaggregated albumin excludes significant shunting to the lungs. **B,** Celiac arteriogram shows multiple vascular masses in the liver. The cystic artery is identified *(arrow)*. **C,** A coaxial microcatheter is used to select the artery, which is then embolized with coils **(D)**. Inadvertent delivery of ^{90}Y to this site could lead to cholecystitis.

Extrahepatic Masses

Neoplasms arising near the major splenic, hepatic, and portal vessels may impinge on these structures. In particular, adenocarcinoma of the pancreas frequently causes vascular encasement, displacement, or occlusion (see Fig. 11-2). Identical findings may be seen with chronic pancreatitis and its sequelae (e.g., pseudocyst formation) (see Fig. 11-6).

Trauma

Etiology and Clinical Features

The liver and spleen are particularly susceptible to injury from blunt or penetrating trauma. Open or laparoscopic surgical procedures are responsible for a significant number of cases.[204] Trauma can produce arterial laceration and parenchymal or peritoneal bleeding, subcapsular hematoma, pseudoaneurysms, or arteriovenous fistulas.[205,206] Although most patients with significant vascular injuries are symptomatic, some show little evidence of massive bleeding.

Imaging

Sonography. In most centers, sonography has replaced diagnostic peritoneal lavage as the screening tool for detecting posttraumatic intra-abdominal hemorrhage.

Computed Tomography. Hemodynamically unstable patients go directly to the operating room. CT is the primary imaging study for stable patients with blunt trauma to the abdomen.

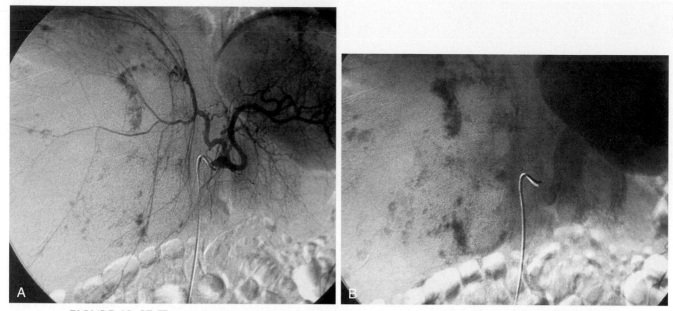

FIGURE 10-37 ■ Cavernous hemangioma of the liver. Early (**A**) and late (**B**) images from a celiac arteriogram demonstrate a huge mass occupying the liver, with displacement of vessels and multiple contrast puddles that persist into the venous phase of the study.

CT can accurately stage the extent of injury to the liver or spleen and detect other abdominal or pelvic injuries.[207]

Angiography. With blunt trauma, arteriography shows extravasation, subcapsular or parenchymal hematomas, arterial occlusion, or diffuse punctate injury (Fig. 10-38). With penetrating trauma, typical findings include extravasation, pseudoaneurysms, and arteriovenous fistulas.

Treatment

Hemodynamically stable patients with blunt hepatic injuries usually are not explored.[208] Most of them do well with close observation. Management of splenic trauma is somewhat more controversial. Although laparotomy and total splenectomy is an option, the significant risk of late sepsis after splenectomy has encouraged more conservative strategies.[209]

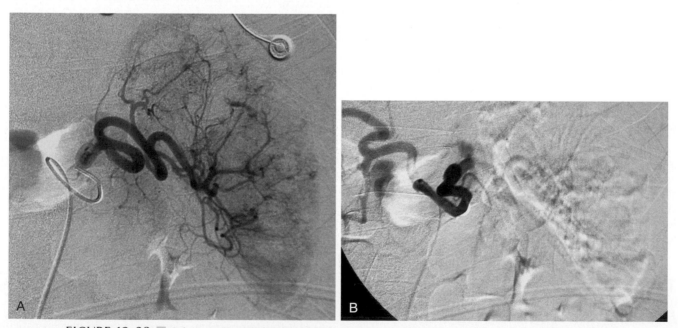

FIGURE 10-38 ■ Splenic artery embolization for abdominal trauma following a motor vehicle accident. **A,** Splenic arteriogram reveals diffuse injury with irregular branch vessels and areas of gross and punctate extravasation. **B,** Following shower embolization with Gelfoam pieces, the artery is occluded and bleeding is no longer seen.

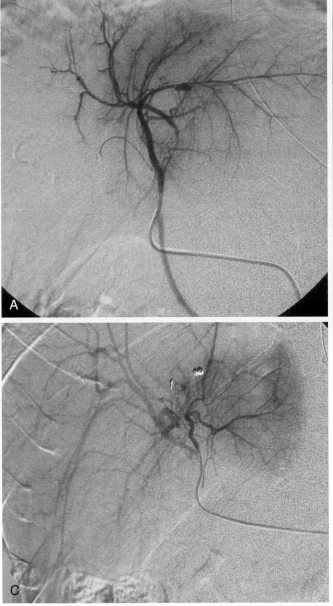

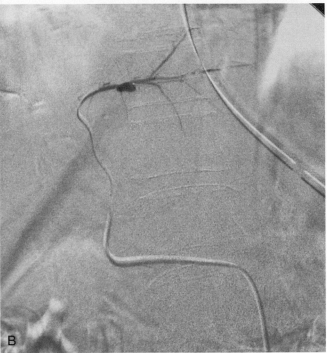

FIGURE 10-39 ■ Peripheral hepatic artery pseudoaneurysm from an abdominal stab wound. **A,** Selective left hepatic arteriogram demonstrates a branch pseudoaneurysm. A coaxial microcatheter was used to select the affected vessel (**B**), which was embolized to prevent further bleeding (**C**).

Endovascular Therapy. Embolization is the first-line treatment for most significant hepatic and splenic arterial injuries.[205,209-212] Embolotherapy is safe in the liver because of its dual blood supply and in the spleen because of the rich collateral circulation. Pseudoaneurysms and fistulas are closed with coils or Gelfoam pledgets (Fig. 10-39). In the liver, embolic material is placed directly at the site of injury to minimize organ ischemia and prevent backflow into the aneurysm through collateral vessels. In the spleen, more proximal embolization with coils often is sufficient to stop hemorrhage; embolic material such as microcoils or Gelfoam pieces also can be deposited in intrasplenic branches that feed a bleeding site (see Fig. 10-38). Embolotherapy is successful in greater than 85% of cases.[205,209,212] Complications include abscess formation (especially in the spleen), tissue infarction (common after splenic embolization and usually self-limited), bleeding, and nontarget embolization.[213]

Surgical Therapy. Operative treatment for liver injuries involves gauze packing, oversewing, or partial hepatic resection. In most patients, splenectomy after abdominal trauma is unnecessary. Operation is reserved for patients who are hemodynamically unstable or who fail embolotherapy.

Vascular Complications After Liver Transplantation

Liver transplantation is the definitive treatment for patients with nonreversible hepatic failure, complications of cirrhosis and portal hypertension, certain metabolic liver diseases, and HCC. The interventionalist has two primary roles in this setting: (1) to provide a bridge to transplantation by portal decompression (e.g., TIPS creation) or tumor ablation, and (2) to help manage vascular complications afterward.[214,215] In the former situation, the goal of interventional procedures is to maintain the patient as a transplant candidate. Extensive preoperative imaging (usually with MR angiography and cholangiography) is necessary to determine the suitability for transplantation with regard to liver size, underlying liver disease, and vascular/biliary anatomic variants.[216,217] Rarely, catheter angiography is required prior to reduced-size transplants to identify arterial variants, segmental blood supply, and the size of the donor artery.[218]

Operative Procedures

In the classic *orthotopic liver transplant procedure*, the hepatic arterial anastomosis is made between the donor celiac axis or common hepatic artery and the recipient common hepatic artery.[214] When the recipient has two arteries supplying the liver (e.g., replaced right hepatic artery), a common trunk is created. Occasionally, an infrarenal iliac artery homograft is used (Fig. 10-40). The PV anastomosis is created in an end-to-end fashion. An iliac vein interposition graft to the SMV may be required if the PV is diseased. The IVC connection can be created with both suprahepatic and infrahepatic anastomoses. However, many transplant surgeons now use the "piggyback technique" in which an end-to-side anastomosis is formed using the suprahepatic donor segment and the hepatic vein confluence of the recipient.

Segmental (reduced or split) liver transplantation allows for pediatric or adult transplants from either cadaveric **or** living donors and increases the overall number of available grafts.[214,219] Surgical options include removal of the left lateral portion (segments II and III), right trisegmentectomy (segments IV to VIII), left lobe (segments II, III, IVa, and IVb), or right lobe (segments V to VIII).[220] Obviously, the interventionalist must understand the precise operative anatomy in a particular case before proceeding with diagnostic or interventional procedures.

Complications

Up to 25% of patients suffer vascular complications after liver transplantation. Because often they are initially silent and the clinical course may be hard to differentiate from graft rejection or primary nonfunction, routine imaging of transplants with noninvasive imaging (contrast ultrasound, CT, or MR) is crucial.[221-223]

Hepatic Artery Thrombosis. The most common and grave complication after liver transplant is hepatic artery thrombosis, which occurs in about 3% to 12% of cases, and more frequently in children.[224-227] The most common causes are operative errors, progressive hepatic artery stenosis, rejection, and arterial kinking. With the exception of some children, no extrahepatic arterial collaterals support the graft in this situation. Coupled with some loss of the normal reciprocal relationship between portal and arterial liver flow, the graft will be in jeopardy. Since the biliary tree is exclusively supplied by the hepatic artery, bile duct ischemia occurs frequently

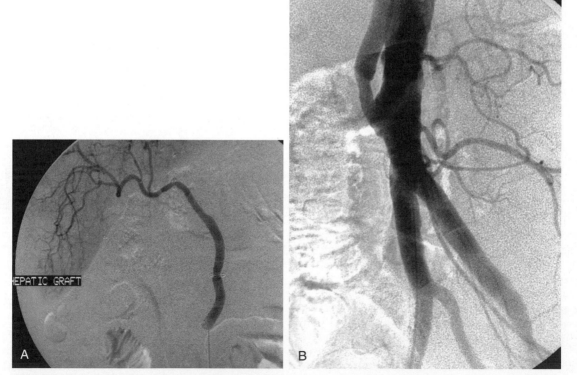

FIGURE 10-40 ▪ Orthotopic liver transplant with the donor hepatic artery (**A**) fed by an iliac artery homograft anastomosed to the recipient's distal abdominal aorta (**B**).

without treatment, resulting in strictures, bilomas, or mucosal sloughing.[227]

Hepatic artery thrombosis usually occurs within 2 to 3 months of transplantation. Patients often show signs of fulminant liver failure, biliary leak, or sepsis. The diagnosis is made with contrast-enhanced ultrasound, CT, or MR. Catheter angiography is virtually never required. While endovascular thrombolysis, angioplasty, and stent placement have been attempted, most patients require immediate revascularization to avoid the need for retransplantation.[224,228,229]

Hepatic Artery Stenosis. Hepatic artery stenosis is less common than frank occlusion (about 4% to 12% of cases).[214,227] Most stenoses occur at the anastomosis and are caused by technical errors, intimal hyperplasia, or graft rejection (see Fig. 2-30). Even when stenoses do not jeopardize graft viability, biliary duct ischemia complicated by stricture formation is common (see above). Sonographic signs of hepatic artery stenosis include a "parvus-et-tardus" waveform, focal peak hepatic artery velocity of greater than 200 to 300 cm/second, a resistive index less than 0.5, and a systolic acceleration time greater than 0.08 seconds in the intrahepatic arteries (Fig. 10-41).[230,231]

Angioplasty of hepatic artery stenoses is technically successful in about 80% of cases.[232] However, stenoses in fresh grafts (<2 weeks old) may rupture if opened with a balloon. Reported rates of restenosis have been highly variable; stents may improve on these results.[233]

Portal Vein Thrombosis/Stenosis. Significant PV stenosis or thrombosis is uncommon (up to 7% of pediatric recipients, 1% to 2% of adults).[214,227,234] PV obstruction is signaled by absence of flow, focal areas of stenosis with increased peak velocity, or alterations in normal flow patterns and phasicity. However, the significance of noninvasive imaging findings must be confirmed with direct catheter-based pressure measurements (>5 mm Hg being significant). Stenoses respond extremely well to angioplasty and selective stent placement as needed.[235-237] However, most thrombotic obstructions require operative repair.

Inferior Vena Cava/Hepatic Vein Obstruction. IVC obstructions are the least common among the various vascular complications after liver transplantation. Hepatic venous obstructions are virtually unheard of after orthotopic liver transplant (in which no hepatic vein anastomosis is created), but they have been reported in 7% to 17% of cases after split liver transplants. Early lesions are related to technical issues such as a tight suture line or venous kinking; late stenoses are a consequence of fibrosis or neointimal hyperplasia around the anastomosis. Symptoms typically include ascites, abdominal pain, and signs of liver graft dysfunction.

These obstructions result in slow or monophasic hepatic venous waveforms on Doppler sonography and nonopacification of hepatic veins on CT angiography. As with suspected portal vein stenoses, direct pressure gradients are needed to confirm cross-sectional imaging findings (gradient >5 to 6 mm Hg). Because reoperation in this situation is technically difficult, most surgeons prefer endovascular treatment. Stent placement usually is necessary for durable results in adults (Fig. 10-42).[238-240]

Hepatic Artery Pseudoaneurysms. These lesions may present some time after transplantation with fever, hemobilia, unexplained bleeding, graft dysfunction, or arterial occlusion.[214] **Extrahepatic** arterial pseudoaneurysms are rare and potentially catastrophic. They occur typically at the hepatic arterial anastomosis and may have an infectious origin. **Intrahepatic** pseudoaneurysms and arteriovenous fistulas usually are caused by a postoperative percutaneous procedure.

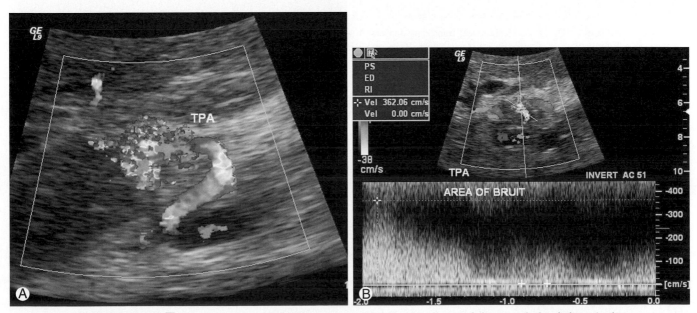

FIGURE 10-41 ■ Liver transplant hepatic artery stenosis. Color Doppler ultrasound shows marked turbulence in the region of the anastomosis (**A**) and elevated velocities (362 cm/second) (**B**).

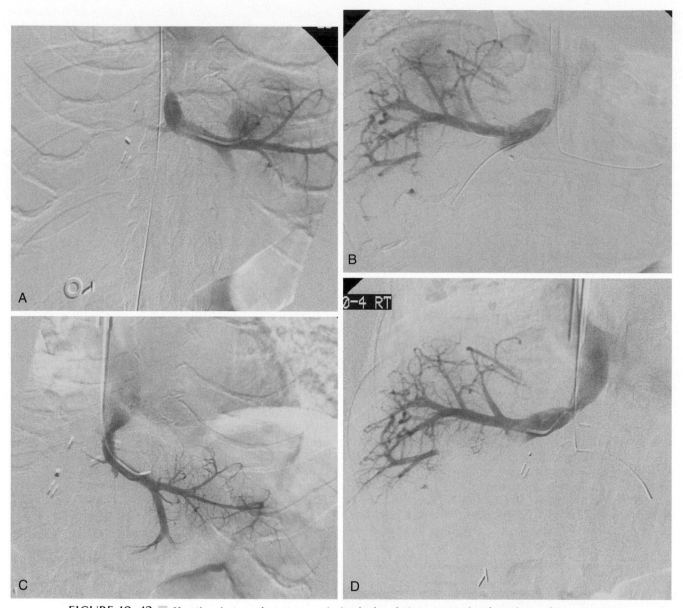

FIGURE 10-42 ▪ Hepatic vein transplant stenoses. A piggyback technique was used to form the caval anastomosis. Tight narrowing of both the left (**A**) and right (**B**) hepatic vein outflow is observed. Following angioplasty (**C** and **D**), luminal diameters are improved and pressure gradients were markedly reduced. However, stent placement may be required for a durable result.

▪ OTHER DISORDERS

Obstructive Arterial Diseases

Atherosclerosis may affect the hepatic and splenic arteries, but clinically significant disease is rare. Several other entities can mimic atherosclerotic plaque (Box 10-10). Marked elongation, tortuosity, and calcification of the splenic artery is a frequent finding in older patients. Atherosclerosis may progress to complete thrombotic occlusion (Box 10-11). However, the extensive collateral pathways to the spleen and the dual blood supply of the liver usually prevent

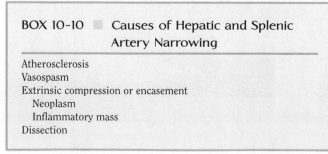

BOX 10-10 ▪ Causes of Hepatic and Splenic
               Artery Narrowing

Atherosclerosis
Vasospasm
Extrinsic compression or encasement
    Neoplasm
    Inflammatory mass
Dissection

BOX 10-11 ■ Causes of Hepatic and Splenic Artery Occlusion

Thrombosis secondary to underlying stenosis
Embolus
Dissection
Trauma
Chemoinfusion
Aneurysm thrombosis

Aneurysms

Visceral artery aneurysms and pseudoaneurysms are uncommon. However, the splenic and hepatic arteries are the most frequently affected vessels.[244,245] Splenic artery aneurysms/pseudoaneurysms are associated most commonly with pancreatitis, trauma, atherosclerosis, or portal hypertension (Box 10-12). Intrahepatic artery aneurysms are usually posttraumatic.

Patients with splenic artery aneurysms typically have abdominal pain or hypotension from bleeding. Hepatic artery aneurysms may present with abdominal pain, hemobilia, or jaundice. At least one half of patients are asymptomatic at the time of detection by cross-sectional imaging.

On noninvasive studies, a focally enlarged, enhancing vessel is seen, sometimes with fluid adjacent to the aneurysm (Fig. 10-44). On angiography, degenerative splenic artery aneurysms are fusiform or saccular, often

organ infarction. Splenic infarction is generally the result of hematologic disorders or embolization (usually from the heart) (Fig. 10-43).[241] Dissection of the hepatic or splenic artery may be posttraumatic or spontaneous (e.g., extension of a celiac artery dissection).[242,243]

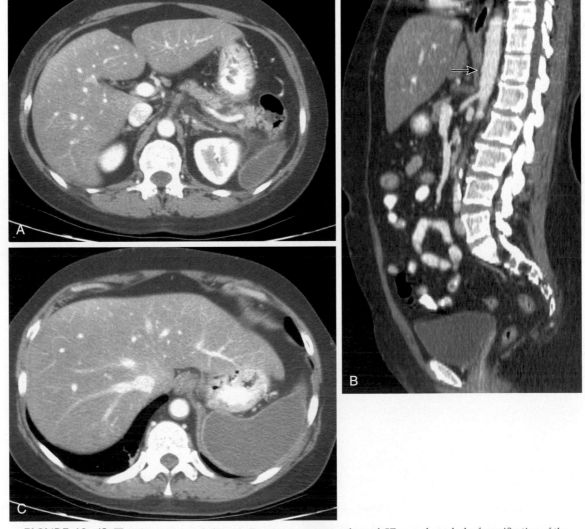

FIGURE 10-43 ■ Celiac artery embolism. **A,** Transverse contrast-enhanced CT scan shows lack of opacification of the celiac axis, which is confirmed on a sagittal reformatted image (**B,** *arrow*). **C,** CT scan shows splenic infarction due to the acute ischemic insult.

BOX 10-12 ■ Causes of Splenic and Hepatic Artery Aneurysms and Pseudoaneurysms

Inflammation
  Pancreatitis
  Infection
Atherosclerosis-associated degeneration
Trauma
Collagen vascular diseases
Portal hypertension
Infusion of chemotherapeutic drugs
Hypersplenism
Congenital disorder
Vasculitis (microaneurysms)

multiple, and may be calcified. Hepatic artery aneurysms usually are solitary and extrahepatic. In patients with polyarteritis nodosa, numerous intrahepatic or intrasplenic microaneurysms are seen (Fig. 10-45).

Although the natural history of some visceral aneurysms is one of persistent growth and eventual rupture, it is difficult to predict which ones will ultimately bleed. Hemorrhage may occur into the peritoneal space, lesser sac (splenic aneurysms), or biliary system (hepatic aneurysms). Degenerative splenic artery aneurysm rupture is uncommon. Treatment is recommended when the aneurysm is large (>2.5 cm), symptomatic, rapidly expanding, or found in a patient who is or could become pregnant. Visceral aneurysms in pregnant women are especially prone to rupture.[246,247] Aneurysm leak with exsanguinating hemorrhage is more common with extrahepatic arterial aneurysms; therefore, most authorities favor early repair in almost all cases.[248]

Transcatheter embolization is the treatment of choice for most *intrahepatic* and splenic artery aneurysms and pseudoaneurysms.[244,245,249] The preferred embolic agent is a coil; Gelfoam pledgets can be used to accelerate thrombosis. Embolization across the aneurysm neck is important to prevent retrograde flow into the aneurysm through collateral vessels feeding the distal artery. For intrahepatic aneurysms, embolization is done as close to the aneurysm neck as possible (see Fig. 10-39).

Surgery (by exclusion, excision, or bypass grafting) is required for some *extrahepatic* artery aneurysms and for failures of embolotherapy. Covered stent placement is an alternative technique.[250] Splenic artery aneurysms rarely require splenectomy and aneurysm removal or proximal and distal ligation.

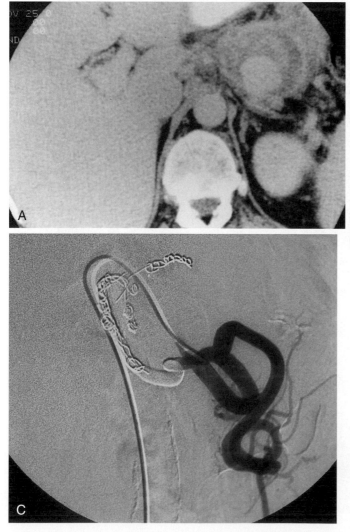

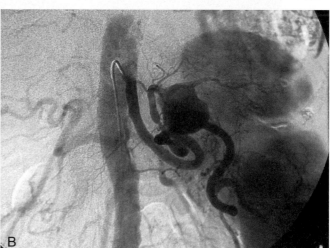

FIGURE 10-44 ■ Splenic artery pseudoaneurysm caused by pancreatitis. **A,** Contrast-enhanced CT scan shows a round, enhancing mass in the tail of the pancreas surrounded by a larger, inhomogeneous soft tissue collection. **B,** Celiac arteriography in another patient shows a large midsplenic artery pseudoaneurysm. **C,** The branch feeding the aneurysm has been embolized with coils, and flow to the spleen was preserved.

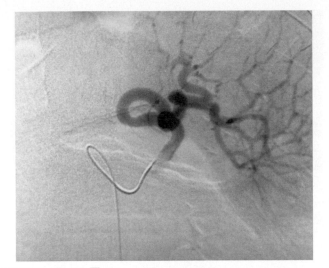

FIGURE 10-45 ■ Polyarteritis nodosa with multiple microaneurysms of intrasplenic arteries.

Vasculitis

Several forms of arteritis can affect the liver and spleen. *Polyarteritis nodosa* and illicit drug use can produce a necrotizing vasculitis that may involve the liver, kidneys, intestinal tract, and extremities (see Fig. 10-45). Liver involvement with giant cell arteritis also has been described.[251]

Arteriovenous Communications

A wide variety of disorders can form or accentuate arteriovenous shunts in the liver (Box 10-13; see Fig. 3-43).[252,253] Massive arterioportal shunting is one of the causes of hyperdynamic portal hypertension. Portohepatic vein fistulas are rare and usually congenital.[254] Intrahepatic fistulas may be closed by transcatheter embolotherapy.[255,256]

Splenic arteriovenous fistulas are rare lesions caused by rupture of a splenic artery aneurysm, a congenital malformation, or previous splenectomy.[257] Hyperdynamic portal hypertension may result.

In a minority of patients with *hereditary hemorrhagic telangiectasia,* liver AVMs predominate and become responsible for abdominal ischemia, heart or liver failure, or portal hypertension. Staged embolization has been used with success, but fatalities from this procedure have also been reported.[258-260]

Hypersplenism

Hypersplenism is a condition in which the normal destruction of cellular blood elements by the spleen is exaggerated because of reticuloendothelial hyperplasia in the organ. The syndrome is associated with cirrhosis and portal hypertension, thalassemia, idiopathic thrombocytopenic purpura, and

several other disorders.[261-263] Signs of the disorder include splenomegaly, anemia, leukopenia, and thrombocytopenia.

Although splenectomy is the traditional therapy for hypersplenism, the risk of postsplenectomy sepsis makes it a less than ideal approach. Splenic artery embolization often is requested before open or laparoscopic splenectomy for this condition to minimize intraoperative blood loss (Fig. 10-46). *Partial splenic embolization* is an accepted method for reducing splenic size and the inhibitory effects on platelets and red blood cells while maintaining some splenic activity to prevent postprocedure sepsis.[261-265] Embolization is performed from the distal splenic artery beyond the pancreatic and gastric branches. Gelfoam pledgets, PVA particles, or microspheres may be used. The goal is to reduce splenic volume by 60% to 80%. Some interventionalists prefer to stage the procedure over several weeks.

Patients are given broad-spectrum antibiotics beforehand and are treated for postembolization syndrome for several days afterward. The spleen shrinks markedly over 3 to 4 months. The procedure increases total blood cell counts and improves qualitative platelet activity.[266] The results are long lasting in many patients, although repeat embolization is often necessary if less than 50% of splenic volume is eliminated initially. Complications, including splenic abscess formation and splenic vein thrombosis, are unlikely if complete organ infarction is avoided.[267]

Peliosis

Peliosis hepatis is a rare disorder in which multiple blood-filled cavities develop within the liver. Although the cause is unknown in many patients, peliosis is associated with androgen hormone-replacement therapy and *Bartonella* infections.[268,269] The diagnosis can be made with cross-sectional imaging.[270] Innumerable lucent spaces are seen on imaging studies.

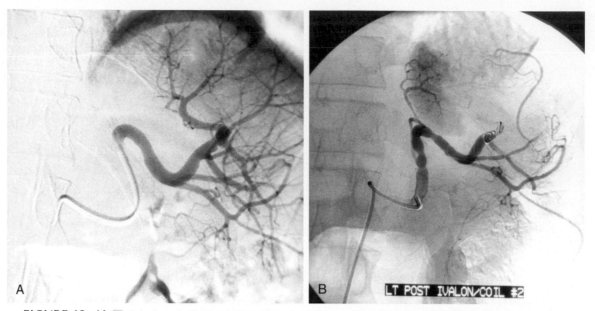

FIGURE 10-46 ■ Splenic embolization before splenectomy in a patient with idiopathic thrombocytopenic purpura. **A,** Arteriography reveals an enlarged spleen. **B,** The spleen is almost completely devascularized after embolization with polyvinyl alcohol particles and coils. Residual filling of splenic tissue from the superior polar artery is seen. (**A,** From Rose SC, Lim GA, Arrellano RS, et al: Temporary splenic artery balloon occlusion for protection of nonsplenic vascular beds during splenic embolization. AJR Am J Roentgenol 1998;170:1186.)

Segmental Arterial Mediolysis

This exceedingly rare disease of unknown etiology is characterized by destruction of arterial medial smooth muscle cells and eventual replacement by fibrin and granulation tissue.[271] Over time, extension to the entire arterial wall can produce multiple spontaneous dissections and/or aneurysms. It has been postulated that segmental arterial mediolysis is related to fibromuscular dysplasia. Segmental arterial mediolysis primarily affects mesenteric, renal, and coronary arteries (see Fig. 9-42).

REFERENCES

1. Brazzini A, Hunter DW, Darcy MD, et al: Safe splenoportography. Radiology 1987;162:607.
2. Burke CT, Weeks SM, Mauro MA, et al: CO_2 splenoportography for evaluating the splenic and portal veins before or after liver transplantation. J Vasc Interv Radiol 2004;15:1161.
3. Caridi JG, Hawkins IF Jr, Cho K, et al: CO_2 splenoportography: preliminary results. AJR Am J Roentgenol 2003;180:1375.
4. Sadler TW, ed: Langman's Medical Embryology. Baltimore, Williams & Wilkins, 1995:254.
5. Sadler TW, ed: Langman's Medical Embryology. Baltimore, Williams & Wilkins, 1995:219.
6. Takahashi S, Murakami T, Takamura M, et al: Multi-detector row helical CT angiography of hepatic vessels: depiction with dual-arterial phase acquisition during single breath hold. Radiology 2002;222:81.
7. Lee VS, Morgan GR, Teperman LW, et al: MR imaging as the sole preoperative imaging modality for right hepatectomy: a prospective study of living adult-to-adult liver donor candidates. AJR Am J Roentgenol 2001;176:1475.
8. Lavelle MT, Lee VS, Rofsky NM, et al: Dynamic contrast-enhanced three-dimensional MR imaging of liver parenchyma: source images and angiographic reconstructions to define hepatic arterial anatomy. Radiology 2001;218:389.
9. Guiney MJ, Kruskal JB, Sosna J, et al: Multi-detector row CT of relevant vascular anatomy of the surgical plane in split-liver transplantation. Radiology 2003;229:401.
10. Liu DM, Salem R, Bui JT, et al: Angiographic considerations in patients undergoing liver-directed therapy: a comprehensive review. J Vasc Interv Radiol 2005;16:911.
11. Sielaff TD, Curley SA: Liver. In: Brunicardi FC, Andersen DK, Dunn DL, et al, eds. Schwartz's Principles of Surgery. New York, McGraw-Hill, 2005:1140.
12. The Terminology Committee of the IHPBA: The Brisbane 2000 terminology of hepatic anatomy and resections. HPB. 2000;2:333.
13. Fasel JH, Selle D, Evertsz CJ, et al: Segmental anatomy of the liver: poor correlation with CT. Radiology 1998;206:151.
14. Pieters PC, Miller WJ, DeMeo JH: Evaluation of the portal venous system: complementary roles of invasive and non-invasive imaging strategies. Radiographics 1997;17:879.
15. Graf O, Boland GW, Kaufman JA, et al: Anatomic variants of mesenteric veins: depiction with helical CT venography. AJR Am J Roentgenol 1997;168:1209.
16. LaBerge JM: Anatomy relevant to the transjugular intrahepatic portosystemic shunt procedure. Semin Intervent Radiol 1995;12:337.
17. Covey AM, Brody LA, Getrajdman GI, et al: Incidence, patterns, and clinical relevance of variant portal vein anatomy. AJR Am J Roentgenol 2004;183:1055.
18. Bannister LH, ed: Alimentary system. In: Williams PL, Bannister LH, Berry MM, et al, eds. Gray's Anatomy, 38th ed. New York, Churchill Livingstone, 1995:1802.
19. Gabella G, ed: Cardiovascular system. In: Williams PL, Bannister LH, Berry MM, et al, eds. Gray's Anatomy, 38th ed. New York, Churchill Livingstone, 1995:1551.
20. Ishigami K, Zhang Y, Rayhill S, et al: Does variant hepatic artery anatomy in a liver transplant recipient increase the risk of hepatic artery complications after transplantation? AJR Am J Roentgenol 2004;183:1577.
21. Koops A, Wojciechowski B, Broering DC, et al: Anatomic variations of the hepatic arteries in 604 selective celiac and superior mesenteric angiographies. Surg Radiol Anat 2004;26:239.
22. Kopka L, Rodenwaldt J, Vosshenrich R, et al: Hepatic blood supply: comparison of optimized dual phase contrast-enhanced three-dimensional MR angiography and digital subtraction angiography. Radiology 1999;211:51.
23. Michels NA: Blood Supply and Anatomy of the Upper Abdominal Organs with Descriptive Atlas. Philadelphia, Lippincott, 1955.

24. Covey AM, Brody LA, Maluccio MA, et al: Variant hepatic arterial anatomy revisited: digital subtraction angiography performed in 600 patients. Radiology 2002;224:542.
25. Gayer G, Zissin R, Apter S, et al: CT findings in congenital anomalies of the spleen. Br J Radiol 2001;74:767.
26. Carr JC, Nemcek AA Jr, Abecassis M, et al: Preoperative evaluation of the entire hepatic vasculature in living liver donors with use of contrast-enhanced MR angiography and true fast imaging with steady-state precession. J Vasc Interv Radiol 2003;14:441.
27. Crawford JM: Liver and biliary tract. In: Kumar V, Abbas AK, Fausto N, eds. Robbins and Cotran Pathologic Basis of Disease, 7th ed. Philadelphia, Saunders, 2005;877.
28. Farzaneh-Far R, Moore K: Nitric oxide and the liver. Liver 2001;21:161.
29. Sharara AI, Rockey DC: Gastroesophageal variceal hemorrhage. N Engl J Med 2001;345:669.
30. Lebrec D, Moreau R: Pathogenesis of portal hypertension. Eur J Gastroenterol Hepatol 2001;13:309.
31. Vaughan RB, Chin-Dusting JP: Current pharmacotherapy in the management of cirrhosis: focus on the hyperdynamic circulation. Expert Opin Pharmacother 2003;4:625.
32. de Franchis R, Primignani M: Natural history of portal hypertension in patients with cirrhosis. Clin Liver Dis 2001;5:645.
33. Sharara AI, Hunt CM, Hamilton JD: Hepatitis C. Ann Intern Med 1996;125:658.
34. Mergo PJ, Ros PR: Imaging of diffuse liver disease. Radiol Clin North Am 1998;36:365.
35. Neuberger J: Primary biliary cirrhosis. Lancet 1997;350:875.
36. Okudaira M, Ohbu M, Okuda K: Idiopathic portal hypertension and its pathology. Semin Liver Dis 2002;22:59.
37. Defreyne L, De Schrijver I, Vanlangenhove P, et al: Detachable balloon embolization of an aneurysmal gastroduodenal arterioportal fistula. Eur Radiol 2002;12:231.
38. Jaffe DL, Chung RT, Friedman LS: Management of portal hypertension and its complications. Med Clin North Am 1996;80:1021.
39. Reynolds TB: Interrelationships of portal pressure, variceal size, and upper gastrointestinal bleeding. Gastroenterology 1980;79:1332.
40. Gines P, Cardenas A, Arroyo V, et al: Management of cirrhosis and ascites. N Engl J Med 2004;350:1646.
41. Benjaminov FS, Prentice M, Sniderman KW, et al: Portopulmonary hypertension in decompensated cirrhosis with refractory ascites. Gut 2003;52:1355.
42. Menon KV, Kamath PS: Regional and systemic hemodynamic disturbances in cirrhosis. Clin Liver Dis 2001;5:617.
43. Wong F, Blendis L: New challenge of hepatorenal syndrome: prevention and treatment. Hepatology 2001;34:1242.
44. Reynolds TB, Ito S, Iwatsuki S: Measurement of portal pressure and its clinical application. Am J Med 1970;49:649.
44. Little AF, Zajko AB, Orons PD: Transjugular liver biopsy: a prospective study in 43 patients with the Quick-Core biopsy needle. J Vasc Interv Radiol 1996;7:127.
45. Gorriz E, Reyes R, Lobrano MB, et al: Transjugular liver biopsy: a review of 77 biopsies using a spring-propelled cutting needle (biopsy gun). Cardiovasc Intervent Radiol 1996;19:442.
46. Wallace MJ, Narvios A, Lichtiger B, et al: Transjugular liver biopsy in patients with hematologic malignancy and severe thrombocytopenia. J Vasc Interv Radiol 2003;14:323.
47. Psooy BJ, Clark TW, Beecroft JR, et al: Transjugular liver biopsy with use of the shark jaw needle: diagnostic yield, complications, and cost-effectiveness. J Vasc Interv Radiol 2001;12:61.
48. Lipchik EO, Cohen EB, Mewissen MW: Transvenous liver biopsy in critically ill patients: adequacy of tissue samples. Radiology 1991;181:497.
49. Banares R, Alonso S, Catalina MV, et al: Randomized controlled trial of aspiration needle versus automated biopsy device for transjugular liver biopsy. J Vasc Interv Radiol 2001;12:583.
50. Lowe RC, Grace ND: Primary prophylaxis of variceal hemorrhage. Clin Liver Dis 2001;5:665.
51. Grace ND: Diagnosis and treatment of gastrointestinal bleeding secondary to portal hypertension: American College of Gastroenterology Practice Parameters Committee. Am J Gastroenterol 1997;92:1081.
52. Cello JP: Endoscopic management of esophageal variceal hemorrhage: injection, banding, glue, octreotide, or a combination? Semin Gastroenterol Dis 1997;8:179.
53. Lui HF, Stanley AJ, Forrest EH, et al: Primary prophylaxis of variceal hemorrhage: a randomized controlled trial comparing band ligation, propranolol, and isosorbide mononitrate. Gastroenterology 2002; 123:735.

54. Villanueva C, Minana J, Ortiz J, et al: Endoscopic ligation compared with combined treatment with nadolol and isosorbide mononitrate to prevent recurrent variceal bleeding. N Engl J Med 2001;345:647.
55. Lunderquist A, Vang J: Transhepatic catheterization and obliteration of the coronary vein in patients with portal hypertension and esophageal varices. N Engl J Med 1974;291:646.
56. L'Hermine CL, Chastanet P, Delemazure O, et al: Percutaneous transhepatic embolization of gastroesophageal varices: results in 400 patients. AJR Am J Roentgenol 1989;152:755.
57. Kiyosue H, Mori H, Matsumoto S, et al: Transcatheter obliteration of gastric varices: Part 2. Strategy and techniques based on hemodynamic features. Radiographics 2003;23:921.
58. Kiyosue H, Mori H, Matsumoto S, et al: Transcatheter obliteration of gastric varices. Part 1. Anatomic classification. Radiographics 2003; 23:911.
59. Hirota S, Matsumoto S, Tomita M, et al: Retrograde transvenous obliteration of gastric varices. Radiology 1999;211:349.
60. Sonomura T, Horihata K, Yamahara K, et al: Ruptured duodenal varices successfully treated with balloon-occluded retrograde transvenous obliteration: usefulness of microcatheters. AJR Am J Roentgenol 2003;181:725.
61. Fukuda T, Hirota S, Sugimura K: Long-term results of balloon-occluded retrograde transvenous obliteration for the treatment of gastric varices and hepatic encephalopathy. J Vasc Interv Radiol 2001;12:327.
62. Warren WD, Millikan WJ Jr, Henderson JM, et al: Ten years portal hypertensive surgery at Emory. Ann Surg 1982;195:530.
63. Orloff MJ, Orloff MS, Orloff SL, et al: Three decades of experience with emergency portacaval shunt for acutely bleeding esophageal varices in 400 unselected patients with cirrhosis of the liver. J Am Coll Surg 1995;180:257.
64. Boyer TD, Haskal ZJ: American association for the study of liver diseases practice guidelines: the role of transjugular intrahepatic portosystemic shunt creation in the management of portal hypertension. J Vasc Interv Radiol 2005;16:615.
65. Shiffman ML, Jeffers L, Hoofnagle JH, et al: The role of transjugular intrahepatic portosystemic shunt for treatment of portal hypertension and its complications: a conference sponsored by the National Digestive Diseases Advisory Board. Hepatology 1995;22:1591.
66. Spencer EB, Cohen DT, Darcy MD: Safety and efficacy of transjugular intrahepatic portosystemic shunt creation for the treatment of hepatic hydrothorax. J Vasc Interv Radiol 2002;13:385.
67. Cosenza CA, Hoffman AL, Friedman ML, et al: Transjugular intrahepatic portosystemic shunt: efficacy for the treatment of portal hypertension and impact on liver transplantation. Am Surgeon 1996;62:835.
68. Menegaux F, Keeffe EB, Baker E, et al: Comparison of transjugular and surgical portosystemic shunts on the outcome of liver transplantation. Arch Surg 1994;129:1018.
69. Haskal ZJ, Scott M, Rubin RA, et al: Intestinal varices: treatment with transjugular intrahepatic portosystemic shunt. Radiology 1994;191:183.
70. Trevino HH, Brady CE 3rd, Schencker S: Portal hypertensive gastropathy. Dig Dis 1996;14:258.
71. Wallace M, Swaim M: Transjugular intrahepatic portosystemic shunts through hepatic neoplasms. J Vasc Interv Radiol 2003;14:501.
72. Shin ES, Darcy MD: Transjugular intrahepatic portosystemic shunt placement in the setting of polycystic liver disease: questioning the contraindication. J Vasc Interv Radiol 2001;12:1099.
73. Ferral H, Patel NH: Selection criteria for patients undergoing transjugular intrahepatic portosystemic shunt procedures: current status. J Vasc Interv Radiol 2005;16:449.
74. Ferral H, Vasan R, Speeg KV, et al: Evaluation of a model to predict poor survival in patients undergoing elective TIPS procedures. J Vasc Interv Radiol 2002;13:1103.
75. Rajan DK, Haskal ZJ, Clark TW: Serum bilirubin and early mortality after transjugular intrahepatic portosystemic shunts: results of a multivariate analysis. J Vasc Interv Radiol 2002;13:155.
76. Schepke M, Roth F, Fimmers R, et al: Comparison of MELD, Child-Pugh, and Emory model for the prediction of survival in patients undergoing transjugular intrahepatic portosystemic shunting. Am J Gastroenterol 2003;98:1167.
77. Walser E, Ozkan OS, Raza S, et al: Hepatic perfusion as a predictor of mortality after transjugular intrahepatic portosystemic shunt creation in patients with refractory ascites. J Vasc Interv Radiol 2003;14:1251.
78. Patel NH, Sasadeusz KJ, Seshadri R, et al: Increase in hepatic arterial blood flow after transjugular intrahepatic portosystemic shunt creation and its potential predictive value of postprocedure encephalopathy and mortality. J Vasc Interv Radiol 2001;12:1279.

79. Walser EM, DeLa Pena R, Villanueva-Meyer J, et al: Hepatic perfusion before and after the transjugular intrahepatic portosystemic shunt procedure: impact on survival. J Vasc Interv Radiol 2000;11:913.

80. Kerlan RK Jr, LaBerge JM, Gordon RL, et al: Transjugular intrahepatic portosystemic shunts: current status. AJR Am J Roentgenol 1995;164:1059.

81. LaBerge JM, Ring EJ, Gordon RL, et al: Creation of transjugular intrahepatic portosystemic shunts with the Wallstent endoprosthesis: results in 100 patients. Radiology 1993;187:413.

82. Darcy MD, Sterling KM: Comparison of portal vein anatomy and bony anatomic landmarks. Radiology 1996;200:707.

83. Rees CR, Niblett RL, Lee SP, et al: Use of carbon dioxide as a contrast medium for transjugular intrahepatic portosystemic shunt procedures. J Vasc Interv Radiol 1994;5:383.

84. Rose SC, Pretorius DH, Nelson TR, et al: Adjunctive 3D US for achieving portal vein access during transjugular intrahepatic portosystemic shunt procedures. J Vasc Interv Radiol 2000;11:611.

85. Schultz SR, LaBerge JM, Gordon RL, et al: Anatomy of the portal vein bifurcation: intra- versus extrahepatic location-implications for transjugular intrahepatic portosystemic shunts. J Vasc Interv Radiol 1994;5:457.

86. Tesdal IK, Filser T, Weiss C, et al: Transjugular intrahepatic portosystemic shunts: adjunctive embolotherapy of gastroesophagel collateral vessels in the prevention of variceal rebleeding. Radiology 2005;236:360.

87. Coldwell DM, Ring EJ, Rees CR, et al: Multicenter investigation of the role of transjugular intrahepatic portosystemic shunt in management of portal hypertension. Radiology 1995;196:335.

88. Barton RE, Roesch J, Saxon RR, et al: TIPS: short- and long-term results: a survey of 1750 patients. Semin Intervent Radiol 1995;12:364.

89. Roessle M, Haag K, Ochs A, et al: The transjugular intrahepatic portosystemic stent-shunt procedure for variceal bleeding. N Engl J Med 1994;330:165.

90. Cabrera J, Maynar M, Granados R, et al: Transjugular intrahepatic portosystemic shunt versus sclerotherapy in the elective treatment of variceal hemorrhage. Gastroenterology 1996;110:832.

91. Ochs A, Roessle M, Haag K, et al: The transjugular intrahepatic portosystemic stent-shunt procedure for refractory ascites. N Engl J Med 1995;332:1192.

92. Ferral H, Bjarnason H, Wegryn SA, et al: Refractory ascites: early experience in treatment with transjugular intrahepatic portosystemic shunt. Radiology 1993;189:795.

93. Crenshaw WB, Gordon FD, McEniff NJ, et al: Severe ascites: efficacy of the transjugular intrahepatic portosystemic shunt in treatment. Radiology 1996;200:185.

94. Freedman AM, Sanyal AJ, Tisnado J, et al: Complications of the transjugular intrahepatic portosystemic shunt: a comprehensive review. Radiographics 1993;13:1185.

95. Darcy MD, Vesely TM, Picus D, et al: Percutaneous revision of an acutely thrombosed transjugular intrahepatic portosystemic shunt. J Vasc Interv Radiol 1992;3:77.

96. Schmitz-Rode T, Vorwerk D, Marschall H-U, et al: Portal vein thrombosis after occlusion of a transjugular intrahepatic portosystemic shunt: recanalization with the impeller catheter. J Vasc Interv Radiol 1994;5:467.

97. Riggio O, Merlli M, Pedretti G, et al: Hepatic encephalopathy after transjugular intrahepatic portosystemic shunt: incidence and risk factors. Dig Dis Sci 1996;41:578.

98. Valji K, Bookstein JJ, Roberts AC, et al: Overdilation of the Wallstent to optimize portal decompression during transjugular intrahepatic portosystemic shunt placement. Radiology 1994;191:173.

99. Lind CD, Malisch TW, Chong WK, et al: Incidence of shunt occlusion or stenosis following transjugular intrahepatic portosystemic shunt placement. Gastroenterology 1994;106:1277.

100. Haskal ZJ, Pentecost MJ, Soulen MC, et al: Transjugular intrahepatic portosystemic shunt stenosis and revision: early and midterm results. AJR Am J Roentgenol 1994;163:439.

101. Sterling KM, Darcy MD: Stenosis of transjugular intrahepatic portosystemic shunts: presentation and management. AJR Am J Roentgenol 1997;168:239.

102. LaBerge JM, Ferrell LD, Ring EJ, et al: Histopathologic study of transjugular intrahepatic portosystemic shunts. J Vasc Interv Radiol 1991;2:549.

103. LaBerge JM, Ferrell LD, Ring EJ, et al: Histopathologic study of stenotic and occluded transjugular intrahepatic portosystemic shunts. J Vasc Interv Radiol 1993;4:779.

104. Saxon RR, Mendel-Hartvig J, Corless CL, et al: Bile duct injury as a major cause of stenosis and occlusion in transjugular intrahepatic portosystemic shunts: comparative histopathologic analysis in humans and swine. J Vasc Interv Radiol 1996;7:487.

105. Hausegger KA, Karnel F, Georgieva B, et al: Transjugular intrahepatic portosystemic shunt creation with the Viatorr expanded polytetrafluoroethylene-covered stent-graft. J Vasc Interv Radiol 2004;15:239.

106. Saxon R: A new era for transjugular intrahepatic portosystemic shunts? J Vasc Interv Radiol 2004;15:217.

107. Charon J-P, Alaeddin FH, Pimpalwar SA, et al: Results of a retrospective multicenter trial of the Viatorr expanded polytetrafluoroethylene-covered stent-graft for transjugular intrahepatic portosystemic shunt creation. J Vasc Interv Radiol 2004;15:1219.

108. Bureau C, Garcia-Pagan JC, Otal P, et al: Improved clinical outcome using polytetrafluoroethylene-coated stents for TIPS: results of a randomized study. Gastroenterology 2004;126:469.

109. Chopra S, Dodd GD III, Chintapalli KN, et al: Transjugular intrahepatic portosystemic shunt: accuracy of helical CT angiography in the detection of shunt abnormalities. Radiology 2000;215:115.

110. Kanterman RY, Darcy MD, Middleton WD, et al: Doppler sonographic findings associated with transjugular intrahepatic portosystemic shunt malfunction. AJR Am J Roentgenol 1997;168:467.

111. Foshager MC, Ferral H, Nazarian GK, et al: Duplex sonography after transjugular intrahepatic portosystemic shunts (TIPS): normal hemodynamic findings and efficacy in predicting shunt patency and stenosis. AJR Am J Roentgenol 1995;165:1.

112. Dodd GD III, Zajko AB, Orons PD, et al: Detection of transjugular intrahepatic portosystemic shunt dysfunction: value of duplex Doppler sonography. AJR Am J Roentgenol 1995;164:1119.

113. Feldstein VA, Patel MD, LaBerge JM: Transjugular intrahepatic portosystemic shunts: accuracy of Doppler US in determination of patency and detection of stenoses. Radiology 1996;201:141.

114. Saxon RR, Barton RE, Keller FS, et al: Prevention, detection, and treatment of TIPS stenosis and occlusion. Semin Intervent Radiol 1995;12:375.

115. Hoxworth JM, LaBerge MM, Gordon RL, et al: Inferior vena cava thrombosis after transjugular intrahepatic portosystemic shunt revision with a covered stent. J Vasc Interv Radiol 2004;15:995.

116. Madoff DC, Wallace MJ, Ahrar K, et al: TIPS-related hepatic encephalopathy: management options with novel endovascular techniques. Radiographics 2004;24:21.

117. Kaufman L, Itkin M, Furth EE, et al: Detachable balloon-modified reducing stent to treat hepatic insufficiency after transjugular intrahepatic portosystemic shunt creation. J Vasc Interv Radiol 2003;14:635.

118. Saket RR, Sze DY, Razavi MK, et al: TIPS reduction with use of stents or stent grafts. J Vasc Interv Radiol 2004;15:745.

119. Paz-Fumagalli R, Crain MR, Mewissen MW, et al: Fatal hemodynamic consequences of therapeutic closure of a transjugular intrahepatic portosystemic shunt. J Vasc Interv Radiol 1994;5:831.

120. Cohen J, Edelman RR, Chopra S: Portal vein thrombosis: a review. Am J Med 1992;92:173.

121. Webster GJ, Burroughs AK, Riordan SM: Portal vein thrombosis—new insights into aetiology and management. Aliment Pharmacol Ther 2005;21:1.

122. Weber SM, Rikkers LF: Splenic vein thrombosis and gastrointestinal bleeding in chronic pancreatitis. World J Surg 2003;27:1271.

123. Bradbury MS, Kavanagh PV, Bechtold RE, et al: Mesenteric venous thrombosis: diagnosis and noninvasive imaging. Radiographics 2002;22:527.

124. Hughes LA, Hartnell GG, Finn JP, et al: Time-of-flight MR angiography of the portal venous system: value compared with other imaging procedures. AJR Am J Roentgenol 1996;166:375.

125. Darcy MD: Portal vein thrombolysis and closure of competitive shunts following liver transplantation: invited commentary. J Vasc Interv Radiol 1994;5:616.

126. Malkowski P, Pawlak J, Michalowicz B, et al: Thrombolytic treatment of portal thrombosis. Hepatogastroenterology 2003;50:2098.

127. Hollingshead M, Burke CT, Mauro MA, et al: Transcatheter thrombolytic therapy for acute mesenteric and portal vein thrombosis. J Vasc Interv Radiol 2005;16:651.

128. Henao EA, Bohannon WT, Silva MB Jr: Treatment of portal venous thrombosis with selective superior mesenteric artery infusion of recombinant tissue plasminogen activator. J Vasc Surg 2003;38:1411.

129. Lopera JE, Correa G, Brazzini A, et al: Percutaneous transhepatic treatment of symptomatic mesenteric venous thrombosis. J Vasc Surg 2002;36:1058.

130. Radosevich PM, Ring EJ, LaBerge JM, et al: Transjugular intrahepatic portosystemic shunts in patients with portal vein occlusion. Radiology 1993;186:523.
131. Blum U, Haag K, Roessle M, et al: Noncavernomatous portal vein thrombosis in hepatic cirrhosis: treatment with transjugular intrahepatic portosystemic shunt and local thrombolysis. Radiology 1995;195:153.
132. McDermott VG, England RE, Newman GE: Case report: bleeding gastric varices secondary to splenic vein thrombosis successfully treated by splenic artery embolization. Br J Radiol 1995;68:928.
133. Klempnauer J, Grothues F, Bektas H, et al: Results of portal thrombectomy and splanchnic thrombolysis for the surgical management of acute mesentericoportal thrombosis. Br J Surg 1997;84:129.
134. Menon KV, Shah V, Kamath PS: The Budd-Chiari syndrome. N Engl J Med 2004;350:578.
135. Smith FO, Johnson MS, Scherer LR, et al: Transjugular intrahepatic portosystemic shunting (TIPS) for treatment of severe hepatic veno-occlusive disease. Bone Marrow Transplant 1996;18:643.
136. Lim JH, Park JH, Auh YH: Membranous obstruction of the inferior vena cava: comparison of findings at sonography, CT and venography. AJR Am J Roentgenol 1992;159:515.
137. Park JH, Han JK, Choi BI, et al: Membranous obstruction of the inferior vena cava with Budd-Chiari syndrome: MR imaging findings. J Vasc Interv Radiol 1991;2:463.
138. Kane R, Eustace S: Diagnosis of Budd-Chiari syndrome: comparison between sonography and MR angiography. Radiology 1995;195:117.
139. Carreras E, Granena A, Navasa M, et al: Transjugular liver biopsy in BMT. Bone Marrow Transplant 1993;11:21.
140. Griffith JF, Mahmoud AE, Cooper S, et al: Radiological intervention in Budd-Chiari syndrome: techniques and outcome in 18 patients. Clin Radiol 1996;51:775.
141. Raju GS, Felver M, Olin JW, et al: Thrombolysis for acute Budd-Chiari syndrome: case report and literature review. Am J Gastroenterol 1996; 91:1262.
142. Park JH, Chung JW, Han JK, et al: Interventional management of benign obstruction of the hepatic inferior vena cava. J Vasc Interv Radiol 1994;5:403.
143. Venbrux AC, Mitchell SE, Savader SJ, et al: Long-term results with the use of metallic stents in the inferior vena cava for treatment of Budd-Chiari syndrome. J Vasc Interv Radiol 1994;5:411.
144. Blum U, Roessle M, Haag K, et al: Budd-Chiari syndrome: technical, hemodynamic, and clinical results of treatment with transjugular intrahepatic portosystemic shunt. Radiology 1995;197:805.
145. Peltzer MY, Ring EJ, LaBerge JM, et al: Treatment of Budd-Chiari syndrome with a transjugular intrahepatic portosystemic shunt. J Vasc Interv Radiol 1993;4:263.
146. Ryu RK, Durham JD, Krysl J, et al: Role of TIPS as a bridge to hepatic transplantation in Budd-Chiari syndrome. J Vasc Interv Radiol 1999;10:799.
147. Srinivasan P, Rela M, Prachalias A, et al: Liver transplantation for Budd-Chiari syndrome. Transplantation 2002;73:973.
148. Hayashi PH, Di Bisceglie AM: The progression of hepatitis B- and C-infections to chronic liver disease and hepatocellular carcinoma: epidemiology and pathogenesis. Med Clin North Am 2005;89:371.
149. Hayashi PH, Di Bisceglie AM: The progression of hepatitis B- and C-infections to chronic liver disease and hepatocellular carcinoma: presentation, diagnosis, screening, prevention, and treatment of hepatocellular carcinoma. Med Clin North Am 2005;89:345.
150. Kaibori M, Matsui Y, Yanagida H, et al: Positive status of alpha-feto-protein and des-gamma-carboxy prothrombin: important prognostic factor for recurrent hepatocellular carcinoma. World J Surg 2004;28:702.
151. Colombo M: Hepatocellular carcinoma. J Hepatol 1992;15:225.
152. Daniele B, Bencivenga A, Megna AS, et al: Alpha-fetoprotein and ultrasonography screening for hepatocellular carcinoma. Gastroenterology 2004;127(5 Suppl 1):S108.
153. Brannigan M, Burns PN, Wilson SR: Blood flow patterns in focal liver lesions at microbubble-enhanced US. Radiographics 2004;24:921.
154. Kamel IR, Bluemke DA: Imaging evaluation of hepatocellular carcinoma. J Vasc Interv Radiol 2002;13(9 Pt 2):S173.
155. Baker ME, Pelley R: Hepatic metastases: basic principles and implications for radiologists. Radiology 1995;197:329.
156. Yu SC, Yeung DT, So NM: Imaging features of hepatocellular carcinoma. Clin Radiol 2004;59:145.
157. Madoff DC, Abdalla EK, Vauthey JN, et al: Portal vein embolization in preparation for major hepatic resection: evolution of a new standard of care. J Vasc Interv Radiol 2005;16:779.
158. Madoff DC, Hicks ME, Abdalla EK, et al: Portal vein embolization with polyvinyl alcohol particles and coils in preparation for major liver resection for hepatobiliary malignancy: safety and effectiveness—study in 26 patients. Radiology 2003;227:251.
159. Madoff DC, Abdalla EK, Gupta S, et al: Transhepatic ipsilateral right portal vein embolization extended to segment IV: improving hypertrophy and resection outcomes with spherical particles and coils. J Vasc Interv Radiol 2005;16:215.
160. Brown KT, Brody LA, Decorato DR, et al: Portal vein embolization with use of polyvinyl alcohol particles. J Vasc Interv Radiol 2001;12:882.
161. Kodama Y, Shimizu T, Endo H, et al: Complications of percutaneous transhepatic portal vein embolization. J Vasc Interv Radiol 2002;13:1233.
162. Ahmed M, Goldberg SN: Thermal ablation therapy for hepatocellular carcinoma. J Vasc Interv Radiol 2002;13(9 Pt 2):S231.
163. Goldberg SN, Dupuy DE: Image-guided radiofrequency tumor ablation: challenges and opportunities—part I. J Vasc Interv Radiol 2001; 12:1021.
164. Kettenbach J, Kostler W, Rucklinger E, et al: Percutaneous saline-enhanced radiofrequency ablation of unresectable hepatic tumors: initial experience in 26 patients. AJR Am J Roentgenol 2003;180:1537.
165. Rossi S, Garbagnati F, Lencioni R, et al: Percutaneous radiofrequency thermal ablation of nonresectable hepatocellular carcinoma after occlusion of tumor blood supply. Radiology 2000;217:119.
166. Pawlik TM, Izzo F, Cohen DS, et al: Combined resection and radiofrequency ablation for advanced hepatic malignancies: results in 172 patients. Ann Surg Oncol 2003;10:1059.
167. Livraghi T, Solbiati L, Meloni F, et al: Percutaneous radiofrequency ablation of liver metastases in potential candidates for resection: the "test-of-time approach." Cancer 2003;97:3027.
168. Rhim H, Goldberg SN, Dodd GD 3rd, et al: Essential techniques for successful radio-frequency thermal ablation of malignant hepatic tumors. Radiographics 2001;21:S17.
169. Dupuy DE, Goldberg SN: Image-guided radiofrequency tumor ablation: challenges and opportunities—part II. J Vasc Interv Radiol 2001;12:1135.
170. Shibata T, Shibata T, Maetani Y, et al: Transthoracic percutaneous radiofrequency ablation for liver tumors in the hepatic dome. J Vasc Interv Radiol 2004;15:1323.
171. Livraghi T, Goldberg SN, Solbiati L, et al: Percutaneous radiofrequency ablation of liver metastases from breast cancer: initial experience in 24 patients. Radiology 2001;220:145.
172. Solbiati L, Livraghi T, Goldberg SN, et al: Percutaneous radiofrequency ablation of hepatic metastases from colorectal cancer: long-term results in 117 patients. Radiology 2001;221:159.
173. Livraghi T, Solbiati L, Meloni MF, et al: Treatment of focal liver tumors with percutaneous radio-frequency ablation: complications encountered in a multicenter study. Radiology 2003;226:441.
174. Vogl TJ, Trapp M, Schroeder H, et al: Transarterial chemoembolization for hepatocellular carcinoma: volumetric and morphologic CT criteria for assessment of prognosis and therapeutic success-results from a liver transplantation center. Radiology 2000;214:349.
175. Brown DB, Fundakowski CE, Lisker-Melman M, et al: Comparison of MELD and Child-Pugh scores to predict survival after chemoembolization for hepatocellular carcinoma. J Vasc Interv Radiol 2004;15:1209.
176. Camma C, Schepis F, Orlando A, et al: Transarterial chemoembolization for unresectable hepatocellular carcinoma: meta-analysis of randomized controlled trials. Radiology 2002;224:47.
177. Rajan DK, Soulen MC, Clark TW, et al: Sarcomas metastatic to the liver: response and survival after cisplatin, doxorubicin, mitomycin-C, Ethiodol, and polyvinyl alcohol chemoembolization. J Vasc Interv Radiol 2001;12:187.
178. Saccheri S, Lovaria A, Sangiovanni A, et al: Segmental transcatheter arterial chemoembolization treatment in patients with cirrhosis and inoperable hepatocellular carcinomas. J Vasc Interv Radiol 2002; 13:995.
179. Touzios JG, Kiely JM, Pitt SC, et al: Neuroendocrine hepatic metastases: does aggressive management improve survival? Ann Surg 2005;241:776.
180. Gee M, Soulen MC: Chemoembolization for hepatic metastases. Tech Vasc Interv Radiol 2002;5:132.
181. Lang EK, Brown CL Jr: Colorectal metastases to the liver: selective chemoembolization. Radiology 1993;189:417.
182. Stokes KR, Stuart K, Clouse ME: Hepatic arterial chemoembolization for metastatic endocrine tumors. J Vasc Interv Radiol 1993;4:341.

183. Bedikian AY, Legha SS, Mavligit G, et al: Treatment of uveal melanoma metastatic to the liver: a review of the M. D. Anderson Cancer Center experience and prognostic factors. Cancer 1995;76:1665.

184. Mavligit GM, Pollock RE, Evans HL, et al: Durable hepatic tumor regression after arterial chemoembolization-infusion in patients with islet cell carcinoma of the pancreas metastatic to the liver. Cancer 1993; 72:375.

185. Therasse E, Breittmayer F, Roche A, et al: Transcatheter chemoembolization of progressive carcinoid liver metastases. Radiology 1993;189:541.

186. Leung DA, Goin JE, Sickles C, et al: Determinants of postembolization syndrome after hepatic chemoembolization. J Vasc Interv Radiol 2001;12:321.

187. Miyayama S, Matsui O, Nishida H, et al: Transcatheter arterial chemoembolization for unresectable hepatocellular carcinoma fed by the cystic artery. J Vasc Interv Radiol 2003;14:1155.

188. Miyayama S, Matsui O, Akakura Y, et al: Hepatocellular carcinoma with blood supply from omental branches: treatment with transcatheter arterial embolization. J Vasc Interv Radiol 2001;12:1285.

189. Miyayama S, Matsui O, Taki K, et al: Transcatheter arterial chemoembolization for hepatocellular carcinoma fed by the reconstructed inferior phrenic artery: anatomical and technical analysis. J Vasc Interv Radiol 2004;15:815.

190. Nakai M, Sato M, Kawai N, et al: Hepatocellular carcinoma: involvement of the internal mammary artery. Radiology 2001;219:147.

191. Groupe D'Etude et de Traitment du Carcinome Hepatocellulaire: A comparison of Lipiodol chemoembolization and conservative treatment for unresectable hepatocellular carcinoma. N Engl J Med 1995; 332:1256.

192. Lo CM, Ngan H, Tso WK, et al: Randomized controlled trial of transarterial lipiodol chemoembolization for unresectable hepatocellular carcinoma. Hepatology 2002;35:1164.

193. Llovet JM, Bruix J: Systematic review of randomized trials for unresectable hepatocellular carcinoma: chemoembolization improves survival. Hepatology 2003;37:429.

194. Llovet JM, Real MI, Montana X, et al: Arterial embolisation or chemoembolisation versus symptomatic treatment in patients with unresectable hepatocellular carcinoma: a randomised controlled trial. Lancet 2002;359:1734.

195. Kim W, Clark TW, Baum RA, et al: Risk factors for liver abscess formation after hepatic chemoembolization. J Vasc Interv Radiol 2001;12:965.

196. Salem R, Thurston KG, Carr BI, et al: Yttrium-90 microspheres: radiation therapy for unresectable liver cancer. J Vasc Interv Radiol 2002;13(9 Pt 2):S223.

197. Goin JE, Salem R, Carr BI, et al: Treatment of unresectable hepatocellular carcinoma with intrahepatic yttrium 90 microspheres: factors associated with liver toxicities. J Vasc Interv Radiol 2005;16:205.

198. Dawson LA: Hepatic arterial yttrium 90 microspheres: another treatment option for hepatocellular carcinoma. J Vasc Interv Radiol 2005; 16:161.

199. Geschwind JF, Salem R, Carr BI, et al: Yttrium-90 microspheres for the treatment of hepatocellular carcinoma. Gastroenterology 2004;127(5 Suppl 1):S194.

200. Stubbs RS, Cannan RJ, Mitchell AW: Selective internal radiation therapy with 90yttrium microspheres for extensive colorectal liver metastases. J Gastrointest Surg 2001;5:294.

201. Siragusa DA, Friedman AC: Imaging-guided percutaneous biopsy of hepatic masses. Tech Vasc Interv Radiol 2001;4:172.

202. Farges O, Daradkeh S, Bismuth H: Cavernous hemangiomas of the liver: are there any indications for resection? World J Surg 1995;19:19.

203. Graham E, Cohen AW, Soulen M, et al: Symptomatic liver hemangioma with intra-tumor hemorrhage treated by angiography and embolization during pregnancy. Obstet Gynecol 1993;81:813.

204. Cassar K, Munro A: Iatrogenic splenic injury. J R Coll Surg Edinb 2002;47:731.

205. Schwartz RA, Teitelbaum GP, Katz MD, et al: Effectiveness of transcatheter embolization in the control of hepatic vascular injuries. J Vasc Interv Radiol 1993;4:359.

206. Sclafani SJA, Shaftan GW, Scalea TM, et al: Nonoperative salvage of computed tomography-diagnosed splenic injuries: utilization of angiography for triage and embolization for hemostasis. J Trauma 1995;39:818.

207. Shanmuganathan K: Multi-detector row CT imaging of blunt abdominal trauma. Semin Ultrasound CT MR 2004;25:180.

208. Pachter HL, Knudson MM, Esrig B, et al: Status of nonoperative management of blunt hepatic injuries in 1995: a multicenter experience with 404 patients. J Trauma 1996;40:31.

209. Haan JM, Bochicchio GV, Kramer N, et al: Nonoperative management of blunt splenic injury: a 5-year experience. J Trauma 2005;58:492.

210. Wahl WL, Ahrns KS, Chen S, et al: Blunt splenic injury: operation versus angiographic embolization. Surgery 2004;136:891.

211. Haan JM, Biffl W, Knudson MM, et al: Splenic embolization revisited: a multicenter review. J Trauma. 2004;56:542.

212. Hagiwara A, Yukioka T, Ohta S, et al: Nonsurgical management of patients with blunt splenic injury: efficacy of transcatheter arterial embolization. AJR Am J Roentgenol 1996;167:159.

213. Killeen KL, Shanmuganathan K, Boyd-Kranis R, et al: CT findings after embolization for blunt splenic trauma. J Vasc Interv Radiol 2001;12:209.

214. Karani JB, Yu DF, Kane PA: Interventional radiology in liver transplantation. Cardiovasc Intervent Radiol 2005;28:271.

215. Fontana RJ, Hamidullah H, Nghiem H, et al: Percutaneous radiofrequency thermal ablation of hepatocellular carcinoma: a safe and effective bridge to liver transplantation. Liver Transpl 2002;8:1165.

216. Lee VS, Morgan GR, Lin JC, et al: Liver transplant donor candidates: associations between vascular and biliary anatomic variants. Liver Transpl 2004;10:1049.

217. Erbay N, Raptopoulos V, Pomfret EA, et al: Living donor liver transplantation in adults: vascular variants important in surgical planning for donors and recipients. AJR Am J Roentgenol 2003;181:109.

218. Kostelic JK, Piper JB, Leef JA, et al: Angiographic selection criteria for living related liver transplant donors. AJR Am J Roentgenol 1996;166:1103.

219. Renz JF, Yersiz H, Reichert PR, et al: Split-liver transplantation: a review. Am J Transplant 2003;3:1323.

220. Renz JF, Emond JC, Yersiz H, et al: Split-liver transplantation in the United States: outcomes of a national survey. Ann Surg 2004;239:172.

221. Crossin JD, Muradali D, Wilson SR: US of liver transplants: normal and abnormal. Radiographics 2003;23:1093.

222. Pandharipande PV, Lee VS, Morgan GR, et al: Vascular and extravascular complications of liver transplantation: comprehensive evaluation with three-dimensional contrast-enhanced volumetric MR imaging and MR cholangiopancreatography. AJR Am J Roentgenol 2001;177:1101.

223. Brancatelli G, Katyal S, Federle MP, et al: Three-dimensional multislice helical computed tomography with the volume rendering technique in the detection of vascular complications after liver transplantation. Transplantation 2002;73:237.

224. Nishida S, Kato T, Levi D, et al: Effect of protocol Doppler ultrasonography and urgent revascularization on early hepatic artery thrombosis after pediatric liver transplantation. Arch Surg 2002;137:1279.

225. Vivarelli M, Cucchetti A, La Barba G, et al: Ischemic arterial complications after liver transplantation in the adult: multivariate analysis of risk factors. Arch Surg 2004;139:1069.

226. Martin SR, Atkison P, Anand R, et al: Studies of Pediatric Liver Transplantation 2002: patient and graft survival and rejection in pediatric recipients of a first liver transplant in the United States and Canada. Pediatr Transplant 2004;8:273.

227. Glockner JF, Forauer AR: Vascular or ischemic complications after liver transplantation. AJR Am J Roentgenol 1999;173:1055.

228. Pinna AD, Smith CV, Furukawa H, et al: Urgent revascularization of liver allografts after early hepatic artery thrombosis. Transplantation 1996;62:1584.

229. Vorwerk D, Guenther RW, Klever P, et al: Angioplasty and stent placement for treatment of hepatic artery thrombosis following liver transplantation. J Vasc Interv Radiol 1994;5:309.

230. Dodd GD III, Memel DS, Zajko AB, et al: Hepatic artery stenosis and thrombosis in transplant recipients: Doppler diagnosis with resistive index and systolic acceleration time. Radiology 1994;192:657.

231. Platt JF, Yutzy GG, Bude RO, et al: Use of Doppler sonography for revealing hepatic artery stenosis in liver transplant recipients. AJR Am J Roentgenol 1997;168:473.

232. Orons PD, Zajko AB, Bron KM, et al: Hepatic artery angioplasty after liver transplantation: experience in 21 allografts. J Vasc Interv Radiol 1995;6:523.

233. Denys AL, Qanadli SD, Durand F, et al: Feasibility and effectiveness of using coronary stents in the treatment of hepatic artery stenoses after orthotopic liver transplantation: preliminary report. AJR Am J Roentgenol 2002;178:1175.

234. Buell JF, Funaki B, Cronin DC, et al: Long-term venous complications after full-size and segmental pediatric liver transplantation. Ann Surg 2002;236:658.

235. Funaki B, Rosenblum JD, Leef JA, et al: Percutaneous treatment of portal venous stenosis in children and adolescents with segmental hepatic transplants: long-term results. Radiology 2000;215:147.

236. Zajko AB, Sheng R, Bron K, et al: Percutaneous transluminal angioplasty of venous anastomotic stenoses complicating liver transplantation: intermediate-term results. J Vasc Interv Radiol 1994;5:121.

237. Haskal ZJ, Naji A: Treatment of portal vein thrombosis after liver transplantation with percutaneous thrombolysis and stent placement. J Vasc Interv Radiol 1993;4:789.

238. Wang SL, Sze DY, Busque S, et al: Treatment of hepatic venous outflow obstruction after piggyback liver transplantation. Radiology 2005;236:352.

239. Ko GY, Sung KB, Yoon HK, et al: Endovascular treatment of hepatic venous outflow obstruction after living-donor liver transplantation. J Vasc Interv Radiol 2002;13:591.

240. Weeks SM, Gerber DA, Jaques PF, et al: Primary Gianturco stent placement for inferior vena cava abnormalities following liver transplantation. J Vasc Interv Radiol 2000;11:177.

241. Frippiat F, Donckier J, Vandenbossche P, et al: Splenic infarction: report of three cases of atherosclerotic embolization originating in the aorta and retrospective study of 64 cases. Acta Clin Belg 1996;51:395.

242. Matsuo R, Ohta Y, Ohya Y, et al: Isolated dissection of the celiac artery—a case report. Angiology 2000;51:603.

243. Yoon DY, Park JH, Chung JW, et al: Iatrogenic dissection of the celiac artery and its branches during transcatheter arterial embolization for hepatocellular carcinoma: outcome in 40 patients. Cardiovasc Intervent Radiol 1995;18:16.

244. Chiesa R, Astore D, Guzzo G, et al: Visceral artery aneurysms. Ann Vasc Surg 2005;19:42.

245. Tessier DJ, Stone WM, Fowl RJ, et al: Clinical features and management of splenic artery pseudoaneurysm: case series and cumulative review of literature. J Vasc Surg 2003;38:969.

246. Asokan S, Chew EK, Ng KY, et al: Post partum splenic artery aneurysm rupture. J Obstet Gynaecol Res 2000;26:199.

247. Mattar SG, Lumsden AB: The management of splenic artery aneurysms: experience with 23 cases. Am J Surg 1995;169:580.

248. Lumsden AB, Mattar SG, Allen RC, et al: Hepatic artery aneurysms: the management of 22 patients. J Surg Res 1996;60:345.

249. McDermott VG, Shlansky-Goldberg R, Cope C: Endovascular management of splenic artery aneurysms and pseudoaneurysms. Cardiovasc Intervent Radiol 1994;17:179.

250. Rami P, Williams D, Forauer A, et al: Stent-graft treatment of patients with acute bleeding from hepatic artery branches. Cardiovasc Intervent Radiol 2005;28:153.

251. Ilan Y, Ben-Chetrit E: Liver involvement in giant cell arteritis. Clin Rheumatol 1993;12:219.

252. Lumsden AB, Allen RC, Sreeram S, et al: Hepatic arterioportal fistula. Am Surgeon 1993;59:722.

253. Park CM, Cha SH, Kim DH, et al: Hepatic arterioportal shunts not directly related to hepatocellular carcinoma: findings on CT during hepatic arteriography, CT arterial portography and dual phase spiral CT. Clin Radiol 2000;55:465.

254. Itai Y, Saida Y, Irie T, et al: Intrahepatic portosystemic venous shunts: spectrum of CT findings in external and internal subtypes. J Comput Assist Tomogr 2001;25:348.

255. Huang MS, Lin Q, Jiang ZB, et al: Comparison of long-term effects between intra-arterially delivered ethanol and Gelfoam for the treatment of severe arterioportal shunt in patients with hepatocellular carcinoma. World J Gastroenterol 2004;10:825.

256. Raghuram L, Korah IP, Jaya V, et al: Coil embolization of a solitary congenital intrahepatic hepatoportal fistula. Abdom Imaging 2001; 26:194.

257. Brothers TE, Stanley JC, Zelenock GB: Splenic arteriovenous fistula. Int Surgery 1995;80:189.

258. Whiting JH Jr, Korzenik JR, Miller FJ Jr, et al: Fatal outcome after embolotherapy for hepatic arteriovenous malformations of the liver in two patients with hereditary hemorrhagic telangiectasia. J Vasc Interv Radiol 2000;11:855.

259. Chavan A, Caselitz M, Gratz KF, et al: Hepatic artery embolization for treatment of patients with hereditary hemorrhagic telangiectasia and symptomatic hepatic vascular malformations. Eur Radiol 2004;14:2079.

260. Larson AM: Liver disease in hereditary hemorrhagic telangiectasia. J Clin Gastroenterol 2003;36:149.

261. Romano M, Giojelli A, Capuano G, et al: Partial splenic embolization in patients with idiopathic portal hypertension. Eur J Radiol 2004;49:268.

262. Kimura F, Itoh H, Ambiru S, et al: Long-term results of initial and repeated partial splenic embolization for the treatment of chronic idiopathic thrombocytopenic purpura. AJR Am J Roentgenol 2002; 179:1323.

263. Stanley P, Shen TC: Partial embolization of the spleen in patients with thalassemia. J Vasc Interv Radiol 1995;6:137.

264. Palsson B, Hallen M, Forsberg AM, et al: Partial splenic embolization: long-term outcome. Langenbecks Arch Surg 2003;387:421.

265. Petersons A, Volrats O, Bernsteins A: The first experience with nonoperative treatment of hypersplenism in children with portal hypertension. Eur J Pediatr Surg 2002;12:299.

266. Noguchi H, Hirai K, Aoki Y, et al: Changes in platelet kinetics after a partial splenic arterial embolization in cirrhotic patients with hypersplenism. Hepatology 1995;22:1682.

267. Sakai T, Shiraki K, Inoue H, et al: Complications of partial splenic embolization in cirrhotic patients. Dig Dis Sci 2002;47:388.

268. Gelfand MM, Wiita B: Androgen and estrogen-androgen hormone replacement therapy: a review of the safety literature, 1941 to 1996. Clin Ther 1997;19:383.

269. Koehler JE, Sanchez MA, Garrido CS, et al: Molecular epidemiology of *Bartonella* infections in patients with bacillary angiomatosis-peliosis. N Engl J Med 1997;337:1876.

270. Vignaux O, Legmann P, de Pinieux G, et al: Hemorrhagic necrosis due to peliosis hepatis: imaging findings and pathological correlation. Eur Radiol 1999;9:454.

271. Ryan JM, Suhocki PV, Smith TP: Coil embolization of segmental arterial mediolysis of the hepatic artery. J Vasc Interv Radiol 2000;11:865.

11

Endocrine, Exocrine, and Reproductive Systems

PANCREAS

ARTERIOGRAPHY

Pancreatic angiography begins with celiac and superior mesenteric arteriography using a 5-French hook, cobra-, or sidewinder-shaped catheter. Evaluation or treatment of intrapancreatic vessels often requires gastroduodenal, splenic, inferior pancreaticoduodenal, and, rarely, dorsal pancreatic catheterization (see Chapters 9 and 10). The major veins surrounding the pancreas are visualized on late-phase superior mesenteric artery (SMA) and celiac artery injections.

ANATOMY AND PHYSIOLOGY

The pancreas is supplied by branches of the celiac and superior mesenteric arteries.[1,2] The head and uncinate process are fed by the *anterior* and *posterior superior pancreaticoduodenal arteries* (arising from the gastroduodenal artery) and the *anterior* and *posterior inferior pancreaticoduodenal arteries* (arising from the SMA) (Fig. 11-1). These arteries form a rich network within the pancreatic head and are an important collateral pathway between the celiac artery and SMA (see Fig. 9-12). The *inferior pancreaticoduodenal artery* occasionally comes off the first or second jejunal artery.

The body and tail of the pancreas are supplied by the *dorsal pancreatic artery* and by numerous smaller branches of the splenic artery, including the *pancreatica magna* and *caudal pancreatic arteries* (see Figs. 11-1 and 10-6). A right branch of the dorsal pancreatic artery communicates with the anterior superior pancreaticoduodenal artery. The left branch becomes the *transverse pancreatic artery* and runs through the inferior portion of the distal pancreas. The dorsal pancreatic artery may arise directly from the celiac artery or from other vessels (e.g., splenic artery).

The venous drainage of the pancreas largely follows the corresponding arteries. The *anterior superior pancreaticoduodenal vein* enters the *gastrocolic vein*, which is a major venous tributary of the superior mesenteric vein (see Fig. 10-3). The other pancreaticoduodenal veins have separate entrances into the portal system. The body and tail of the pancreas drain into the *splenic* and *inferior pancreatic veins.* The latter may empty into the inferior mesenteric vein, superior mesenteric vein, or splenic vein.

The head and neck of the pancreas lie in front of the portal and superior mesenteric vein junction and the SMA. The splenic artery and vein run behind the body and tail of the pancreas. The celiac axis and common hepatic artery are just superior to the gland. A replaced right or common hepatic artery may course behind the head and neck of the pancreas. Inflammatory or neoplastic diseases of the pancreas often encroach on one or more of these vessels.

The pancreas has both endocrine and exocrine functions.[3] Digestive proteins are produced by epithelial cells that form the pancreatic acini, which ultimately drain into the pancreatic ducts. Cells of the islets of Langerhans produce various hormones, including glucagon (alpha cells), insulin (beta cells), somatostatin, pancreatic polypeptide, and vasoactive intestinal polypeptide (VIP) (delta cells and other cell types).

MAJOR DISORDERS

Nonendocrine Tumors

Etiology

The pancreas is affected by a variety of benign and malignant tumors (Box 11-1). *Adenocarcinoma* arising from the ductal epithelium is the most common pancreatic neoplasm. The tumor grows primarily by local infiltration and invasion. More than 50% of these tumors occur in the pancreatic head.[4] Even a small mass at this site can cause symptomatic biliary duct obstruction. Tumors in the body and tail often reach a large size before they become symptomatic.

Gastroduodenal artery

Posterior
superior
pancreatico-
duodenal
artery

Anterior
superior
pancreatico-
duodenal
artery

A

Right gastroepiploic artery

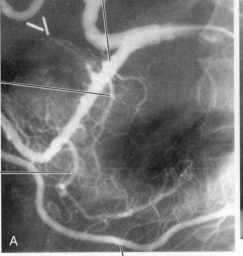

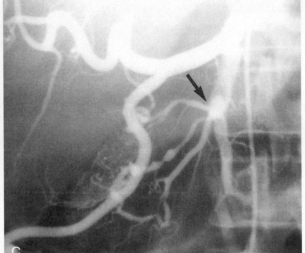

Dorsal pancreatic artery

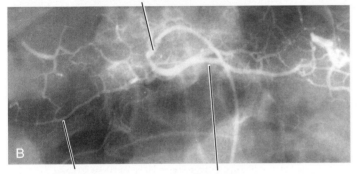

B

Pancreatic
head arcades

Transverse
pancreatic artery

FIGURE 11-1 ■ Pancreatic arterial anatomy. **A,** Gastroduodenal arteriogram. **B,** Dorsal pancreatic arteriogram from the undersurface of the celiac artery. **C,** Common hepatic arteriogram shows filling of pancreatic arcades with retrograde filling of inferior arcades and the inferior pancreaticoduodenal artery *(arrow)* arising from the superior mesenteric artery. Small intrapancreatic artery aneurysms alternating with narrowed segments are indicative of chronic pancreatitis.

Islet cell (endocrine) tumors are considered later. *Microcystic adenomas* (serous cystadenomas) consist of multiple small cysts with calcification and a central scar.[5] They occur with an even distribution throughout the gland. *Mucinous cystic neoplasms* (cystadenocarcinomas) contain several large cysts. They frequently are found in the tail of the gland and can be benign or malignant.

BOX 11-1 ■ Major Neoplasms of the Pancreas

Ductal adenocarcinoma
Endocrine (islet cell) tumors
Cystic epithelial tumors
    Microcystic adenoma
    Mucinous cystic neoplasm
    Intraductal papillary mucinous neoplasm
Solid and papillary epithelial tumors
Metastases
Lymphoma

Clinical Features

When a nonendocrine pancreatic tumor is detected in the early stages, it usually has caused biliary obstruction and jaundice. Otherwise, the tumor must become large before vague symptoms of fatigue, abdominal pain, and weight loss have developed. Microcystic adenomas and mucinous cystic neoplasms typically are seen in middle-aged or elderly women.[5] Patients with endocrine neoplasms usually present with distinctive clinical syndromes (see later).

Imaging

The detection and staging of pancreatic tumors is done entirely by cross-sectional techniques. The major goal of imaging is to avoid extensive surgery in patients with local spread or metastatic disease. Signs of unresectability include tumor extension to the boundary of the gland or to adjacent structures, extracapsular involvement, major extrapancreatic vascular involvement, and distant metastases.[6] However, absolute criteria for unresectability differ

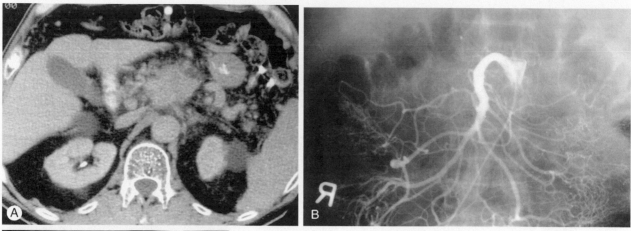

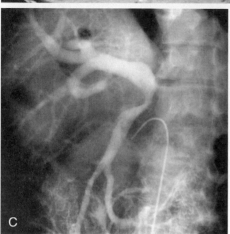

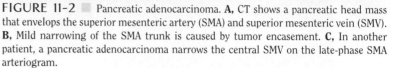

FIGURE 11-2 ▪ Pancreatic adenocarcinoma. **A,** CT shows a pancreatic head mass that envelops the superior mesenteric artery (SMA) and superior mesenteric vein (SMV). **B,** Mild narrowing of the SMA trunk is caused by tumor encasement. **C,** In another patient, a pancreatic adenocarcinoma narrows the central SMV on the late-phase SMA arteriogram.

among institutions. Unfortunately, most patients have unresectable disease at the time of presentation.

Cross-sectional Techniques. CT, MR imaging, and endoscopic sonography are the most widely used methods for staging nonendocrine pancreatic tumors.[6-9] CT is almost 100% specific in showing unresectability but tends to understage some neoplasms (Fig. 11-2) .

Angiography. Although arteriography accurately shows vascular involvement in 80% to 90% of cases, it clearly is less sensitive than other techniques and is unable to identify other signs of unresectability.[4]

The angiographic findings of pancreatic adenocarcinoma are those of arterial or venous compression, encasement, and occlusion (see Fig. 11-2).[10-12] Serrated arterial encasement is said to be diagnostic of tumor. Neovascularity is common, but hypervascularity is rare.

Treatment

An operation is performed to palliate symptoms or for potential cure in patients without evidence for unresectability. Surgical options include the *Whipple procedure* (i.e., radical pancreaticoduodenectomy, cholecystectomy, choledochojejunostomy, and gastrojejunostomy), total pancreatectomy, and palliative diversion for biliary obstruction (i.e., choledochojejunostomy) or duodenal obstruction (i.e., gastrojejunostomy). Preoperative or postoperative adjuvant radiation therapy and chemotherapy

are used in some centers.[13] Mean survival is about 1 year; the 5-year survival rate is less than 10% in most series.[14]

Islet Cell (Neuroendocrine) Tumors

Etiology

Islet cells in and around the pancreas are the source of a variety of rare neuroendocrine tumors. These neoplasms release excess amounts of one or more hormones that are normal products of the pancreas (e.g., insulin) or normally found in the fetal pancreas or other glands (e.g., gastrin).[15-17] Neuroendocrine tumors generally are slow growing and small and they produce symptoms from hormone imbalance rather than mass effect. About 15% are "nonfunctioning," although they may liberate certain hormones that are not responsible for the clinical picture.

Insulinomas are the most common islet cell tumor of the pancreas. These tumors usually are quite small (<1 cm) when discovered.[18] They are evenly distributed throughout the pancreas. About 10% are multiple, and 10% are malignant.[15] Rarely, insulinoma is part of the *multiple endocrine neoplasia (MEN 1) syndrome*, which features adenomas of the pancreas, parathyroid, and pituitary. Most patients are women with symptoms related to episodic hypoglycemia, including weakness, shaking, tachycardia, lightheadedness, and fatigue. Serum levels of insulin and C-peptide are elevated.

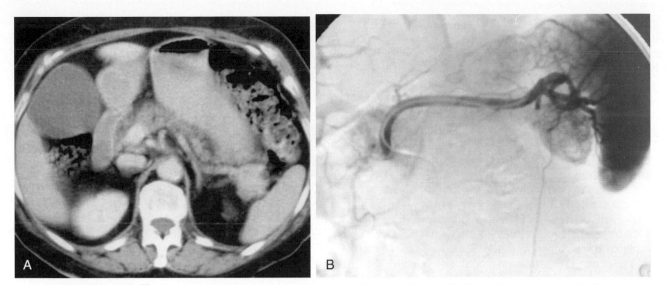

FIGURE 11-3 ■ Glucagonoma. A CT scan (**A**) and late phase splenic arteriogram (**B**) show a hyperdense mass in the tail of the pancreas.

Gastrinomas cause *Zollinger-Ellison syndrome*, which is characterized by hypersecretion of gastric acid, upper gastrointestinal tract ulcers, and diarrhea. They are frequently malignant and usually small (<1 cm).[17] About one third of cases is associated with the MEN 1 syndrome and have multiple lesions. Most tumors are located within the "gastrinoma triangle," which is bordered by the cystic and common bile ducts, the junction between the pancreatic head and neck, and the second and third portions of the duodenum.[19] They often are found in the duodenal wall.

Carcinoids are the most common neuroendocrine tumors of the gastrointestinal system, but they arise far more often in the gut than in the pancreas.[15]

Most of several other exceedingly rare islet cell tumors are malignant:

■ *VIPomas* cause watery diarrhea, hypokalemia, hypotension, and skin flushing (WDHA or *Verner-Morrison syndrome*).
■ *Glucagonomas* produce a migratory rash, weight loss, diabetes, and anemia.
■ *Somatostatinomas* are associated with gallstones, diabetes, and weight loss.
■ *Nonfunctioning tumors* (some of which release pancreatic polypeptide or other hormones) cause symptoms by mass effect (jaundice, abdominal pain) and are, therefore, quite large at presentation. They usually are solitary and malignant but slow growing.

Imaging

The diagnosis itself is made with hormonal testing. The goal of imaging is **localization** of primary and metastatic lesions. Detection of these tumors has undergone a revolution over the past several decades, and a wide variety of techniques is in use.[15,17,18,20-22] Each institution must find its own approach to these unusual cases. Preoperative localization can be accomplished in greater than 90% of patients.[15]

Noninvasive Imaging. Considerable enthusiasm exists for the use of endoscopic sonography and somatostatin receptor scintigraphy (SRS) in this setting.[23-25] SRS entails injection of ^{111}In-labeled octreotide, a synthetic somatostatin analogue, which is taken up by somatostatin receptors expressed on most of these tumors (with the exception of some insulinomas). Primary and metastatic tumors are then detected by single photon emission tomographic imaging. Overall sensitivity is perhaps somewhat less with CT and MR imaging and selective arteriography and venous sampling.[20,22-25] Positron emission tomography recently has been used in this setting.

Most islet cell tumors are high signal on T2-weighted MR images and hyperdense on contrast-enhanced CT images, although hypodense lesions have been described (Figs. 11-3 and 11-4).

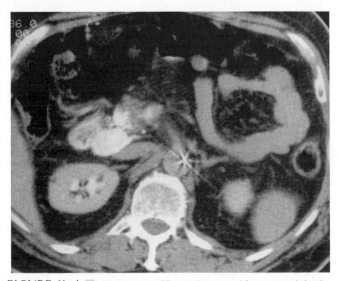

FIGURE 11-4 ■ Gastrinoma. CT arteriogram with contrast injection into the celiac artery shows a densely enhancing mass adjacent to the duodenum and pancreatic head.

Angiography. Noninvasive imaging is less sensitive for islet cell tumor detection than for most other solid tumors. For this reason, angiography continues to have a role (albeit small) in tumor localization.[17,18,26]

■ Selective arteriography (superior mesenteric, celiac, splenic, gastroduodenal, and dorsal pancreatic arteries)
■ Arteriography after intra-arterial injection of a secretagogue that stimulates hormone production
■ Transhepatic portal venous sampling, in which blood samples are obtained at various sites in the splenic, superior mesenteric, portal, and pancreatic veins. A focal step-up in hormone concentration can identify the tumor.[26,27]
■ Arterial stimulation with hepatic venous sampling, in which a secretagogue is injected into various arteries supplying the pancreas and hepatic venous blood samples are obtained for hormonal analysis[28]

The angiographic appearance of most islet cell tumors is that of a round, well-circumscribed, hypervascular mass within the substance of the pancreas or an adjacent organ (Fig. 11-5; see also Fig. 11-3). Rarely, these lesions are hypovascular.[29] Neuroendocrine tumors should not be confused with an accessory spleen, hypervascular region of normal pancreatic tissue, or nodal metastases. Injection of the secretagogues *calcium* or *secretin*, followed by selective arteriography or venous sampling, may allow detection

of occult insulinomas or gastrinomas, respectively (see Fig. 11-5).[28,30,31]

Treatment

The usual treatment for neuroendocrine tumors of the pancreas is surgical resection or chemotherapy.[16] Medical therapy includes administration of somatostatin analogues such as octreotide.[32] Interferon is also used in this setting. Embolotherapy has been reported as an alternative definitive treatment.[33] Radiofrequency ablation (RFA) and chemoembolization have a role in management of symptomatic metastatic disease to the liver, particularly with carcinoid (see Chapter 10).[34-39]

Surgical cure can be expected with small, solitary, non-metastatic lesions; otherwise, most patients are managed with medical therapy.

Inflammatory Diseases

Etiology

Acute pancreatitis is the result of autodigestion of the gland after release of proteolytic enzymes into the tissue.[40] An intense inflammatory reaction follows, leading to hemorrhage

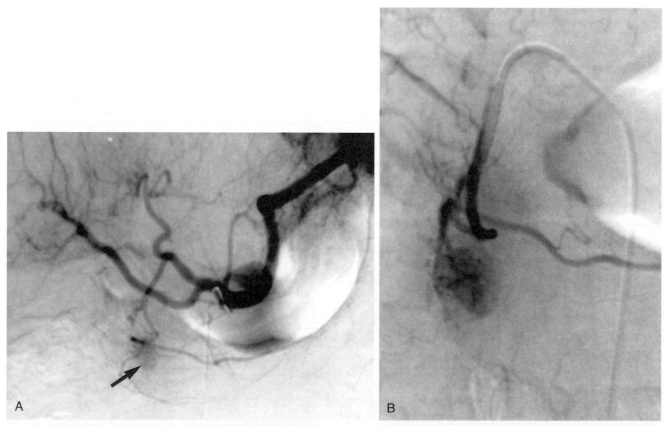

FIGURE 11-5 ■ Insulinoma. **A,** A region of hypervascularity in the pancreatic head is identified by celiac arteriography *(arrow).* **B,** After intra-arterial injection of 1 mEq of calcium gluconate, the islet cell tumor is readily seen during gastroduodenal artery injection.

and fat necrosis. If the patient survives the acute event, the disease can progress to phlegmon, abscess, or pseudocyst formation. The most common risk factors for acute and chronic pancreatitis are alcohol abuse and biliary tract obstruction (e.g., gallstones). Other causes include trauma, surgery, biliary cirrhosis, infection, drugs, hyperparathyroidism, and hyperlipidemia. *Chronic pancreatitis* follows repeated bouts of acute pancreatitis or chronic pancreatic duct obstruction and is characterized by diffuse fibrosis, gland calcification, and pseudocyst formation.

Vascular complications of pancreatitis include splenic vein thrombosis, formation of small intrapancreatic or large vessel pseudoaneurysms from enzymatic destruction or severe inflammation, pseudoaneurysm rupture, and pseudocyst hemorrhage.[41] Blood may leak into the gastrointestinal tract (through the biliary system *[hemosuccus pancreaticus]* or directly into bowel), retroperitoneum, or peritoneal cavity. Penetration of a pseudoaneurysm or pseudocyst into the portal vein can lead to hyperdynamic portal hypertension.

Clinical Features

Acute pancreatitis often becomes a medical emergency, with severe abdominal pain, jaundice, and shock. There is an early rise in serum amylase levels and a later rise in the serum lipase concentration. About 10% of patients with severe pancreatitis suffer bleeding complications signaled by gastrointestinal bleeding, hypotension, or a falling hematocrit.[42]

Imaging

Angiography. Hemorrhagic complications of pancreatitis often are first identified by CT or sonography. Arteriography may be needed for transcatheter therapy. The pancreas appears hypervascular in the acute and subacute stages of the disease. The angiographic findings in chronic pancreatitis can mimic those of pancreatic carcinoma, with effacement,

narrowing, smooth encasement, or frank occlusion of large vessels, most notably the gastroduodenal artery, splenic artery, and splenic vein (Fig. 11-6). Multiple small aneurysms of intrapancreatic arteries alternating with irregular stenoses are quite characteristic (see Fig. 11-1). Large pseudoaneurysms, bleeding pseudocysts, and free extravasation are readily seen at angiography.

Treatment

Endovascular Therapy. Embolization is the treatment of choice for most hemorrhagic complications, particularly because many of these patients are poor surgical candidates.[43-47] The most popular embolic agents are coils and Gelfoam pledgets, although other materials and routes have been used, including direct percutaneous thrombin injection. Exclusion across the neck of a pseudoaneurysm is necessary to prevent backfilling from the distal segment of the damaged artery (Fig. 11-7). Embolization generally is safe in the upper gastrointestinal tract. However, embolization of small or large bowel branches (e.g., jejunal arteries, middle colic artery arising from the dorsal pancreatic artery) poses some risk of bowel infarction. Permanent control of hemorrhage is achieved in about 75% of cases.

■ OTHER DISORDERS

Aneurysms

Aneurysms of the pancreatic and pancreaticoduodenal arteries are rare, and most are pseudoaneurysms caused by pancreatitis (Box 11-2; see also Figs. 11-1 and 11-7).[44,48] Erosion into the gastrointestinal tract with gastrointestinal bleeding may occur and often is the presenting symptom. An unusual

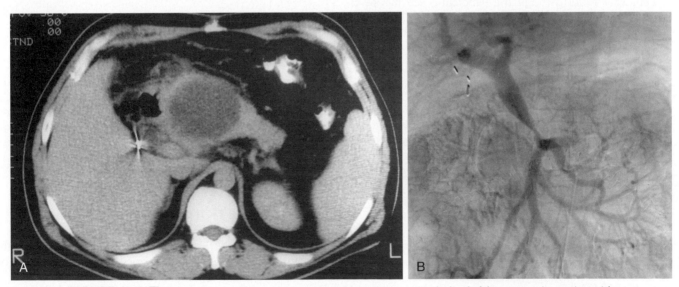

FIGURE 11-6 ■ Pancreatic pseudocyst. **A,** A large, hypodense mass occupies the head of the pancreas in a patient with a history of acute pancreatitis. **B,** Smooth narrowing of the portal vein is seen on the late-phase superior mesenteric artery arteriogram.

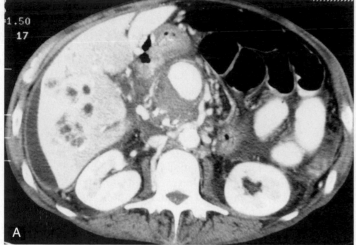

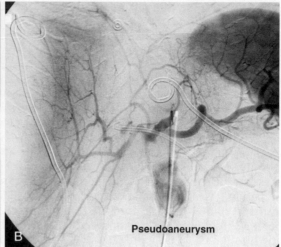

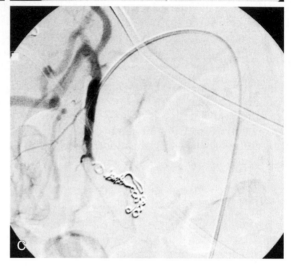

FIGURE 11-7 ■ Gastroduodenal artery pseudoaneurysm. **A,** CT scan shows a large mass in the head of the pancreas with central dense enhancement. Subcapsular fluid and numerous cystic hepatic lesions are also seen. **B,** Celiac arteriogram shows the gastroduodenal artery pseudoaneurysm. Subcapsular hepatic fluid has compressed the parenchyma. **C,** Microcoils were placed distal and proximal to the aneurysm neck to exclude it.

but noteworthy cause of pancreaticoduodenal aneurysms is obstruction of the celiac artery or SMA. Massive dilation of the collateral route through the pancreatic bed has been reported to produce frank aneurysm formation.[49] Treatment of certain types of pancreatic artery aneurysms was discussed previously.[50]

Trauma

Injury to the pancreas can be the result of blunt trauma, criminal penetrating trauma, or medical procedures.

BOX 11-2 ■ Causes of Aneurysms of Pancreatic Arteries

Inflammation (i.e., pancreatitis)
Trauma
Infection
Degenerative (atherosclerosis-related) causes
High-flow state with celiac or superior mesenteric artery obstruction
Tumor
Vasculitis

Blunt trauma and most cases of penetrating trauma are evaluated initially by CT imaging.[51,52]

Arteriovenous Malformations

Arteriovenous malformations of the pancreas are exceedingly rare. They may manifest as incidental findings or with rupture into the gastrointestinal tract.[53] These lesions are diagnosed by CT, MR, or color Doppler sonography. Angiography is required occasionally to confirm the diagnosis. The usual treatment is operative removal.

Transplantation Complications

Transplantation of the pancreas (often combined with kidney transplantation) is performed for selected patients with type 1 diabetes. In one operative approach, the donor's iliac artery is harvested along with the pancreas and its arterial supply from the splenic artery and SMA. The transplant splenic artery and SMA are connected to the graft internal and external iliac artery stumps, respectively.[54] The common iliac artery trunk of the Y graft is then anastomosed to the recipient's external iliac artery. The donor portal vein is connected to the recipient external iliac vein.

Vascular complications of pancreatic transplantation, although uncommon, can jeopardize the graft.[55,56] The most important of these are venous thrombosis, arterial thrombosis, and pseudoaneurysm formation. Early arterial thrombosis usually is caused by improper formation of the anastomosis or graft damage after harvesting. Gadolinium-enhanced MR imaging and color Doppler sonography are the preferred methods for imaging these patients.[54,57,58] Angiography is rarely needed for diagnosis.

ADRENAL GLANDS

■ ARTERIOGRAPHY, VENOGRAPHY, AND VENOUS SAMPLING

The only remaining indication for adrenal arteriography is percutaneous ablation of tumors. Several catheter shapes may be used; a reverse-curve catheter (sidewinder or Simmons shape) is the most versatile.

Given the sensitivity of CT, scintigraphy, and adrenal venous sampling in the diagnosis of adrenal gland neoplasms, adrenal venography is required only to document location during sampling. The major risk of adrenal venography is extravasation with infarction from overinjection of contrast, which can lead to complete nonfunction of the gland.[59]

Adrenal venous sampling is an important technique (though rarely performed) for evaluating hormonally active tumors of the gland. The procedure must be performed with meticulous attention to detail. An endhole catheter should be used and a blood sample obtained **before** a **small** contrast injection is made to document catheter position. The right adrenal gland is catheterized with a spinal or sidewinder catheter by searching the posterolateral aspect of the inferior vena cava (IVC) near the upper pole of the right kidney. The right adrenal vein must be differentiated from small, upwardly directed hepatic veins. The left adrenal vein, which is much easier to engage, is sampled with a headhunter catheter. The catheter tip is advanced well into the left renal vein and then withdrawn slowly with the tip pointing up until it enters the left phrenicoadrenal trunk.

■ ANATOMY

Classically, three arteries feed each of the adrenal glands[60]:

- *Superior adrenal artery* from the inferior phrenic artery (Fig. 11-8)
- *Middle adrenal artery* directly from the aorta above the renal artery (see Fig. 5-1)
- *Inferior adrenal artery* from the proximal renal artery

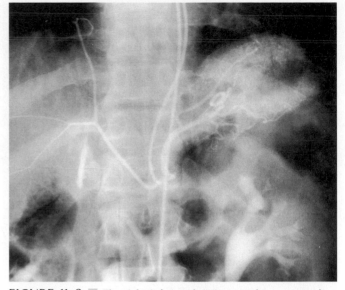

FIGURE 11-8 ■ The right inferior phrenic artery has an anomalous origin from the left gastric artery. The right adrenal gland, which is densely stained, is partially supplied by the superior adrenal branch of the inferior phrenic artery.

The right adrenal gland has three main venous tributaries that merge into a main trunk that enters the posterolateral IVC above the right renal vein (Fig. 11-9). A central vein runs through the substance of the left adrenal gland. It joins the left inferior phrenic vein to form a common trunk, which then empties into the upper surface of the left renal vein just lateral to the vertebrae.

Anomalous origins of the adrenal arteries are relatively common. The right adrenal vein may join a hepatic vein or enter directly into the right renal vein.

■ MAJOR DISORDERS

Cushing Syndrome

Etiology

Hypercortisolism has several causes[61]:

- Bilateral adrenal hyperplasia resulting from excess corticotropin (ACTH) production by a pituitary tumor or other source
- Benign adrenal adenoma
- Malignant adrenal carcinoma
- Excess cortisol intake

Excluding exogenous Cushing syndrome, adrenal tumors account for about 30% of cases. Benign adenomas tend to be small, but functioning adrenal carcinomas often are quite large.

Clinical Features

Patients typically present with hypertension, hirsutism, abdominal striae, obesity, diabetes, and mental disturbances.

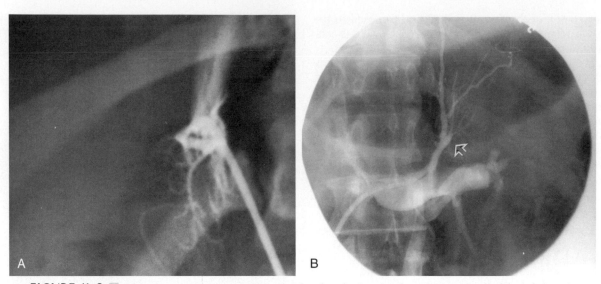

FIGURE 11-9 ■ Adrenal venous anatomy. **A,** Normal right adrenal vein arises from the lateral wall of the infrahepatic inferior vena cava. **B,** Normal left adrenal vein *(arrow)* joins the inferior phrenic vein and then drains into the left renal vein.

The disease occurs in adults and children.[61] The serum cortisol level is elevated. A dexamethasone suppression test may discriminate between ACTH-dependent adrenal hyperplasia and an ACTH-independent adrenal tumor.

Imaging

An adrenal mass is sought with sonography, CT, or MR, although the latter two methods are more sensitive.[62-65] Adrenal cortical scintigraphy with NP-59 (iodomethylnorcholesterol) may also be useful in detection. If routine imaging studies are nondiagnostic, adrenal venous sampling should be performed. This procedure is extremely accurate for the diagnosis.[66] A unilateral cortisol gradient is diagnostic of adrenal adenoma or adenocarcinoma. Venography shows bilaterally enlarged glands in some cases of adrenal hyperplasia, but they may appear normal.[67,68] An adenoma produces draping of venules about a rounded mass (Fig. 11-10). The contralateral gland is shrunken. Adrenal carcinoma often invades and obliterates adrenal venules.

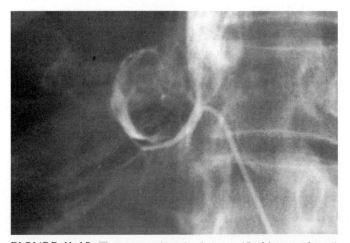

FIGURE 11-10 ■ Benign adrenal adenoma (Cushing syndrome) causes draping of venules about a rounded mass.

Aldosteronism

Etiology

Primary aldosteronism has several major causes:

- Adrenal adenoma *(Conn's syndrome)*
- Bilateral adrenal hyperplasia
- Adrenal carcinoma
- Ectopic tissue

A hyperfunctioning adrenal adenoma is the culprit in 50% to 75% of cases.[69,70] These adenomas tend to be smaller than those seen with Cushing syndrome (<2 cm). **Secondary** aldosteronism usually is caused by renal artery stenosis or, rarely, by a *reninoma* (a tumor of the juxtaglomerular apparatus), both of which elevate renin levels and accelerate the renin-angiotensin-aldosterone system.

Clinical Features

Patients with primary or secondary aldosteronism are hypertensive. Hypokalemia, metabolic alkalosis, low serum renin levels, high serum aldosterone levels, and elevated urinary aldosterone metabolites are characteristic. The reported incidence of aldosteronism in hypertensive populations is 1% to 2%, although some series have found much higher numbers.[69,71]

Imaging

The distinction between a functioning tumor and bilateral adrenal hyperplasia is important, because the former is treated with surgery for cure and the latter is treated medically with aldosterone antagonists. CT and MR imaging are the primary imaging modalities.[62,72,73] Scintigraphy with NP-59 is probably as sensitive as CT. If an adenoma is found, adrenalectomy usually is performed. However, nonfunctioning adrenal adenomas may occur in hypertensive patients and confound the diagnosis.

Adrenal venous sampling is helpful when CT or MR fails to detect an adenoma or reveals bilateral adrenal masses, one of which may be an "incidentaloma."[65] Sampling is accurate in differentiating hyperplasia from adenoma and for localization of tumor in greater than 90% of cases.[66,74-77] Blood aliquots are obtained from the right and left adrenal veins and the IVC for aldosterone and cortisol analysis. An aldosterone/cortisol ratio greater than 1.5 is diagnostic of a tumor.[26] A small contrast injection is made after sampling to document the catheter position.

Treatment

Functioning adenomas and adrenal carcinomas are treated by open adrenalectomy or with laparoscopic techniques. Bilateral hyperplasia is managed with drug therapy. Percutaneous ablation by arterial embolotherapy (e.g., with alcohol sometimes admixed with contrast material) or radiofrequency ablation (RFA) have been effective and durable in selected cases.[78-80]

▪ OTHER DISORDERS

Adrenogenital Syndromes

Virilization, or, less frequently, feminization, in adults usually is the result of adrenal disease (i.e., adenoma, carcinoma, or bilateral hyperplasia) or a gonadal tumor. Ovarian tumors usually produce testosterone, whereas adrenal tumors typically produce dehydroepiandrosterone (DHEA) and dehydroepiandrosterone sulfate.[81] Urinary 17-ketosteroid levels are markedly elevated in either case. Affected women complain of hirsutism, menstrual problems, acne, and obesity.

CT and MR are the imaging procedures of choice. If the results are equivocal, bilateral adrenal and ovarian venous sampling should be performed.[26,82] Various hormonal levels are measured, including testosterone, DHEA, and androstenedione. Virilizing adrenal or ovarian tumors are associated with an abnormally high hormone ratio between the ipsilateral vein and a peripheral blood sample.

Pheochromocytoma

These rare tumors of chromaffin cells of the sympathetic nervous system originate in the adrenal medulla *(pheochromocytoma)* or extra-adrenal sites *(paraganglionomas* or *chemodectomas).*[83] The tumor has been described by the "10% rule," whereby 10% of lesions are extra-adrenal, metastatic, bilateral, cystic, or associated with multiple endocrine adenoma syndromes. Symptoms are related to excess production of catecholamines (including epinephrine and norepinephrine) and other hormones from the abnormal tissue.

The diagnosis of pheochromocytoma or paraganglionoma usually is made with metaiodobenzylguanidine (MIBG) scintigraphy, MR imaging, or CT scanning. Angiography is almost never required. Iodinated contrast material given by any route may precipitate a potentially lethal hypertensive crisis.[85] Patients with suspected disease should be pretreated with alpha-adrenergic and possibly beta-adrenergic antagonists. A typical regimen includes phenoxybenzamine for several days before the procedure and phentolamine as needed during the procedure.

CT-guided RFA or percutaneous ethanol injection (PEI) have been employed for treatment of these lesions.[80,86]

Nonfunctioning Tumors

A variety of nonendocrine neoplasms affects the adrenal gland, including metastases, adrenal carcinoma, adenoma, myelolipoma, neuroblastoma, and lymphoma. The diagnosis of these entities does not require angiography. However, transcatheter embolization has been used successfully to reduce tumor size and relieve pain.[87] In addition, PEI and RFA are being studied as alternative treatment methods.[80,88]

PARATHYROID GLANDS

▪ ARTERIOGRAPHY AND VENOGRAPHY

Parathyroid arteriography includes bilateral subclavian arteriography (for road mapping), followed by bilateral thyrocervical, internal thoracic, and common carotid arteriography. Arch aortography is needed sometimes to identify a *thyroidea ima artery* supplying an ectopic parathyroid gland in the mediastinum. Rare complications of parathyroid arteriography include stroke and spinal cord injury. The latter has been reported with inadvertent overinjection of the costocervical artery, which has branches to the spinal cord. The thyrocervical trunk rarely supplies the spinal cord.

The technique for parathyroid venous sampling is complex.[26] A complete procedure requires selective catheterization of inferior, superior, and middle thyroid veins and the thymic and internal jugular veins. Large vein sampling (i.e., bilateral internal jugular and brachiocephalic veins) is simpler but far less accurate. Small contrast injections are made after obtaining blood samples to document catheter position. In postoperative patients, the vertebral veins also are sampled at several sites.

▪ ANATOMY

The paired superior parathyroid glands are small, ovoid structures that lie deep in the thyroid capsule. Although the paired inferior glands normally are located in the lower portion of the capsule, they may reside well into the mediastinum. Some patients have more than four glands. The arterial supply includes[26,89,90]:

- ▪ *Inferior thyroid branch* of the thyrocervical artery (Fig. 11-11)
- ▪ *Superior thyroid branch* of the external carotid artery
- ▪ *Thymic branch* of the internal thoracic artery (Fig. 11-12)
- ▪ *Thyroidea ima artery* from the undersurface of the aortic arch

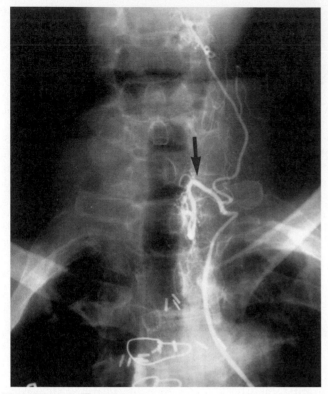

FIGURE 11-11 ■ The inferior thyroid artery *(arrow)* arises from the left thyrocervical artery.

The primary venous drainage routes are

■ *Inferior thyroid vein* to the upper surface of the left brachiocephalic or right internal jugular vein (see Fig. 15-4)
■ *Superior* and *middle thyroid veins* to the internal jugular vein
■ *Thymic vein* to the undersurface of the left brachiocephalic vein (see Fig. 11-12)

During surgery for parathyroid disease, the thyroidal veins often are ligated. The thyroid bed then drains through collateral channels that join the vertebral veins.

■ MAJOR DISORDERS

Hyperparathyroidism

Etiology and Clinical Features

Primary hyperparathyroidism is a disorder of excess secretion of parathyroid hormone (PTH) from solitary or multiple parathyroid adenomas, bilateral hyperplasia, or parathyroid carcinoma.[91] Adenomas account for about 80% of cases. The resulting hypercalcemic state is responsible for kidney stones, abdominal pain, renal dysfunction, and dehydration seen with this disease. The treatment usually is surgical resection of the adenoma or subtotal parathyroidectomy for glandular hyperplasia. In a few patients, symptoms persist or recur after surgery because of ectopic or supernumerary glands or incomplete initial removal of tissue. Residual tumors usually are found in the tracheoesophageal groove

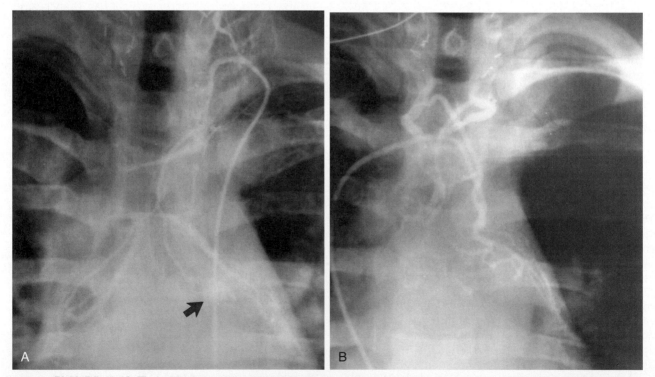

FIGURE 11-12 ■ Mediastinal parathyroid adenoma. **A,** A hypervascular nodule is detected in the mediastinum *(arrow).* The adenoma is supplied by a thymic branch of the left internal thoracic artery. **B,** Venous sampling from the thymic tributary of the left brachiocephalic vein confirmed the diagnosis.

of the superior mediastinum, in the thymus, or within the thyroid gland.

Imaging

Noninvasive Imaging. Patients are first evaluated with sonography, CT, MR, or ^{99m}Tc-sestamibi scintigraphy of the neck and mediastinum.[91,92] If symptoms persist after surgery or parathormone levels remain elevated, additional studies may be needed to confidently localize the residual tumor before reoperation.[93] Scintigraphy appears to be more sensitive than other modalities in this regard.[94] Percutaneous aspiration and PTH assay of suspicious lesions also has been done to confirm the diagnosis.[95]

Angiography. In rare cases, noninvasive studies fail to detect residual tissue after surgery. These patients may benefit from selective parathyroid angiography with venous sampling.[26,96] The arteriogram shows the tumor or provides a road map for venous sampling. An adenoma appears as a sharp, round, densely staining mass anywhere from the upper neck to the superior mediastinum (see Fig. 11-12). Opacification of the thyroid gland or a lymph node can mimic an adenoma. Likewise, normal thyroid tissue can hide an adenoma. With venous sampling, a 2:1 PTH ratio between a sampled site and a peripheral vein is diagnostic. In experienced hands, the sensitivity of arteriography is about 60% to 70% and that of selective venous sampling is about 80% to 90%.[97,98]

Treatment

Medical Therapy. A distinct set of patients with asymptomatic hyperparathyroidism can be treated conservatively.[99]

Surgical Therapy. Repeated exploration of the neck or mediastinum is based on imaging studies. Repeat operation is curative in greater than 90% of cases.[93,94]

Endovascular Therapy. Transcatheter arterial ablation of residual parathyroid adenomas has been described.[93,100] Injection of a high-osmolar contrast agent or alcohol is usually sufficient to destroy the lesion. The procedure should be performed only if some parathyroid tissue is preserved to prevent hypoparathyroidism. The reported cure rate is about 70%.

MALE REPRODUCTIVE SYSTEM

■ ARTERIOGRAPHY AND VENOGRAPHY

In the evaluation of men with suspected high-flow priapism or penile trauma, a pelvic arteriogram serves as a road map for selective catheterization. The internal pudendal artery is easily catheterized using an ultralong reverse-curve (Bookstein or Roberts) catheter.

Cavernosography is performed by injecting dilute, isosmolar contrast material at a rate of 1 to 2 mL/second through a small butterfly needle inserted into one corpus cavernosum just proximal to the glans. Both corpora fill because of normal perforations in the intercavernosal septum.

For varicocele embolization, many experts favor access through the right internal jugular vein rather than the femoral vein. From the neck, a sheath is inserted and a headhunter catheter is advanced into the IVC. A left renal venogram may be performed with the patient partially upright or during a Valsalva maneuver to encourage reflux into the left internal spermatic vein. The right internal spermatic vein is engaged with a sidewinder or Simmons catheter from the groin or a reshaped headhunter catheter from the neck. The terminal valve is crossed with a hydrophilic guidewire, and selective venography is done to map the vein and other collateral routes. Lead shielding of the testes is important.

■ ANATOMY

The penis is fed by the *internal pudendal artery*, which is a major branch of the anterior division of the internal iliac artery. However, the penile arteries are sometimes supplied by collateral vessels or anomalous routes such as the obturator, inferior gluteal, external pudendal, or inferior epigastric artery.[101,102] The internal pudendal gives off scrotal branches, after which it becomes the *common penile artery* (Fig. 11-13). The *artery to the bulb* supplies the corpus spongiosum and the urethra. The penile artery has two terminal branches. The *dorsal penile artery* runs in the superficial fascia of the penis; the *cavernosal artery* enters the substance of

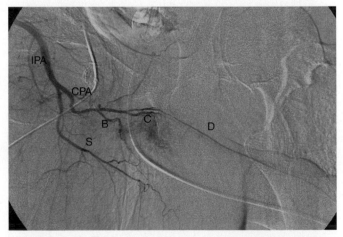

FIGURE 11-13 ■ Right internal pudendal arteriogram in a patient with peroneal trauma and possible arteriocavernosal fistula causing priapism. The cavernosal artery is truncated beyond its origin. Staining of the bulb of the corpus spongiosum is normal. B, artery to the bulb; C, cavernosal artery; CPA, common penile artery; D, dorsal penile artery; IPA, internal pudendal artery; S, scrotal branches.

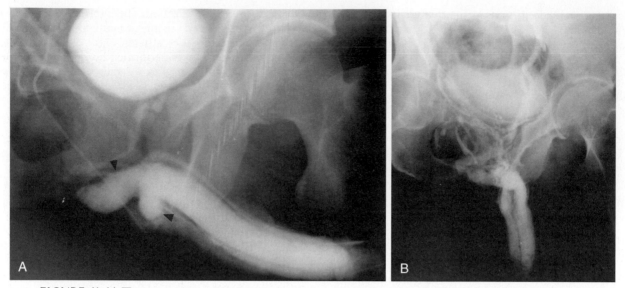

FIGURE 11-14 ■ Normal cavernosography. **A,** Both corpora cavernosa are filled to the crura *(arrowheads)*, and the deep dorsal vein is filled. **B,** The intercavernosal septum is seen in another patient. The cavernosa drain into the preprostatic plexus and then into internal pudendal and other deep pelvic veins.

the corpus cavernosum. Helicine arterioles directly supply the lacunar spaces of the corpora.

The testes are fed by the *testicular arteries*, which arise from the anterolateral surface of the aorta just at or below the renal artery origins.

The corpora cavernosa drain through a deep system (i.e., *deep dorsal vein*) and a superficial system (i.e., *superficial dorsal vein*) into the crural and preprostatic plexuses and finally into the internal pudendal and other deep pelvic veins (Fig. 11-14).

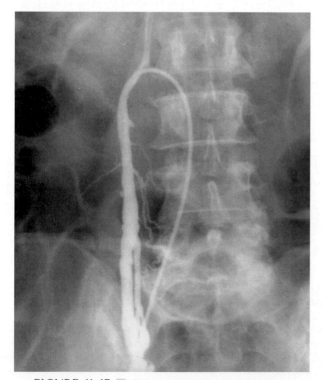

FIGURE 11-15 ■ Right internal spermatic venogram.

The physiology of penile erection is complex. The critical hemodynamic event is relaxation of the smooth muscle of the corpora cavernosa, which is mediated naturally through neurogenic impulses that result in nitric oxide release (and can be enhanced with phosphodiesterase-5 inhibitors).[103,104] With expansion of the lacunar spaces, arterial inflow increases rapidly. As the lacunae become engorged with blood, small perforating venules are compressed against the rigid tunica albuginea surrounding the corpora. Venous drainage is impeded, and the penis becomes erect.

Blood drains from the testis and epididymis through the *pampiniform plexus*.[104] At the superficial inguinal ring, this complex forms three or four tributaries that enter the pelvis (Fig. 11-15). These veins eventually merge into two and then into a single internal spermatic vein running in front of the ureter and alongside the gonadal artery. It is common for the main venous channel to have medial and lateral components; the lateral branch often terminates in renal capsular, mesenteric, colonic, or retroperitoneal veins. The *right internal spermatic vein* enters the IVC just below the right renal vein. The *left internal spermatic vein* enters the undersurface of the left renal vein lateral to the vertebral column (see Fig. 8-4). Variant anatomy is seen in about 20% of cases.[105] Important anomalies include drainage of the right internal spermatic vein into the right renal vein (8%) and multiple terminal gonadal veins (15% to 20%). Valves are present in most but not all veins.

■ MAJOR DISORDERS

Varicocele and Infertility

Etiology

Varicocele is a dilation of the pampiniform plexus with or without central venous dilation.[106] The disorder affects about 15% of the adult male population, with most cases occurring on the left side. The right side is affected in up to 10% of cases, although some reports suggest a much higher frequency.[107,108]

The origin of **primary** varicocele is still debated. Various theories have been proposed, including absence or abnormal formation of internal spermatic vein valves and compression of the left renal vein, causing internal spermatic vein hypertension. Regardless of the cause, venous reflux and chronic venous hypertension are the result.

Secondary varicocele is caused by abdominal or pelvic masses that impede drainage of the pampiniform plexus. The sudden onset of varicocele in an older man or the presence of a right-sided varicocele should raise the suspicion of a neoplasm (e.g., left renal vein invasion from renal cell carcinoma).

Clinical Features

Although many patients with varicocele are asymptomatic and do not have a fertility problem (>80%), the disorder can be responsible for infertility, scrotal pain, or disfigurement.[109] Up to 40% of men evaluated in infertility clinics are found to have a varicocele.[110] The leading theories for the association between varicocele and infertility invoke elevations in scrotal temperature or backflow of renal or adrenal metabolites as a cause for testicular dysfunction and suboptimal sperm production. Abnormalities of total sperm count, sperm density, and sperm motility are found in many patients with varicocele.

Imaging

Most varicoceles can be detected by physical examination. When the diagnosis is questioned or a subclinical varicocele is suspected (i.e., infertility with abnormal sperm activity but a nonpalpable varicocele), the scrotum is evaluated with duplex sonography.[111] Spermatic venography is reserved for patients undergoing embolotherapy.

Treatment

Varicocele Embolization

Patient Selection. The indications for treatment of varicocele include infertility with laboratory evidence for sperm dysfunction, failures of surgical ligation, scrotal pain, massive size, and testicular hypoplasia in adolescent boys.[112-114] However, some investigators have failed to show a true benefit with regard to fertility (see below).

Technique. Embolization is performed from the jugular or femoral vein approach using a guiding catheter. Catheterization of the gonadal veins may be difficult if variant anatomy is present.[115] A diagnostic venogram is obtained to document valvular incompetence, reflux of contrast, venous dilation, and filling of collateral tributaries (Fig. 11-16). The preferred embolic agents are coils (with or without adjuvant sclerosing agent such as polidocanol or sodium morrhuate), detachable balloons, and glue.

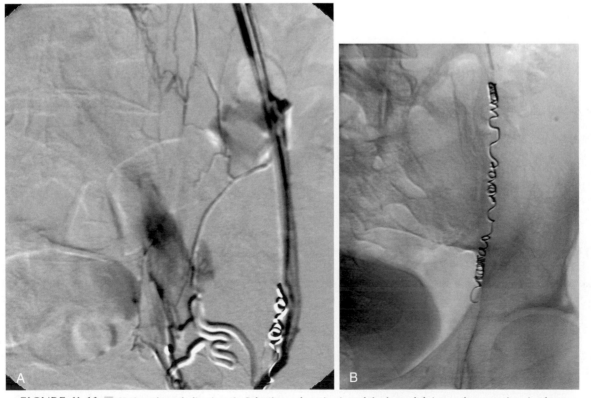

FIGURE 11-16 ■ Varicocele embolization. **A,** Selective catheterization of the lower left internal spermatic vein about the inguinal ligament. Several platinum coils and Gelfoam pieces were placed. Because several collateral channels opacified, sodium morrhuate was injected as a liquid sclerosant. **B,** Additional platinum coils sandwiched around Gelfoam pieces were deposited along the course of the vein up to its orifice at the left renal vein.

The internal spermatic vein is first occluded around the level of the superior pubic ramus. Occlusion is then continued upward to the renal vein, taking care not to allow coil springs to extend into the renal vein or IVC. Venography is repeated periodically to identify collateral channels that also may require embolization. Nitroglycerin (100 to 200 μg) is given to relieve venospasm. In patients with left-sided varicocele, right-sided embolization is performed only if the right internal spermatic vein is incompetent.

Results. Embolotherapy is technically successful in greater than 80% to 90% of cases.[113,114,116-119] The most common reasons for failure are inability to cannulate the internal spermatic vein or traverse a competent valve, venospasm, and the presence of multiple central collateral veins. The late recurrence rate is 4% to 12%, primarily because of the development of collateral channels.[113,117,120] A significant improvement in sperm density and motility is observed in most patients; about one third of couples become pregnant in follow-up studies.[113,117,121-123] Similar results are achieved for embolization of recurrent varicocele after failed surgical ligation.[124] However, some studies have failed to show increased likelihood of pregnancy or association of pregnancy with improved sperm quality after varicocele embolization.[125,126]

Complications. Minor flank or scrotal pain, low-grade fever, and transient numbness over the anterior thigh are minor side effects of the procedure. Vein rupture with extravasation usually is self-limited. Complications specific to the procedure are uncommon (5% to 10%) and include embolization of coils to the lung, thrombosis of the pampiniform plexus, and aspermia.

Surgical Therapy

Operation for varicocele entails surgical ligation of the internal spermatic vein and collateral vessels. Classically, ligation is performed at the retroperitoneal, internal inguinal ring (Ivanissevich procedure), or subinguinal level (Marmor procedure). A laparoscopic approach is favored by many surgeons.[127] In most reports, the results of embolotherapy and surgical ligation are comparable in terms of technical success, improvement in sperm density and function, pregnancy outcome, and complications.[121-123,128] However, recurrence rates are higher after surgery.

■ OTHER DISORDERS

Penile Diseases

Several disorders affecting the penis may require vascular imaging:

■ *Peyronie's disease* is characterized by buildup of fibrotic plaques in the tunica albuginea and corpora cavernosa that cause penile deviation with erection and, less often, impotence.[129] The usual treatment is surgical plaque excision. Patients often require evaluation with cavernosography and dynamic cavernosometry before operation.[130,131]

■ Penile fracture, which can result from vigorous sexual activity, leads to cavernosal laceration, penile deformity, urethral injury, or impotence.[132-134]
■ Blunt perineal or penile trauma also can cause arteriocavernous fistulas and priapism or arteriovenous fistulas and erectile dysfunction.[135,136]

FEMALE REPRODUCTIVE SYSTEM

■ ARTERIOGRAPHY AND VENOGRAPHY

Angiography of the female reproductive organs is analogous to evaluation of the male reproductive system (see earlier).

■ ANATOMY

The ovaries are fed by the *ovarian arteries*, which arise from the anterolateral surface of the aorta below the renal arteries (see Fig. 5-1). The vessels descend into the pelvis and then enter the broad ligament of the uterus. The *right ovarian vein* empties directly into the IVC below the right renal vein. The *left ovarian vein* drains into the undersurface of the left renal vein. Variant anatomy is seen in a minority of cases.[137]

The uterus is primarily supplied by the *uterine arteries*, which usually take off as separate branches of the anterior divisions of the internal iliac arteries.[137] They course medially in the broad ligament and then ascend along the lateral border of the uterus. These vessels have anastomoses with branches of the ovarian arteries (see below).

■ MAJOR DISORDERS

Uterine Leiomyomas

Etiology

Uterine leiomyomas (fibroids) are the most common tumor affecting the female reproductive organs and occur in about 20% to 25% of all women.[138] Histologically, they are benign tumors composed primarily of whorls of smooth muscle cells and fibrous stroma. These discrete lesions are classified by location as *intramural, subserosal,* or *submucosal.* Many uterine fibroids remain asymptomatic and do not require treatment. When they do cause symptoms, they are usually multiple. As the tumors enlarge, cystic degeneration and calcific deposits can result. Fibroids also may become pedunculated, with long stalks that allow them to migrate into the cervix, vagina, or abdomen. Degeneration into *leiomyosarcoma* is rare but is described. Leiomyomas must be distinguished from their malignant relative and from *adenomyosis,* which is benign growth of endometrial gland tissue into the myometrium that causes generalized uterine enlargement. Isolated foci of adenomyosis also can mimic leiomyoma.

Clinical Features

Fibroids are up to three times more common in African-American women than in Caucasian women. Most symptomatic patients are between the ages of 35 and 50. Because they are hormonally sensitive, fibroids enlarge rapidly during pregnancy and usually regress after menopause. Development and growth of these lesions is attributed to both genetic and hormonal factors.

Most fibroids do not produce symptoms. When they do, it is primarily by mass effect on the bladder, ureters, and adjacent pelvic structures. Women may suffer from pain, pressure, or heaviness in the pelvis, back, perineum, or legs; heavy menstrual bleeding; abdominal bloating and distention; urinary frequency or incontinence; and ureteral obstruction.[139] Submucosal fibroids can interfere with normal endometrial activity and lead to prolonged menses or infertility or prolapse into the cervix. Other diseases (including gynecologic malignancies such as ovarian cancer) may cause similar symptoms; they must be excluded by imaging studies or other means.

Imaging

Transabdominal or transvaginal sonography is sensitive in depicting uterine fibroids and in identifying other possible causes for symptoms or concurrent disease. However, MR imaging is superior in assessing the number, size, and location of fibroids; internal architecture and vascularity; effect on adjacent structures; and the presence of coexisting adenomyosis or other pathology. For most experienced practitioners, it is the preferred study before and after uterine artery embolization (UAE) procedures (see below).

Fibroids appear as discrete round masses with heterogeneous low signal on T2-weighted images and isointense with myometrium on T1-weighted images.[140] Lesions enhance variably on T1-weighted images after gadolinium (Fig. 11-17). In one study, favorable tumor shrinkage after UAE was predicted by lower signal intensity on T1-weighted images and higher intensity on T2-weighted images.[141] Adenomyosis appears as widening of the junctional zone with bright signals in the myometrium on T2-weighted images.

Treatment

Uterine Artery Embolization

The rationale behind UAE is that bland small vessel occlusion of the feeding arteries causes tumor infarction and eventual shrinkage, resulting in abatement of symptoms. Because of the rich collateral circulation that is usually present, normal uterine tissue remains viable.

Patient Selection. The choice between endovascular and operative treatment should be made jointly by the patient, gynecologist, and interventionalist after the current status of all available treatment modalities has been considered and presented in a forthright fashion. Only **symptomatic** patients in whom other causes for disease have been excluded (including a recent Papanicolaou test) should undergo this treatment. The interventionalist is obligated to become the primary physician caring for the patient in pre-procedure consultation, hospital recovery, and all outpatient management. Adenomyosis also may respond to UAE.[142]

Absolute or relative contraindications include pregnancy, active or chronic pelvic infection, gynecologic malignancy (unless palliative or as an adjunct to operation), uncorrectable coagulopathy, severe contrast allergy, and prior pelvic surgery or radiation therapy.[139] The effect of UAE on fertility has not been established, although pregnancy can occur after the procedure. Gonadotropin-releasing hormones that may have been prescribed as medical therapy for the condition should be stopped at least 3 months before procedure; these drugs cause uterine artery constriction and can make catheterization difficult. Pedunculated fibroids with relatively narrow stalks are prone to detachment after UAE and may require operative removal.

Technique. UAE for fibroids was first reported by Ravina and coworkers.[143] A thorough consultation with the interventionalist is mandatory well before the procedure. Because pain is to be expected after the embolization is accomplished, moderate sedation and patient-controlled anesthesia should be used liberally. Although there is no consensus about prophylactic antibiotics in this setting, many practitioners choose to use them (e.g., cephazolin 1 g IV). Radiation exposure should be kept to a minimum by limiting use of prolonged acquisition, magnification, oblique projections, and wide fields of view. Fluoroscopy time (or preferably peak skin dose) must be measured and recorded.

A Foley catheter is inserted. The common femoral artery is the usual access route.[144] A pelvic arteriogram with the catheter positioned in the infrarenal abdominal aorta is obtained as a road map. Selective catheterization of the anterior divisions of the internal iliac arteries is performed with a cobra or ultra-long reverse-curve (e.g., Roberts) catheter (see Fig. 11-17). Once the uterine artery is identified and selected, angiography shows the markedly dilated *spiral arteries* feeding the uterus. Tumor hypervascularity and vessel displacement is seen. In some cases, the descending portion of the uterine artery can be engaged with the 5-French diagnostic catheter. However, vasospasm may be a problem, so that coaxial placement of a microcatheter directed well into the uterine artery often is required.

The preferred agents for embolization are small-caliber particulate matter, including polyvinyl alcohol (PVA) particles (350 to 500 or 500 to 700 µm), tris-acryl gelatin microspheres (Embospheres, 700 to 900 µm), and Gelfoam pieces. Most practitioners use one of the former two materials.[145-147] There does not appear to be any significant difference in clinical efficacy between the two agents. Proximal embolization (e.g., with coils) is inadvisable, because collateral vessels are sure to develop and continue to feed the tumors.

Embolization with particulate slurry (made with diluted contrast material) is continued until there is static flow in uterine artery branches ("pruned-tree" appearance). Regardless of the location of fibroids, bilateral embolization

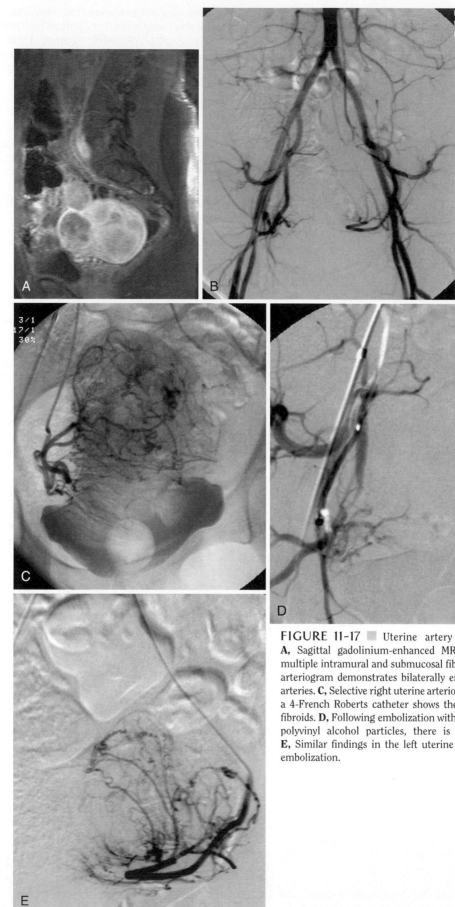

FIGURE 11-17 ■ Uterine artery embolization. **A,** Sagittal gadolinium-enhanced MR image shows multiple intramural and submucosal fibroids. **B,** Pelvic arteriogram demonstrates bilaterally enlarged uterine arteries. **C,** Selective right uterine arteriography through a 4-French Roberts catheter shows the hypervascular fibroids. **D,** Following embolization with 300 to 500-μm polyvinyl alcohol particles, there is stasis of flow. **E,** Similar findings in the left uterine artery prior to embolization.

is necessary to prevent recruitment of collateral vessels. Bilateral completion internal iliac arteriograms are obtained to identify any additional vessels feeding the tumors.

The interventionalist should be observant of variant arterial anatomy and important collateral vessels. In most cases, the ovarian arteries contribute to fibroids through anastomoses with the main uterine artery. In about 10% of patients, the uterine artery is the major blood supply to the ovary, or the ovarian artery has significant direct communication with the fibroid (Fig. 11-18).[148] Of course, embolization of these vessels theoretically increases the risk of ovarian infarction and infertility. Any other collateral vessels that feed the tumor must also be occluded. This is particular true in women who have undergone prior pelvic surgery, had other tubal pathology, or have fundal fibroids.[149]

Postprocedure care should be directed by the interventionalist who performed the UAE. A postembolization syndrome consisting of pain, nausea and vomiting, and low-grade fever is to be expected. Most patients are hospitalized overnight, although discharge later in the day is possible in some cases. Pain must be aggressively managed with IV and then oral narcotics.[150] Antiemetics are given prophylactically or as needed. Discharge medications include anti-inflammatory drugs (e.g., ketorolac) and potent oral narcotics. Follow-up is done by the interventionalist, including routine clinic evaluation at 1 to 3 weeks after the procedure.

Results. Bilateral UAE is successful in about 95% of cases. Incomplete infarction of fibroids may be associated with the potential for continued growth.[151] Clinical success with substantial improvement in symptoms is seen in about 80% to 90% of women.[152,154,156] Submucosal lesions and small lesions seem to respond better than other tumors.[157] Failure or recurrence is noted in about 6% of cases.[152] The primary reasons for failure are outlined in Box 11-3. If symptoms continue and leiomyomas persist or enlarge on imaging studies, repeat UAE (with aggressive search for collateral vessels including the ovarian arteries) is often warranted (see Fig. 11-18).

Complications. Intra- and postprocedure pain is a common problem after UAE.[158] The most important complications after UAE are intrauterine infection, uterine ischemia and necrosis, pulmonary embolism, and expulsion of pedunculated submucosal lesions.[159] The overall complication rate is about 5%; major complications occur about 1% of the time.[160] Most patients do not have a significant change in follicle stimulating hormone afterward, although this is more likely in women older than 45 years of age.[161] Amenorrhea

(which is often transient) occurs in less than 10% of cases, but it is much more likely in patients older than 45 to 50 years of age.[152,154,156] Serious infectious complications are observed in 1% of treated women. Less than 2% require subsequent hysterectomy for any complications of UAE.[162]

Other Percutaneous Methods

Studies are underway to evaluate MR- and ultrasound-focused "surgery" to ablate uterine fibroids. In addition, ultrasound-guided cryoablation has been attempted.

Surgical Therapy

The standard treatment is open myomectomy. UAE and myomectomy are comparable in terms of symptom relief, but the risk of complications is higher with the operative approach.[163-165]

Obstetric and Gynecologic Postoperative Bleeding

Etiology

Massive intrapelvic or vaginal bleeding is a rare but serious complication of vaginal and cesarean deliveries.[166] Significant hemorrhage may occur also after hysterectomy and spontaneous or therapeutic abortion. The major causes of postpartum bleeding are retained products of conception, lacerations, uterine atony, and uterine rupture. Women with placental disorders, coexisting leiomyomas, or ectopic pregnancy are at particularly high risk for significant bleeding. Abnormalities of placentation include *placenta accreta* (penetration into the uterine wall), *placenta increta* (penetration through the myometrium), and *placenta percreta* (penetration to the serosa).[167] Some of these patients have disseminated intravascular coagulation because of release of tissue thromboplastin, which further predisposes them to hemorrhage.

Clinical Features

Massive obstetric bleeding usually is associated with tachycardia and hypotension. Bleeding may be vaginal or intra-abdominal.

Treatment

Medical Therapy. Initial management of postpartum bleeding includes uterine massage, drug therapy (e.g., oxytocin), vaginal packing, closure of lacerations, and curettage for retained products. In most cases, bleeding stops with these maneuvers.

Surgical Therapy. The original operative treatment was bilateral internal iliac artery ligation (which is ineffective in many cases) or bilateral uterine artery ligation (which is usually effective). Hysterectomy is required for life-threatening hemorrhage after delivery.

BOX 11-3 ■ Causes of Uterine Artery Embolization Failure

Inability to catheterize uterine arteries
Incomplete embolization
Presence of important collaterals (e.g., ovarian arteries)
Large fibroids
Recanalization of embolized arteries
Coexisting adenomyosis or leiomyosarcoma

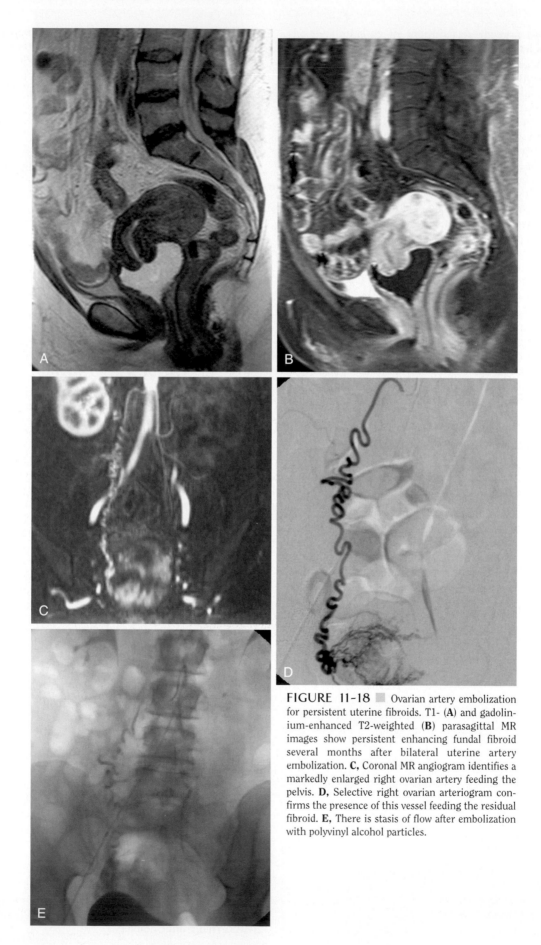

FIGURE 11-18 ▇ Ovarian artery embolization for persistent uterine fibroids. T1- (**A**) and gadolinium-enhanced T2-weighted (**B**) parasagittal MR images show persistent enhancing fundal fibroid several months after bilateral uterine artery embolization. **C,** Coronal MR angiogram identifies a markedly enlarged right ovarian artery feeding the pelvis. **D,** Selective right ovarian arteriogram confirms the presence of this vessel feeding the residual fibroid. **E,** There is stasis of flow after embolization with polyvinyl alcohol particles.

Endovascular Therapy. Embolotherapy is extremely effective for most cases of pregnancy-related or posthysterectomy bleeding.[166-171] The procedure begins with pelvic and then bilateral internal iliac arteriography. Embolization of the branches causing the bleeding is accomplished with microcoils or Gelfoam pledgets (Fig. 11-19). The ovarian arteries should be examined if no extravasation is found from pelvic arteries. Collateral vessels (i.e., lumbar, femoral circumflex, inferior epigastric, and inferior mesenteric arteries) are other potential sources of bleeding, particularly in postoperative patients. After embolization, bilateral internal iliac arteriography is repeated to confirm that bleeding has stopped. Hemorrhage can be controlled in almost every patient.

Complications, including pelvic abscess, organ ischemia, and nerve damage, are reported in less than 10% of cases. The risk of permanent nerve injury is negligible if small particulate agents are avoided. Embolization does not appear to affect fertility and subsequent pregnancy significantly because distal embolization with particulate or liquid agents is avoided.[171,172]

In women with abnormal placentation, the standard operation at the time of delivery is cesarean hysterectomy,

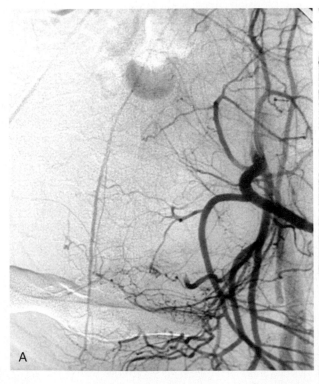

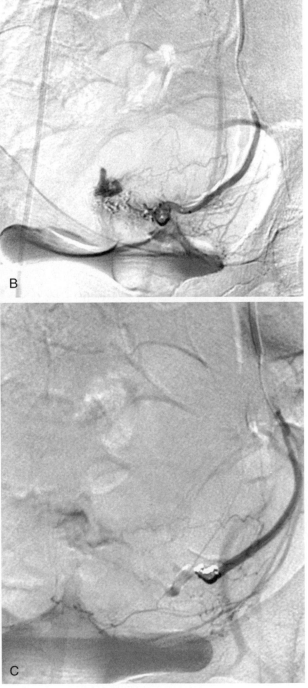

FIGURE 11-19 ■ Massive pelvic bleeding after a vaginal hysterectomy. **A,** The initial left internal iliac arteriogram failed to identify a bleeding site. **B,** Selective injection of a small branch of the anterior division through a coaxial microcatheter shows extravasation. **C,** Bleeding ceased after placement of several microcoils in the vessel.

which is often associated with massive blood loss and significant associated mortality. When antenatal diagnosis is made (as is usually the case), some obstetricians elect to have occlusion balloons placed in the proximal internal iliac arteries preoperatively through bilateral femoral artery access. The volume of fluid needed to distend each balloon and completely obstruct flow is recorded by the interventionalist, and balloons are inflated in the operating room, if necessary. However, there is no incontrovertible evidence that this method is associated with reduced bleeding or decreased morbidity or mortality.[167,173,174]

■ OTHER DISORDERS

Malignant Gynecologic Tumors

Women with pelvic malignancies, particularly of the uterus and cervix, occasionally develop massive hemorrhage from vascular invasion, after radiation therapy, or during surgery. Bleeding may be transvaginal or intra-abdominal. Embolotherapy is extremely effective in controlling bleeding.[175-178] Because of the progressive nature of the disease, occlusions must be bilateral, and the embolic agent must be permanent and small (e.g., PVA particles). Rebleeding is a common problem, although many patients die soon after the procedure from the underlying malignancy. The major potential complications are pelvic organ

ischemia, skin necrosis, and nerve damage (e.g., sciatic neuropathy).

Pelvic Congestion Syndrome

Ovarian vein varices increasingly are being recognized as an important cause of unexplained pelvic pain in women of childbearing age. Hormonal and hemodynamic factors are believed to be responsible for the condition. In a minority of patients, compression of the left renal vein between the aorta and superior mesenteric artery ("nutcracker syndrome") is responsible; many of these women also complain of hematuria.[179] Symptoms include lower abdominal or perineal pain and fullness, menorrhagia, dyspareunia, and polymenorrhea.[180,181] Pain is worse usually with prolonged standing, after intercourse, and just before menses. Superficial varicosities often are found on the vulva and thigh.

Unlike male varicocele, the diagnosis requires imaging studies such as MR or color Doppler sonography.[179,180] A significant number of asymptomatic women, however, demonstrates ovarian vein enlargement and reflux on imaging studies obtained for unrelated reasons.[182] Operative treatment (open or laparoscopic) involves ovarian vein ligation along with obliteration of collateral pathways.[183] Ovarian vein embolization is an attractive alternative to surgery.[184-187] At venography, incompetent ovarian vein valves, venous dilation, reflux, and cross-pelvic collateral drainage are characteristic (Fig. 11-20).

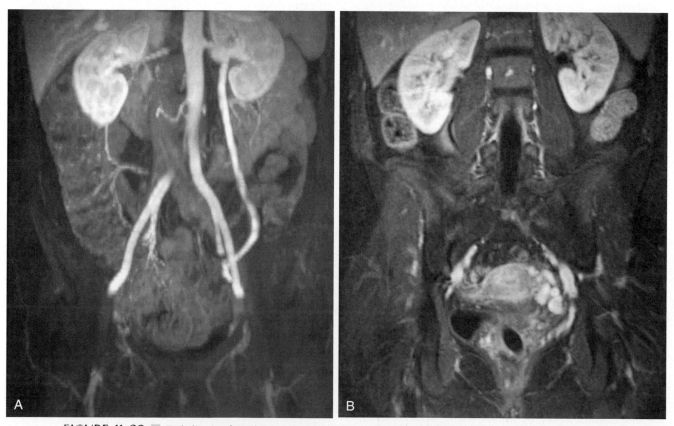

FIGURE 11-20 ■ Embolization for pelvic congestion syndrome. **A** and **B,** Gadolinium-enhanced MR venography with maximum intensity coronal projection shows reflux down a markedly dilated left ovarian vein with numerous left-sided pelvic varicosities.

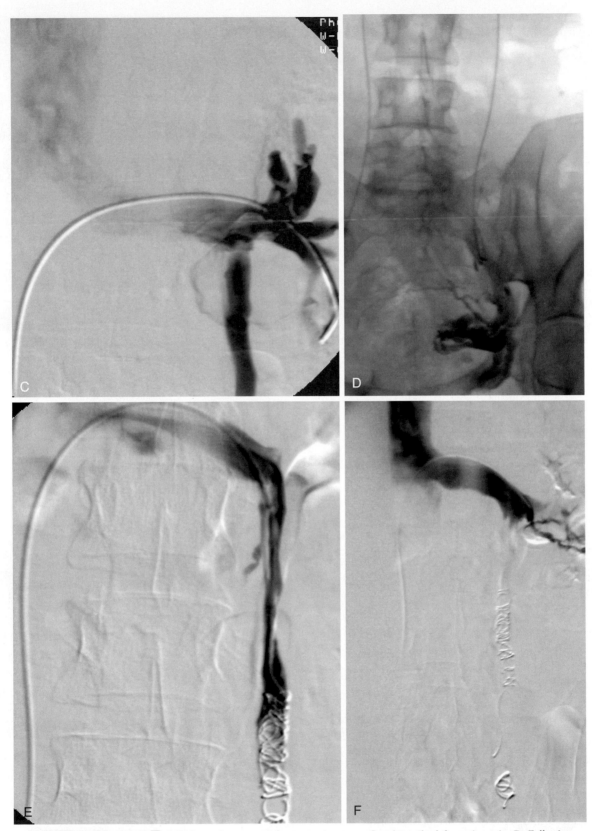

FIGURE 11-20 *Cont'd* ■ **C,** Left renal venogram shows spontaneous reflux down the left ovarian vein. **D,** Following deep catheterization of the vein, an 8-mL slurry of sodium morrhuate and Gelfoam pieces was slowly infused with patient in near upright position. **E,** Coil embolization now has been achieved almost to the level of the ovarian vein orifice. **F,** No further reflux is seen.   *Continued*

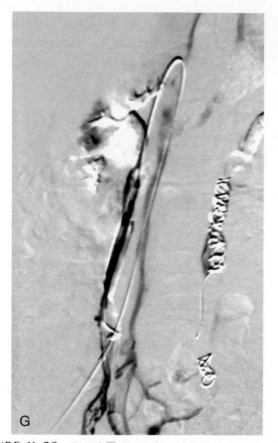

FIGURE 11-20 *Cont'd* ■ **G,** Right ovarian venography shows filling of collateral channels but small caliber vein and no spontaneous reflux.

Occlusion is accomplished with a variety of agents, including coils, sclerosing agents, and glue. Most patients notice improvement or resolution of symptoms after the procedure.

Uterine and Cervical Vascular Malformations

Pelvic arteriovenous malformations (AVMs) are rare lesions that can affect the female reproductive organs (see Chapter 6) (Fig. 11-21).[188,189] Many so-called uterine AVMs are actually acquired complex arteriovenous fistulas that are related to prior pelvic surgery or gestational trophoblastic disease, although the bizarre angiographic appearance is similar to that of an AVM. Vaginal or intraabdominal bleeding may occur. Surgical resection of symptomatic lesions is extremely difficult. Percutaneous embolotherapy is indicated for palliation of symptoms.[190,191] Repeat procedures may be necessary to largely eradicate the lesion.

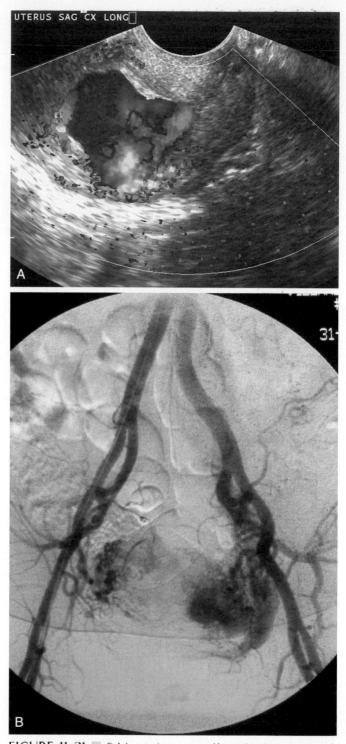

FIGURE 11-21 ■ Pelvic arteriovenous malformation in a woman with prior gynecologic instrumentation and massive vaginal bleeding. **A,** Sagittal color Doppler sonography reveals a huge vascular mass within the uterus and extending into the cervix. **B,** Pelvic arteriogram shows the massively dilated inflow arteries and early venous shunting.

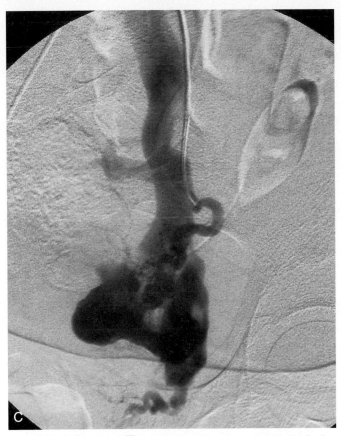

FIGURE 11-21 *Cont'd* ■ **C,** Selective left uterine arteriography further confirms the massive shunt.

REFERENCES

1. Gabella G, ed: Cardiovascular system. In: Williams PL, Bannister LH, Berry MM, et al, eds. Gray's Anatomy, 38th ed. New York, Churchill Livingstone, 1995:1549.
2. Skandalakis LJ, Rowe JS Jr, Gray SW, et al: Surgical embryology and anatomy of the pancreas. Surg Clin North Am 1993;73:661.
3. Jensen RT: Endocrine neoplasms of the pancreas. In: Yamada T, Alpers DH, Laine L, eds. Textbook of Gastroenterology, 4th ed. Philadelphia, Lippincott, Williams and Wilkins, 2003:2108.
4. Freeny PC, Traverso LW, Ryan JA: Diagnosis and staging of pancreatic adenocarcinoma with dynamic computed tomography. Am J Surg 1993;165:600.
5. Brugge WR, Lauwers GY, Sahani D, et al: Cystic neoplasms of the pancreas. N Engl J Med 2004;351:1218.
6. Horton KM, Fishman EK: Adenocarcinoma of the pancreas: CT imaging. Radiol Clin North Am 2002;40:1263.
7. Ly JN, Miller FH: MR imaging of the pancreas: a practical approach. Radiol Clin North Am 2002;40:1289.
8. Ingram M, Arregui ME: Endoscopic ultrasonography. Surg Clin North Am 2004;84:1035.
9. Muller MF, Meyenberger C, Bertschinger P, et al: Pancreatic tumors: evaluation with endoscopic US, CT, and MR imaging. Radiology 1994; 190:745.
10. Biehl TR, Traverso LW, Hauptmann E, et al: Preoperative visceral angiography alters intraoperative strategy during the Whipple procedure. Am J Surg 1993;165:607.
11. Mackie CR, Lu CT, Noble HG, et al: Prospective evaluation of angiography in the diagnosis and management of patients suspected of having pancreatic cancer. Ann Surg 1979;189:11.
12. Goldstein HM, Neiman HL, Bookstein JJ: Angiographic evaluation of pancreatic disease. A further appraisal. Radiology 1974;112:275.
13. Ghaneh P, Neoptolemos JP: Conclusions from the European Study Group for Pancreatic Cancer adjuvant trial of chemoradiotherapy and chemotherapy for pancreatic cancer. Surg Oncol Clin N Am 2004;13:567.
14. Cameron JL, Crist DW, Sitzmann JV, et al: Factors influencing survival after pancreaticoduodenectomy for pancreatic cancer. Am J Surg 1991; 161:120.
15. Modlin IM, Tang LH: Approaches to the diagnosis of gut neuroendocrine tumors: the last word (today). Gastroenterology 1997;112:583.
16. Mansour JC, Chen H: Pancreatic endocrine tumors. J Surg Res 2004;120:139.
17. Somogyi L, Mishra G: Diagnosis and staging of islet cell tumors of the pancreas. Curr Gastroenterol Rep 2000;2:159.
18. Buetow PC, Miller DL, Parrino TV, et al: Islet cell tumors of the pancreas: clinical, radiologic, and pathologic correlation in diagnosis and localization. Radiographics 1997;17:453.
19. Norton JA, Jensen RT: Current surgical management of Zollinger-Ellison syndrome (ZES) in patients without multiple endocrine neoplasia-type 1 (MEN1). Surg Oncol 2003;12:145.
20. Kalra MK, Maher MM, Mueller PR, et al: State-of-the-art imaging of pancreatic neoplasms. Br J Radiol 2003;76:857.
21. Nino-Murcia M, Jeffrey RB Jr: Multidetector-row CT and volumetric imaging of pancreatic neoplasms. Gastroenterol Clin North Am 2002; 31:881.
22. Becherer A, Szabo M, Karanikas G, et al: Imaging of advanced neuroendocrine tumors with (18)F-FDOPA PET. J Nucl Med 2004;45:1161.
23. Gibril F, Reynolds JC, Doppman JL, et al: Somatostatin receptor scintigraphy: its sensitivity compared with that of other imaging methods in detecting primary and metastatic gastrinomas—a prospective study. Ann Intern Med 1996;125:26.
24. Roesch T, Lightdale CJ, Botet JF, et al: Localization of pancreatic endocrine tumors by endoscopic ultrasonography. N Engl J Med 1992;326:1721.
25. Zimmer T, Stolzel U, Bader M, et al: Endoscopic ultrasonography and somatostatin receptor scintigraphy in the preoperative localisation of insulinomas and gastrinomas. Gut 1996;39:562.
26. Miller DL: Endocrine angiography and venous sampling. Radiol Clin North Am 1993;31:1051.
27. Miller DL, Doppman JL, Metz DC, et al: Zollinger-Ellison syndrome: technique, results, and complications of portal venous sampling. Radiology 1992;182:235.
28. Wiesli P, Brändle M, Schmid C, et al: Selective arterial calcium stimulation and hepatic venous sampling in the evaluation of hyperinsulinemic hypoglycemia: potential and limitations. J Vasc Interv Radiol 2004;15:1251.
29. Fink IJ, Krudy AG, Shawker TH, et al: Demonstration of an angiographically hypovascular insulinoma with intraarterial dynamic CT. AJR Am J Roentgenol 1985;144:555.
30. Brandle M, Pfammatter T, Spinas GA, et al: Assessment of selective arterial calcium stimulation and hepatic venous sampling to localize insulin-secreting tumours. Clin Endocrinol (Oxf) 2001;55:357.
31. Doppman JL, Miller DL, Chang R, et al: Gastrinomas: localization by means of selective intraarterial injection of secretin. Radiology 1990; 174:25.
32. Oberg K, Kvols L, Caplin M, et al: Consensus report on the use of somatostatin analogs for the management of neuroendocrine tumors of the gastroenteropancreatic system. Ann Oncol 2004;15:966.
33. Uflacker R: Arterial embolization as definitive treatment for benign insulinoma of the pancreas. J Vasc Interv Radiol 1992;3:639.
34. Kress O, Wagner HJ, Wied M, et al: Transarterial chemoembolization of advanced liver metastases of neuroendocrine tumors—a retrospective single-center analysis. Digestion 2003;68:94.
35. Yao KA, Talamonti MS, Nemcek A: Indications and results of liver resection and hepatic chemoembolization for metastatic gastrointestinal neuroendocrine tumors. Surgery 2001;130:677.
36. Chamberlain RS, Canes D, Brown KT, et al: Hepatic neuroendocrine metastases: does intervention alter outcomes? J Am Coll Surg 2000; 190:432.
37. Brown KT, Koh BY, Brody LA, et al: Particle embolization of hepatic neuroendocrine metastases for control of pain and hormonal symptoms J Vasc Interv Radiol 1999;10:397.
38. Fiorentini G, Rossi S, Bonechi F, et al: Intra-arterial hepatic chemoembolization in liver metastases from neuroendocrine tumors: a phase II study. J Chemother 2004;16:293.
39. Gee M, Soulen MC: Chemoembolization for hepatic metastases. Tech Vasc Interv Radiol 2002;5:132.
40. Glasbrenner B, Adler G: Pathophysiology of acute pancreatitis. Hepatogastroenterology 1993;40:517.

41. Boudghene F, L'Hermine C, Bigot J-M: Arterial complications of pancreatitis: diagnostic and therapeutic aspects in 104 cases. J Vasc Interv Radiol 1993;4:551.
42. Stabile BE, Wilson SE, Debas HT: Reduced mortality from bleeding pseudocysts and pseudoaneurysms caused by pancreatitis. Arch Surg 1983;118:45.
43. Mauro MA, Jacques P: Transcatheter management of pseudoaneurysms complicating pancreatitis. J Vasc Interv Radiol 1991;2:527.
44. Messina LM, Shanley CJ: Visceral artery aneurysms. Surg Clin North Am 1997;77:425.
45. Tessier DJ, Stone WM, Fowl RJ, et al: Clinical features and management of splenic artery pseudoaneurysm: case series and cumulative review of literature. J Vasc Surg 2003;38:969.
46. Beattie GC, Hardman JG, Redhead D, et al: Evidence for a central role for selective mesenteric angiography in the management of the major vascular complications of pancreatitis. Am J Surg 2003; 185:96.
47. Carr JA, Cho JS, Shepard AD, et al: Visceral pseudoaneurysms due to pancreatic pseudocysts: rare but lethal complications of pancreatitis. J Vasc Surg 2000;32:722.
48. Paty PS, Cordero JA Jr, Darling RC 3rd, et al: Aneurysms of the pancreaticoduodenal artery. J Vasc Surg 1996;23:710.
49. Uher P, Nyman U, Ivancev K, et al: Aneurysms of the pancreaticoduodenal artery associated with occlusion of the celiac artery. Abdom Imaging 1995;20:470.
50. Chiang KS, Johnson CM, McKusick MA, et al: Management of inferior pancreaticoduodenal artery aneurysms: a 4-year single center experience. Cardiovasc Intervent Radiol 1994;17:217.
51. Siegel MJ, Sivit CJ: Pancreatic emergencies. Radiol Clin North Am 1997;35:815.
52. Lane MJ, Mindelzun RE, Jeffrey RB: Diagnosis of pancreatic injury after blunt abdominal trauma. Semin Ultrasound CT MR 1996;17:177.
53. Chang S, Lim HK, Lee WJ, et al: Arteriovenous malformation of the pancreas in a patient with gastrointestinal bleeding: helical CT findings. Abdom Imaging 2004;29:259.
54. Krebs TL, Daly B, Wong JJ, et al: Vascular complications of pancreatic transplantation: MR evaluation. Radiology 1995;196:793.
55. Spiros D, Christos D, John B, et al: Vascular complications of pancreas transplantation. Pancreas 2004;28:413.
56. Ciancio G, Cespedes M, Olson L, et al: Partial venous thrombosis of the pancreatic allografts after simultaneous pancreas-kidney transplantation. Clin Transplant 2000;14:464.
57. Boeve WJ, Kok T, Tegzess AM, et al: Comparison of contrast enhanced MR-angiography-MRI and digital subtraction angiography in the evaluation of pancreas and/or kidney transplantation patients: initial experience. Magn Reson Imaging 2001;19:595.
58. Pozniak MA, Propeck PA, Kelcz F, et al: Imaging of pancreatic transplants. Radiol Clin North Am 1995;33:581.
59. Bookstein JJ, Conn J, Reuter SR: Intra-adrenal hemorrhage as a complication of adrenal venography in primary aldosteronism. Radiology 1968;90:778.
60. Gabella G, ed: Cardiovascular system. In: Williams PL, Bannister LH, Berry MM, et al, eds. Gray's Anatomy, 38th ed. New York, Churchill Livingstone, 1995:1556.
61. Tsigos C, Chrousos GP: Differential diagnosis and management of Cushing's syndrome. Ann Rev Med 1996;47:443.
62. Hussain HK, Korobkin M: MR imaging of the adrenal glands. Magn Reson Imaging Clin N Am 2004;12:515.
63. Rockall AG, Babar SA, Sohaib SA, et al: CT and MR imaging of the adrenal glands in ACTH-independent Cushing syndrome. Radiographics 2004;24:435.
64. Ng L, Libertino JM: Adrenocortical carcinoma: diagnosis, evaluation and treatment. J Urol 2003;169:5.
65. Dunnick NR, Korobkin M: Imaging of adrenal incidentalomas: current status. AJR Am J Roentgenol 2002;179:559.
66. Dedrick CG: Adrenal arteriography and venography. Urol Clin North Am 1989;16:515.
67. Reuter SR, Blair AJ, Schteingart DE, et al: Adrenal venography. Radiology 1967;89:805.
68. Mitty HA, Nicolis GL, Gabrilove JL: Adrenal venography: clinical-roentgenographic correlation in 80 patients. AJR Am J Roentgenol 1973;119:564.
69. Gordon RD, Stowasser M, Tunny TJ, et al: High incidence of primary aldosteronism in 199 patients referred with hypertension. Clin Exp Pharmacol Physiol 1994;21:315.
70. Abdelhamid S, Muller-Lobeck H, Pahl S, et al: Prevalence of adrenal and extra-adrenal Conn syndrome in hypertensive patients. Arch Intern Med 1996;156:1190.
71. Thakkar RB, Oparil S: Primary aldosteronism: a practical approach to diagnosis and treatment. J Clin Hypertens (Greenwich) 2001;3:189.
72. Mayo-Smith WW, Boland GW, Noto RB, et al: State-of-the-art adrenal imaging. Radiographics 2001;21:995.
73. Dunnick NR, Leight GS Jr, Roubidoux MA, et al: CT in the diagnosis of primary aldosteronism: sensitivity in 29 patients. AJR Am J Roentgenol 1993;160:321.
74. Takasaki I, Shionoiri H, Yasuda G, et al: Preoperative lateralisation of aldosteronomas by aldosterone/cortisol ratios in adrenal venous plasma. J Hum Hypertens 1987;1:95.
75. Young WF Jr, Hogan MJ, Klee GG, et al: Primary aldosteronism: diagnosis and treatment. Mayo Clin Proc 1990;65:96.
76. Dunnick NR, Doppman JL, Mills SR, et al: Preoperative diagnosis and localization of aldosteronomas by measurement of corticosteroids in adrenal venous blood. Radiology 1979;133:331.
77. Wheeler MH, Harris DA: Diagnosis and management of primary aldosteronism. World J Surg 2003;27:627.
78. Inoue H, Nakajo M, Miyazono N, et al: Transcatheter arterial ablation of aldosteronomas with high-concentration ethanol: preliminary and long-term results. AJR Am J Roentgenol 1997;168:1241.
79. Hokotate H, Inoue H, Baba Y, et al: Aldosteronomas: experience with superselective adrenal arterial embolization in 33 cases. Radiology 2003;227:401.
80. Mayo-Smith WW, Dupuy DE: Adrenal neoplasms: CT-guided radiofrequency ablation-preliminary results. Radiology 2004;231:225.
81. Del Gaudio A, Del Gaudio GA: Virilizing adrenocortical tumors in adult women: report of 10 patients, 2 of whom each had a tumor secreting only testosterone. Cancer 1993;72:1997.
82. Bricaire C, Raynaud A, Benotmane A, et al: Selective venous catheterization in the evaluation of hyperandrogenism. J Endocrinol Invest 1991;14:949.
83. Francis IR, Korobkin M: Pheochromocytoma. Radiol Clin North Am 1996;34:1101.
84. Berglund AS, Hulthen UL, Manhem P, et al: Metaiodobenzylguanidine (MIBG) scintigraphy and computed tomography (CT) in clinical practice. Primary and secondary evaluation for localization of phaeochromocytomas. J Intern Med 2001;249:247.
85. Konen E, Konen O, Katz M, et al: Are referring clinicians aware of patients at risk from intravenous injection of iodinated contrast media? Clin Radiol 2002;57:132.
86. Wang P, Zuo C, Qian Z, et al: Computerized tomography guided percutaneous ethanol injection for the treatment of hyperfunctioning pheochromocytoma. J Urol 2003;170:1132.
87. O'Keeffe FN, Carrasco CH, Charnsangavej C, et al: Arterial embolization of adrenal tumors: results in nine cases. AJR Am J Roentgenol 1988;151:819.
88. Shibata T, Maetani Y, Ametani F, et al: Percutaneous ethanol injection for treatment of adrenal metastasis from hepatocellular carcinoma. AJR Am J Roentgenol 2000;174:333.
89. Nobori M, Saiki S, Tanaka N, et al: Blood supply of the parathyroid gland from the superior thyroid artery. Surgery 1994;115:417.
90. Norton JA: Reoperation for missed parathyroid adenoma. Adv Surg 1997;31:273.
91. Akerstrom G, Hellman P: Primary hyperparathyroidism. Curr Opin Oncol 2004;16:1.
92. Weber AL, Randolph G, Aksoy FG: The thyroid and parathyroid glands. CT and MR imaging and correlation with pathology and clinical findings. Radiol Clin North Am 2000;38:1105.
93. McIntyre RC Jr, Kumpe DA, Liechty RD: Reexploration and angiographic ablation for hyperparathyroidism. Arch Surg 1994;129:499.
94. Jaskowiak N, Norton JA, Alexander HR, et al: A prospective trial evaluating a standard approach to reoperation for missed parathyroid adenoma. Ann Surg 1996;224:308.
95. Sacks BA, Pallotta JA, Cole A, et al: Diagnosis of parathyroid adenomas: efficacy of measuring parathormone levels in needle aspirates of cervical masses. AJR Am J Roentgenol 1994;163:1223.
96. Seehofer D, Steinmuller T, Rayes N, et al: Parathyroid hormone venous sampling before reoperative surgery in renal hyperparathyroidism: comparison with noninvasive localization procedures and review of the literature. Arch Surg 2004;139:1331.
97. Sugg SL, Fraker DL, Alexander R, et al: Prospective evaluation of selective venous sampling for parathyroid hormone concentration in

patients undergoing reoperations for primary hyperparathyroidism. Surgery 1993;114:1004.

98. Miller DL, Chang R, Doppman JL, et al: Localization of parathyroid adenomas: superselective arterial DSA versus superselective conventional arteriography. Radiology 1989;170:1003.

99. Silverberg SJ, Bilezikian JP: Asymptomatic primary hyperparathyroidism: a medical perspective. Surg Clin North Am 2004;84:787.

100. Miller DL, Doppman JL, Chang R, et al: Angiographic ablation of parathyroid adenomas: lessons from a ten-year experience. Radiology 1987;165:601.

101. Bookstein JJ, Valji K: Penile vascular catheterization in diagnosis and therapy of erectile dysfunction. In: Baum S, Pentecost MJ, eds. Abram's Angiography: Interventional Radiology. Boston, Little, Brown, 1997:705.

102. Bookstein JJ: Penile angiography: the last angiographic frontier. AJR Am J Roentgenol 1988;150:47.

103. Gonzalez-Cadavid NF, Rajfer J: Therapy of erectile dysfunction: potential future treatments. Endocrine 2004;23:167

104. Gabella G, ed: Cardiovascular system. In: Williams PL, Bannister LH, Berry MM, et al, eds. Gray's Anatomy, 38th ed. New York, Churchill Livingstone, 1995:1600.

105. Lechter A, Lopez G, Martinez C, et al: Anatomy of the gonadal veins: a reappraisal. Surgery 1991;109:735.

106. Male Infertility Best Practice Policy Committee of the American Urological Association; Practice Committee of the American Society for Reproductive Medicine. Report on varicocele and infertility. Fertil Steril 2004;82(Suppl 1):S142.

107. Shuman L, White RI Jr, Mitchell SE, et al: Right-sided varicocele: technique and clinical results of balloon embolotherapy from the femoral approach. Radiology 1986;158:787.

108. Gat Y, Bachar GN, Zukerman Z, et al: Varicocele: a bilateral disease. Fertil Steril 2004;81:424.

109. Bong GW, Koo HP: The adolescent varicocele: to treat or not to treat. Urol Clin North Am 2004;31:509.

110. Meacham RB, Townsend RR, Rademacher D, et al: The incidence of varicoceles in the general population when evaluated by physical examination, gray scale sonography, and color Doppler sonography. J Urol 1994;151:1535.

111. Petros JA, Andriole GL, Middleton WD, et al: Correlation of testicular color Doppler ultrasonography, physical examination, and venography in the detection of left varicoceles in men with infertility. J Urol 1991;145:785.

112. Lord DJ, Burrows PE: Pediatric varicocele embolization. Tech Vasc Interv Radiol 2003;6:169.

113. Shlansky-Goldberg RD, Van Arsdalen KN, Rutter CM, et al: Percutaneous varicocele embolization versus surgical ligation for the treatment of infertility: changes in seminal parameters and pregnancy outcomes. J Vasc Interv Radiol 1997;8:759.

114. Reyes BL, Trerotola SO, Venbrux AC, et al: Percutaneous embolotherapy of adolescent varicocele: results and long-term follow-up. J Vasc Interv Radiol 1994;5:131.

115. Tay KH, Martin ML, Mayer AL, et al: Selective spermatic venography and varicocele embolization in men with circumaortic left renal veins. J Vasc Interv Radiol 2002;13:739.

116. Di Bisceglie C, Fornengo R, Grosso M, et al: Follow-up of varicocele treated with percutaneous retrograde sclerotherapy: technical, clinical and seminal aspects. J Endocrinol Invest 2003;26:1059.

117. Zuckerman AM, Mitchell SE, Venbrux AC, et al: Percutaneous varicocele occlusion: long-term follow-up. J Vasc Interv Radiol 1994;5:315.

118. Mazzoni G, Fiocca G, Minucci S, et al: Varicocele: a multidisciplinary approach in children and adolescents. J Urol 1999;162:1755.

119. Ferguson JM, Gillespie IN, Chalmers N, et al: Percutaneous varicocele embolization in the treatment of infertility. Br J Radiol 1995;68:700.

120. Marsman JWP: The aberrantly fed varicocele: frequency, venographic appearance, and results of transcatheter embolization. AJR Am J Roentgenol 1995;164:649.

121. Sayfan J, Soffer Y, Orda R: Varicocele treatment: prospective randomized trial of 3 methods. J Urol 1992;148:1447.

122. Yavetz H, Levy R, Papo J, et al: Efficacy of varicocele embolization versus ligation of the left internal spermatic vein for improvement of sperm quality. Int J Androl 1992;15:338.

123. Schlesinger MH, Wilets IF, Nagler HM: Treatment outcome after varicocelectomy: a critical analysis. Urol Clin North Am 1994;21:517.

124. Punekar SV, Prem AR, Ridhorkar VR, et al: Post-surgical recurrent varicocele: efficacy of internal spermatic venography and steel-coil embolization. Br J Urol 1996;77:124.

125. Evers JL, Collins JA: Assessment of efficacy of varicocele repair for male subfertility: a systematic review. Lancet 2003;361:1849.

126. Nabi G, Asterlings S, Greene DR, et al: Percutaneous embolization of varicoceles: outcomes and correlation of semen improvement with pregnancy. Urology 2004;63:359.

127. Miersch WD, Schoeneich G, Winter P, et al: Laparascopic varicocelectomy: indications, technique, and surgical results. Br J Urol 1995;76:636.

128. Dewire DM, Thomas AJ Jr, Falk RM, et al: Clinical outcome and cost comparison of percutaneous embolization and surgical ligation of varicocele. J Androl 1994;15(Suppl):38S.

129. Somers KD, Dawson DM: Fibrin deposition in Peyronie's disease plaque. J Urol 1997;157:311.

130. Lopez JA, Jarow JP: Penile vascular evaluation of men with Peyronie's disease. J Urol 1993;149:53.

131. Jordan GH, Angermeier KW: Preoperative evaluation of erectile function with dynamic infusion cavernosometry/cavernosography in patients undergoing surgery for Peyronie's disease: correlation with postoperative results. J Urol 1993;150:1138.

132. Lurie AL, Bookstein JJ, Kessler WO: Posttraumatic impotence: angiographic evaluation. Radiology 1987;165:115.

133. Kowalczyk J, Athens A, Grimaldi A: Penile fracture: an unusual presentation with lacerations of bilateral corpora cavernosa and partial disruption of the urethra. Urology 1994;44:599.

134. Munarriz RM, Yan QR, Nehra A, et al: Blunt trauma: the pathophysiology of hemodynamic injury leading to erectile dysfunction. J Urol 1995;153:1831.

135. Bastuba MD, Saenz de Tejada I, Dinlenc CZ, et al: Arterial priapism: diagnosis, treatment, and long-term follow-up. J Urol 1994;151:1231.

136. Savoca G, Pietropaolo F, Scieri F, et al: Sexual function after highly selective embolization of cavernous artery in patients with high flow priapism: long-term followup. J Urol 2004;172:644.

137. Bannister LH, Dyson M, eds: Reproductive system. In: Williams PL, Bannister LH, Berry MM, et al, eds. Gray's Anatomy, 38th ed. New York, Churchill Livingstone, 1995:1873.

138. Wallach EE, Vlahos NF: Uterine myomas: an overview of development, clinical features, and management. Obstet Gynecol 2004;104:393.

139. Andrews RT, Spies JB, Sacks D, et al: Patient care and uterine artery embolization for leiomyomata. J Vasc Interv Radiol 2004;15:115.

140. Szklaruk J, Tamm EP, Choi H, et al: MR imaging of common and uncommon pelvic masses. Radiographics 2003;23:403.

141. Burn PR, McCall JM, Chinn RJ, et al: Uterine fibroleiomyoma: MR imaging appearances before and after embolization of uterine arteries. Radiology 2000;214:729.

142. Siskin GP, Tublin ME, Stainken BF, et al: Uterine artery embolization for the treatment of adenomyosis: clinical response and evaluation with MR imaging. AJR Am J Roentgenol 2001;177:297.

143. Ravina JH, Herbreteau D, Ciraru-Vigneron N, et al: Arterial embolisation to treat uterine myomata. Lancet 1995;346:671.

144. Worthington-Kirsch RL, Andrews RT, et al: Uterine fibroid embolization: technical aspects. Tech Vasc Interv Radiol 2002;5:17.

145. Banovac F, Ascher SM, Jones DA, et al: Magnetic resonance imaging outcome after uterine artery embolization for leiomyomata with use of tris-acryl gelatin microspheres. J Vasc Interv Radiol 2002;13:681.

146. Pelage JP, Le Dref O, Beregi JP, et al: Limited uterine artery embolization with tris-acryl gelatin microspheres for uterine fibroids. J Vasc Interv Radiol 2003;14:15.

147. Pelage JP, Le Dref O, Soyer P, et al: Arterial anatomy of the female genital tract: variations and relevance to transcatheter embolization of the uterus. AJR Am J Roentgenol 1999;172:989.

148. Razavi MK, Wolanske KA, Hwang GL, et al: Angiographic classification of ovarian artery-to-uterine artery anastomoses: initial observations in uterine fibroid embolization. Radiology 2002;224:707.

149. Pelage JP, Walker WJ, Le Dref O, et al: Ovarian artery: angiographic appearance, embolization and relevance to uterine fibroid embolization. Cardiovasc Intervent Radiol 2003;26:227.

150. Siskin GP, Bonn J, Worthington-Kirsch RL, et al: Uterine fibroid embolization: pain management. Tech Vasc Interv Radiol 2002;5:35.

151. Pelage JP, Guaou NG, Jha RC, et al: Uterine fibroid tumors: long-term MR imaging outcome after embolization. Radiology 2004;230:803.

152. Pelage JP, Le Dref O, Soyer P, et al: Fibroid-related menorrhagia: treatment with superselective embolization of the uterine arteries and midterm follow-up. Radiology 2000;215:428.

153. Spies JB, Ascher SA, Roth AR, et al: Uterine artery embolization for leiomyomata. Obstet Gynecol 2001;98:29.

154. Walker WJ, Pelage JP: Uterine artery embolisation for symptomatic fibroids: clinical results in 400 women with imaging follow up. BJOG 2002;109:1262.

155. Goodwin SC, McLucas B, Lee M, et al: Uterine artery embolization for the treatment of uterine leiomyomata: midterm results. J Vasc Interv Radiol 1999;10:1159.

156. Pron G, Bennett J, Common A, et al: The Ontario Uterine Fibroid Embolization Trial. Part 2. Uterine fibroid reduction and symptom relief after uterine artery embolization for fibroids. Fertil Steril 2003;79:120.

157. Spies JB, Roth AR, Jha RC, et al: Leiomyomata treated with uterine artery embolization: factors associated with successful symptom and imaging outcome. Radiology 2002;222:45.

158. Pron G, Mocarski E, Bennett J, et al: Tolerance, hospital stay, and recovery after uterine artery embolization for fibroids: the Ontario Uterine Fibroid Embolization Trial. J Vasc Interv Radiol 2003; 14:1243.

159. Pelage JP, Walker WJ, Dref OL: Uterine necrosis after uterine artery embolization for leiomyoma. Obstet Gynecol 2002;99:6767.

160. Spies JB, Spector A, Roth AR, et al: Complications after uterine artery embolization for leiomyomas. Obstet Gynecol 2002;100:873.

161. Spies JB, Roth AR, Gonsalves SM, et al: Ovarian function after uterine artery embolization for leiomyomata: assessment with use of serum follicle stimulating hormone assay. J Vasc Interv Radiol 2001;12:437.

162. Pron G, Mocarski E, Cohen M, et al: Hysterectomy for complications after uterine artery embolization for leiomyoma: results of a Canadian multicenter clinical trial. J Am Assoc Gynecol Laparosc 2003;10:99.

163. Spies JB, Cooper JM, Worthington-Kirsch R, et al: Outcome of uterine embolization and hysterectomy for leiomyomas: results of a multicenter study. Am J Obstet Gynecol 2004;191:22.

164. Razavi MK, Hwang G, Jahed A, et al: Abdominal myomectomy versus uterine fibroid embolization in the treatment of symptomatic uterine leiomyomas. AJR Am J Roentgenol 2003;180:1571.

165. Pinto I, Chimeno P, Romo A, et al: Uterine fibroids: uterine artery embolization versus abdominal hysterectomy for treatment—a prospective, randomized, and controlled clinical trial. Radiology 2003;226:425.

166. Vedantham S, Goodwin SC, McLucas B, et al: Uterine artery embolization: an underused method of controlling pelvic hemorrhage. Am J Obstet Gynecol 1997;176:938.

167. Kidney DD, Nguyen AM, Ahdoot D, et al: Prophylactic perioperative hypogastric artery balloon occlusion in abnormal placentation. AJR Am J Roentgenol 2001;176:1521.

168. Mitty HA, Sterling KM, Alvarez M, et al: Obstetric hemorrhage: prophylactic and emergency arterial catheterization and embolotherapy. Radiology 1993;188:183.

169. Pelage JP, Soyer P, Repiquet D, et al: Secondary postpartum hemorrhage: treatment with selective arterial embolization. Radiology 1999;212:385.

170. Pelage JP, Le Dref O, Mateo J, et al: Life-threatening primary postpartum hemorrhage: treatment with emergency selective arterial embolization. Radiology 1998;208:359.

171. Ornan D, White R, Pollak J, et al: Pelvic embolization for intractable postpartum hemorrhage: long-term follow-up and implications for fertility. Obstet Gynecol 2003;102:904.

172. Stancato-Pasik A, Mitty HA, Richard HM, et al: Obstetric embolotherapy: effect on menses and pregnancy. Radiology 1997;204:791.

173. Levine AB, Kuhlman K, Bonn J: Placenta accreta: comparison of cases managed with and without pelvic artery balloon catheters. J Matern Fetal Med 1999;8:173.

174. Dubois J, Garel L, Grignon A, et al: Placenta percreta: balloon occlusion and embolization of the internal iliac arteries to reduce intraoperative blood losses. Am J Obstet Gynecol 1997;176:723.

175. Pisco JM, Martins JM, Correia MG: Internal iliac artery: embolization to control hemorrhage from pelvic neoplasms. Radiology 1989; 172:337.

176. Yamashita Y, Harada M, Yamamoto H, et al: Transcatheter arterial embolization of obstetric and gynaecological bleeding: efficacy and clinical outcome. Br J Radiol 1994;67:530.

177. Salai M, Garniek A, Rubinstein Z, et al: Preoperative angiography and embolization of large pelvic tumors. J Surg Oncol 1999;70:41.

178. de Baere T, Ousehal A, Kuoch V, et al: Endovascular management of bleeding iliac artery pseudoaneurysms complicating radiation therapy for pelvic malignancies. AJR Am J Roentgenol 1998; 170:349.

179. Scultetus AH, Villavicencio JL, Gillespie DL: The nutcracker syndrome: its role in the pelvic venous disorders. J Vasc Surg 2001; 34:812.

180. Park SJ, Lim JW, Ko YT, et al: Diagnosis of pelvic congestion syndrome using transabdominal and transvaginal sonography. AJR Am J Roentgenol 2004;182:683.

181. Mathis BV, Miller JS, Lukens ML, et al: Pelvic congestion syndrome: a new approach to an unusual problem. Am Surg 1995;61:1016.

182. Nascimento AB, Mitchell DG, Holland G: Ovarian veins: magnetic resonance imaging findings in an asymptomatic population. J Magn Reson Imaging 2002;15:551.

183. Grabham JA, Barrie WW: Laparoscopic approach to pelvic congestion syndrome. Br J Surg 1997;84:1264.

184. Venbrux AC, Chang AH, Kim HS, et al: Pelvic congestion syndrome (pelvic venous incompetence): impact of ovarian and internal iliac vein embolotherapy on menstrual cycle and chronic pelvic pain. J Vasc Interv Radiol 2002;13(2 Pt 1):171.

185. Sichlau MJ, Yao JST, Vogelzang RL: Transcatheter embolotherapy for the treatment of pelvic congestion syndrome. Obstet Gynecol 1994;83:892.

186. Capasso P, Simons C, Trotteur G, et al: Treatment of symptomatic pelvic varices by ovarian vein embolization. Cardiovasc Intervent Radiol 1997;20:107.

187. Maleux G, Stockx L, Wilms G, et al: Ovarian vein embolization for the treatment of pelvic congestion syndrome: long-term technical and clinical results. J Vasc Interv Radiol 2000;11:859.

188. Calligaro KD, Sedlacek TV, Savarese RP, et al: Congenital pelvic arteriovenous malformations: long term follow-up in two cases and a review of the literature. J Vasc Surg 1992;16:100.

189. Vogelzang RL, Nemcek AA Jr, Skrtic Z, et al: Uterine arteriovenous malformations: primary treatment with therapeutic embolization. J Vasc Interv Radiol 1991;2:517.

190. Lim AK, Agarwal R, Seckl MJ, et al: Embolization of bleeding residual uterine vascular malformations in patients with treated gestational trophoblastic tumors. Radiology 2002;222:640.

191. Ghai S, Rajan DK, Asch MR, et al: Efficacy of embolization in traumatic uterine vascular malformations. J Vasc Interv Radiol 2003; 14:1401.

12

Pulmonary and Bronchial Arteries

◼ ARTERIOGRAPHY

Pulmonary Arteriography

The primary indication for pulmonary arteriography is the diagnosis of acute pulmonary embolism when noninvasive studies such as CT angiography are equivocal. Catheter angiography also is used to evaluate patients with suspected chronic pulmonary thromboembolic disease, pulmonary artery hypertension, vasculitis, arteriovenous malformations, and hemoptysis. Before angiography, the interventionalist should evaluate several items:

- Duplex sonograms of the lower extremity veins (if available) to exclude thrombosis at the planned access site
- A recent electrocardiogram to exclude a left bundle branch block. Right heart catheterization can induce complete heart block in such a case, and a temporary pacemaker may be required before angiography.
- The need for an inferior vena cava (IVC) filter if the angiogram shows acute emboli

Pulmonary arteriography is performed from the femoral, internal jugular, or brachial vein; catheterization is somewhat more difficult from the latter approach.[1] The pulmonary artery may be catheterized in several ways:

- *Omniflush catheter.* The 5-French catheter is advanced into the right atrium. When a stiff hydrophilic guidewire is inserted, it opens the curve and the wire tip can be directed into the right ventricular outflow tract (Fig. 12-1).[2]
- *Grollman catheter.* The preshaped 7-French Grollman catheter is designed for easy manipulation into the right ventricle and then into the pulmonary artery (Fig. 12-2). When the right atrium is enlarged, a tip-deflecting wire may be needed to advance the catheter fully into the right ventricle.
- *Pigtail and deflecting wire technique.* A 6- or 7-French pigtail catheter is advanced with a tip-deflecting wire (Fig. 12-3).
- *Balloon flotation catheter.* A flow-directed balloon catheter (with multiple distal side holes) is inserted through a femoral or internal jugular vein sheath and directed from the right atrium into the pulmonary artery with the balloon inflated.

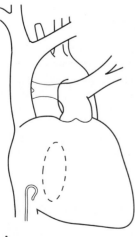 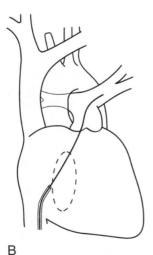

A   B   C

FIGURE 12-1 ◼ Pulmonary arteriography using an Ominflush catheter. **A,** The catheter is positioned in the middle of the right atrium. **B,** When a stiff hydrophilic wire is inserted, the catheter curve opens and points the guidewire toward the right ventricular outflow tract. **C,** The catheter is then advanced into the pulmonary artery. (Adapted from Velling TE, Brennan FJ, Hall LD: Pulmonary angiography with use of the 5 French omniflush catheter: a safe and efficient procedure with a common catheter. J Vasc Interv Radiol 2000;11:1005.)

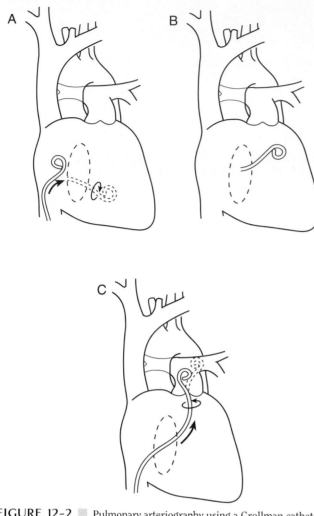

FIGURE 12-2 ■ Pulmonary arteriography using a Grollman catheter. **A,** The catheter is directed through the tricuspid valve into the right ventricle. **B,** The catheter is then turned 180 degrees so that the pigtail points up toward the right ventricular outflow tract. **C,** The catheter is then advanced into the main pulmonary artery and directed to the right or left. (Adapted from Kadir S: Diagnostic Angiography. Philadelphia, WB Saunders, 1986:591.)

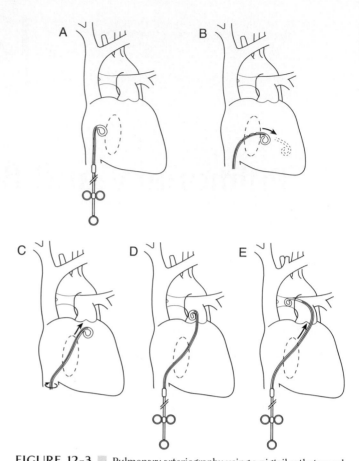

FIGURE 12-3 ■ Pulmonary arteriography using a pigtail catheter and deflecting wire. **A,** The pigtail is advanced to the right atrium. **B,** While a bend is placed on the tip-deflecting wire, the catheter is fed off into the right ventricle. **C,** The deflection is released, straightening the catheter. **D,** The catheter is then rotated and advanced through the right ventricular outflow tract into the main pulmonary artery. **E,** The catheter can be directed into the right or left pulmonary artery by rotating the pigtail toward the desired side and feeding it off the deflected wire. (Adapted from Kadir S: Diagnostic Angiography. Philadelphia, WB Saunders, 1986:590.)

Extreme care should be taken while traversing the right heart chambers. Cardiac dysrhythmias may occur during manipulation of the catheter or guidewire. Short bursts of ventricular tachycardia almost always stop by repositioning the catheter or guidewire. For sustained or recurrent ventricular tachycardia, *amiodarone* (150 mg IV over 10 minutes) or *lidocaine* (1 mg/kg IV bolus, followed by 1 to 4 mg/minute infusion) may be required. Cardiac perforation can be avoided by gentle catheter manipulation.

When catheterization is difficult, a J-tipped guidewire or tip-deflecting wire may be used to direct the catheter into the right ventricular outflow tract. Inability to advance the catheter from the right atrium to the right ventricle may result from inadvertent entry into the *coronary sinus* (Fig. 12-4). After the catheter has engaged the main pulmonary artery, it is directed to the right or left lung using a standard guidewire or stiff hydrophilic guidewire. The side holes of the catheter should rest in the distal main left or right pulmonary artery.

Selective catheterization of lobar or segmental branches usually is performed by exchanging the pigtail catheter for a preshaped headhunter or hockey stick–shaped catheter over a stiff exchange guidewire.

In patients with suspected thromboembolic disease or pulmonary artery hypertension, pulmonary artery pressures are obtained before contrast injection. Normal right heart pressures are given in Table 12-1.[3] The pulmonary artery pressure may be elevated for a variety of reasons (Box 12-1). Contrary to previous teaching, recent studies show no increased risk from pulmonary angiography in patients with elevated right heart pressures.[4,5] However, it is still wise to minimize the number and volume of contrast injections in such patients. Isosmolar contrast material (which produces less reflex elevation in pulmonary artery pressures than other agents) should always be used.

Interventionalists have different preferences for the initial projections for pulmonary arteriography. In general, lower lobe vessels are displayed best in the ipsilateral **posterior** oblique projection.

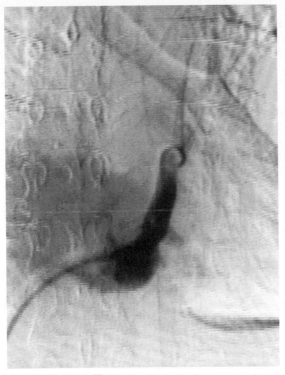

FIGURE 12-4 ■ Pigtail catheter in the coronary sinus.

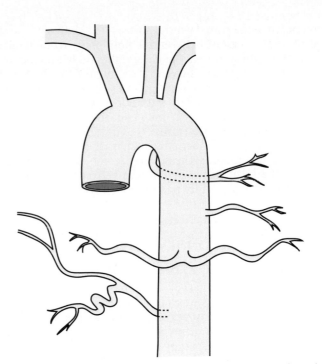

FIGURE 12-5 ■ Common origins of the bronchial arteries from the thoracic aorta.

TABLE 12-1 NORMAL RIGHT HEART PRESSURES

Anatomic Site	Systolic (mm Hg)	Diastolic (mm Hg)	Mean (mm Hg)
Right atrium			0–8
Right ventricle	15–30	0–8	
Pulmonary artery	15–30	3–12	9–16

When pulmonary arteriography is performed in patients with suspected pulmonary embolism, the risks of minor complications, major complications, and death are about 5%, 1%, and 0.2% to 0.5%, respectively.[4] Complications include contrast reaction, transient renal dysfunction, access site hematoma, dysrhythmias, and respiratory distress.

BOX 12-1 ■ Causes of Pulmonary Artery Hypertension

Acute or chronic thromboembolic disease
Obstructive or restrictive parenchymal lung disease
Chronic hypoventilation
Elevated left atrial or pulmonary venous pressure
Left-to-right shunt
Primary pulmonary hypertension
Pulmonary veno-occlusive disease
Pulmonary capillary hemangiomatosis
Vasculitis

Cardiac perforation is rare when appropriate catheters are used.

Bronchial Arteriography

Selective catheterization of the bronchial arteries can be performed with forward-seeking catheters (e.g., spinal catheter) or reverse-curve catheters (e.g., Simmons or Shetty). In either case, the catheter tip must abut the aortic wall to engage the bronchial arteries. Forward-seeking catheters are easier to maneuver but may be more difficult to seat within the vessel. Reverse-curve catheters can be more difficult to maneuver, particularly near the aortic arch, but they engage the artery more securely. The bronchial arteries are found by scraping the catheter tip along the aortic wall in the anticipated location of the vessels (level of the 4th to 6th thoracic vertebrae), which corresponds to the position of the left main stem bronchus (Fig. 12-5).

High-quality images are important to identify small bronchial artery branches that may supply the anterior spinal artery. Nonionic contrast material should be used in all cases.

■ ANATOMY

Development

Early in fetal development, the lung buds are supplied by a network of vessels arising from the aortic sac, which itself is composed of the paired ventral aortae.[6] The sixth aortic arch becomes the conduit between the pulmonary trunk (which arises from the aortic sac) and the right and left pulmonary arteries (see Fig. 4-1). The ventral segment of the **right** sixth aortic arch becomes the right pulmonary artery origin. The ventral segment of the **left** sixth aortic arch develops into part of the pulmonary trunk, and the dorsal segment becomes the ductus arteriosus.

Immediately after birth, the ductus arteriosus constricts. Within several months, the ductus is completely obstructed, leaving the ligamentum arteriosum between the origin of the left pulmonary artery and the aortic arch.

Normal Pulmonary Vascular Anatomy and Physiology

The pulmonary artery arises from the base of the right ventricle.[7] The vessel courses superiorly to the left of the ascending aorta. The artery divides below the aortic arch into right and left pulmonary arteries (Fig. 12-6). The bifurcation is located inferior, anterior, and to the left of the tracheal bifurcation.

The *right pulmonary artery* courses horizontally behind the ascending aorta and superior vena cava (SVC) and in front of the tracheal bifurcation and esophagus to reach the hilum of the right lung (Fig. 12-7). It divides behind the SVC into an ascending branch *(truncus anterior)* supplying the right upper lobe and the descending right pulmonary artery supplying the middle and lower lobes. The ascending trunk usually has three branches to the segments of the right upper lobe: apical, posterior, and anterior. Occasionally, two segmental branches arise in a common trunk. The descending right pulmonary artery courses behind the bronchus intermedius. This artery commonly

gives off an accessory branch to some portion of the right upper lobe. The descending pulmonary artery then provides an anterior branch supplying the right middle lobe and a posterior branch supplying the superior segment of the right lower lobe. The descending pulmonary artery continues inferiorly and gives off branches to the segments of the right lower lobe. Although the branching pattern is somewhat variable, the terminal position of the segmental branches (i.e., anterior, lateral, posterior, and medial) is relatively constant on a frontal pulmonary arteriogram going from lateral to medial.

The *left pulmonary artery* courses upward and posteriorly in front of the aorta and the left main stem bronchus (Fig. 12-8). The ascending branch of the left pulmonary artery divides into apical posterior and anterior segmental arteries. The first one or two branches of the descending left pulmonary artery are the superior and inferior segmental arteries, which supply the lingula. The left pulmonary artery then divides into several vessels supplying the segments of the left lower lobe. The relative location of the terminal portions of the left lower lobe vessels is the mirror image of the pattern just described for the right lung.

Because the venous drainage of the lungs is located within the interlobular septa, the pulmonary veins do not run with the pulmonary arteries and bronchi.[8] The right and left lungs are drained by superior and inferior pulmonary veins (Fig. 12-9). On each side, the vessels usually enter the left atrium separately, anterior and inferior to the pulmonary arteries. In some cases, they form a confluence before draining into the left atrium. The superior pulmonary veins drain the upper and middle (or lingular) lobes of each lung. The inferior pulmonary veins drain the lower lobes.

The pulmonary circulation is a high-flow, low-pressure system with a total resistance that is about one eighth that of the systemic circulation.[9] While standing, blood flows preferentially to the lower lobes. When supine, blood flow is more evenly distributed between the lung bases and apices. Because the system is so distensible and has a large number of reserve vessels, sudden obstruction of one half of the pulmonary circulation in a patient without preexisting cardiopulmonary disease only slightly elevates pulmonary artery pressure. However, in patients with preexisting cardiac or pulmonary disease, which may be associated with elevated right heart pressures and right ventricular dysfunction, acute obstruction of even a small portion of the pulmonary circulation may cause a significant rise in pulmonary artery pressure.

Normal Bronchial Artery Anatomy

The bronchial arteries supply the trachea, bronchi, esophagus, and posterior mediastinum, and they also act as the vasa vasorum of the pulmonary arteries. The bronchial arteries usually are not visible at thoracic aortography in patients without lung disease. However, they become markedly enlarged and serve as an important collateral pathway in patients with certain congenital heart diseases, chronic lung infections, lung tumors, and obstruction of pulmonary arteries or veins.[10]

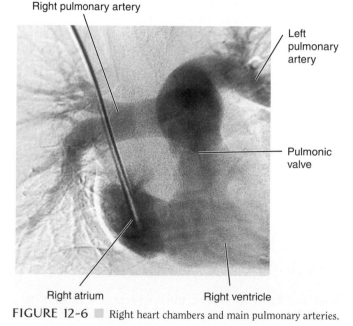

Right pulmonary artery

Left pulmonary artery

Pulmonic valve

Right atrium

Right ventricle

FIGURE 12-6 ■ Right heart chambers and main pulmonary arteries.

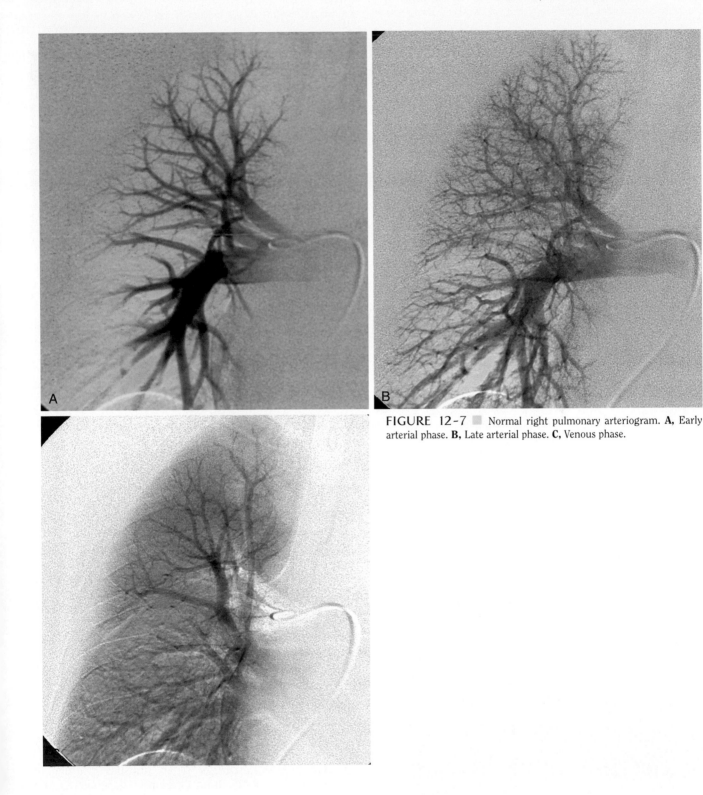

FIGURE 12-7 ■ Normal right pulmonary arteriogram. **A,** Early arterial phase. **B,** Late arterial phase. **C,** Venous phase.

Bronchial artery anatomy is extremely variable.[11-13] Anatomic and angiographic studies differ in the reported pattern and distribution of bronchial artery origins. As a rule, one or two bronchial arteries supply each lung; however, up to four bronchial arteries may supply one lung. Several patterns are commonly observed (Fig. 12-10; see also Fig. 12-5):

■ Right intercostal-bronchial trunk from the posterolateral surface of the aorta

■ Left bronchial artery from the anterolateral surface of the aorta

■ Common right and left bronchial artery trunk from the anterior surface of the aorta

Rarely, a right intercostal-bronchial artery trunk gives rise to a left bronchial artery. Unusual bronchial artery origins include a left bronchial artery takeoff from the right posterior aortic wall and a bronchial artery originating from

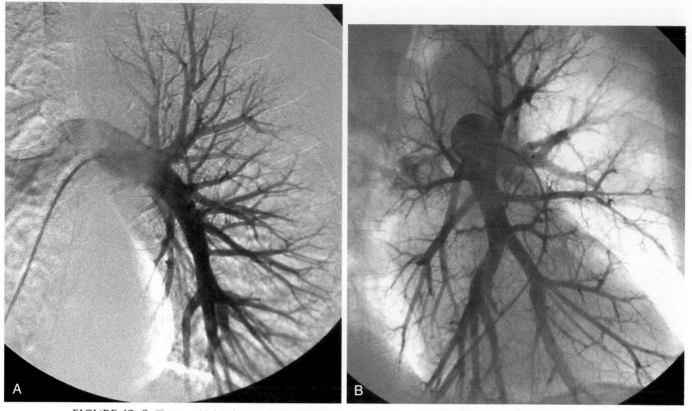

FIGURE 12-8 ■ Normal left pulmonary arteriogram. **A,** Frontal projection. **B,** Left posterior oblique projection lays out lower lobe branches.

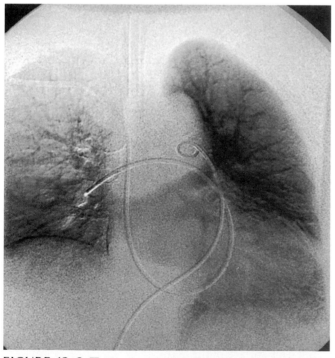

FIGURE 12-9 ■ The late-phase pulmonary arteriogram shows pulmonary veins entering the left atrium.

the under- or upper surface of the aortic arch or near the left subclavian artery ostium.

Bronchial arteries may have branches to the anterior spinal artery, which supplies the spinal cord. In a few patients, a right bronchointercostal artery (and rarely a right or left bronchial artery) feeds the great anterior radicular artery *(artery of Adamkiewicz)* or a smaller radiculomedullary branch[14] (Fig. 12-11). Very rarely, transverse myelitis with paraplegia may be caused by bronchial arteriography or embolization if this anatomy is present.

Variant Anatomy

A variety of congenital anomalies may affect the pulmonary vasculature (Box 12-2).[15,16]

Pulmonary sequestration is an unusual disorder in which a portion of the lung develops independently and derives its blood supply from a systemic artery.[17] In *intralobar sequestration,* the abnormal tissue lies within the visceral pleura of the adjacent lung. The sequestered segment usually is found in the posterior portion of the lower lobe, more commonly on the left side. The systemic blood supply to the sequestration comes from the descending thoracic or abdominal aorta (Fig. 12-12). The venous drainage usually is through the pulmonary veins; IVC and azygous drainage also have been described. In *extralobar sequestration,* the abnormal segment is contained within its own pleural membrane.

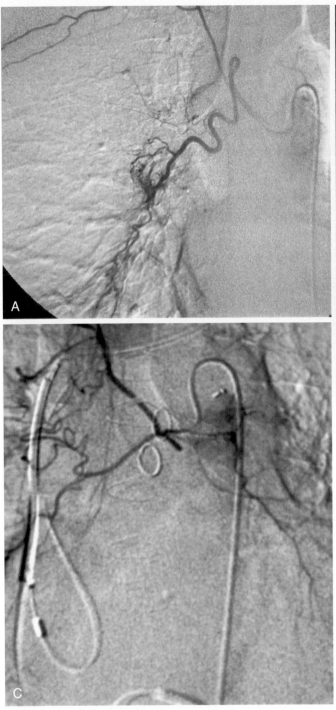

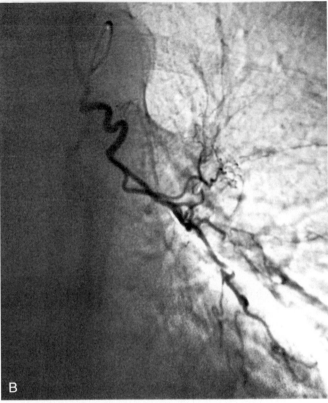

FIGURE 12-10 ■ Bronchial artery patterns. **A,** Right bronchointercostal trunk. **B,** Left bronchial artery. **C,** Common right and left bronchial trunk arising from the anterior surface of the thoracic aorta.

The anomaly occurs when splanchnic branches of the aorta that supply the developing lung buds fail to involute. The sequestered segment develops in the left chest in 90% of cases. The systemic arterial supply is from the descending thoracic or abdominal aorta. The sequestration drains into the IVC, azygous veins, or portal venous system. Embolization of the sequestered lung has been performed successfully in neonates.[18]

Hypogenetic lung (scimitar) syndrome occurs with hypoplasia of the right lung and drainage of blood from all or part of the lung into the IVC (or rarely other systemic veins) at the level of the diaphragm.[19] The abnormal lung tissue is fed by branches of the lower thoracic or abdominal aorta. The large draining vein from the mid–right lung to the right cardiophrenic angle produces a C-shaped density on chest radiographs that has been likened to a Turkish sword (scimitar).

Collateral Circulation

The pulmonary artery collateral circulation becomes active with obstruction of a portion of the pulmonary arteries, as a

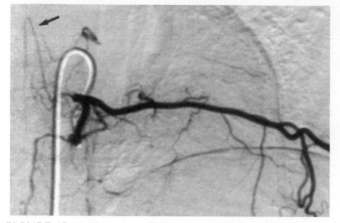

FIGURE 12-11 ■ Spinal artery branch *(arrow)* arising from a left posterior intercostal artery.

reaction to inflammatory or neoplastic processes in the lung, and in response to regional hypoxia. This situation may occur with acute or chronic emboli, right ventricular outflow or pulmonary artery obstruction (often associated with congenital heart diseases), lung tumors, infections, and vasculitis.[10]

The major collateral pathways to the pulmonary arteries are the bronchial arteries, small descending thoracic aortic branches (e.g., intercostal arteries), and vessels from major aortic branches (Fig. 12-13).[20] These pathways may fill the pulmonary artery centrally or peripherally.

BOX 12-2 ■ **Congenital Anomalies of the Pulmonary Vessels**

Main Pulmonary Artery
Pulmonary valve stenosis
Pulmonary artery stenosis
Idiopathic pulmonary artery dilation
Pulmonary artery aneurysm
Unilateral absence of pulmonary artery
Persistent truncus arteriosus
Pulmonary atresia
Aorticopulmonary window
Absent pulmonic valve

Proximal Pulmonary Arteries
Patent ductus arteriosus
Pulmonary artery stenosis
Pulmonary artery aneurysm
Anomalous origin of coronary artery from pulmonary artery
Absence of right or left pulmonary artery
Crossed pulmonary artery

Distal Pulmonary Arteries
Peripheral pulmonary artery stenosis

Pulmonary Arteries and Veins
Arteriovenous malformation
Pulmonary sequestration
Hypogenetic lung syndrome
Anomalous pulmonary venous drainage

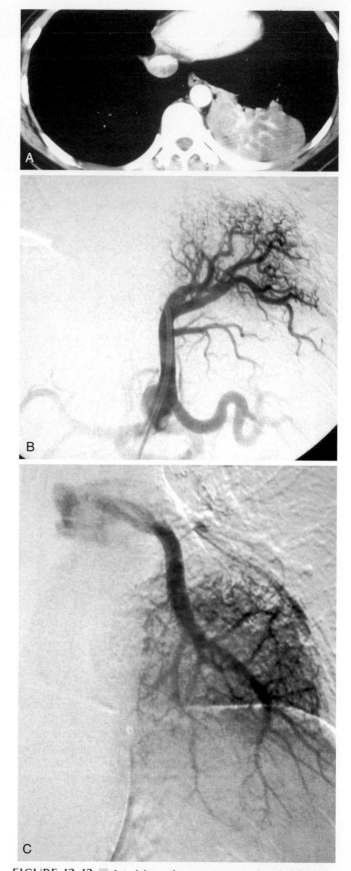

FIGURE 12-12 ■ Intralobar pulmonary sequestration. **A,** A hypervascular multicystic mass in the left lower lobe is identified by CT. **B,** Celiac arteriogram shows a massively enlarged left inferior phrenic artery crossing the hemidiaphragm to supply the sequestration. **C,** The late-phase arteriogram shows venous drainage into the pulmonary veins.

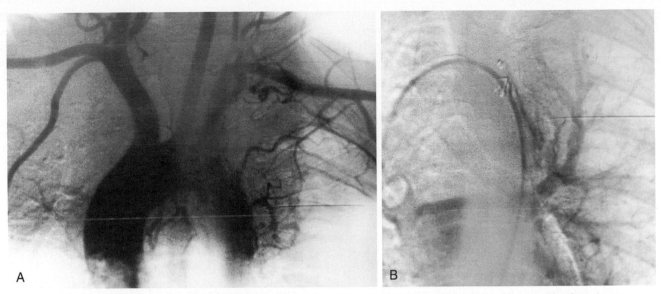

FIGURE 12-13 ■ Complete left pulmonary artery obstruction with bronchial collateral circulation. **A,** The thoracic aortogram shows enlarged collateral vessels around the upper descending thoracic aorta. **B,** The late-phase arteriogram shows collateral filling of the left pulmonary artery and its branches.

■ MAJOR DISORDERS

Acute Pulmonary Embolism

Etiology and Natural History

Pulmonary embolism is a common disorder and one of the leading causes of in-hospital mortality.[21] Pulmonary embolism is part of the spectrum of venous thromboembolic disease. It is estimated that 80% to 90% of pulmonary emboli arise from the deep veins of the legs.[22] The remainder come from pelvic veins, the IVC and its tributaries, and upper extremity veins. The last is recognized as an increasingly common source of pulmonary embolism, often because of thrombosis associated with vascular access devices. Lower extremity venous clots usually originate in the soleal sinuses of the deep veins of the calf. In patients with one or more risk factor for thrombosis (Box 12-3), clot may propagate into

---

BOX 12-3 ■ **Risk Factors for Venous Thrombosis and Pulmonary Embolism**

Immobilization or bed rest
Recent surgery
Major trauma
Prior history of venous thromboembolic disease
Cancer
Advanced age
Obesity
Use of oral contraceptives or estrogen therapy
Pregnancy
Primary hypercoagulable states
Cerebrovascular accident
Congestive heart failure

---

the calf, popliteal, and femoral veins (see Chapter 13). The risk of pulmonary embolism with untreated "proximal" (femoropopliteal) deep vein thrombosis approaches 50%.[23] When embolization occurs, the clot usually shatters while in transit and produces multiple, bilateral occlusions of pulmonary artery branches.

Clots directly obstruct pulmonary blood flow and also cause the release of a variety of humoral vasospastic activators that intensify the obstruction. The clinical effect of pulmonary embolism depends on the extent of preexisting cardiopulmonary disease.[24] In patients with normal heart and lungs, small emboli produce little effect. However, when the clot burden overwhelms the pulmonary circulation reserve, right ventricular and pulmonary artery pressures rise sharply. This situation may lead to right ventricular dilation, ventricular failure, and, ultimately, cardiogenic shock. The overall mortality of patients who present with hemodynamic compromise is 20% to 30%.[25] Although this picture usually is associated with massive pulmonary embolism, even small emboli can start such a chain of events in patients with underlying heart or lung disease. In some patients, inadequate bronchial artery collateral circulation to the obstructed region results in pulmonary infarction.

The natural history of pulmonary emboli in patients who survive is usually endogenous lysis of clot over a period of weeks.[26] About one half of patients have complete resolution of clot; the remainder have partial resolution or chronic obstruction.[27]

Other nonthrombotic causes of pulmonary embolism include medical devices (e.g., catheter fragments), septic foci, fat, air, amniotic fluid, and intravascular tumor deposits.[28-30]

Clinical Features

Pulmonary embolism is a grossly underdiagnosed problem. Physicians must remain alert to the possibility in any patient with cardiopulmonary symptoms and risk factors for venous thromboembolic disease. The most common symptoms are chest pain, shortness of breath, cough, tachypnea, and tachycardia. With massive pulmonary embolism, patients may present with syncope, dysrhythmias, or cardiogenic shock. The clinical picture often mimics acute myocardial infarction, pneumonia, exacerbation of chronic obstructive lung disease, or congestive heart failure.

Diagnosis

Because pulmonary embolism is a common disease and symptoms are nonspecific, screening of patients before requesting imaging studies is useful. Many experts rely on **both** clinical probability and laboratory/imaging tests to evaluate patients with suspected pulmonary embolism.

D-dimer Test. D-dimer is a breakdown product of cross-linked fibrin. Serum levels are elevated in the setting of vascular thrombosis among many other conditions (advanced age, trauma, pregnancy, operation, inflammation, neoplasms).[25] The D-dimer test has become a popular screening tool in patients with suspected pulmonary embolism. The variability in reported accuracy is largely a function of differences in assay methods and thresholds for diagnosis.[21] Using higher thresholds (e.g., >500 μg/L), the negative predictive value of the test approaches 100%.

Imaging[31,32]

Chest Radiography. Chest radiographs are useful for excluding other diseases (e.g., pneumonia or congestive heart failure) and are critical for interpretation of radionuclide lung scans. However, plain radiographs are almost useless for the specific diagnosis of pulmonary embolism. Many patients have nonspecific abnormalities, such as vague parenchymal densities, areas of atelectasis, or pleural effusions.[33] Findings that are more suggestive of pulmonary embolism are rounded or wedge-shaped pleural-based opacities reflecting pulmonary infarction *(Hampton's hump),* local oligemia *(Westermark's sign),* and central pulmonary artery enlargement (Fig. 12-14). However, these radiographic signs are uncommon and are not entirely specific for pulmonary embolism.

Computed Tomographic Angiography. In most centers, CT angiography is now the principal imaging modality for the diagnosis of acute pulmonary embolism. The reported sensitivity and specificity for detection of central emboli with helical single detector row scanners is 86% to 100% and 92% to 100%, respectively.[34-36] Even though the accuracy of multidetector row CT angiography compared with catheter angiography (the gold standard for many decades) has not been thoroughly proven, it is considered at least as and perhaps more sensitive and specific for the diagnosis. Accurate evaluation even to the level of the subsegmental pulmonary arteries may be achieved[37-39] (Fig. 12-15). In addition, CT provides thorough evaluation of the lungs and mediastinum to allow diagnosis of many other entities that can mimic pulmonary embolism.

The clinical significance of isolated subsegmental or distal clots (which account for only 6% to 30% of diagnosed cases) is controversial.[25,40-42] This is fortunate because accurate detection is more problematic. The negative predictive value of CT angiography reportedly approaches 99%.[31,43-46]

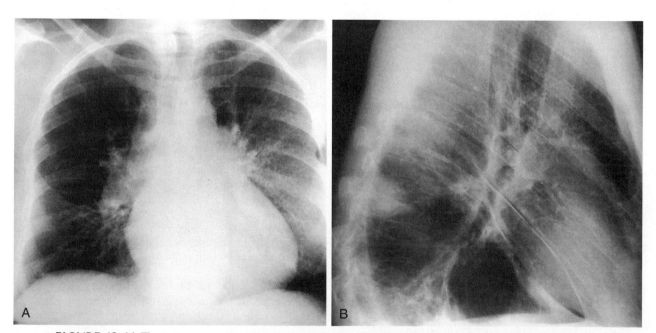

FIGURE 12-14 ■ Classic chest radiographic findings for pulmonary embolism. **A,** Diminished vascularity in the right lung (i.e., Westermark's sign) and enlargement of the right pulmonary artery suggest pulmonary embolism. **B,** The wedge-shaped, pleural-based density with the apex toward the hilum (i.e., Hampton's hump) suggests pulmonary embolism with infarction.

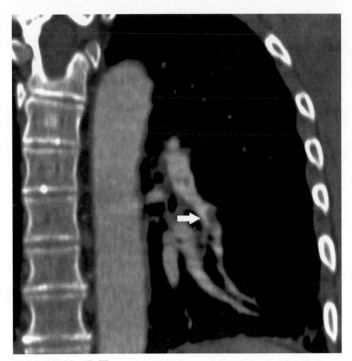

FIGURE 12-15   Multiplanar reformatted CT angiography displays a segmental pulmonary embolus *(arrow)*.

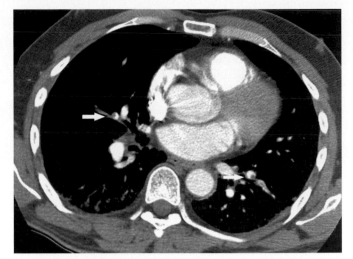

FIGURE 12-17   Several subsegmental pulmonary emboli *(arrows)* are identified on chest CT angiography.

Specific protocols are used for CT pulmonary angiography. In some centers, chest imaging is followed by CT venography of the lower extremities.[47,48] Lung, mediastinal, and embolism-specific displays must be evaluated.[49] Multiplanar reformatted constructions are useful in confirming the diagnosis of clot or the presence of artifacts (see Fig. 12-15). Pulmonary arteries are followed from their origins through the subsegmental branches. Pulmonary artery branches follow their respective bronchi; in the basal segments, medially running pulmonary veins should not be confused with arterial branches.

Acute emboli appear as complete, partial, or peripheral filling defects sometimes surrounded by contrast (Figs. 12-16 and 12-17). The affected vessels are often enlarged. These findings must be distinguished from chronic thromboembolic disease (see below). A peripheral wedge-shaped density may represent an infarct (Fig. 12-18). Signs of right ventricular failure (right ventricular dilation or deviation of the intraventricular septum) should be sought. Potential pitfalls in diagnosis are outlined in Table 12-2.[49]

Radionuclide Lung Scanning. Ventilation-perfusion (V/Q) lung scanning once was widely used for evaluating patients

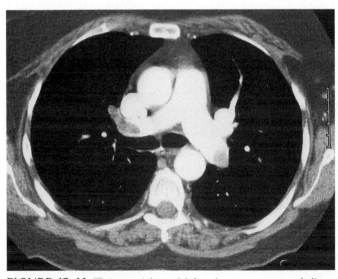

FIGURE 12-16   Acute right and left pulmonary artery emboli are identified by CT angiography.

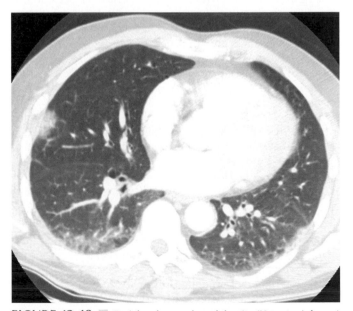

FIGURE 12-18   Peripheral parenchymal density (Hampton's hump) distal to segmental pulmonary emboli identified on embolus windows.

TABLE 12-2   MISDIAGNOSIS OF PULMONARY EMBOLISM ON COMPUTED TOMOGRAPHIC ANGIOGRAPHY

Cause	Evidence or Response
Simulate Bland Acute Pulmonary Embolism	
Respiratory motion artifact	"Seagull sign" from vessel motion
Image noise	Increase detector width in obese patients
Pulmonary artery catheter	Evaluate bone windows
Flow-related artifacts	>78 HU
Lung algorithm artifact	Inspect standard algorithms
Partial volume effect	Evaluate vessels in contiguous images
Partial voluming with lymph nodes	Sagittal and coronal reformatted images
Luceny in peripheral pulmonary veins	Connection with central pulmonary veins
Mucous plug in airway	Note adjacent normal pulmonary artery
Perivascular edema	Other signs of heart failure
Slow flow (e.g., atelectasis)	
Primary pulmonary sarcoma	Lobulated, enhancing, extravascular spread
Tumor emboli (RCC, HCC)	
Chronic pulmonary embolism	(See text)
Mask Pulmonary Embolism	
Window settings	Window width/level: 700 HU/100 HU
Streak artifact (especially near SVC)	Nonanatomic morphology

HCC, hepatocellular carcinoma; HU, Hounsfield units; RCC, renal cell carcinoma; SVC, superior vena cava.

BOX 12-4   ▪   PIOPED Criteria for Ventilation-Perfusion Lung Scanning

High Probability
Two or more large segmental perfusion defects with absent or substantially smaller (mismatched) ventilation or radiographic defects
Two or more moderate segmental mismatched perfusion defects *and* one large mismatched segmental defect
Four or more moderate mismatched segmental defects

Low Probability
Perfusion defects without segmental shape
One moderate segmental mismatched perfusion defect
Perfusion defect with substantially larger chest radiograph defect
Four or fewer large or moderate matched perfusion defects in one lung
Four or more small segmental perfusion defects with normal chest radiograph

Very Low Probability
Three or fewer small perfusion defects with normal chest radiograph

Intermediate Probability
Perfusion defect pattern not belonging in high or low probability category

Normal
No perfusion defects

PIOPED, Prospective Investigation of Pulmonary Embolism Diagnosis.

with suspected pulmonary embolus. Because it is less specific than CT angiography and a definitive diagnosis cannot be made in most patients with pulmonary embolism, it has assumed a lesser role in most centers.

Lung perfusion scans are performed by intravenous injection of technetium 99m (^{99m}Tc)-labeled, macroaggregated albumin particles.[50] Pulmonary emboli produce localized perfusion defects (Fig. 12-19). Perfusion defects also may be seen in areas of lung consolidation, lung collapse, vasoconstriction due to hypoxia (e.g., chronic obstructive pulmonary disease), and for other reasons. Ventilation scanning is performed to exclude such entities. One of several agents, including ^{133}Xe gas and ^{99m}Tc-diethylenetriamine-penta-acetic acid (^{99m}Tc-DTPA) aerosol, are used for this purpose.

Several classification schemes have been proposed for interpreting V/Q scans. One of the most widely accepted is the system established in the Prospective Investigation of Pulmonary Embolism Diagnosis trial (PIOPED-I), which evaluated the diagnostic usefulness of V/Q scanning for acute pulmonary embolism[51] (Box 12-4). Several important conclusions can be drawn from the results of the PIOPED study (Table 12-3):

▪ Interpretation of V/Q scans should not be done in a vacuum. The diagnostic utility is improved by correlation with the clinical likelihood of disease.
▪ The likelihood of pulmonary embolus in patients with normal scans (4%) and in patients with low-probability scans plus a low clinical index of suspicion (4%) effectively excludes the diagnosis.

▪ The likelihood of pulmonary embolus in patients with high-probability scans (87%) supports definitive treatment if there is no risk factor for anticoagulation.
▪ Other combinations of clinical suspicion and radionuclide scanning results (which constitute about 75% of cases) are not useful in making or excluding the diagnosis, and these patients should undergo further evaluation.

Lower Extremity Duplex Sonography. Because most pulmonary emboli arise from the legs and because treatment of pulmonary embolism is aimed at prevention of recurrent embolism, some practitioners initially perform leg duplex sonography to detect potential sources of recurrent emboli.[52] However, up to half of patients with **proven** pulmonary embolism have no sonographic evidence of proximal clot at the time of examination.[25] Deep vein thrombosis

TABLE 12-3   RESULTS OF LUNG SCANNING IN PIOPED STUDY

Lung Scan Category	Scans (%)	Positive Arteriogram (%)
Normal/near normal	14	4
Low probability	34	14
Intermediate probability	39	30
High probability	13	87

PIOPED, Prospective Investigation of Pulmonary Embolism Diagnosis.

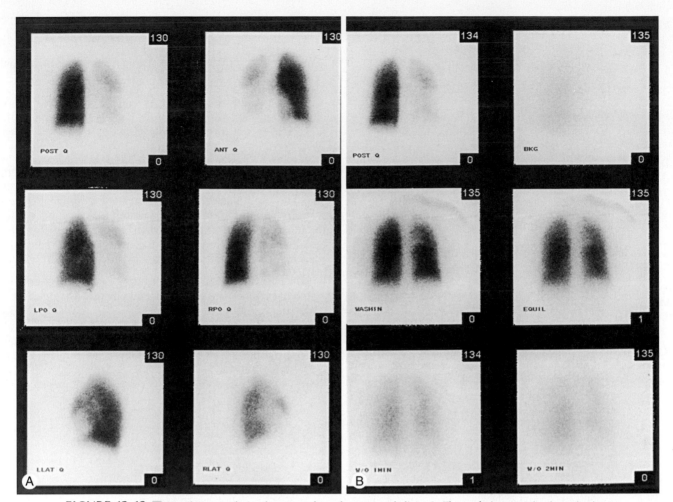

FIGURE 12-19 ▪ Ventilation-perfusion lung scan for pulmonary embolism. **A,** The perfusion scan in six projections shows large segmental defects in the right lower lobe. **B,** The ventilation scan in the posterior projection shows that defects are mismatched.

of the leg is detected in patients with **suspected** pulmonary embolism less than 25% of the time.[53-55] Sonography may be most useful in patients with equivocal or low probability V/Q scans when clinical signs of deep venous thrombosis or risks factors for venous thromboembolic disease are present.

Magnetic Resonance Imaging. Promising results have been obtained with the use of MR angiography for pulmonary embolism diagnosis. The reported sensitivity and specificity of gadolinium-enhanced MR angiography is 77% to 100% and 95% to 98%, respectively.[56-58] However, thrombi in segmental or subsegmental vessels are more difficult to assess with current MR techniques. Multidetector row CT appears to be more accurate than MR imaging because of its better spatial resolution and fewer artifacts.[31]

Catheter Angiography. For decades, pulmonary arteriography was considered the final arbiter in pulmonary embolism diagnosis, but this is no longer true. Multidetector row CT angiography is probably as accurate; in fact, even experienced angiographers misdiagnose isolated subsegmental emboli in up to one third of cases.[41,42] Because it is invasive, expensive, and requires experienced operators,

pulmonary arteriography is now relegated to a secondary role in diagnosis of equivocal cases or when treatment of massive embolism is contemplated.

The only reliable angiographic sign of acute pulmonary embolism is an intraluminal filling defect at least partially surrounded by contrast material (Fig. 12-20). Secondary signs of an acute embolus include abrupt vessel cutoff, regional hypoperfusion, slow flow, pruning of vessels, and filling of collateral vessels. Emboli are often multiple and bilateral. They tend to lodge in the lower lobes more often than in the upper lobes.[59] The accuracy of pulmonary arteriography can be optimized by adhering to the following principles:

▪ Because some pulmonary emboli lyse rapidly, angiography should be performed without delay.[60]
▪ Exclusion of pulmonary embolism requires evaluation of both lungs with enough projections to resolve all pulmonary artery branches.
▪ Because up to one third of patients with pulmonary embolism have only subsegmental clots, careful evaluation of small vessels (particularly in the lower lobes) is critical.
▪ Emboli often are missed because of overlapping vessels, small size, or suboptimal imaging from respiratory or

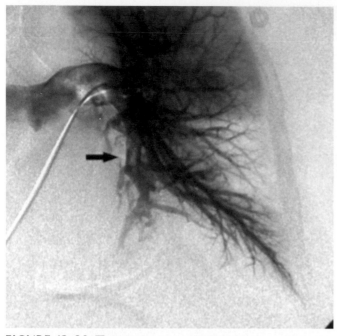

FIGURE 12-20 ■ Embolus *(arrow)* identified in the posterior segmental branch of the left lower lobe on catheter pulmonary arteriography. Note diminished overall vascularity to this region.

patient motion. Selective oblique magnification views may be necessary to adequately exclude clots (Fig. 12-21).

■ Emboli often are misdiagnosed because of overlapping vessels, cystic air spaces, or poorly opacified vessels.

Several other disorders can cause pulmonary artery obstruction, and some may be identified at angiography (e.g., chronic thromboembolic disease, tumor, arteritis) (Box 12-5).

Diagnostic Algorithm. The optimal approach to studying patients with suspected pulmonary embolism is controversial. The old algorithm (i.e., chest radiography, V/Q lung scanning, and pulmonary arteriography) is no longer valid. In most centers, patients with suspected pulmonary embolism are referred for CT angiography. The radiologist then may face the following scenarios:

■ Low clinical probability. A negative D-dimer test effectively excludes the diagnosis and obviates the need for further imaging.
■ Equivocal or uninterpretable CT angiography
  ■ If there is evidence for lower extremity deep venous thrombosis (see Chapter 13), consider duplex sonography.

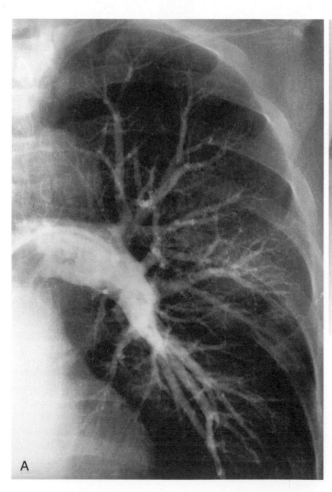

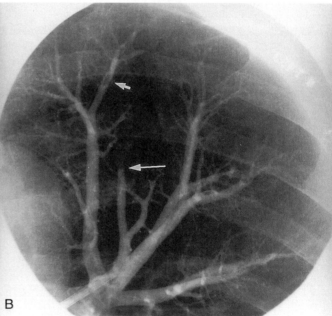

FIGURE 12-21 ■ The value of selective magnification pulmonary arteriography is demonstrated. **A,** The left pulmonary arteriogram shows no definite emboli. **B,** A selective magnification view of the left upper lobe reveals several intraluminal clots *(short arrow)* and truncation of a branch to the apex of the lung *(long arrow)*.

BOX 12-5 ■ Causes of Pulmonary Artery
Obstruction

Central Arteries
Acute or chronic embolus
Neoplasm (extra- or intravascular)
Mediastinal lymphadenopathy
Fibrosing mediastinitis
Congenital disorders

Peripheral Arteries
Acute or chronic embolic disease
Neoplasm
Inflammatory disease
Vasculitis
Takayasu's arteritis
Thrombosed aneurysm
Radiation therapy

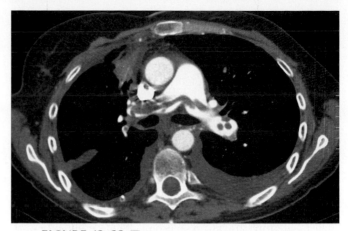

FIGURE 12-22 ■ Massive pulmonary artery embolism.

■ If no parenchymal lung disease is identified, a negative
V/Q scan may exclude the diagnosis.
■ Otherwise, consider repeat CT angiography (if the
first study was equivocal) or catheter angiography.

Treatment

Medical Therapy. Because many pulmonary emboli
undergo spontaneous lysis and most patients survive a
single episode of pulmonary embolism, the primary goal of
treatment is prevention of recurrent embolism and progression of thrombosis in the pulmonary arteries. Anticoagulation
with intravenous unfractionated heparin followed by oral
warfarin (Coumadin) for 3 to 6 months was the standard
therapy for decades. Now, treatment with subcutaneous low-
molecular-weight heparin compounds (for about 5 days)
with concurrent treatment with a vitamin K antagonist (for
3 months or more) is recommended (see Chapter 2).[61] With
proper treatment, the mortality rate from pulmonary
embolism is reduced from about 30% to less than 5%.[61,62]

Endovascular Therapy. Patients with a contraindication to
anticoagulants or who fail anticoagulation should undergo
placement of an IVC filter.[63] This technique is highly effective in preventing further pulmonary embolism (see
Chapter 14). The recurrent embolism rate (regardless of the
type of filter used) is about 3% to 5%.[63,64]

The role of systemic thrombolytic infusion or local transcatheter therapy for acute pulmonary embolism is controversial. Current practice is to reserve aggressive endovascular
therapy for patients with cardiopulmonary instability, usually
because of massive pulmonary embolism (Fig. 12-22).[61]
Catheter-directed thrombolysis, thromboaspiration, mechanical clot fragmentation, or stent placement has been quite
effective in selected patients with large clot burden.[65-70]

Surgical Therapy. Open pulmonary embolectomy has a
substantial mortality rate and is usually a last resort in
patients with cardiopulmonary collapse who do not respond
rapidly to transcatheter techniques.[61,71]

Hemoptysis and Bronchial Artery Embolization

Etiology

Mild to moderate hemoptysis is a common problem that
usually responds to treatment of the underlying condition.
However, several diseases can produce massive hemoptysis
that requires more aggressive therapy (Box 12-6).[13,72]
Patients with moderate but recurrent bleeding (e.g., in
cystic fibrosis) also may present for angiographic diagnosis
and transcatheter therapy. The following bleeding sources
should be considered:

■ The bronchial arteries are the source of bleeding in
most cases.
■ Nonbronchial systemic collateral arteries have been
shown to be partially or largely responsible for massive
hemoptysis in 30% to 50% of cases.[73-75]

BOX 12-6 ■ Causes of Massive Hemoptysis

Infection
  Tuberculosis
  Fungus (e.g., mycetoma)
  Chronic pneumonia
  Abscess
Cystic fibrosis
Bronchiectasis
Neoplasm
Bronchovascular fistula
Pulmonary artery aneurysm
Iatrogenic (e.g., pulmonary artery balloon catheter)
Pulmonary arteriovenous malformation
Pulmonary embolus
Pulmonary hypertension
Mitral stenosis
Idiopathic causes

■ The pulmonary artery is rarely the source of bleeding. Unusual conditions include a *Rasmussen's aneurysm* (classically, erosion of a tuberculosis cavity into a pulmonary artery branch), traumatic pseudoaneurysm (e.g., from a Swan-Ganz catheter), and pulmonary arteriovenous malformation.[76,77]

Clinical Features

By convention, massive hemoptysis is present when the bleeding rate exceeds 300 mL in a 24-hour period. Localization of the region of bleeding is useful before arteriography. Serial changes in chest radiographs or CT scans may suggest the involved lobes. Fiberoptic bronchoscopy often is used to identify the site of bleeding, guide embolotherapy, and, in some cases, coagulate the culprit lesion.[72] Blood transfusion and correction of coagulation deficiencies should be under way at the time of angiography. Airway protection may be necessary if the bleeding is exuberant. Because of the remote possibility of spinal cord injury from bronchial artery embolization, a complete neurologic examination should be documented in the medical record.

Imaging

Angiography is the procedure of choice. The technique for bronchial arteriography was outlined earlier. An empiric search is made for the bronchial arteries on the affected side (see Fig. 12-5). Bronchial arteries arise from the aorta and pass to the hilus of the lung, where they become tortuous and then give off numerous branches. If a bleeding source cannot be found, a descending thoracic aortogram with the catheter placed near the left subclavian artery to identify bronchial or nonbronchial system collaterals vessels (especially intercostal or inferior phrenic arteries) may be helpful (Fig. 12-23).[78] Occasionally, CT angiography with multiplanar reformatting may be useful in localizing ectopic origins of culprit vessels.[79]

The classic findings in patients with bronchial artery bleeding include enlargement of the main artery (>3 mm), hypervascularity, parenchymal stain, and bronchial to pulmonary artery shunting (Fig. 12-24). Frank extravasation, which is uncommon, need not be present to proceed with embolization. It is critical to look for small branches to the anterior spinal artery, which usually arise from the proximal portion of the vessel and take a characteristic hairpin turn as they pass superiorly and then inferiorly into the anterior spinal cord in the midline (see Fig. 12-11).

After one or more bronchial arteries supplying the bleeding site is identified and embolized, potential nonbronchial systemic collaterals should be studied (Fig. 12-25). The more common sources are[74,78]:

■ Internal thoracic (mammary) artery
■ Thyrocervical trunk of the subclavian artery
■ Lateral branches of the subclavian or axillary artery
■ Intercostal arteries
■ Inferior phrenic artery

As a rule, collaterals arise from vessels in proximity to the bleeding site (e.g., lower lobe lesions may be fed by an inferior phrenic artery). Rarely, collateral vessels arising on the opposite side are responsible for bleeding. If neither a bronchial nor nonbronchial systemic arterial source can be found, a pulmonary angiogram is performed to exclude a pulmonary artery lesion (Fig. 12-26).

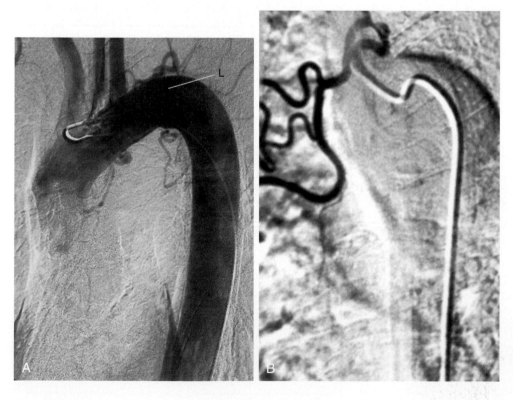

FIGURE 12-23 ■ Unusual origin of a bronchial artery. **A,** Right posterior oblique thoracic aortogram shows an enlarged vessel arising from the upper surface of the descending thoracic aorta. **B,** Selective catheterization proves this vessel is a bronchial artery supplying bleeding in the right lung.

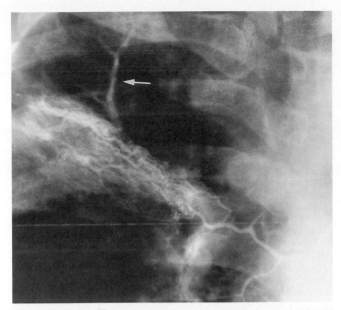

FIGURE 12-24 ■ Right bronchial arteriogram in a patient with massive hemoptysis from actinomycosis. Characteristic findings include bronchial artery enlargement, hypervascularity, and shunting to the pulmonary artery branches *(arrow)*. The parenchymal stain is prominent.

Treatment

Bronchial Artery Embolization

Patient Selection. Embolotherapy is the first-line treatment for massive hemoptysis or recurrent intractable hemoptysis.[80,81] Presence of a major spinal artery branch or radiculomedullary branch from the bronchial artery is considered to be a contraindication to embolotherapy by some interventionalists, but others perform embolization if a microcatheter can be negotiated well beyond such a vessel.

Technique. If the diagnostic catheter (without side holes) can be advanced deep into the artery, embolotherapy is performed directly without a significant risk of refluxing material into the aorta. Usually, however, a coaxial microcatheter system is advanced well into the bronchial artery beyond intercostal or mediastinal branches (Fig. 12-27).

Although a variety of materials has been used for bronchial artery embolization, the most common agents are polyvinyl alcohol (PVA) and Gelfoam pledgets.[13,82-86] PVA foam particles cause long-term occlusion of distal arteries and prevent recruitment of collateral arteries that may result in rebleeding. Particle sizes between 250 and 700 μm are used. Smaller particles could pass through small spinal artery branches or bronchial-pulmonary artery shunts and then potentially through small arteriovenous shunts into the systemic circulation.

Patients with extremely large bronchopulmonary artery shunts may require larger emboli to avoid pulmonary infarction or systemic embolization. If spherical microspheres

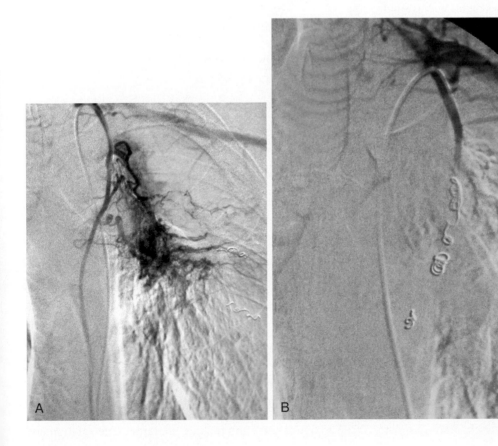

FIGURE 12-25 ■ Nonbronchial systemic collateral arteries. **A,** The left internal thoracic artery supplies numerous hilar vessels. **B,** The distal artery was embolized with coils to prevent nontarget embolization of polyvinyl alcohol particles, which were then delivered to pulmonary branches to complete the occlusion.

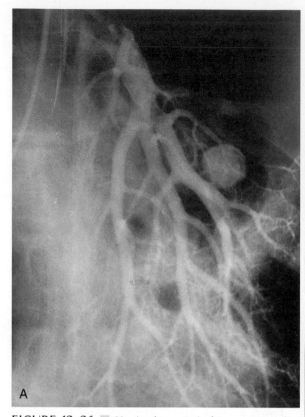

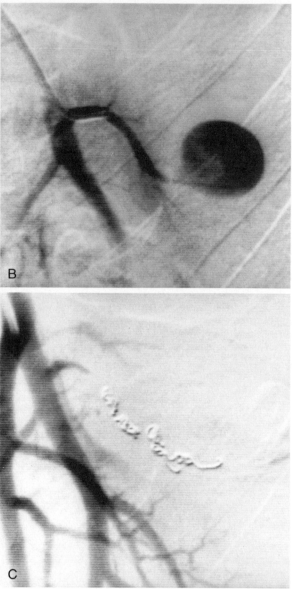

FIGURE 12-26 ■ Massive hemoptysis from a ruptured Rasmussen's aneurysm in a patient with disseminated tuberculosis. No bronchial or nonbronchial systemic collateral arteries were identified as a source of the bleeding. **A,** A pseudoaneurysm of a lingular branch of the left pulmonary artery is identified. **B,** Selective catheterization of the feeding branch shows the aneurysm neck. **C,** Embolization with coils across the neck of the pseudoaneurysm led to complete occlusion.

are chosen, it may be prudent to upsize the material to prevent coronary or cerebral embolization.[87] PVA particles are delivered as a slurry made with diluted contrast material. Small aliquots (1 to 2 mL) are injected slowly to avoid reflux into the aorta. Gelfoam pledgets also have been used successfully by some interventionalists, although this material is resorbed over a period of weeks.

Contrast is injected after each delivery to follow the progress of embolization, which is continued until blood flow is static. Delayed filling of branches to the anterior spinal artery should be sought. Small pledgets of Gelfoam sometimes are deployed to complete the embolization.

Embolization of a pulmonary artery aneurysm or pseudoaneurysm may be accomplished using coils to cover the neck of the aneurysm (see Fig. 12-26).[77,88]

Results. Bronchial artery embolization can be accomplished in greater than 90% of cases. Technical failure usually results from an inability to identify bronchial arteries or to successfully catheterize such vessels. Bleeding stops in about 70% to 95% of cases.[13,80-85,89] On the whole, better immediate results have been achieved with PVA foam than with Gelfoam pledgets. Early or late recurrent bleeding affects about 20% to 30% of patients.[76,82,84,85] The principal reasons are incomplete initial embolization, recruitment of collateral vessels, recanalization of embolized vessels, unidentified bleeding arteries, and progression of disease. If rebleeding occurs, a second trial of embolotherapy is warranted. The previously treated vessels are again studied, and other bronchial and nonbronchial sources of hemorrhage are sought. In some series, early or late rebleeding is particularly common in patients with cystic fibrosis.[86]

Complications. Some patients develop a postembolization syndrome consisting of fever, chest wall pain, and, rarely, dysphagia. Symptoms may be severe and can last for up to 1 week. Complications from embolotherapy occur in about 2% to 5% of cases and include nontarget embolization and

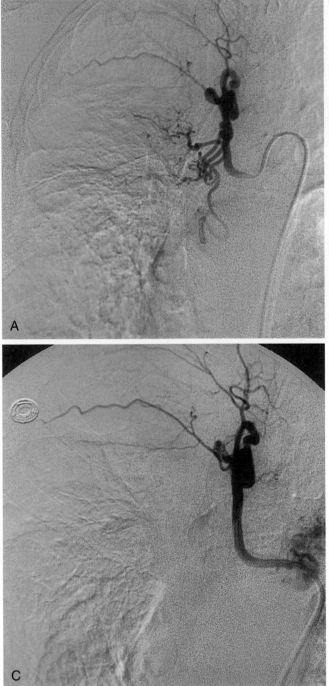

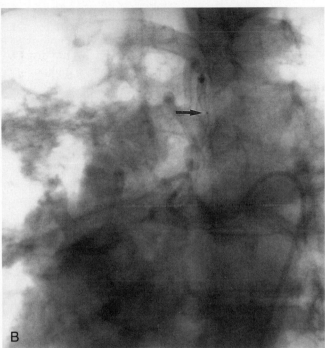

FIGURE 12-27 ■ Bronchial artery embolization. **A,** An enlarged right bronchointercostal artery feeds hypervascular vessels in the right hilum. **B,** Through the 5-French Shetty catheter, a 3-French Tracker catheter was placed coaxially into the bronchial artery beyond the intercostal branches (*arrow* indicates the tip). **C,** After embolization with 300- to 500-μm polyvinyl alcohol particles and Gelfoam pledgets, the bronchial branches are occluded but the intercostal arteries are preserved.

bronchial or esophageal necrosis. There is a risk of pulmonary infarction if bronchial embolization is performed in the presence of pulmonary artery (or branch) occlusion.[90] The most feared but rare complication is transverse myelitis from embolization of a branch to the anterior spinal artery.[91]

Surgical Therapy

An operation to stop bleeding is performed if one or two trials of bronchial artery embolization are unsuccessful. Elective operation is performed after bleeding is controlled in patients who require definitive treatment of disease.

■ OTHER DISORDERS

Chronic Pulmonary Thromboembolic Disease

Most patients who survive an episode of acute pulmonary embolism have partial or complete resolution of the emboli, usually within 1 to 3 weeks after the event.[92] In some cases, however, emboli do not resolve. It was widely believed that about 0.2% of patients with pulmonary embolism eventually develop chronic pulmonary artery hypertension as a result of one or more episodes of unresolved pulmonary embolism, and that symptoms usually begin many years after the insult(s).[93] However, a recent study suggests that upward of 4% of patients may develop symptomatic chronic disease (elevated pulmonary artery pressures, normal pulmonary capillary wedge pressure, and classic imaging findings) within 2 years after a first episode.[94] No specific coagulation abnormality has been identified in this group. There is a greater risk of this disorder with recurrent pulmonary embolism.

Patients with chronic pulmonary thromboembolic disease often present with progressive dyspnea and fatigue. Almost one half of them have no documented history of pulmonary embolism or lower extremity deep venous thrombosis. The disorder is generally progressive and often fatal. The only successful treatment is pulmonary thromboendarterectomy, which leads to excellent hemodynamic, angiographic, and functional improvement in most patients.[95] Lifelong therapy with certain prostanoids (e.g., epoprostenol [Flolan]) delivered by inhalation or continuous intravenous infusion (through a tunneled central venous catheter) has shown significant clinical benefit in inoperable patients.[96,97]

Imaging studies are critical to make the diagnosis and determine the extent and sites of resectable disease.[98] Lung V/Q scanning shows multiple bilateral segmental mismatched defects in most patients, although the scan almost always underestimates the extent of disease.[99] High-resolution helical CT and (to a lesser extent) gadolinium-enhanced MR angiography are extremely accurate in differentiating this disorder from other causes of chronic pulmonary artery hypertension and in postoperative follow-up.[100-103]

The presence of central disease with minimal small vessel involvement is a reliable predictor of a favorable outcome after operation.[104] The spectrum of findings at CT angiography include complete vessel occlusion, vessel narrowing, peripheral crescentic filling defects, diffuse wall thickening, and webs or flaps (Fig. 12-28).[49] A "mosaic" parenchymal pattern also is typical. The central pulmonary arteries are markedly enlarged.

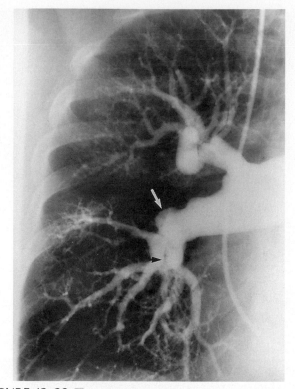

FIGURE 12-29 ■ Chronic pulmonary thromboembolic disease. The classic findings include webs *(black arrow)*, pouches *(white arrow)*, mural irregularity, branch occlusions, areas of diminished perfusion, and central pulmonary artery dilation.

Catheter angiography usually is performed prior to surgery. The findings are characteristic and differ from those of acute pulmonary embolism, primary pulmonary hypertension, or Takayasu's arteritis.[105] The disease is virtually always bilateral. The main pulmonary arteries usually are dilated. Chronic, partially resolved emboli produce webs, luminal irregularities, "pouches," segments of abrupt vessel narrowing, and frank obstructions (Fig. 12-29). The mean pulmonary artery pressure typically is in the range of 35 to 60 mm Hg, and pulmonary vascular resistance is markedly elevated.

Primary Pulmonary Hypertension

Primary pulmonary hypertension (PPH) is a rare disease in which pulmonary artery pressure is elevated significantly (mean pressure > 25 mm Hg) without evidence for an underlying cause.[106] The disorder must be distinguished from other causes of pulmonary hypertension. The precise etiology of PPH is unknown, but several factors have been implicated.[107] The prominent pathologic finding is thickening or fibrosis of small pulmonary arteries. PPH is more common in women than men, and most patients present in the fourth decade of life. Typical symptoms include dyspnea, fatigue, chest pain, and syncope. The disease often is progressive and fatal. Treatment includes pulmonary artery vasodilator therapy (including inhaled nitric oxide, phosphodiesterase-5 inhibitors, and prostacyclin analogues, such as epoprostenol) and lung transplantation.[96,108]

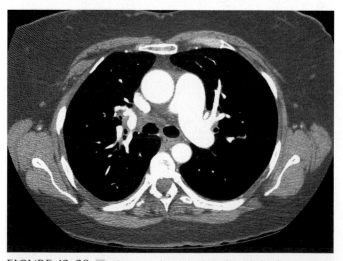

FIGURE 12-28 ■ Chronic pulmonary thromboembolic disease on CT angiography. Bilateral recanalization with narrowed lumens and thickened walls is characteristic.

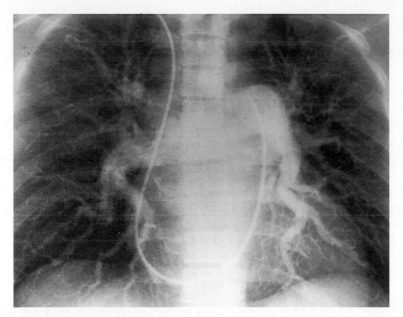

FIGURE 12-30 ■ Primary pulmonary hypertension. Main pulmonary arteriogram shows enlarged central arteries and tortuous distal branches. The pulmonary artery pressure was markedly elevated.

Lung V/Q scans usually are interpreted as normal or low probability.[109,110] CT and MR imaging findings are not particularly diagnostic.[111,112] When angiography is performed, it shows high pulmonary artery pressures, dilation of the central pulmonary arteries, and widespread tortuosity and severe tapering of distal arterial branches (Fig. 12-30); acute or organized thrombus usually is not seen. Angiograms may be normal in a small percentage of patients.

Vasculitis

A wide variety of vasculitides may affect the pulmonary arteries (Box 12-7).[113-115] *Takayasu's arteritis* is an inflammatory vasculitis of large- and medium-sized elastic arteries (see Chapter 3).[116,117] The disease normally is seen in young to middle-aged women. Although involvement of the thoracic and abdominal aorta is universal, the pulmonary arteries are affected in about 50% of cases.[118] Pulmonary Takayasu's arteritis is usually bilateral and most commonly targets the segmental branches, producing wall thickening and enhancement, luminal stenoses and frank occlusions, or aneurysms and patchy areas of parenchymal low attenuation (Fig. 12-31). When the disease is segmental, there may be a predilection for upper lobe branches.

The *collagen-vascular diseases* are associated with a pulmonary vasculitis with fibrotic proliferation in small pulmonary vessels.[119] Pulmonary hypertension may result.

Behçet's disease is a multisystem disorder characterized by aphthous ulcers of the mouth and genital area and by ocular involvement.[120] A small percentage of patients with Behçet's disease (particularly young men) develop multiple hilar or parahilar pulmonary artery aneurysms.[121-123] Complications of aneurysm formation include thrombosis and rupture.

Aneurysms

Aneurysms and pseudoaneurysms of the pulmonary arteries have many causes (Box 12-8; see also Fig 12-26).[124,125]

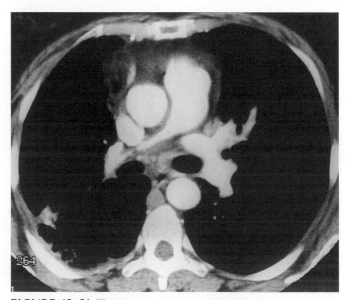

FIGURE 12-31 ■ Takayasu's arteritis of the right pulmonary artery. Notice the long, smooth luminal narrowing and wall thickening.

BOX 12-7 ■ Causes of Pulmonary Vasculitis

Takayasu's arteritis
Connective tissue disorders
  Scleroderma
  Rheumatoid arthritis
  Systemic lupus erythematosus
Behçet's disease
Wegener's granulomatosis
Allergic angiitis and granulomatosis

identified on imaging studies. Transcatheter embolization is the treatment of choice and is almost always successful.[129] The mortality rate without treatment is extremely high.

Bronchial artery aneurysms are rare lesions that may be congenital or caused by inflammation, atherosclerosis, or trauma. Rupture into the mediastinum or an airway is the most serious complication. Endovascular treatment with a variety of agents has been successful.[130-132]

Arteriovenous Malformations

Pulmonary arteriovenous malformations (AVMs) may occur sporadically, but most are seen in patients with *hereditary hemorrhagic telangiectasia* (HHT), also known as *Osler-Weber-Rendu* syndrome.[133,134] HHT is an autosomal dominant genetic disorder characterized by telangiectasias of the mouth and telangiectasias or AVMs of the gastrointestinal tract, brain, liver, and lung. About 20% to 50% of patients with HHT have pulmonary AVMs, and about 60% have multiple lesions.[135] Many patients present with epistaxis. Family members should be evaluated, because about one third of them also have pulmonary AVMs. Screening is done with contrast (echo-bubble) echocardiography, arterial blood gas measurements, and helical CT scanning.[136] Posttraumatic pulmonary AVMs also have been reported.

About 90% of pulmonary AVMs are **simple** (single segmental arterial supply), and 10% are **complex** (multiple segmental arterial supply).[137,138] They are most commonly found in the lower lobes. The AVM causes a right-to-left shunt and provides an open pathway between the venous and arterial circulations. Patients commonly present with dyspnea, fatigue, hemoptysis, stroke, or brain abscess. A primary reason to treat symptomatic and asymptomatic patients is to prevent neurologic complications.

AVMs often are detected incidentally on chest radiographs. CT angiography is exquisitely sensitive for detecting lesions that require treatment (usually >3 mm) (Fig. 12-32).

Dilation of the main pulmonary artery usually is caused by left-to-right shunts (Eisenmenger physiology) or pulmonary artery hypertension. Post-stenotic dilation from pulmonary valve or root disease can mimic an aneurysm. Central right or left pulmonary artery aneurysms usually are caused by congenital disorders or vasculitis. Multiple aneurysms may be seen with infection (e.g., septic emboli) and arteritis.[126] Typically, large pulmonary artery aneurysms manifest with hemoptysis, dyspnea, or chest pain, or they may be an incidental finding on chest radiographs or CT scans.

Distal arterial rupture with pseudoaneurysm formation may occur as a rare complication of Swan-Ganz catheter placement.[77,127,128] Several mechanisms of injury have been postulated, including vessel perforation by the catheter tip and overinflation of the wedge balloon. Pseudoaneurysms usually are found in the right middle or lower lobe arteries. The presenting sign is hemoptysis or a new lung mass

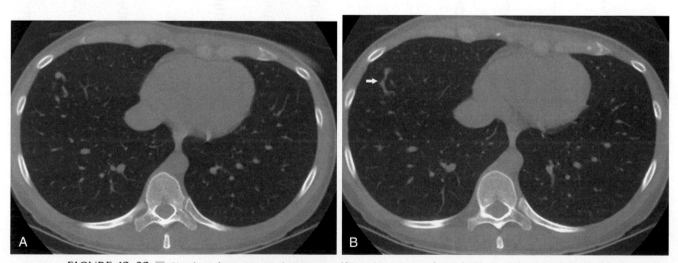

FIGURE 12-32 ■ Simple pulmonary arteriovenous malformation on unenhanced CT. **A,** Enlarged subsegmental branch feeds the nidus. **B,** Enlarged draining vein is noted *(arrow).*

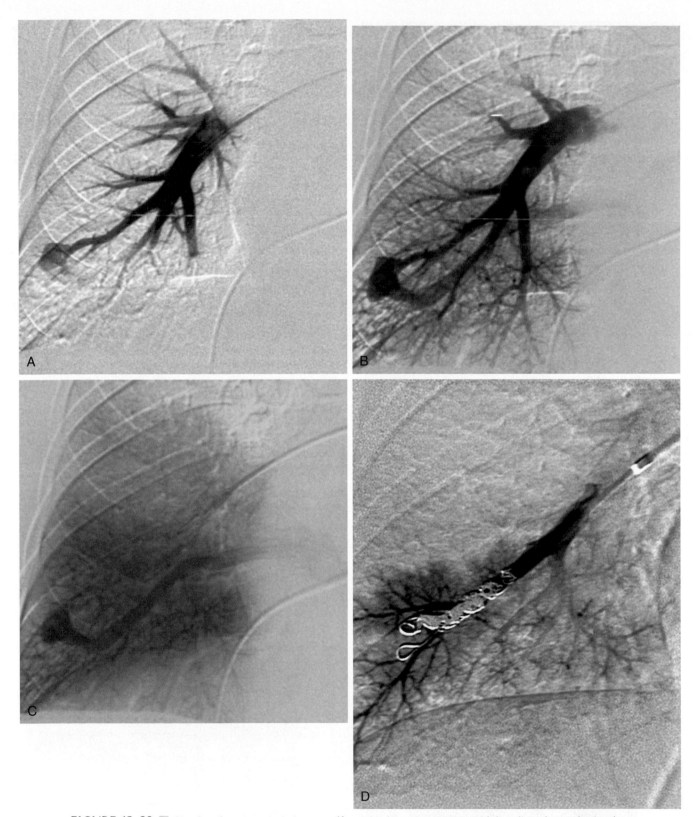

FIGURE 12-33 ■ Simple pulmonary arteriovenous malformation in a young woman with hereditary hemorrhagic telangiectasia. **A,** Single enlarged segmental artery feeds the lesion. **B** and **C,** Later phases of angiogram show rapid washout into enlarged draining pulmonary vein. **D,** Lesion is occluded with densely compacted Nester platinum coils.

Pulmonary angiography is performed for evaluation and embolotherapy, which is the treatment of choice.[80,138,139] Selective arteriography in multiple projections is necessary to map out the arterial supply. Great care must be taken to avoid allowing room air into the catheter after it is in a selective position in the segmental artery feeding the malformation. Angiography shows one or more dilated segmental arteries (often with several subsegmental branches) feeding an aneurysmally dilated sac with rapid venous outflow (Figs. 12-33 and 12-34).

Many devices have been used for occlusion, including coils and detachable balloons. Coils are chosen to be 1 to 2 mm larger than the artery being embolized and should be deposited as close as possible to the aneurysmal enlargement near the nidus of the malformation. Nester platinum coils are preferred by many experts; these long, highly radiopaque coils can be packed densely into the feeding vessel to prevent recanalization.[140] Detachable balloons may be preferable to coils in small feeding arteries (<5 mm diameter) because they can be placed more precisely. Patients with numerous lesions may require multiple treatment sessions.

Embolization is successful in almost every case, and occlusion is permanent in greater than 90% of patients.[80,138,139,141] A postembolization syndrome with fever or pleuritic chest pain is common. Complications occur in 10% to 20% of cases, but most are minor. Serious complications, including paradoxical embolization of coils, balloons, or air (which may produce coronary ischemia), occur in less than 5% of procedures. Long-term follow-up with chest radiography and CT is important to ensure persistent closure and to detect growth of additional AVMs.

Neoplasms

Arteriography has no role in the diagnosis and staging of lung tumors. Occasionally, a mediastinal or lung malignancy mimics another disease, such as pulmonary embolism (Fig. 12-35). Lung neoplasms typically produce vascular encasement, displacement, or obstruction.

Radiofrequency ablation has shown promise in treating patients with unresectable primary and secondary malignancies of the lung.[142-145] It may be used as an alternative or adjunct to chemotherapy and radiation therapy. In a substantial number of cases, lesions stabilize or regress for significant periods of time. However, complications are common, including pneumothorax, pleural effusion, hemoptysis, and lung abscess.

Primary and secondary tumors of the pulmonary arteries are rare. The most common primary tumor is *pulmonary artery sarcoma,* which usually arises in the main, right, or left pulmonary artery and often is contained within the lumen (Fig. 12-36).[146,147] Differentiation from bland thrombus may be difficult. Transvenous biopsy has been used to make the diagnosis.[148]

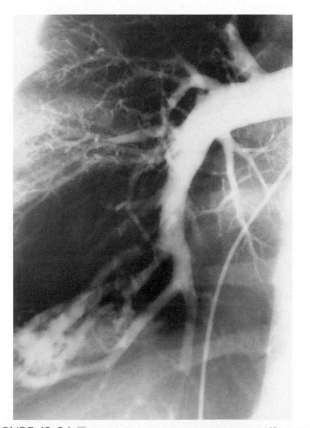

FIGURE 12-34 ▪ A complex pulmonary arteriovenous malformation is fed by several segmental arterial branches of the descending right pulmonary artery.

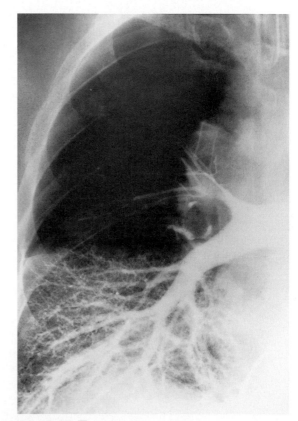

FIGURE 12-35 ▪ Encasement of the right upper lobe pulmonary artery by a mediastinal tumor.

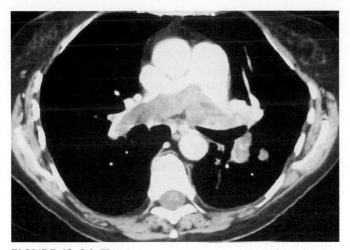

FIGURE 12-36 ■ Pulmonary artery sarcoma extends from the main pulmonary artery into both the right and left sides.

REFERENCES

1. Grollman JH Jr: Pulmonary arteriography. Cardiovasc Intervent Radiol 1992;15:166.
2. Velling TE, Brennan FJ, Hall LD: Pulmonary angiography with use of the 5-F omniflush catheter: a safe and efficient procedure with a common catheter. J Vasc Interv Radiol 2000;11:1005.
3. Grossman W: Cardiac catheterization. In: Braunwald E, ed. Heart Disease: A Textbook of Cardiovascular Medicine, 4th ed. Philadelphia, WB Saunders, 1992:180.
4. Stein PD, Athanasoulis C, Alavi A, et al: Complications and validity of pulmonary angiography in acute pulmonary embolism. Circulation 1992;85:462.
5. Mills SR, Jackson DC, Older RA, et al: The incidence, etiologies, and avoidance of complications of pulmonary angiography in a large series. Radiology 1980;136:295.
6. Collins P, ed: Embryology and development. In: Williams PL, Bannister LH, Berry MM, et al, eds. Gray's Anatomy, 38th ed. New York, Churchill Livingstone, 1995:312.
7. Gabella G, ed: Cardiovascular system. In: Williams PL, Bannister LH, Berry MM, et al, eds. Gray's Anatomy, 38th ed. New York, Churchill Livingstone, 1995:1504.
8. Gabella G, ed: Cardiovascular system. In: Williams PL, Bannister LH, Berry MM, et al, eds. Gray's Anatomy, 38th ed. New York, Churchill Livingstone, 1995:1574.
9. Fishman AP: The pulmonary circulation. In: Fishman AP, ed. Pulmonary Diseases and Disorders, 3rd ed. New York, McGraw-Hill, 1998:1233.
10. Tadavarthy SM, Klugman J, Castaneda-Zuniga WR, et al: Systemic-to-pulmonary collaterals in pathological states. A review. Radiology 1982;144:55.
11. Cauldwell EW, Siekert RG, Linninger RE, et al: The bronchial arteries: an anatomic study of 150 human cadavers. Surg Gynecol Obstet 1948;86:395.
12. Liebow AA: Patterns of origin and distribution of the major bronchial arteries in man. J Anat 1965;117:19.
13. Uflacker R, Kaemmerer A, Picon PD, et al: Bronchial artery embolization in the management of hemoptysis: technical aspects and long-term results. Radiology 1985;157:637.
14. Kardjiev V, Symeonov A, Chankov I: Etiology, pathogenesis, and prevention of spinal cord lesions in selective angiography of the bronchial and intercostal arteries. Radiology 1974;112:81.
15. Rose AG: Diseases of the pulmonary circulation. In: Silver MD, Gotlieb AI, Schoen FJ, eds. Cardiovascular Pathology. New York, Churchill Livingstone, 2001:166.
16. Ellis K: Developmental abnormalities in the systemic blood supply to the lungs. AJR Am J Roentgenol 1991;156:669.
17. Berrocal T, Madrid C, Novo S, et al: Congenital anomalies of the tracheobronchial tree, lung, and mediastinum: embryology, radiology, and pathology. Radiographics 2004;24:e17.
18. Lee K-H, Sung K-B, Yoon H-K, et al: Transcatheter arterial embolization of pulmonary sequestration in neonates: long-term follow-up results. J Vasc Interv Radiol 2003;14:363.
19. Zylak CJ, Eyler WR, Spizarny DL, et al: Developmental lung anomalies in the adult: radiologic-pathologic correlation. Radiographics 2002; 22:S25.
20. Lois JF, Gomes AS, Smith DC, et al: Systemic-to-pulmonary collateral vessels and shunts: treatment with embolization. Radiology 1988; 169:671.
21. Smith TP: Pulmonary embolism: what's wrong with this diagnosis? AJR Am J Roentgenol 2000;174:1489.
22. Browse NL, Thomas ML: Source of nonlethal pulmonary emboli. Lancet 1974;1:258.
23. Huisman MV, Bueller HR, ten Cate JW, et al: Unexpected high prevalence of silent pulmonary embolism in patients with deep venous thrombosis. Chest 1989;95:498.
24. Palevsky TE, Kelley MA, Fishman AP: Pulmonary thromboembolic disease. In: Fishman AP, ed. Pulmonary Diseases and Disorders, 3rd ed. New York, McGraw-Hill, 1998:1297.
25. Fedullo PF, Tapson VF: The evaluation of suspected pulmonary embolism. New Engl J Med 2003;349:1247.
26. Carlson JL, Kelley MA, Duff A, et al: The clinical course of pulmonary embolism. New Engl J Med 1992;326:1240.
27. Remy-Jardin M, Louvegny S, Remy J, et al: Acute central thromboembolic disease: posttherapeutic follow-up with spiral CT angiography. Radiology 1997;203:173.
28. Rossi SE, Goodman PC, Franquet T: Nonthrombotic pulmonary emboli. AJR Am J Roentgenol 2000;174:1499.
29. Brecher CW, Lang EV: Tumor thromboembolism masquerading as bland pulmonary embolism. J Vasc Interv Radiol 2004;15:293.
30. Vesely T: Air embolism during insertion of central venous catheters. J Vasc Interv Radiol 2001;12:1291.
31. Schoepf UJ, Costello P: CT angiography for diagnosis of pulmonary embolism: state of the art. Radiology 2004;230:329.
32. Johnson MS: Current strategies for the diagnosis of pulmonary embolism. J Vasc Interv Radiol 2002;13:13.
33. Stein PD, Terrin ML, Hales CA, et al: Clinical, laboratory, roentgenographic, and electrocardiographic findings in patients with acute pulmonary embolism and no pre-existing cardiac or pulmonary disease. Chest 1991;100:598.
34. van Rossum AB, Pattynama PMT, Ton ER, et al: Pulmonary embolism: validation of spiral CT angiography in 149 patients. Radiology 1996;201:467.
35. Teigen CL, Maus TP, Sheedy PF II, et al: Pulmonary embolism: diagnosis with contrast enhanced electron beam CT and comparison with pulmonary angiography. Radiology 1995;194:313.
36. Goodman LR, Curtin JJ, Mewissen MW, et al: Detection of pulmonary embolism in patients with unresolved clinical and scintigraphic diagnosis: helical CT versus angiography. AJR Am J Roentgenol 1995;164:1369.
37. Schoepf U, Holzknecht N, Helmberger TK, et al: Subsegmental pulmonary emboli: improved detection with thin-collimation multidetector row spiral CT. Radiology 2002;222:483.
38. Raptopoulos V, Boiselle PM: Multi-detector row spiral CT pulmonary angiography: comparison with single-detector row spiral CT. Radiology 2001;221:606.
39. Patel S, Kazerooni EA, Cascade PN: Pulmonary embolism: optimization of small pulmonary artery visualization at mult-detector row CT. Radiology 2003;227:455.
40. Stein PD, Henry JW, Gottshalk A: Reassessment of pulmonary angiography for the diagnosis of pulmonary embolism: relation of interpreter agreement to the order of the involved pulmonary branch. Radiology 1999;210:689.
41. Diffin DC, Leyendecker JR, Johnson SP, et al: Effect of anatomic distribution of pulmonary emboli on interobserver agreement in the interpretation of pulmonary angiography. AJR Am J Roentgenol 1998;171:1085.
42. deMonye W, van Strijen MJL, Hulsman MV, et al: Suspected pulmonary embolism: prevalence and anatomic distribution in 487 consecutive patients. Radiology 2000;215:184.
43. Goodman LR, Lipchik RJ, Kuzo RS, et al: Subsequent pulmonary embolism: risk after negative helical CT pulmonary angiogram—prospective comparison with scintigraphy. Radiology 2000;215:535.
44. Garg K, Sieler H, Welsh CH, et al: Clinical validity of helical CT being interpreted as negative for pulmonary embolism: implications for patient treatment. AJR Am J Roentgenol 1999;172:1627.

45. Tillie-Leblond I, Mastora I, Radenne F, et al: Risk of pulmonary embolism after a negative spiral CT angiogram in patients with pulmonary disease: 1-year clinical follow-up study. Radiology 2002;223:461.
46. Lomis NN, Moran AG, Miller FJ: Clinical outcomes of patients after negative spiral CT pulmonary arteriogram in the evaluation of acute pulmonary embolism. J Vasc Interv Radiol 1999;10:707.
47. Coche EE, Hamoir XL, Hammer FD, et al: Using dual-detector helical CT angiography to detect deep venous thrombosis in patients with suspicion of pulmonary embolism: diagnostic value and additional findings. AJR Am J Roentgenol 2001;176:1035.
48. Loud PA, Katz DS, Klippenstein DL, et al: Combined CT venography and pulmonary angiography in suspected thromboembolic disease: diagnostic accuracy for deep venous evaluation. AJR Am J Roentgenol 2000;174:61.
49. Wittram C, Maher MM, Yoo AJ, et al: CT angiography of pulmonary embolism: diagnostic criteria and causes of misdiagnosis. Radiographics 2004;24:1219.
50. Worsley DF, Alavi A: Radionuclide imaging of acute pulmonary embolism. Semin Nucl Med 2003;33:259.
51. PIOPED Investigators: Value of the ventilation/perfusion scan in acute pulmonary embolism: results of the Prospective Investigation of Pulmonary Embolism Diagnosis (PIOPED). JAMA 1990;263:2753.
52. Goodman LR, Lipchik RJ: Diagnosis of acute pulmonary embolism: time for a new approach. Radiology 1996;199:25.
53. Rosen MP, Sheiman RG, Weintraub J, et al: Compression sonography in patients with indeterminate or low-probability lung scans: lack of usefulness in the absence of both symptoms of deep-vein thrombosis and thromboembolic risk factors. AJR Am J Roentgenol 1996;166:285.
54. Beecham RP, Dorfman GS, Cronan JJ, et al: Is bilateral lower extremity compression sonography useful and cost-effective in the evaluation of suspected pulmonary embolism? AJR Am J Roentgenol 1993;161:1289.
55. Smith LL, Iber C, Sirr S: Pulmonary embolism: confirmation with venous duplex US as adjunct to lung scanning. Radiology 1994;191:143.
56. van Beek EJ, Wild JM, Fink C, et al: MRI for the diagnosis of pulmonary embolism. J Magn Reson Imaging 2003;18:627.
57. Gupta A, Frazer CK, Ferguson JM, et al: Acute pulmonary embolism: diagnosis with MR angiography. Radiology 1999;210:353.
58. Stein PD, Woodard PK, Hull RD, et al: Gadolinium-enhanced magnetic resonance angiography for detection of acute pulmonary embolism: an in-depth review. Chest 2003;124:2324.
59. Oser RF, Zuckerman DA, Gutierrez FR, et al: Anatomic distribution of pulmonary emboli at pulmonary angiography: implications for cross-sectional imaging. Radiology 1996;199:31.
60. Fred HL, Axelrad MA, Lewis JM et al: Rapid resolution of pulmonary thromboemboli in man: an angiographic study. JAMA 1966;196:1137.
61. Bueller HR, Agnelli G, Hull RD, et al: Antithrombotic therapy for venous thromboembolic disease. The seventh ACCP conference on antithrombotic and thrombolytic therapy. Chest 2004;126:401S.
62. Barritt DW, Jordan SC: Anticoagulant drugs in the treatment of pulmonary embolism: a controlled trial. Lancet 1960;1:1309.
63. Kinney TB: Update on inferior vena cava filters. J Vasc Interv Radiol 2003;14:425.
64. Ferris EJ, McCowan TC, Carver DK, et al: Percutaneous inferior vena caval filters: follow-up of seven designs in 320 patients. Radiology 1993;188:851.
65. Haskal ZJ, Soulen MC, Huettl EA, et al: Life-threatening pulmonary emboli and cor pulmonale: treatment with percutaneous pulmonary artery stent placement. Radiology 1994;191:473.
66. Uflacker R, Strange C, Vujic I: Massive pulmonary embolism: preliminary results of treatment with the Amplatz thrombectomy device. J Vasc Interv Radiol 1996;7:519.
67. Schmitz-Rode T, Guenther RW, Pfeffer JG, et al: Acute massive pulmonary embolism: use of a rotatable pigtail catheter for diagnosis and fragmentation therapy. Radiology 1995;197:157.
68. Uflacker R: Interventional therapy for pulmonary embolism. J Vasc Interv Radiol 2001;12:147.
69. Zeni PT, Blank BG, Peeler DW: Use of rheolytic thrombectomy in treatment of acute massive pulmonary embolism. J Vasc Interv Radiol 2003;14:1511.
70. deGregorio MA, Gimeno AJ, Mainar A, et al: Mechanical and enzymatic thrombolysis for massive pulmonary embolism. J Vasc Interv Radiol 2002;13:163.
71. Gray HH, Morgan JM, Paneth M, et al: Pulmonary embolectomy for acute massive pulmonary embolism: an analysis of 71 cases. Br Heart J 1988;60:196.
72. Jean-Baptiste E: Clinical assessment and management of massive hemoptysis. Crit Care Med 2000;28:1642.
73. Jardin M, Remy J: Control of hemoptysis: systemic angiography and anastomoses of the internal mammary artery. Radiology 1988;168:377.
74. Keller FS, Rosch J, Loflin TG, et al: Nonbronchial systemic collateral arteries: significance in percutaneous embolotherapy for hemoptysis. Radiology 1987;164:687.
75. Yu-Tang Goh P, Lin M, Teo N, et al: Embolization for hemoptysis: a six-year review. Cardiovasc Intervent Radiol 2002;25:17.
76. Rabkin JE, Astafjev VI, Gothman LN, et al: Transcatheter embolization in the management of pulmonary hemorrhage. Radiology 1987;163:361.
77. Ferretti GR, Thony F, Link KM, et al: False aneurysm of the pulmonary artery induced by a Swan-Ganz catheter: clinical presentation and radiologic management. AJR Am J Roentgenol 1996;167:941.
78. Chun HJ, Byun JY, Yoo SS, et al: Added benefit of thoracic aortography after transarterial embolization in patients with hemoptysis. AJR Am J Roentgenol 2003;180:1577.
79. Remy-Jardin M, Bouaziz N, Dumont P, et al: Bronchial and non-bronchial systemic arteries at multi-detector row CT angiography: comparison with conventional angiography. Radiology 2004;233:741.
80. Saluja S, Henderson KJ, White RI Jr: Embolotherapy in the bronchial and pulmonary circulations. Radiol Clin North Am 2000;38:425.
81. Yoon W, Kim JK, Kim YH, et al: Bronchial and nonbronchial systemic artery embolization for life-threatening hemoptysis: a comprehensive review. Radiographics 2002;22:1395.
82. Katoh O, Kishikawa T, Yamada H, et al: Recurrent bleeding after arterial embolization in patients with hemoptysis. Chest 1990;97:541.
83. Cohen AM, Doershuk CF, Stern RC: Bronchial artery embolization to control hemoptysis in cystic fibrosis. Radiology 1990;175:401.
84. Hayakawa K, Tanaka F, Torizuka T, et al: Bronchial artery embolization for hemoptysis: immediate and long-term results. Cardiovasc Intervent Radiol 1992;15:154.
85. Swanson KL, Johnson CM, Prakash UB, et al: Bronchial artery embolization: experience with 54 patients. Chest 2002;121:789.
86. Barben JU, Ditchfield M, Carlin JB, et al: Major haemoptysis in children with cystic fibrosis: a 20-year retrospective study. Cyst Fibros 2003;2:105.
87. Vinaya KN, White RI Jr, Sloan JM: Reassessing bronchial artery embolotherapy with newer spherical embolic materials. J Vasc Interv Radiol 2004;15:304.
88. Santelli ED, Katz DS, Goldschmidt AM, et al: Embolization of multiple Rasmussen aneurysms as a treatment of hemoptysis. Radiology 1994;193:396.
89. Ramakantan R, Bandekar VG, Gandhi MS, et al: Massive hemoptysis due to pulmonary tuberculosis: control with bronchial artery embolization. Radiology 1996;200:691.
90. Remy-Jardin M, Wattinne L, Remy J: Transcatheter occlusion of pulmonary arterial circulation and collateral supply: failures, incidents, and complications. Radiology 1991;180:699.
91. Fraser KL, Grosman H, Hyland RH, et al: Transverse myelitis: a reversible complication of bronchial artery embolisation in cystic fibrosis. Thorax 1997;52:99.
92. Benotti JR, Dalen JE: The natural history of pulmonary embolism. Clin Chest Med 1984;5:403.
93. Fedullo PF, Auger WR, Kerr KM, et al: Chronic thromboembolic pulmonary hypertension. N Engl J Med 2001;345:1465.
94. Pengo V, Lensing AW, Prins MH, et al: Incidence of chronic thromboembolic pulmonary hypertension after pulmonary embolism. New Engl J Med 2004;350:2257.
95. Thistlethwaite PA, Madani M, Jamieson SW: Pulmonary thromboendarterectomy surgery. Cardiol Clin 2004;22:467.
96. Galie N, Manes A, Branzi A: Prostanoids for pulmonary arterial hypertension. Am J Respir Med 2003;2:123.
97. Nagaya N, Sasaki N, Ando M, et al: Prostacyclin therapy before pulmonary thromboendarterectomy in patients with chronic thromboembolic pulmonary hypertension. Chest 2003;123:338.
98. McGoon M, Gutterman D, Steen V, et al: Screening, early detection, and diagnosis of pulmonary arterial hypertension: ACCP evidence-based clinical practice guidelines. Chest 2004;126(1 Suppl):14S.
99. Bergin CJ, Hauschildt J, Rios G, et al: Accuracy of MR angiography compared with radionuclide scanning in identifying the cause of pulmonary arterial hypertension. AJR Am J Roentgenol 1997;168:1549.
100. Bergin CJ, Rios G, King MA, et al: Accuracy of high-resolution CT in identifying chronic pulmonary thromboembolic disease. AJR Am J Roentgenol 1996;166:1371.

101. Filipek MS, Gosselin MV: Multidetector pulmonary CT angiography: advances in the evaluation of pulmonary arterial diseases. Semin Ultrasound CT MR 2004;25:83.

102. Kreitner KF, Ley S, Kauczor HU, et al: Chronic thromboembolic pulmonary hypertension: pre- and postoperative assessment with breath-hold MR imaging techniques. Radiology 2004;232:535.

103. Ley S, Kauczor HU, Heussel CP, et al: Value of contrast-enhanced MR angiography and helical CT angiography in chronic thromboembolic pulmonary hypertension. Eur Radiol 2003;13:2365.

104. Bergin CJ, Sirlin C, Deutsch R, et al: Predictors of patient response to pulmonary thromboendarterectomy. AJR Am J Roentgenol 2000; 174:509.

105. Auger WR, Fedullo PF, Moser KM, et al: Chronic major-vessel thromboembolic pulmonary artery obstruction: appearance at angiography. Radiology 1992;182:393.

106. Peacock AJ: Primary pulmonary hypertension. Thorax 1999;54:1107.

107. Mandegar M, Thistlethwaite PA, Yuan JX et al: Molecular biology of primary pulmonary hypertension. Cardiol Clin 2004;22:417.

108. Leuchte HH, Schwaiblmair M, Baumgartner RA, et al: Hemodynamic response to sildenafil, nitric oxide, and iloprost in primary pulmonary hypertension. Chest 2004;125:580.

109. Worsley DF, Palevsky HI, Alavi A: Ventilation-perfusion lung scanning in the evaluation of pulmonary hypertension. J Nucl Med 1994; 35:793.

110. Chapman PJ, Bateman ED, Benatar SR: Primary pulmonary hypertension and thromboembolic pulmonary hypertension-similarities and differences. Respir Med 1990;84:485.

111. Ley S, Kreitner KF, Fink C, et al: Assessment of pulmonary hypertension by CT and MR imaging. Eur Radiol 2004;14:359.

112. Hansell DM: Small-vessel diseases of the lung: CT-pathologic correlates. Radiology 2002;225:639.

113. Leavitt RY, Fauci AS: Pulmonary vasculitis. Am Rev Respir Dis 1986;134:149.

114. Seo JB, Im JG, Chung JW, et al: Pulmonary vasculitis: the spectrum of radiological findings. Br J Radiol 2000;73:1224.

115. Nastri MV, Baptista LP, Baroni RH, et al: Gadolinium-enhanced three-dimensional MR angiography of Takayasu arteritis. Radiographics 2004;24:773.

116. Liu Y-Q, Jin B-L, Ling J: Pulmonary artery involvement in aortoarteritis: an angiographic study. Cardiovasc Intervent Radiol 1994;17:2.

117. Yamada I, Shibuya H, Matsubara O, et al: Pulmonary artery disease in Takayasu's arteritis: angiographic findings. AJR Am J Roentgenol 1992; 159:263.

118. Yamada I, Nakagawa T, Himeno Y, et al: Takayasu arteritis: diagnosis with breath-hold contrast-enhanced three-dimensional MR angiography. J Magn Reson Imaging 2000;11:481.

119. Hunninghake GW, Fauci AS: Pulmonary involvement in the collagen vascular diseases. Am Rev Respir Dis 1979;119:471.

120. Erkan F, Gul A, Tasali E, et al: Pulmonary manifestations of Behçet's disease. Thorax 2001;56:572.

121. Tunaci A, Berkmen YM, Gokmen E: Thoracic involvement in Behçet's disease: pathologic, clinical, and imaging features. AJR Am J Roentgenol 1995;164:51.

122. Hamuryudan V, Er T, Seyahi E, et al: Pulmonary artery aneurysms in Behçet syndrome. Am J Med 2004;117:867.

123. Hiller N, Lieberman S, Chajek-Shaul T, et al: Thoracic manifestations of Behçet disease at CT. Radiographics 2004;24:801.

124. Bartter T, Irwin RS, Nash G: Aneurysms of the pulmonary arteries. Chest 1988;94:1065.

125. Donaldson B, Ngo-Nonga B: Traumatic pseudoaneurysm of the pulmonary artery: case report and review of the literature. Am Surg 2002;68:414.

126. SanDretto MA, Scanlon GT: Multiple mycotic pulmonary artery aneurysms secondary to intravenous drug abuse. AJR Am J Roentgenol 1984;142:89.

127. Abreu AR, Campos MA, Krieger BP: Pulmonary artery rupture induced by a pulmonary artery catheter: a case report and review of the literature. J Intensive Care Med 2004;19:291.

128. Poplausky MR, Rozenblit G, Rundback JH, et al: Swan-Ganz catheter-induced pulmonary artery pseudoaneurysm formation: three case reports and a review of the literature. Chest 2001;120:2105.

129. Ray CE Jr, Kaufman JA, Geller SC, et al: Embolization of pulmonary catheter-induced pulmonary artery pseudoaneurysms. Chest 1996; 110:1370.

130. Tanaka K, Ihaya A, Horiuci T, et al: Giant mediastinal bronchial artery aneurysm mimicking benign esophageal tumor: a case report and review of 26 cases from literature. J Vasc Surg 2003;38:1125.

131. Pugnale M, Portier F, Lamarre A, et al: Hemomediastinum caused by rupture of a bronchial artery aneurysm: successful treatment by embolization with N-butyl-2-cyanoacrylate. J Vasc Interv Radiol 2001;12:1351.

132. Sakuma K, Takase K, Saito H, et al: Bronchial artery aneurysm treated with percutaneous transluminal coil embolization. Jpn J Thorac Cardiovasc Surg 2001;49:330.

133. Guttmacher AE, Marchuk DA, White RI Jr: Hereditary hemorrhagic telangiectasia. N Engl J Med 1995;333:918.

134. van den Driesche S, Mummery CL, Westermann CJ: Hereditary hemorrhagic telangiectasia: an update on transforming growth factor beta signaling in vasculogenesis and angiogenesis. Cardiovasc Res 2003;58:20.

135. Jaskolka J, Wu L, Chan RP, et al: Imaging of hereditary hemorrhagic telangiectasia. AJR Am J Roentgenol 2004;183:307.

136. Cottin V, Plauchu H, Bayle JY, et al: Pulmonary arteriovenous malformations in patients with hereditary hemorrhagic telangiectasia. Am J Respir Crit Care Med 2004;169:994.

137. Remy J, Remy-Jardin M, Giraud F, et al: Angioarchitecture of pulmonary arteriovenous malformations: clinical utility of three-dimensional helical CT. Radiology 1994;191:657.

138. White RI Jr, Pollak JS, Wirth JA: Pulmonary arteriovenous malformations: diagnosis and transcatheter embolotherapy. J Vasc Interv Radiol 1996;7:787.

139. Mager JJ, Overtoom TT, Blauw H, et al: Embolotherapy of pulmonary arteriovenous malformations: long-term results in 112 patients. J Vasc Interv Radiol 2004;15:451.

140. Prasad V, Chan RP, Faughnan ME: Embolotherapy of pulmonary arteriovenous malformations: efficacy of platinum versus stainless steel coils. J Vasc Interv Radiol 2004;15:153.

141. Remy J, Remy-Jardin M, Wattinne L, et al: Pulmonary arteriovenous malformations: evaluation with CT of the chest before and after treatment. Radiology 1992;182:809.

142. Belfiore G, Moggio G, Tedeschi E, et al: CT-guided radiofrequency ablation: a potential complementary therapy for patients with unresectable primary lung cancer—a preliminary report of 33 patients. AJR Am J Roentgenol 2004;183:1003.

143. Akeboshi M, Yamakado K, Nakatsuka A, et al: Percutaneous radiofrequency ablation of lung neoplasms: initial therapeutic response. J Vasc Interv Radiol 2004;15:463.

144. Yasui K, Kanazawa S, Sano Y, et al: Thoracic tumors treated with CT-guided radiofrequency ablation: initial experience. Radiology 2004;231:850.

145. King J, Glenn D, Clark W, et al: Percutaneous radiofrequency ablation of pulmonary metastases in patients with colorectal cancer. Br J Surg 2004;91:217.

146. Yi CA, Lee KS, Choe YH, et al: Computed tomography in pulmonary artery sarcoma: distinguishing features from pulmonary embolic disease. J Comput Assist Tomogr 2004;28:34.

147. Kaplinsky EJ, Favaloro RR, Pombo G, et al: Primary pulmonary artery sarcoma resembling chronic thromboembolic pulmonary disease. Eur Respir J 2000;16:1202.

148. Winchester PA, Khilnani NM, Trost DW, et al: Endovascular catheter biopsy of a pulmonary artery sarcoma. AJR Am J Roentgenol 1996; 167:657.

13

Lower Extremity Veins

■ DUPLEX SONOGRAPHY

Color Doppler sonography is the principal imaging tool used for evaluation of acute and chronic diseases of the lower extremity veins. The scanning protocol varies with the clinical situation (e.g., acute deep venous thrombosis versus venous insufficiency).

For detection of acute or chronic deep venous thrombosis, a high frequency linear transducer (5 to 10 MHz) with color Doppler capability is used. The patient is placed supine; the leg is externally rotated and the knee slightly flexed. Starting at the groin, the deep veins of the thigh are compressed in 1-cm increments with the transducer perpendicular to the vessel (Fig. 13-1). The popliteal vein is examined with the patient prone or in the lateral decubitus position. The study then is continued into the calf to assess the three paired tibial veins in the same fashion, preferably with the leg hanging over the examination table. Color Doppler imaging helps to identify the course of the veins and any luminal defects; Doppler waveform analysis is used to evaluate flow characteristics (see Fig 13-1).

Similar equipment is used for evaluation of patients with suspected chronic venous insufficiency or varicose veins. However, the study is performed with the patient standing and bearing weight on the opposite leg. The leg is slightly flexed at the knee. The great saphenous vein is interrogated from the groin to the level of the lowest varicosity.[1] The vein diameter is measured, and the location of tributaries feeding any varicosities is noted. Venous reflux is sought from the saphenofemoral junction through peripheral perforating veins with color imaging and Doppler waveform analysis following manual compression and release of calf veins (Fig. 13-2). The short saphenous vein and associated tributaries are examined from a posterior approach.

■ ASCENDING CONTRAST VENOGRAPHY

The patient lies on a tilting fluoroscopic table with the foot of the unaffected leg resting on a box to support the body. The affected leg does not bear weight in order to prevent muscular contraction and premature emptying of the calf veins during the procedure.

After tourniquets are wrapped around the ankle, a vein is chosen on the dorsum of the foot as peripheral and lateral as possible. Ultrasound may be used to identify an appropriate vessel. Superficial veins become more prominent when warm, damp towels are placed around the dependent foot. Edema can be relieved temporarily by placing an elastic wrap around the foot before venipuncture. The vein is cannulated with a 21- or 23-gauge butterfly needle or 22- to 24-gauge Angiocath. Once the needle is in place, a small volume of saline is injected to exclude extravasation.

Using leg tourniquets during venography is controversial. Some practitioners do not use tourniquets at all. Others prefer to place several around the ankle (and sometimes the lower thigh) to force contrast into the deep venous system. The table is tilted upright 45 to 75 degrees. Nonionic contrast material is injected manually at about 1 mL/second while the foot is inspected for extravasation.

As the contrast column is followed from the ankle to the groin, digital images are obtained in multiple projections (particularly in the calf). After the upper thigh is imaged, the patient is asked to compress the groin manually to slow venous outflow from the leg. The fluoroscopy table then is placed in a horizontal position, groin pressure is released, and the calf is gently squeezed to propel a bolus of contrast into the iliac veins and inferior vena cava for pelvic imaging.

Complications of ascending venography include contrast material reaction, contrast-induced nephropathy, local extravasation, and venous thrombosis (which occurs in less than 5% to 10% of cases).[2] Mild contrast extravasation can be managed with leg elevation and wet compresses. Large-volume extravasation should be evaluated by a surgeon.

■ ANATOMY

Normal Anatomy and Physiology

The leg is drained by superficial and deep venous systems. The deep veins, which are dominant, run alongside their corresponding arteries. The superficial veins are located in

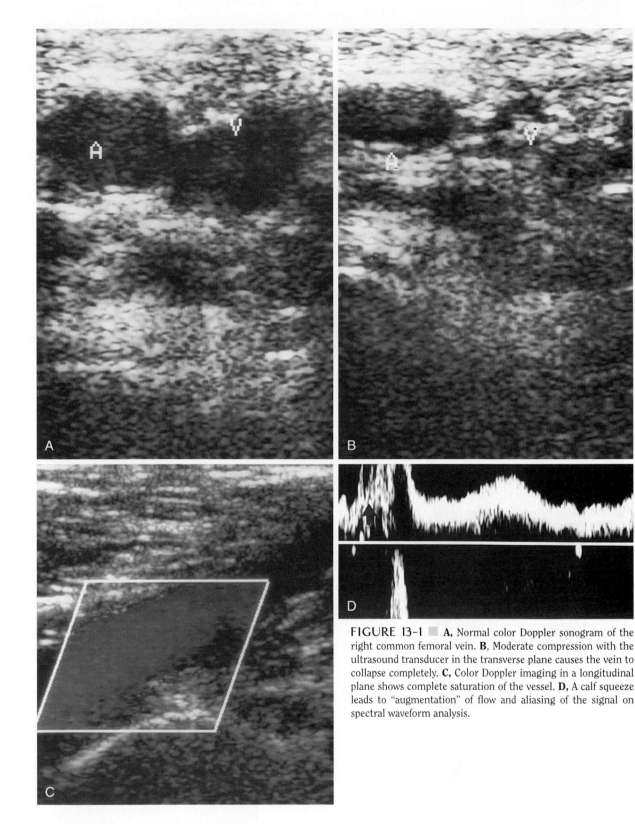

FIGURE 13-1 ■ **A,** Normal color Doppler sonogram of the right common femoral vein. **B,** Moderate compression with the ultrasound transducer in the transverse plane causes the vein to collapse completely. **C,** Color Doppler imaging in a longitudinal plane shows complete saturation of the vessel. **D,** A calf squeeze leads to "augmentation" of flow and aliasing of the signal on spectral waveform analysis.

the superficial fascia. A network of perforating veins connects these two venous beds.

In the foot, the deep plantar arch is formed by the plantar metatarsal veins.[3] The arch forms the medial and lateral plantar veins, which give off branches to the saphenous system and also contribute to formation of the tibial veins. The paired *posterior tibial, anterior tibial,* and *peroneal veins* form the deep system of the calf (Fig. 13-3). The tibial veins merge below the knee to form the *popliteal vein,* which is usually superficial to the popliteal artery. Multiple muscular *soleal* and *gastrocnemius veins* also drain into the tibial and popliteal veins. The popliteal vein becomes the *superficial femoral vein* (SFV) at the adductor canal (Fig 13-4). It runs posterolateral to the artery above the knee and then posteromedial to the artery

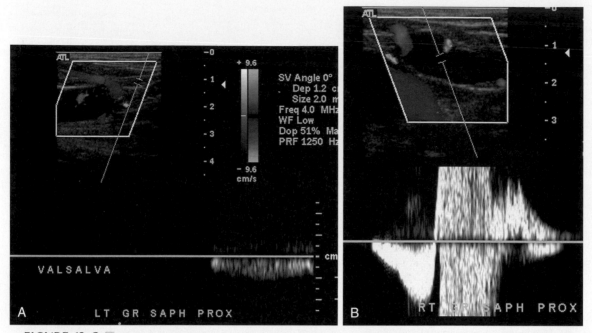

FIGURE 13-2 ■ Chronic venous reflux study by duplex sonography. **A,** With a calf squeeze there is forward flow but no retrograde flow in the left great saphenous vein. **B,** With a calf squeeze a burst of forward flow is followed by reversed flow greater than 0.5 seconds in duration in the right great saphenous vein, indicating venous reflux.

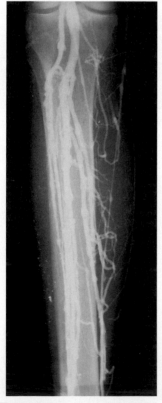

FIGURE 13-3 ■ Normal right lower extremity ascending venography. Three paired tibial veins follow the expected course of the tibial arteries.

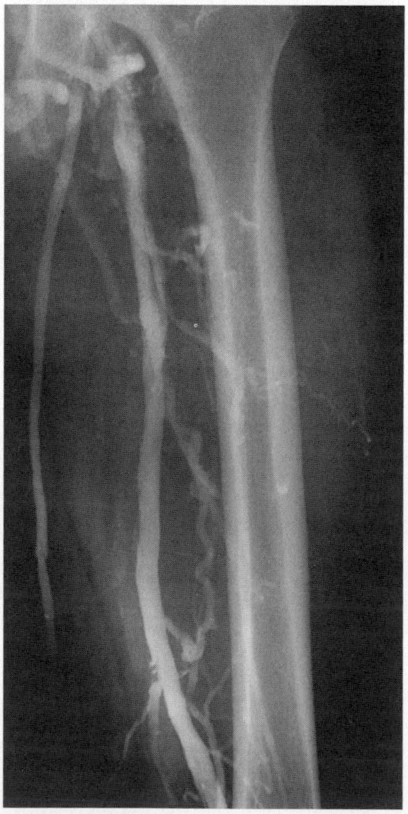

FIGURE 13-4 ■ Ascending venogram of the left leg shows the superficial femoral vein (laterally) and great saphenous vein (medially). They join at the saphenofemoral junction in the groin.

near the inguinal ligament. The *deep femoral vein* passes alongside the deep femoral artery and joins the SFV at a variable distance below the inguinal ligament.

The superficial venous system is composed of the *great (long) saphenous vein* (GSV) and the *small (short, lesser) saphenous vein* (SSV) and their numerous tributaries.[4] The GSV begins anterior to the medial malleolus. The vessel ascends along the medial aspect of the calf and thigh superficial to the muscular fascia (Fig. 13-5). It then passes through the saphenous opening of the deep fascia and enters the medial side of the superficial femoral vein (also receiving several pelvic venous tributaries) at the *saphenofemoral junction* (SFJ) (see Fig. 13-4). The SSV originates posterior to the lateral malleolus. It runs behind the heads of the gastrocnemius muscle bundles and, in most cases, joins the popliteal vein around the knee at the *saphenopopliteal junction* (SPJ). In about one third of the population, the SSV communicates with the GSV directly (via the vein of Giacomini) or through another tributary.[1]

Numerous *perforating (communicating) veins* connect the superficial and deep veins in the calf and thigh. The most important of these are the Hunterian perforator (mid-thigh), Dodd perforator (lower thigh), Boyd perforator (around the knee), and Cockett perforator (calf). Bicuspid valves are present throughout the superficial, perforating, and deep veins of the leg up to the common femoral vein. They are oriented to direct blood from the superficial to the deep system.

At the inguinal ligament, the *common femoral vein* becomes the *external iliac vein*, which runs medial to the iliac artery (Fig. 13-6). Its tributaries include the pubic, deep circumflex iliac, and inferior epigastric veins. The external iliac vein courses over the pelvic brim to the level of the sacroiliac joint, where it joins the *internal iliac vein* to form the *common iliac vein*. The right common iliac vein is first posterior and then lateral to the iliac artery. The left common iliac vein has a more horizontal course and lies between the right common iliac artery and the spine. Mild extrinsic compression normally may be present at this site (see Fig. 13-6). *Ascending lumbar veins* arise from the upper surface of the common iliac veins. The iliac veins merge at the L4-L5 level to form the *inferior vena cava* (IVC).

The essential elements required for normal blood return from the leg against substantial hydrodynamic resistance are an intact muscular pump, competent valves, and unobstructed outflow. Although the walls of the superficial and muscular leg veins contain smooth muscle and are capable of constriction, blood return depends largely on extrinsic compression by leg muscles, particularly the "calf pump." At rest, blood flows from the superficial system into the deep veins. Competent valves prevent retrograde flow. With muscular contraction, blood is propelled centrally by forceful emptying of the deep veins.

Variant Anatomy

Duplication of segments of the lower extremity veins is common. Accessory saphenous veins (which run in the extrafascial compartment) are described in 20% to 35% of the general population.[5,6] Duplicated or multiple superficial femoral or popliteal veins are reported in about one third of cases (Fig. 13-7).[7] However, some studies suggest that these figures are exaggerated.[8]

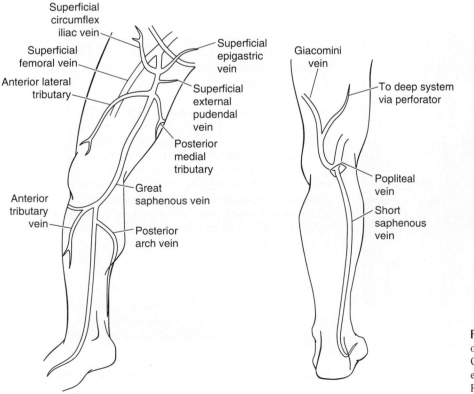

FIGURE 13-5 ■ Superficial venous system of the leg. (Adapted from Min RJ, Khilnani NM, Golia P: Duplex ultrasound evaluation of lower extremity venous insufficiency. J Vasc Interv Radiol 2003;14:1233.)

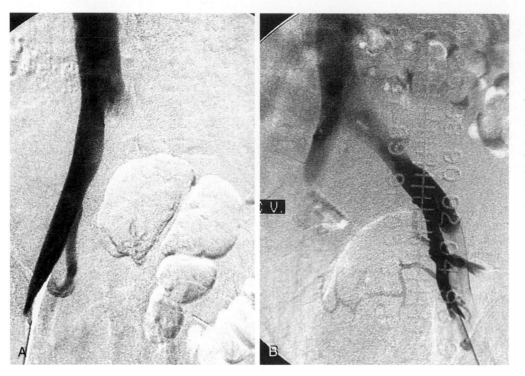

FIGURE 13-6 ■ Normal right (**A**) and left (**B**) pelvic venograms. Retrograde flow is seen in both internal iliac veins, as is apparent narrowing of the right external iliac vein above the catheter tip due to coaptation of vein walls from the high-pressure fluid jet (i.e., Venturi effect). Diminished contrast density at the junction of the left common iliac vein and inferior vena cava is caused by mild extrinsic compression between the right common iliac artery and spine. Lucency in the left external iliac vein results from unopacified blood entering the vessel.

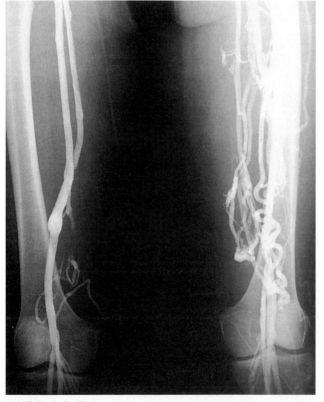

FIGURE 13-7 ■ Partial duplication of the right superficial femoral vein. Also note acute left deep venous thrombosis superimposed on chronic disease. Numerous deep collaterals bypass a chronically occluded left superficial femoral vein.

Klippel-Trénaunay syndrome is a rare congenital disorder that features markedly abnormal lower extremity veins (varicosities and venous malformations), bone and soft tissue enlargement, and cutaneous hemangiomas.[9-11] When accompanied by arteriovenous malformations, it is called *Klippel-Trénaunay-Weber* syndrome or simply *Parkes Weber syndrome*. There is some evidence that the disease results from genetic mutations in the angiogenic protein VG5Q.[12] Plain films show limb hypertrophy, phleboliths, and, occasionally, other osseous abnormalities (Fig. 13-8). Sonography and MR venography are useful in mapping the bizarre, disordered venous channels.[13] Sonographic studies have identified deep veins in almost all patients, challenging the traditional belief that hypoplasia or aplasia of the deep venous system is a central feature of this disorder. A large superficial vein may be identified on the lateral aspect of the thigh. Sclerotherapy and embolotherapy are used to treat the abnormal venous channels and arteriovenous malformations associated with this syndrome. Surgery is reserved for patients with functional disabilities or severe bleeding or ulcerations.[14]

Persistent sciatic vein is a very rare congenital anomaly in which a remnant of the embryologic vessel serves as the primary venous drainage between the adductor canal and the internal iliac vein.[15] The vein is markedly dilated and tortuous. The disorder may be an isolated condition but often is associated with Klippel-Trénaunay syndrome.

Collateral Circulation

When superficial or deep veins become occluded, the companion system operates as the main collateral pathway

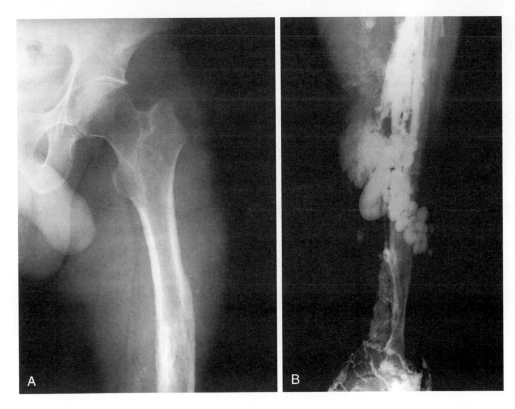

FIGURE 13-8 ◾ Klippel-Trénaunay syndrome. **A,** Plain radiograph shows massive limb enlargement, sclerotic changes in the middle left femur, and phleboliths. **B,** Bizarre, dilated venous collaterals fill on an ascending venogram in place of a normal deep venous system.

(see Fig. 13-7). With partial or total iliac vein obstruction, transpelvic and ascending lumbar veins serve as the chief collateral channels (Fig. 13-9).

◾ MAJOR DISORDERS

Acute Deep Venous Thrombosis

Etiology and Natural History

Acute lower extremity deep venous thrombosis (DVT) is part of the spectrum of *venous thromboembolic disease*, which also includes pulmonary embolism and *chronic venous insufficiency* (CVI, sometimes called *postthrombotic* or *postphlebitic syndrome*).[16,17] Acute DVT is a common disorder, with an overall lifetime risk of about 2% to 5%.[18]

In the normal population, thrombi frequently form in the valve sinuses of the muscular calf veins. The endogenous fibrinolytic system usually dissolves these small clots. Thrombus remains confined to the calf veins in about 75% of untreated patients.[19] The risk of symptomatic pulmonary embolism in this situation is low.[20] In the remaining cases, thrombus extends to the "proximal" (femoropopliteal) veins. Most of these patients have one or more predisposing factors to clot formation, such as sluggish blood flow, vessel injury, or hypercoagulability (i.e., *Virchow's triad*) (see Box 12-3).[21] In the legs, DVT is seen most frequently with surgery, prolonged immobilization, malignancy, prior venous thrombosis, or a thrombophilic disorder (see Box 3-5). Iliac vein thrombosis usually results from further propagation of femoropopliteal vein clot. Isolated *iliofemoral venous*

thrombosis accounts for no more than 20% of cases of lower extremity DVT and usually can be attributed to local factors (Fig. 13-10 and Box 13-1). Left iliac vein compression (May-Thurner) syndrome frequently is responsible for left-sided iliofemoral thrombosis (see below).

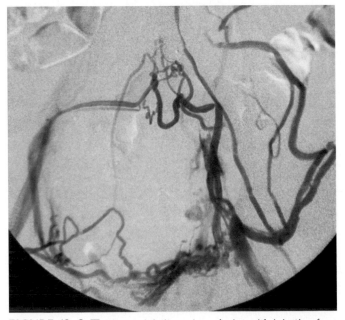

FIGURE 13-9 ◾ Chronic left iliac vein occlusion with injection from the left common femoral vein. Transpelvic and circumflex iliac venous collaterals drain the leg.

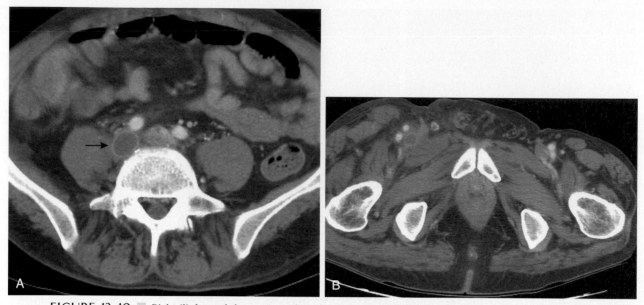

FIGURE 13-10 ■ Right iliofemoral deep venous thrombosis *(arrow)* caused by posttraumatic right thigh and groin hematoma. Contrast-enhanced CT scans through the upper pelvis (**A**) and inguinal region (**B**). The more peripheral veins were normal.

In a minority of patients, extensive peripheral and iliofemoral thrombosis occurs, leading to an edematous, painful white leg *(phlegmasia alba dolens)*. If obstruction of collateral channels ensues, venous drainage is almost completely blocked and the patient presents with a markedly swollen, painful cyanotic leg, sometimes with diminished arterial pulses *(phlegmasia cerulea dolens)*.[22] This grave condition (which requires immediate intervention) may lead to *venous gangrene*, massive pulmonary embolism, or death.

The true incidence of pulmonary embolism after an episode of acute lower extremity DVT is unknown. However, the risk is considerably greater with thrombus in proximal veins and may approach 35% to 50% in untreated patients.[21,23] Valvular incompetence (the precursor to CVI) is a late sequela of acute lower extremity DVT in up to two thirds of cases.[24]

Clinical Features

The symptoms and signs of lower extremity DVT are notoriously unreliable. Many patients (particularly in the postoperative setting) with proven DVT are asymptomatic, and many others with classic features do not have the disease. Patients may complain of the acute onset of leg pain, swelling, or tenderness. Less common signs include distention of superficial veins, cyanosis, erythema, palpable calf cords, or Homans' sign (calf pain with forced dorsiflexion of the foot). Pulmonary embolism can be the first indicator of acute DVT. When isolated iliofemoral DVT occurs, symptoms initially may be confined to the pelvis and thigh. Iliofemoral DVT occurs more frequently in the left leg than the right and more frequently in women than men.

Diagnostic Tests

Acute lower extremity DVT is a common disease. Clinical features often are misleading, and the consequences of a missed diagnosis and withheld treatment can be life threatening. For these reasons, screening of high-risk asymptomatic patients and accurate diagnosis of symptomatic patients is critical and must depend on objective diagnostic tests or imaging studies. Although clinical signs and symptoms alone are inaccurate, a combined assessment of physical findings and risk factors may help determine how aggressively one should pursue the diagnosis (Box 13-2)

D-dimer Test. D-dimer is a byproduct of endogenous fibrin degradation, and plasma levels are elevated in patients with venous thrombosis or pulmonary embolism. The D-dimer radioimmunoassay has been useful in excluding the disease, particularly in conjunction with risk factor analysis.[18,25] Although the test is very sensitive, its specificity can be extremely low.[18,26]

BOX 13-1 ■ **Causes of Isolated Pelvic Vein Thrombosis**

Iliac vein compression (May-Thurner) syndrome
Malignancy
Pregnancy
Surgery
Prior iliocaval deep venous thrombosis
Inferior vena cava filter
Indwelling catheter
Hypercoagulable disorder
Trauma
  Accidental
  Iatrogenic (e.g., prior catheterization)
Benign extrinsic compression
  Retroperitoneal fibrosis
Radiation therapy

Impedance Plethysmography. Impedance plethysmography (IPG) has been touted widely for the evaluation of patients at risk for or suspected to have lower extremity DVT. A blood pressure cuff is placed around the thigh. Inflation of the cuff increases the blood volume in the calf, which is measured as reduced impedance between two calf electrodes. In a patient with normal central veins, rapid outflow of blood with deflation of the cuff is accompanied by increased impedance between the electrodes. With downstream venous obstruction, the impedance pattern is altered. Less blood accumulates in the calf when the cuff is inflated, and blood loss from the calf is sluggish when the cuff is deflated. IPG generally does not detect calf thrombi or nonocclusive proximal clots. In symptomatic patients, the sensitivity of the test for detecting **proximal** DVT is reported to be 85% to 95% in some series.[16,27] However, the sensitivity is much lower in asymptomatic populations.[28,29]

Imaging

Sonography. Because duplex sonography is extremely accurate, easy to perform, relatively inexpensive, and completely safe, it is the principal imaging study in both symptomatic and asymptomatic groups. Several factors are evaluated[30]:

- *Compressibility.* Moderate compression of a normal vein with the ultrasound transducer in the **transverse** plane completely coapts the vein walls (see Fig. 13-1). The lumen of a clot-filled vein is incompressible or barely so (Fig. 13-11). This finding is the cardinal sign of acute DVT.

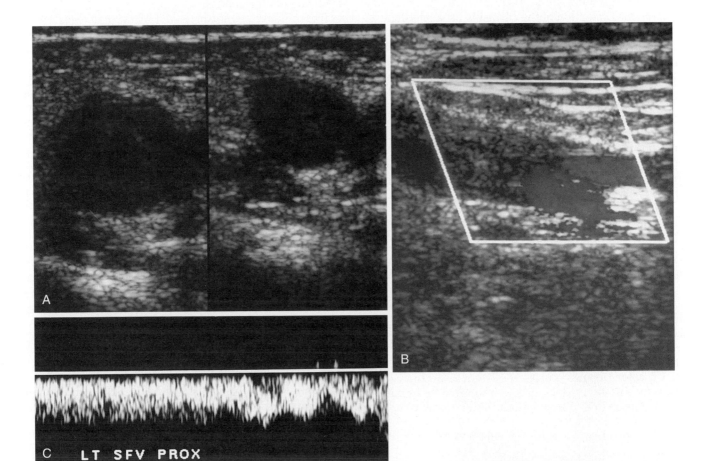

FIGURE 13-11 ▪ Acute left common femoral vein thrombosis. **A,** The vein is enlarged *(left).* There is minimal deformity of the vein with compression *(right).* **B,** Color saturation ends at the lower end of the common femoral vein. **C,** A relatively flat spectral tracing in the superficial femoral vein is further evidence of a more central obstruction. The tracing remained flat with the Valsalva maneuver.

As a rule, acute thrombus also causes venous distention, whereas chronic disease leads to vein contraction. Most of the deep veins of the leg (up to the common femoral vein) are accessible to transducer compression. This sign is less useful at relative blind spots (e.g., superficial femoral vein at the adductor canal in some patients) and inaccessible sites (e.g., overlying hematoma or bandage).

■ *Color flow saturation.* The deep veins are examined in the longitudinal plane with color Doppler imaging.[30-32] DVT can be excluded when there is complete saturation of the entire deep venous system (see Fig. 13-1). Absence of color flow and nonocclusive filling defects are signs of thrombus (see Fig. 13-11).

■ *Phasicity.* Doppler flow in the upper leg veins shows phasic variation with respiration: decreased flow with inspiration and increased flow with expiration. A monotonous waveform may be a sign of obstruction somewhere between the sampled vein and the heart (see Fig. 13-11).

■ *Provocative maneuvers.* Flow in the femoral vein normally increases with calf compression (i.e., augmentation) and decreases with the Valsalva maneuver (see Fig. 13-1). An abnormal response to these measures should raise the suspicion of obstruction peripheral or central to the femoral vein, respectively.

■ *Thrombus echogenicity.* The presence or absence of echogenic material within the lumen is **not** a reliable sign of the presence or age of DVT.

■ *Calf veins.* Evaluation of the calf veins usually is done with color Doppler imaging. Longitudinal color flow saturation in the three paired deep tibial veins (and gastrocnemius and soleal branches when visible) and coaptation of vein walls with transverse compression can exclude thrombus. Often it is difficult to visualize the anterior tibial veins.

■ *Saphenous vein.* The risk of significant pulmonary embolism from isolated saphenous vein clot is unknown. However, upper saphenous vein clot frequently propagates into the femoral vein, and thrombus extension into the iliofemoral system with subsequent pulmonary embolism can occur.[33]

■ *Ancillary findings.* Sonography detects other causes for leg symptoms, such as a Baker's cyst, lymphadenopathy, hematoma, or popliteal artery aneurysm.

In *symptomatic* patients, compression and color Doppler sonography are about as accurate as contrast venography in the diagnosis of acute proximal DVT, with a sensitivity of greater than 95% and specificity of greater than 98%.[30-32,34] Outcome analysis of a large cohort of patients with suspected DVT estimated the negative predictive value of a normal compression sonogram as greater than 99.5%.[35]

In screening of *asymptomatic* patients with risk factors for DVT, color Doppler sonography is not as accurate. The reasons for this discrepancy largely are related to the nature of the occlusion in this setting (localization to calf veins and presence of smaller, nonocclusive, segmental thrombi).[30] Misdiagnosis may occur for several reasons[36]:

■ Underlying chronic venous disease
■ Isolated clot in the iliac vein, calf veins, deep femoral vein, or one limb of a duplicated femoral or popliteal vein
■ Technical errors

TABLE 13-1	SONOGRAPHIC DISTINCTION BETWEEN ACUTE AND CHRONIC DEEP VENOUS THROMBOSIS (DVT)

Feature	Acute DVT	Chronic DVT
Lumen	Dilated	Narrowed or normal caliber
Luminal flow	Absent or minimal	Residual flow, reflux
Vein wall	Thin	Thickened
Collaterals	Poorly developed	Well developed
Compression resistance	Spongy	Firm

Acute and chronic DVT can be confused at sonography. Certain features are used to differentiate between these entities (Table 13-1).[30,36] Sometimes, however, it is impossible to distinguish among an acute clot in a previously normal vein, a chronic organized clot, and acute clot superimposed on chronic disease (Fig 13-12). It is for this reason that some experts recommend follow-up sonograms as a baseline study for all patients with acute DVT in the event that symptoms recur. Contrast venography occasionally is helpful in sorting out difficult cases (see below). Recently, scintigraphic imaging with the ^{99m}Tc platelet glycoprotein IIb/IIIa receptor antagonist *apcitide* (which only binds to fresh thrombus) has shown promise in distinguishing between fresh and old thrombus.[37]

The clinical significance of isolated *calf vein* DVT is controversial.[23,38,39] Compression sonography and color Doppler flow imaging are fairly accurate in detecting calf vein clot.[40-42] In some series, the sensitivity of color Doppler sonography is comparable in the calf veins and proximal veins. But, in routine practice, technically inadequate studies of the calf are relatively common.[32,43] Some practitioners opt to obtain serial examinations of the proximal veins to detect propagation of clot into the femoropopliteal system.

Computed Tomography. While CT venography of the lower extremities is feasible and relatively accurate, it is rarely employed by itself in routine cases. Some centers advocate combined CT venography and CT pulmonary angiography in patients with suspected venous thromboembolic disease.[44] CT venography is more accurate than sonography in the pelvic veins and IVC.[45,46] Typical findings include luminal filling defect, vein wall enhancement, and filling of collateral veins (see Fig 13-10).[46,47] Incomplete opacification of the vein and beam-hardening artifacts can mimic intraluminal clot.

Magnetic Resonance Imaging. The accuracy of MR venography in the diagnosis of DVT in the leg is similar to contrast venography and duplex sonography.[48-52] However, an MR examination is more costly and time consuming than a sonogram. MR is superior to ascending venography and sonography for pelvic vein and IVC thrombus (Fig. 13-13).

Ascending Venography. Although contrast venography was once considered the gold standard in the diagnosis of acute and chronic DVT, it is not always reliable.[53] One autopsy study revealed a sensitivity and specificity of 89% and 97%, respectively.[54] Interobserver variability is about

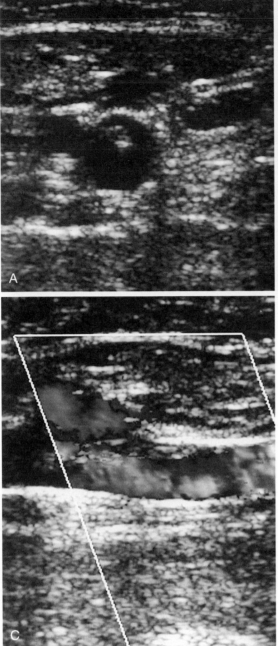

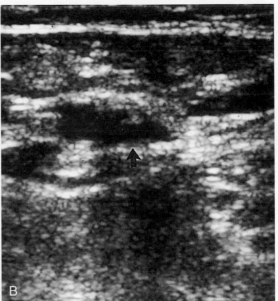

FIGURE 13-12 ▪ Chronic deep venous thrombosis detected by sonography. **A,** The right common femoral vein has internal echoes along its anterior aspect. **B,** There is incomplete compression of the vein *(arrow)*. **C,** Longitudinal color Doppler image shows narrowing of the lumen and thickening of the vein wall.

10% to 15%.[55] The procedure is uncomfortable for the patient, and it has a small risk of significant complications. For these reasons, it rarely is used for diagnosis except to distinguish acute from chronic disease when less invasive studies are equivocal.

A fresh clot produces an intraluminal, wormlike filling defect (Fig. 13-14). Several projections of the calf veins may be required to detect thrombi accurately in this location. Abrupt occlusion of a vein can reflect acute or chronic thrombosis (see Fig. 13-7). Nonfilling of deep veins, preferential filling of superficial veins, and opacification of collateral veins may occur with acute or chronic DVT. Clot may be confused with other causes for nonfilling of parts of the deep venous system (Box 13-3; see also Fig. 13-6).

Imaging Strategy

Every physician must develop his or her own algorithm for assessing symptomatic and high-risk patients for acute DVT using a combination of risk-factor analysis, lab testing (D-dimer), duplex sonography, and other imaging studies. Periodic surveillance of at-risk populations has uncovered lower extremity DVT in up to 28% of patients, about 80% of whom were asymptomatic.[56-58] Many centers perform follow-up exams after a normal ultrasound in all cases or at least in those with moderate to high clinical probability of disease. However, only 1% to 2% of patients with initially negative studies subsequently are shown to have developed proximal DVT.[59,60] D-dimer results (if they have been validated for

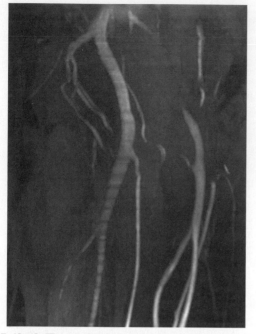

FIGURE 13-13 ■ Chronic left common and external iliac vein thrombosis on oblique sagittal gadolium-enhanced MR venogram.

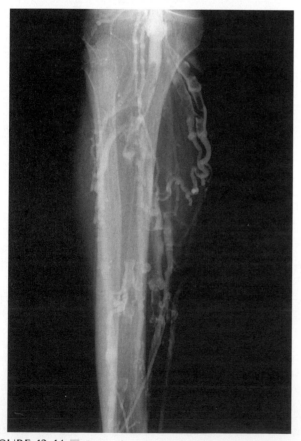

FIGURE 13-14 ■ Acute thrombosis of tibial, gastrocnemius, and popliteal veins.

diagnosis in this setting) may be used to withhold ultrasound in patients with low clinical probability or to guide follow-up imaging.[30] A late follow-up study after completion of treatment may be valuable in higher-risk patients in the event that symptoms recur in order to distinguish chronic disease from recurrent acute DVT.

Treatment

Patients with acute DVT are treated to relieve symptoms and to prevent or limit the major sequelae of venous thrombosis: pulmonary embolism, CVI, and recurrent DVT.[23,61]

Medical Therapy. The cornerstone of treatment is anticoagulation. Anticoagulation does not directly promote fibrinolysis, but it allows endogenous lysis to occur and reduces the likelihood of pulmonary embolism by limiting clot propagation. If there is a contraindication to or complication from anticoagulation, an IVC filter should be placed instead (see Chapter 14). For many decades, treatment for DVT consisted of unfractionated intravenous heparin (3 to 5 days) and oral warfarin (at least 3 to 6 months).[23] Now, the standard therapy for acute DVT (or prophylaxis of DVT) is low-molecular-weight (LMW) heparin (e.g., enoxaparin, tinzaparin), which has a more predictable response, longer duration of action, and can be given at home once or twice daily as a subcutaneous injection (see Chapter 2). Monitoring of drug levels is unnecessary except in certain situations (e.g., obesity, pregnancy, heart or liver failure).

Therapeutic anticoagulation substantially reduces the likelihood of pulmonary embolism. However, recurrent DVT still occurs in up to 25% of cases, and up to 50% of patients can still develop CVI (see below).[61-63]

Treatment of isolated calf vein DVT is controversial, because there is a 20% to 30% risk of clot propagation, a small risk of significant pulmonary embolism, and about a 30% risk of CVI.[58,61-64] Short-term anticoagulation probably is warranted in most patients. Those not treated should undergo follow-up Doppler sonography to exclude clot propagation.

Endovascular Therapy. The rationale for using aggressive measures to remove clot directly is rapid relief of symptoms and prevention of CVI and recurrent DVT in patients with proximal acute disease. There is ample evidence that the likelihood of retaining normal valve function largely is related to the speed with which the thrombus is cleared.[65,66]

The frequency of chronic obstruction and valve dysfunction may be reduced with **systemic** thrombolysis, but bleeding complications can be significant.[67-69] Catheter-directed thrombolysis with or without adjunctive mechanical thrombectomy offers the possibility of faster and safer treatment for acute *iliofemoral thrombosis*.[70-72] However, because the long-term benefit of this approach has not been firmly established, careful patient selection is important (Box 13-4).

■ Patients with subacute or chronic venous thrombosis (>2 to 4 weeks) generally do not benefit from thrombolysis and should be treated directly with angioplasty and stent placement (Fig. 13-15).

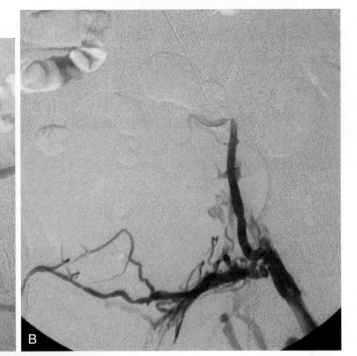
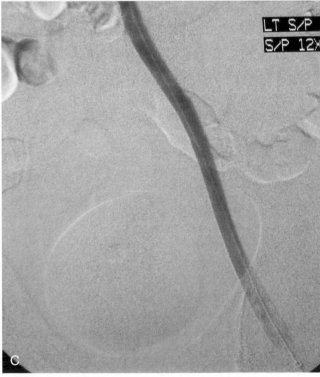

FIGURE 13-15 ■ Chronic iliac vein venous thrombosis unresponsive to thrombolysis (same patient as Figure 13-9). **A,** After overnight infusion with tissue plasminogen activator, some lysis is noted. **B,** After about 48 hours of thrombolytic infusion, persistent occlusion is noted. **C,** Following angioplasty and Wallstent placement, the vein is widely patent.

- Most interventionalists do not place prophylactic IVC filters before thrombolysis unless the consequence of even small pulmonary emboli is great or large free-floating iliac or IVC clot is found.
- Single, dual, or triple access through the right internal jugular, popliteal, or femoral vein is used (Fig. 13-16). Calf veins can be accessed, if necessary, through direct ultrasound-guided posterior tibial, soleal, or retrograde popliteal vein puncture.
- After determining the extent of thrombosis, the occlusion is crossed with a guidewire, and catheters with multiple side holes are placed. Anticoagulation with heparin is initiated. Thrombolysis alone often requires large doses of a fibrinolytic agent and 2 to 3 days of infusion.[71,73-81]
- Recanalization often is incomplete when enzymatic lysis or mechanical thrombectomy devices (MTD) are used alone (see Chapter 2). MTD may be used initially to reduce the clot burden or to remove residual clots after enzymatic lysis. A variety of devices has been used off-label for this purpose. Care should be taken to limit vein wall or valve damage by avoiding retrograde passage through veins.
- After most of the clot has been removed, balloon angioplasty and self-expandable stent placement (as needed in the iliac veins) are performed to treat residual disease.
- Following the procedure, patients are maintained on aggressive anticoagulation for 6 months to 1 year (or indefinitely if a thrombophilic disorder is identified).

Technical success is achieved in about 80% to 95% of cases when the disease is acute. Bleeding complications occurred in 10% of cases in a multi-institution series.[71] The likelihood of long-term improvement or resolution of symptoms has not been established. In some studies, 1-year patency is reported to be about 90%.[75,76]

Surgical Therapy. Endovascular methods largely have replaced open operative thrombectomy procedures unless venous gangrene is imminent. Operative techniques for treating iliofemoral DVT include Fogarty embolectomy, thrombectomy, and venovenous bypass. Occasionally, a temporary distal arteriovenous fistula is constructed to improve flow through the newly recanalized vessels.[82]

Varicose Veins and Primary Venous Insufficiency

Etiology and Natural History

Lower extremity venous insufficiency manifested by telangiectasias and varicose veins afflicts 15% of men and 25% of women in the United States.[1] In most individuals, the cause is *primary* incompetence of the superficial venous valves of the legs unrelated to prior DVT. In a minority of cases, obstruction and valve incompetence in the deep veins is responsible. The most common pattern is SFJ incompetence with GSV reflux; less often, reflux at the SPJ into the SSV is found. Primary superficial venous incompetence can progress to chronic venous insufficiency with associated skin changes, although many of those patients have chronic deep vein disease (see below).

The underlying cause for the disorder is unknown, although varicose veins are more common in some families, in women, and with advancing age.[83] Regardless of the etiology of valve dysfunction, both hydrostatic forces (column of blood acting unopposed on superficial veins) and hydrodynamic ones (calf muscle pump acting on subcutaneous veins in the absence of functional perforating valves) are responsible for the disease. Insufficiency of perforating veins also may be secondary to increased flow from superficial vein insufficiency rather than primary incompetence.[1]

Clinical Features

The obvious visual signs of the disease are small telangiectasias, reticular varicosities, and large varicose veins. Patients also may complain of leg aching, pain, or "heaviness." Symptoms become worse with prolonged standing and at the beginning of the menstrual period. In a minority of cases, chronic skin changes develop (see below).

Imaging

Duplex Sonography. Ultrasound is the primary modality for assessing patients with superficial venous incompetence and associated symptoms.[1] Marked enlargement of the GSV (>4 mm) or SSV (>3 mm) is noted. At the level of major valves, prolonged reversal of flow (>0.5 seconds) is observed with Doppler waveform analysis after manual compression of distal venous beds (see Fig. 13-2). Reflux in the main channels is traced to the level of incompetent tributaries and superficial varicosities. In particular, the anteriolateral and posteriomedial channels should be assessed. Even following saphenous vein ligation, one may identify persistent refluxing segments of the GSV or enlarged major tributaries. The most common patterns are SFJ insufficiency and GSV reflux, insufficiency of the Hunterian perforator with lower GSV reflux, external pudendal vein reflux leading to GSV reflux, and incompetence of the vein of Giacomini leading to GSV and SSV reflux.

Treatment

Surgical Therapy. For many years, the standard treatment for superficial venous insufficiency was high ligation of the saphenous vein and local treatment of varicosities. Unfortunately, patients often develop recurrent symptoms after this procedure. Saphenous vein stripping (usually above the knee) combined with stab avulsion or sclerotherapy of varicosities is more likely to lead to permanent elimination of hydrodynamic and hydrostatic forces causing the deformities.

Endovascular Therapy. Recently, endovascular techniques have become popular in treatment of this common disorder. Two methods have emerged as alternatives to surgery for obliteration of the GSV. Radiofrequency (RF) thermal ablation of the saphenous vein has a high degree of success and durability, though it is associated with a small risk of skin burns, nerve injury, or thrombophlebitis.[84,85]

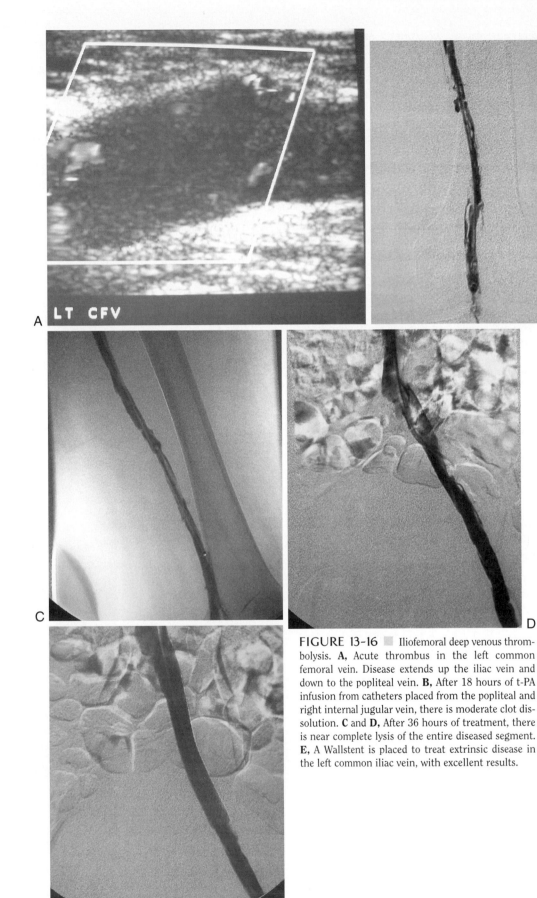

FIGURE 13-16 ■ Iliofemoral deep venous thrombolysis. **A,** Acute thrombus in the left common
femoral vein. Disease extends up the iliac vein and
down to the popliteal vein. **B,** After 18 hours of t-PA
infusion from catheters placed from the popliteal and
right internal jugular vein, there is moderate clot dissolution. **C** and **D,** After 36 hours of treatment, there
is near complete lysis of the entire diseased segment.
E, A Wallstent is placed to treat extrinsic disease in
the left common iliac vein, with excellent results.

Some practitioners now favor *endovenous laser therapy* followed by compression sclerotherapy for this condition. Laser energy heats the vein and causes wall thickening with eventual fibrosis of the vessel. Patients with DVT, tortuous GSV, or inability to walk should **not** be treated in this way.[86]

After ultrasound interrogation of the entire great saphenous vein, access is gained to the GSV around the knee. An 810 or 940 nanometer wavelength laser device is inserted through a guiding sheath, which has been advanced to the SFJ. Using ultrasound guidance and multiple injections, 60 to 120 mL of 0.2% lidocaine with bicarbonate is applied along the entire extravascular course of the GSV ("tumescent anesthesia"). In addition to providing pain relief, this important step compresses the vein wall around the laser tip and creates a "heat-sink" that protects surrounding vital structures. The exposed activated tip of the device and guiding sheath then are slowly withdrawn through the length of the vein. Peripheral varicose tributaries are treated locally by sclerotherapy. Patients are asked to wear a fitted support stocking for 1 week after the procedure.

Early results are extremely promising, with over 90% persistent obliteration at 2-year follow-up.[86,87] Local complications seem to occur less frequently than with RF ablation, particularly when lower energy laser devices are used.

Chronic Venous Insufficiency

Etiology and Natural History

Once acute DVT occurs, the fate of the thrombus is variable[88]:

- Embolization
- Complete clot resolution
- Incomplete clot resolution
- Persistent occlusion

If the clot does not embolize, it becomes attached to the vein wall within several weeks. If endogenous fibrinolysis occurs at all, it begins in the center of the lumen. Over time, the clot may lyse completely and leave intact vein walls and relatively normal valves. If clot resolution is incomplete, the result is residual vein wall thickening, an irregular intraluminal channel, and incompetence of deep and perforating vein valves (see Fig. 13-12).

Chronically diseased veins remain in one half to two thirds of patients with iliofemoral DVT.[88-90] The unifying feature of symptomatic CVI is *venous hypertension*. In most cases, it is caused by incompetent valves and abnormal reflux of blood from the deep to the superficial venous system.[91] Less often, venous hypertension is the result of central outflow obstruction (e.g., iliac vein occlusion) or, rarely, inadequate function of the calf pump (e.g., paralyzed patients).

The pathophysiology of CVI has been postulated but not proven. Venous hypertension leads to trapping of white blood cells in subcutaneous capillaries.[92] Capillaries are damaged, and leakage of fibrinogen produces a "fibrin cuff" that contributes to the classic skin changes associated with the disease (see below). Fibrin accumulation and edema in subcutaneous tissue ultimately causes local hypoxia, inflammation, and tissue loss.

Clinical Features

Symptoms usually develop months to many years after the acute episode.[93] Some patients give no history of acute DVT. Early signs of CVI include leg "heaviness" or aching and skin thickening, edema, and erythema, particularly around the medial malleolus. These abnormalities may progress to skin induration and hyperpigmentation *(lipodermatosclerosis)*. In the late stages, the skin becomes fibrotic and venous ulcers develop. When caused by prior thrombotic disease, the symptoms often are unilateral. When caused by primary valve dysfunction, the symptoms usually are bilateral.

Imaging

Imaging is important in the management of patients with chronic lower extremity venous disease. The most important questions to address are patency of the deep venous system, valvular incompetence in superficial, deep, and perforating veins, the extent of reflux, and the exact site(s) of incompetent veins.

Sonography. Color Doppler sonography is the standard tool for studying patients with CVI when invasive therapy is

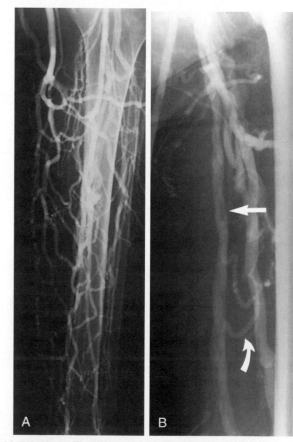

FIGURE 13-17 ▪ Chronic lower extremity deep venous thrombosis. **A,** Deep veins of the calf remain completely occluded, and venous drainage is entirely through superficial channels. **B,** Recanalization of a previously occluded left superficial femoral vein. The vein is irregular, contains several webs *(straight arrow)*, is devoid of normal appearing valves, and communicates with the deep femoral vein *(curved arrow)*.

being considered.[94,95] With the aid of provocative measures (e.g., compression of calf veins, Valsalva maneuver), venous reflux, valvular dysfunction, and incompetent perforating veins are detected and mapped (see above). Sonography also identifies persistently occluded or partially recanalized deep veins.

CT and MR Imaging. CT or MR venography can be a useful adjunct to duplex sonography, particularly in the evaluation of chronic pelvic venous disease.

Contrast Venography. Ascending venography rarely is needed in this setting. The appearance of chronic DVT can vary from recanalized veins with narrow, irregular, web-filled lumens, distorted valves, and incompetent perforators to nonopacification of deep veins with preferential filling of superficial veins and collateral channels (Figs. 13-17 and 13-18; see also Figs. 3-47 and 13-7).

Treatment

Medical Therapy. The mainstay of therapy for CVI is leg elevation, exercise, and compressive stockings.

Endovascular Therapy. Patients with CVI primarily due to venous outflow obstruction may benefit from endovascular treatment, particularly when disease is confined to the iliocaval segment.[96,97] Fibrinolysis and mechanical devices generally have no role in this situation. The obstruction is crossed with a guidewire from the internal jugular, ipsilateral, or contralateral femoral vein. After starting a heparin infusion,

angioplasty is performed, followed by placement of self-expanding stents (see Fig. 13-15). Endovascular recanalization of chronic femoropopliteal disease is generally not durable.

Surgical Therapy. CVI from deep vein incompetence can be treated with vein transplant (if caused by chronic DVT) or with closed external valvuloplasty of the deep thigh veins. Iliac vein obstruction can be managed with a femorofemoral vein crossover graft (Dale-Palma procedure).[98]

Iliofemoral Venous Stenoses

Etiology

Clinically significant stenoses of the lower extremity veins are uncommon. Obstructions usually develop at sites of extrinsic compression or intimal injury (Box 13-5). Most symptomatic stenoses are found in the iliac veins. Some of these patients suffer from pelvic (especially gynecologic) malignancies and have undergone local treatment with surgery or irradiation.

Mild narrowing of the upper left common iliac vein as it passes between the right common iliac artery and the spine is a frequent finding in the normal population (see Fig. 13-6). Severe compression may lead to *iliac vein compression (May-Thurner* or *Cockett) syndrome* (Fig. 13-19)[99-101] In this disorder, the venous intima has been injured from

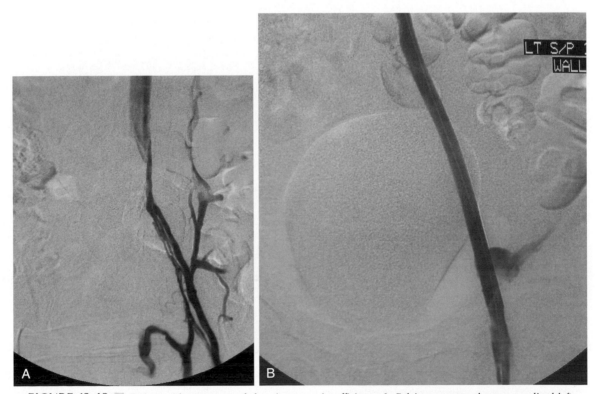

FIGURE 13-18 ■ Patient with symptoms of chronic venous insufficiency. **A,** Pelvic venogram shows recanalized left external and common iliac veins and lower inferior vena cava with luminal irregularity. Ascending lumbar venous collaterals also are present. **B,** After angioplasty with a 10-mm balloon and placement of a 14-mm diameter Wallstent, the vein is widely patent.

BOX 13-5 ▓ **Causes of Iliofemoral Vein Narrowing**

Iliac vein compression (May-Thurner) syndrome
Pelvic surgery
Pelvic neoplasm or mass
Chronic deep venous thrombosis
Trauma
Pregnancy
Retroperitoneal fibrosis
Venospasm
Radiation therapy
Idiopathic causes

---

long-standing compression; webs (bands, "spurs") form in the lumen and obstruct venous flow. Stenosis can progress to complete thrombosis. Mild compression at this site can be found in up to 20% of the population, but symptomatic disease is much less common.[101]

Clinical Features

Typical symptoms are leg swelling and pain. Associated DVT of the leg is common. Unilateral left-sided complaints, particularly in a young woman without a history of pelvic malignancy or trauma, should raise the possibility of May-Thurner syndrome.

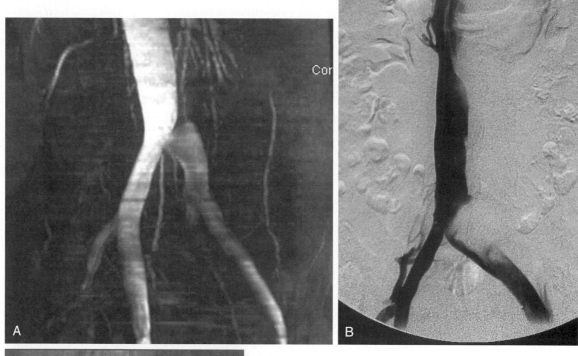

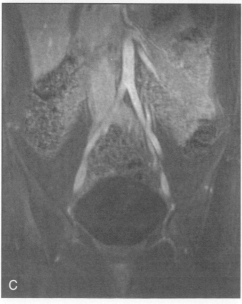

FIGURE 13-19 ▓ May-Thurner syndrome. MR (**A**) and catheter (**B**) pelvic venograms (in different patients) show narrowing of the left common iliac vein due to compression between the spine and the right common iliac artery (**C**).

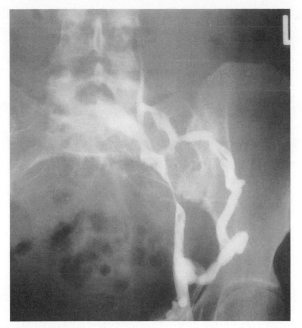

FIGURE 13-20 ■ Left iliac vein stenosis from pelvic malignancy. A focal stenosis of the left iliac vein is associated with collateral flow around the obstruction

Imaging

Although duplex sonography may suggest the presence of iliac vein obstruction, MR or catheter venography usually are required to make a definitive diagnosis. Stenoses usually are smooth and short (Fig. 13-20) but may be long and irregular, particularly when they are caused by chronic DVT. Signs of hemodynamic significance include filling of collateral channels or a focal pressure gradient of 3 to 4 mm Hg or more.[99] Several conditions can mimic fixed narrowing, including coaptation of the iliac vein walls from the high-pressure contrast jet at the catheter tip (i.e., Venturi effect) (see Fig. 13-6) and venospasm from catheter or guidewire manipulation.

Treatment

Endovascular Therapy. Generally, iliac vein stenoses require stent placement in addition to balloon angioplasty to achieve a durable result. Obstructions may be approached from the right internal jugular vein or either common femoral vein. The jugular route avoids damage and possible thrombosis of the inflow vein, which could jeopardize the results of the procedure. Patients are heparinized during the procedure. Predilation with an angioplasty balloon usually is performed. Self-expanding stents generally are preferred because many of these lesions have a component of extrinsic compression that could cause permanent plastic deformation and crushing of a balloon-expandable device. Typically, a 10- or 12-mm-diameter stent is required.

Some experts favor anticoagulation with warfarin after stent placement. Recanalization is successful in greater than 90% of cases.[99,102-104] The 1-year primary patency rate ranges from about 50% to 80%. Malignant obstructions are more prone to late occlusion than are benign strictures.

Major complications are reported in up to 7% of cases and include access site bleeding, stent malposition, and stent migration.

Surgical Therapy. For patients who fail to respond to transcatheter techniques, surgical options includes thrombectomy, crossover vein bypass grafts, and direct venous repair.

Preoperative Vein Mapping

Superficial veins of the legs and arms are the most common conduits for coronary artery and infrainguinal bypass grafts. Mapping of potential donor veins is done with duplex sonography.[105,106] Both legs are studied for exclusionary criteria, such as intrinsic saphenous vein disease, small caliber, or coexistent deep venous disease. The normal diameter of the great saphenous vein is 2.5 to 4.5 mm. Veins less than 2.0 mm in diameter may be unsuitable for bypass. If the great saphenous veins are unusable, the short saphenous veins or superficial arm veins may be considered.

■ OTHER DISORDERS

Trauma

Lower extremity venous trauma requires specific therapy far less often than does arterial trauma, and imaging is rarely needed to evaluate potential injuries. However, occult venous damage is relatively common and ultimately can lead to DVT or pulmonary embolism. Color Doppler sonography is an excellent tool for screening this population; its accuracy is similar to that of contrast venography.[107] Unsuspected venous trauma may be discovered at the time of surgery for an associated arterial injury. The vein is treated by direct repair, bypass grafting, or ligation.

Venous Malformations

Congenital venous malformations of the legs are considered in Chapter 6.

Aneurysms

Aneurysms of extremity veins are exceedingly rare. By far, the most common site is the popliteal vein.[108] The diagnosis usually is made by color Doppler sonography.[109] Because of the likelihood for clot formation and subsequent pulmonary embolism, venous reconstruction often is performed.

REFERENCES

1. Min RJ, Khilnani NM, Golia P: Duplex ultrasound evaluation of lower extremity venous insufficiency. J Vasc Interv Radiol 2003;14:1233.

2. Bettman MA, Robbins A, Braun SD, et al: Contrast venography of the leg: diagnostic efficacy, tolerance, and complication rates with ionic and nonionic contrast media. Radiology 1987;165:113.

3. Gabella G, ed: Cardiovascular system. In: Williams PL, Bannister LH, Berry MM, et al, eds. Gray's Anatomy, 38th ed. New York, Churchill Livingstone, 1995:1595.

4. Caggiati A, Bergan JJ: The saphenous vein: derivations of its name and its relevant anatomy. J Vasc Surg 2002;35:172.

5. Ricci S, Caggiati A: Does a double long saphenous vein exist? Phlebology 1999;14:59.

6. Shah DM, Chang BB, Leopold PW, et al: The anatomy of the greater saphenous venous system. J Vasc Surg 1986;3:273.

7. Liu G-C, Ferris EJ, Reifsteck JR, et al: Effect of anatomic variations on deep venous thrombosis of the lower extremity. AJR Am J Roentgenol 1986;146:845.

8. Kerr TM, Smith JM, McKenna P, et al: Venous and arterial anomalies of the lower extremities diagnosed by duplex scanning. Surg Gynecol Obstet 1992;175:309.

9. Kanterman RY, Witt PD, Hsieh PS, et al: Klippel-Trénaunay syndrome: imaging findings and percutaneous intervention. AJR Am J Roentgenol 1996;167:989.

10. Roebuck DJ, Howlett DC, Frazer CK, et al: Pictorial review: the imaging features of lower limb Klippel-Trénaunay syndrome. Clin Radiol 1994;49:346.

11. Howlett DC, Roebuck DJ, Frazer CK, et al: The use of ultrasound in the venous assessment of lower limb Klippel-Trénaunay syndrome. Eur J Radiol 1994;18:224.

12. Tian XL, Kadaba R, You SA, et al: Identification of an angiogenic factor that when mutated causes susceptibility to Klippel-Trenaunay syndrome. Nature 2004;427:640.

13. Peirce RM, Funaki B: Direct MR venography of persistent sciatic vein in a patient with Klippel-Trenaunay-Weber syndrome. AJR Am J Roentgenol 2002;178:513.

14. Noel AA, Gloviczki P, Cherry KJ Jr, et al: Surgical treatment of venous malformations in Klippel-Trenaunay syndrome. J Vasc Surg 2000;32:840.

15. Cherry KJ Jr, Gloviczki P, Stanson AW: Persistent sciatic vein: diagnosis and treatment of a rare condition. J Vasc Surg 1996;23:490.

16. American Thoracic Society: The diagnostic approach to acute venous thromboembolism. Am J Respir Crit Care Med 1999;160:1043.

17. Hyers TM: Management of venous thromboembolism. Arch Intern Med 2003;163:759.

18. Wells PS, Anderson DR, Rodger M, et al: Evaluation of D-dimer in the diagnosis of suspected deep-vein thrombosis. N Engl J Med 2003;349:1227.

19. Philbrick JT, Becker DM: Calf deep venous thrombosis. A wolf in sheep's clothing? Arch Intern Med 1988;148:2131.

20. Moser KM, LeMoine JR: Is embolic risk conditioned by location of deep venous thrombosis? Ann Intern Med 1981;94:439.

21. Piccioli A, Prandoni P, Goldhaber SZ: Epidemiologic characteristics, management, and outcome of deep venous thrombosis in a tertiary-care hospital: the Brigham and Women's Hospital DVT registry. Am Heart J 1996;132:1010.

22. Hood DB, Weaver FA, Modrall JG, et al: Advances in the treatment of phlegmasia cerulea dolens. Am J Surg 1993;166:206.

23. Bates SM, Ginsberg JS: Treatment of deep-vein thrombosis. New Engl J Med 2004;351:268.

24. Markel A, Manzo RA, Bergelin RO, et al: Incidence and time of occurrence of valvular incompetence following deep vein thrombosis. Wien Med Wochenschr 1994;144:216.

25. Stein PD, Hull RD, Patel KC, et al: D-dimer for the exclusion of acute venous thromboembolism and pulmonary embolism: a systematic review. Ann Intern Med 2004;140:589.

26. Caprini JA, Glase CJ, Anderson CB, et al: Laboratory markers in the diagnosis of venous thromboembolism. Circulation 2004;109(Suppl 1):I4.

27. Huisman MV, Bueller HR, ten Cate JW, Vreeken J: Serial impedance plethysmography for suspected deep venous thrombosis in outpatients. The Amsterdam General Practitioner Study. N Engl J Med 1986;314:823.

28. Heijboer H, Bueller HR, Lensing AW, et al: A comparison of real-time compression ultrasonography with impedance plethysmography for the diagnosis of deep-vein thrombosis in symptomatic outpatients. N Engl J Med 1993;329:1365.

29. Ginsberg JS, Wells PS, Hirsh J, et al: Reevaluation of the sensitivity of impedance plethysmography for the detection of proximal deep vein thrombosis. Arch Intern Med 1994;154:1930.

30. Fraser JD, Anderson DR: Deep venous thrombosis: recent advances and optimal investigation with US. Radiology 1999;211:9.

31. Lewis BD, James EM, Welch TJ, et al: Diagnosis of acute deep venous thrombosis of the lower extremities: prospective evaluation of color duplex flow imaging versus venography. Radiology 1994;192:651.

32. Rose SC, Zwiebel WJ, Nelson BD, et al: Symptomatic lower extremity deep venous thrombosis: accuracy, limitations, and role of color duplex flow imaging in diagnosis. Radiology 1990;175:639.

33. Chengelis DL, Bendick PJ, Glover JL, et al: Progression of superficial venous thrombosis to deep venous thrombosis. J Vasc Surg 1996;24:745.

34. Baxter GM, McKechnie S, Duffy P: Colour Doppler ultrasound in deep venous thrombosis: a comparison with venography. Clin Radiol 1990;42:32.

35. Vaccaro JP, Cronan JJ, Dorfman GS: Outcome analysis of patients with normal compression US examinations. Radiology 1990;175:645.

36. Wright DJ, Shepard AD, McPharlin M, et al: Pitfalls in lower extremity venous duplex scanning. J Vasc Surg 1990;11:675.

37. Bates SM, Lister-James J, Julian JA, et al: Imaging characteristics of a novel technetium Tc 99m-labeled platelet glycoprotein IIb/IIIa inhibitor antagonist in patients with acute deep vein thrombosis or a history of deep vein thrombosis. Arch Intern Med 2003;163:452.

38. Cornuz J, Pearson SD, Polak JF: Deep venous thrombosis: complete lower extremity venous US evaluation in patients without known risk factors—outcome study. Radiology 1999;211:637.

39. Gottlieb RH, Voci SL, Syed L, et al: Randomized prospective study comparing routine versus selective use of sonography of the complete calf in patients with suspected deep venous thrombosis. AJR Am J Roentgenol 2003;180:241.

40. Polak JF, Culter SS, O'Leary DH: Deep veins of the calf: assessment with color Doppler flow imaging. Radiology 1989;171:481.

41. Baxter GM, Duffy P, Partridge E: Colour flow imaging of calf vein thrombosis. Clin Radiol 1992;46:198.

42. Yucel EK, Fisher JS, Egglin TK, et al: Isolated calf venous thrombosis: diagnosis with compression US. Radiology 1991;179:443.

43. Rose SC, Zwiebel WJ, Murdock LE, et al: Insensitivity of color Doppler flow imaging for detection of acute calf deep venous thrombosis in asymptomatic post-operative patients. J Vasc Interv Radiol 1993;4:111.

44. Katz DS, Loud PA, Bruce D, et al: Combined CT venography and pulmonary angiography: a comprehensive review. Radiographics 2002;22:S3.

45. Garg K, Mao J: Deep venous thrombosis: spectrum of findings and pitfalls in interpretation on CT venography. AJR Am J Roentgenol 2001;177:319.

46. Ghaye B, Szapiro D, Willems V, et al: Pitfalls in CT venography of lower limbs and abdominal veins. AJR Am J Roentgenol 2002;178:1465.

47. Baldt MM, Zontsich T, Stuempflen A, et al: Deep venous thrombosis of the lower extremity: efficacy of spiral CT venography compared with conventional venography in diagnosis. Radiology 1996;200:423.

48. Fraser DG, Moody AR, Davidson IR, et al: Deep venous thrombosis: diagnosis by using venous enhanced subtracted peak arterial MR venography versus conventional venography. Radiology 2003;226:812.

49. Spritzer CE, Arata MA, Freed KS: Isolated pelvic deep venous thrombosis: relative frequency as detected with MR imaging. Radiology 2001;219:521.

50. Carpenter JP, Holland GA, Baum RA, et al: Magnetic resonance venography for the detection of deep venous thrombosis: comparison with contrast venography and duplex Doppler ultrasonography. J Vasc Surg 1993;18:734.

51. Evans AJ, Sostman HD, Knelson MH, et al: Detection of deep venous thrombosis: prospective comparison of MR imaging with contrast venography. AJR Am J Roentgenol 1993;161:131.

52. Laissy J-P, Cinqualbre A, Loshkajian A, et al: Assessment of deep venous thrombosis in the lower limbs and pelvis: MR venography versus duplex Doppler sonography. AJR Am J Roentgenol 1996;167:971.

53. Redman HC: Deep venous thrombosis: is contrast venography still the diagnostic "gold standard"? Radiology 1988;168:277.

54. Lund F, Diener L, Ericsson JL: Postmortem intraosseous phlebography as an aid in studies of venous thromboembolism. Angiology 1969;20:155.

55. McLachlan MS, Thomson JG, Taylor DW, et al: Observer variation in the interpretation of lower limb venograms. AJR Am J Roentgenol 1979;132:227.

56. Headrick JR Jr, Barker DE, Pate LM, et al: The role of ultrasonography and inferior vena cava filter placement in high-risk trauma patients. Am Surgeon 1997;63:1.

57. Flinn WR, Sandager GP, Silva MB Jr, et al: Prospective surveillance for perioperative venous thrombosis: experience in 2643 patients. Arch Surg 1996;131:472.

58. Hirsch DR, Ingenito EP, Goldhaber SZ: Prevalence of deep venous thrombosis among patients in medical intensive care. JAMA 1995;274:335.

59. Cogo A, Lensing AW, Koopman MM, et al: Compression ultrasonography for diagnostic management of patients with clinically suspected deep vein thrombosis: prospective cohort study. Br Med J 1998;316:17.

60. Heijboer H, Ginsberg JS, Buller HR, et al: The use of the D-dimer test in combination with non-invasive testing versus serial non-invasive testing alone for the diagnosis of deep-vein thrombosis. Thromb Haemost 1992;67:510.

61. Ginsberg JS: Management of venous thromboembolism. N Engl J Med 1996;335:1816.

62. Sharafuddin MJ, Sun S, Hoballah JJ, et al: Endovascular management of venous thrombotic and occlusive disease of the lower extremities. J Vasc Interv Radiol 2003;14:405.

63. Prandoni P, Lensing AW, Cogo A, et al: The long-term clinical course of acute deep venous thrombosis. Ann Intern Med 1996;125:1.

64. Lindner DJ, Edwards JM, Phinney ES, et al: Long-term hemodynamic and clinical sequelae of lower extremity deep vein thrombosis. J Vasc Surg 1986;4:436.

65. van Bemmelen PS, Bedford G, Beach K, et al: Functional status of the deep venous system after an episode of deep venous thrombosis. Ann Vasc Surg 1990;4:455.

66. O'Shaughnessy AM, FitzGerald DE: The patterns and distribution of residual abnormalities between the individual proximal venous segments after an acute deep vein thrombosis. J Vasc Surg 2001;33:379.

67. Comerota AJ, Aldridge SC: Thrombolytic therapy for deep venous thrombosis: a clinical review. Can J Surg 1993;36:359.

68. Meyerovitz MF, Polak JF, Goldhaber SZ: Short-term response to thrombolytic therapy in deep venous thrombosis: predictive value of venographic appearance. Radiology 1992;184:345.

69. Turpie AG, Levine MH, Hirsh J, et al: Tissue plasminogen activator (rt-PA) vs. heparin in deep vein thrombosis: results of a randomized trial. Chest 1990;97(Suppl 4):172S.

70. Semba CP, Dake MD: Iliofemoral deep venous thrombosis: aggressive therapy with catheter directed thrombolysis. Radiology 1994;191:487.

71. Mewissen MW, Seabrook GR, Meissner MH, et al: Catheter-directed thrombolysis for lower extremity deep venous thrombosis: report of a national multicenter registry. Radiology 1999;211:39.

72. Robinson DL, Teitelbaum GP: Phlegmasia cerulea dolens: treatment by pulse-spray and infusion thrombolysis. AJR Am J Roentgenol 1993;160:1288.

73. Grunwald MR, Hofmann LV: Comparison of urokinase, alteplase, and reteplase for catheter-directed thrombolysis of deep venous thrombosis. J Vasc Interv Radiol 2004;15:347.

74. Castaneda F, Li R, Young K, et al: Catheter-directed thrombolysis in deep venous thrombosis with use of reteplase: immediate results and complications from a pilot study. J Vasc Interv Radiol 2002;13:577.

75. O'Sullivan GJ, Semba CP, Bittner CA, et al: Endovascular management of iliac vein compression (May-Thurner) syndrome. J Vasc Interv Radiol 2000;11:823.

76. Patel NH, Stookey KR, Ketcham DB, et al: Endovascular management of acute extensive iliofemoral deep venous thrombosis caused by May-Thurner syndrome. J Vasc Interv Radiol 2000;11:1297.

77. Vedantham S, Vesely TM, Parti N, et al: Lower extremity venous thrombolysis with adjunctive mechanical thrombectomy. J Vasc Interv Radiol 2002;13:1001.

78. Vedantham S, Vesely TM, Sicard GA, et al: Pharmacomechanical thrombolysis and early stent placement for iliofemoral deep vein thrombosis. J Vasc Interv Radiol 2004;15:565.

79. Kasirajan K, Gray B, Ouriel K: Percutaneous Angiojet thrombectomy in the management of extensive deep venous thrombosis. J Vasc Interv Radiol 2001;12:179.

80. Wells PS, Forster AJ: Thrombolysis in deep vein thrombosis: is there still an indication. Thromb Haemost 2001;86:499.

81. Comerota AJ, Throm RC, Mathias SD, et al: Catheter-directed thrombolysis for iliofemoral deep venous thrombosis improves health-related quality of life. J Vasc Surg 2000;32:130.

82. Comerota AJ, Aldridge SC, Cohen G, et al: A strategy of aggressive regional therapy for acute iliofemoral venous thrombosis with contemporary venous thrombectomy or catheter-directed thrombolysis. J Vasc Surg 1994;20:244.

83. Bergan JJ, Kumins NH, Owens EL, et al: Surgical and endovascular treatment of lower extremity venous insufficiency. J Vasc Interv Radiol 2002;13:563.

84. Rautio TT, Perala JM, Wiik HT, et al: Endovenous obliteration with radiofrequency-resistive heating for greater saphenous vein insufficiency: a feasibility study. J Vasc Interv Radiol 2002;13:569.

85. Pichot O, Kabnick LS, Creton D, et al: Duplex ultrasound scan findings two years after great saphenous vein radiofrequency endovenous obliteration. J Vasc Surg 2004;39:189.

86. Min RJ, Khilnani N, Zimmet SE: Endovenous laser treatment of saphenous vein reflux: long-term results. J Vasc Interv Radiol 2003;14:991.

87. Perkowski P, Ravi R, Gowda RC, et al: Endovenous laser ablation of the saphenous vein for treatment of venous insufficiency and varicose veins: early results from a large single-center experience. J Endovasc Ther 2004;11:132.

88. Murphy TP, Cronan JJ: Evolution of deep venous thrombosis: a prospective evaluation with US. Radiology 1990;177:543.

89. Strandness DE Jr, Langlois Y, Cramer M, et al: Long-term sequelae of acute venous thrombosis. JAMA 1983;250:1289.

90. Akesson H, Brudin L, Dahlstrom JD, et al: Venous function assessed during a 5-year period after acute iliofemoral venous thrombosis treated with anticoagulation. Eur J Vasc Surg 1990;4:43.

91. Jamieson WG: State of the art of venous investigation and treatment. Can J Surg 1993;36:119.

92. Ibrahim S, MacPherson DR, Goldhaber SZ: Chronic venous insufficiency: mechanisms and management. Am Heart J 1996;132:856.

93. Tran NT, Meissner MH: The epidemiology, pathophysiology, and natural history of chronic venous disease. Semin Vasc Surg 2002;15:5.

94. Gaitini D, Torem S, Pery M, et al: Image-directed Doppler ultrasound in the diagnosis of lower-limb venous insufficiency. J Clin Ultrasound 1994;22:291.

95. Baldt MM, Bohler K, Zontsich T, et al: Preoperative imaging of lower extremity varicose veins: color-coded duplex sonography or venography. J Ultrasound Med 1996;15:143.

96. Neglen P, Thrasher TL, Raju S: Venous outflow obstruction: an underestimated contributor to chronic venous disease. J Vasc Surg 2003;38:879.

97. Blattler W, Blattler IK: Relief of obstructive pelvic venous symptoms with endoluminal stenting. J Vasc Surg 1999;29:484.

98. Eklof BG, Kistner RL, Masuda EM: Venous bypass and valve reconstruction: long-term efficacy. Vasc Med 1998;3:157.

99. Nazarian GK, Bjarnason H, Dietz CA Jr, et al: Iliofemoral venous stenoses: effectiveness of treatment with metallic endovascular stents. Radiology 1996;200:193.

100. Binkert CA, Schoch E, Stuckmann G, et al: Treatment of pelvic venous spur (May Thurner syndrome) with self expanding metallic endoprostheses. Cardiovasc Intervent Radiol 1998;21:22.

101. Baron HC, Shams J, Wayne M: Iliac vein compression syndrome: a new method of treatment. Am Surg 2000;66:653.

102. Vorwerk D, Guenther RW, Wendt G, et al: Iliocaval stenosis and iliac venous thrombosis in retroperitoneal fibrosis: percutaneous treatment by use of hydrodynamic thrombectomy and stenting. Cardiovasc Intervent Radiol 1996;19:40.

103. Lamont JP, Pearl GJ, Patetsios P, et al: Prospective evaluation of endoluminal venous stents in the treatment of the May-Thurner syndrome. Ann Vasc Surg 2002;16:61.

104. Hurst DR, Forauer AR, Bloom JR, et al: Diagnosis and endovascular treatment of iliocaval compression syndrome. J Vasc Surg 2001;34:106.

105. Head HD, Brown MF: Preoperative vein mapping for coronary artery bypass operations. Ann Thorac Surg 1995;59:144.

106. van Dijk LC, Wittens CH, Pieterman H, et al: The value of preoperative ultrasound mapping of the greater saphenous vein before "closed" in situ bypass operations. Eur J Radiol 1996;23:235.

107. Gagne PJ, Cone JB, McFarland D, et al: Proximity penetrating extremity trauma: the role of duplex ultrasound in the detection of occult venous injuries. J Trauma 1995;39:1157.

108. Calligaro KD, Ahmad S, Dandora R, et al: Venous aneurysms: surgical indications and review of the literature. Surgery 1995;117:1.

109. Fernando C, Vallance S: Retrograde venography and colour Doppler imaging of a popliteal venous aneurysm. Australas Radiol 1993;37:323.

Inferior Vena Cava

■ INFERIOR VENACAVOGRAPHY

Inferior venacavography is performed from the common femoral or (right) internal jugular vein approach. The jugular route must be taken in patients with bilateral common femoral, iliac vein, or inferior vena cava thrombosis. Real-time sonographic guidance is required for internal jugular vein puncture and may be helpful for groin puncture. In some patients, the common femoral vein lies posterior or posteromedial to the common femoral artery (see Fig. 2-8). To avoid traversing the artery, a single-wall needle is slowly inserted through the skin toward the vein with continuous aspiration on the needle hub.

Number 4- or 5-French pigtail (or similarly shaped) catheters are used for venacavography with the side holes placed at the common iliac vein confluence. Sizing catheters with radiopaque markers assist in determining true caval diameter in patients undergoing inferior vena cava filter placement. When iodinated contrast must be avoided because of renal insufficiency or history of severe contrast allergy, CO_2 or gadolinium-based agents (the latter providing superior imaging) are used.[1,2] A typical injection rate with iodinated contrast is 15 mL/second for 2 seconds. With CO_2 venography, rapid injection of 60 mL is necessary for adequate opacification. CO_2 should **not** be chosen if the patient has a known right-to-left shunt.

■ ANATOMY

Development

The posterior cardinal veins drain the caudal portion of the fetus during the first weeks of development.[3,4] By the seventh week of gestation, these veins begin to involute, and the subcardinal and supracardinal venous systems emerge (Fig. 14-1). In the middle of the abdomen, these two paired systems fuse into a vascular sinus, the *subcardinal-supracardinal*

anastomosis. The normal right-sided inferior vena cava and the azygous and hemiazygous venous systems are formed from these vessels.

Normal Anatomy

The *inferior vena cava* (IVC) begins at the confluence of the common iliac veins, which corresponds to the L4-L5 level (Figs. 14-1 and 14-2).[3,5] The left common iliac vein and IVC course between the right common iliac artery and the spine at this site. The IVC ascends in the retroperitoneum to the right of the aorta. In the mid-abdomen, the IVC passes behind the head of the pancreas, the superior portion of the duodenum, and the portal vein. The vessel then runs in a groove on the posterior surface of the liver. As it traverses the diaphragm, it passes through the pericardium and then enters the inferoposterior aspect of the right atrium. The *eustachian valve* is located on the right lateral side of the IVC at its junction with the right atrium. Otherwise, the IVC has no valves.

The *ascending lumbar veins* arise from the common iliac veins and run alongside the vertebral bodies (Fig. 14-3). Four pairs of *lumbar veins* draining the ascending lumbar veins enter the IVC (Fig. 14-4). Above the L2 level, they drain into the azygos system (see below).

The *renal veins* enter the IVC at the L1-L2 level (see Figs. 14-2 and 14-4). Renal vein anomalies (e.g., multiple veins, circumaortic or retroaortic left renal vein) are seen in up to 30% of patients (Fig. 14-5; see also Chapter 8).[6,7] The *right gonadal vein* enters the IVC just below the right renal vein, and the *left gonadal vein* drains into the undersurface of the left renal vein lateral to the vertebral column (see Fig. 14-4). The *right adrenal vein* enters the IVC in a horizontal plane directly above the right renal vein; the *left adrenal vein* joins the left renal vein in a vertical plane as a common trunk with the *left inferior phrenic vein* (see Fig. 11-9).

The *right, middle,* and *left hepatic veins* merge into the IVC just below the diaphragm (see Fig. 10-4). In many

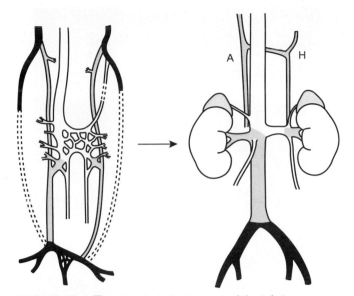

FIGURE 14-1 ■ Embryologic development of the inferior vena cava. Shading indicates the posterior cardinal origin *(black)*, supracardinal origin *(gray)*, and subcardinal origin *(white)*. A, azygous vein; H, hemiazygous vein. (Adapted from Lundell C, Kadir S: Inferior vena cava and spinal veins. In: Kadir S, ed: Atlas of Normal and Variant Angiographic Anatomy. Philadelphia, WB Saunders, 1991:187.)

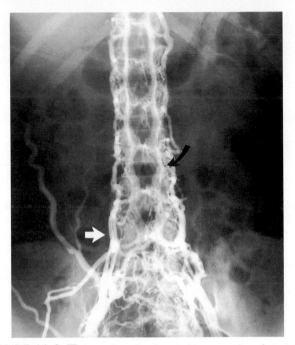

FIGURE 14-3 ■ Ascending lumbar *(white arrow)* and vertebral *(curved arrow)* venous system in a patient with complete inferior vena cava occlusion.

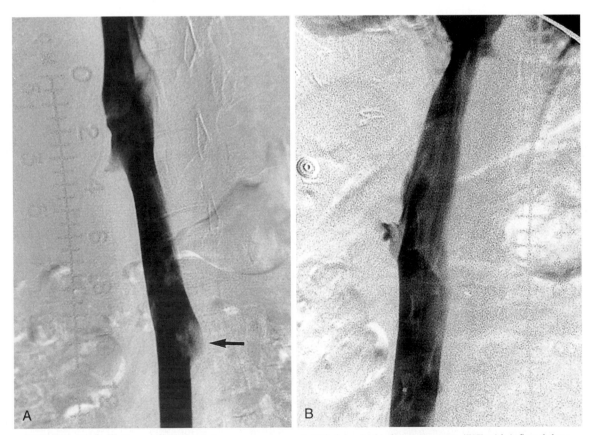

FIGURE 14-2 ■ Normal frontal inferior venacavograms. **A,** Mid-abdominal inferior vena cava (IVC) with inflow defects from the left common iliac vein *(arrow)* and both renal veins. **B,** Upper abdominal IVC with mild compression of the intrahepatic segment below the right atrium.

patients, accessory hepatic veins drain portions of the right or caudate lobes below these vessels. However, in about 3% of the population, the right lobe of the liver is **primarily** drained through a large *inferior right hepatic vein* that enters the IVC well below the other hepatic veins (see Fig. 14-4).[8] Inflow defects at cavography caused by unopacified blood from the renal, hepatic, and contralateral iliac veins (see Fig. 14-2) should not be confused with clot, which does not change in appearance on sequential images.

The *azygous venous system* drains the posterior chest wall, esophagus, mediastinum, and pericardium. It also provides a potential collateral circulation for the IVC and tributaries when they become obstructed (Fig. 14-6). The *azygous vein* originates at about the L1-L2 level as an indirect continuation of the right ascending lumbar veins. It then ascends through the abdomen and chest on the right lateral aspect of the spine. At about the T4-T5 level, it arches anteriorly to join the superior vena cava. The *hemiazygous vein* also originates about the L1-L2 level and runs on the left lateral side of the spine. It crosses the midline to join the azygous vein at about the 8th thoracic vertebra. The *accessory hemiazygous vein*, which arises from the left brachiocephalic vein, joins the superior vena cava just above the hemiazygous connection.

The IVC often appears elliptical rather than round in the transverse plane. Below the renal veins, its mean transverse diameter in adults is about 19 mm.[6,9] The diameter usually decreases during inspiration and with a Valsalva maneuver, and it usually increases during expiration.[10] Mild or moderate narrowing of the intrahepatic IVC is common (see Fig. 14-2B).

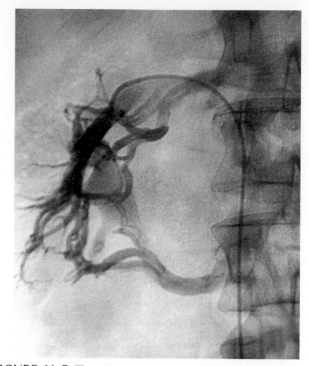

FIGURE 14-5 ■ Multiple right renal veins communicate in the hilum. The accessory vein was not suspected on the inferior vena-cavogram.

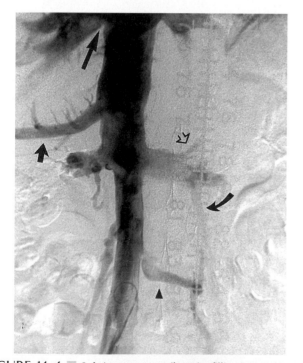

FIGURE 14-4 ■ Inferior vena cava tributaries filling in a patient with elevated right-sided heart pressures. Notice the main hepatic vein confluence *(long arrow)*, anomalous inferior right hepatic vein *(short arrow)*, left gonadal vein *(curved arrow)*, left adrenal vein *(open arrow)*, and lumbar veins *(arrowhead)*.

Variant Anatomy

The major IVC anomalies can be explained by errors in normal fetal development of the major veins of the abdomen and pelvis (see Fig. 14-1).[4,5]

Duplication of the IVC results from persistence of the inferior portion of the **left supracardinal** vein. This anomaly is identified in 2% to 3% of autopsy specimens, but it is observed much less frequently (0.3%) on imaging studies.[5,11] Each iliac vein drains into its corresponding vena cava (Fig. 14-7). The left IVC usually joins the right IVC at the level of the left renal vein. The right and left common iliac veins sometimes communicate. At venacavography performed from the right femoral vein, IVC duplication may be suspected by the absence of an inflow defect from the left iliac vein and by the small caliber of the infrarenal IVC. However, it can go undetected on routine cavograms obtained from the right groin; attempts at direct catheterization of the left iliac vein may be necessary.

Left (transposed) IVC results from persistence of the inferior portion of the **left supracardinal** vein with involution of the inferior portion of the **right supracardinal** vein. In autopsy series, left IVC is found in 0.2% to 0.5% of cases; a similar frequency (0.2%) has been reported in imaging studies.[5,11] Usually, the left IVC joins the suprarenal IVC at or just inferior to the left renal vein (Fig. 14-8). Occasionally, it may join the azygous or hemiazygous system.[12] Rarely, it connects with a left superior vena cava and drains into the coronary sinus.[13]

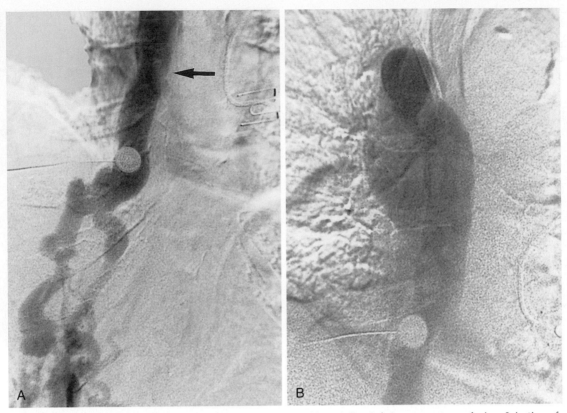

FIGURE 14-6 ▮ Ascending lumbar collaterals in a patient with complete inferior vena cava occlusion. Injection of the right iliac vein fills the ascending lumbar collaterals, which drain into the azygous vein (**A,** *arrow*) and then into the superior vena cava (**B**).

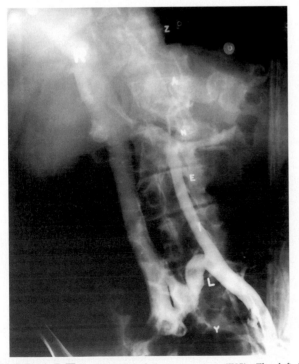

FIGURE 14-7 ▮ Duplicated inferior vena cava (IVC). The left IVC communicates with the right IVC in the upper pelvis and drains into the left renal vein.

Interruption of the IVC with azygous or hemiazygous continuation occurs when the **right subcardinal** vein fails to join the intrahepatic venous complex. In this case, blood flows from the lower IVC into the azygous or hemiazygous vein and then into the heart (Fig. 14-9). With IVC interruption, which is found in 0.6% of autopsy specimens, the hepatic veins drain directly into the right atrium.[3,5] The anomaly often is associated with congenital heart disease and with abnormalities of the spleen (i.e., asplenia or polysplenia), cardiac position, and abdominal situs.[14,15]

Other exceedingly rare caval variants include double IVC with retroaortic right renal vein and hemiazygous continuation of the IVC, double IVC with retroaortic left renal vein and azygous continuation of the IVC, and absent infrarenal IVC with preserved suprarenal segment.[5]

Collateral Circulation

Several collateral pathways return blood to the heart when there is severe stenosis or occlusion of the IVC.[16] The most common collateral network in IVC obstruction is the ascending lumbar venous plexus (see Fig. 14-3). These vessels communicate freely with an extensive vertebral venous network. Blood flows cephalad through these veins into the azygous or hemiazygous systems and then into the *superior vena cava (SVC)* (see Fig. 14-6).

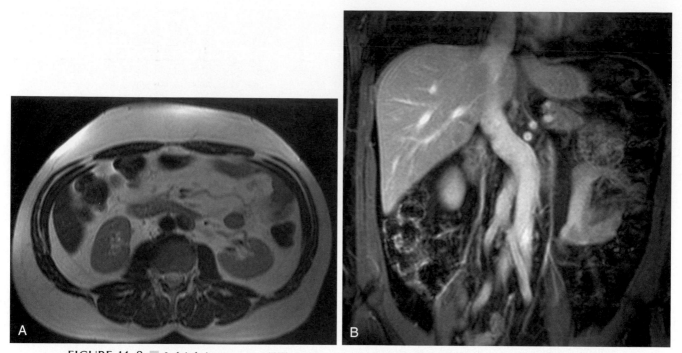

FIGURE 14-8 ■ Left inferior vena cava (IVC). **A,** T1-weighted MR image shows IVC to the left of the aorta at the level of the kidneys. **B,** Coronal maximum intensity projection MR angiogram shows the left IVC crossing the midline to join the orthotopic suprarenal IVC.

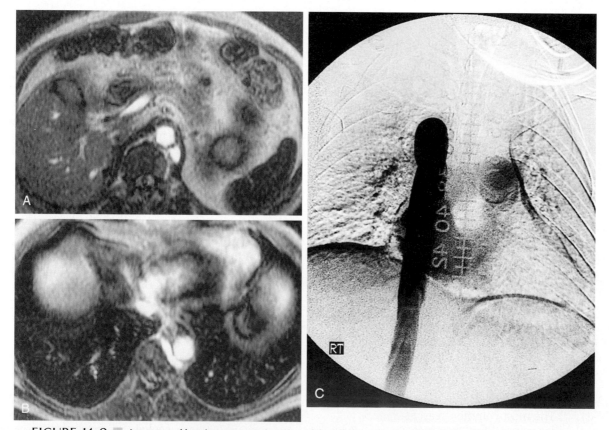

FIGURE 14-9 ■ Azygous and hemiazygous continuation of the inferior vena cava (IVC). **A,** The IVC is absent on a transverse gradient-echo MR image of the mid-abdomen; the hemiazygous vein (to the left of the aorta) is enlarged. **B,** In the lower chest, the hemiazygous vein passes behind the aorta en route to the azygous vein. **C,** In another patient, injection of the abdominal IVC shows azygous continuation into the chest.

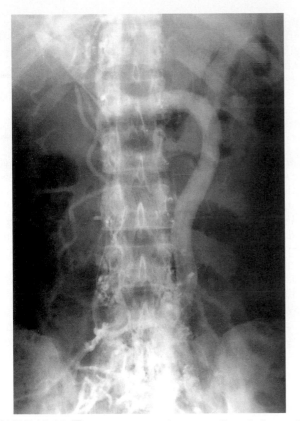

FIGURE 14-10 ■ Systemic to portal venous collaterals in a patient with inferior vena cava occlusion. Injection of the right common femoral vein fills internal iliac collaterals that enter the hemorrhoidal venous system and ultimately drain into a massively dilated inferior mesenteric vein.

Blood from the pelvic veins also may bypass the IVC through periureteric and gonadal venous communications. The external iliac vein can drain through the inferior epigastric vein; superficial vessels then merge with the internal thoracic and subclavian veins. Alternatively, blood may flow from the superficial epigastric and circumflex iliac veins into the lateral thoracic vein and then into the axillary vein. A systemic to portal venous pathway runs from the internal iliac veins through the hemorrhoidal plexus, then into the inferior mesenteric vein, and ultimately into the portal vein (Fig. 14-10). Superficial abdominal wall veins also may communicate with paraumbilical veins that enter the left portal vein.

■ MAJOR DISORDERS

Inferior Vena Cava Thrombosis

Etiology

Thrombotic occlusion of the IVC has numerous causes (Box 14-1).[17-19] The most common reasons are extension of clot from the iliac veins, IVC catheters, transvenous spread of tumor thrombus from abdominal or pelvic neoplasms, and thrombosis of IVC filters. In infants and children, IVC obstruction usually is caused by thrombosis from indwelling

---

BOX 14-1 ■ Causes of Obstruction of the Inferior Vena Cava
Thrombosis
Extension of iliac vein thrombus
Inferior vena cava filter or surgical interruption
Indwelling catheter
Trauma
Thrombophilic state
Aneurysm
Tumor extension
Intraluminal growth
Direct invasion
Severe extrinsic compression
Membranous webs
Idiopathic causes

venous catheters, thrombophilic states, or intra-abdominal tumors.[20]

Clinical Features

If the collateral circulation has sufficient time to develop, IVC thrombosis may be clinically silent. Otherwise, patients develop bilateral leg edema, dilated superficial veins over the legs and abdomen, and skin changes resulting from chronic venous stasis. When the occlusion involves both renal veins, the nephrotic syndrome can occur. Acute IVC thrombosis associated with severe iliofemoral thrombosis may lead to the rare syndrome of *phlegmasia cerulea dolens*.[21] These patients suffer massive leg swelling, severe pain, cyanosis, and (sometimes) arterial ischemia. A substantial number of cases ends in amputation, massive pulmonary embolism, or death.

Imaging

Cross-sectional Techniques. IVC thrombosis is usually diagnosed by CT or MR angiography or by color Doppler sonography.[22,23] On contrast-enhanced CT, the IVC is enlarged, and collateral vessels may opacify. A low-density filling defect with enhancement of the caval wall is seen (Fig. 14-11). Heterogenous enhancement of the lumen (from mixing of unopacified blood) can mimic intraluminal clot in the early phases of dynamic scanning. Intraluminal extension of tumor thrombus (typically from renal cell or hepatocellular carcinoma) can cause IVC thrombosis (see Fig. 8-38).

Angiography. Catheter venacavography is reserved for patients about to undergo IVC filter placement or thrombolysis. A thrombus produces a discrete filling defect (Fig. 14-12). In cases of complete or long-standing occlusion, the IVC does not opacify, and only collateral vessels are seen (see Fig. 14-3). The pattern of collateral circulation depends on the level and extent of occlusion. In low IVC occlusion, the cava often remains patent at and above the entry of the renal veins. Venography from the internal jugular vein approach may be necessary to determine the upper extent of the occlusion.

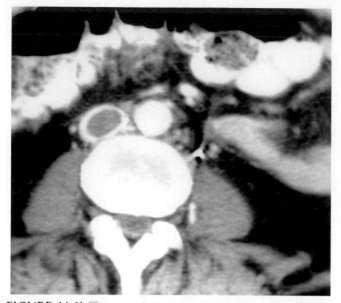

FIGURE 14-11 ■ Acute inferior vena cava thrombosis detected by CT. A markedly enhancing caval wall surrounds a low-density thrombus.

The major goals of treatment are to prevent pulmonary embolism, limit clot propagation that may cause renal vein and hepatic vein thrombosis, and potentially prevent chronic venous insufficiency. However, this regimen is contraindicated in certain cases, including patients with risk factors for bleeding from anticoagulants and those who have had a previous adverse reaction to heparin or warfarin. In such cases, placement of a suprarenal IVC filter may be appropriate (see below).

Endovascular Therapy. Catheter-directed thrombolysis has been used to treat acute IVC thrombosis from a variety of causes, including IVC filter occlusion, Budd-Chiari syndrome, nephrotic syndrome, indwelling central venous catheters, and spontaneous causes.[25-30] Thrombolysis should be considered in patients with severe symptoms (e.g., phlegmasia cerulea dolens) and in those who fail to respond to anticoagulant therapy (see Chapters 2 and 13). Complete clot lysis usually requires prolonged infusions (>2 days), large doses of fibrinolytic agent, or adjunctive mechanical thrombectomy Initial treatment with pulse-spray techniques may accelerate the lytic process. The need for temporary/retrievable filter placement above the clot before thrombolysis to prevent pulmonary embolism is controversial (see below).

Treatment

Medical Therapy. The standard therapy for IVC thrombosis is identical to management of lower extremity deep venous thrombosis: intravenous heparin (or low-molecular-weight heparin) followed by a course of oral warfarin (Coumadin).[24]

Venous Thromboembolic Disease and Permanent IVC Filter Placement

Insertion of an IVC filter is performed: to prevent clinically relevant pulmonary embolism in patients with documented

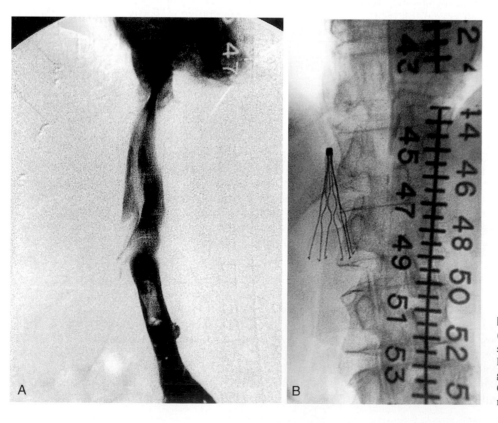

FIGURE 14-12 ■ Inferior vena cava (IVC) thrombus. **A,** Inferior venacavogram shows a filling defect in the infrarenal IVC. Lucency must be differentiated from bowel gas and inflow defects. **B,** A suprarenal Greenfield filter was placed through the right internal jugular vein.

venous thrombosis of the legs or pelvis or as prophylaxis in selected patients at high risk for the disease. However, IVC filters should **not** replace standard medical therapy for lower extremity venous thrombosis or documented pulmonary embolism in patients who are reasonable candidates for anticoagulant therapy (see Chapter 13). There is almost universal acceptance of this intervention in appropriate patients, although a few experts still remain skeptical about the evidence that significant pulmonary embolism will be prevented or that overall mortality is improved compared with more conservative treatment.[31-34]

Patient Selection

The primary indications for filter insertion are outlined in Box 14-2.[35-38] In certain situations, placement of a retrievable filter may be more appropriate (see below).[39,40] SVC filters are placed in selected cases, although the current devices are not specifically indicated for that use (see Fig. 15-17).[41,42] For some patients, both IVC filter insertion **and** anticoagulation are necessary to adequately reduce the risk of pulmonary embolism (e.g., chronic pulmonary thromboembolic disease before surgical thromboendarterectomy).

Contraindications include severe uncorrectable coagulopathy, absence of a suitable access route to the IVC, and chronic thrombosis of the cava. Although some interventionalists are reluctant to place IVC filters in septic patients, it is unclear whether the risk of filter seeding is real.[35,43]

Staging

Inferior venacavography is performed to guide filter selection and placement.

Inferior Vena Cava Diameter and Length. About 2% of the population has a *megacava*, in which the true transverse diameter (corrected for magnification) exceeds 28 to 29 mm.[44,45] Diameter measurements should be based on a calibrated catheter using angiographic equipment software. With all but one device, filter embolization could occur during or sometime after release. In this instance, the Bird's nest filter (which expands to 40 mm) must be used (Fig. 14-13).[46] Alternatively, smaller filters are placed in each common iliac vein. The Bird's nest filter system is longer than other devices (7 cm or greater) and may not be suitable if the infrarenal IVC length is short.

Location and Number of Renal Veins. By convention, IVC filters are deployed with the most superior point immediately below the level of the renal veins. If the filter clots spontaneously or becomes filled with emboli, rapid flow

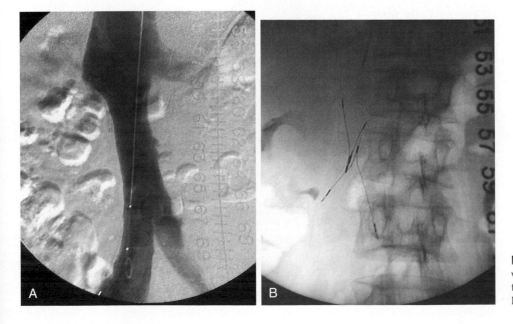

FIGURE 14-13 ■ Megacava. **A,** Inferior venacavogram shows caval diameter greater than 29 mm (based on catheter markers). **B,** Bird's nest filter was placed.

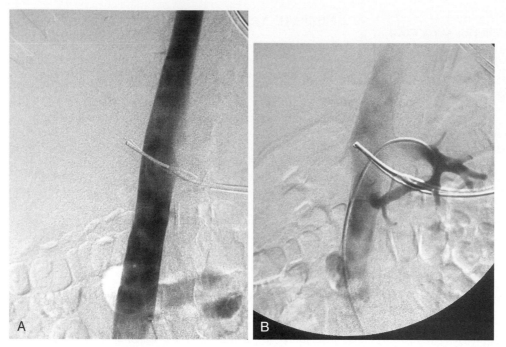

from the renal veins should prevent thrombosis above the filter if no dead space is left. The main renal veins are identified by inflow defects on the venacavogram (see Fig. 14-2). However, **accessory** renal veins are present in up to 25% to 30% of cases (more frequently on the right than the left). These vessels are not always detected by venacavography alone, and selective catheterization often is necessary to identify them (Fig. 14-14).[6] Accessory renal veins must be differentiated from lumbar veins. In patients with multiple renal veins (circumaortic or otherwise), the filter is deposited below the inferiormost vein to prevent this vessel from acting as a conduit for clots if the lower IVC becomes occluded.

Inferior Vena Cava Anomalies. Variants in IVC anatomy are sought. A duplicated IVC requires placement of filters in each moiety or suprarenal insertion of a single device.

Intrinsic Disease. If thrombus is found in the IVC, the filter is inserted above the clot through the internal jugular vein (see Fig. 14-12). Chronic total occlusion of the IVC possibly obviates the need for filter placement, although clots still can pass through enlarged collaterals. Filter location may be influenced by the presence of chronic mural disease or extrinsic compression.

Extension of clot from IVC tributaries may be caused by occult malignancy. If suprarenal filter placement is required, it is critical to identify an appropriate landing site and be certain that the nondiseased caval segment is long enough to accommodate the filter without extension into the right atrium.

Devices

Before endoluminal IVC filtration devices were developed, operative interruption was achieved by ligation, stapling, plication, or clipping (Fig. 14-15). However, IVC thrombosis was a frequent problem after these procedures.[47,48]

Several permanent IVC filters are commercially available (Figs. 14-16 and 14-17 and Table 14-1). The most popular ones are discussed below.[36] All devices have elements on the legs that attach to the caval wall to prevent filter migration.

■ *Stainless-steel Greenfield filter.* The Greenfield IVC filter has gone through several iterations since the initial designs that allowed operative insertion (in 1973)

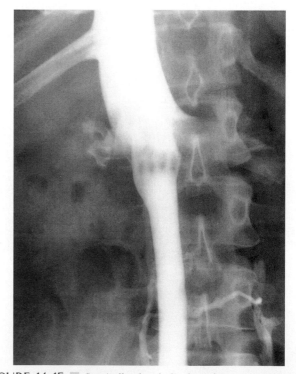

FIGURE 14-15 ■ Surgically placed clip for inferior vena cava interruption causes a deformity of the caval lumen.

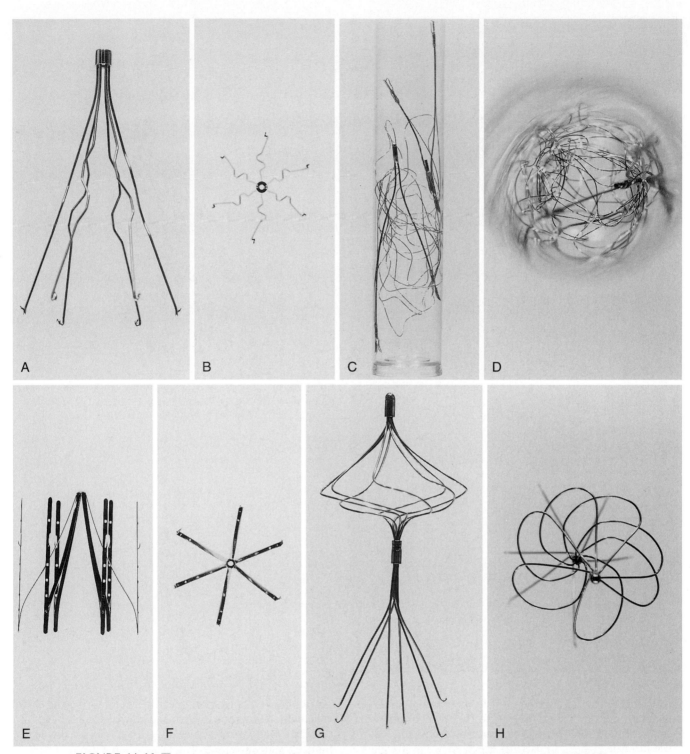

FIGURE 14-16 ■ Frontal and aerial views of inferior vena cava filter designs. **A** and **B,** Stainless-steel Greenfield filter (Boston Scientific, Natick, Mass.). **C** and **D,** Bird's nest filter (Cook Inc., Bloomington, Ind.). **E** and **F,** Vena-Tech LGM filter (B. Braun, Evanston, Ill.). **G** and **H,** Simon nitinol filter (Bard, Inc., Tempe, Ariz.).

and then percutaneous placement (in 1984).[49,50] A lower profile (12-French) titanium version replaced the massive 24-French system and greatly simplified the insertion process. The most recent device is an over-the-wire design that is placed through a 12-French sheath. The central wire helps to orient the filter along the caval axis during deployment.

■ *Bird's nest filter.* This unique design incorporates two V-shaped struts that are placed in opposing directions and secure the device to the IVC wall. Multiple stainless-steel microwires emanate from the strut joints and upon deployment create a random mesh that traps clot.
■ *Simon nitinol filter.* The thermal memory of the nickel-titanium alloy permits the device to be compressed into

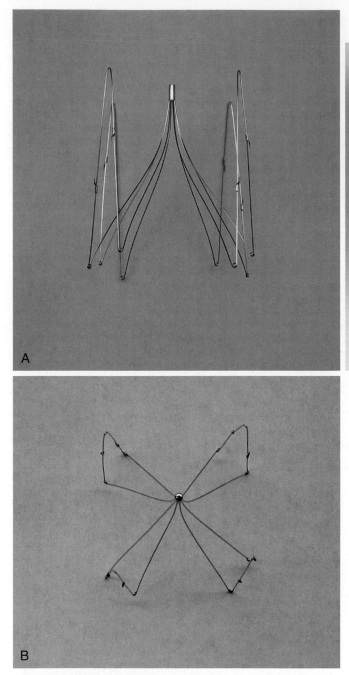

FIGURE 14-17 ■ Frontal and aerial views of newer inferior vena cava filter designs. **A** and **B,** Low-profile Vena-Tech LGM (**B,** Braun, Evanston, Ill.). **C,** TrapEase filter (Cordis Corp., Miami Lakes, Fla.)

the delivery carrier and then regain its nominal form when exposed to body temperature. To prevent postinsertion migration, the manufacturer recommends that the filter be avoided in patients expected to require general anesthesia within several weeks of placement.

■ *Vena-Tech LGM low-profile filter.* Eight Phynox wires form a conical shape and merge centrally to an apical joint. The side rails appose the caval wall and center the device along the caval axis.

■ *TrapEase filter.* Two baskets with diamond-shaped openings are connected by struts that align the filter with the IVC. The dual filtration system makes it especially efficient in trapping thrombi.

The most important factors in filter design are clot-trapping efficiency, IVC and access vein occlusion rates, risk of filter migration or embolization, mechanical integrity, and ease of placement. Numerous in vitro and animal studies have compared the relative efficacy of IVC filters; none of the devices holds a clear advantage.[51-54] The Simon nitinol, TrapEase, and Bird's nest filters seem to have superior clot-trapping ability (the former two because of the two-level filtration system).[55-57] This property may be associated with higher rates of caval thrombosis, but it may make these devices more suitable for patients who cannot tolerate even small pulmonary emboli.

Insertion Technique

IVC filters usually are placed from the right internal jugular or right common femoral vein. Access to these vessels is

TABLE 14-1   INFERIOR VENA CAVA FILTERS

Device/Manufacturer	Material	Length	Sheath
Permanent			
Bird's nest filter (Cook, Inc.)	Stainless steel	>70 mm	12 Fr
Greenfield filter (Boston Scientific)	Stainless steel	49 mm	12 Fr
Simon nitinol filter (Bard, Inc.)	Nitinol	45 mm	7 Fr
TrapEase filter (Cordis Corp.)	Nitinol	50–62 mm	6 Fr
Vena-Tech LGM low profile (B. Braun)	Phynox	43 mm	7 Fr
Retrievable or Permanent			
Guenther-Tulip filter (Cook, Inc.)	Elgiloy	45 mm	8.5 Fr
Recovery filter (Bard, Inc.)	Nitinol		7 Fr
OptEase filter (Cordis, Corp.)	Nitinol	50–62 mm	6 Fr
Temporary			
Tempofilter II (B. Braun)	Phynox	43 mm	7Fr

BOX 14-3 ■ Indications for Suprarenal Inferior Vena Cava (IVC) Filter Placement

Renal or gonadal vein thrombosis
IVC thrombosis
Pregnancy and women of childbearing age
Thrombus above a previously inserted infrarenal IVC filter

explained in Chapters 2 and 16. From the groin, one must avoid accidental puncture of the femoral artery (which may be anterior to the vein) and subsequent development of an arteriovenous fistula. The left common femoral vein may be used if right common femoral vein thrombus is identified

on the right side by sonography. However, the steeper angle between the left iliac vein and IVC may cause exaggerated tilting of some filters. Marked narrowing of the iliac vein, often from chronic wall thickening due to prior thromboembolic disease, can make insertion of the filter difficult or impossible (Fig. 14-18).

If infrarenal IVC thrombus is found, the filter is placed through the right internal jugular vein. In the rare circumstance in which both femoral and internal jugular veins are occluded or unavailable, the external jugular vein can be used.[58] Alternatively, one of the lower profile devices is placed through an antecubital or upper arm vein.[59]

Filters are deposited in the infrarenal IVC unless a thrombus is present in this segment (see Fig. 14-12). Indications for **suprarenal** IVC filter placement are outlined in Box 14-3.[35,60-62] Suprarenal insertion is recommended in pregnant women to avoid compression of the device by the gravid uterus and to prevent pulmonary embolism if ovarian vein thrombosis develops.

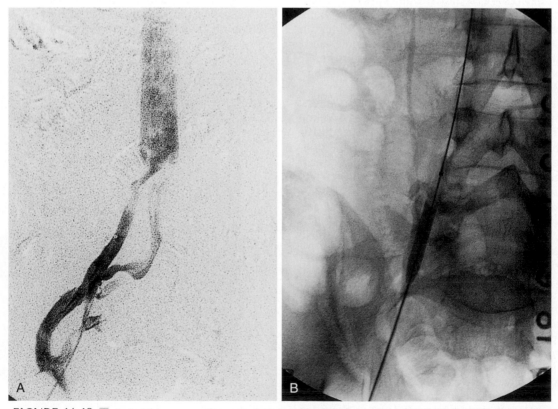

FIGURE 14-18 ■ **A,** A right common iliac vein stenosis is identified before filter placement. **B,** A 5-mm angioplasty balloon was used to dilate the stenosis and allow passage of the filter delivery sheath.

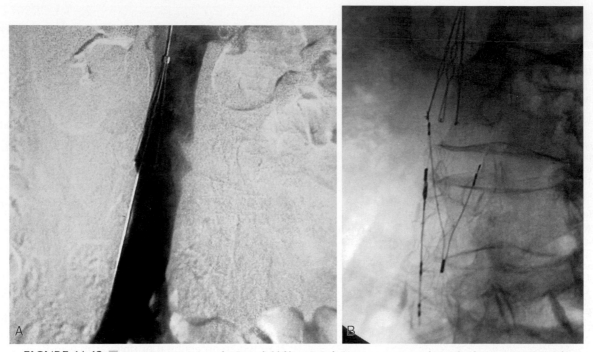

FIGURE 14-19 ■ Improper expansion of a Greenfield filter. **A,** Inferior venacavogram shows the device protecting only the right lateral side of the inferior vena cava. With the guidewire in place and the tip in the superior vena cava, multiple unsuccessful attempts were made using several catheters (placed in tandem through the delivery sheath) to reposition the legs. **B,** A Bird's nest filter was placed below the first device to adequately prevent pulmonary embolism.

Filters are delivered through 6- to 12-French sheaths. Details of filter insertion and deployment vary with each device.[63] Some devices are asymmetric and require different delivery systems for jugular and femoral deployment. Bedside placement of permanent (or retrievable) filters in unstable patients in the intensive care unit is feasible, albeit more difficult than insertion in the interventional suite.[64,65] Portable fluoroscopy or intravascular ultrasound is used for imaging guidance.

Suboptimal expansion can occur with any of the filters. The most common problems are incomplete opening or tilting of the Vena-Tech LGM filter,[66] tilting or asymmetric distribution of filter legs with the 12-French titanium or stainless-steel Greenfield filter (Fig. 14-19),[67,68] prolapse of wire mesh with the Bird's nest filter,[69] and tilting or migration of the Simon nitinol filter (Fig. 14-20).[70]

Most filters align themselves properly with the long axis of the IVC to provide optimal protection from clinically significant pulmonary embolism. The stainless-steel Greenfield filter is particularly different in this regard in that significant filter tilting off axis, asymmetric leg opening, or even failed expansion are observed. The impact of leg asymmetry or filter tilting on recurrent pulmonary embolism is controversial.[67,71] However, some interventionalists attempt to improve the leg orientation or filter axis if it is grossly asymmetric, even though this practice is **not** recommended by the manufacturers or some experts.[36,68,72,73] Instead, a second filter can be placed (see Fig. 14-19).

Very rarely, the filter fails to open, making the device useless and at risk for embolization to the heart. In this rare circumstance, attempts should be made to open the filter, although the interventionalist should consider placement of a temporary or retrievable filter superior to the failed device in the event that embolization occurs with manipulations.[74]

Prolapse of the wire mesh of the Bird's nest filter into the suprarenal IVC is relatively common. Wire prolapse

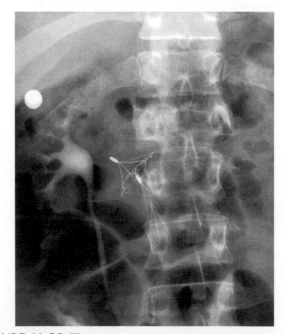

FIGURE 14-20 ■ Migration of a Simon nitinol filter into the right renal vein.

TABLE 14-2	COMPLICATIONS FROM INFERIOR VENA CAVA (IVC) FILTER PLACEMENT

Event	Frequency (%)
Access site thrombosis	2–28
IVC thrombosis	0–28
IVC perforation (almost always inconsequential)	9–24
Filter migration (almost always inconsequential)	3–69
Filter embolization	<1
Filter fracture	1
Dislodgement or entrapment by catheters or guidewires	<1
Other complications	4–11
Infection	
Air embolism (to right heart chambers)	
Bleeding	
Pneumothorax	
Stroke (from paradoxical embolism of air or clot)	
Failed deployment	

is minimized by putting three 360-degree twists on the catheter-sheath unit during deployment.[75] However, several studies have shown that wire prolapse has no effect on the efficiency of the filter.[69,76]

Results

Using fluoroscopic guidance, IVC filters can be placed successfully in almost every case.[35,36,77] Historical case series (with wide-ranging methodology) have failed to show a clear overall advantage of any of the available devices, hence the wide choice of IVC filters.[34,36,78] Technical failures usually result from inability to place a filter in a diseased vena cava.

The recurrent pulmonary embolism rate of 2% to 5% is strikingly similar for all available filters.[34,79-83] The risk of subsequent **fatal** pulmonary embolism is estimated at about 0.7%.[36] Recurrent pulmonary emboli have several causes, including device failure, propagation of thrombus above the filter, and embolization from other sources (e.g., upper extremity, gonadal or renal vein). Such cases may require placement of an additional filter or anticoagulation.

Complications

Immediate and long-term complications of IVC filter placement are outlined in Table 14-2.[36,84-86] The major complication rate is about 0.3%. There is no significant difference in success or adverse outcomes between suprarenal and infrarenal placement.[34] Less than 0.2% of patients die as a direct result of the procedure.

Access site thrombosis is the most common complication of IVC filter insertion.[87] With 12- to 14-French delivery systems, the frequency of occlusive thrombosis is about 2% to 10%.[36,77,80,82,87] Nonocclusive femoral vein thrombosis develops in about 25% of patients and probably is less frequent with the internal jugular vein approach.

IVC thrombosis is a serious and potentially life-threatening complication of filter placement (Fig. 14-21). Thrombosis may occur from spontaneous clotting of the filter or from thrombi trapped within the filter. The thrombus may extend above the filter and cause pulmonary embolism. IVC occlusion usually is tolerated because obstruction is gradual and

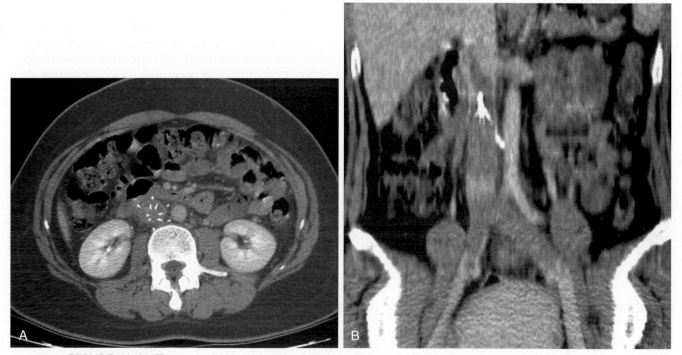

FIGURE 14-21 ■ Inferior vena cava thrombosis after placement of a Recovery filter. **A,** Axial CT angiogram shows thrombus within the cone of the filter. Note that some of the filter legs have penetrated the caval wall. **B,** Reformatted coronal CT image documents the thrombus, which extends above the filter.

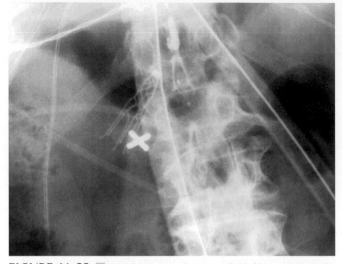

FIGURE 14-22 ■ Malplacement of a Greenfield filter in the right renal vein from operative insertion through the right internal jugular vein.

collateral circulation has time to develop. The reported frequency of symptomatic IVC occlusion varies from 0 to 28%, although it is generally in the 2% to 12% range.[55,77,82,88-90] In patients with profound or life-threatening symptoms from IVC thrombosis (e.g., phlegmasia cerulea dolens), catheter-directed thrombolysis may be indicated (see Chapter 13).[28,91]

Minor degrees of late filter migration are relatively common and usually of little consequence. However, embolization of an IVC filter to the heart or pulmonary artery is potentially lethal.[92,93] Significant filter migration after image-guided placement has been reported but is far less common than **malplacement** from inadequate or nonexistent imaging during insertion (Fig. 14-22). If an IVC filter becomes lodged in the heart, pericardial tamponade, acute myocardial infarction, arrhythmias, and tricuspid valve injury can result. Transvenous retrieval or repositioning has been performed successfully with a variety of techniques, including use of a large sheath system and looped guidewire or snare.[94,95]

Penetration of the caval wall by device legs or hooks is common (see Fig. 14-21). However, perforation into various neighboring structures (e.g., aorta, bowel, ureter) can be problematic.[85,96,97] Dislodgement of the filter or guidewire entrapment can occur when a wire is advanced into the IVC during a subsequent procedure such as central line placement (see Fig. 16-22).

BOX 14-4 ■ Indications for Retrievable Inferior Vena Cava (IVC) Filter Placement

Young patient
Prophylaxis after major trauma, in intensive care unit setting, or before high-risk operations
Before nephrectomy with IVC thrombosis
During lower extremity deep vein thrombolysis, especially with IVC involvement

Retrievable and Temporary Inferior Vena Cava Filters

Patient Selection

The development of retrievable and temporary IVC filters was prompted by growing concerns about the long-term effects of device placement (particularly in young patients) and the existence of subsets of patients with a limited, predictable period of increased risk for venous thromboembolic disease and pulmonary embolism. A *temporary IVC filter* is intended for use over a very short interval (e.g., during lower extremity venous thrombolysis) and **must** be ultimately removed. *Retrievable IVC filters* are meant to be removed when the risk factors for venous thromboembolic disease that warranted filter insertion have resolved or anticoagulation is considered safe; however, they also may be permanently left in place.

The primary indications for retrievable filter placement are outlined in Box 14-4.[98] Prophylactic placement, which generally has been avoided with permanent filters, has become a reasonable treatment option in certain clinical settings (e.g., major trauma, patients in the intensive care unit).[36,40,99]

Before a retrievable filter is removed, imaging studies are performed to exclude lower extremity deep venous thrombosis. In some cases, anticoagulation should be started immediately before or after retrieval. The feasibility of removing a filter is largely a function of dwell time and the presence of residual thrombus within the filter (Table 14-3).[100] If the anticipated period required for embolic protection is longer than the accepted dwell time of the filter, one option is to partially retrieve the filter and move it to a slightly different location in the IVC every 2 weeks or so until permanent removal is permissible.[101,102] Some retrievable filters can be removed safely after much longer periods than recommended by the manufacturers, although the safety of this maneuver has not been proven.[99,103-106]

TABLE 14-3   MANUFACTURERS' GUIDELINES FOR INFERIOR VENA CAVA FILTER REMOVAL

Filter	Retrieval Interval	Percentage of Thrombus Allowing Removal	Access Site
Guenther-Tulip	<2 wk	25% of cone	Jugular
Recovery	<4 mo	No recommendation	Jugular
Optease	<2 wk	No recommendation	Femoral
Tempofilter II	<12 wk		Jugular

Devices (Fig. 14-23)

■ *Guenther-Tulip filter.* Four wires joined at the superior apex extend in the shape of a cross.
■ *Recovery filter.* The device has two levels of filtration, with six diverging nitinol arms and six legs that all join at the filter apex.[107]
■ *OptEase filter.* This device is a retrievable version of the TrapEase filter with a capture hook on the inferior apex. As such, it must be removed from a **femoral** route.[64]
■ *Tempofilter II.* By removing the side rails with hooks from the permanent Vena-Tech filter, a retrievable device was created.[36,108] The apex is attached to a 6-French tethering catheter, which terminates in an anchoring "olive" that is implanted subcutaneously adjacent to the insertion site in the right internal jugular vein. This device is only temporary and **must** eventually be removed.

Retrieval Technique

A pigtail catheter is negotiated carefully with a guidewire through the filter (or placed just below in the case of the OptEase device) to perform inferior venacavography. This step is necessary to identify thrombus within or extending above the filter, because large volumes of trapped clot may preclude removal or make the risk of pulmonary embolism with removal unacceptable (see Table 14-3). In some cases, catheter-directed thrombolysis must be considered. Another option is to place a second retrievable filter above the thrombus-filled device to capture any clot that showers centrally during removal of the original filter. The second filter then may be retrieved.[109]

Assuming a minimal clot burden, the Guenther-Tulip filter apex is captured with an Amplatz gooseneck snare (see Chapter 2) advanced through a long 11-French sheath from the right internal jugular vein. The sheath is then slid over the filter, compressing the legs and disengaging the device from the caval wall.

The Recovery filter removal can be somewhat more problematic. Ideally, the filter should be aligned precisely with the longitudinal axis of the IVC. If the filter is even slightly tilted, often it is necessary to minimize the tilt by inserting a stiff guidewire from above or below through the filter legs. Alternatively, a tip-deflecting wire is used to center the filter apex with the IVC lumen.[110] The urethane-covered retrieval device then is inserted from the right internal jugular vein through a long 7-French sheath and centered over the apex of the filter (as confirmed by multiple fluoroscopic projections) in order to engage it (Fig. 14-24). Even with extraordinary effort, capturing the filter apex and removing the filter may be impossible (Fig. 14-25).

The OptEase filter is withdrawn through a 6-French sheath from the femoral vein using an Amplatz gooseneck snare.

Results and Complications

Retrievable IVC filters are placed successfully in 95% to 100% of cases.[107,108,111-113] The subsequent pulmonary embolism rate is less than 1%, although most of these devices have not been in use long enough to allow long-term longitudinal studies. In reported series, **attempted** retrieval is accomplished in 90% to 100% of patients.[99,102,107,113-115] The most common reasons for failure are the presence of substantial thrombus within the filter (precluding safe withdrawal), inability to capture the device (especially with the Recovery filter), and incorporation into the IVC wall.

IVC filter occlusion is described in 1% to 5% of cases (see Fig. 14-21); thrombolysis has been performed to remove fresh thrombus.[102,112] It is possible to recanalize some chronically thrombosed IVC filters that are causing incapacitating or life-threatening symptoms by crushing the filter with a stent.[116]

Postinsertion migration of retrievable filters has been described.[117,118] There is recent concern that some of these devices may be particularly prone to late embolization (possibly precipitated by sudden large clot embolization into the device) that has led to fatal cardiac hemorrhage or dysrhythmias. Retrieval techniques in this situation are analogous to those employed for permanent filters (see above and Chapter 16).

Neoplasms

Etiology

Abdominal and pelvic tumors can involve the IVC by intraluminal extension, direct invasion through the caval wall, or extrinsic compression. Tumors that often spread intraluminally include renal cell carcinoma, hepatocellular carcinoma, adrenal carcinoma, and some gynecologic and testicular neoplasms.[119] Tumors that typically attack the IVC by mural invasion include pancreatic neoplasms and retroperitoneal sarcomas.

Renal cell carcinoma is the most common neoplasm to involve the IVC, which occurs in approximately 10% of cases.[120] Identification of renal vein or IVC invasion (Robson stage IIIA) is important in determining prognosis and guiding operative therapy. Hepatoma invades the IVC in about 10% of patients.[121] In such cases, extension of tumor thrombus into the right atrium is common.

Primary malignancies of the IVC are rare. *Leiomyosarcoma* is the most common neoplasm to afflict the IVC, and the IVC is the most common **vascular** site for leiomyosarcoma.[122,123] Primary leiomyosarcoma of the IVC may be impossible to differentiate from the more common retroperitoneal leiomyosarcoma. Both neoplasms may extend into or outside the lumen of the cava. Extraluminal growth occurs in most cases; intraluminal growth alone is seen in about one fourth of patients. Leiomyosarcoma has a fairly uniform distribution throughout the IVC, although the segment from the renal veins to the hepatic veins is most commonly involved.

Clinical Features

Luminal obstruction or extrinsic compression of the IVC by tumor can be asymptomatic or cause leg swelling and distention of superficial veins, abdominal pain or bloating, and deep venous thrombosis. The Budd-Chiari syndrome may develop if intrahepatic IVC occlusion is complete. Patients with leiomyosarcoma also may present with abdominal pain or a palpable abdominal mass. Classically, this extremely rare disease occurs in women in the fifth or sixth decade of life.

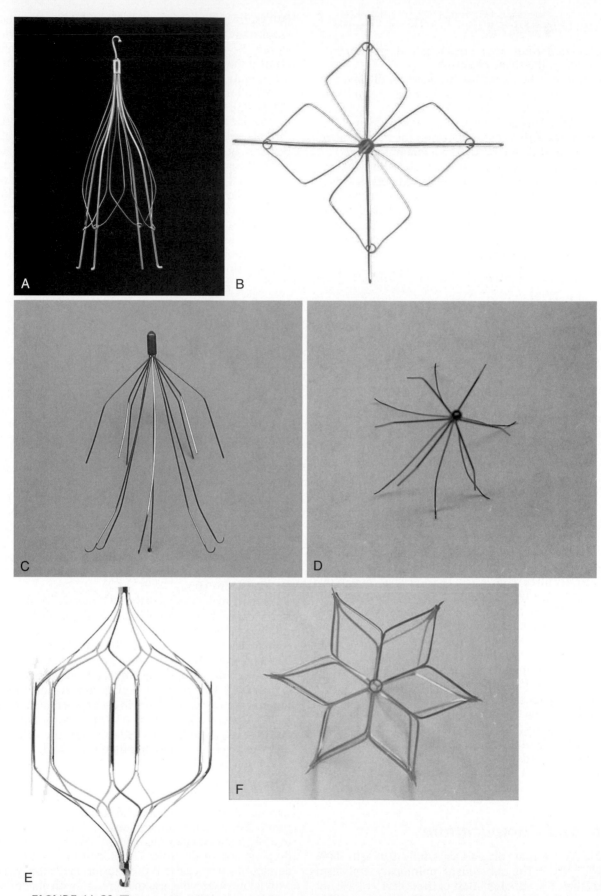

FIGURE 14-23 ▮ Retrievable inferior vena cava filters. **A** and **B,** Guenther-Tulip filter (Cook, Inc., Bloomington, Ind.) **C** and **D,** Recovery filter (Bard, Inc., Tempe, Ariz.). **E** and **F,** OptEase filter (Cordis Corp., Miami Lakes, Fla.).

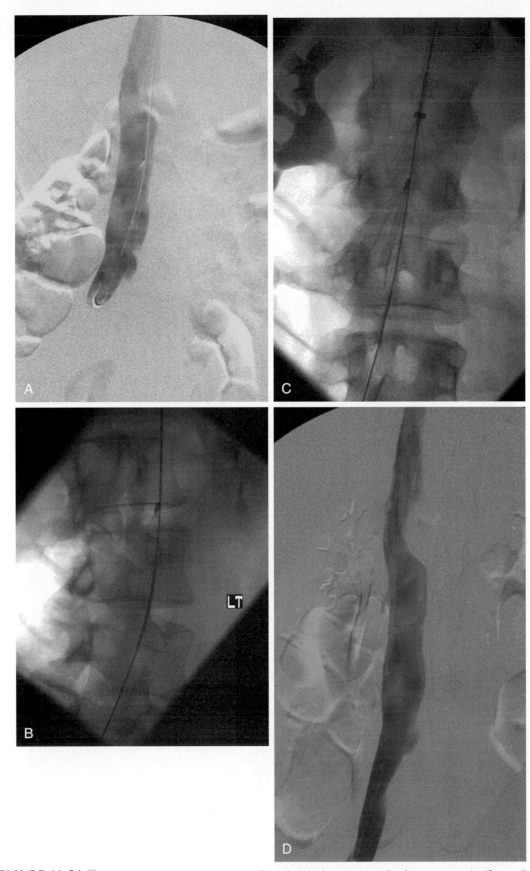

FIGURE 14-24 ■ Successful retrieval of a Recovery filter. **A,** Initial venacavography demonstrates significant tilting of the filter and no thrombus. **B,** A guidewire and catheter are used to better align the filter with the inferior vena cava. **C,** The retrieval cone is advanced through the sheath and used to engage the filter apex. **D,** After filter removal, repeat venacavography shows minimal mural deformity.

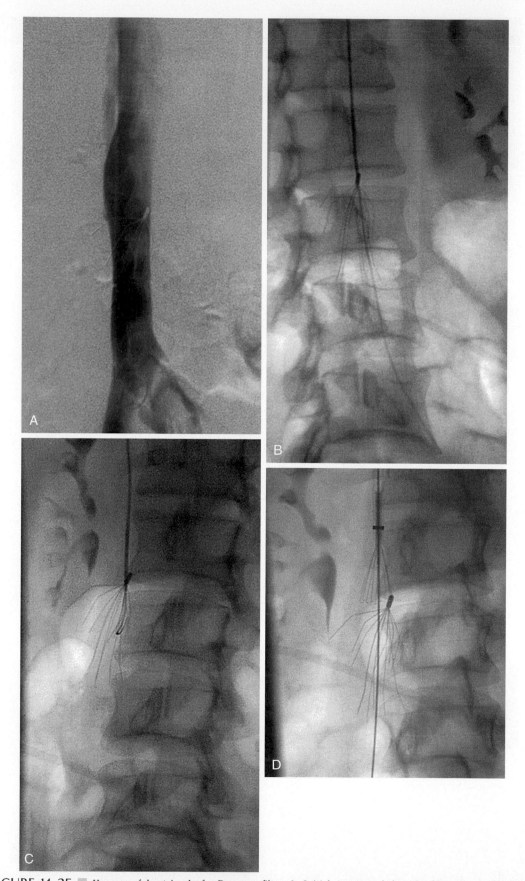

FIGURE 14-25 ■ Unsuccessful retrieval of a Recovery filter. **A,** Initial cavogram below the filter shows significant device tilting. **B,** A stiff guidewire is placed from above to straighten the filter. **C,** A gooseneck snare is used to engage the filter apex and align it with the inferior vena cava. **D,** Multiple unsuccessful attempts were made to engage the filter apex with the retrieval device. The filter ultimately was left in place.

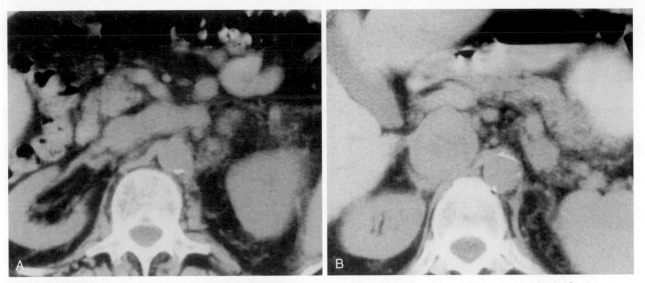

FIGURE 14-26 ■ Left renal cell carcinoma with left renal vein (**A**) and inferior vena cava (**B**) tumor invasion is identified by CT.

Imaging

Cross-sectional Techniques. CT, MR, and sonography are ideal for assessing patients with known or suspected IVC invasion from a malignancy.[124-128] CT and MR findings include enlargement of the IVC, intraluminal filling defects, extension of tumor thrombus to the right atrium, and complete IVC occlusion with opacification of collateral vessels (Fig. 14-26). Occasionally, neovascularity within the tumor thrombus is seen.

Leiomyosarcoma appears as an inhomogeneous mass replacing or filling the IVC (Fig. 14-27).[128] MR findings are variable, with the mass typically showing intermediate signal intensity on T1-weighted sequences and increased signal on T2-weighted sequences.

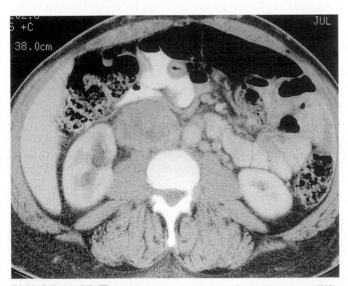

FIGURE 14-27 ■ Leiomyosarcoma of the inferior vena cava (IVC). Notice the marked enlargement of the IVC and inhomogeneous density of the tumor.

Angiography. CT and MR have replaced venacavography in the diagnosis and staging of IVC tumors. However, endovascular biopsy of suspected luminal IVC tumors may be performed when the pathologic diagnosis is unknown.[129,130] Bleeding complications are less likely through an intraluminal route than a percutaneous approach.

Treatment

Radical surgery is favored in some patients with primary or secondary tumor, even when the disease has spread to the intrahepatic IVC.[131,132] Operative techniques include caval wall resection with patching or segmental caval resection with prosthetic grafting.

Chronic Inferior Vena Cava Compression, Stenosis, and Obstruction

Focal or diffuse narrowing of the IVC is common (Box 14-5). **Normal** extrinsic compression of the IVC may be caused by the right common iliac artery (on the bifurcation), right renal artery (on the posterior cava), or the spine (see Fig. 13-19). The most frequent cause of **pathologic** extrinsic compression is liver disease (e.g., severe hepatomegaly, caudate lobe enlargement, hepatic masses, massive ascites) (Figs. 14-28 and 14-29). Large abdominal aortic aneurysms (among other extrinsic masses [Fig. 14-30]) also may efface the vena cava, and severe obstruction of the IVC by an abdominal aortic aneurysm can lead to thrombosis.[133]

Mural thickening from resolved thrombosis can cause mild or moderate caval narrowing. The IVC can appear severely narrowed if the patient performs a vigorous Valsalva maneuver during imaging.

Intravascular stents are placed for certain IVC obstructions with some success. In most cases, stents are inserted

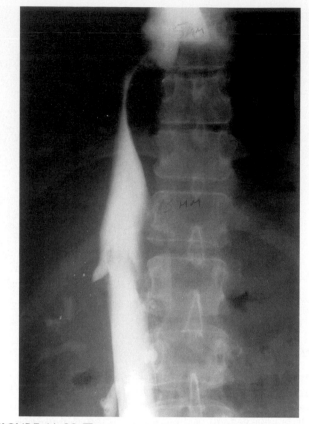

FIGURE 14-29 ■ Severe narrowing of the intrahepatic inferior vena cava is caused by ascites and hepatomegaly. An 8-mm Hg pressure gradient was detected.

for palliative treatment of IVC obstruction caused by malignancy, particularly neoplasms of the liver.[134-137] They have been used also to treat posttransplant IVC stenoses.[138] Gianturco Z-stents and Wallstents have been used, among others, for this purpose (Fig. 14-31). Stents are inserted successfully in virtually every reported case; the device usually remains patent for the life of the patient. The major concern is stent migration, which can have disastrous consequences. Therefore, oversized stents are routinely chosen.

■ OTHER DISORDERS

Retroperitoneal Fibrosis

Retroperitoneal fibrosis is a rare chronic inflammatory disorder of unclear cause. Genetic and autoimmune origins

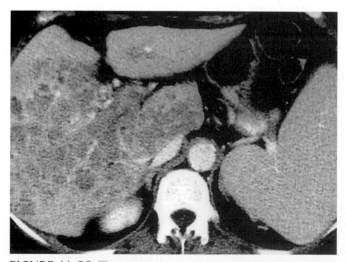

FIGURE 14-28 ■ Massive hepatocellular carcinoma produces extrinsic compression of the intrahepatic inferior vena cava.

have been proposed; in a few cases, it is the result of tumor, infection, or chronic use of certain drugs, such as ergot derivatives.[139] The fibrosis often extends from the level of the kidneys into the pelvis. Symptomatic involvement of the IVC occurs in only 2% of cases.

CT or MR imaging reveals encasement of the IVC, iliac veins, or both (Fig. 14-32).[140,141] In symptomatic patients, complete occlusion of the IVC may be seen. The soft tissue process also can involve the aorta, ureters, and small bowel, particularly the duodenum.

Membranous Obstruction

Membranous obstruction of the IVC is a set of conditions of unknown origin in which a fibromuscular membrane develops within the IVC just below the right atrium (type 1) or a fibrous band completely replaces the intrahepatic IVC for a variable distance (type 2).[142] Hepatic vein involvement is common. Membranous IVC obstruction is most commonly seen in Korea, Japan, India, and South Africa; the disease is rare in non-Asian populations in the United States. Patients often present with symptoms of chronic liver disease and large truncal collateral veins but usually do not have classic features of Budd-Chiari syndrome.

The diagnosis is made by cross-sectional imaging.[143,144] Sonography is useful for detecting and characterizing the IVC obstruction. Hepatic vein involvement and patterns of

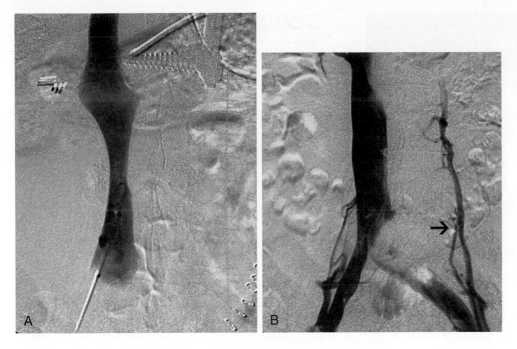

FIGURE 14-30 ■ Extrinsic compression of the inferior vena cava by massive hydronephrosis (**A**) and a known pelvic mass (**B**). Opacification of collateral vessels *(arrow)* proves the hemodynamic significance of the obstruction.

collateral flow also can be evaluated by ultrasound. CT is superior to sonography in detecting occult hepatoma. Venacavography is used only to guide therapy.

Balloon angioplasty, stent placement, and thrombolysis have been used to recanalize the IVC in cases of incomplete or complete obstruction.[145,146] The short-term results of these procedures have been excellent. The long-term results in a large series of patients have not been determined. Surgical options include transcardiac membranectomy, decompression of the liver with a portosystemic shunt, or bypass procedure with a cavoatrial shunt or IVC to SVC graft.

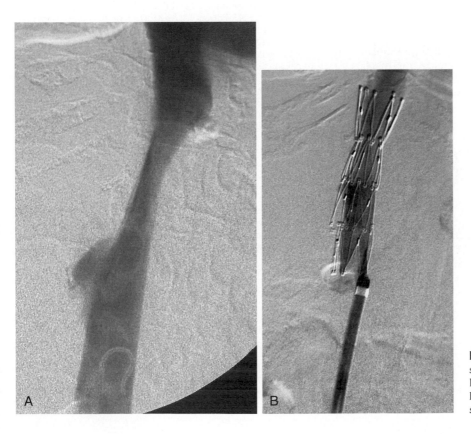

FIGURE 14-31 ■ Inferior vena cava (IVC) stent placement. **A,** Intrahepatic IVC narrowing following liver transplant with a 14-mm Hg gradient. **B,** Widely patent vessel following placement of several Gianturco Z stents.

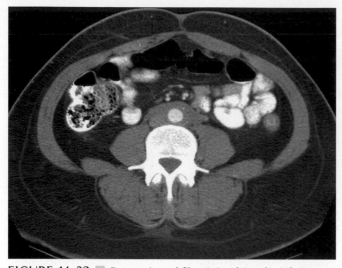

FIGURE 14-32 ■ Retroperitoneal fibrosis involving the inferior vena cava and aorta.

Aortocaval Fistula

Aortocaval fistula is rare; most cases are caused by erosion from an abdominal aortic aneurysm. In the absence of an aortic aneurysm, aortocaval fistula is either spontaneous or secondary to infection or trauma (blunt, penetrating, or lumbar spine surgery).[147-149] The diagnosis is made by sonography, CT angiography, or MR angiography (see Fig. 5-17). The communication most frequently develops between the distal aorta and IVC. Stent-grafts have been used to manage these lesions.

Trauma

Injury to the IVC may occur from blunt or penetrating trauma to the abdomen or chest. Preoperative imaging rarely is performed in such cases.[150] Most patients undergo immediate exploratory laparotomy because they are hemodynamically unstable or show evidence of bleeding on peritoneal lavage or ultrasound. With blunt abdominal trauma, the most common site of laceration is the retrohepatic portion of the IVC. The location of injury varies widely with penetrating injuries.

Aneurysms

Aneurysms of the IVC are exceedingly rare.[151-153] The clinical picture includes abdominal pain, acute IVC occlusion, and pulmonary embolism. IVC aneurysm can mimic IVC occlusion from other causes. Surgical treatment involves partial or complete excision of the aneurysm.

REFERENCES

1. Dewald CL, Jensen CC, Park YH, et al: Vena cavography with CO_2 versus with iodinated contrast material for inferior vena cava filter placement: a prospective evaluation. Radiology 2000;216:752.

2. Brown DB, Pappas JA, Vedantham S, et al: Gadolinium, carbon dioxide, and iodinated contrast material for planning inferior vena cava filter placement: a prospective trial. J Vasc Interv Radiol 2003;14:1017.

3. Gabella G, ed: Cardiovascular system. In: Williams PL, Bannister LH, Berry MM, et al, eds. Gray's Anatomy, 38th ed. New York, Churchill Livingstone, 1995:1600.

4. Collin P, ed: Embryology and development. In: Williams PL, Bannister LH, Berry MM, et al, eds. Gray's Anatomy, 38th ed. New York, Churchill Livingstone, 1995:324.

5. Bass JE, Redwine MD, Kramer LA, et al: Spectrum of congenital anomalies of the inferior vena cava: cross-sectional imaging findings. Radiographics 2000;20:639.

6. Hicks ME, Malden ES, Vesely TM, et al: Prospective anatomic study of the inferior vena cava and renal veins: comparison of selective renal venography with cavography and relevance in filter placement. J Vasc Interv Radiol 1995;6:721.

7. Beckmann CF, Abrams HL: Renal venography: anatomy, technique, applications: analysis of 132 venograms, and a review of the literature. Cardiovasc Intervent Radiol 1980;3:45.

8. LaBerge JM, Ring EJ, Gordon RL: Percutaneous intrahepatic portosystemic shunt created via a femoral vein approach. Radiology 1991; 181:679.

9. Kaufman JA, Waltman AC, Rivitz SM, et al: Anatomical observations on the renal veins and inferior vena cava at magnetic resonance angiography. Cardiovasc Intervent Radiol 1995;18:153.

10. Grant E, Rendano F, Sevinc E, et al: Normal inferior vena cava: caliber changes observed by dynamic ultrasound. AJR Am J Roentgenol 1980;135:335.

11. Mayo J, Gray R, St Louis E, et al: Anomalies of the inferior vena cava. AJR Am J Roentgenol 1983;140:339.

12. Munechika H, Cohan RH, Baker ME, et al: Hemiazgyous continuation of a left inferior vena cava: CT appearance. J Comput Assist Tomogr 1988;12:328.

13. Brickner ME, Eichhorn EJ, Netto D, et al: Left-sided inferior vena cava draining into the coronary sinus via persistent left superior vena cava: case report and review of the literature. Cathet Cardiovasc Diagn 1990;20:189.

14. Sheley RC, Nyberg DA, Kapur R: Azygous continuation of the interrupted inferior vena cava: a clue to prenatal diagnosis of the cardiosplenic syndromes. J Ultrasound Med 1995;14:381.

15. Fulcher AS, Turner MA: Abdominal manifestations of situs anomalies in adults. Radiographics 2002;22:1439.

16. Sonin AH, Mazer MJ, Powers TA: Obstruction of the inferior vena cava: a multiple modality demonstration of causes, manifestations, and collateral pathways. Radiographics 1992;12:309.

17. Kim HL, Zisman A, Han KR, et al: Prognostic significance of venous thrombus in renal cell carcinoma. Are renal vein and inferior vena cava involvement different? J Urol 2004;171:588.

18. Okuda K: Membranous obstruction of the inferior vena cava. J Gastroenterol Hepatol 2001;16:1179.

19. Kaushik S, Federle MP, Schur PH, et al: Abdominal thrombotic and ischemic manifestations of the antiphospholipid antibody syndrome: CT findings in 42 patients. Radiology 2001;218:768.

20. Hausler M, Hubner D, Delhaas T, et al: Long term complications of inferior vena cava thrombosis. Arch Dis Child 2001;85:228.

21. Harris EJ Jr, Kinney EV, Harris EJ Sr, et al: Phlegmasia complicating prophylactic percutaneous inferior vena caval interruption: a word of caution. J Vasc Surg 1995;22:606.

22. Umeoka S, Koyama T, Togashi K, et al: Vascular dilatation in the pelvis: identification with CT and MR imaging. Radiographics 2004;24:193.

23. Katz DS, Loud PA, Bruce D, et al: Combined CT venography and pulmonary angiography: a comprehensive review. Radiographics 2002; 22:S3.

24. Bates SM, Ginsberg JS: Treatment of deep-vein thrombosis. New Engl J Med 2004;351:268.

25. Hansen ME, Miller GL III, Starks KC: Pulse spray thrombolysis of inferior vena cava thrombosis complicating filter placement. Cardiovasc Intervent Radiol 1994;17:38.

26. Robinson DL, Teitelbaum GP: Phlegmasia cerulea dolens: treatment by pulse-spray and infusion thrombolysis. AJR Am J Roentgenol 1993; 160:1288.

27. Ishiguchi T, Fukatsu H, Itoh S, et al: Budd-Chiari syndrome with long segmental inferior vena cava obstruction: treatment with thrombolysis, angioplasty, and intravascular stents. J Vasc Interv Radiol 1992; 3:421.

28. Sharafuddin MJ, Sun S, Hoballah JJ, et al: Endovascular management of venous thrombotic and occlusive disease of the lower extremities. J Vasc Interv Radiol 2003;14:405.

29. Anderson BJ, Keeley SR, Johnson ND: Caval thrombolysis in neonates using low doses of recombinant human tissue-type plasminogen activator. Anaesth Intensive Care 1991;19:22.

30. Wilson JJ, Balsys A, Newman H, et al: IVC thrombosis: successful treatment with low dose streptokinase. J Cardiovasc Surg 1992;33:109.

31. Decousus H, Leizorovicz A, Parent F, et al: A clinical trial of vena caval filters in the prevention of pulmonary embolism in patients with proximal deep-vein thrombosis. Prevention du Risque d'Embolie Pulmonaire par Interruption Cave Study Group. N Engl J Med 1998Feb; 338:409.

32. Girard P, Stern JB, Parent F: Medical literature and vena cava filters: so far so weak. Chest 2002;122:963.

33. Kazmers A, Jacobs LA, Perkins AJ: Pulmonary embolism in Veterans Affairs Medical Centers: is vena cava interruption underutilized? Am Surg 1999;65:1171.

34. Athanasoulis CA, Kaufman JA, Halpern EF, et al: Inferior vena caval filters: review of a 26-year single-center clinical experience. Radiology 2000;216:54.

35. Grassi CJ, Swan TL, Cardella JF, et al: Quality improvement guidelines for percutaneous permanent inferior vena cava filter placement for the prevention of pulmonary embolism. SCVIR Standards of Practice Committee. J Vasc Interv Radiol 2001;12:137.

36. Kinney TB: Update on inferior vena cava filters. J Vasc Interv Radiol 2003;14:425.

37. Rogers FB, Shackford SR, Wilson J, et al: Prophylactic vena cava filter insertion in severly injured trauma patients: indications and preliminary results. J Trauma 1993;35:637.

38. Winchell RJ, Hoyt DB, Walsh JC, et al: Risk factors associated with pulmonary embolism despite routine prophylaxis: implications for improved protection. J Trauma 1994;37:600.

39. Gosin JS, Graham AM, Ciocca RG, et al: Efficacy of prophylactic vena cava filters in high-risk trauma patients. Ann Vasc Surg 1997;11:100.

40. Hoff WS, Hoey BA, Wainwright GA, et al: Early experience with retrievable inferior vena cava filters in high-risk trauma patients. J Am Coll Surg 2004;199:869.

41. Spence LD, Gironta MG, Malde HM, et al: Acute upper extremity deep venous thrombosis: safety and effectiveness of superior vena caval filters. Radiology 1999;210:53.

42. Ascher E, Hingorani A, Tsemekhin B, et al: Lessons learned from a 6-year clinical experience with superior vena cava Greenfield filters. J Vasc Surg 2000;32:881.

43. Greenfield LJ, Proctor MC: Vena caval filter use in patients with sepsis: results in 175 patients. Arch Surg 2003;138:1245.

44. Danetz JS, McLafferty RB, Ayerdi J, et al: Selective venography versus nonselective venography before vena cava filter placement: evidence for more, not less. J Vasc Surg 2003;38:928.

45. Patil UD, Ragavan A, Nadaraj, et al: Helical CT angiography in evaluation of live kidney donors. Nephrol Dial Transplant 2001;16:1900.

46. Reed RA, Teitelbaum GP, Taylor FC, et al: Use of the Bird's nest filter in oversized inferior vena cavae. J Vasc Interv Radiol 1991;2:447.

47. Mansour M, Chang AE, Sindelar WF: Interruption of the inferior vena cava for the prevention of recurrent pulmonary embolism. Am Surgeon 1985;51:375.

48. Miles RM, Richardson RR, Wayne L, et al: Long term results with the serrated Teflon vena caval clip in the prevention of pulmonary embolism. Ann Surg 1969;169:881.

49. Greenfield LJ, McCrudy JR, Brown PP, et al: A new intracaval filter permitting continued flow and resolution of thrombi. Surgery 1973; 73:599.

50. Tadavarthy SM, Castaneda-Zuniga W, Salomonowitz E, et al: Kimray-Greenfield vena cava filter: percutaneous introduction. Radiology 1984; 151:525.

51. Katsamouris AA, Waltman AC, Delichatsios MA, et al: Inferior vena cava filters: in vitro comparison of clot trapping and flow dynamics. Radiology 1988;166:361.

52. Hammer FD, Rousseau HP, Joffre FG, et al: In vitro evaluation of vena cava filters. J Vasc Interv Radiol 1994;5:869.

53. Simon M, Rabkin DJ, Kleshinski S, et al: Comparative evaluation of clinically available inferior vena cava filters with an in vitro physiologic simulation of the vena cava. Radiology 1993;189:769.

54. Korbin CD, Reed RA, Taylor FC, et al: Comparison of filters in an oversized vena caval phantom: intracaval placement of a Bird's nest filter

55. Grassi CJ, Matsumoto AH, Teitelbaum GP: Vena caval occlusion after Simon nitinol filter placement: identification with MR imaging in patients with malignancy. J Vasc Interv Radiol 1992;3:535.

56. Lorch H, Dallmann A, Zwaan M, et al: Efficacy of permanent and retrievable vena cava filters: experimental studies and evaluation of a new device. Cardiovasc Intervent Radiol 2002;25:193.

57. Leask RL, Johnston KW, Ojha M: Hemodynamic effects of clot entrapment in the TrapEase inferior vena cava filter. J Vasc Interv Radiol 2004;15:485.

58. McCowan TC, Ferris EJ, Carver DK, et al: Use of external jugular vein as a route for percutaneous inferior vena caval filter placement. Radiology 1990;176:527.

59. Davison BD, Grassi CJ: TrapEase inferior vena cava filter placed via the basilic arm vein: a new antecubital access. J Vasc Interv Radiol 2002;13:107.

60. Streiff MB: Vena caval filters: a comprehensive review. Blood 2000; 95:3669.

61. Matchett WJ, Jones MP, McFarland DR, et al: Suprarenal vena caval filter placement: follow-up of four filter types in 22 patients. J Vasc Intervent Radiol 1998;9:588.

62. Greenfield LJ, Proctor MC: Suprarenal filter placement. J Vasc Surg 1998;28:432.

63. Kaufman JA, Geller SC, Rivitz SM, et al: Operator errors during percutaneous placement of vena cava filters. AJR Am J Roentgenol 1995; 165:1281.

64. Rosenthal D, Wellons ED, Levitt AB, et al: Role of prophylactic temporary inferior vena cava filters placed at the ICU bedside under intravascular ultrasound guidance in with multiple trauma. J Vasc Surg 2004;40:958.

65. Rose SC, Kinney TB, Valji K, et al: Placement of inferior vena caval filters in the intensive care unit. J Vasc Interv Radiol 1997;8:61.

66. Reed RA, Teitelbaum GP, Taylor FC, et al: Incomplete opening of LGM (Vena Tech) filters inserted via the transjugular approach. J Vasc Interv Radiol 1991;21:441.

67. Kinney TB, Rose SC, Weingarten KW, et al: IVC filter tilt and asymmetry: comparison of over-the-wire stainless-steel and titanium Greenfield IVC filters. J Vasc Intervent Radiol 1997;8:1029.

68. Moore BS, Valji K, Roberts AC, et al: Transcatheter manipulation of asymmetrically opened titanium Greenfield filters. J Vasc Interv Radiol 1993;4:687.

69. Shlansky-Goldberg R, Wing CM, LeVeen RF, et al: Effectiveness of a prolapsed Bird's nest filter. J Vasc Interv Radiol 1993;4:505.

70. LaPlante JS, Contractor FM, Kiproff PM, et al: Migration of the Simon nitinol vena cava filter to the chest. AJR Am J Roentgenol 1993; 160:385.

71. Thompson BH, Cragg AH, Smith TP, et al: Thrombus-trapping efficiency of the Greenfield filter in vivo. Radiology 1989;172:979.

72. Sweeney TJ, Van Aman ME: Deployment problems with the titanium Greenfield filter. J Vasc Interv Radiol 1993;4:691.

73. Dorfman GS: Risks and benefits of manipulation of the titanium Greenfield inferior vena cava filter after deployment: filter facts and filter fantasies. J Vasc Interv Radiol 1993;4:617.

74. Wang WY, Cooper SG, Eberhardt SC: Use of a nitinol gooseneck snare to open an incompletely expanded over-the-wire stainless steel Greenfield filter. AJR Am J Roentgenol 1999;172:499.

75. Roehm JO Jr, Thomas JW: The twist technique: a method to minimize wire prolapse during Bird's nest filter placement. J Vasc Interv Radiol 1995;6:455.

76. Carlson JE, Yedlicka JW Jr, Castaneda-Zuniga WR, et al: Acute clot-trapping efficiency in dogs with compacted versus elongated wires in Bird's nest filters. J Vasc Interv Radiol 1993;4:513.

77. Cho KJ, Greenfield LJ, Proctor MC, et al: Evaluation of a new percutaneous stainless steel Greenfield filter. J Vasc Interv Radiol 1997;8:181.

78. Joels CS, Sing RF, Heniford BT: Complications of inferior vena cava filters. Am Surg 2003;69:654.

79. Ferris EJ, McCowan TC, Carver DK, et al: Percutaneous inferior vena caval filters: follow-up of seven designs in 320 patients. Radiology 1993; 188:851.

80. Wojtowycz MM, Stoehr T, Crummy AB, et al: The Bird's nest inferior vena caval filter: review of a single-center experience. J Vasc Interv Radiol 1997;8:171.

81. Becker DM, Philbrick JT, Selby JB: Inferior vena cava filters: indications, safety, effectiveness. Arch Intern Med 1992;152:1985.

82. Neuerburg JM, Guenther RW, Vorwerk D, et al: Results of a multicenter study of the retrievable Tulip Vena Cava Filter: early clinical experience. Cardiovasc Intervent Radiol 1997;20:10.

83. Streiff MB: Vena caval filters: a review for intensive care specialists. J Intensive Care Med 2003;18:59.

84. Kinney TB, Rose SC, Lim GW, et al: Fatal paradoxic embolism occurring during IVC filter insertion in a patient with chronic pulmonary thromboembolic disease. J Vasc Interv Radiol 2001;12:770.

85. Putterman D, Niman D, Cohen G: Aortic pseudoaneurysm after penetration by a Simon nitinol inferior vena cava filter. J Vasc Interv Radiol 2005;16:535.

86. Ray CE Jr, Kaufman JA: Complications of inferior vena cava filters. Abdom Imaging 1996;21:368.

87. Molgaard CP, Yucel EK, Geller SC, et al: Access site thrombosis after placement of inferior vena cava filters with 12-14F delivery sheaths. Radiology 1992;185:257.

88. Millward SF, Marsh JI, Peterson RA, et al: LGM (Vena Tech) vena cava filter: clinical experience in 64 patients. J Vasc Interv Radiol 1991; 2:429.

89. Engmann E, Asch MR: Clinical experience with the antecubital Simon nitinol IVC filter. J Vasc Intervent Radiol 1998;9:774.

90. Crochet DP, Brunel P, Trogrlic S, et al: Long-term follow-up of Vena Tech-LGM filter: predictors and frequency of caval occlusion. J Vasc Interv Radiol 1999;10:137.

91. Vedantham S, Vesely TM, Parti N, et al: Endovascular recanalization of the thrombosed filter-bearing inferior vena cava. J Vasc Interv Radiol 2003;14:893.

92. Friedell ML, Goldenkranz RJ, Parsonnet V, et al: Migration of a Greenfield filter to the pulmonary artery: a case report. J Vasc Surg 1986;3:929.

93. Rogoff PA, Hilgenberg AD, Miller SL, et al: Cephalic migration of the Bird's nest inferior vena caval filter: report of two cases. Radiology 1992;184:819.

94. Malden ES, Darcy MD, Hicks ME, et al: Transvenous retrieval of misplaced stainless steel Greenfield filters. J Vasc Interv Radiol 1992; 3:703.

95. Deutsch LS: Percutaneous removal of intracardiac Greenfield vena caval filter. AJR Am J Roentgenol 1988;151:677.

96. Chintalapudi UB, Gutierrez OH, Azodo MV: Greenfield filter caval perforation causing an aortic mural thrombus and femoral artery occlusion. Cathet Cardiovasc Diagn 1997;41:53.

97. Goldman HB, Hanna K, Dmochowski RR: Ureteral injury secondary to an inferior vena caval filter. J Urol 1996;156:1763.

98. Wellons E, Rosenthal D, Schoborg T, et al: Renal cell carcinoma invading the inferior vena cava: use of a "temporary" vena cava filter to prevent tumor emboli during nephrectomy. Urology 2004;63:380.

99. Morris CS, Rogers FB, Najarian KE, et al: Current trends in vena caval filtration with the introduction of a retrievable filter at a level I trauma center. J Trauma 2004;57:32.

100. Kerlan RK Jr, Laberge JM, Wilson MW, et al: Residual thrombus within a retrievable IVC filter. J Vasc Interv Radiol 2005;16:555.

101. de Gregorio MA, Gamboa P, Gimeno MJ, et al: The Gunther Tulip retrievable filter: prolonged temporary filtration by repositioning within the inferior vena cava. J Vasc Interv Radiol 2003;14:1259.

102. Tay KH, Martin ML, Fry PD, et al: Repeated Gunther Tulip inferior vena cava filter repositioning to prolong implantation time. J Vasc Interv Radiol 2002;13:509.

103. Binkert CA, Bansal A, Gates JD: Inferior vena cava filter removal after 317-day implantation. J Vasc Interv Radiol 2005;16:395.

104. Reekers JA, Hoogeveen YL, Wijnands M, et al: Evaluation of the retrievability of the OptEase IVC filter in an animal model. J Vasc Interv Radiol 2004;15:261.

105. Terhaar OA, Lyon SM, Given MF, et al: Extended interval for retrieval of Gunther Tulip filters. J Vasc Interv Radiol 2004;15:1257.

106. Millward SF, Oliva VL, Bell SD, et al: Guenther Tulip retrievable vena cava filter: results from the Registry of the Canadian Interventional Radiology Association. J Vasc Interv Radiol 2001;12:1053.

107. Asch MR: Initial experience in humans with a new retrievable inferior vena cava filter. Radiology 2002;225:835.

108. Bovyn G, Gory P, Reynaud P, et al: The Tempofilter: a multicenter study of a new temporary caval filter implantable for up to six weeks. Ann Vasc Surg 1997;11:520.

109. Yavuz K, Geyik S, Barton RE, et al: Retrieval of a malpositioned vena cava filter with embolic protection with use of a second filter. J Vasc Interv Radiol 2005;16:531.

110. Hagspiel KD, Leung DA, Aladdin M, et al: Difficult retrieval of a Recovery IVC filter. J Vasc Interv Radiol 2004;15:645.

111. Rosenthal D, Wellons ED, Lai KM, et al: Retrievable inferior vena cava filters: early clinical experience. J Cardiovasc Surg (Torino) 2005; 46:163.

112. Schutzer R, Ascher E, Hingorani A, et al: Preliminary results of the new 6F TrapEase inferior vena cava filter. Ann Vasc Surg 2003;17:103.

113. Oliva VL, Szatmari F, Giroux M-F, et al: The Jonas study: evaluation of the retrievability of the Cordis Optease™ inferior vena cava filter. J Vasc Interv Radiol 2005;16:1439.

114. Stein PD, Alnas M, Skaf E, et al: Outcome and complications of retrievable inferior vena cava filters. Am J Cardiol 2004;94:1090.

115. Offner PJ, Hawkes A, Madayag R, et al: The role of temporary inferior vena cava filters in critically ill surgical patients. Arch Surg 2003; 138:591.

116. Joshi A, Carr J, Chrisman H, et al: Filter-related, thrombotic occlusion of the inferior vena cava treated with a Gianturco stent. J Vasc Interv Radiol 2003;14:381.

117. Bochenek KM, Aruny JE, Tal MG: Right atrial migration and percutaneous retrieval of a Gunther Tulip inferior vena cava filter. J Vasc Interv Radiol 2003;14:1207.

118. Porcellini M, Stassano P, Musumeci A, et al: Intracardiac migration of nitinol TrapEase vena cava filter and paradoxical embolism. Eur J Cardiothorac Surg 2002;22:460.

119. Concepcion RS, Koch MO, McDougal WS, et al: Management of primary nonrenal parenchymal malignancies with vena caval thrombus. J Urol 1991;145:243.

120. Vaidya A, Ciancio G, Soloway M: Surgical techniques for treating a renal neoplasm invading the inferior vena cava. J Urol 2003;169:435.

121. Kanematsu M, Imaeda T, Minowa H, et al: Hepatocellular carcinoma with tumor thrombus in the inferior vena cava and right atrium. Abdom Imaging 1994;19:313.

122. Mingoli A, Feldhaus RJ, Cavallaro A, et al: Leiomyosarcoma of the inferior vena cava: analysis and search of world literature on 141 patients and report of three new cases. J Vasc Surg 1991;14:688.

123. Hollenbeck ST, Grobmyer SR, Kent KC, et al: Surgical treatment and outcomes of patients with primary inferior vena cava leiomyosarcoma. J Am Coll Surg 2003;197:575.

124. Habboub HK, Abu-Yousef MM, Williams RD, et al: Accuracy of color Doppler sonography in assessing venous thrombus extension in renal cell carcinoma. AJR Am J Roentgenol 1997;168:267.

125. Hallscheidt PJ, Fink C, Haferkamp A, et al: Preoperative staging of renal cell carcinoma with inferior vena cava thrombus using multidetector CT and MRI: prospective study with histopathological correlation. J Comput Assist Tomogr 2005;29:64.

126. Sheth S, Scatarige JC, Horton KM, et al: Current concepts in the diagnosis and management of renal cell carcinoma: role of multidetector CT and three-dimensional CT. Radiographics 2001;21:S237.

127. Goldfarb DA, Novick AC, Lorig R, et al: Magnetic resonance imaging for assessment of vena caval tumor thrombi: a comparative study with venacavography and computerized tomography scanning. J Urol 1990;144:1100.

128. Hartman DS, Hayes WS, Choyke PL, et al: Leiomyosarcoma of the retroperitoneum and inferior vena cava: radiologic-pathologic correlation. Radiographics 1992;12:1203.

129. Fidias P, Fan CM, McGovern FJ, et al: Intracaval extension of germ cell carcinoma: diagnosis via endovascular biopsy and a review of the literature. Eur Urol 1997;31:376.

130. Armstrong PJ, Franklin DP: Pararenal vena cava leiomyosarcoma versus leiomyomatosis: difficult diagnosis. J Vasc Surg 2002; 36:1256.

131. Hemming AW, Langham MR, Reed AI, et al: Resection of the inferior vena cava for hepatic malignancy. Am Surg 2001;67:1081.

132. Blute ML, Leibovich BC, Lohse CM, et al: The Mayo Clinic experience with surgical management, complications and outcome for patients with renal cell carcinoma and venous tumour thrombus. BJU Int 2004; 94:33.

133. Palmer MA: Inferior vena cava occlusion secondary to aortic aneurysm. J Cardiovasc Surg 1990;31:372.

134. Irving JD, Dondelinger RF, Reidy JF, et al: Gianturco self-expanding stents: clinical experience in the vena cava and large veins. Cardiovasc Intervent Radiol 1992;15:328.

135. Furui S, Sawada S, Irie T, et al: Hepatic inferior vena cava obstruction: treatment of two types with Gianturco expandable metallic stents. Radiology 1990;176:665.

136. Brountzos EN, Binkert CA, Panagiotou IE, et al: Clinical outcome after intrahepatic venous stent placement for malignant inferior vena cava syndrome. Cardiovasc Intervent Radiol 2004;27:129.

137. Razavi MK, Hansch EC, Kee ST, et al: Chronically occluded inferior venae cavae: endovascular treatment. Radiology 2000;214:133.

138. Borsa JJ, Daly CP, Fontaine AB, et al: Treatment of inferior vena cava anastomotic stenoses with the Wallstent endoprosthesis after orthotopic liver transplantation. J Vasc Interv Radiol 1999;10:17.

139. Rhee RY, Gloviczki P, Luthra HS, et al: Iliocaval complications of retroperitoneal fibrosis. Am J Surg 1994;168:179.

140. Kottra JJ, Dunnick NR: Retroperitoneal fibrosis. Radiol Clin North Am 1996;34:1259.

141. Vorwerk D, Guenther RW, Wendt G, et al: Iliocaval stenosis and iliac vein thrombosis in retroperitoneal fibrosis: percutaneous treatment by use of hydrodynamic thrombectomy and stenting. Cardiovasc Intervent Radiol 1996;19:40.

142. Okuda K: Membranous obstruction of the inferior vena cava (obliterative hepatocavopathy, Okuda). J Gastroenterol Hepatol 2001;16:1179.

143. Kim TK, Chung JW, Han JK, et al: Hepatic changes in benign obstruction of the hepatic inferior vena cava: CT findings. AJR Am J Roentgenol 1999;173:1235.

144. Lee DH, Ko YT, Yoon Y, et al: Sonography and color Doppler imaging of Budd-Chiari syndrome of membranous obstruction of the inferior vena cava. J Uultrasound Med 1994;13:159.

145. Zhang C, Fu L, Zhang G, et al: Ultrasonically guided inferior vena cava stent placement: experience in 83 cases. J Vasc Interv Radiol 1999;10:85.

146. Yang XL, Cheng TO, Chen CR: Successful treatment by percutaneous balloon angioplasty of Budd-Chiari syndrome caused by membranous obstruction of inferior vena cava: 8-year follow-up study. J Am Coll Cardiol 1996;28:1720.

147. Torigian DA, Carpenter JP, Roberts DA: Mycotic aortocaval fistula: efficient evaluation by bolus-chase MR angiography. J Magn Reson Imaging 2002;15:195.

148. Rajmohan B: Spontaneous aortocaval fistula. J Postgrad Med 2002;48:203.

149. Lau LL, O'reilly MJ, Johnston LC, et al: Endovascular stent-graft repair of primary aortocaval fistula with an abdominal aortoiliac aneurysm. J Vasc Surg 2001;33:425.

150. Klein SR, Baumgartner FJ, Bongard FS: Contemporary management strategy for major inferior vena caval injuries. J Trauma 1994; 37:35.

151. Calligaro KD, Ahmad S, Dandora R, et al: Venous aneurysms: surgical indications and review of the literature. Surgery 1995;117:1.

152. Sullivan VV, Voris TK, Borlaza GS, et al: Incidental discovery of an inferior vena cava aneurysm. Ann Vasc Surg 2002;16:513.

153. Sweeney JP, Turner K, Harris KA: Aneurysms of the inferior vena cava. J Vasc Surg 1990;12:25.

15

Upper Extremity Veins and Superior Vena Cava

◼ VENOGRAPHY

Most clinically significant venous disease of the upper extremity involves the axillary, subclavian, and brachiocephalic veins. A plastic cannula is placed in a vein in the forearm. When an antecubital vein is used, it may be necessary to place a tourniquet above the elbow if contrast flows preferentially into the cephalic vein. Contrast material is injected while digital images are obtained. Superior venacavography is performed directly with a straight or pigtail catheter from the common femoral vein or internal jugular vein.

◼ ANATOMY

Development

In the embryo, the upper limb buds are drained by marginal veins.[1] The deep veins develop along with their corresponding arteries. The preaxial and postaxial portions of the marginal vein become the cephalic and basilic veins, respectively.

The central thoracic veins are formed from the precardinal (anterior) and common cardinal vessels (Fig. 15-1).[1] The upper segment of the precardinal vein becomes the internal jugular vein. The subclavian vein enters from the arm and joins the lower portion of the precardinal vein. An interprecardinal anastomosis connects the two precardinal veins and develops into the left brachiocephalic vein. The lower right precardinal vein becomes the upper superior vena cava. A remnant of the left precardinal vein becomes the left superior intercostal vein.

Normal Anatomy

The arms are drained by superficial and deep venous systems. Numerous perforators connect these systems. Unlike the situation in the lower extremities, the superficial system is dominant. It arises from two complex venous plexuses on the dorsal and palmar surfaces of the hand.[2] The cephalic and basilic veins originate from the dorsal venous network and run on the radial and ulnar sides of the forearm, respectively. The median vein of the forearm drains the palmar venous plexus and joins the basilic vein near the elbow. The *median cubital vein* connects the basilic and cephalic veins at the elbow (Fig. 15-2). In the upper arm, the *basilic vein* lies medial to the biceps muscle and forms the axillary vein at the lateral border of the scapula (see Fig. 15-2). The *cephalic vein* runs superficial and lateral to the biceps muscle, into the deltopectoral groove, through the infraclavicular fossa, and into the upper surface of the axillary vein (Fig. 15-3). The deep veins of the forearm follow the radial and ulnar arteries. They unite and then divide at the elbow to form paired *brachial veins*. These vessels run alongside the brachial artery and then join the basilic vein to become the axillary vein.

The *axillary vein* begins at the confluence of the brachial and basilic veins. Several branches of the brachial plexus

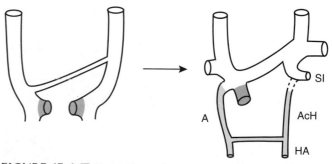

FIGURE 15-1 ◼ Embryologic development of the major thoracic veins. Shading indicates common cardinal vein origin *(dark)*, supracardinal vein origin *(gray)*, and azygous line vein origin *(white)*. A, azygous vein; AcH, accessory hemiazygous vein; HA, hemiazygous vein; SI, superior intercostal vein. (Adapted from Collin P, ed: Embryology and development. In: Williams PL, Bannister LH, Berry MM, et al, eds. Gray's Anatomy, 38th ed. London, Churchill Livingstone, 1995:327.)

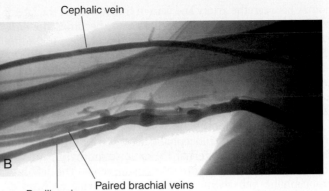
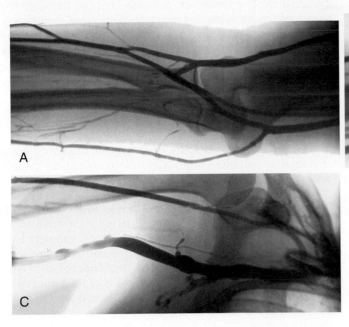

FIGURE 15-2 ■ Venous anatomy of the right arm at the elbow (**A**), upper arm (**B**), and shoulder (**C**).

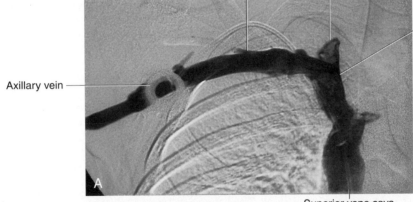

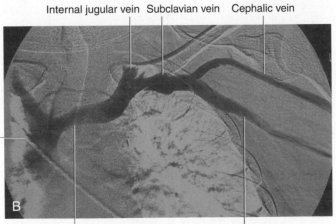

FIGURE 15-3 ■ Normal right (**A**) and left (**B**) central thoracic veins.

course between the artery and vein in this region. At the lateral border of the first rib, the axillary vein becomes the *subclavian vein* (see Fig. 15-3). Several tributaries, including the external jugular vein, enter the subclavian vein. The vein runs in front of the anterior scalene muscle. At the medial edge of the anterior scalene muscle, the *internal jugular vein* joins the subclavian vein to form the *brachiocephalic (innominate) vein.*

The right brachiocephalic vein runs almost vertically in front of the right brachiocephalic artery. Tributaries include the right vertebral, internal thoracic (mammary), inferior thyroid, and first posterior intercostal veins. The left brachiocephalic vein (which is more than twice as long as the right) passes inferomedially in front of the left subclavian and left carotid arteries. Branches are comparable to those on the right with the addition of the left superior intercostal and thymic veins (Fig. 15-4). In most cases, the former vessel is the continuation of the accessory hemiazygous vein (see Fig. 15-1). The major lymphatic ducts (including the thoracic duct on the left) enter the venous circulation near the junction of the left subclavian and jugular veins (see Fig. 18-5).

The brachiocephalic veins merge to form the *superior vena cava* (SVC), which is valveless. The SVC enters the right atrium at about the level of the third costal cartilage. The azygous vein ascends from the abdomen into chest through the right crus of the diaphragm. It arches anteriorly to enter the back wall of the SVC above the right main stem bronchus (Fig. 15-5; see also Fig. 15-1). The main trunk of the *azygous vein* drains the right posterior and superior intercostal veins. The *hemiazygous vein* ascends to the left of the thoracic aorta. At about the T7-T8 level, it gives off a large branch to the azygous vein and then becomes the *accessory hemiazygous vein.*

Valves are present in the superficial and deep veins from the hand to the subclavian veins. Changes in intrathoracic pressure during inspiration and expiration produce a corresponding increase or decrease in flow through the upper extremity veins, respectively. With rapid inspiration, the subclavian vein may collapse. The Doppler ultrasound flow patterns in the subclavian, internal jugular, and axillary veins reflect both atrial and respiratory activity.

Variant Anatomy

The most common anomaly of the upper extremity veins is partial or complete duplication. Rare anomalies include separate drainage of the brachiocephalic veins into the right atrium and absence of the left brachiocephalic vein with blood return through the left superior intercostal vein.[3] MR imaging is ideally suited to evaluating such variants.

Duplication of the SVC is an uncommon anomaly that results from persistence of the left precardinal vein, with or without a maldeveloped left brachiocephalic vein (Fig. 15-6).[3,4] It is found in less than 1% of the population but is more common in patients with congenital heart disease. The left-sided component usually empties into the coronary sinus.

Isolated left SVC, which is a less common variant, occurs when there is persistence of the left precardinal vein **and** regression of the right precardinal vein.

Variations in azygous and hemiazygous venous anatomy are common. In particular, the accessory hemiazygous vein may drain into the azygous, hemiazygous, or left brachiocephalic veins.[2]

Collateral Circulation

With axillosubclavian vein thrombosis, muscular and superficial veins around the shoulder and thorax are recruited as

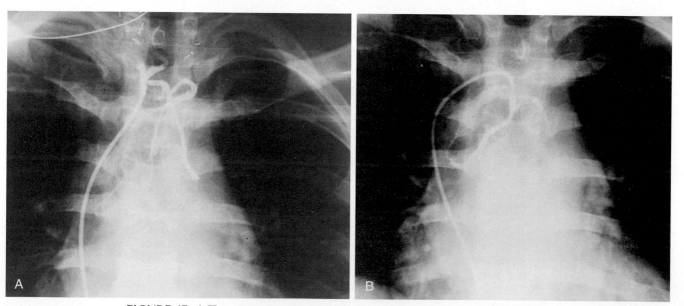

FIGURE 15-4 ■ **A,** Right thyroidal vein with reflux into thymic branches. **B,** Thymic vein.

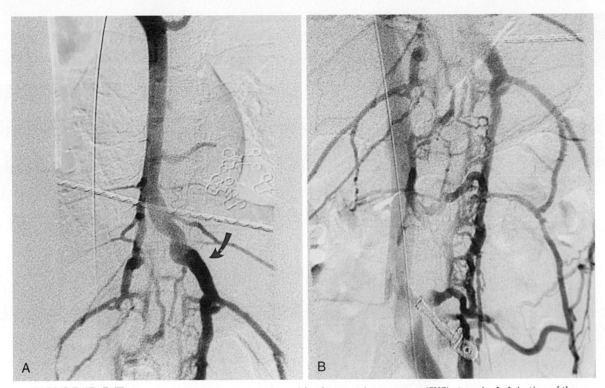

FIGURE 15-5 ■ Azygous venous system in a patient with a low superior vena cava (SVC) stenosis. **A,** Injection of the azygous vein directly from the SVC shows retrograde flow down the vein, with filling of the hemiazygous vein *(arrow)* and numerous lumbar collaterals. **B,** Late phase of the run with imaging over the mid-abdomen shows filling of the left iliac vein and inferior vena cava through lumbar and vertebral collaterals.

collateral pathways, which empty into the brachiocephalic, jugular, or azygous veins. With brachiocephalic vein occlusion, the principal collateral pathway is up the ipsilateral jugular vein to the contralateral jugular or brachiocephalic veins through multiple head and neck channels (Fig. 15-7).

With partial or complete obstruction of the SVC, the major collateral routes are through the azygous-hemiazygous system, internal thoracic veins, lateral thoracic veins, and the vertebral venous plexus.[5,6] With **low** SVC obstruction below the azygous insertion, blood flows down the azygous and hemiazygous veins into the lumbar veins and into the iliac veins and inferior vena cava (IVC) (see Fig. 15-5). With **high** SVC obstruction above or at the azygous arch, collateral flow is mainly through right and left superior intercostal branches and the left brachiocephalic vein and then into the azygous system (Figs. 15-8 and 15-9). If the obstruction engulfs the SVC and the brachiocephalic and azygous veins, drainage is through superficial chest wall, lateral thoracic, and internal thoracic veins into the iliac veins and IVC (Fig. 15-10).

■ MAJOR DISORDERS

Upper Extremity Venous Thrombosis

Etiology

Symptomatic venous thrombosis is much less common in the upper extremity than in the lower extremity. The major causes are outlined in Box 15-1.[7] Prior or existing central venous catheters of various types are the culprits in many patients. Subclavian vein catheters are much more prone to stenosis or occlusion than internal jugular vein catheters.[8] In some populations, stenoses or complete occlusions (often asymptomatic) have been found in up to 50% of patients with a history of subclavian vein catheters.[8-10] Most symptomatic patients have obstruction of the axillary or subclavian veins, with or without more central (brachiocephalic or SVC) occlusion.[7] Hemodialysis catheters present a particular problem as many of these patients require repeated periodic placement of these large caliber devices.[11-13] Presence of a maturing or mature dialysis shunt only exacerbates the problem due to nonphysiologic high blood flow through the outflow veins.

Primary thrombosis (i.e., spontaneous or "effort" thrombosis), also known as *Paget-Schroetter disease,* is a less common cause of upper extremity venous occlusion. In this venous form of the *thoracic outlet syndrome,* the subclavian or axillary vein is compressed by a musculoskeletal structure, most often between the first rib and subclavius tendon or the costoclavicular ligament. Unlike the subclavian artery, the vein runs in *front* of the anterior scalene muscle and is not compressed at this site. Chronic intimal injury, which is worsened by strenuous shoulder activity and slow flow, can lead to thrombosis.

The natural history of acute upper extremity venous thrombosis is different from the disease in the lower extremity. Upper extremity clots account for only 10% to 15% of cases of pulmonary embolism. Likewise, symptomatic pulmonary embolism develops in about 3% to 15% of patients with upper extremity or internal jugular deep

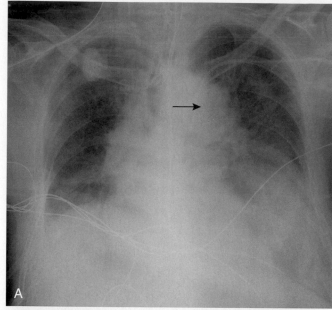

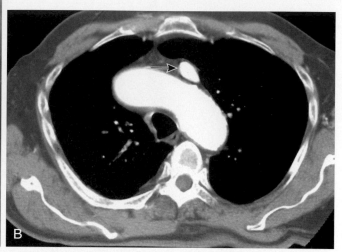

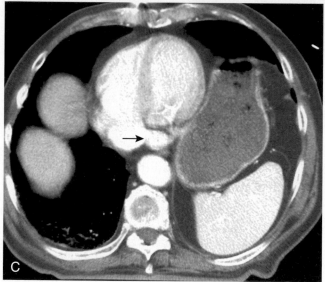

FIGURE 15-6 ■ Left superior vena cava (SVC). **A,** Chest radiograph shows left subclavian central venous catheter passing to the left of the spine *(arrow).* **B,** CT angiogram shows left SVC. **C,** At a more inferior level, the left SVC enters the coronary sinus *(arrow).*

venous thrombosis (DVT).[14-16] Even with anticoagulation, recanalization of thrombosed upper extremity veins is uncommon. Instead, clots organize over time, leaving a fibrotic lumen and scarred vein wall. Postthrombotic syndrome and functional disability can result in 25% to 40% of cases, particularly in those who are not treated with direct therapy.[17]

Clinical Features

Some patients with acute venous thrombosis are asymptomatic. Others complain of arm swelling, pain, cyanosis, coolness, and distended superficial veins. These symptoms can mimic infection, lymphatic obstruction, or blunt trauma. With chronic occlusion, arm fatigue after exercise may be experienced. In less than 5% of patients (most of whom have an underlying malignancy), widespread venous thrombosis leads to the syndrome of *phlegmasia cerulea dolens*

and arterial insufficiency.[18] The typical patient with Paget-Schroetter disease is a young person complaining of sudden onset of arm swelling and pain. A history of vigorous physical activity (e.g., weight lifting) can often be elicited.

Imaging

Sonography. Color Doppler sonography is the chief imaging tool for detecting axillosubclavian and central venous stenosis and thrombosis.[19,20] Unfortunately, the clavicle and sternum hide most of the central brachiocephalic veins and the SVC from direct visualization. Sonography includes study of the accessible portions of the axillary, subclavian, brachiocephalic, and internal jugular veins; upper arm veins are occasionally evaluated. Color Doppler imaging is used to detect stenoses, occlusions, and collateral channels, and Doppler waveform analysis is used to identify physiologic signs of more central obstruction. Normally, a triphasic atrial

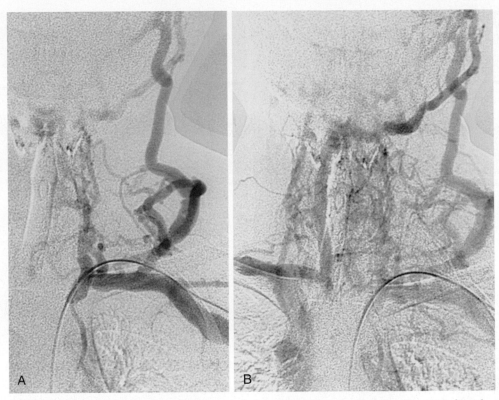

FIGURE 15-7 ■ Left brachiocephalic vein occlusion. **A,** There is retrograde flow up the external jugular vein and into small collateral channels. The left internal jugular vein was occluded. **B,** On delayed images, contrast flows into right-sided neck and thoracic veins and then into the superior vena cava.

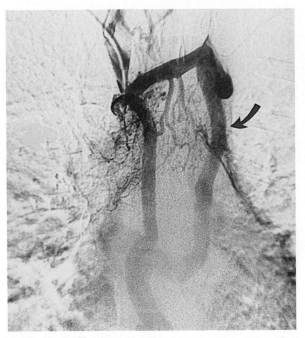

FIGURE 15-8 ■ High superior vena cava obstruction. Contrast flows down the azygous vein and up the left brachiocephalic vein into the accessory hemiazygous vein *(arrow)*. Note the thymic tributaries on the undersurface of the left brachiocephalic vein.

waveform with superimposed respiratory variation is present (Fig. 15-11). Absent or monophasic waveforms or asymmetry between sides is a sign of central obstruction.[21] The subclavian vein dilates with a Valsalva maneuver and collapses with rapid inspiration (i.e., sniff test).

Signs of venous thrombosis include an intraluminal filling defect, absent flow, or an abnormal Doppler tracing (Figs. 15-11 and 15-12). The latter finding can be confirmed with contrast venography. Sonography is very accurate in detecting upper extremity DVT.[19,22] Studies with false-positive results are rare. Thrombosis may be missed in several situations[23]:

- Nonocclusive thrombus
- Short-segment occlusion
- Central occlusions
- Collateral channels mistaken for normal vessels

Indwelling venous catheters do not seem to alter the accuracy of the technique.[24]

Computed Tomography and Magnetic Resonance Imaging. Because duplex sonography is simple to perform, accurate, and relatively inexpensive, more complex cross-sectional techniques rarely are indicated for diagnosing patients with suspected upper extremity DVT. However, MR or CT venography may be useful for suspected central

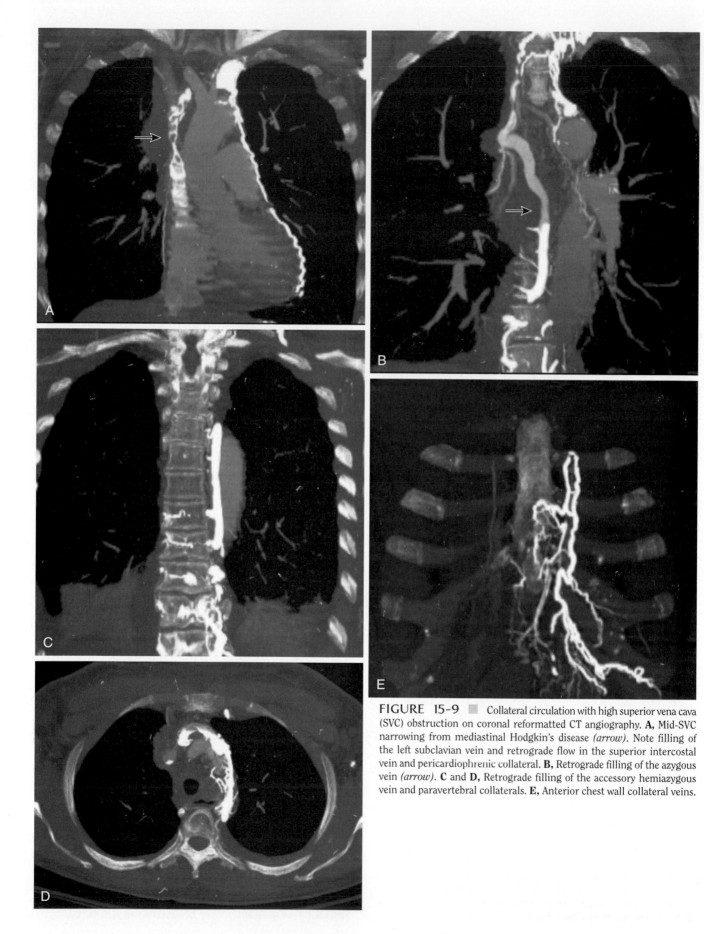

FIGURE 15-9 ▪ Collateral circulation with high superior vena cava (SVC) obstruction on coronal reformatted CT angiography. **A,** Mid-SVC narrowing from mediastinal Hodgkin's disease *(arrow)*. Note filling of the left subclavian vein and retrograde flow in the superior intercostal vein and pericardiophrenic collateral. **B,** Retrograde filling of the azygous vein *(arrow)*. **C** and **D,** Retrograde filling of the accessory hemiazygous vein and paravertebral collaterals. **E,** Anterior chest wall collateral veins.

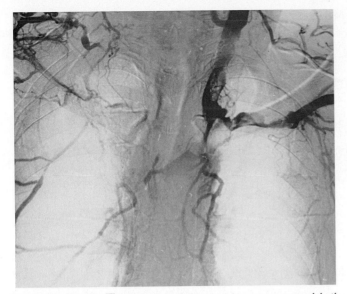

FIGURE 15-10 ■ Occlusion of the superior vena cava and both brachiocephalic veins. Collateral circulation occurs primarily through superficial chest wall veins.

obstruction or for identifying potential vascular access sites in patients with extensive venous disease.[25-31]

Venography. Catheter venography is used to confirm the diagnosis or plan endovascular or surgical treatment of venous thrombosis of the upper extremity. In the acute stage, intraluminal filling defects may be seen (Fig. 15-13). In the subacute or chronic stages, long-segment scarring or stenosis is sometimes evident. Otherwise, the clotted vessels do not opacify and multiple collateral channels are seen (Fig. 15-14; see also Fig. 15-7). If the brachiocephalic vein or SVC is difficult to visualize from a peripheral arm injection because of slow flow in the arm veins or washout from the internal jugular vein, a catheter should be placed centrally.

FIGURE 15-11 ■ Duplex sonography of the subclavian veins. **A,** Normal spectral tracing with reflected atrial activity and superimposed respiratory variation. **B,** Abnormal flat tracing suggests a more central occlusion. In this case, the brachiocephalic vein was occluded.

Treatment

Medical Therapy. The standard treatment for upper extremity venous thrombosis is anticoagulation, bed rest, and elevation of the arm. Anticoagulation limits clot propagation and enables recruitment of collateral vessels. Most patients respond to these measures without further intervention. Patients with indwelling central venous devices may require catheter removal or long-term anticoagulation.

BOX 15-1 ■ Causes of Upper Extremity Venous Thrombosis

Catheter-related causes
    Vascular access devices (prior or existing)
    Transvenous cardiac pacemakers
    Transvenous monitoring devices
Thrombophilic state (see Box 3-5)
Extrinsic compression
    Primary
        Spontaneous (effort) thrombosis (Paget-Schroetter disease)
    Secondary
        Malignancy/adenopathy
        Thoracic masses
        Fibrosing mediastinitis
Trauma/surgery
Intravenous drug abuse
Toxic agents (e.g., chemotherapeutic drugs)
Heart failure
Radiation therapy

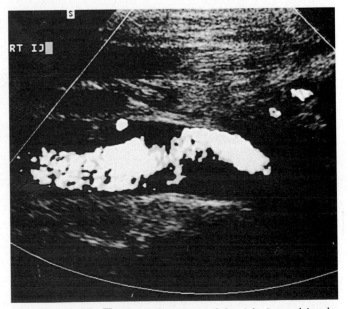

FIGURE 15-12 ■ Partial thrombosis of the right internal jugular vein is identified by color Doppler sonography.

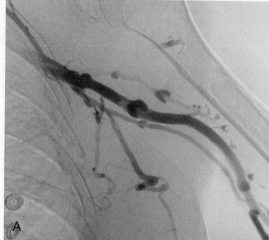

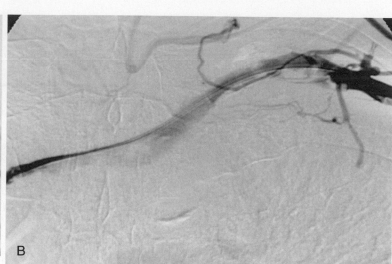

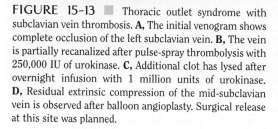

FIGURE 15-13 ▨ Thoracic outlet syndrome with subclavian vein thrombosis. **A,** The initial venogram shows complete occlusion of the left subclavian vein. **B,** The vein is partially recanalized after pulse-spray thrombolysis with 250,000 IU of urokinase. **C,** Additional clot has lysed after overnight infusion with 1 million units of urokinase. **D,** Residual extrinsic compression of the mid-subclavian vein is observed after balloon angioplasty. Surgical release at this site was planned.

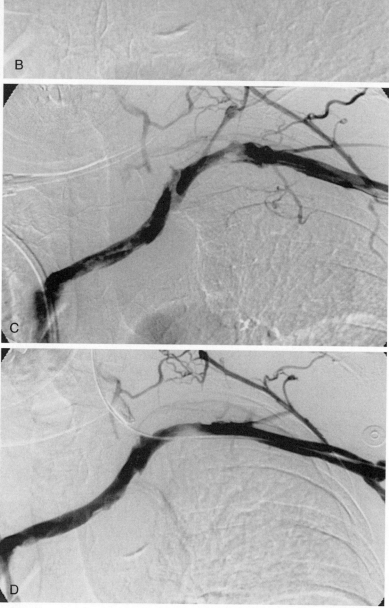

Endovascular Therapy. Thrombolytic therapy should be considered in several situations. Enzymatic fibrinolysis and mechanical thrombectomy devices usually are reserved for acute thrombosis.[17] Subacute and chronic disease (>10 to 14 days old) are much less responsive and usually are treated with angioplasty (and sometimes stent placement)

alone (Fig. 15-15).[32] Consider thrombolytic therapy in the following circumstances:

- Poor response to medical treatment
- Suspected spontaneous (effort) thrombosis
- Widespread venous occlusion (phlegmasia cerulea dolens)

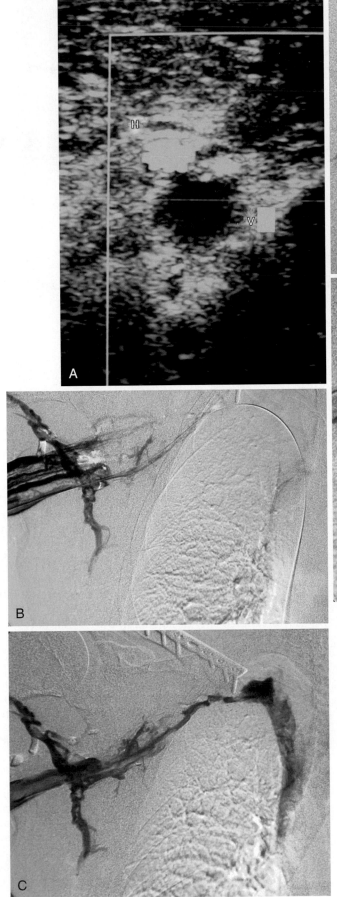

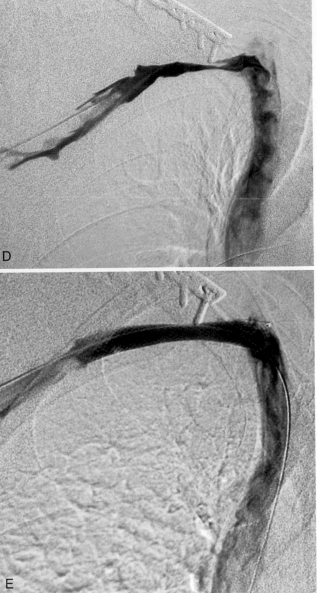

FIGURE 15-14 ■ Acute right subclavian vein thrombosis from shoulder surgery treated with thrombolysis and stent placement. **A,** Transverse color Doppler image shows right subclavian vein thrombosis. **B,** Arm venogram shows complete occlusion of the right axillary and subclavian veins. A guidewire has been passed into the superior vena cava (SVC). **C,** After intrathrombic injection of 5 mg of recombinant tissue–type plasminogen activator (t-PA), there is partial lysis with some flow into the brachiocephalic vein and SVC. **D,** After overnight infusion of a total of 23 mg of t-PA, there is some residual clot and a tight stenosis of the mid SCV. **E,** After placement of a 14-mm Wallstent and 12-mm balloon dilation, the vessel is widely patent.

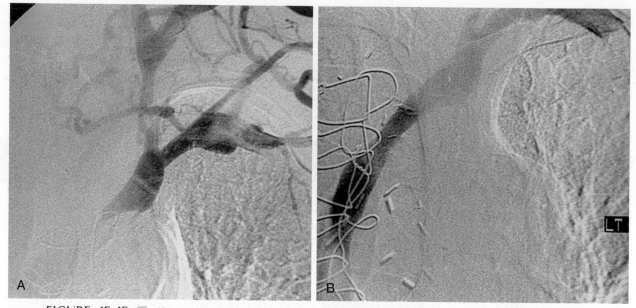

FIGURE 15-15 ■ Chronic left brachiocephalic vein occlusion with collateral filling (**A**) was treated with a 12-mm angioplasty balloon (**B**).

If a central venous catheter or device is present, it is preferable to remove it. However, patients who are dependent on such catheters may have them left in place. Although systemic infusion can be used, the preferred method is catheter-directed local thrombolysis (see Chapter 2 for technical details). Access is gained usually through an ipsilateral basilic or brachial vein. If necessary, the common femoral or internal jugular vein may be used. Therapy may require several days of infusion and relatively large doses of fibrinolytic agents (see Fig. 15-14). Mechanical thrombectomy devices often are used instead of or as adjuncts to enzymatic lysis.[33]

Patients are vigorously anticoagulated during the procedure and may require long-term anticoagulation. Underlying stenoses are treated with balloon angioplasty. The role of stents in this setting is controversial.[34,35] They are generally avoided in thoracic outlet syndrome, although some reports describe good long-term results after stent placement.[36] Stents are used selectively in other cases. If reasonable results can be obtained without one, periodic surveillance and repeat angioplasty may be preferable. Disadvantages of stents in the upper extremity and torso include frequent in-stent restenosis, stent migration, shortening or fracture, and "jailing" of important tributaries such as the internal jugular vein.[37]

Short-term results of thrombolysis with or without mechanical devices are excellent in about 75% to 85% of cases; thrombolysis is clearly superior to anticoagulation alone for reestablishing flow in fresh occlusions.[36,38-41] Late reocclusion is a common problem, particularly when the underlying cause of thrombosis (e.g., indwelling catheter, hypercoagulable state, extrinsic compression) is not eliminated.

For subacute and chronic upper extremity venous occlusions, primary angioplasty with or without stent placement is recommended. Chronic organized occlusions can be notoriously difficult to cross (see Fig. 15-14). If antegrade traversal is impossible, retrograde entry from the common femoral vein may work (Fig. 15-16). If standard guidewires and catheters don't work, the back end of a hydrophilic wire can be tried, or "sharp recanalization" can be attempted with a transjugular intrahepatic portosystemic shunt set.[43]

In primary axillosubclavian thrombosis (venous thoracic outlet syndrome), an integrated approach that combines catheter-directed therapy with delayed surgery is now a widely accepted plan and includes the following features[36,44-46]:

■ Thrombolysis as initial treatment
■ Angioplasty if flow-limiting obstruction is found; stents are not used[47]
■ A short course of anticoagulation with warfarin (Coumadin)
■ Conservative therapy if no extrinsic compression is detected after thrombolysis
■ Immediate or delayed surgical decompression (e.g., first rib resection and subclavius tendon release with patch venoplasty) for axillary or subclavian vein compression detected after thrombolysis; venous reconstruction or venovenous bypass if the underlying vein is not suitable[48]
■ Angioplasty (with or without stent placement) or surgery for residual postoperative stenoses

Patients with a large volume of fresh upper extremity venous clot who are not candidates for anticoagulation can have a filter inserted in the SVC to prevent pulmonary embolism (Fig. 15-17).[49-51] However, this is an off-label use of the device and completely investigational. Care must be taken to delineate the SVC and select a filter of appropriate length. The jugular version of asymmetric filters must be used from the femoral approach.

FIGURE 15-16 ■ Right brachiocephalic vein (BCV) occlusion reduced flow in an ipsilateral arteriovenous dialysis fistula. **A,** Complete chronic occlusion of the right BCV is noted. There is aneurysmal dilation just above the obstruction. **B,** Attempts to cross the lesion from above were unsuccessful. **C,** Superior vena cava injection from a femoral approach. **D,** Traversal from below was successful with an angled catheter and hydrophilic wire. **E,** Angioplasty of the lesion with a 14-mm balloon. **F,** Final result shows good flow through the vessel.

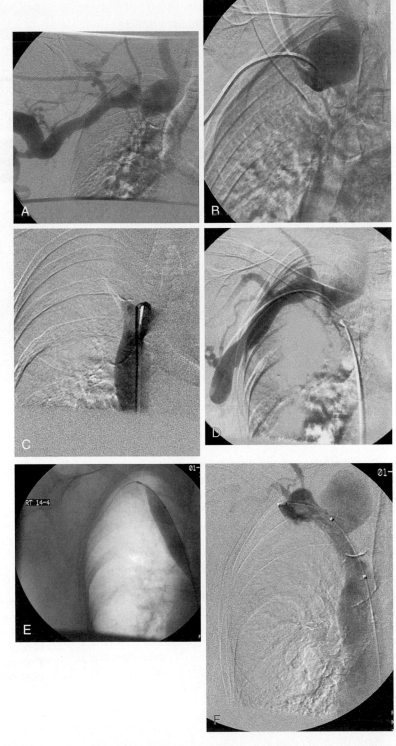

Upper Extremity Venous Stenoses

Etiology

In the upper extremity, the most common causes for venous stenosis are prior or existing central venous catheters, intimal hyperplasia related to ipsilateral hemodialysis access, and extrinsic compression by musculoskeletal structures (Box 15-2). Mild extrinsic compression of the axillosubclavian veins can be identified in 10% to 50% of the normal population on imaging studies when provocative arm maneuvers are performed.[52,53] The most common site is the subclavian vein in the costoclavicular space (Fig. 15-18). Because stenoses develop slowly and the collateral circulation often is adequate, many patients tolerate these lesions as long as the vessel does not become completely occluded. A small percentage of patients becomes symptomatic from the existing stenosis or subsequent thrombosis.

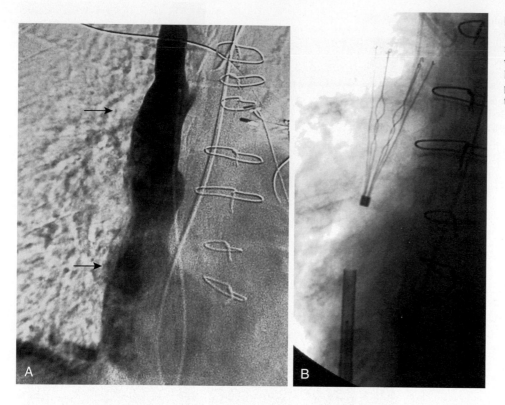

FIGURE 15-17 ■ Superior vena cava (SVC) filter in a patient with recurrent pulmonary embolism from upper extremity venous thrombosis. **A,** SVC diameter and length *(arrows)* are outlined. **B,** Post–filter placement from a femoral approach using the jugular version of the Greenfield filter.

Symptomatic upper extremity vein stenosis occurs most notably in patients with hemodialysis grafts. About 50% of dialysis patients with prior subclavian vein catheters develop significant stenoses or occlusions, which have been attributed to direct vein injury, venous turbulence and supraphysiologic blood flow, and catheter motion within the vessel.[9,54] Extrinsic compression also can be identified in a substantial number of dialysis patients without a history of indwelling catheters.[55] The increased flow exaggerates the pressure gradient (and therefore the significance) of even moderate stenoses. Although these stenoses are most common near the venous anastomosis and at sites of prior temporary catheters, they may occur in any of the outflow veins.

BOX 15-2   ■   Causes of Upper Extremity Venous Narrowing

Vascular access devices (prior or existing)
Extrinsic compression
   Musculoskeletal structures
   Neoplasm/adenopathy
Intimal hyperplasia
   Outflow veins of dialysis grafts
Trauma/surgery
Radiation therapy
Vasospasm

Clinical Features

Many patients have arm swelling, pain, and superficial varicosities. Hemodialysis graft dysfunction is common, including elevated venous pressures at dialysis, poor shunt flow, or graft thrombosis.

Imaging

Cross-sectional Techniques. Stenoses of the central upper extremity veins are detected by color Doppler sonography or MR venography. However, some patients require catheter venography prior to endovascular or surgical treatment. Provocative maneuvers may be required to delineate the obstruction.[53,56]

Contrast Venography. Upper extremity venous stenoses usually are smooth and focal (Fig. 15-19). It may be difficult to differentiate **extrinsic** compression (caused by musculoskeletal structures or tumor) from **intrinsic** mural disease (see Fig. 15-15). Several conditions can mimic fixed obstruction, including vasospasm from catheter or guidewire manipulation or trauma (Fig. 15-20) and external compression from an overlying surgical drape or compression between the humerus and ribs in arm adduction (Fig. 15-21).

The presence of an extensive collateral network around a stenosis is an indicator of hemodynamic significance. Moderate stenoses can be assessed by measuring a focal pressure gradient (3 to 5 mm Hg) across the lesion (Fig. 15-22).

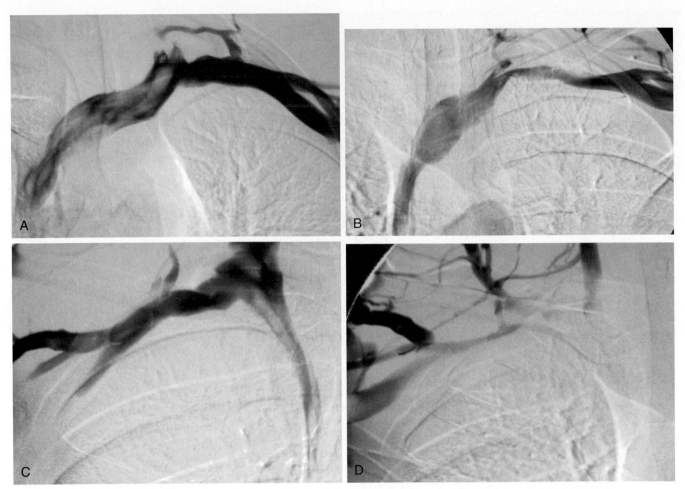

FIGURE 15-18 ■ Extrinsic compression of both subclavian veins from thoracic outlet syndrome. **A,** Patent left subclavian vein (SCV). Lucency in the vessel is due to inflow from the unopacified internal jugular vein. **B,** With arm abduction, there is mild narrowing of the left SCV with few collaterals. **C,** Right SCV in neutral position. **D,** With arm abduction, near-complete occlusion of the right SCV is seen with exuberant filling of collateral channels.

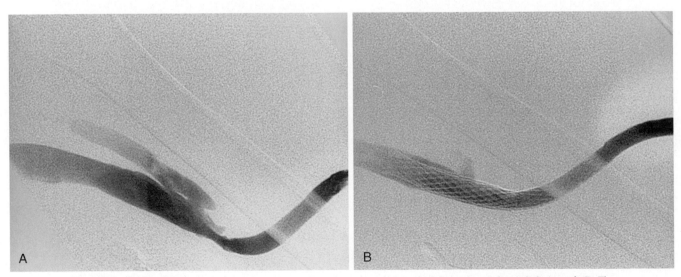

FIGURE 15-19 ■ **A,** Smooth focal stenosis at the venous anastomosis of a left upper arm hemodialysis graft. **B,** The stenosis is relieved with a 6-mm Wallstent.

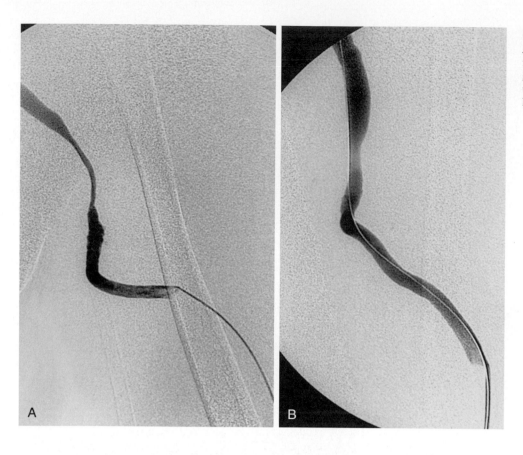

FIGURE 15-20   ■   Venospasm.
A, Long-segment narrowing of the outflow vein of an upper arm hemodialysis graft is identified after guidewire manipulations. **B,** Ten minutes later, the spasm has resolved.

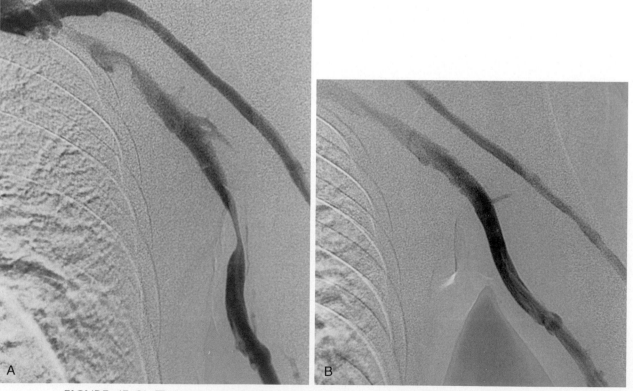

FIGURE 15-21   ■   External compression of the left basilic vein. **A,** Narrowing of the vein is seen with the initial contrast injection. **B,** After releasing the overlying surgical drape and abducting the arm, the compression is resolved.

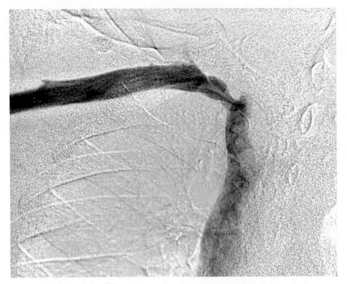

FIGURE 15-22 ■ Nonsignificant right brachiocephalic vein stenosis. No collateral vessels are seen, and the pressure gradient was 2 mm Hg.

Treatment

Endovascular Therapy. Balloon angioplasty is the first-line therapy for hemodynamically significant venous stenoses. Obstructions can be approached directly from an antecubital, upper arm, or common femoral vein or through a dialysis graft, if present. Typically, the axillary and subclavian veins require 8- to 12-mm angioplasty balloons, and the brachiocephalic vein requires up to 14-mm balloons (Fig. 15-23). It is prudent to start with an undersized balloon. Multiple, prolonged inflations and high-pressure balloons may be needed to open resistant stenoses. For completely resistant lesions, cutting balloons can be used to weaken the vein wall, making it more amenable to angioplasty. Patients usually experience mild discomfort during balloon inflation. Severe pain is a sign of overdilation or vein rupture.

The results of balloon angioplasty in this setting have been mixed. In central upper extremity stenoses, technical success (<30% residual stenosis) is achieved in about 75% of cases.[57] However, 6-month primary patency is often less than 30%.[58,59] Most treated stenoses fail before 2 years without reintervention.[60] However, repeated dilations allow respectable primary assisted patency rates that approach surgical results (e.g., 2-year patency of 66%) and may extend the useful life of dialysis grafts.[60] Complications (including vein rupture) occur in less than 10% of cases, and most are minor. Vein rupture is managed with repeat prolonged balloon inflation or placement of a bare or covered stent, if necessary.

Intravascular stents have shown some promise in the treatment of upper extremity venous obstructions. However, stents are reserved for cases of failed angioplasty (elastic stenoses, acute vein rupture, or rapid restenosis) (Fig. 15-24). Stents should **not** be placed within very fibrotic lesions that cannot be fully dilated with a balloon. Stents are avoided in patients with obstructions from thoracic outlet syndrome. Stent selection is critical.[61] The nitinol stents and the Wallstent are favored by many interventionists (see Figs. 15-14 and 15-19). If possible, the stent should not be placed across the internal jugular vein orifice. Nominal stent diameter should be at least 2 mm greater than the largest target vessel diameter to prevent stent migration. The patient and referring physician should understand that the device may interfere with future placement of central venous access devices.

In some series, primary patency rates have surpassed those with angioplasty alone (e.g., 50% at 6 months).[62,63]

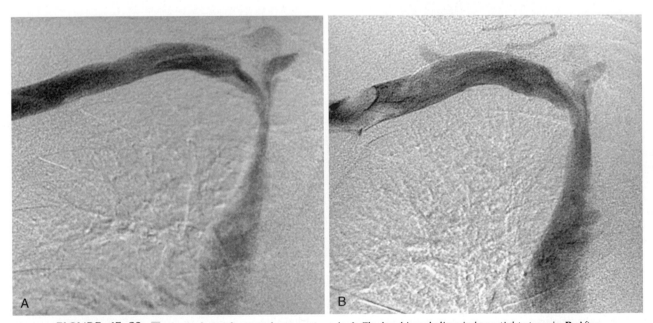

FIGURE 15-23 ■ Angioplasty of a central venous stenosis. **A,** The brachiocephalic vein has a tight stenosis. **B,** After angioplasty with a 12-mm balloon, the lumen is widened.

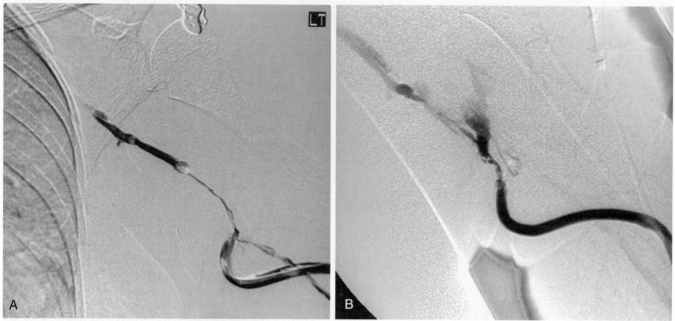

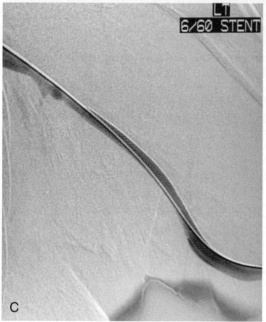

FIGURE 15-24 ■ Stent placement for angioplasty-induced vein rupture. **A,** Atretic outflow vein distal to a recanalized left arm hemodialysis graft. **B,** Angioplasty with a 6-mm balloon ruptured the vein. **C,** A 6-mm Wallstent was placed across the torn vein to reestablish flow through the vessel.

One study found comparable long-term results with surgical bypass and angioplasty plus stenting.[64] However, others report dismal results for angioplasty or stenting of central venous stenoses, with a 6-month primary patency rate of less than 31% for central and peripheral lesions.[65] Stent restenosis may be relieved with balloon angioplasty, with or without placement of additional stents (Fig. 15-25). Primary assisted patency rates with angioplasty are excellent in most series. Periodic maintenance of these lesions should be anticipated. Complications of stent placement include vein rupture and stent migration, which can be disastrous (Fig. 15-26).

Surgical Therapy. For brachiocephalic vein occlusions, direct bypass with prosthetic material or jugular-jugular bypass may be performed.[60] For central subclavian vein occlusions, internal jugular to subclavian vein transposition is effective.

For peripheral subclavian and axillary venous occlusions, direct axillary-jugular bypass is advocated.

Superior Vena Cava Obstruction

Etiology

Obstruction of the SVC is the result of luminal disease (i.e., thrombus or tumor), extrinsic compression (tumor or adenopathy), or mural disease (i.e., intimal hyperplasia or tumor invasion). A variety of underlying diseases is responsible (Box 15-3).[66-68] The obstruction may be stenotic or frankly occlusive. In older series, malignancy (particularly lung cancer) was the cause in at least 90% of cases. However, indwelling vascular devices (e.g., infusion

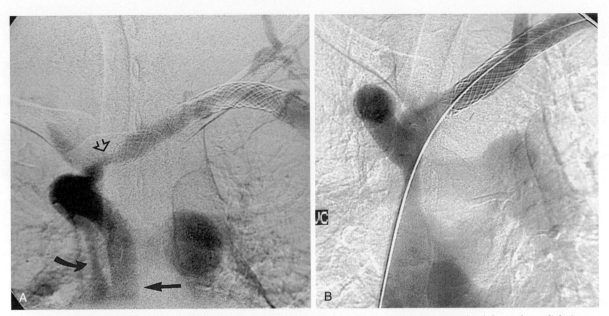

FIGURE 15-25 ■ Left subclavian and brachiocephalic vein stent restenosis in a patient with a left arm hemodialysis graft. **A,** There is narrowing of the lumen of the subclavian vein and at the mouth of the brachiocephalic vein stent *(open arrow)*. A tight superior vena cava stenosis *(curved arrow)* causes retrograde flow into a dilated azygous vein *(arrow)*. **B,** The left brachiocephalic vein and superior vena cava are opened after 12-mm balloon angioplasty.

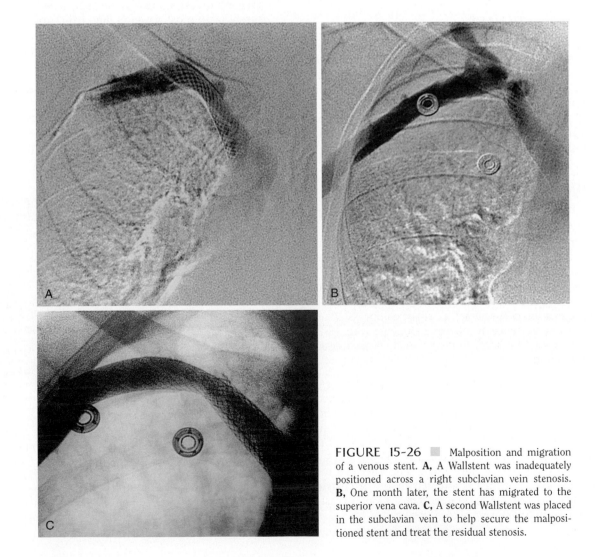

FIGURE 15-26 ■ Malposition and migration of a venous stent. **A,** A Wallstent was inadequately positioned across a right subclavian vein stenosis. **B,** One month later, the stent has migrated to the superior vena cava. **C,** A second Wallstent was placed in the subclavian vein to help secure the malpositioned stent and treat the residual stenosis.

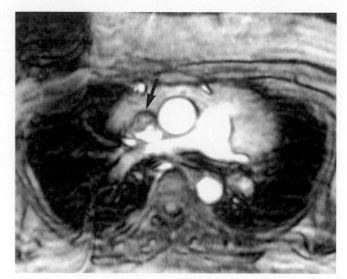

FIGURE 15-27 ■ Thrombus *(arrow)* in the superior vena cava is identified by MR imaging.

catheters, pacemaker wires) are an increasingly common cause of SVC stenosis. *Fibrosing mediastinitis* is a localized or diffuse infiltrative disease of the mediastinum that may be idiopathic or caused by chronic infection such as histoplasmosis.[69] The SVC is affected in more than one third of cases; the pulmonary artery and bronchi also may be involved.

Clinical Features

Significant SVC or bilateral brachiocephalic vein stenosis or obstruction can lead to the *SVC syndrome*. This rare entity is marked by facial and neck swelling, bilateral arm swelling, cyanosis, distention of superficial veins, shortness of breath, hoarseness, and headache. Left untreated, severe laryngeal edema or cerebral congestion with altered mental status and, eventually, coma can develop. The condition may be life-threatening.

Imaging

Cross-sectional Techniques. Although sonography cannot directly evaluate the SVC, alterations in spectral waveform from both subclavian veins (e.g., lack of normal reflected atrial activity and respiratory phasicity or response to provocative maneuvers) should raise suspicion. CT and MR angiography are extremely effective in the diagnosis of SVC obstruction.[26,27,70] Findings include intraluminal defects, nonopacification of the vessel, extrinsic compression or mass invasion, and presence of collateral channels (Fig. 15-27; see also Fig. 15-9). The latter finding usually is associated with symptomatic disease.

Venography. Catheter venography is reserved for cases in which cross-sectional studies are equivocal or transcatheter treatment is being considered. The SVC can be imaged from one or both antecubital veins, the internal jugular vein, or the femoral vein (see Fig. 15-25). Stenoses caused by indwelling or prior devices usually are long and smooth. Extrinsic masses efface the lumen (Fig. 15-28). Collateral vessels fill when contrast is injected above the obstruction. Associated narrowing of the brachiocephalic (and, occasionally, the internal jugular) vein is common.

Treatment

Catheter-directed therapy should be considered only in patients with moderate to severe symptoms who fail to respond to less aggressive measures. SVC occlusion itself is rarely fatal; most patients die of the underlying malignant disease. The purpose of treatment in these patients is short-term palliation of symptoms. Long-term patency is the goal in patients with benign SVC obstruction.

Medical Therapy. For malignant obstructions, urgent chemotherapy and/or radiotherapy is used to treat the underlying cause of disease. Intravenous corticosteroids and diuretics also have been used. Patients may notice transient worsening of symptoms with the onset of radiation therapy as the tumor swells. Heparin is given to limit clot progression.

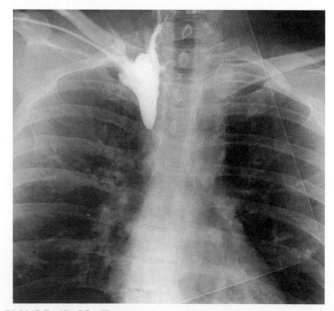

FIGURE 15-28 ■ Chronic superior vena cava occlusion is caused by fibrosing mediastinitis after histoplasmosis infection.

Endovascular Therapy. Although balloon angioplasty alone is effective in some benign SVC obstructions, it is rarely durable in malignant disease.[71,72] However, intravascular stents are extremely effective in both benign and malignant SVC obstructions, whether stenotic or occlusive.[73-81] The primary indication is moderate to severe SVC syndrome. Thrombolysis precedes angioplasty if acute or subacute clot exists in the vena cava or central thoracic veins (Fig. 15-29). Otherwise, angioplasty and stent placement may be used alone (Fig. 15-30). Stents may be placed safely over pacemaker wires.[82] Central venous catheters may be repositioned and then reinserted after the stent is deployed.[83]

Stents can be placed through venous access from above or below the occlusion. If the obstruction can be traversed only from above, a snare placed from the femoral vein can be used to capture the guidewire. The procedure is then continued from below. The stenosis often is predilated with an angioplasty balloon to ensure it opens and to delineate its length. Heparin is given during the procedure.

A variety of different devices has been used for this purpose, including nitinol stents, Gianturco Z-stent, Palmaz stent, and the Wallstent.[71,84-86] Large stent, diameters (>16 mm) are required; stents are purposely oversized to ensure that they remain well secured to the SVC wall after deployment.

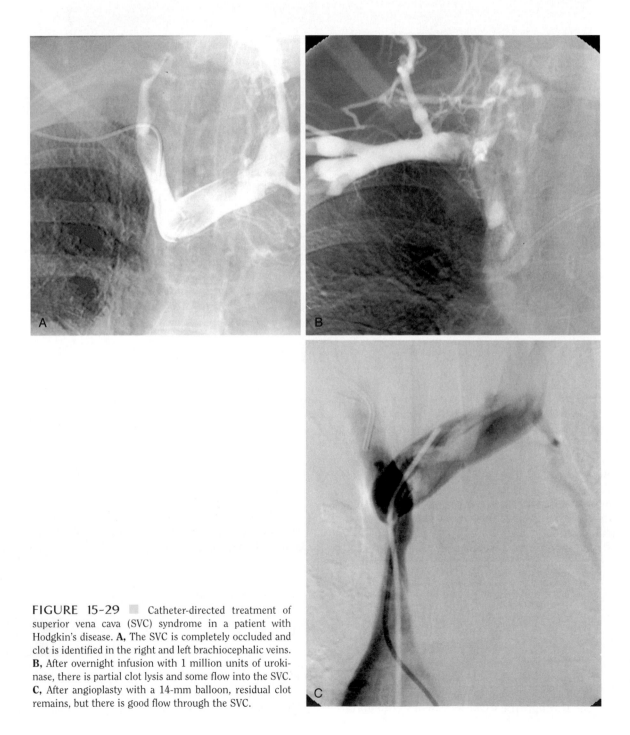

FIGURE 15-29 ■ Catheter-directed treatment of superior vena cava (SVC) syndrome in a patient with Hodgkin's disease. **A,** The SVC is completely occluded and clot is identified in the right and left brachiocephalic veins. **B,** After overnight infusion with 1 million units of urokinase, there is partial clot lysis and some flow into the SVC. **C,** After angioplasty with a 14-mm balloon, residual clot remains, but there is good flow through the SVC.

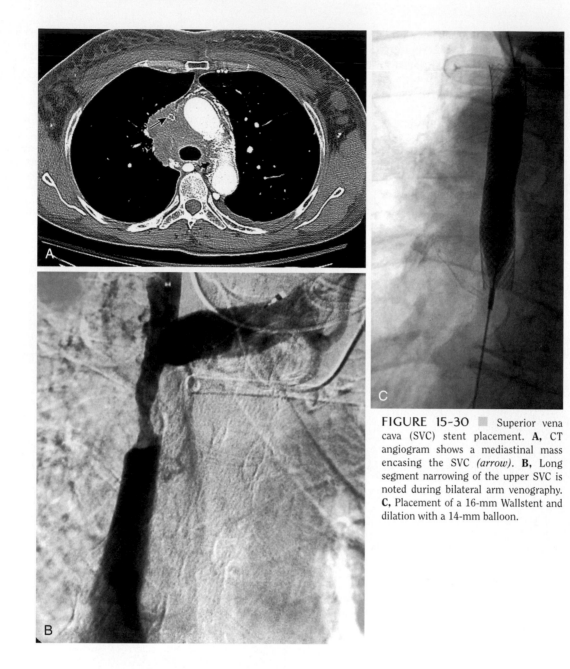

FIGURE 15-30 ▪ Superior vena cava (SVC) stent placement. **A,** CT angiogram shows a mediastinal mass encasing the SVC *(arrow)*. **B,** Long segment narrowing of the upper SVC is noted during bilateral arm venography. **C,** Placement of a 16-mm Wallstent and dilation with a 14-mm balloon.

If the occlusion involves the confluence of the brachio-cephalic veins, stents may be extended into one vessel across the ostium of the other. Alternatively, a Y-shaped stent configuration may be created by laying stents into each brachiocephalic vein.

SVC obstructions can be relieved in almost every case, with dramatic and rapid relief of symptoms. Most patients with malignant disease die of the underlying disease with a patent stent. Major complications are rare and include stent migration or shortening (which may be delayed), early or late stent thrombosis, bleeding, and vein rupture.

A rare but devastating complication of SVC stent placement is immediate or delayed massive bleeding into the mediastinum or pericardium.[87-89] Hemorrhage may occur from venous rupture at delivery (more likely with a fragile wall in malignant obstructions) or puncture by the ends of the stent through the caval wall or into the aorta.

Appropriately sized covered stents should be available immediately, if necessary.

Surgical Therapy. Operations rarely are indicated for SVC obstruction. Bypass grafting can be performed with autologous vein or synthetic material. Venous transposition is possible.[90]

▪ OTHER DISORDERS

Trauma

Traumatic injuries to the upper extremity veins may be criminal, iatrogenic, or accidental. Iatrogenic injuries related to catheterization were discussed previously. Significant venous trauma that requires specific therapy is far less common than arterial injury, and venography is rarely indicated. Color Doppler sonography is an excellent tool for screening this population; it has a high degree of accuracy compared with contrast venography.[91] Unsuspected venous trauma often is detected during surgery for an associated arterial injury. The injured vein is then treated by direct repair, bypass grafting, or ligation. Balloon catheter tamponade of life-threatening large vein trauma also has been described.[92]

Neoplasms

Almost all tumors that affect the SVC arise from the lung or mediastinum. Primary tumors of the SVC are a rare cause of SVC syndrome.[93,94] Most are *leiomyosarcomas*. The diagnosis is usually made by CT or MR imaging, and transvenous biopsy may be performed to assist in the diagnosis.

Aneurysms of upper extremity and thoracic veins are rare.[95,96] The most common sites are the jugular and brachiocephalic veins. The diagnosis often is made by color Doppler sonography. Because of the great propensity for thrombus formation and pulmonary embolism, venous reconstruction is advisable.

REFERENCES

1. Collin P, ed: Embryology and development. In: Williams PL, Bannister LH, Berry MM, et al, eds. Gray's Anatomy, 38th ed. New York, Churchill Livingstone, 1995:327.
2. Gabella G, ed: Cardiovascular system. In: Williams PL, Bannister LH, Berry MM, et al, eds. Gray's Anatomy, 38th ed. New York, Churchill Livingstone, 1995:1589.
3. White CS, Baffa JM, Haney PJ, et al: MR imaging of congenital anomalies of the thoracic veins. Radiographics 1997;17:595.
4. Sarodia BD, Stoller JK: Persistent left superior vena cava: case report and literature review. Respir Care 2000;45:411.
5. Stanford W, Jolles H, Ell S, et al: Superior vena cava obstruction: a venographic classification. AJR Am J Roentgenol 1987;148:259.
6. Bashist B, Parisi A, Frager DH, et al: Abdominal CT findings when the superior vena cava, brachiocephalic vein, or subclavian vein is obstructed. AJR Am J Roentgenol 1996;167:1457.
7. Trerotola SO, Kuhn-Fulton J, Johnson MS, et al: Tunneled infusion catheters: increased incidence of symptomatic venous thrombosis after subclavian versus internal jugular venous access. Radiology 2000;217:89.
8. Balestreri L, De Cicco M, Matovic M, et al: Central venous catheter-related thrombosis in clinically asymptomatic oncologic patients: a phlebographic study. Eur J Radiol 1995;20:108.
9. Schillinger F, Schillinger D, Montagnac R, et al: Postcatheterisation vein stenosis in haemodialysis: comparative angiographic study of 50 subclavian and 50 internal jugular accesses. Nephrol Dial Transplant 1991;6:722.
10. Horne MK, May DJ, Alexander HR, et al: Venographic surveillance of tunneled venous access devices in adult oncology patients. Ann Surg Oncol 1995;2:174.
11. Vesely T, Hovsepian D, Pilgram T, et al: Upper extremity central venous obstruction in hemodialysis patients: treatment with Wallstents. Radiology 1997;204:343.
12. Lumsden AB, MacDonald MJ, Isiklar H, et al: Central venous stenosis in the hemodialysis patient: incidence and efficacy of endovascular treatment. Cardiovasc Surg 1997;5:504.
13. Mickley V, Gorich J, Rilinger N, et al: Stenting of central venous stenoses in hemodialysis patients: long-term results. Kidney Int 1997; 51:277.
14. Hingorani A, Ascher E, Lorenson E, et al: Upper extremity deep venous thrombosis and its impact on morbidity and mortality rates in a hospital-based population. J Vasc Surg 1997;26:853.
15. Monreal M, Raventos A, Lerma R, et al: Pulmonary embolism in patients with upper extremity DVT associated to [sic] venous central lines—a prospective study. Thromb Haemost 1994;72:548.
16. Sheikh MA, Topoulos AP, Deitcher SR: Isolated internal jugular vein thrombosis: risk factors and natural history. Vasc Med 2002;7:177.
17. Sharafuddin MJ, Sun S, Hoballah JJ: Endovascular management of venous thrombotic disease of the upper torso and extremities. J Vasc Interv Radiol 2002;13:975.
18. Kammen BF, Soulen MC: Phlegmasia cerulea dolens of the upper extremity. J Vasc Interv Radiol 1995;6:283.
19. Longley DG, Finlay DE, Letourneau JG: Sonography of the upper extremity and jugular veins. AJR Am J Roentgenol 1993;160:957.
20. Gooding GA, Woodruff A: Color Doppler imaging in the subclavian-axillary region and upper extremity. Clin Imaging 1994;18:165.
21. Rose SC, Kinney TB, Bundens WP, et al: Doppler analysis of transmitted atrial waveforms, respiratory variation, and flow symmetry for detection of thoracic central veno-occlusive disease missed by sonographic imaging. Radiology 1997;205(P):499.
22. Knudson GJ, Wiedmeyer DA, Erickson SJ, et al: Color Doppler sonographic imaging in the assessment of upper-extremity deep venous thrombosis. AJR Am J Roentgenol 1990;154:399.
23. Haire WD, Lynch TG, Lund GB, et al: Limitations of magnetic resonance imaging and ultrasound-directed (duplex) scanning in the diagnosis of subclavian vein thrombosis. J Vasc Surg 1991;13:391.
24. Burbidge SJ, Finlay DE, Letourneau JG, et al: Effects of central venous catheter placement on upper extremity duplex US findings. J Vasc Interv Radiol 1993;4:399.
25. Charon JP, Milne W, Sheppard DG, et al: Evaluation of MR angiographic technique in the assessment of thoracic outlet syndrome. Clin Radiol 2004;59:588.
26. Kim HC, Chung JW, Yoon CJ, et al: Collateral pathways in thoracic central venous obstruction: three-dimensional display using direct spiral computed tomography venography. J Comput Assist Tomogr 2004;28:24.
27. Lawler LP, Corl FM, Fishman EK: Multi-detector row and volume-rendered CT of the normal and accessory flow pathways of the thoracic systemic and pulmonary veins. Radiographics 2002;22:S45.
28. Shinde TS, Lee VS, Rofsky NM, et al: Three-dimensional gadolinium-enhanced MR venographic evaluation of patency of central veins in the thorax: initial experience. Radiology 1999;213:555.
29. Thornton MJ, Ryan R, Varghese JC, et al: A three-dimensional gadolinium-enhanced MR venography technique for imaging central veins. AJR Am J Roentgenol 1999;173:999.
30. Dymarkowski S, Bosmans H, Marchal G, et al: Three-dimensional MR angiography in the evaluation of thoracic outlet syndrome. AJR Am J Roentgenol 1999;173:1005.
31. Rose SC, Gomes AS, Yoon HC: MR angiography for mapping potential central venous access sites in patients with advanced venous occlusive disease. AJR Am J Roentgenol 1996;166:1181.
32. Kalman PG, Lindsay TF, Clarke K, et al: Management of upper extremity central venous obstruction using interventional radiology. Ann Vasc Surg 1998;12:202.
33. Kasirajan K, Gray B, Ouriel K: Percutaneous AngioJet thrombectomy in the management of extensive deep venous thrombosis. J Vasc Interv Radiol 2001;12:179.
34. Hall LD, Murray JD, Boswell GE: Venous stent placement as an adjunct to the staged multimodal treatment of Paget-Schroetter syndrome. J Vasc Interv Radiol 1995;6:565.
35. Meier GH, Pollak JS, Rosenblatt M, et al: Initial experience with venous stents in exertional axillary-subclavian vein thrombosis. J Vasc Surg 1996;24:974.
36. Kreienberg PB, Chang BB, Darling RC III, et al: Long-term results in patients treated with thrombolysis, thoracic inlet decompression, and subclavian vein stenting for Paget-Schroetter syndrome. J Vasc Surg 2001;33(Suppl):S100.
37. Verstandig AG, Bloom AI, Sasson T, et al: Shortening and migration of Wallstents after stenting of central venous stenoses in hemodialysis patients. Cardiovasc Intervent Radiol 2003;26:58.
38. Chang R, Horne MK III, Mayo DJ, et al: Pulse-spray treatment of subclavian and jugular venous thrombi with recombinant tissue plasminogen activator. J Vasc Interv Radiol 1996;7:845.
39. Rutherford RB: Primary subclavian-axillary vein thrombosis: the relative roles of thrombolysis, percutaneous angioplasty, stents, and surgery. Semin Vasc Surg 1998;11:91.
40. Sheeran S, Hallisey M, Murphy T, et al: Local thrombolytic therapy as part of a multidisciplinary approach to acute axillosubclavian vein thrombosis (Paget-Schroetter syndrome). J Vasc Interv Radiol 1997;8:253.

41. Adelman MA, Stone DH, Riles TS, et al: A multidisciplinary approach to the treatment of Paget-Schroetter syndrome. Ann Vasc Surg 1997; 11:149.

42. Lokanathan R, Salvian AJ, Chen JC, et al: Outcome after thrombolysis and selective thoracic outlet decompression for primary axillary vein thrombosis. J Vasc Surg 2001;33:783.

43. Farrell T, Lang EV, Barnhart W: Sharp recanalization of central venous occlusions. J Vasc Interv Radiol 1999;10:149.

44. Machleder HI: Thrombolytic therapy and surgery for primary axillosubclavian vein thrombosis: current approach. Semin Vasc Surg 1996;9:46.

45. Rutherford RB, Hurlbert SN: Primary subclavian-axillary vein thrombosis: consensus and commentary. Cardiovasc Surg 1996;4:420.

46. Hall LD, Murray JD, Boswell GE: Venous stent placement as an adjunct to the staged, multimodal treatment of Paget-Schroetter syndrome. J Vasc Interv Radiol 1995;6:565.

47. Urschel HC Jr, Patel AN: Paget-Schroetter syndrome therapy: failure of intravenous stents. Ann Thorac Surg 2003;75:1693.

48. Angle N, Gelabert HA, Farooq MM, et al: Safety and efficacy of early surgical decompression of the thoracic outlet Paget-Schroetter syndrome. Ann Vasc Surg 2001;15:37.

49. Ascher E, Gennaro M, Lorensen E, et al: Superior vena caval Greenfield filters: indications, techniques, and results. J Vasc Surg 1996;23:498.

50. Spence LD, Gironta MG, Malde HM, et al: Acute upper extremity deep venous thrombosis: safety and effectiveness of superior vena caval filters. Radiology 1999;210:53.

51. Ascher E, Hingorani A, Tsemekhin B, et al: Lessons learned from a 6-year clinical experience with superior vena caval Greenfield filters. J Vasc Surg 2000;32:881.

52. Rayan GM, Jensen C: Thoracic outlet syndrome: provocative examination maneuvers in a typical population. J Shoulder Elbow Surg 1995; 4:113.

53. Longley DG, Yedlicka JW, Molina EJ, et al: Thoracic outlet syndrome: evaluation of the subclavian vessels by color duplex sonography. AJR Am J Roentgenol 1992;158:623.

54. Barrett N, Spencer S, McIvor J, et al: Subclavian stenosis: a major complication of subclavian dialysis catheters. Nephrol Dial Transplant 1988;3:423.

55. Itkin M, Kraus MJ, Trerotola SO: Extrinsic compression of the left innominate vein in hemodialysis patients. J Vasc Interv Radiol 2004;15:51.

56. Demondion X, Boutry N, Drizenko A, et al: Thoracic outlet: anatomic correlation with MR imaging. AJR Am J Roentgenol 2000;175:417.

57. Criado E, Marston WA, Jaques PF, et al: Proximal venous outflow obstruction in patients with upper extremity arteriovenous dialysis access. Ann Vasc Surg 1994;8:530.

58. Kovalik EC, Newman GE, Suhocki P, et al: Correction of central venous stenoses: use of angioplasty and vascular Wallstents. Kidney Int 1994; 45:1177.

59. Beathard GA: Percutaneous transvenous angioplasty in the treatment of vascular access stenosis. Kidney Int 1992;42:1390.

60. Wisselink W, Money SR, Becker MO, et al: Comparison of operative reconstruction and percutaneous balloon dilatation for central venous obstruction. Am J Surg 1993;166:200.

61. Bjarnason H, Hunter DW, Crain MR, et al: Collapse of a Palmaz stent in the subclavian vein. AJR Am J Roentgenol 1993;160:1123.

62. Gray RJ, Horton KM, Dolmatch BL, et al: Use of Wallstents for hemodialysis access-related venous stenoses and occlusions untreatable with balloon angioplasty. Radiology 1995;195:479.

63. Vorwerk D, Guenther RW, Mann H, et al: Venous stenosis and occlusion in hemodialysis shunts: follow-up results of stent placement in 65 patients. Radiology 1995;195:140.

64. Bhatia DS, Money SR, Ochsner JL, et al: Comparison of surgical bypass and percutaneous balloon dilatation with primary stent placement in the treatment of central venous obstruction in the dialysis patient: one-year follow-up. Ann Vasc Surg 1996;10:452.

65. Quinn SF, Schuman ES, Demlow TA, et al: Percutaneous transluminal angioplasty versus endovascular stent placement in the treatment of venous stenoses in patients undergoing hemodialysis: intermediate results. J Vasc Interv Radiol 1995;6:851.

66. Chen JC, Bongard F, Klein SR: A contemporary perspective on superior vena cava syndrome. Am J Surg 1990;160:207.

67. Puel V, Caudry M, Le Metayer P, et al: Superior vena cava thrombosis related to catheter malposition in cancer chemotherapy given through implanted ports. Cancer 1993;72:2248.

68. Tovar-Martin E, Tovar-Pardo AE, Marini M, et al: Intraluminal leiomyosarcoma of the superior vena cava: a cause of superior vena cava syndrome. J Cardiovasc Surg 1997;38:33.

69. Sherrick AD, Brown LR, Harms GF, et al: The radiographic findings of fibrosing mediastinitis. Chest 1994;106:484.

70. Kim HJ, Kim HS, Chung SH: CT diagnosis of superior vena cava syndrome: importance of collateral vessels. AJR Am J Roentgenol 1993;161:539.

71. Elson JD, Becker GJ, Wholey MH, et al: Vena caval and central venous stenoses: management with Palmaz balloon-expandable intraluminal stents. J Vasc Interv Radiol 1991;2:215.

72. Capek P, Cope C: Percutaneous treatment of superior vena cava syndrome. AJR Am J Roentgenol 1989;152:183.

73. Kee ST, Kinoshita L, Razavi MK, et al: Superior vena cava syndrome: treatment with catheter-directed thrombolysis and endovascular stent placement. Radiology 1998;206:187.

74. Qanadli SD, El Hajjam M, Mignon F, et al: Subacute and chronic benign superior vena cava obstructions: endovascular treatment with self-expanding metallic stents. AJR Am J Roentgenol 1999;173:159.

75. Lanciego C, Chacon JL, Julian A, et al: Stenting as first option for endovascular treatment of malignant superior vena cava syndrome. AJR Am J Roentgenol 2001;177:585.

76. Yim CD, Sane SS, Bjarnason H: Superior vena cava stenting. Radiol Clin North Am 2000;38:409.

77. Petersen BD, Uchida BT: Long-term results of treatment of benign central venous obstructions unrelated to dialysis with expandable Z stents. J Vasc Interv Radiol 1999;10:757.

78. Miller JH, McBride K, Little F, et al: Malignant superior vena cava obstruction: stent placement via the subclavian route. Cardiovasc Intervent Radiol 2000;23:155.

79. Sasano S, Onuki T, Mae M, et al: Wallstent endovascular prosthesis for the treatment of superior vena cava syndrome. Jpn J Thorac Cardiovasc Surg 2001;49:165.

80. Tanigawa N, Sawada S, Mishima K, et al. Clinical outcome of stenting in superior vena cava syndrome associated with malignant tumors: comparison with conventional treatment. Acta Radiol 1998;39:669.

81. Schindler N, Vogelzang RL: Superior vena cava syndrome: experience with endovascular stents and surgical therapy. Surg Clin North Am 1999;79:683.

82. Slonim SM, Semba CP, Sze DY, et al: Placement of SVC stents over pacemaker wires for the treatment of SVC syndrome. J Vasc Interv Radiol 2000;11:215.

83. Stockx L, Raat H, Donck J, et al: Repositioning and leaving in situ the central venous catheter during percutaneous treatment of associated superior vena cava syndrome: a report of eight cases. Cardiovasc Intervent Radiol 1999;22:224.

84. Furui S, Sawada S, Kuramoto K, et al: Gianturco stent placement in malignant caval obstruction: analysis of factors for predicting the outcome. Radiology 1995;195:147.

85. Kishi K, Sonomura T, Mitsuzane K, et al: Self-expandable metallic stent therapy for superior vena cava syndrome: clinical observations. Radiology 1993;189:531.

86. Gross CM, Kraemer J, Waigand J, et al: Stent implantation in patients with superior vena cava syndrome. AJR Am J Roentgenol 1997;169:429.

87. Smith SL, Manhire AR, Clark DM: Delayed spontaneous superior vena cava perforation associated with a SVC Wallstent. Cardiovasc Intervent Radiol 2001;24:286.

88. Martin M, Baumgartner I, Kolb M, et al: Fatal pericardial tamponade after Wallstent implantation for malignant superior vena cava syndrome. J Endovasc Ther 2002;9:680.

89. Recto MR, Bousamra M, Yeh T Jr: Late superior vena cava perforation and aortic laceration after stenting to treat superior vena cava syndrome secondary to fibrosing mediastinitis. J Invasive Cardiol 2002;14:624.

90. Moore WM Jr, Hollier LH, Pickett TK: Superior vena cava and central venous reconstruction. Surgery 1991;110:35.

91. Gagne PJ, Cone JB, McFarland D, et al: Proximity penetrating extremity trauma: the role of duplex ultrasound in the detection of occult venous injuries. J Trauma 1995;39:1157.

92. DiGiacomo JC, Rotondo MF, Schwab CW: Transcutaneous balloon catheter tamponade for definitive control of subclavian venous injuries: case reports. J Trauma 1994;37:111.

93. Spaggiari L, Regnard JF, Nottin R, et al: Leiomyosarcoma of the superior vena cava. Ann Thorac Surg 1996;62:274.

94. Levett JM, Meffert WG, Strong WW, et al: Leiomyosarcoma of the superior vena cava and azygous vein. Ann Thorac Surg 1995;60:1415.

95. Calligaro KD, Ahmad S, Dandora R, et al: Venous aneurysms: surgical indications and review of the literature. Surgery 1995;117:1.

96. Picou MA, Antonovic R, Holden WE: Position-dependent mediastinal mass: aneurysm of the superior vena cava. AJR Am J Roentgenol 1993;161:1110.

16

Vascular Access Placement and Foreign Body Retrieval

The demand for central venous catheters (CVCs) has increased dramatically over the last two decades. CVCs are used for infusion of drugs (e.g., antibiotics, chemotherapeutic agents, narcotics), administration of blood products, blood sampling, hyperalimentation, and temporary dialysis and apheresis. In the past, CVCs were placed by surgeons in the operating room. Interventional radiologists have assumed the major role in the insertion of these catheters.[1,2] In some hospitals, vascular access placement is the most commonly performed procedure in the interventional radiology suite.

Image-guided placement of a CVC has several advantages over blind insertion.[3-5] The risk of immediate complications such as pneumothorax, arterial puncture, and catheter malposition is diminished. Precise positioning of the catheter tip is guaranteed. Imaging is critical when placing catheters through occluded thoracic veins or outside the chest (e.g., into the inferior vena cava [IVC]). Finally, procedure costs are reduced.

ACCESS PLANNING

Devices

Tunneled external infusion catheters are made of silicone or polyurethane and are available with one, two, or three lumens in sizes from 4 to 12 French (Fig. 16-1). The device is inserted into a large vein and travels through a subcutaneous tunnel before exiting the skin. A Dacron cuff embedded on the shaft incites a fibrotic reaction that ultimately secures the catheter in place and reduces the risk of infection spreading from the exit site to the circulation. Some catheters have a silver ion-impregnated cuff or silver coating that is meant to serve as an instant antimicrobial barrier; however, the value of this feature is debated.[6,7] Infusion catheters have end holes or side valves (e.g., Groshong catheter). Valves are meant to allow fluid injection and blood aspiration but prevent blood or air from entering the catheter when it is not in use (Fig. 16-2). In theory, the risks of catheter occlusion and air embolism are reduced. Although valved catheters require less frequent flushing, they may be just as likely to malfunction as endhole catheters.[8,9]

Tunneled hemodialysis and *apheresis catheters* are short, large-bore (11.5 to 16 French), dual-lumen devices capable of handling high flow rates (e.g., 300 to 500 mL/minute) (Fig. 16-3). These catheters have staggered or nonstaggered end holes or split lumens.[10,11] Tunneled hemodialysis catheters must be distinguished from nontunneled temporary catheters (usually placed by nephrologists) for several sessions of acute, emergent dialysis. No single device convincingly has been proven to be most effective, although there is some evidence that split catheters are more durable and have fewer complications than other designs.[12,13] Some separation of the uptake and return lumens is necessary to prevent recirculation, which can significantly diminish the efficacy of dialysis.[14]

Implantable ports are constructed from a variety of materials, including titanium and plastic (Fig. 16-4). Small ports are designed for children, patients with minimal subcutaneous fat, or arm placement. The catheter is connected to a reservoir with a silicon window that is accessed through the skin using a noncoring (Huber) needle. The system is buried in the subcutaneous tissue of the chest or arm. These devices are available in single- and double-lumen configurations. Ports provide central venous access without the need for an external catheter. Although it is widely believed that infections are less common with implanted

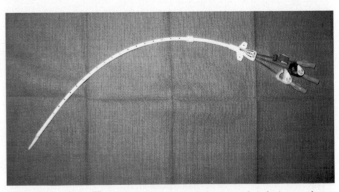

FIGURE 16-1 ■ Triple-lumen tunneled external infusion catheter (Bard Access Systems, Salt Lake City, Utah). Dacron cuff is mounted on the proximal portion of the catheter shaft.

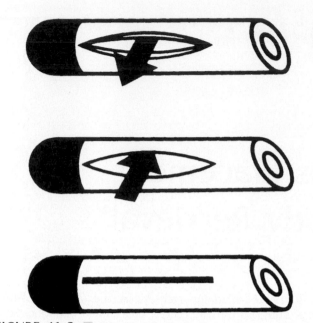

FIGURE 16-2 ■ Side slits in catheter allow aspiration of blood or infusion of fluids but prevent blood from entering the catheter when not in use. (Courtesy of Bard Access Systems, Salt Lake City, Utah.)

ports than with external catheters, some studies have found no such difference.[15-17]

Hemodialysis ports are implantable systems for use in patients who have no more usable sites for dialysis access fistulas or grafts. They are essentially dual-lumen ports that can accommodate large flows required for dialysis. Early reports suggest that rates of infection and catheter dysfunction are improved compared with tunneled dialysis catheters.[18,19]

Peripherally inserted central catheters (PICCs) are essentially long intravenous lines placed from a peripheral arm vein into the central venous system (Fig. 16-5). Single-, double-, and triple-lumen configurations are available in sizes from 3.0 to 7.0 French. Some of the designs are capable

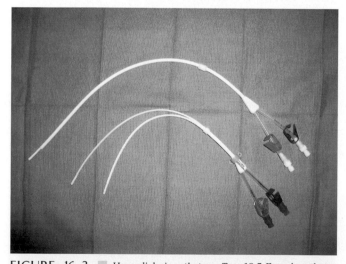

FIGURE 16-3 ■ Hemodialysis catheters. *Top*, 13.5-French catheter with staggered lumens (proximal end hole is the arterial lumen) (Bard Access Systems, Salt Lake City, Utah). *Bottom*, split dialysis catheter (Medcomp, Harleysville, Penn.).

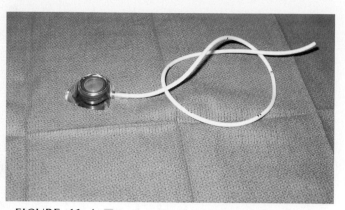

FIGURE 16-4 ■ Implantable chest port with catheter attached.

of handling high flows required during power injection of contrast material for CT scanning.

Device Selection

The selection of the most appropriate catheter in an individual case should be made jointly by the referring physician, interventional radiologist, and patient. Several factors are important, including intended purpose, frequency and duration of use, and patient preference for an external or implanted device (Table 16-1). Tunneled infusion catheters and implantable ports are indicated only when continuous vascular access is needed for several months or longer. Otherwise, a PICC line is sufficient.

■ VENOUS ACCESS

Access Route

CVCs typically are usually inserted through the internal jugular vein, upper arm vein, axillary (subclavian) vein, or common femoral vein. The subclavian vein should be avoided if at all possible, because symptomatic or asymptomatic stenosis or thrombosis is much more likely to occur with this route.[20-23] The **right** internal jugular vein is preferred over the **left.** Standard teaching is to avoid placement on the side of the body that has undergone (or will undergo) mastectomy, radiation therapy, or axillary lymph node dissection, all of which may compromise lymphatic or venous drainage.

If an occluded central vein can be recanalized or simply traversed with a guidewire (from above or below), catheter insertion still may be possible.[24] If not, the external jugular vein, enlarged collateral veins (e.g., intercostal vein), or the common femoral vein is used.[24,25] Practically, this situation mostly occurs in patients requiring chronic hemodialysis. The femoral vein is avoided when possible because of the higher rates of infection and catheter malfunction.[26] As a last resort, central venous access is obtained directly into the IVC through a translumbar or transhepatic approach.[27,28]

FIGURE 16-5 ■ Single-lumen peripherally inserted central catheter *(right)* with inner stiffening guidewire *(left)* and peel-away sheath and dilator *(top)* (Cook, Inc., Bloomington, Ind.).

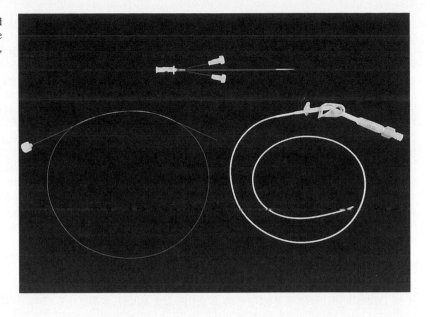

Patient Preparation

Access insertion (except for PICCs) in an interventional suite demands the same aseptic environment found in an operating room.[29,30] All procedures should begin with antibacterial cleaning of surfaces that may come in contact with the patient, wide surgical preparation of the operating field, surgical scrub by all operators, and maintenance of strict aseptic technique during the procedure. Some interventionalists give prophylactic antibiotics (e.g., 1 g of cephazolin IV) within 1 hour of placement of tunneled catheters or ports, even though there is no objective support for this precaution.[31] Sepsis is a relative contraindication to placement of tunneled catheters and implantable ports.[32] Coagulation parameters should be checked and corrected before the procedure (see Chapter 1).

Venous Entry

Duplex sonography or injection of contrast through a peripheral vein can confirm that the intended access vein is patent

and that the route to the superior vena cava (SVC) is open. In the internal jugular and axillary veins, Doppler spectral analysis normally shows a triphasic waveform with respiratory variation (see Fig. 15-11). Dampening of the waveform suggests a central obstruction. Sonographic guidance reduces the risk of inadvertent arterial puncture or pneumothorax and the number of needle passes required for venous entry.[33]

Many interventionalists prefer to gain access with a 21-gauge micropuncture needle with an 0.018-inch guidewire and transitional 4- or 5-French dilator (see Fig. 2-3). Continuous suction is applied to a saline-filled syringe and tubing is connected to the needle until blood returns. If the needle coapts and then punctures the front and back walls of the vein, blood return occurs with needle withdrawal.

For *internal jugular vein puncture*, a site on the lower neck above the clavicle is selected. The vessel is visualized with the transducer in a transverse plane while the needle is advanced from the side or from above (Fig. 16-6).

TABLE 16-1	GUIDELINES FOR ACCESS DEVICE SELECTION
Device	**Purpose or Situation**
External, tunneled catheter	Continuous use Multiple, simultaneous uses Patient preference
Implantable port	Intermittent use Immunocompromised patient Patient preference
High-flow catheter	Hemodialysis Apheresis
PICC	Short-term use (<2–3 mo) Infrequent blood drawing

PICC, peripherally inserted central catheter.

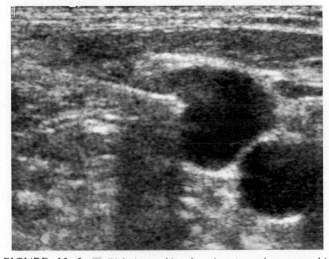

FIGURE 16-6 ■ Right internal jugular vein entry under sonographic guidance in the transverse plane. Needle enters from a lateral approach; carotid artery is medial to the vein.

The transverse orientation ensures that the carotid artery is monitored at all times.

For *axillary vein puncture,* the entry should be lateral to the ribs in the subcoracoid region. This position almost completely eliminates the possibility of pneumothorax. It ensures also that the catheter is well within the subclavian vein as it passes through the costoclavicular space. If the catheter is extravascular at that site, chronic compression may occur and lead to catheter erosion and fracture ("pinch-off" syndrome) (Fig. 16-7).[34,35] The axillary vein lies just inferior to the axillary artery (Fig. 16-8). During sonography, the vein is identified by its color flow pattern, changes with respiration, and lack of pulsatility. After application of local anesthesia, the transducer is oriented parallel to the vessel while the needle is advanced with real-time imaging.

For *upper arm vein puncture,* the basilic vein is preferred, followed by the brachial and cephalic veins (Fig. 16-9). Venospasm is particularly problematic with the latter route. It is helpful to place a tourniquet around the upper arm to distend the vein before puncture. The vein is entered with a 21-gauge needle from a micropuncture set or a 21- to 22-gauge sheath needle. Care must be taken to avoid puncturing the brachial artery. Because the veins are small and tend to go into spasm, it is wise to start peripherally on the vein and avoid a double wall puncture. After blood is aspirated, an 0.018-inch guidewire is inserted. If the guidewire does not advance despite needle adjustment, a more central site on the vein is used. Sometimes, the guidewire hangs up because it has entered a small collateral channel. In this case, contrast injection may outline the more direct route to the central circulation.

For *common femoral vein puncture,* blind puncture based on the arterial pulse or sonographic guidance may be used.[36] Catheters are tunneled laterally onto the thigh or lower abdomen (see below).

Inferior vena cava puncture may be required if all potential access sites in the chest, arms, and thigh are exhausted.[28,37,38] Prior CT scans should be evaluated to identify obstacles or contraindications to the selected route. Initially, a sheath, guidewire, or catheter is placed into the IVC from the groin, although this is not absolutely necessary and bony landmarks alone may be used (Fig. 16-10). The patient is placed prone on the interventional table, and a site for venous entry is chosen on the right flank above the iliac crest just lateral to the vertebral column. The IVC is demarcated by the indwelling guidewire or catheter or by contrast injection through the groin sheath. The vessel is punctured under fluoroscopic guidance using a long 18- to 20-gauge needle. After the needle enters the IVC, the remainder of the procedure is similar to catheter placement from other access routes. A stiff guidewire should be inserted before placement of the peel-away sheath. It is important to create a cephalic track into the IVC to avoid a sharp right angle as the needle enters the vein, which can make it difficult to place the sheath and catheter.

Transhepatic venous access has been described for patients whose only patent central vein is the suprarenal IVC. While this route is feasible in most cases, catheter durability is a serious problem.[27,39] Finally, *transrenal venous access* into the IVC has been described for patients with end stage renal disease who require temporary dialysis catheters.[40]

After the vein is entered, a guidewire is placed followed by a transitional dilator or 5-French catheter. The guidewire

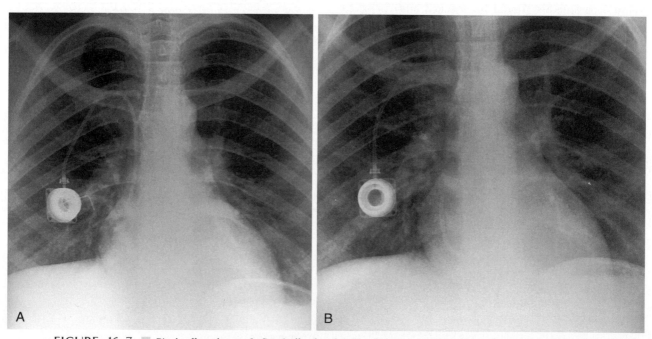

FIGURE 16-7 ■ Pinch-off syndrome. **A,** Surgically placed right subclavian vein port. The catheter runs in the costoclavicular space before entering the vein. **B,** Six months after port placement, chest radiograph shows catheter fracture with a fragment lying in the right atrium.

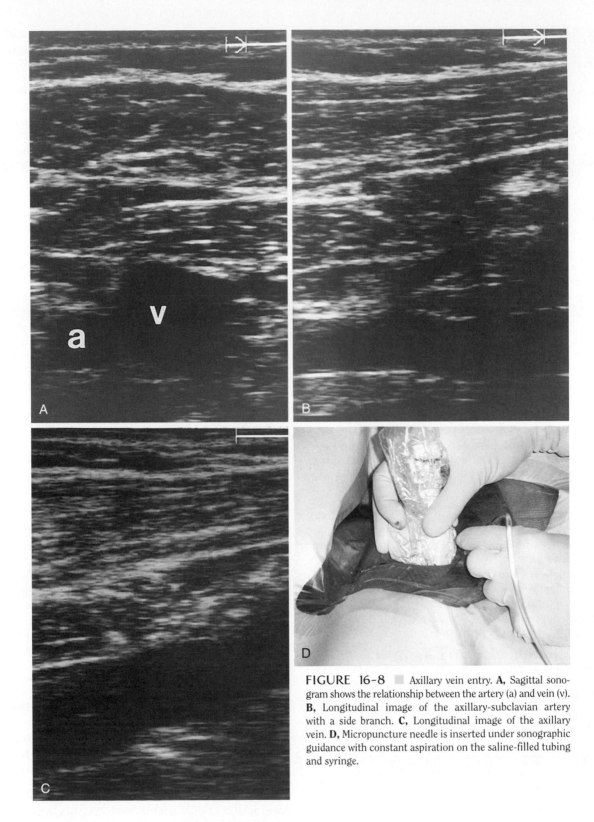

FIGURE 16-8 ▪ Axillary vein entry. **A,** Sagittal sonogram shows the relationship between the artery (a) and vein (v). **B,** Longitudinal image of the axillary-subclavian artery with a side branch. **C,** Longitudinal image of the axillary vein. **D,** Micropuncture needle is inserted under sonographic guidance with constant aspiration on the saline-filled tubing and syringe.

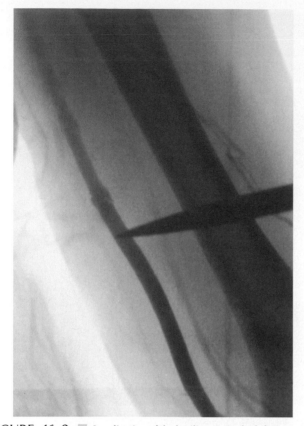

FIGURE 16-9 ■ Localization of the basilic vein in the left upper arm for peripherally inserted central catheter placement by injection of contrast through a peripheral intravenous line.

is advanced into the right atrium (or IVC) to confirm that venous rather than arterial access has been achieved. If the guidewire does not advance, a contrast injection may show a central venous obstruction.

The *intravascular catheter length* is estimated by placing the tip of a guidewire in the right atrium with the patient in deep inspiration. The wire is clamped at the catheter hub, and the exposed hub length is subtracted from the clamped guidewire length.

- If the catheter **can** be trimmed to size (PICCs, and tunneled infusion catheters), an appropriate catheter length (tip to hub) is determined based on the intravascular length (plus additional catheter segment added to allow for a 7- to 10-cm tunnel when appropriate).
- If the catheter **cannot** be trimmed to size because of the tip configuration (hemodialysis and apheresis catheter, Groshong catheters), an appropriately sized device is chosen based on the intravascular length and the desired tunnel length.

A guidewire is readvanced into the SVC or IVC to prevent accidental loss of access while the subcutaneous tunnel or pocket is being created.

Catheter Tip Position

The manufacturers of most vascular access devices recommend positioning of the catheter tip in the SVC.

Nonetheless, because most CVCs (with the possible exception of PICCs) routinely migrate 3 to 4 cm upward after insertion, it is now standard practice to place the catheter tip in the mid-right atrium.[41-45] In this position, the catheter end holes cannot become obstructed by fibrin sheaths that plaster the catheter against the caval wall. Because all of these devices are composed of soft polyurethane or silicone material, puncture of the right atrium in this position should not occur. Placement in the **low** right atrium runs the theoretical risk of cardiac perforation or atrial arrhythmias, but these events are extremely rare.

■ DEVICE PLACEMENT

Tunneled Infusion Catheters

Nonvalved catheters may be cut to size (see above). The Dacron cuff should be located about 2 to 3 cm from the skin exit site (to allow for easier removal) and the subcutaneous tunnel should be about 7 to 10 cm long. A skin exit site is chosen on the anterior chest wall below the clavicle, away from the axilla and breast tissue.[46,47] A medial location is better for women to avoid interference with clothing or bra straps. The exit site and subcutaneous tissues along the tunnel track are infiltrated with lidocaine. A stab incision is made with a blade large enough to accommodate the catheter but small enough to ensure a snug fit to prevent the catheter from falling out. The catheter is pulled through the tunnel with a tunneling device until the cuff is near the vein entry site. The catheter should form a gentle curve as it enters the vein.

The vein is dilated to accommodate the delivery sheath. In some patients, serial dilation, a stiff guidewire, or both may be necessary to advance the sheath through the subcutaneous tissues. Laceration of the vein wall by the dilator or guidewire can occur if this step is not followed under fluoroscopy. The guidewire and inner dilator are removed while the patient is in deep inspiration to avoid air embolism. For some devices, valved sheaths are available to possibly avoid this problem. The catheter is immediately inserted into the sheath and then advanced into the right atrium.

If the catheter does not pass easily because the sheath has kinked (usually at the brachiocephalic vein junction), it is carefully withdrawn until it lies in the straight portion of the subclavian vein, and the catheter is readvanced. Alternatively, a hydrophilic guidewire is inserted through the catheter into the SVC. The catheter is then advanced over the guidewire. If the catheter tip enters the internal jugular, azygous, or contralateral brachiocephalic vein, it may be directed into the SVC by buckling it with a guidewire, withdrawing the sheath slightly and readvancing the catheter, or advancing the catheter over a guidewire.

The sheath is peeled away while the catheter is held in position at the venous entry site. The catheter is then withdrawn at the skin exit site until the tip is in the desired location in the mid-right atrium. The catheter lumen(s) is flushed with heparin lock solution (100 units/mL). The device is secured to the skin to avoid early dislodgement before the Dacron cuff is incorporated.

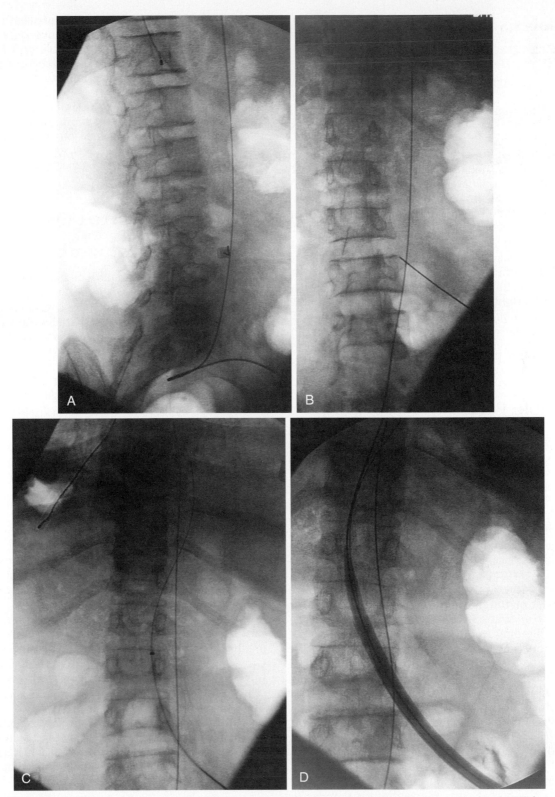

FIGURE 16-10 ■ Inferior vena cava (IVC) vascular access placement. **A,** A guidewire has been placed in the IVC from the right common femoral vein. In an oblique prone position, a 22-gauge, 15-cm Chiba needle is directed toward the guidewire from the right flank. **B,** The image intensifier is rotated away from the operator, and the needle is advanced to the IVC along a cephalad track. **C,** A 6-French, tapered access set is advanced into the IVC over an 0.018-inch guidewire. **D,** The peel-away sheath for the hemodialysis catheter is inserted over a heavy-duty guidewire. Catheter placement followed.

Hemodialysis and Apheresis Catheters

Up to 50% of chronic hemodialysis patients develop sub-clavian vein stenoses or frank occlusions after placement of temporary or tunneled venous catheters through this route.[20-23,48,49] In addition to causing disabling symptoms, these obstructions can interfere with function of future hemodialysis access. For this reason, CVC in patients on chronic hemodialysis should be placed in the right (or left) internal jugular vein whenever possible.

From an accessible site on the chest wall, the catheter is tunneled over the clavicle. Generous dissection of the subcutaneous tissues at the venotomy site and a somewhat low internal jugular vein puncture can prevent kinking of the catheter as it makes a U-turn out of the vein and toward the chest.[50] For catheters with staggered lumens, the arterial lumen (proximal port) is positioned with the end hole **away** from the right atrial wall for optimal function.[49] The catheter tip should be readjusted if rapid aspiration of blood is not possible after placement. Some dialysis units prefer to fill catheters with high-dose heparin (1000 or 5000 units/mL) to prevent thrombosis.

Implantable Ports

Ports may be placed in the chest or arm, depending on the patient's lifestyle and preference.[51-56] Chest ports are somewhat easier to access. The port site must have enough subcutaneous fat to accommodate the device easily to avoid wound dehiscence or skin breakdown. However, a port can be difficult to access if there is too much surrounding adipose tissue or if it is poorly supported by underlying bone. Ideally, the port septum should be about 0.5 to 2.0 cm below the skin surface. The device should not be placed in breast tissue or the axilla.

After venous access is obtained, a 3- to 5-cm transverse incision is made on the anterior chest wall using a No. 10 or 15 blade after infiltration with lidocaine and epinephrine (Fig. 16-11). Bleeding from small arterial branches always stops with manual compression or clamp occlusion. A pocket is created below the incision using blunt dissection. The pocket should be large enough to accommodate the port and allow easy closure of the wound. Some interventionalists place two sutures in the fascial plane below the incision to secure the port after it is inserted into the pocket.

The catheter is tunneled through the subcutaneous track and then inserted into the internal jugular vein using a peel-away sheath. The catheter tip is positioned in the mid-right atrium. The catheter is cut to size and connected to the port. Some interventionalists prefer to insert the catheter into the vein after it is attached to the port. The fascial stay sutures (if used) are run through the front eyelets of the port base, the port is placed in the pocket, and the sutures are tied. The device is accessed with a noncoring (Huber) needle and flushed with heparin lock solution (100 units/mL) to ensure that it is functional. Under fluoroscopy, the entire course of the catheter is examined for kinks. The incision is closed with interrupted absorbable sutures in the subcutaneous layer to approximate tissues and continuous absorbable suture in the subcuticular layer. Steri-Strips and a sterile dry dressing are placed over the incision. The venotomy may be closed with Steri-Strips or suture material.

Arm ports are inserted in a similar fashion above the elbow. The tunnel can be very short, allowing the catheter to be pulled from the skin incision to the venotomy site using forceps rather than a tunneling device. Care must be taken to avoid damaging the brachial artery.

Peripherally Inserted Central Catheters

PICCs are suitable for patients who need short-term central vascular access, typically for antibiotics, chemotherapy, or hyperalimentation.[57-61] It is more cost-effective for PICCs to be placed at the bedside by specially trained nurses.[60,62] Radiologic placement is indicated when bedside insertion is unsuccessful or unavailable. The dilator or sheath is inserted into the accessed vein. The catheter is cut to size and inserted through the peel-away sheath with the accompanying stylet to assist with catheter passage. It is then advanced into the mid-right atrium and flushed with heparin lock solution. The hub is secured to the skin with nonabsorbable suture material or an adhesive appliance.

■ ACCESS MANAGEMENT

Catheter and Exit Site Care

Meticulous catheter and exit site care is the most important step in limiting CVC-related complications. Patient or care-giver education is done before and after device placement by a specially trained nurse.

Protocols for catheter and wound care and for catheter flushing vary somewhat among institutions. Most catheters are flushed with heparin solution weekly and after each use. Groshong catheters may be filled with saline and require less frequent flushing. A sterile, dry gauze dressing or occlusive plastic dressing is kept over the fresh incision or exit site. The incision must be kept completely dry for about 3 days. The exit site, incision, and tunnel track are examined daily by the patient or caregiver for signs of infection, catheter withdrawal, catheter fracture, wound dehiscence, or skin breakdown. The site also should be examined by a physician or nurse within 5 to 7 days of placement.

Device Removal

To remove tunneled catheters, the exit site is sterilized and the tunnel track anesthetized. Using blunt dissection, the catheter is separated from the subcutaneous tissues.

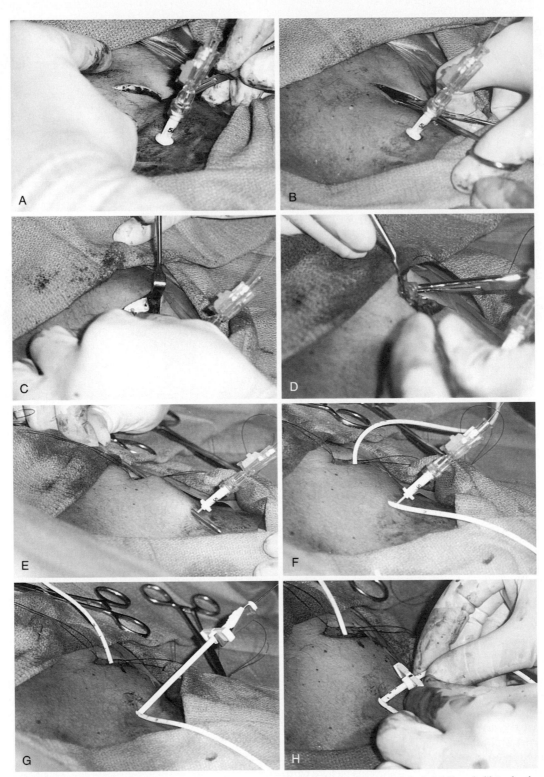

FIGURE 16-11 ■ Placement of an implantable chest port. The patient's head is on the left. **A,** A 5-French dilator has been inserted in the right axillary vein. In this case, both internal jugular veins were unsuitable for access. An incision is made below the venotomy site. **B,** A pocket is created with blunt dissection. **C,** The pocket is made large enough to accommodate the port. **D,** Two nonabsorbable sutures are placed in the fascial layer. **E,** After applying local anesthesia, a tunneling device is run through the subcutaneous tissues from the incision to the venotomy. **F,** The catheter is pulled through the tunnel. **G,** The peel-away sheath is inserted into the vein. **H,** The catheter is fed through after the guidewire and dilator have been removed.

Continued

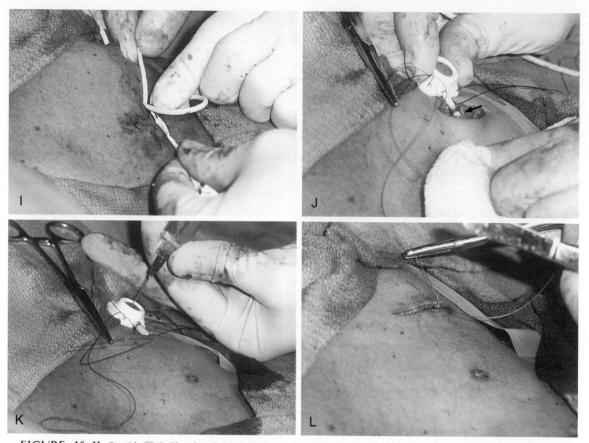

FIGURE 16-11 *Cont'd* ■ **I,** The sheath is peeled away after the catheter tip has been positioned in the right atrium. **J,** The catheter is cut to size and connected to the port. A plastic sleeve *(arrow)* is slid up the catheter to the reservoir. The fascial stay sutures have been run through the front eyelets of the port base. **K,** The port is accessed with a noncoring needle and flushed with heparin lock solution. **L,** After the port is placed in the pocket and secured with stay sutures, the subcutaneous layer is closed with interrupted absorbable suture. The skin is closed with a continuous subcuticular suture line.

Sharp dissection may be needed to release the cuff. If the cuff is far from the skin exit site, it is sometimes necessary to perform a cutdown over the cuff to release the catheter. The catheter may fracture if excessive force is applied to remove it. Retention of the polyester cuff is not associated with an increased risk of later infection.[63]

To remove implanted ports, an incision is made over the original scar after local anesthesia is applied. Using sharp and blunt dissection, the port and catheter hub are separated from the surrounding tissue. The fibrous capsule around the port is incised with a dissecting scissors or scalpel to release the device. The stay sutures (if present) are cut, and the port and attached catheter are removed. The incision is closed in an identical manner to port placement. If there is any evidence of infection, the pocket is packed with iodoform gauze and allowed to close by secondary intention.

■ COMPLICATIONS

Immediate Complications

The overall complication rate for CVC placement is about 4% to 7%.[32,47,55,60,64] Immediate complications occur less

frequently with image-guided placement than without (Table 16-2 and Fig. 16-12).[3,5,49,52,54-56,65] With the exception of venous thrombosis, procedure-related complication rates generally are lower for PICCs and peripheral ports than for devices placed in the chest or neck.

Air embolism can occur during the interval between removing the dilator and peeling away the sheath. This event usually can be avoided by immediately crimping the sheath or removing the dilator and guidewire with the patient in suspended deep inspiration. Valved sheaths are available to help prevent this complication. If air embolism occurs,

TABLE 16-2   EARLY COMPLICATIONS FROM IMAGE-GUIDED VASCULAR ACCESS PLACEMENT

Event	Frequency (%)
Pneumothorax	0–1
Arterial puncture	<1
Hemorrhage or hematoma	0–2
Air embolism	1
Catheter malposition	0
Venous perforation	<1

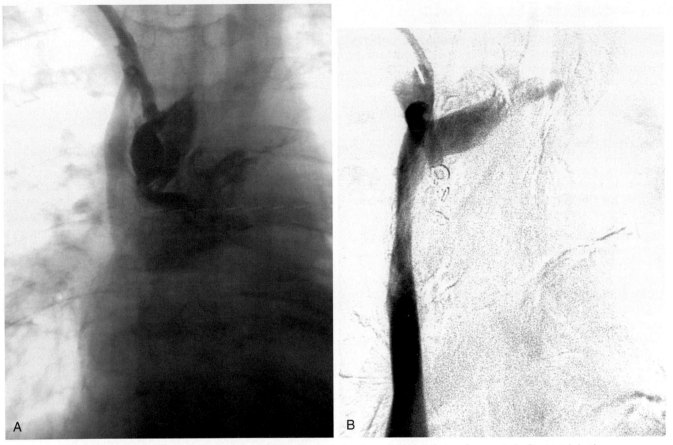

FIGURE 16-12 ■ Superior vena cava (SVC) rupture during hemodialysis catheter placement. **A,** Contrast injection shows extravasation outside the SVC. **B,** Several large stainless-steel coils were used to close the leak. Subsequently, a tunneled catheter was placed into the SVC.

the chest is examined with fluoroscopy. Conventional teaching is to place the patient in the left lateral decubitus position immediately to keep the air in the right heart chambers and prevent "air lock." In reality, the air bolus almost always has traveled to the pulmonary artery by the time the embolism is recognized. Supplemental oxygen and intravenous fluids are given, and the patient is carefully monitored. In this situation, air embolism is usually self-limited, although fatal events have been reported.[66]

Persistent blood oozing from the skin exit site is a problem occasionally. Prolonged gentle pressure usually resolves the bleeding. Coagulation parameters should be checked. If necessary, Gelfoam pledgets or collagen plug from an arterial closure device may be helpful. Silver nitrate can be applied (to the subcutaneous tissue only) to achieve hemostasis.

Fatalities during vascular access placement have been reported from laceration of the central veins or heart by the tip of the dilator or guidewire.[67] This catastrophe is avoided by advancing the sheath or dilator with careful fluoroscopic monitoring.

Late Complications

The primary late complications of CVC placement are infection, catheter occlusion or malfunction, venous thrombosis,

and catheter migration (Table 16-3).[3,5,49,52,54,55,60,65] The frequency of infections and catheter occlusion are substantially greater for tunneled hemodialysis catheters than for small-bore infusion catheters.

Infectious complications include bacteremia, exit site infection, port pocket or subcutaneous tunnel infection, and septic thrombophlebitis. The incidence of infections after image-guided radiologic placement is comparable to (and perhaps better than) surgical placement.[3-5,54] Bacteremia and ascending infections usually are related to the *biofilm* that forms on all intravascular devices. This layer provides a

TABLE 16-3 LATE COMPLICATIONS FROM IMAGE-GUIDED VASCULAR ACCESS PLACEMENT

Event	Frequency (%)
Catheter occlusion	1–10
Catheter or device migration	0–3
Catheter dislodgement	2–9
Catheter fracture	1
Wound dehiscence	1
Central venous thrombosis	0–10 (0.01–0.03/100 catheter days)
Local infection	1–7
Catheter-related bacteremia	1–4
Overall infection	0.01–0.30/100 catheter days

relative sanctuary for microorganisms. Thus, almost all infections are related to intraluminal spread.[68]

There are established criteria for diagnosing catheter-related bloodstream infections. Fever alone is not usually sufficient. As a rule, two positive blood cultures (one obtained from a peripheral vein) are required. The offending organism is typically coagulase-negative *Staphylococcus* or *Staphylococcus aureus*. In patients with fever and positive blood cultures, it is often difficult to determine whether the device is responsible for bacteremia. Left untreated, catheter-related bacteremia can lead to septic shock or endocarditis.

The management of catheter-related infections depends largely on the site of infection, the offending organism, and the patient's underlying immunologic state.

■ Patients with skin infections or fever from unknown source are initially treated with broad-spectrum intravenous antibiotics and local wound care. Skin, catheter lumen, and blood cultures are obtained to guide antibiotic choice. If the patient responds to treatment, the catheter is left in place or exchanged over a guidewire for a new device.[69,70]

■ Patients with tunnel infections, port pocket infections, septic thrombophlebitis, or septic shock require intravenous antibiotics and immediate removal of the device. The catheter tip or infected site is cultured and antibiotics adjusted based on culture sensitivity results. After removing an infected port, the pocket is irrigated and packed with iodoform gauze. The packing is changed every few days and then allowed to heal by secondary intention.

■ For certain microorganisms, there is a general consensus that resolution of bacteremia requires catheter removal (Box 16-1).[68]

■ Patients with markedly compromised immune systems warrant catheter removal in most cases.

The timing for reinsertion of a new tunneled catheter is highly controversial.[68] Ideally, the interventionalist should wait until the entire course of antibiotics has been given, but this is often impractical. At the very least, the patient should become afebrile, have a normal white blood cell count and negative blood cultures, and have received at least 2 days of intravenous antibiotics.

Catheter malfunction is a vexing problem in patients with central venous access devices. The best approach is prevention: positioning of the catheter tip in the mid-right atrium. Malfunction can occur for several reasons:

■ Fibrin or clot occluding the end hole
■ Catheter malposition or migration
■ Catheter kinks
■ Catheter tip abutting or eroding into the vessel wall
■ Catheter fracture

With 1 week of placement, all CVCs are covered by a layer of fibrin.[71] At some point, this *fibrin sheath (sleeve)* may obstruct the catheter end hole (Fig. 16-13). Fluid usually can be injected, but blood cannot be aspirated. Hemodialysis catheter dysfunction often is signaled by diminished blood flow rates or inefficient dialysis. With catheter-related thrombosis, obstructive clots or complete occlusion is seen. Malfunctioning catheters can be managed in several ways.[72] It is not entirely clear which method is preferable, although catheter exchange is more durable than fibrin stripping (see below).[73-77]

■ *Low-dose fibrinolytic agent.* The catheter lumens are filled with 2 mg of Cathflo Activase (alteplase, Genentech, South San Francisco, Calif.). The solution is left to dwell for up to 90 minutes, after which aspiration is attempted. If unsuccessful, the maneuver should be repeated. This technique temporarily salvages about 90% of catheters, but the results may not be lasting.[74,78]

■ *Catheter exchange.* The malfunctioning catheter is exchanged over a guidewire for a new catheter using the existing tunnel and venous entry site.[75] Some interventionalists use a large-caliber (e.g., 12-mm) angioplasty

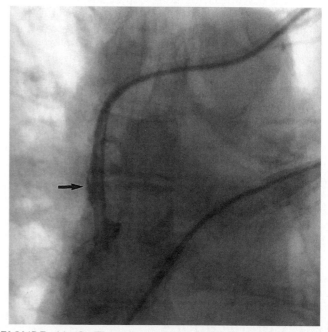

FIGURE 16-13 ■ Fibrin sheath. Contrast injected through the catheter lumen runs back along the catheter shaft *(arrow)* rather than exiting the catheter freely.

BOX 16-1 ■ **Organisms that Generally Require Catheter Removal**

Acinetobacter baumannii
Agrobacterium species
Aspergillus species
Bacillus species
Candida species
Corynebacterium jeikeium
Malassezia furfur
Mycobacterium species
Pseudomonas aeruginosa
Other *Pseudomonas* species
Staphylococcus aureus
Stenotrophomonas species
Other gram-negative rods

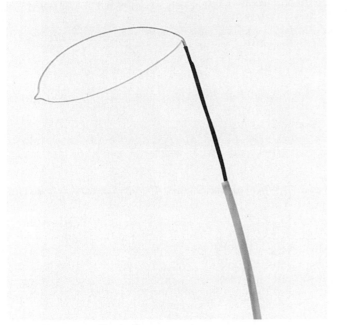

FIGURE 16-14 ■ Amplatz nitinol gooseneck snare (Microvena, White Bear Lake, Minn.) with outer 6-French guiding catheter.

balloon to disrupt the fibrin sheath in the SVC. This maneuver must be avoided if there is any evidence of infection at the skin exit site.

■ *Fibrin sheath stripping.*[75,77] With positioning of the catheter tip in the right atrium, the fibrin sheath is much less likely to interfere with catheter function. From the femoral vein, a 25- to 35-mm Amplatz nitinol gooseneck snare (Microvena, White Bear Lake, Minn.) is advanced to the SVC through a 6-French guiding catheter (Fig. 16-14). The open snare is used to encircle the tip and then advanced up the catheter shaft (Fig. 16-15). The snare is cinched snugly around the catheter and then withdrawn to strip off the fibrin coat. This procedure is repeated several times. Often, the catheter tip is stuck to the venous wall and cannot be engaged by the snare. In this situation, a guidewire is inserted through the distal lumen of the catheter. The snare is looped around the wire and then advanced up and over the catheter. The stripping maneuver reestablishes flow in most cases.

Venous thrombosis (either partial or complete) can cause disabling arm or head and neck symptoms and occasionally interferes with vascular access function (Fig. 16-16).[79,80] Up to two thirds of patients with an underlying malignancy

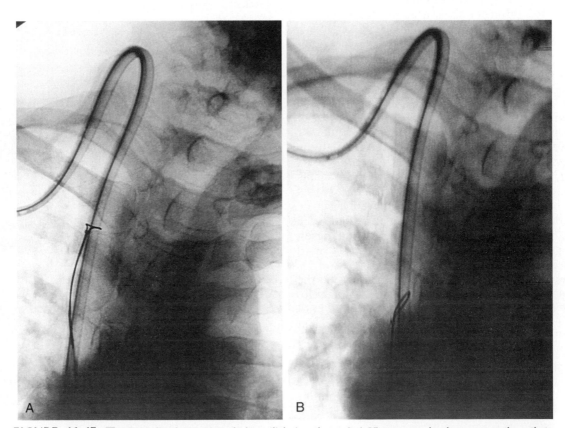

FIGURE 16-15 ■ Fibrin sheath stripping of a hemodialysis catheter. **A,** A 25-mm snare has been run up the catheter shaft and cinched around the catheter. **B,** The fibrin sheath is stripped off the catheter by withdrawing the snare device and guiding catheter at the groin.

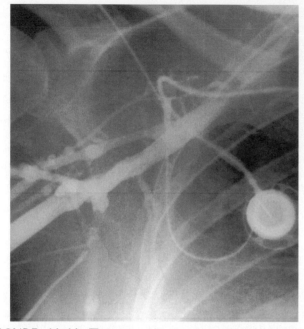

FIGURE 16-16 ■ Right subclavian vein thrombosis from an indwelling vascular access de]vice.

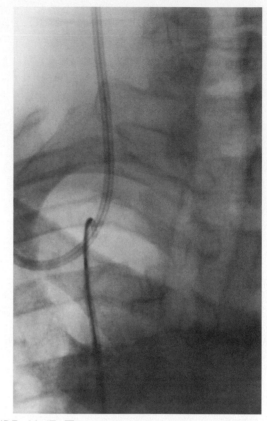

FIGURE 16-17 ■ Repositioning of a central venous catheter. The catheter had spontaneously migrated from the superior vena cava to the right internal jugular vein. A pigtail catheter and tip-deflecting wire were used to engage the catheter and pull it back into the vena cava.

develop venous thrombosis from CVCs.[81] The diagnosis is made by duplex sonography or contrast venography from a peripheral arm vein. For symptomatic central venous thrombosis, the initial treatment is anticoagulation. Catheter-directed thrombolysis is used for severe or persistent symptoms despite anticoagulation. If symptoms fail to improve within several days or there is evidence for septic thrombophlebitis, the device should be removed. Thrombotic complications from CVCs may be reduced by maintaining patients on daily low-dose warfarin (1 mg).[82,83]

Catheter migration can occur despite correct initial positioning. The catheter tip may end up in a variety of sites, most often the brachiocephalic, internal jugular, or azygous vein.[84] Rarely, the catheter tip erodes through the vein wall and becomes extravascular.[85] This scenario occurs most often when the tip of a left-sided catheter abuts the right lateral wall of the SVC. Catheters that are placed or migrate into the low right atrium may have inadequate flow or produce dysrhythmias. Malpositioned catheters are detected by poor function or as an incidental finding on chest radiography. The catheter should not be used until an intravascular location is confirmed.

Catheters can be repositioned in several ways.[86-88] If the catheter tip has migrated into the internal jugular vein, a guidewire is inserted into one lumen and advanced until the catheter buckles into the SVC. Alternatively, a pigtail catheter (with or without a tip-deflecting wire) inserted in the femoral vein is used to engage the shaft and pull the catheter back into the right atrium (Fig. 16-17). A snare is inserted from the femoral vein, placed around the free end of the catheter, cinched down, and pulled centrally. If these efforts fail, the catheter must be exchanged for a new one.

For catheter malposition with ports, the internal jugular or common femoral vein is accessed. From this position, the catheter can be repositioned (Fig. 16-18). If the port

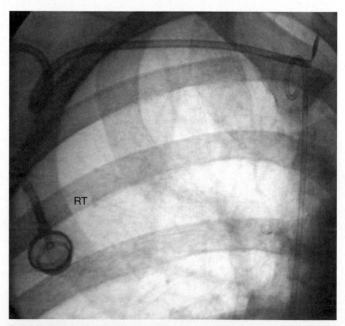

FIGURE 16-18 ■ A right chest port catheter has withdrawn since placement. A pigtail catheter has been introduced through the right common femoral vein to engage the catheter tip, free it from the vein wall, and allow a gooseneck snare to engage the tip and pull it back into the right atrium.

catheter is too long, it is snared and withdrawn through a sheath at the access site. A short segment of the catheter is cut off, and the catheter end is then reinserted and positioned properly.

If the catheter falls out, it should be replaced immediately if the tract is mature by probing the subcutaneous tunnel with a guidewire or catheter.[89] Kits are available to repair the external portion of damaged or fractured catheters.

■ FOREIGN BODY RETRIEVAL

Sources

A wide variety of objects can become lodged in the vascular system, including catheter and guidewire fragments, coils, stents, balloon fragments, IVC filters, and bullets.[90] The ultimate destination of a foreign body depends on its shape, size, and stiffness and on the hemodynamics of the local circulation. In some cases, catheter fracture (e.g., from pinch-off syndrome) is detected days to weeks after the event (see Fig. 16-7). Guidewires may become entrapped within IVC filters, usually during blind central venous catheter insertion. Potential complications of intravascular foreign bodies include dysrhythmias, clot formation and embolization, sepsis, and vascular or heart perforation with ensuing hemorrhage or cardiac tamponade. For this reason, these objects should be removed unless they are well incorporated into the vascular wall. Most intravascular foreign bodies can be retrieved by endovascular means.

Technique

Several devices are available for transcatheter retrieval, including vascular retrieval forceps and baskets (Cook Inc., Bloomington, Ind.). However, the most popular and versatile device is the Amplatz nitinol gooseneck snare (Microvena, White Bear Lake, Minn.) (see Fig. 16-14).[91,92] The catheter is available in a wide range of loop diameters (5 to 35 mm). Larger snares (25 to 35 mm) are used for retrieval in the SVC and right atrium. An 8- to 10-French (or larger) vascular sheath is inserted in the common femoral or internal jugular vein. Ideally, the sheath should be large enough to accommodate the collapsed foreign body and snare so as to minimize trauma to the access vein as the object is removed.

A guiding catheter is advanced through the sheath up to the foreign body, and the snare is inserted and opened. The snare is manipulated around a free end (or loop) of the fragment (Fig. 16-19). Often, both ends of the fragment abut the vein wall. In this case, the midsection of the fragment is engaged with a pigtail catheter and tip-deflecting wire (Fig. 16-20). The pigtail is withdrawn at the access site to reposition the fragment and free one of the ends. After the fragment is snared (preferably near the tip), the snare is cinched around it tightly by withdrawing the snare wire while holding the guiding catheter stationary. The object then is pulled through the IVC or SVC into the sheath and out of the vein. Larger foreign bodies (e.g., IVC filters, stents) may require more complex techniques for removal (Fig. 16-21).[92-94] In some instances, the device must be withdrawn into the external iliac or

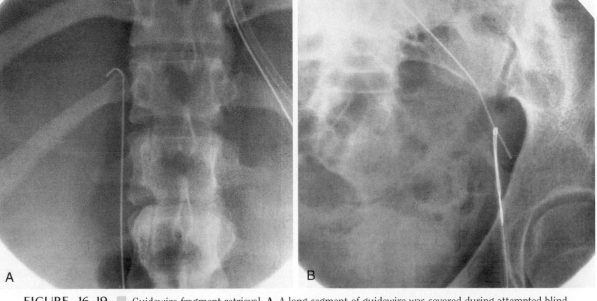

FIGURE 16-19 ■ Guidewire fragment retrieval. **A,** A long segment of guidewire was severed during attempted blind placement of a central venous access device. The wire became lodged in the inferior vena cava. **B,** A nitinol gooseneck snare was inserted from the left femoral vein and used to grab the free end of the guidewire.   *Continued*

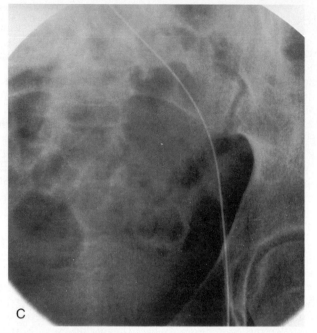

FIGURE 16-19 *Cont'd* ▪ **C,** The guidewire and snare are removed through a femoral vein sheath.

common femoral vein and removed through a simple surgical cutdown.

There are several ways to approach guidewires that have become trapped within IVC filters.[95,96] If the guidewire is still exiting the skin, a sheath may be placed over the wire and advanced into the IVC (Fig. 16-22). Gentle pressure may allow the wire to become dislodged from the catheter, which is then snared and removed. Otherwise, a loop snare is introduced from the femoral vein to capture the end of the wire and dislodge it from the filter.

Results and Complications

Percutaneous foreign body retrieval is successful in greater than 95% of attempts.[90,91] Even large devices such as intravascular stents and IVC filters can be removed safely (see Fig. 16-21). Cardiac dysrhythmias may develop during snare manipulation in the heart. Although percutaneous removal of catheter and guidewire fragments generally is quite safe, removal of large objects with sharp edges poses greater risk. In some cases, surgical removal is preferable.

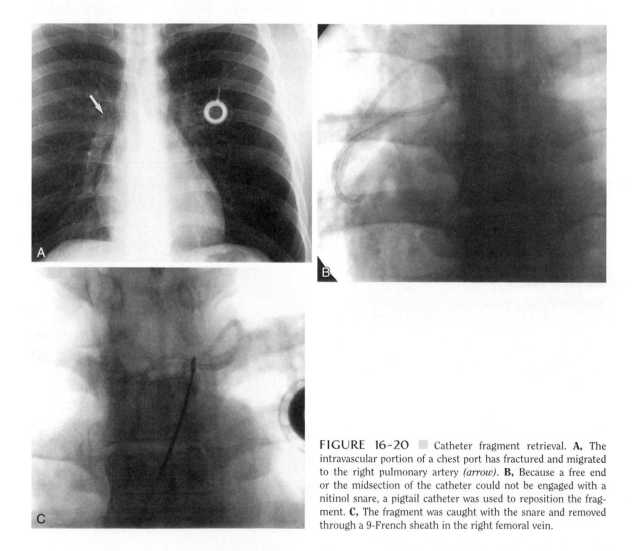

FIGURE 16-20 ▪ Catheter fragment retrieval. **A,** The intravascular portion of a chest port has fractured and migrated to the right pulmonary artery *(arrow)*. **B,** Because a free end or the midsection of the catheter could not be engaged with a nitinol snare, a pigtail catheter was used to reposition the fragment. **C,** The fragment was caught with the snare and removed through a 9-French sheath in the right femoral vein.

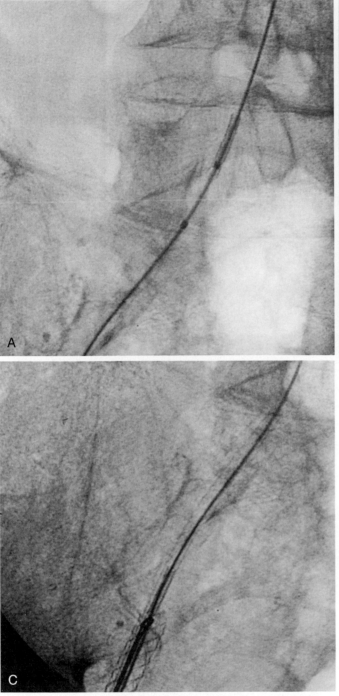

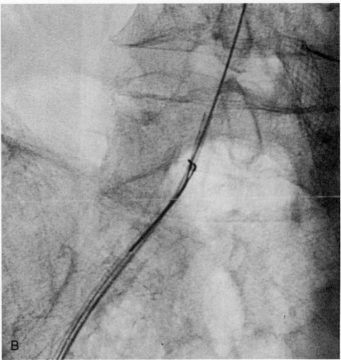

FIGURE 16-21 ▪ Retrieval of a Palmaz stent. **A,** Stent has slipped off an angioplasty balloon during renal artery treatment. **B,** A nitinol snare was placed around the lower end of the collapsed stent after the angioplasty balloon was removed. **C,** The stent was pulled into an 8-French sheath and removed.

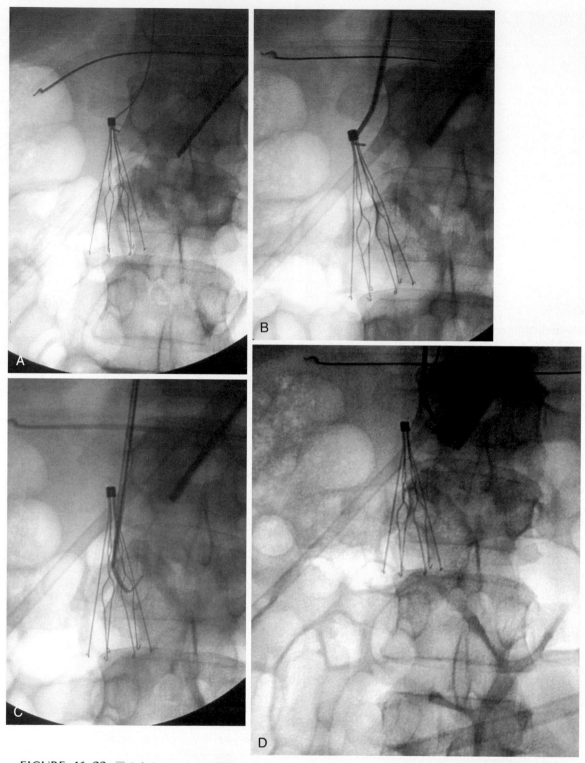

FIGURE 16-22 ■ Inferior vena cava (IVC) guidewire entrapment. **A,** During bedside placement of a central venous line, the house officer felt resistance upon guidewire withdrawal from the subclavian vein. Image shows guidewire trapped in the legs of a Greenfield filter. **B,** A 5-French catheter was advanced over the wire into the IVC. **C,** A long vascular sheath was introduced over the catheter for stability. **D,** After advancing the entire system from the filter neck, the guidewire was dislodged and ultimately removed.

REFERENCES

1. Mauro MA, Jaques PF: Insertion of long-term hemodialysis catheters by interventional radiologists: the trend continues. Radiology 1996; 198:316.
2. Reeves AR, Seshadri R, Trerotola SO: Recent trends in central venous catheter placement: a comparison of interventional radiology with other specialties. J Vasc Interv Radiol 2001;12:1211.
3. McBride KD, Fisher R, Warnock N, et al: A comparative analysis of radiological and surgical placement of central venous catheters. Cardiovasc Intervent Radiol 1997;20:17.
4. Nosher JL, Shami MM, Siegel RL, et al: Tunneled central venous access catheter placement in the pediatric population: comparison of radiologic and surgical results. Radiology 1994;192:265.
5. Foley MJ: Radiologic placement of long-term central venous peripheral access system ports (PAS port): results in 150 patients. J Vasc Interv Radiol 1995;6:255.
6. Maki DG, Cobb L, Garman JK, et al: An attachable silver-impregnated cuff for prevention of infection with central venous catheters: a prospective randomized multicenter trial. Am J Med 1988;85:307.
7. Trerotola SO, Johnson MS, Shah H, et al: Tunneled hemodialysis catheters: use of a silver-coated catheter for prevention of infection— a randomized study. Radiology 1998;207:491.
8. Pasquale MD, Campbell JM, Magnant CM: Groshong versus Hickman catheters. Surg Gynecol Obstet 1992;174:408.
9. Biffi R, De Braud F, Orsi F, et al: A randomized, prospective trial of central venous ports connected to standard open-ended or Groshong catheters in adult oncology patients. Cancer 2001;92:1204.
10. Jean G, Chazot C, Vanel T, et al: Central venous catheters for haemodialysis: looking for optimal blood flow. Nephrol Dial Transplant 1997; 12:1689.
11. Prabhu PN, Kerns SR, Sabatelli FW, et al: Long-term performance and complications of the Tesio twin catheter system for hemodialysis access. Am J Kidney Dis 1997;30:213.
12. Trerotola SO, Kraus M, Shah H, et al: Randomized comparison of split tip versus step tip high-flow hemodialysis catheters. Kidney Int 2002; 62:282.
13. Richard HM 3rd, Hastings GS, Boyd-Kranis RL, et al: A randomized, prospective evaluation of the Tesio, Ash split, and Opti-flow hemodialysis catheters. J Vasc Interv Radiol 2001;12:431.
14. Senecal L, Saint-Sauveur E, Leblanc M: Blood flow and recirculation rates in tunneled hemodialysis catheters. ASAIO J 2004;50:94.
15. Ross MN, Haase GM, Poole MA, et al: Comparison of a totally implanted reservoir with external catheters as venous access devices in pediatric oncologic patients. Surg Gynecol Obstet 1988;167:141.
16. Keung Y-K, Watkins K, Chen S-C, et al: Comparative study of infectious complications of different types of chronic central venous access devices. Cancer 1994;73:2832.
17. Mueller BU, Skelton J, Callender DPE, et al: A prospective randomized trial comparing the infectious and noninfectious complications of an externalized catheter versus a subcutaneously implanted device in cancer patients. J Clin Oncol 1992;10:1943.
18. Schwab SJ, Weiss MA, Rushton F, et al: Multicenter clinical trial results with the LifeSite hemodialysis access system. Kidney Int 2002;62:1026.
19. Rayan SS, Terramani TT, Weiss VJ, et al: The LifeSite Hemodialysis Access System in patients with limited access. J Vasc Surg 2003;38:714.
20. Wilkin TD, Kraus MA, Lane KA, et al: Internal jugular vein thrombosis associated with hemodialysis catheters. Radiology 2003;228:697.
21. Trerotola SO, Kuhn-Fulton J, Johnson MS, et al: Tunneled infusion catheters: increased incidence of symptomatic venous thrombosis after subclavian versus internal jugular venous access. Radiology 2000; 217:89.
22. Schillinger F, Schillinger D, Montagnac R, et al: Post catheterisation vein stenosis in haemodialysis: comparative angiographic study of 50 subclavian and 50 internal jugular accesses. Nephrol Dial Transplant 1991;6:722.
23. Lowell JA, Bothe A Jr: Central venous catheter-related thrombosis. Surg Oncol Clin North Am 1995;4:479.
24. Funaki B, Zaleski GX, Leef JA, et al: Radiologic placement of tunneled hemodialysis catheters in occluded neck, chest, or small thyrocervical collateral veins in central venous occlusion. Radiology 2001;218:471.
25. Kaufman JA, Kazanjian SA, Rivitz SM, et al: Long-term central venous catheterization in patients with limited access. AJR Am J Roentgenol 1996;167:1327.
26. Contreras G, Liu PY, Elzinga L, et al: A multicenter, prospective randomized comparative evaluation of dual- versus triple-lumen catheters for hemodialysis and apheresis in 485 patients. Am J Kidney Dis 2003;42:315.
27. Smith TP, Ryan JM, Reddan DN: Transhepatic catheter access for hemodialysis. Radiology 2004;232:246.
28. Lund GB, Lieberman RP, Haire WD, et al: Translumbar inferior vena cava catheters for long-term venous access. Radiology 1990;174:31.
29. Mauro MA, Jaques PF: Radiologic placement of long-term central venous catheters: a review. J Vasc Interv Radiol 1993;4:127.
30. Denny DF Jr: Placement and management of long-term central venous access catheters and ports. AJR Am J Roentgenol 1993;161:385.
31. Ryan JM, Ryan BM, Smith TP: Antibiotic prophylaxis in interventional radiology. J Vasc Interv Radiol 2004;15:547.
32. Lewis CA, Allen TE, Burke DR, et al: Quality improvement guidelines for central venous access. J Vasc Interv Radiol 1997;8:475.
33. Gordon AC, Saliken JC, Johns D, et al: US-guided puncture of the internal jugular vein: complications and anatomic considerations. J Vasc Interv Radiol 1998;9:333.
34. Hinke DH, Zandt-Stastny DA, Goodman LR, et al: Pinch-off syndrome: a complication of implantable subclavian venous access devices. Radiology 1990;177:353.
35. Punt CJ, Strijk S, van der Hoeven JJ, et al: Spontaneous fracture of implanted central venous catheters in cancer patients: report of two cases and retrospective analysis of the "pinch-off sign" as a risk factor. Anticancer Drugs 1995;6:594.
36. Zaleski GX, Funaki B, Lorenz JM, et al: Experience with tunneled femoral hemodialysis catheters. AJR Am J Roentgenol 1999;172:493.
37. Markowitz DG, Rosenblum DI, Newman JS, et al: Translumbar inferior vena caval Tesio catheter for hemodialysis. J Vasc Interv Radiol 1998; 9:145.
38. Elduayen B, Martinez-Cuesta A, Vivas I, et al: Central venous catheter placement in the inferior vena cava via the direct translumbar approach. Eur Radiol 2000;10:450.
39. Stavropoulos SW, Pan JJ, Clark TWI, et al: Percutaneous transhepatic venous access for hemodialysis. J Vasc Interv Radiol 2003;14:1187.
40. Murthy R, Arbabzadeh M, Lund G, et al: Percutaneous transrenal hemodialysis catheter insertion. J Vasc Interv Radiol 2002;13:1043.
41. Nazarian GK, Bjarnason H, Dietz CA Jr, et al: Changes in tunneled catheter tip position when a patient is upright. J Vasc Interv Radiol 1997;8:437.
42. Schutz JC, Patel AA, Clark TW, et al: Relationship between chest port catheter tip position and port malfunction after interventional radiologic placement. J Vasc Interv Radiol 2004;15:581.
43. Kowalski CM, Kaufman JA, Rivitz SM, et al: Migration of central venous catheters: implications for initial catheter tip positioning. J Vasc Interv Radiol 1997;8:443.
44. Vesely TM: Central venous catheter tip position: a continuing controversy. J Vasc Interv Radiol 2003;14:527.
45. Forauer AR, Alonzo M: Change in peripherally inserted central catheter tip position with abduction and adduction of the upper extremity. J Vasc Interv Radiol 2000;11:1315.
46. Robertson LJ, Mauro MA, Jaques PF: Radiologic placement of Hickman catheters. Radiology 1989;170:1007.
47. Hull JE, Hunter CS, Luiken GA: The Groshong catheter: initial experience and early results of imaging-guided placement. Radiology 1992;185:803.
48. Cimochowski GE, Worley E, Rutherford WE, et al: Superiority of the internal jugular over the subclavian access for temporary hemodialysis. Nephron 1990;54:154.
49. Trerotola SO, Johnson MS, Harris VJ, et al: Outcome of tunneled hemodialysis catheters placed via the right internal jugular vein by interventional radiologists. Radiology 1997;203:489.
50. Silberzweig JE, Mitty HA: Central venous access: low internal jugular vein approach using imaging guidance. AJR Am J Roentgenol 1998; 170:1617.
51. Lorenz JM, Funaki B, Van Ha T, et al: Radiologic placement of implantable chest ports in pediatric patients. AJR Am J Roentgenol 2001;176:991.
52. Simpson KR, Hovsepian DM, Picus D: Interventional radiologic placement of chest wall ports: results and complications in 161 consecutive placements. J Vasc Interv Radiol 1997;8:189.
53. Morris SL, Jaques PF, Mauro MA: Radiology-assisted placement of implantable subcutaneous infusion ports for long-term venous access. Radiology 1992;184:149.

54. Funaki B, Szymski GX, Hackworth CA, et al: Radiologic placement of subcutaneous infusion chest ports for long-term central venous access. AJR Am J Roentgenol 1997;169:1431.

55. Hills JR, Cardella JF, Cardella K, et al: Experience with 100 consecutive central venous access arm ports placed by interventional radiologists. J Vasc Interv Radiol 1997;8:983.

56. Shetty PC, Mody MK, Kastan DJ, et al: Outcome of 350 implanted chest ports placed by interventional radiologists. J Vasc Interv Radiol 1997; 8:991.

57. Andrews JC, Marx MV, Williams DM, et al: The upper arm approach for placement of peripherally inserted central catheters for protracted venous access. AJR Am J Roentgenol 1992;158:427.

58. Crowley JJ, Pereira JK, Harris LS, et al: Peripherally inserted central catheters: experience in 523 children. Radiology 1997;204:617.

59. Dubois J, Garel L, Tapiero B, et al: Peripherally inserted central catheters in infants and children. Radiology 1997;204:622.

60. Cardella JF, Cardella K, Bacci N, et al: Cumulative experience with 1,273 peripherally inserted central catheters at a single institution. J Vasc Interv Radiol 1996;7:5.

61. Polak JF, Anderson D, Hagspiel K, et al: Peripherally inserted central venous catheters: factors affecting patient satisfaction. AJR Am J Roentgenol 1998;170:1609.

62. Neuman ML, Murphy BD, Rosen MP: Bedside placement of peripherally inserted central catheters: a cost-effectiveness analysis. Radiology 1998;206:423.

63. Kohli MD, Trerotola SO, Namyslowski J, et al: Outcome of polyester cuff retention following traction removal of tunneled central venous catheters. Radiology 2001;219:651.

64. Tseng M, Sadler D, Wong J, et al: Radiologic placement of central venous catheters: rates of success and immediate complications in 3412 cases. Can Assoc Radiol J 2001;52:379.

65. Damascelli B, Patelli G, Frigerio LF, et al: Placement of long-term central venous catheters in outpatients: study of 134 patients over 24,596 catheter days. AJR Am J Roentgenol 1997;168:1235.

66. Vesely TM: Air embolism during insertion of central venous catheters. J Vasc Interv Radiol 2001;12:1291.

67. Spies JB, Berlin L: Complications of central venous catheter placement. AJR Am J Roentgenol 1997;169:339.

68. Hall K, Farr B: Diagnosis and management of long-term central venous catheter infections. J Vasc Interv Radiol 2004;15:327.

69. Capdevila JA, Segarra A, Planes AM, et al: Successful treatment of haemodialysis catheter-related sepsis without catheter removal. Nephrol Dial Transplant 1993;8:231.

70. Shaffer D: Catheter-related sepsis complicating long-term, tunneled central venous dialysis catheters: management by guidewire exchange. Am J Kidney Dis 1995;25:593.

71. Haskal ZJ, Leen VH, Thomas-Hawkins C, et al: Transvenous removal of fibrin sheaths from tunneled hemodialysis catheters. J Vasc Interv Radiol 1996;7:513.

72. Knelson MH, Hudson ER, Suhocki PV, et al: Functional restoration of occluded central venous catheters: new interventional techniques. J Vasc Interv Radiol 1995;6:623.

73. Angle JF, Shilling AT, Schenk WG, et al: Utility of percutaneous intervention in the management of tunneled hemodialysis catheters. Cardiovasc Intervent Radiol 2003;26:9.

74. Semba CP, Deitcher SR, Li X, et al: Treatment of occluded central venous catheters with alteplase: results in 1,064 patients. J Vasc Interv Radiol 2002;13:1199.

75. Merport M, Murphy TP, Egglin TK, et al: Fibrin sheath stripping versus catheter exchange for the treatment of failed tunneled hemodialysis catheters: randomized clinical trial. J Vasc Interv Radiol 2000;11:1115.

76. Duszak R Jr, Haskal ZJ, Thomas-Hawkins C, et al: Replacement of failing tunneled hemodialysis catheters through pre-existing subcutaneous tunnels: a comparison of catheter function and infection rates for de novo placements and over-the-wire exchanges. J Vasc Interv Radiol 1998;9:321.

77. Gray RJ, Levitin A, Buck D, et al: Percutaneous fibrin sheath stripping versus transcatheter urokinase infusion for malfunctioning well-positioned tunneled central venous dialysis catheters: a prospective, randomized trial. J Vasc Interv Radiol 2000;11:1121.

78. Savader SJ, Haikal LC, Ehrman KO, et al: Hemodialysis catheter-associated fibrin sheaths: treatment with a low-dose rt-PA infusion. J Vasc Interv Radiol 2000;11:1131.

79. Allen AW, Megargell JL, Brown DB, et al: Venous thrombosis associated with the placement of peripherally inserted central catheters. J Vasc Interv Radiol 2000;11:1309.

80. Kuriakose P, Colon-Otero G, Paz-Fumagalli R: Risk of deep venous thrombosis associated with chest versus arm central venous subcutaneous port catheters: a 5-year single-institution retrospective study. J Vasc Interv Radiol 2002;13:179.

81. DeCicco M, Matovic M, Balestreri L, et al: Central venous thrombosis: an early and frequent complication in cancer patients bearing long-term Silastic catheter: a prospective study. Thromb Res 1997;86:101.

82. Bern MM, Lokich JJ, Wallach SR, et al: Very low doses of warfarin can prevent thrombosis in central venous catheters. A randomized prospective trial. Ann Intern Med 1990;112:423.

83. Klerk CP, Smorenburg SM, Buller HR: Thrombosis prophylaxis in patient populations with a central venous catheter: a systematic review. Arch Intern Med 2003;163:1913.

84. Krutchen AE, Bjarnason H, Stackhouse DJ, et al: The mechanisms of positional dysfunction of subclavian venous catheters. Radiology 1996;200:159.

85. Duntley P, Siever J, Korwes ML, et al: Vascular erosion by central venous catheters: clinical features and outcome. Chest 1992;101:1633.

86. Hartnell GG, Gates J, Suojanen JN, et al: Transfemoral repositioning of malpositioned central venous catheters. Cardiovasc Intervent Radiol 1996;19:329.

87. Bessoud B, de Baere T, Kuoch V, et al: Experience at a single institution with endovascular treatment of mechanical complications caused by implanted central venous access devices in pediatric and adult patients. AJR Am J Roentgenol 2003;180:527.

88. Stockx L, Raat H, Donck J, et al: Repositioning and leaving in situ the central venous catheter during percutaneous treatment of associated superior vena cava syndrome: a report of eight cases. Cardiovasc Intervent Radiol 1999;22:224.

89. Egglin TKP, Rosenblatt M, Dickey KW, et al: Replacement of accidentally removed tunneled venous catheters through existing subcutaneous tracts. J Vasc Interv Radiol 1997;8:197.

90. Egglin TK, Dickey KW, Rosenblatt M, Pollak JS: Retrieval of intravascular foreign bodies: experience in 32 cases. AJR Am J Roentgenol 1995;164:1259.

91. Cerkirge S, Weiss JP, Foster RG, et al: Percutaneous retrieval of foreign bodies: experience with the nitinol goose neck snare. J Vasc Interv Radiol 1993;4:805.

92. Gabelmann A, Kramer S, Gorich J: Percutaneous retrieval of lost or misplaced intravascular objects. AJR Am J Roentgenol 2001; 176:1509.

93. Saeed M, Knowles HJ Jr, Brems JJ, et al: Percutaneous retrieval of a large Palmaz stent from the pulmonary artery. J Vasc Interv Radiol 1993;4:811.

94. Bochenek KM, Aruny JE, Tal MG: Right atrial migration and percutaneous retrieval of a Guenther Tulip inferior vena cava filter. J Vasc Interv Radiol 2003;14:1207.

95. Loehr SP, Hamilton C, Dyer R: Retrieval of entrapped guide wire in an IVC filter facilitated with use of a myocardial biopsy forceps and snare device. J Vasc Interv Radiol 2001;12:1116.

96. Duong MH, Jensen WA, Kirsch CM, et al: An unusual complication during central venous catheter placement. J Clin Anesth 2001;13:131.

17

Hemodialysis Access

Anne C. Roberts, MD

ACCESS CONSTRUCTION

The ideal hemodialysis access is an endogenous fistula created by surgical anastomosis of an artery and vein. The Dialysis Outcomes Quality Initiative (DOQI) clinical practice guidelines have set a goal of primary arteriovenous fistula being constructed in at least 50% of all new kidney failure patients, with ultimately 40% of hemodialysis patients having a native fistula.[1] The Brescia-Cimino fistula is a side-to-side anastomosis of the radial artery and the cephalic vein at the wrist (Fig. 17-1); it is the first choice for a permanent access.[1] A native fistula also can be constructed between the brachial artery and the cephalic vein. This brachiocephalic fistula is the second choice for a fistula.[1] This type of access may be more likely to result in arm swelling or distal ischemia than with other approaches. Less common fistulas include connections between the brachial artery and basilic vein (brachiobasilic fistula), a brachial artery to median antecubital vein (brachiomedian antecubital fistula), and between the femoral artery and saphenous vein.[2] If a fistula can be created and is functional, it can be expected to have excellent patency and a low rate of complications.[1] Although this is the ideal access, it may be difficult or impossible to create in a significant number of patients.

The fistula must be established early enough to be functional at the time the patient needs to be dialyzed. The fistula ideally should be allowed to mature for 3 to 4 months.[1,3] The veins in the arm must not have been damaged by previous venipunctures. For the fistula to become functional, the veins must mature properly, become large enough, and have sufficient blood flow to allow dialysis to take place. These constraints are such that failure rates from 10% to 65% have been reported, although most authors suggest that 15% to 20% is a usual figure.[4,5] Failures are common particularly in elderly and diabetic patients, which are considered high-risk groups, but with careful evaluation even these high-risk patients may be able to get successful fistulas.[5] If an endogenous fistula can be constructed and matures properly, it should have excellent long-term patency.

A synthetic graft is the alternative to an endogenous fistula. These grafts are commonly made of polytetrafluoroethylene (PTFE). They may be placed in the forearm in a straight configuration from the radial artery to a brachial vein, but a looped configuration from the brachial artery to a brachial vein (Fig. 17-2) usually is preferred.[1] Grafts also may be constructed in the upper arm, usually in a looped configuration from the brachial or axillary artery to a high brachial vein. If all possible sites in the arm and chest are exhausted, a loop graft can be placed in the thigh from the common femoral artery to the common femoral vein.

PTFE grafts may be used much earlier than native fistulas, usually within 14 days of placement.[1] However, they do not have the longevity that can be achieved with an endogenous fistula. Primary patency rate at 1 year is reported to be approximately 40%.[4,6] Secondary patency rate ranges from 60% to 90%.[1,7] The most common reason for failure is development of a stenosis in the outflow vein, leading to thrombosis of the graft.[1]

It is crucial to extend the functional life of each access for as long as possible, because the sites available for dialysis

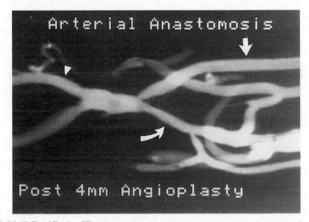

FIGURE 17-1 ■ Hemodialysis access. Endogenous radiocephalic arteriovenous fistula. Note the inflow radial artery *(upper right arrow)*, efferent radial artery *(arrowhead)*, and outflow cephalic vein *(curved arrow)*.

463

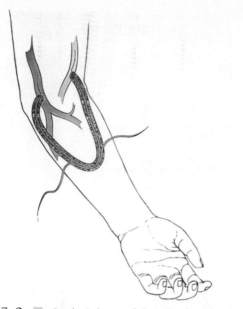

FIGURE 17-2 ■ Synthetic loop graft from the distal brachial artery to the cephalic vein. Crossed catheters are in place for pulse-spray thrombolysis. (From Valji K: Pharmacomechanical thrombolysis of thrombosed hemodialysis access grafts. Semin Dialysis 1998;11:374.)

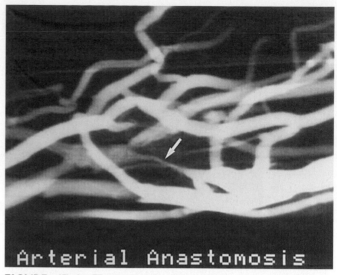

FIGURE 17-3 ■ Arteriovenous shunt stenosis. Narrowing occurs just beyond the arteriovenous anastomosis *(arrow)*. Note the extensive filling of collateral veins caused by obstruction of the main venous outflow. After balloon angioplasty, the anastomosis is patent, and collateral flow has diminished (see Fig. 17-1).

fistulas are limited and patients are dependent on dialysis for survival.

■ MAJOR DISORDERS

Failing Dialysis Grafts

Etiology

Veins that are subjected to the high flows, high pressures, and turbulence created by an arteriovenous fistula are prone to develop stenoses from neointimal hyperplasia. Intimal hyperplasia may be a response to turbulent blood flow, vibratory effects from the placement of the graft,[8] compliance mismatch between the graft material and the vein,[9] or angulation and stretching of the vein.[10] Regardless of the cause, the venous stenoses progressively worsen until blood flow is markedly reduced and thrombosis occurs. These venous outflow lesions usually recur (again and again) at the same site.

Endogenous arteriovenous fistulas may have decreased inflow because of a stenosis of the vein just beyond the arteriovenous anastomosis. They also may have venous outflow stenoses that produce large collateral veins, arm swelling, high venous pressures, and low flows in the dialysis circuit (Fig. 17-3).

Surveillance and Imaging

The National Kidney Foundation-DOQI (NKF-DOQI) document recommends an organized monitoring program to identify grafts in jeopardy of thrombosis by regular assessment of several clinical and functional dialysis parameters.[1] Monitoring may include intra-access flow,[11-13] static venous

dialysis pressure, and dynamic venous pressure.[1,3,14] Other studies that are used to detect arteriovenous graft stenosis include measurement of access recirculation,[15] decreases in the measured amount of hemodialysis delivered, or elevated negative arterial pre-pump pressures that prevent increasing to acceptable blood flow.[1,16,17] Normal flow in a graft should be in excess of 800 to 1000 mL/minute, and if flows decrease to less than 400 to 600 mL/minute, risk of failure is increased. Clinical indicators include changes in the physical characteristics of the graft thrill, difficulty with needle placement, prolonged bleeding after needle removal, swelling of the arm, or, ultimately, clotting of the graft.[1,18-20]

Persistent abnormalities in any of these parameters suggest graft dysfunction and should prompt venographic evaluation of the graft. Venography can be performed easily after dialysis through the indwelling needles or can be performed at a separate session, usually prior to dialysis. If a stenosis is discovered at the time of the venogram, angioplasty can be performed immediately. Early correction of venous stenoses reduces thrombosis rates. In a number of studies, a 50% to 90% decrease in the thrombosis rate can occur when monitoring is instituted (Table 17-1)[21,22] and prolongs access viability (Table 17-2).[1,3,12,23,24]

Surveillance for arteriovenous fistulas depends on many of the same methods as those used for grafts. Physical examination is very helpful and is even more informative than

TABLE 17-1

Study	No. of Patients	Reduction in Thrombosis
Schwab[21]	168	1.45 → 0.15 pt/yr
Besarab[112]	107	0.58 → 0.19 pt/yr
Roberts[113]	121	1.0 → 0.5 pt/yr
Safa[54]	57	48% → 17%/yr
Martin[114]	21	0.44 → 0.10 pt/yr

TABLE 17-2

Study	No. of Patients	Increased Graft Survival
Schwab[21]	168	26 → 7% replace pt/yr
Besarab[112]	107	2.0 → 3.0 yr
Roberts[113]	121	6.3 → 15.8 mo
Lumsden[115]	64	47% → 51% at 1 yr

with grafts. Ultrasound can be used both preoperatively to increase the rate of successful fistula placements[25] and to evaluate fistula maturation.[26] The other measures of graft function, recirculation, increased static venous pressures, decreased flow rates, are also evidence of fistula malfunction, but the thresholds for abnormality are not worked out as well in fistulas as they are for grafts. There are multiple outflow collaterals in the majority of arteriovenous fistulas, not just the main draining vein. As a result of the low resistance and presence of the collateral veins, a venous stenosis causes a reduction in blood flow, but without the corresponding increase in access pressure.[27]

Treatment

Percutaneous Therapy

Patient Selection. Disagreement continues regarding the relative benefits of surgical revision and balloon angioplasty for patients with failing dialysis grafts. One study reported a 36% patency rate at 6 months and a 25% patency rate at 12 months for a group of patients treated operatively, compared with 11% and 9% patency rates at 6 and 12 months, respectively, in a group treated percutaneously.[28] However, another study found comparable patency rates—17% and 28% at 6 months, for surgery and angioplasty, respectively.[29] An additional study showed approximately the same primary patency rate at 12 months, and assisted primary patency rate, but showed a higher expense for percutaneous therapy.[30] The NKF-DOQI advises that each dialysis center determine which procedure is best for an individual patient based on local expertise. Surgical revision is held to a higher standard than percutaneous transluminal angioplasty, because surgical revision usually extends the access further up the extremity by the use of a jump graft.[1] More vein is used in surgical revision than in percutaneous transluminal angioplasty.

Balloon angioplasty for venous and other graft-related stenoses has been popular for many years. Although angioplasty is plagued with the same problems with recurrent stenosis as surgery therapy, it does have some advantages. Patients accept percutaneous balloon angioplasty better than they do a surgical procedure. The angioplasty procedure avoids using a site further up the venous outflow, leaving it available for subsequent revision when it becomes necessary. The graft is immediately available for dialysis, avoiding the need for temporary dialysis catheters. Redilations allow easy and safe graft salvage for months or years.[18]

In arteriovenous fistulas, failure of maturation is the most common problem. This may be manifest by a fistula that has not developed a major venous outflow and instead has multiple outflow veins, none of which is large enough to

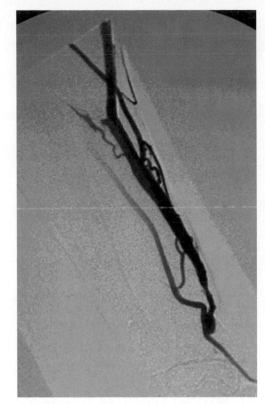

FIGURE 17-4 ■ Arteriovenous fistula with a stenosis at the arterial anastomosis. Fistula is not functional for dialysis.

support dialysis. In other cases, the fistula may have developed but may have decreased flow and the fistula may appear flat, which indicates an arterial/anastomotic inflow problem (Fig. 17-4). If the vein is dilated in one area but then becomes flat further up the arm, an outflow problem is indicated. With palpation, it may be possible to delineate the area of stenosis, either by the change in caliber of the vein or the change in the quality of the pulse/thrill. Dialysis grafts tend to have a majority of the stenoses at the venous anastomosis, but arteriovenous fistulas more commonly have multiple, tandem stenoses in various aspects of the outflow. Ultrasound may be very helpful in evaluating the fistulas and identifying the source of the problem. There is even less enthusiasm for surgically revising poorly functioning fistulas, and angioplasty usually is the first therapy attempted.

Technique

Dialysis graft/fistula venography always should include a complete evaluation from the inflow artery to the superior vena cava. There are several critical areas where problems can be expected to occur.

Venous anastomotic stenoses are the most common reason for malfunction of dialysis grafts. They usually occur in the vein within a few centimeters of the graft-vein anastomosis (Fig. 17-5). At times, multiple venous channels may overlap and conceal important stenosis. Several oblique views may be required to visualize the narrowing. After the stenosis is found, it is dilated with an appropriately sized angioplasty balloon catheter. In the forearm hand near the elbow, a 6-mm balloon typically is used initially. On occasion, veins may

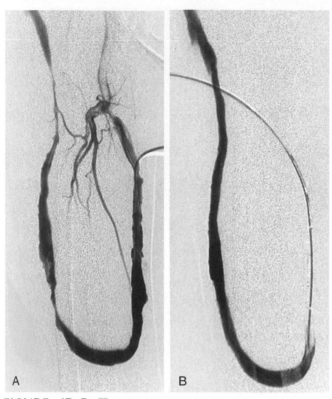

FIGURE 17-5 ▪ Venous anastomotic and intragraft stenoses. **A,** Initial fistulogram through a catheter placed in the arterial limb of the graft shows both lesions responsible for elevated venous pressures at dialysis. **B,** After angioplasty with a 7-mm balloon, the stenoses are relieved.

require 5- to 8-mm balloons. High-pressure balloons (burst pressures 20 to 30 mm Hg) often are required to dilate these lesions. Multiple, prolonged inflations (e.g., 5 minutes) are thought to be useful in resistant lesions.

If the stenosis does not respond to the initial dilation, repeated inflations may be required to open the vessel. Cutting balloons have been used for extremely resistant stenoses (Fig. 17-6).[31-36] Inflation of the cutting balloon is done across the stenosis, and then balloon angioplasty is repeated. The cutting balloon, which has small blades imbedded in the balloon, presumably weakens the wall, allowing the angioplasty to succeed. In other cases, the balloon may completely inflate, but the stenosis remains following the inflation (elastic lesion). However, in some cases, this represents underdilation of the lesion. If the patient has no pain with the angioplasty, the balloon may not have been large enough to dilate the stenosis. In this situation, using a larger balloon achieves a better result. Of course, if the patient has experienced significant pain with the initial angioplasty, balloon size should not be increased. In these cases, cutting balloons have been used to try to correct the elastic recoil.

Stent placement has been used for venous stenoses, but the use of stents should be very selective. Some indications for stents include vein rupture (probably the best indication), elastic recoil, and restenosis (Fig. 17-7). Stents may improve the immediate results of angioplasty, but their long-term benefit often is less favorable. Intimal hyperplasia commonly develops within the stent as well as at the ends of the stent. The stenosis that develops requires treatment with further

balloon angioplasty and, occasionally, further stenting. Veins that could be used for a new graft or venous anastomosis should not be stented because it limits potential revision. Areas of bending, such as at the elbow joint, usually are not stented because of increased strain on the stent. The DOQI guidelines indicate that stents generally should be reserved for surgically inaccessible stenoses that fail angioplasty, because the unassisted patency of the stents in hemodialysis access is no better than that of angioplasty, with the exception of truly elastic lesions.[1]

Stents are used also to salvage vein rupture after balloon angioplasty (Fig. 17-8). The reported primary patency rates in this setting are 52% at 60 days, 26% at 6 months, and 11% at 1 year.[37] There are now reports of patients being treated with covered stents.[38-40] The stent grafts that are available presently are approved by the U.S. Food and Drug Administration (FDA) for tracheal/bronchial applications, but they are used "off label" in the vascular system. The usual indication is rupture of the vein following angioplasty,[40,41] but covered stents also have been used to treat pseudoaneurysms in experimental models[39] and in patients with aging, degenerating grafts.[38,42,43] It is unclear what the long-term success of covered stents will be in the patient with dialysis, and in most cases uncovered stents can salvage a case of vein rupture without resorting to a covered stent.

Evaluation of fistulas requires a different technique than evaluation of grafts. Fistulas may have problems with lack of maturation or with developing dysfunction. It is important to evaluate the fistula in its entirety; it may be difficult to perform this by directly accessing the fistula. A variety of techniques can be used to help with a difficult access. A tourniquet can be used to impede outflow and increase the size of the draining veins. Ultrasound can be used to better identify the largest draining vein and guide access. For a forearm fistula, the brachial artery can be punctured at the elbow with a micropuncture needle and the smaller (3 French) inner dilator of the micropuncture set placed in the artery. Angiography/fistulography then can be performed. This also allows evaluation of the palmar arch and antegrade or retrograde filling of the distal segment of the artery feeding the fistula.[41] After the diagnostic study has been performed, the fistula can be cannulated by a retrograde approach. If this is unsuccessful, the antegrade cannulation of the brachial artery and selective catheterization of the feeding artery can be performed.[41] Turmel-Rodrigues believes that venous stenoses must be dilated to at least 5 mm in order to obtain adequate flows.[41] However, in a poorly developed fistula, it may be important to perform serial dilations, starting with small balloons (3 to 4 mm) in order to avoid rupturing a small, undilated vein. If the vein is not well developed, dilation with a small balloon during one procedure and a repeat evaluation in 1 to 3 weeks with dilation using a larger balloon may allow for development of the venous outflow and maturation of the fistula.

Arterial stenoses have been reported as being responsible for graft problems in up to 28% of cases,[44] although others feel the incidence is less than 15%.[45,46] Construction of the dialysis access creates a low-resistance/high-flow circuit that may unmask a significant arterial inflow stenosis.[44,47] The inflow artery and arterial anastomosis are visualized by direct injection at this site, manually compressing the mid-portion of the graft during injection, or inflating a balloon

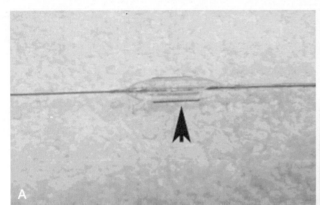

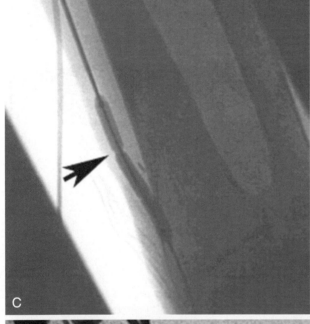

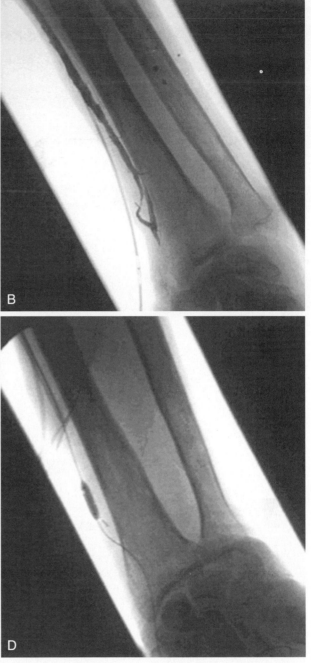

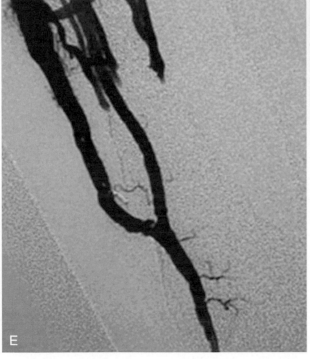

FIGURE 17-6   **A,** Cutting balloon has small blades incorporated into the wall of the balloon that may help treat resistant lesions. **B** and **C,** Venous stenosis, resistant to balloon dilation. The arrow in C demonstrates resistant stenosis. **D** and **E,** Cutting balloon in place in the lesion. The lesion can now be dilated. **E,** Post angioplasty result.

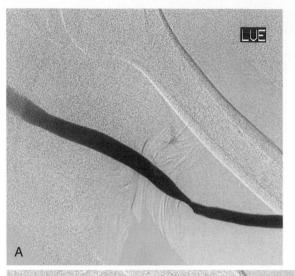

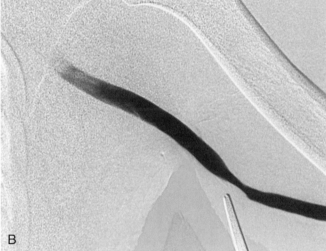

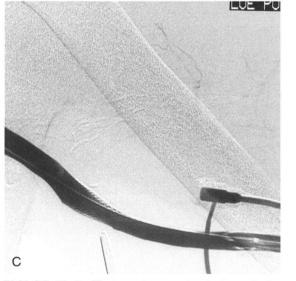

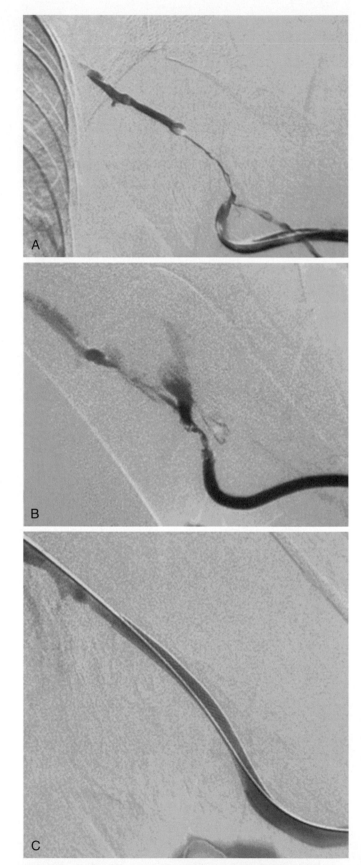

FIGURE 17-7   ■   Stent placement for elastic recoil of a venous out-flow stenosis. **A,** Stenosis in the left basilic vein just beyond the venous anastomosis. The overlying surgical drape was not responsible for the narrowing. **B,** Although a 7-mm balloon inflated fully, the lesion has significant elastic recoil. **C,** After placement of a Wallstent, the stenosis is relieved.

FIGURE 17-8   ■   **A,** Marked venous stenosis in dialysis graft outflow. The stenosis is long and very tight. **B,** Following balloon dilation, rupture of vein has occurred with extravasation of contrast. **C,** Rupture treated with uncovered stent placement.

catheter with the end hole directed toward the anastomosis. Several projections may be required to adequately delineate the arterial inflow. If a significant arterial stenosis is identified, angioplasty usually is indicated. The lesion often can be accessed through the graft. Otherwise, a direct brachial (or common femoral) arterial puncture is necessary. In some cases the arterial lesion is in the inflow vessels, so arteriography should be considered during the evaluation of a dysfunctional access, particularly if the patient has recurring graft dysfunction without an evident cause.[44,48] Measuring of the flow during percutaneous procedures may lead to increased detection of arterial stenoses.[44]

Intragraft stenoses are relatively uncommon. These stenoses usually respond well to angioplasty (see Fig. 17-5). Balloon sizing in the graft should take into account that these grafts are most commonly 6 mm in diameter. Occasionally the grafts also are tapered (4 to 6 mm or 4 to 7 mm). In most cases a balloon that is 1 mm larger than the graft diameter is an appropriate size. If there is graft

degeneration, it is particularly important that a larger balloon not be used because the graft can be ruptured.

Central venous stenoses are an important, although less frequent, problem with hemodialysis grafts. Stenosis of the subclavian and innominate veins usually is caused by venous injury from prior dialysis catheters. The importance of these obstructions is their potential to compromise future dialysis access sites and to cause significant arm swelling. If the lesion is not causing symptoms, it should be left alone. It is uncommon for central stenoses to cause graft thrombosis. If a patient has a thrombosed graft, the most likely culprit is a stenosis at the venous anastomosis. Unless the outflow is thrombosed up to the level of the central vein, the central venous stenosis probably is not responsible for thrombosis. Outflow stenoses should be treated with angioplasty only if they are considered to be responsible for graft dysfunction (Fig. 17-9). Near the shoulder and in the central veins, 10- to 12-mm balloons (or larger) may be necessary. Unfortunately, the results of stent placement are not

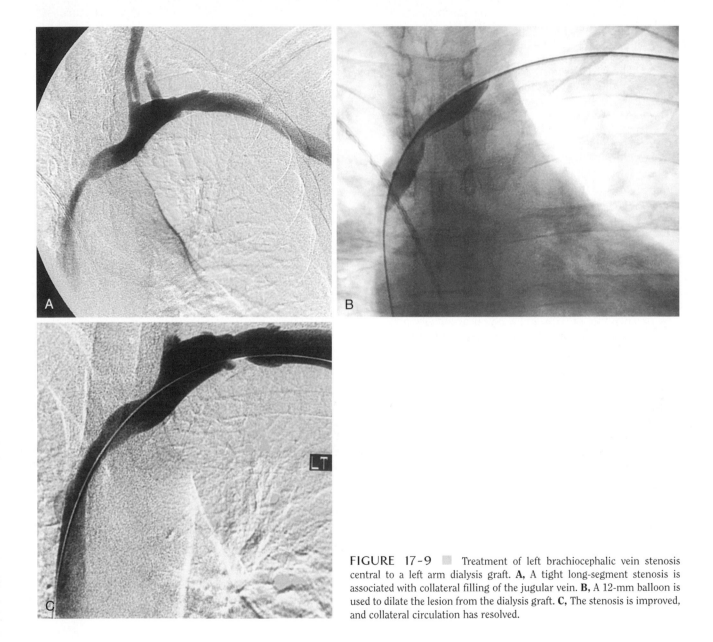

FIGURE 17-9 ■ Treatment of left brachiocephalic vein stenosis central to a left arm dialysis graft. **A,** A tight long-segment stenosis is associated with collateral filling of the jugular vein. **B,** A 12-mm balloon is used to dilate the lesion from the dialysis graft. **C,** The stenosis is improved, and collateral circulation has resolved.

markedly better than those of balloon angioplasty. The DOQI guidelines recommend transluminal angioplasty as the preferred treatment for central vein stenosis, and stent placement is indicated only with elastic lesions, when stenosis recurs within 3 months, or with occluded vessels.[1,49] The stent needs to be carefully oversized to avoid migration.[50-53] The primary problem with stenting is intimal hyperplasia, which causes recurrent stent stenosis. Stents should not be placed across the internal jugular or contralateral innominate veins, which may be needed for future dialysis catheters.

Results

In one study, 106 grafts suspected of having a venous stenosis on clinical examination were evaluated.[54] Grafts were studied angiographically, and any venous stenosis was treated with balloon angioplasty. The technical success for angioplasty was 98%. The primary patency rates at 6 months and 1 year were 43% and 23% for PTFE grafts, respectively. Repeated angioplasty enabled a primary assisted patency of 68% at 1 year and 51% at 2 years. The secondary patency rate (allowing for intercurrent thrombolysis and angioplasty) was 82% at 1 year and 65% at 2 years. Although these patency rates seem low, they are comparable to results of operative treatment. The DOQI recommendations are that the cumulative patency rate of all dialysis arteriovenous grafts should be at least 70% at 1 year, 60% at 2 years, and 50% at 3 years. They indicate also that the angioplasty primary unassisted patency (time from one intervention to the next or loss of the graft) should be 50% at 6 months.[1]

It is not quite as clear what the results should be for arteriovenous fistulas. One study of dysfunctional fistulas had a primary, assisted primary, and secondary patency rates in 53 dysfunctional fistulas after intervention at 3 months of 84% ± 5%, 88% ± 5%, and 90% ± 4%, respectively. At 6 months, the patency rates were 55% ± 8%, 80% ± 6%, and 82% ± 6%. At 12 months the rates were 26% ± 11%, 80% ± 6%, and 82% ± 6%.[55] Turmel-Rodrigues reported a primary patency rate of 39% and a secondary patency rate of 79% at 12 months in dysfunctional forearm fistulas,[41] and a rate of 57% in patients with upper arm fistulas.[56] Others have reported a 1-year secondary patency rate of 64% and a 2-year secondary patency rate of 53%, with fewer procedures to keep the fistulas functioning in comparison with grafts (Fig. 17-10).[4]

For stents placed in the central veins (20 patients), primary patency rates of 90% at 1 month, 67% at 3 months, 42% at 6 months, and 25% at 1 year have been reported. Assisted primary patency (additional angioplasty, stenting, or both) were 88% at 3 months, 62% at 6 months, and 47% at 1 year in that series.[57] Another study (22 patients) with a mix of stents showed primary patency rates after 3, 6, 9, and 12 months of 82%, 73%, 56%, and 43%, respectively. The primary assisted patency rates at the same time periods was 91%, 90%, 88%, and 83%, respectively.[58]

Complications

Fortunately, complications resulting from recanalization of venous outflow or arterial inflow lesions are quite rare. Minor complications such as bleeding, hematoma, and contrast reactions are similar to those of any angiographic procedure. Occasionally, damage to the veins may occur,

including rupture. Ruptures appear to be somewhat more common in autologous fistulas. One series reported a 1.8% complication rate in grafts and a 4.1% complication rate in fistulas, with 70% of the complication being some degree of rupture.[59] The significance of the vein rupture is variable depending on the extent of the rupture. Because the angioplasty balloon should already be in place, the balloon can be placed across the rupture to seal the leak. If prolonged balloon inflation does not seal the rupture, a stent or covered stent can be used.[41] Small ruptures may be clinically insignificant while large ruptures may cause a large, rapidly expanding hematoma. Smaller, more stable ruptures may be stented. Large ruptures need to be treated either with placement of a covered stent or with occlusion of the graft. If stenting (with or without a covering) is not an option, control of the rupture should be maintained by simply compressing the graft until clotting occurs. Because grafts are superficial, they are easily compressed. If this should happen, the patient may require a new graft, which is what would have been required if no percutaneous therapy was available. The complication of vascular rupture should occur only in 2% to 4% of cases, and perforation requiring blood transfusion, emergent surgery, or limb-threatening ischemia should occur in less than 0.5% of cases.[49]

Surgical Therapy

Several surgical options are available for obstructions that fail to respond to percutaneous interventions, including revision with patch grafting,[29] a jump graft with extension of the graft further up along the venous outflows,[28,60] or complete graft replacement. Revision is preferred over a new graft when feasible. Replacement has the disadvantage of exhausting access sites much more rapidly. The 1-year primary patency rate after surgical revision is as low as 25%, with secondary patency rate reported at 60% to 70%.[28,61] Most grafts require multiple additional procedures to maintain patency. Long-segment stenoses have significantly worse patency rates than do focal ones.

Thrombosed Dialysis Grafts

Etiology

In most cases, graft thrombosis occurs because of progressive stenosis in the graft circuit (usually at the venous end). Avoiding this ultimate outcome, caused by stenosis, is the reason for carefully monitoring patient's flow rates and venous pressures. It is much easier and less expensive to correct a venous stenosis than to have to declot the graft/fistula and then correct the venous stenosis that caused the thrombosis. Occasionally, graft may clot because of hypotension, graft infection, trauma, or a hypercoagulable state.

Imaging and Treatment

Percutaneous Therapy

Unique characteristics of dialysis grafts make them particularly amenable to percutaneous therapy. They are easy to

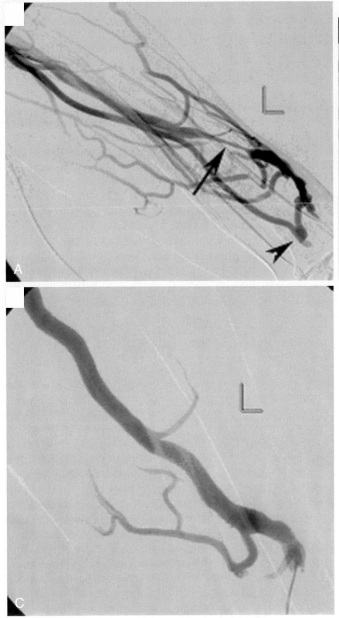

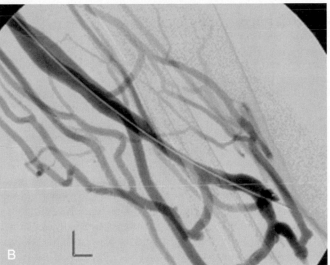

FIGURE 17-10 ■ **A,** Poorly developed fistula, which cannot be used for dialysis. Arterial anastomosis *(arrowhead)* and stenosis within the major outflow vein *(arrow)* are shown. Note the multiple collateral veins that are filling. **B,** Fistula immediately following 4-mm balloon angioplasty. Appearance is improved. **C,** Same fistula 18 months later. The vein has developed well, and the fistula is being used for dialysis.

access because of their superficial location, they contain fresh clot (usually not more than 48 to 72 hours old), and they are a closed system with only a single inflow and (usually) outflow. The percutaneous approach to the dialysis graft allows thrombolytic (either pharmacologic or mechanical) therapy and allows angiographic evaluation of all aspects of the graft. The proximal arterial inflow, graft body, and the entire venous outflow can be evaluated. Abnormalities usually can be treated percutaneously, and the complete therapy takes place in a single session.

Patient Selection. Virtually all patients with clotted dialysis grafts are candidates for percutaneous therapy. The criteria for rejecting patients for pharmacologic graft thrombolysis are similar to those for other thrombolysis procedures. If pharmacologic therapy is not appropriate,

mechanical thrombolysis can be used. Absolute contraindications to pharmacologic therapy include any cerebrovascular process/disease/procedure (tumor, recent stoke, trauma, surgery) within 2 months, or active gastrointestinal bleeding. Relative contraindications include major surgery or organ biopsy within 2 weeks, recent serious trauma, preexisting uncorrectable coagulation defects, uncontrolled severe hypertension, and pregnancy or postpartum period. Dialysis graft infection is an important contraindication to any type of thrombolysis. Lysis of infected clot can precipitate bacteremia and lethal sepsis. Determining if a graft is infected can be difficult.[62] Classic signs of infection (i.e., redness, tenderness, warmth, swelling, and fever) may be subtle or absent in patients with chronic renal failure. Definite signs of infection, such as a purulent discharge or skin breakdown over the graft, are rare. Needle aspirates of graft clot or fluid collections around the graft can be sent for Gram stain and culture.[63] Infection of the graft requires treatment with antibiotics and referral for surgical removal.

Small pulmonary emboli are produced during most percutaneous dialysis grafts declotting procedures.[64-66] Although most patients tolerate these emboli, patients with significant pulmonary hypertension or severe underlying lung disease may not. A known right-to-left cardiac shunt (which could result in embolic stroke) is a strict contraindication to any type of lysis procedure.

Grafts that fail within days to several weeks of placement usually have a technical problem responsible for thrombosis. Although the graft may not be salvageable with percutaneous therapy, thrombolysis or simple contrast injection of the venous anastomosis and outflow veins may help guide surgical revision. Although some risk of hemorrhage from the anastomoses exists, manual compression usually controls such bleeding.

Pharmacologic Thrombolysis. There are several methods for administering thrombolytic agents into dialysis grafts. One of the techniques described relatively early in experience of treating dialysis grafts with thrombolysis is pulse-spray pharmacomechanical thrombolysis (PSPMT). Although perhaps supplanted by more recently described thrombolytic approaches, PSPMT remains a good technique, particularly for operators who are just gaining experience in grafts thrombolysis. If for some reason one of the other thrombolytic approaches does not work, this technique can be used to salvage the situation. Many of the principles important to dialysis graft thrombolysis are well demonstrated with this system, making it an appropriate technique to describe before going on to describe other techniques. Dialysis graft thrombolysis also is an excellent system in which to gain experience that can then be used for cases of arterial thrombolysis.

Several catheter systems are suitable for PSPMT, including infusion catheters (Cook, Inc., Bloomington, Ind.) and side-slit catheters (Angiodynamics, Inc., Glen Falls, NY). These catheters have multiple side holes or slits over lengths of 4 to 30 cm. A tip-occluding wire is used to obstruct the catheter endhole. All of the devices allow a high-pressure fluid spray to be delivered into the substance of the clot. Injections are made through a hemostatic valve (Touhy-Borst or Y adapter), which goes over the wire.

To lyse the entire clot and treat the arterial and venous ends of the grafts, a crossed catheter technique is used (Fig. 17-11).[45,67,68] A single-wall, 18-gauge needle or micropuncture needle (Cook, Inc., Bloomington, Ind.) is used to access the graft. The first puncture is made toward the venous anastomosis. Puncturing the graft sometimes is difficult because of scar tissue from repeated dialysis needle puncture. It is helpful to hold the graft firmly between the thumb and fingers of one hand while puncturing the graft with the needle held in the other hand. When the needle passes through the graft material, usually there is a "popping" sensation or loss of resistance, although if scar has developed, this sensation may be diminished. There usually is little or no blood return when a thrombosed graft is entered. When the needle is in the graft, a guidewire normally passes easily. Occasionally, the guidewire seems to pass relatively smoothly even though it is not intraluminal. If the patient

complains of pain with the guidewire passage or the wire fails to go around a bend in a loop graft or past a joint space, the guidewire probably is extraluminal. Fluoroscopy and "feel" are very important for determining that the wire is within the graft. It is tempting to inject contrast to determine if the graft has been entered. This temptation should be resisted. It is often not helpful. By the time enough contrast is injected to demonstrate that the needle is not within the graft, the soft tissues become full of contrast, obscuring the graft for the remainder of the procedure.

The needle is removed and a 5-French dilator is placed over the guidewire. The guidewire is then advanced beyond the venous anastomosis and into the venous outflow. An angled Glidewire (Terumo, Inc., Boston Scientific, Watertown, Mass.) may be useful to overcome difficulty in traversing the anastomosis. If the guidewire and catheter cannot be manipulated into the venous outflow, the procedure should be terminated. Attempting thrombolysis in the face of an impassable venous obstruction leads to bleeding when inflow is reestablished. In this situation, the patient is referred for thrombectomy and surgical revision of the venous anastomosis.

A small amount of contrast is injected through the catheter, and the catheter is withdrawn until the venous end of the thrombus is identified. The length of the thrombosed segment, from the venous end of the clot to the entrance site into the graft, is determined. A pulse-spray catheter with appropriate length of side holes is placed into the graft.

The arterial end of the graft is approached in a similar manner. The needle is placed into the graft a short distance away from the venous end of the graft and directed toward the arterial end. A pulse-spray catheter is positioned with the end hole just beyond the arterial anastomosis. It is important to manipulate guidewires and catheters gently at the arterial end of the graft. Forceful, vigorous motion of the wire or injection of contrast may dislodge clot into the feeding artery.

When the catheters are in place, the end holes are occluded with tip-occluding wires, and a Y adapter is fitted on the catheter. The thrombolytic solution is divided equally between two syringes, which are attached to one of the side ports of a one-way valve system connected to the Y adapter. A tuberculin (TB) syringe is connected to the other side port. The TB syringe is filled with 1 mL of the thrombolytic solution and infused to fill the catheter. The pulse-spray procedure then begins. The TB syringe is filled with 0.2 to 0.3 mL of thrombolytic solution, which is forcefully injected into the catheter. The forceful injection allows the homogenous and simultaneous distribution of concentrated thrombolytic agent throughout the entire length of the occluded graft. This enhances the diffusion of the thrombolytic agent into the clot and produces some mechanical disruption of the clot matrix, increasing the surface area exposed to the thrombolytic agent.[69]

The entire dose of thrombolytic solution is given over approximately 10 minutes (approximately two to four pulses/minute). If the length of clot being treated is longer than the length of side holes, the catheter is repositioned to treat the remainder of the clot when approximately one half of the thrombolytic solution has been delivered. One mL of saline is then pulsed through the catheters in 0.2-mL aliquots to clear the remaining thrombolytic solution.

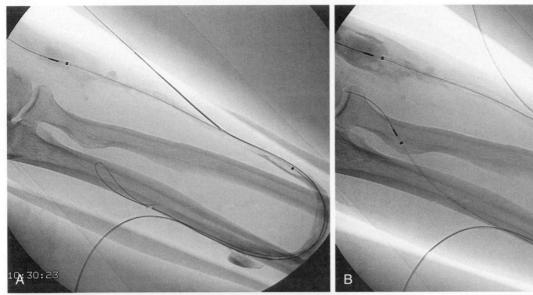

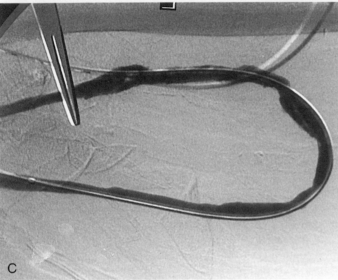

FIGURE 17-11 ▪ Crossed catheter technique is used for pulse-spray pharmacomechanical thrombolysis of a forearm loop dialysis graft. **A,** The pulse-spray catheter is already in place across the venous limb of a graft. A guidewire has been inserted through a single-wall needle that is directed toward the arterial anastomosis. **B,** Both pulse-spray catheters are in place. **C,** Graft is free of clot after treatment with thrombolytic.

A relatively gentle injection of contrast can be made through the arterial catheter with the tip-occluding wire removed to assess the degree of clot lysis. The graft may have only a weak pulse despite near complete lysis because of resistant clot at the arterial anastomosis. One dose of thrombolytic solution is sufficient to treat most hemodialysis grafts. Small to moderate volumes of residual clot do not require further thrombolytic therapy. Large amounts of residual clot may indicate incomplete treatment of the entire clot, insufficient heparinization, or infected thrombus resistant to thrombolytic agents. An activated clotting time can be obtained to evaluate the anticoagulation status. Occasionally, loop grafts with great clot volumes require additional thrombolytic solution.

Contrast injection through the venous catheter, which has been withdrawn below the anastomosis, demonstrates a stenosis in about 90% of cases. The venous stenosis is treated with balloon angioplasty to provide graft outflow before graft inflow is addressed. Improving the outflow prior

to improving the inflow helps to prevent bleeding from catheter entry sites.

In many cases, a lysis-resistant clot remains at the arterial anastomosis (Fig. 17-12). This arterial "plug" is probably composed of densely packed layers of platelets and fibrin.[70,71] Because these plugs are relatively resistant to thrombolysis, further thrombolytic treatment is of little value. Mechanical dislodgement and maceration of the plug is much more effective. Thrombectomy is performed using compliant balloons that can exert force and traction on the plug as it is pulled out of the arterial anastomosis. These balloons include an 8.5-mm occlusion balloon catheter (Boston Scientific, Watertown, Mass.) or an over-the-wire Fogarty balloon catheter (Baxter, Irvine, Calif.). Maceration with a dilation balloon at the arterial anastomosis is avoided because of the risk of arterial embolization or injury. A guidewire is carefully positioned beyond the plug in the inflow artery (Fig. 17-13). The occlusion balloon is then placed over the wire and situated beyond the plug in the

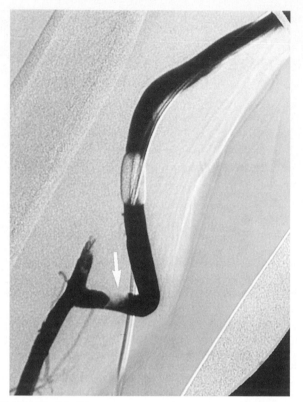

FIGURE 17-12 ■ Lysis-resistant "plug" on the graft side of the arterial anastomosis *(arrow)*. Contrast has been injected into the proximal graft and feeding radial artery after inflating the occlusion balloon.

inflow artery (see Fig. 17-13). The balloon is inflated gently with dilute contrast material until it conforms to the artery and is then pulled back into the graft. It is important to avoid overinflation of the balloon in the native artery. If the balloon is overexpanded, the balloon may rupture or damage to the artery may result. Three to four passes may be necessary to completely remove the clot. When the plug is displaced from the anastomosis, it may become trapped in the graft, usually at the site where the catheters enter the graft. In this situation, an angioplasty balloon is used to fragment the clot, because there is no longer any risk of arterial embolization. Any other residual clot in the graft also is macerated with an angioplasty balloon.

After the flow has been established, the entire graft circuit from the arterial inflow to the superior vena cava is studied with venography for other obstructions. If the patient is going to dialysis immediately, 7-French dialysis sheaths (Hemo-caths, Angiodynamics, Glens Falls, NY; Check-Flo Performer, Cook, Inc., Bloomington, Ind.) are placed. Otherwise, an activated clotting time is obtained to assess the patient's anticoagulation status before removing the catheters. After hemostasis is obtained, the patient can be discharged home or to the dialysis unit.

A popular alternative method for thrombolysis is the "lyse and wait" technique or a variation known as "lyse and go." The "lysis and wait" technique was described by Cynamon[72,73] as an injection of thrombolytic agent through a standard intravenous angiocatheter inserted within the venous limb of the graft. The graft is manually compressed at the arterial and venous anastomoses while the thrombolytic mixture

is infused over 1 minute into the graft. This portion of the procedure could be performed in a holding area outside the interventional radiology suite. After at least 30 minutes, the patient is transferred to the interventional radiology suite, and the declotting procedure is continued with venography, angioplasty of the venous stenosis, and mobilization of the arterial plug as described for the pulse-spray technique. Introducing the thrombolytic mixture into the graft before bringing the patient into the interventional radiology suite resulted in the declotting portion of the procedure, requiring little or no room time and avoiding the expense of an infusion catheter.[69] This technique has been described using urokinase in the initial papers, and then using tissue plasminogen activator (TPA) as the thrombolytic agent. The articles describe using 2 to 5 mg of TPA,[73-75] although now the usual dose would be 2 mg because the higher doses may increase hemorrhagic complications. The "lysis and go" variation is very similar, but the thrombolytic is injected when the patient is in the angiographic room, and the patient is prepped and draped and the procedure started without any waiting period.

Fibrinolytic Agents. The fibrinolytic agents are those described in Chapter 2. Urokinase (UK) was the primary fibrinolytic agent used for dialysis grafts until it was recalled by the FDA in 1999. It was reintroduced in the U.S. market, but the manufacturer has since decided to withdraw it from the United States. In countries where urokinase is available, a 250,000-unit vial is dissolved in 9 mL of sterile water. One mL of heparin (5000 units/mL) is added to the vial to give a concentration of 25,000 units of UK and 500 units of heparin per 1 mL of solution.

The most commonly used thrombolytic in the United States for dialysis grafts is TPA (alteplase, Genentech, San Francisco, Calif.).[74-76] The other modifications of TPA (rPA, reteplase and TNK, tenecteplase) also have been used in dialysis graft thrombolysis.[77,78] The dosage of TPA usually is 2 mg dissolved in 5 to 10 mL of normal saline. Although the manufacturer states that heparin should not be combined with TPA because of the concern for possible precipitation, many clinicians feel that the benefit of intrathrombic heparin is outweighed by the theoretical concern for precipitation, and 3000 to 5000 units of heparin can be combined with the TPA to make a final volume of 5 to 10 mL of thrombolytic solution.[74] If heparin is not given as an intrathrombic agent, it needs to be given intravenously. Reteplase usually is used in a dose of 1 to 3 units of RPA and 3000 to 5000 units of heparin, again diluted with normal saline to make a volume of 5 to 10 mL.[77]

Adjuvant medications can improve the results of thrombolysis. Animal and clinical studies support the value of intrathrombic heparin in speeding lysis.[79,80] If intrathrombic heparin is not administered, intravenous heparin should be given. Aspirin (325 mg PO) is given before the procedure to inhibit platelet activity, assuming that the patient has no contraindications to aspirin and is not taking aspirin. Soluble aspirin is rapidly absorbed in the stomach, with significant plasma concentrations in less than 30 minutes and a peak value at about 2 hours.[81] Enteric-coated aspirin requires hours for absorption, which may be incomplete. Other antiplatelet agents can be given, but they are expensive and it is not clear that they are any more effective than aspirin.

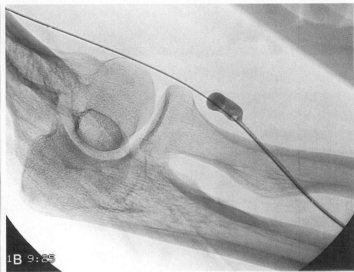

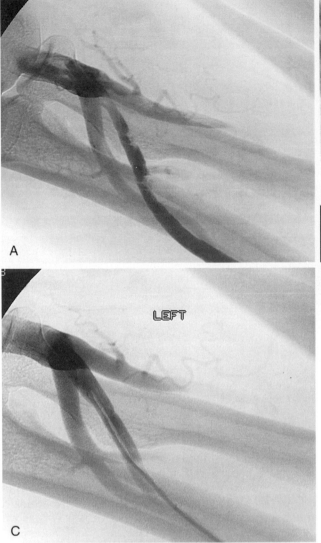

FIGURE 17-13 ▪ Treatment of arterial plug. **A,** Arterial end of the graft after pulse-spray thrombolysis shows residual clot. **B,** An occlusion balloon has been inflated in the inflow artery and then pulled into the graft to dislodge the thrombus. **C,** The arterial anastomosis is widely patent.

Mechanical Thrombectomy. There are now multiple mechanical thrombectomy devices that are available for treating dialysis grafts. The aim is to mechanically remove clot within dialysis grafts. The devices include the Amplatz Thrombectomy Device (ATD), also know as the Helix Clot Buster (Microvena, White Bear Lake, Minn.); the Angio-Jet (Possis Medical, Minneapolis, Minn.); and the Arrow-Trerotola Percutaneous Thrombectomy Device (PTD) (Arrow International, Reading, Pa.). The Cragg and Castaneda thrombolytic brushes (Microtherapeutics, San Clemente, Calif.), the Oasis catheter (Boston Scientific, Natick, Mass.), the X-Sizer (EV3, Plymouth, Minn.), the Hydrolyser (Cordis, Miami, Fla.), and other devices are available for treating dialysis grafts. Thrombectomy devices have a variety of methods for removal of clot. Some cause clot fragmentation by producing a vortex created by a high-speed rotating impeller or basket.[82] Others work by a Venturi effect, in which thrombus is sucked into the aperture of the device and macerated by high local shear forces. The fragments are removed through an exhaust lumen.[82] Whatever device is chosen, the operator should be familiar with the device and understand its capabilities, characteristics, and problems.

The approach to using these devices is similar to the approach for pulse-spray thrombolysis. The initial needle puncture is made into the arterial limb directed toward the venous end of the graft. An angiographic catheter is advanced through the venous anastomosis and a diagnostic venogram is performed to evaluate the graft and the venous outflow, including the central veins. Some operators do not open the venous stenosis until after performing the thrombectomy, whereas others angioplasty the venous end to allow outflow and to try to decrease the risk of increased pressure in the graft leading to arterial emboli.[83] After the venogram, the angiographic catheter is replaced with a sheath to provide access for the mechanical device. The device is then used as indicated in the graft. Contrast can be injected through the sheath to visualize the clot. After the clot is removed from the venous end, the venous stenosis is dilated. After the venous angioplasty, the venous end of the graft is punctured directed toward the arterial end. The thrombectomy device is then advanced to clear the clot at the arterial end. An occlusion balloon is placed to dislodge the arterial plug. Following this maneuver the graft is assessed with contrast to determine if the procedure

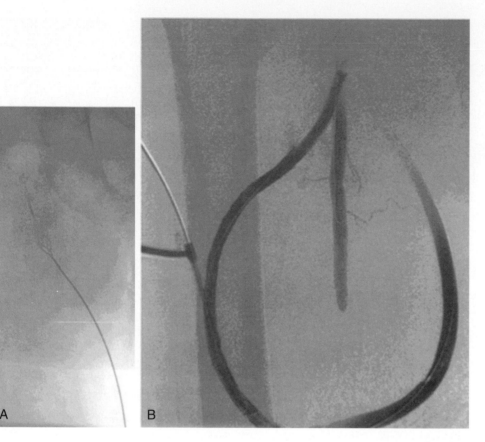

A
B

FIGURE 17-14   ■   **A,** Arrow-Trerotola device in a looped graft in thigh. **B,** Following activation of the device, the graft is largely free of clot.

is complete or if there are other areas that require therapy (Fig. 17-14).

There are some modifications of this basic technique. Some operators prefer to use a single approach using the apex of a loop graft as their access point, then directing the catheters/thrombectomy devices/balloons toward whichever part of the graft requires treatment. Other operators pull the arterial plug back into the graft early in the procedure, before treating the venous stenosis, so the plug can be fragmented by the mechanical device.[83]

Heparin and aspirin also are important adjuncts to these devices. Heparin (2000 to 5000 units) is commonly infused through the sheath prior to placement of the thrombectomy device.[83] If it is not given through the sheath, it should be given intravenously. It is very important to give aspirin since the use of devices in the clot, as well as the lysis of clot, leads to platelet aggregation and clot formation.

Arteriovenous Fistula Thrombosis. Arteriovenous (AV) fistula thrombosis is considered to be much more challenging than graft thrombosis. There is a commonly held perception that autogenous fistulas, when thrombosed, cannot be percutaneously salvaged.[84,85] Part of this reflects the relative infrequency of thrombosis in AV fistulas and, consequently, the lack of experience treating these thromboses. Although AV fistulas have more complicated anatomy making thrombolysis somewhat more complicated, they can be treated successfully and attempts should be made to restore flow to the fistula percutaneously.[84,86]

It is important to determine that the fistula is actually thrombosed, rather than have a stenosis that is causing poor

flow and subsequent flattening of the fistula. In many cases there may be only a very short segment of thrombus near the anastomosis or a small amount of thrombus within the outflow vein. If thrombosis is identified, pharmacological thrombolysis is very appropriate and may have less of a risk of damaging the venous endothelium.[87] Access into the fistula may be aided by using ultrasound guidance or placement of a tourniquet.[41] The fistulas may be approached using an antegrade or retrograde approach depending on the anatomy. Occasionally, as described above in the section on failing fistulas, a puncture in the brachial artery may be required to better demonstrate the anatomy. If an arterial puncture is required, the access should be kept as small as possible to avoid bleeding if thrombolytics are being used. As in grafts, pulse-spray and "lyse and wait" techniques have been used.[84] Thrombectomy devices also have been used for thrombosed AV fistulas.[88-90]

In some cases, direct thromboaspiration of the fistula may be successful.[41,90,91] This can be performed with 7- or 8-French, thin-walled aspiration catheters and a 20-mL syringe to provide the aspiration suction.[82,84]

Results. PSPMT is very effective for treatment of clotted dialysis grafts, with initial clinical success (i.e., ability to undergo at least one session of dialysis) of greater than 90%. The overall procedure time is usually less than 2 hours. The different mechanical thrombectomy devices seem to be relatively comparable in their reported success rates; they all remove clot, and differences may be more in operator experience.[83,92,93] The technical success results are comparable between devices and pharmacologic thrombolysis and the patency rates at 1 month, 3 months, and 6 months also are comparable.[75,92,94-96] The mechanical thrombectomy devices tend to be quite expensive, approximately $500 to $600 for the catheters, with some devices requiring very expensive drive pumps. Because the procedure still requires angioplasty balloons, occlusion balloons, and angiographic catheter(s), the expense of the devices has to be measured against the expense of the thrombolytic catheters and the thrombolytics. The thrombolytic catheters are relatively inexpensive ($100 to $150), and TPA in the doses used for dialysis grafts runs approximately $50 to $100 (costs, not charges).

Long-term primary patency of thrombosed dialysis grafts is relatively poor whether grafts are treated by PSPMT, mechanical devices, or surgical thrombectomy and revision. For enzymatic thrombolysis, the primary patency rate at 1 year is 11% to 26% and secondary patency rate at 1 year is 51% to 69%. Studies directly comparing surgical thrombectomy with thrombolysis and angioplasty demonstrate similar patency rates. However, reocclusion rates are similar following multiple declotting procedures, regardless of the technique used, so continual percutaneous managements should be undertaken to preserve each graft for as long as possible.[61] Even if grafts rethrombose early (within 1 month), aggressive retreatment of these grafts, commonly using a larger angioplasty balloon, or occasionally stent placement allowed salvage of the grafts without significantly decreased patency rates.[97]

Treatment of thromboses fistulas is quite good, with technical success rates for declotting of fistulas ranging from 75% to 100%. Primary patency rates are reported to be 36% to 70% and 18% to 60% at 3 and 6 months, respectively, with 60% to 80% assisted primary patency rates at 6 months.[84] Declotting of fistulas may involve multiple modalities such as thrombolytics, thromboaspiration, mechanical thrombectomy, balloon thrombectomy, and angioplasty.

Complications. Major and minor complications of thrombolysis for dialysis grafts occur in about 1% and 10% of cases, respectively.[49] Most of the complications involve perigraft bleeding, arterial embolization, and vein rupture from angioplasty.[98] The complication rates for most of the mechanical devices are similar. Bleeding from previous needle punctures is seen occasionally, particularly when the venous outflow stenosis is not treated before flow is reestablished. In this situation, pressure is applied to the bleeding site, and the venous outflow is opened expeditiously.

Embolization into the arterial system occurs in up to 10% of procedures.[49] Further thrombolysis of these emboli (which usually arise from the arterial plug) is often ineffective, and mechanical removal is required. After determining the location of the embolus, a wire is placed past the arterial anastomosis and past the embolus. An occlusion balloon catheter is placed from the graft into the artery beyond the clot, and the clot is pulled back into the graft. If the graft is patent, another technique known as the "back-bleeding" technique can be tried.[99] A balloon catheter is placed into the arterial inflow, just above the anastomosis, on the upstream side. The balloon is inflated, and the patient exercises the hand for about 1 minute. The balloon is deflated and an arteriogram is performed to evaluate the results. A successful procedure dislodges the embolus from its position in the artery below the anastomosis and moves it into the graft.[59]

Small pulmonary emboli are produced with all percutaneous declotting techniques.[64-66,100-102] Symptomatic pulmonary embolism is rare. However, fatal pulmonary embolism has been reported after mechanical thrombectomy in which the entire clot burden of a graft was delivered to the lungs.[100,103]

■ OTHER DISORDERS

Ischemia and Steal Syndrome

Dialysis fistulas/grafts create a low-resistance circuit between the arterial and venous systems. Most patients tolerate this physiology without difficulty, but some patients may develop distal ischemia. The incidence of ischemic complications ranges between 1% and 10%.[104-106] The most common cause is high resistance in the arterial bed beyond the arteriovenous anastomosis, with shunting of blood into the graft. A "steal" from the ulnar artery through the palmar arches causes reversed flow in the distal radial artery, shunting of blood away from the peripheral tissues, and resultant hand ischemia (Fig. 17-15). This situation is most common in patients with coexisting small vessel disease such as diabetes, vasculitis, or peripheral vascular disease.[106] In these patients even mild degrees of arterial flow reversal may result in a clinically significant steal. A second cause for distal ischemia is occlusive disease in the inflow arteries.[48] The combination of decreased inflow and shunting of blood through the graft leads to ischemic hand symptoms.

A patient with dialysis graft-related ischemia has a cool, pale extremity. Trophic changes of the skin and nails or muscle wasting may develop. The patient may complain of numbness, tingling, impairment of motor function, or pain on exertion of the hand. The symptoms often are worse during dialysis.[104] In more severe cases, numbness and pain progress, with diminished sensation, muscle and nerve paralysis, ischemic ulcers, and progressive dry gangrene of one or more affected digits.[104]

The diagnosis of ischemia can be made in several ways, including digital plethysmography, pulse oximetry, and segmental pressure measurements.[106] A significant drop in blood pressure along the extremity indicates an obstruction in the arterial circulation at this site. Pulse volume recordings documenting digital pressures less than 50 mm Hg and augmentation of the pulse wave with fistula compression are diagnostic of vascular steal.[104,106] Digital pulse oximetry also has proven useful in diagnosing vascular access-associated steal. Oxygen saturations are low, but they rise to normal levels when the fistula is compressed.[104] Angiography can be performed to identify proximal or distal arterial obstruction that may be responsible for ischemia.

Angioplasty may be performed for arterial stenoses proximal to the arteriovenous access. This may augment blood flow to the peripheral tissues with relief of pain and healing of ulcers.[48,106] Operative intervention may be required in patients with symptomatic vascular insufficiency. In forearm grafts, ligation of the radial artery immediately distal to the fistula abolishes the steal and may improve flow to the hand. Coil embolization of the radial artery distal to the graft

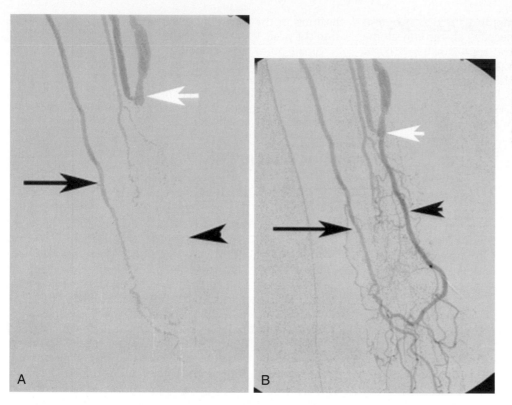

can be performed, which accomplishes the same function as surgical ligation.[105,107] Fistula banding reduces steal through the graft but may jeopardize graft patency.[106] In severe cases, graft takedown is required.

Another serious ischemic complication is ischemic monomelic neuropathy, which is a complication of vascular access seen almost exclusively in diabetic patients, particularly those with preexisting peripheral neuropathy and/or peripheral vascular disease.[104] It is not commonly seen by the interventional radiologist because it usually occurs within minutes to hours after placement of an arteriovenous access. It results from the sudden diversion of blood supply from the nerves of the forearm and hand, this acute ischemic insult being severe enough to damage nerves but not sufficient enough to produce necrosis of the other tissues.[104] It may result in a claw-hand deformity with profound loss of function and, often, severe neuropathic pain.

Venous Hypertension

Obstruction of the venous outflow may lead to retrograde, high-pressure flow through collateral veins and result in venous hypertension. This situation is most common with upper arm fistulas when there is occlusion of the subclavian vein. Patients suffering from venous hypertension have edema, cyanotic discoloration, and, with long-standing hypertension, pigmentation changes of the skin.[108] Dilated, tortuous collateral veins are observed in the extremity and often across the chest. Swelling of the extremity causes pain and impaired function and may lead to ischemic ulceration.[108]

Patients should be evaluated before graft placement if they have preexisting arm edema, collateral vein development, history of subclavian vein catheters or pacemaker placement,[109] or trauma to the extremity. Imaging is done with contrast venography, duplex ultrasound, or MR imaging.[110,111]

If symptoms of venous hypertension occur after graft placement, a venogram should be performed. If there is a central venous stenosis or occlusion, angioplasty and possibly stenting (for an occlusion) should be attempted. In many cases, angioplasty resolves the arm swelling at least for 3 to 6 months, then repeated angioplasty can be performed, which can prolong the use of the access sometimes for years.[18]

Aneurysms and Pseudoaneurysms

Aneurysms and pseudoaneurysms are detected as pulsatile masses within synthetic dialysis grafts or arteriovenous fistulas. Large aneurysms may result in skin breakdown, bleeding, or rupture.

Aneurysms usually occur in arteriovenous fistulas from repeated dialysis needle puncture at the same site. Occasionally, they occur in the outflow vein away from puncture sites. These aneurysms are thought to be associated with venous hypertension and are more likely to occur in long-established fistulas. Surgical intervention is not required unless the aneurysm involves the anastomosis. However, venipuncture of the aneurysm should be avoided because hemostasis may be difficult.

Pseudoaneurysms result from graft degeneration at sites when repeated punctures have been made and occur in

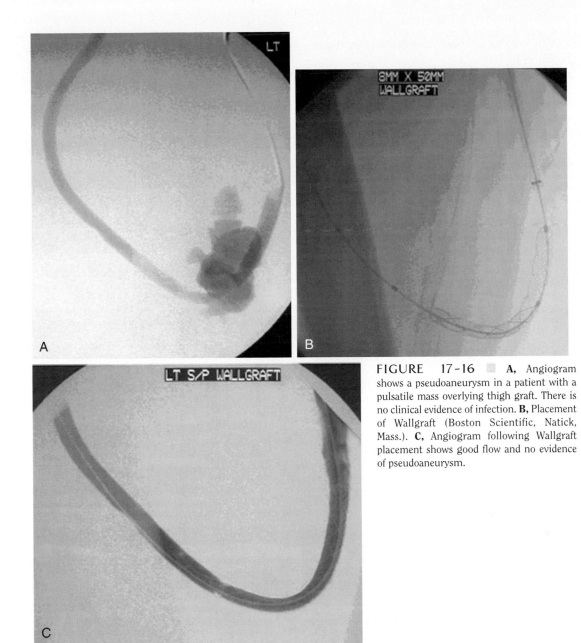

FIGURE 17-16 ■ **A,** Angiogram shows a pseudoaneurysm in a patient with a pulsatile mass overlying thigh graft. There is no clinical evidence of infection. **B,** Placement of Wallgraft (Boston Scientific, Natick, Mass.). **C,** Angiogram following Wallgraft placement shows good flow and no evidence of pseudoaneurysm.

2% to 10% of dialysis access grafts.[42] When these pseudoaneurysm defects become large, they may compromise graft function. Surgical intervention is warranted for skin breakdown, rapid expansion, massive dilation (i.e., more than twice the diameter of the graft), spontaneous bleeding, or infection. Surgery usually involves resection of the pseudoaneurysm and interposition or bypass grafting around the lesion. More recently stent grafts have been used to treat patients with pseudoaneurysms of their dialysis grafts and aneurysms of AV fistulas (Fig. 17-16).[42,43]

REFERENCES

1. III. NKF-K/DOQI Clinical Practice Guidelines for Vascular Access: update 2000. Am J Kidney Dis 2001;37:S137.

2. Chin AI, Chang W, Fitzgerald JT, et al: Intra-access blood flow in patients with newly created upper-arm arteriovenous native fistulae for hemodialysis access. Am J Kidney Dis 2004;44:850.

3. D'Cunha PT, Besarab A: Vascular access for hemodialysis: 2004 and beyond. Curr Opin Nephrol Hypertens 2004;13:623.

4. Perera GB, Mueller MP, Kubaska SM, et al: Superiority of autogenous arteriovenous hemodialysis access: maintenance of function with fewer secondary interventions. Ann Vasc Surg 2004;18:66.

5. Lok CE, Bhola C, Croxford R, Richardson RM: Reducing vascular access morbidity: a comparative trial of two vascular access monitoring strategies. Nephrol Dial Transplant 2003;18:1174.

6. Huber TS, Buhler AG, Seeger JM: Evidence-based data for the hemodialysis access surgeon. Semin Dial 2004;17:217.

7. Huber TS, Carter JW, Carter RL, Seeger JM: Patency of autogenous and polytetrafluoroethylene upper extremity arteriovenous hemodialysis accesses: a systematic review. J Vasc Surg 2003;38:1005.

8. Fillinger M, Reinitz E, Schwartz R, et al: Graft geometry and venous intimal-medial hyperplasia in arteriovenous loop grafts. J Vasc Surg 1990;11:556.

9. Windus DW: Permanent vascular access: a nephrologist's view. Am J Kidney Dis 1993;21:457.

10. Malchesky P, Koshino I, Pennza P, et al: Analysis of the segmental venous stenosis in blood access. Trans Amer Soc Artif Int Organs 1975;21:310.

11. Sullivan KL, Besarab A, Bonn J, et al: Hemodynamics of failing dialysis grafts. Radiology 1993;186:867.

12. Schwarz C, Mitterbauer C, Boczula M, et al: Flow monitoring: performance characteristics of ultrasound dilution versus color Doppler ultrasound compared with fistulography. Am J Kidney Dis 2003; 42:539.

13. Roberts A, Valji K: Screening and assessment of dialysis graft function. Tech Vasc Interv Radiol 1999;2:186.

14. Besarab A, Lubkowski T, Frinak S, et al: Detection of access strictures and outlet stenoses in vascular accesses. Which test is best? ASAIO J 1997;43:M543.

15. Basile C, Ruggieri G, Vernaglione L, et al: A comparison of methods for the measurement of hemodialysis access recirculation. J Nephrol 2003;16:908.

16. Lopot F, Nejedly B, Valek M: Vascular access monitoring: methods and procedures—something to standardize? Blood Purif 2005;23:36.

17. Lopot F, Nejedly B, Sulkova S, Blaha J: Comparison of different techniques of hemodialysis vascular access flow evaluation. Int J Artif Organs 2003;26:1056.

18. Ziegler TW, Safa A, Amarillis K, et al: Prolonging the life of difficult hemodialysis access using thrombolysis, angiography and angioplasty. Adv Renal Replace Ther 1995;2:52.

19. Beathard GA: Physical examination of AV grafts. Semin Dial 1996;5:74.

20. Trerotola SO, Scheel PJ Jr, Powe NR, et al: Screening for dialysis access graft malfunction: comparison of physical examination with US. J Vasc Interv Radiol 1996;7:15.

21. Schwab SJ, Raymond JR, Saeed M, et al: Prevention of hemodialysis fistula thrombosis. Early detection of venous stenoses. Kidney Int 1989;36:707.

22. Besarab A, Lubkowski T, Frinak S, et al: Detecting vascular access dysfunction. ASAIO J 1997;43:M539.

23. McCarley P, Wingard RL, Shyr Y, et al: Vascular access blood flow monitoring reduces access morbidity and costs. Kidney Int 2001; 60:1164.

24. Cayco AV, Abu-Alfa AK, Mahnensmith RL, Perazella MA: Reduction in arteriovenous graft impairment: results of a vascular access surveillance protocol. Am J Kidney Dis 1998;32:302.

25. Robbin ML, Gallichio MH, Deierhoi MH, et al: US vascular mapping before hemodialysis access placement. Radiology 2000;217:83.

26. Robbin ML, Chamberlain NE, Lockhart ME, et al: Hemodialysis arteriovenous fistula maturity: US evaluation. Radiology 2002;225:59.

27. Polkinghorne KR, Kerr PG: Predicting vascular access failure: a collective review. Nephrology (Carlton) 2002;7:170.

28. Marston WA, Criado E, Jaques PF, et al: Prospective randomized comparison of surgical versus endovascular management of thrombosed dialysis access grafts. J Vasc Surg 1997;26:373.

29. Bitar G, Yang S, Badosa F: Balloon versus patch angioplasty as an adjuvant treatment to surgical thrombectomy of hemodialysis grafts. Am J Surg 1997;174:140.

30. Dougherty MJ, Calligaro KD, Schindler N, et al: Endovascular versus surgical treatment for thrombosed hemodialysis grafts: a prospective, randomized study. J Vasc Surg 1999;30:1016.

31. Sreenarasimhaiah VP, Margassery SK, Martin KJ, Bander SJ: Cutting balloon angioplasty for resistant venous anastomotic stenoses. Semin Dial 2004;17:523.

32. Vorwerk D, Adam G, Muller-Leisse C, Guenther RW: Hemodialysis fistulas and grafts: use of cutting balloons to dilate venous stenoses. Radiology 1996;201:864.

33. Bittl JA, Feldman RL: Cutting balloon angioplasty for undilatable venous stenoses causing dialysis graft failure. Catheter Cardiovasc Interv 2003;58:524.

34. Funaki B: Cutting balloon angioplasty in arteriovenous fistulas. J Vasc Interv Radiol 2005;16:5.

35. Song HH, Kim KT, Chung SK, et al: Cutting balloon angioplasty for resistant venous stenoses of Brescia-Cimino fistulas. J Vasc Interv Radiol 2004;15:1463.

36. Singer-Jordan J, Papura S: Cutting balloon angioplasty for primary treatment of hemodialysis fistula venous stenoses: preliminary results. J Vasc Interv Radiol 2005;16:25.

37. Funaki B, Szymski GX, Leef JA, et al: Wallstent deployment to salvage dialysis graft thrombolysis complicated by venous rupture: early and intermediate results. AJR Am J Roentgenol 1997;169:1435.

38. Silas AM, Bettmann MA: Utility of covered stents for revision of aging failing synthetic hemodialysis grafts: a report of three cases. Cardiovasc Intervent Radiol 2003;26:550.

39. Lin PH, Johnson CK, Pullium JK, et al: Transluminal stent graft repair with Wallgraft endoprosthesis in a porcine arteriovenous graft pseudoaneurysm model. J Vasc Surg 2003;37:175.

40. Quinn SF, Kim J, Sheley RC: Transluminally placed endovascular grafts for venous lesions in patients on hemodialysis. Cardiovasc Intervent Radiol 2003;26:365.

41. Turmel-Rodrigues L, Mouton A, Birmele B, et al: Salvage of immature forearm fistulas for haemodialysis by interventional radiology. Nephrol Dial Transplant 2001;16:2365.

42. Najibi S, Bush RL, Terramani TT, et al: Covered stent exclusion of dialysis access pseudoaneurysms. J Surg Res 2002;106:15.

43. Ryan JM, Dumbleton SA, Doherty J, Smith TP: Technical innovation. Using a covered stent (wallgraft) to treat pseudoaneurysms of dialysis grafts and fistulas. AJR Am J Roentgenol 2003;180:1067.

44. Khan FA, Vesely TM: Arterial problems associated with dysfunctional hemodialysis grafts: evaluation of patients at high risk for arterial disease. J Vasc Interv Radiol 2002;13:1109.

45. Roberts AC, Valji K, Bookstein JJ, Hye RJ: Pulse-spray pharmacomechanical thrombolysis for treatment of thrombosed dialysis access grafts. Am J Surg 1993;166:221.

46. Saeed M, Newman GE, McCann RL, et al: Stenoses in dialysis fistulas: treatment with percutaneous angioplasty. Radiology 1987; 164:693.

47. Huber TS, Seeger JM: Approach to patients with "complex" hemodialysis access problems. Semin Dial 2003;16:22.

48. Guerra A, Raynaud A, Beyssen B, et al: Arterial percutaneous angioplasty in upper limbs with vascular access devices for haemodialysis. Nephrol Dial Transplant 2002;17:843.

49. Aruny JE, Lewis CA, Cardella JF, et al: Quality improvement guidelines for percutaneous management of the thrombosed or dysfunctional dialysis access. J Vasc Interv Radiol 2003;14:S247.

50. Verstandig AG, Bloom AI, Sasson T, et al: Shortening and migration of Wallstents after stenting of central venous stenoses in hemodialysis patients. Cardiovasc Intervent Radiol 2003;26:58.

51. Sharma AK, Sinha S, Bakran A: Migration of intra-vascular metallic stent into pulmonary artery. Nephrol Dial Transplant 2002; 17:511.

52. Fernandez-Juarez G, Letosa RM, Mirete JO: Pulmonary migration of a vascular stent. Nephrol Dial Transplant 1999;14:250.

53. Yao L, Veytsman AM, Dhamee MS: Images in anesthesia: a right atrial foreign body. Can J Anaesth 2004;51:173.

54. Safa AA, Valji K, Roberts AC, et al: Detection and treatment of dysfunctional hemodialysis access grafts: effect of a surveillance program on graft patency and the incidence of thrombosis. Radiology 1996; 199:653.

55. Clark TW, Hirsch DA, Jindal KJ, et al: Outcome and prognostic factors of restenosis after percutaneous treatment of native hemodialysis fistulas. J Vasc Interv Radiol 2002;13:51.

56. Turmel-Rodrigues L, Pengloan J, Baudin S, et al: Treatment of stenosis and thrombosis in haemodialysis fistulas and grafts by interventional radiology. Nephrol Dial Transplant 2000;15:2029.

57. Vesely TM, Hovsepian DM, Pilgram TK, et al: Upper extremity central venous obstruction in hemodialysis patients: treatment with Wallstents. Radiology 1997;204:343.

58. Maskova J, Komarkova J, Kivanek J, et al: Endovascular treatment of central vein stenoses and/or occlusions in hemodialysis patients. Cardiovasc Intervent Radiol 2003;26:27.

59. Beathard GA: Management of complications of endovascular dialysis access procedures. Semin Dial 2003;16:309.

60. Marston WA, Beathard GA: Surgical management of thrombosed dialysis access grafts. Am J Kidney Dis 1998;32:168.

61. Mansilla AV, Toombs BD, Vaughn WK, Zeledon JI: Patency and lifespans of failing hemodialysis grafts in patients undergoing repeated percutaneous de-clotting. Tex Heart Inst J 2001;28:249.

62. Davis GB, Dowd CF, Bookstein JJ, et al: Thrombosed dialysis grafts: efficacy of intrathrombic deposition of concentrated urokinase, clot maceration, and angioplasty. AJR Am J Roentgenol 1987;149:177.

63. Valji K, Roberts A, Bookstein J: Thrombosed hemodialysis access grafts: management with pulse-spray thrombolysis and balloon angioplasty. In: Strandness D, Van Breda A, eds. Vascular Diseases: Surgical and Interventional Therapy. New York, Churchill Livingstone, 1994:1087.

64. Kinney TB, Valji K, Rose SC, et al: Pulmonary embolism from pulse-spray pharmacomechanical thrombolysis of clotted hemodialysis grafts: urokinase versus heparinized saline. J Vasc Interv Radiol 2000;11: 1143.
65. Smits HF, Van Rijk PP, Van Isselt JW, et al: Pulmonary embolism after thrombolysis of hemodialysis grafts. J Am Soc Nephrol 1997; 8:1458.
66. Petronis JD, Regan F, Briefel G, et al: Ventilation-perfusion scintigraphic evaluation of pulmonary clot burden after percutaneous thrombolysis of clotted hemodialysis access grafts. Am J Kidney Dis 1999;34:207.
67. Bookstein J, Fellmeth B, Roberts A, et al: Pulsed-spray pharmacomechanical thrombolysis: preliminary clinical results. AJR Am J Roentgenol 1989;152:1097.
68. Valji K, Bookstein JJ, Roberts AC, Davis GB: Pharmacomechanical thrombolysis and angioplasty in the management of clotted hemodialysis grafts: early and late clinical results. Radiology 1991;178:243.
69. Roberts AC, Silberzweig JE: Hemodialysis access management. In: Bakal CW, Silberzweig JE, Cynamon J, Sprayregen S, eds. Vascular and Interventional Radiology: Principles and Practice. New York, Thieme, 2002:459.
70. Etheredge E, Haid S, Maeser M, et al: Salvage operations for malfunctioning polytetrafluroethylene hemodialysis access grafts. Surgery 1983;94:464.
71. Winkler TA, Trerotola SO, Davidson DD, Milgrom ML: Study of thrombus from thrombosed hemodialysis access grafts. Radiology 1995; 197:461.
72. Cynamon J, Lakritz PS, Wahl SI, et al: Hemodialysis graft declotting: description of the "lyse and wait" technique. J Vasc Interv Radiol 1997;8:825.
73. Cynamon J, Pierpont CE: Thrombolysis for the treatment of thrombosed hemodialysis access grafts. Rev Cardiovasc Med 2002;3 Suppl 2:S84.
74. Falk A, Mitty H, Guller J, et al: Thrombolysis of clotted hemodialysis grafts with tissue-type plasminogen activator. J Vasc Interv Radiol 2001;12:305.
75. Vogel PM, Bansal V, Marshall MW: Thrombosed hemodialysis grafts: lyse and wait with tissue plasminogen activator or urokinase compared to mechanical thrombolysis with the Arrow-Trerotola Percutaneous Thrombolytic Device. J Vasc Interv Radiol 2001;12:1157.
76. Sofocleous CT, Hinrichs CR, Weiss SH, et al: Alteplase for hemodialysis access graft thrombosis. J Vasc Interv Radiol 2002;13:775.
77. Falk A, Guller J, Nowakowski FS, et al: Reteplase in the treatment of thrombosed hemodialysis grafts. J Vasc Interv Radiol 2001;12:1257.
78. Boobes Y, al Hassan H, Neglen P, et al: Recombinant tissue plasminogen activator to declot dialysis fistulas. J Nephrol 1997;10:107.
79. Valji K, Bookstein JJ: Efficacy of adjunctive intrathrombic heparin with pulse spray thrombolysis in rabbit inferior vena cava thrombosis. Invest Radiol 1992;27:912.
80. Harrell DS, Kozlowski M, Katz MD, Hanks SE: Admixture of heparin with urokinase to decrease thrombolysis time and urokinase dose in polytetrafluoroethylene dialysis graft recanalization. J Vasc Interv Radiol 1996;7:193.
81. Flower R, Moncada S, Vane J: Analgesic-antipyretics and anti-inflammatory agents; drugs employed in the treatment of gout. In: Gilman A, Goodman L, Rall T, Murad F, eds. The Pharmacological Basis of Therapeutics. New York, Macmillan, 1985:674.
82. Morgan R, Belli AM: Percutaneous thrombectomy: a review. Eur Radiol 2002;12:205.
83. Vesely TM: Techniques for using mechanical thrombectomy devices to treat thrombosed hemodialysis grafts. Tech Vasc Interv Radiol 1999;2:208.
84. Rajan DK, Clark TW, Simons ME, et al: Procedural success and patency after percutaneous treatment of thrombosed autogenous arteriovenous dialysis fistulas. J Vasc Interv Radiol 2002;13:1211.
85. Kumpe DA, Cohen MA: Angioplasty/thrombolytic treatment of failing and failed hemodialysis access sites: comparison with surgical treatment. Prog Cardiovasc Dis 1992;34:263.
86. Zaleski GX, Funaki B, Kenney S, et al: Angioplasty and bolus urokinase infusion for the restoration of function in thrombosed Brescia-Cimino dialysis fistulas. J Vasc Interv Radiol 1999;10:129.
87. Cooper SG, Gaetz H, Sofocleous CT, et al: Hemodialysis graft mechanical thrombolysis with use of the Amplatz Thrombectomy Device: histopathologic evaluation of extracted myointimal tissue. J Vasc Interv Radiol 1999;10:285.

88. Pattynama PM, van Baalen J, Verburgh CA, et al: Revascularization of occluded haemodialysis fistulae with the Hydrolyser thrombectomy catheter: description of the technique and report of six cases. Nephrol Dial Transplant 1995;10:1224.
89. Rocek M, Peregrin JH, Lasovickova J, et al: Mechanical thrombolysis of thrombosed hemodialysis native fistulas with use of the Arrow-Trerotola percutaneous thrombolytic device: our preliminary experience. J Vasc Interv Radiol 2000;11:1153.
90. Overbosch EH, Pattynama PM, Aarts HJ, et al: Occluded hemodialysis shunts: Dutch multicenter experience with the hydrolyser catheter. Radiology 1996;201:485.
91. Turmel-Rodrigues L, Sapoval M, Pengloan J, et al: Manual thromboaspiration and dilation of thrombosed dialysis access: mid-term results of a simple concept. J Vasc Interv Radiol 1997;8:813.
92. Gibbens DT, Triolo J, Yu T, et al: Contemporary treatment of thrombosed hemodialysis grafts. Tech Vasc Interv Radiol 2001; 4:122.
93. Smits HF, Smits JH, Wust AF, et al: Percutaneous thrombolysis of thrombosed haemodialysis access grafts: comparison of three mechanical devices. Nephrol Dial Transplant 2002;17:467.
94. Sofocleous CT, Cooper SG, Schur I, et al: Retrospective comparison of the Amplatz thrombectomy device with modified pulse-spray pharmacomechanical thrombolysis in the treatment of thrombosed hemodialysis access grafts. Radiology 1999;213:561.
95. Barth KH, Gosnell MR, Palestrant AM, et al: Hydrodynamic thrombectomy system versus pulse-spray thrombolysis for thrombosed hemodialysis grafts: a multicenter prospective randomized comparison. Radiology 2000;217:678.
96. Trerotola SO, Vesely TM, Lund GB, et al: Treatment of thrombosed hemodialysis access grafts: Arrow-Trerotola percutaneous thrombolytic device versus pulse-spray thrombolysis. Arrow-Trerotola Percutaneous Thrombolytic Device Clinical Trial. Radiology 1998;206:403.
97. Murray SP, Kinney TB, Valji K, et al: Early rethrombosis of clotted hemodialysis grafts: graft salvage achieved with an aggressive approach. AJR Am J Roentgenol 2000;175:529.
98. Sofocleous CT, Schur I, Koh E, et al: Percutaneous treatment of complications occurring during hemodialysis graft recanalization. Eur J Radiol 2003;47:237.
99. Tretotola SO, Johnson MS, Shah H, Namyslowski J: Backbleeding technique for treatment of arterial emboli resulting from dialysis graft thrombolysis. J Vasc Interv Radiol 1998;9:141.
100. Swan TL, Smyth SH, Ruffenach SJ, et al: Pulmonary embolism following hemodialysis access thrombolysis/thrombectomy. J Vasc Interv Radiol 1995;6:683.
101. Trerotola SO, Johnson MS, Schauwecker DS, et al: Pulmonary emboli from pulse-spray and mechanical thrombolysis: evaluation with an animal dialysis-graft model. Radiology 1996;200:169.
102. Beathard GA, Welch BR, Maidment HJ: Mechanical thrombolysis for the treatment of thrombosed hemodialysis access grafts. Radiology 1996;200:711.
103. Soulen MC, Zaetta JM, Amygdalos MA, et al: Mechanical declotting of thrombosed dialysis grafts: experience in 86 cases. J Vasc Interv Radiol 1997;8:563.
104. Miles AM: Upper limb ischemia after vascular access surgery: differential diagnosis and management. Semin Dial 2000;13:312.
105. Morsy AH, Kulbaski M, Chen C, et al: Incidence and characteristics of patients with hand ischemia after a hemodialysis access procedure. J Surg Res 1998;74:8.
106. Tordoir JH, Dammers R, van der Sande FM: Upper extremity ischemia and hemodialysis vascular access. Eur J Vasc Endovasc Surg 2004;27:1.
107. Valji K, Hye RJ, Roberts AC, et al: Hand ischemia in patients with hemodialysis access grafts: angiographic diagnosis and treatment. Radiology 1995;196:697.
108. Neville RF, Abularrage CJ, White PW, Sidawy AN: Venous hypertension associated with arteriovenous hemodialysis access. Semin Vasc Surg 2004;17:50.
109. Teruya TH, Abou-Zamzam AM Jr, Limm W, et al: Symptomatic subclavian vein stenosis and occlusion in hemodialysis patients with transvenous pacemakers. Ann Vasc Surg 2003;17:526.
110. Paksoy Y, Gormus N, Tercan MA: Three-dimensional contrast-enhanced magnetic resonance angiography (3-D CE-MRA) in the evaluation of hemodialysis access complications, and the condition of central veins in patients who are candidates for hemodialysis access. J Nephrol 2004;17:57.

111. Laissy JP, Menegazzo D, Debray MP, et al: Failing arteriovenous hemodialysis fistulas: assessment with magnetic resonance angiography. Invest Radiol 1999;34:218.
112. Besarab A, Sullivan KL, Ross RP, Moritz MJ: Utility of intra-access pressure monitoring in detecting and correcting venous outlet stenoses prior to thrombosis. Kidney Int 1995;47:1364.
113. Roberts AB, Kahn MB, Bradford S, et al: Graft surveillance and angioplasty prolongs dialysis graft patency. J Am Coll Surg 1996;183:486.

114. Martin LG, MacDonald MJ, Kikeri D, et al: Prophylactic angioplasty reduces thrombosis in virgin ePTFE arteriovenous dialysis grafts with greater than 50% stenosis: subset analysis of a prospectively randomized study. J Vasc Interv Radiol 1999;10:389.
115. Lumsden AB, McDonald MJ, Kikeri D, et al. Prophylatic balloon angioplasty fails to prolong the patency of expanded polytetrafluoroethylene arteriovenous grafts: Results of a prospective randomized study. J Vasc Surg 1997;26:382.

18

Lymphatic System

LYMPHOGRAPHY

Intraluminal Lymphangiography

The technique of lymphangiography is described in detail elsewhere.[1,2] For most indications, lymphography is performed by cannulating a superficial lymphatic channel in the foot. Evaluation of the upper extremity lymphatic system can be done by catheterizing a channel on the dorsum of the hand.

After sterile preparation of the foot, 0.5 to 1.0 mL of a vital dye (e.g., methylene blue, isosulfan blue [Lymphazurin]) diluted with 1% lidocaine is injected intradermally into several interdigital web spaces using a 25-gauge tuberculin syringe. Within about 5 minutes, superficial lymphatic channels appear over the dorsum of the foot.

After applying 1% lidocaine to the tissue overlying visualized channels, a 3-cm transverse incision is made. The subcutaneous fat is bluntly dissected, and a lymphatic channel is isolated. Silk ties are placed around each end of the lymphatic vessel. Connective tissue must be completely teased away before cannulation is attempted.

The proximal suture is taped to the adjacent skin to partially distend the channel. A 27- to 30-gauge lymphangiography needle is advanced into the lymphatic, and saline is injected to confirm an intraluminal location. The needle is carefully secured with a Steri-Strip. The proximal suture may be tied around the needle if there is minor leakage of injected fluid. The patient must keep the foot motionless after this point.

Iodized poppy seed oil (e.g., Ethiodol) is then slowly infused through the needle at a rate of about 0.1 mL/min. The total injection volume is 5 to 8 mL. Fluoroscopy of the foot and calf ensures that the contrast is entering the lymphatic system. When the injection is finished, the needle is removed, and the skin is closed with absorbable suture material.

A series of plain films of the pelvis, abdomen, and chest in several projections is taken at the completion of the injection (*channel* or *lymphatic phase*) and 24 hours later (*nodal phase*). For the evaluation of lymphedema, early and delayed films of the legs also are obtained. Spot films, such as radiographs of a suspected site of lymphatic leak, may be useful.

Lymphography is a relatively safe and well-tolerated procedure, if somewhat time-consuming and technically challenging. Patients should be warned that the vital dye discolors the urine for several days. Lymphography causes a foreign body reaction, with enlargement of the lymph nodes lasting for several weeks. Complications, which are uncommon, include allergic reaction to contrast material or vital dye, wound infection, contrast extravasation, pulmonary oil embolism, chemical pneumonitis, and, rarely, hepatic or cerebral embolization.[1,2] Most of the contrast material is taken up within lymph nodes. A small quantity embolizes to the capillaries of the lung after passing through the thoracic duct and venous circulation. Although embolization is expected, symptoms are rare (<1%).[3] Significant dyspnea or hypoxia is more likely in patients with preexisting lung disease. In these patients, lymphography should be avoided, or the total contrast volume should be limited.

Interstitial Lymphography

Interstitial lymphography evaluates the peripheral lymphatics at almost any site on the body.[4,5] Lymph nodes are not adequately visualized with this method. A 27-gauge butterfly needle is inserted into the subcutaneous tissue of a web space on the foot. Nonionic water-soluble contrast material is injected at 0.1 mL/minute, up to a dose of 2 mL. Images of the lymphatic system are obtained periodically during infusion.

ANATOMY AND PHYSIOLOGY

The lymphatic system has a variety of functions, most notably the uptake of excess fluid and plasma proteins that diffuse out of capillaries into interstitial tissues.[6] Unlike blood vessels, peripheral lymphatic vessels are quite permeable to macromolecules and cellular material. Lymphatics begin as blind-ending tubes, called *end-bulbs* in the periphery and *lacteals* in the intestinal tract. Lymphatic capillaries merge to form lymphatic channels. These channels, which contain numerous valves, pass through a series of lymph node groups before entering a major lymph duct (Fig. 18-1). During the early channel phase of a lymphangiogram, contrast is seen in lymphatic vessels and lymph nodes. Three or more hours after injection, the lymph channels clear, and contrast collects in the lymph nodes (nodal phase).

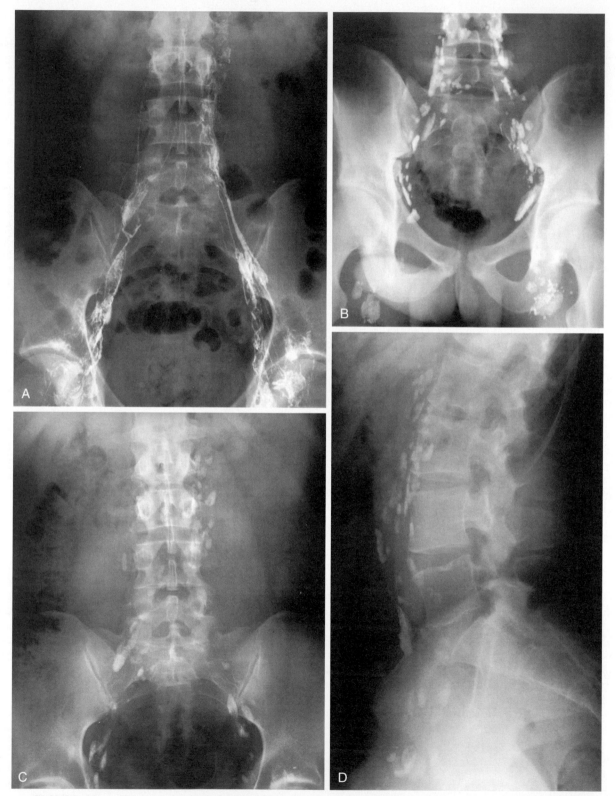

FIGURE 18-1 ■ Normal lymphangiogram. **A,** Channel phase in the pelvis and abdomen. **B,** Nodal phase (24 hours later) in the pelvis. **C** and **D,** Frontal and lateral projections of nodal phase in the abdomen in another patient.

Rich communications exist between lymph channels and lymph nodes. Lymph ducts ultimately drain into the venous circulation near the junction of the internal jugular and subclavian veins. Movement of lymph centrally depends on spontaneous contraction of lymphatic channels, the presence of one-way valves, and muscular or visceral organ activity.

Lymph nodes are composed of numerous lymphoid follicles separated by fibrous trabeculae and sinuses.[7] Multiple **afferent** lymphatic channels enter each node (Fig. 18-2). Lymph fluid percolates through the sinuses and leaves through **efferent** channels clustered at the hilum of the node. Small lymph nodes are spherical; larger truncal nodes are almond shaped (Fig. 18-3). At lymphography, a normal node is well circumscribed and has a fine, homogeneous, mottled internal architecture. A central hilar defect often is seen on the efferent side. Larger or multiple defects are common in the femoral nodes because of age-related fatty infiltration (fibrolipomatosis) or previous foot infections.

The lower extremities have superficial and deep lymphatic systems.[7] The deep channels follow their corresponding veins. The superficial channels, which are opacified during pedal lymphography, bifurcate as they ascend up the leg. For this reason, injection of a single superficial channel in the foot opacifies 12 to 20 channels in the upper thigh (see Fig. 18-2). The *node of Rosenmüller* is medial to the upper femoral vein. Several deep and numerous (9 to 12) superficial nodes are located around the inguinal ligament. Three external and common iliac lymph chains (i.e., lateral,

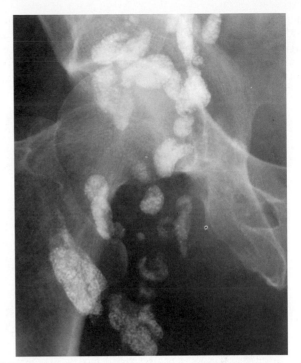

FIGURE 18-3 ■ Internal architecture of inguinal lymph nodes. Most of the nodes appear normal, with a homogeneous, mottled texture. Central hilar defects are seen on the efferent side of some nodes. Areas of mild inhomogeneity and node deformity represent benign hyperplasia.

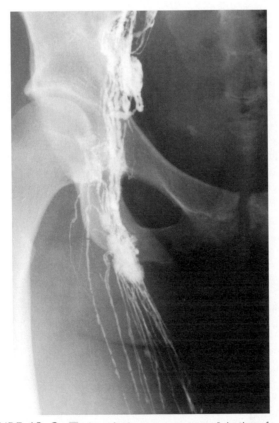

FIGURE 18-2 ■ Lymphatic system anatomy. Injection of a single lymphatic vessel in the foot fills multiple channels in the inguinal region. Afferent channels enter the large node of Rosenmüller, and several efferent channels exit at the hilum of the node. The vessels contain multiple valves.

middle, and medial) follow the iliac vessels (see Fig. 18-1). The iliac chains continue as preaortic and paired lateral aortic chains. Normally, aortic lymph nodes extend no more than 3 cm in front of the anterior border of the lumbar vertebrae and no further than the lateral transverse processes.[1]

The preaortic nodes also drain the organs supplied by the anterior branches of the abdominal aorta, including most of the intestinal tract. The lateral aortic nodes also drain organs supplied by the lateral aortic branches, including the kidneys, gonads, pelvic viscera, and adrenal glands. The testes and ovaries drain to lateral aortic nodes at the level of the renal veins and to external iliac nodes. The cervix drains to external and internal iliac nodes.

In most cases, the aortic channels merge into lumbar trunks at about the L1-L2 level. The intestinal lymph trunks also drain into a confluence at this level. When the confluence is fusiform and unilocular, it is known as the *cisterna chyli* (Fig. 18-4). The *thoracic duct* arises from the cisterna chyli and ascends into the chest between the aorta and the azygous vein. Portions of the duct may be duplicated or multiple (Fig. 18-5). At about the T5 level, it passes to the left behind the aortic arch and then empties into the venous circulation at the notch of the left subclavian and jugular vein junction or into either of these vessels. Three other lymphatic trunks draining the left side of the head, neck, and thorax and the left arm also enter near this site. The right lymphatic trunks drain into a comparable location on the right side.

The upper extremity also has superficial and deep lymphatic systems. The deep system follows the corresponding blood vessels. Both systems drain into the axillary lymph nodes, which are arranged in five groups: lateral, anterior,

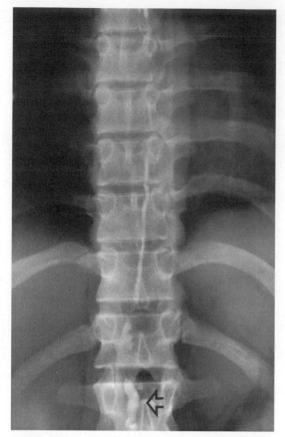

FIGURE 18-4 ■ Cisterna chyli *(arrow)* and thoracic duct.

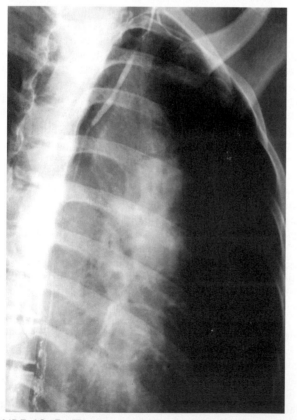

FIGURE 18-5 ■ The lower thoracic duct is composed of multiple channels. The duct entrance is at the left subclavian-jugular vein junction.

posterior, central, and apical. Much of the superficial system (seen at lymphography) drains into the lateral group. The breast, chest, and upper abdominal wall also drain into these nodes. The subclavian lymphatic trunks then enter the venous system near the entrance of the right lymphatic duct or thoracic duct.

The composition of lymph fluid varies with its source. All lymph fluid has a high protein content (>3 g/dL).[8] Peripheral lymphatic fluid is clear and colorless. Lymph fluid draining the intestinal lacteals *(chyle)* has a milky appearance due to neutral fat, cholesterol, and free fatty acid content. About 60% to 70% of ingested fat is delivered to the circulation through lymphatics. Chyle is made turbid by absorbed chylomicrons from the intestinal tract.

■ MAJOR DISORDERS

Lymphedema

Etiology

Lymphedema is a common condition in which a congenital or acquired lymphatic disorder causes buildup of proteins and fluids in interstitial tissue, usually in the extremities. If this state persists, chronic inflammation and soft tissue fibrosis occur. With time, chronic lymphedema may result in massive enlargement of the extremity, cutaneous fistulas, and, rarely, lymphangiosarcoma *(Stewart-Treves syndrome)*.[9]

Lymphedema may be congenital (primary) or acquired (secondary) (Box 18-1).[10] Most children with lymphedema have a congenital cause. Primary lymphedema may manifest at birth (congenita), in childhood or young adulthood (praecox), or later in life (tarda). *Milroy's disease* is a hereditary, autosomal dominant form of primary lymphedema presenting in infancy or later in life. The pathologic defect in primary lymphedema is aplasia, hypoplasia, or hyperplasia of some portion of the *superficial* lymphatic system. The disease often is bilateral, although symptoms may be unilateral. Chylothorax or chylous ascites may be present. Numerous genetic syndromes also are associated with primary lymphedema.

BOX 18-1 ■ **Causes of Lymphedema**

Congenital or Primary Causes
Aplasia or hypoplasia of the superficial lymphatic system
Lymphatic hyperplasia (lymphangiectasis)
Lymphangioma

Acquired or Secondary Causes
Cardiac, renal, or hepatic failure (causing widespread edema)
Malignancy
Hypoproteinemia
Infection or inflammation (e.g., filariasis)
Trauma
Radiation therapy

Clinical Features

Initially, lymphedema is pitting. In the chronic phase, the tissues become thickened and firm. Most patients with primary lymphedema present with the praecox form, and most are female. The disease can be unilateral or bilateral. The presentation ranges from almost imperceptible swelling to elephantiasis.

Imaging

Lymphedema must be distinguished from acquired or (rarely) congenital venous disease. Other unusual causes of chronic extremity swelling include lipedema, hemihypertrophy, macrodystrophia lipomatosa, and mixed vascular disorders (e.g., Klippel-Trénaunay syndrome).[10] After other diseases have been excluded by clinical features, color Doppler venous sonography, and other cross-sectional studies, imaging of the lymphatic system is performed to confirm the diagnosis.

Lymphoscintigraphy. At most centers, this technique has become the procedure of choice for evaluation of lymphedema.[11-13] A variety of scintigraphic agents is used, including ^{99m}Tc-labeled antimony-trisulfide colloid, human serum albumin, and dextran.[11] These particulate agents (10 to 100 nm in diameter) are absorbed by the lymphatic, but not venous, system after subcutaneous injection in a web space on the foot or hand. Static images give morphologic information about the status of the lymphatic system. Dynamic studies also provide flow data that can detect mild cases and can be used to grade the disease. In patients without lymphedema, the agent is rapidly taken up in lymphatic channels, followed by concentration in pelvic and abdominal nodes. In patients with lymphedema, delayed or absent lymphatic filling and slow transit are seen (Fig. 18-6). Regional lymph nodes may not be visualized. Other findings include tracer extravasation into interstitial tissues and retrograde flow into collaterals in the skin (i.e., dermal backflow).

Lymphography. Intraluminal lymphangiography occasionally is used to diagnose primary lymphedema. Imaging findings depend on the pathologic type of lymphedema, but they can include several features (Fig. 18-7)[10]:

■ Reduced caliber and number of lymphatic channels
■ Filling of collateral vessels, including dermal lymphatics and lymphovenous connections
■ Hypoplastic truncal lymphatics with distended extremity lymphatics
■ Enlarged, valveless channels with shrunken lymph nodes
■ Absence or hypoplasia of the thoracic duct with hyperplasia of peripheral lymphatic channels and lymph nodes

Findings at interstitial lymphography include lymphatic hypoplasia or hyperplasia, a reticular pattern, and retrograde flow.[5]

Treatment

Conservative therapy (i.e., exercise, elevation, and compressive devices) is the mainstay of therapy, because lymphedema

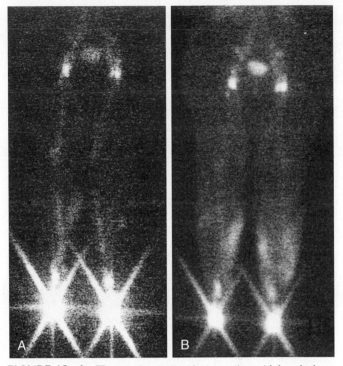

FIGURE 18-6 ■ Lymphoscintigraphy in a patient with lymphedema. **A,** Imaging 30 minutes after injection of 1 MCi of ^{99m}Tc-labeled human serum albumin shows delayed flow in the lymphatic channels in both legs. **B,** Imaging at 2 hours shows filling of the inguinal and pelvic lymph nodes. Soft tissue activity in both calves suggests dermal backflow from lymphatic obstruction.

eventually stabilizes in many patients. The results of surgical therapy often are disappointing.[14]

Neoplasms

Hodgkin's and non-Hodgkin's lymphoma were once routinely staged and monitored with lymphangiography.[15] Lymphography is extremely accurate in Hodgkin's disease and somewhat less so in non-Hodgkin's lymphoma. Classic findings include lymph node enlargement and displacement, central or marginal (cookie bite) filling defects, diffuse and foamy appearance of the internal architecture, or nonopacification due to complete replacement with tumor (Fig. 18-8). With the advent of CT, early comparative studies suggested that the two modalities were comparable for the evaluation of Hodgkin's disease.[16]

The major advantage of lymphography was the ability to assess the internal architecture of lymph glands, allowing subtle malignant changes in normal size nodes to be identified. In theory, lymph nodes enlarged by tumor could be distinguished from *benign reactive hyperplasia*, which is associated with a variety of infectious and inflammatory processes and with a nonneoplastic response to adjacent malignant nodes (see Fig. 18-3). The major advantage of CT is the ability to visualize enlarged nodes away from the path of lymph contrast, such as internal iliac nodes. CT often shows a greater extent of disease than lymphography. In reality, several benign entities can be confused with lymphoma at

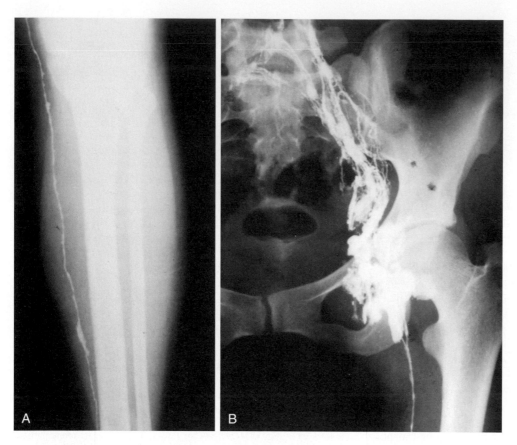

FIGURE 18-7 ■ Primary lymphedema (Milroy's disease) delineated by lymphangiography. **A** and **B,** The early phase of the study shows marked hypoplasia of lymphatic channels in the leg and distorted inguinal lymph nodes.

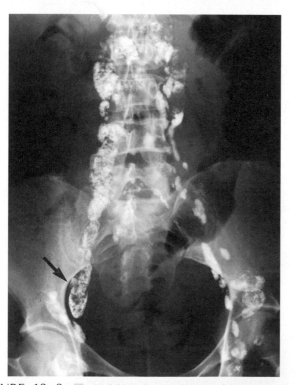

FIGURE 18-8 ■ Hodgkin's disease. The lymphangiogram shows enlarged iliac and para-aortic lymph nodes, some of which have multiple internal defects or a diffuse, "foamy" appearance caused by tumor replacement *(arrow).*

lymphography, including reactive hyperplasia, carcinomatosis, and fat infiltration.[17] State-of-the-art CT is more accurate than lymphography in staging Hodgkin's disease.[1,18] It is debatable whether lymphography is useful for patients with biopsy-proven disease but normal abdominal or chest CT scans or for guiding pelvic node irradiation.[19,20] In practice, the use of lymphography in this population has been all but abandoned at most centers in the United States.

Metastatic disease from pelvic malignancies, particularly of the testes, ovary, and cervix, was once staged and followed with lymphography. CT and MR (sometimes with lymphatic contrast agents) has virtually replaced lymphography in this setting.[21-25]

■ OTHER DISORDERS

Lymphatic Leak

Spillage of lymphatic fluid (chylous or nonchylous) into body cavities is an infrequent complication of a variety of disorders.[26] Fluid analysis is used to make the diagnosis. For the most part, lymphoscintigraphy or lymphangiography is required only in some congenital and posttraumatic cases. In addition to confirming the site of leak, accessory ducts and the course of the thoracic duct are identified.

Chylothorax is the leakage of lymphatic fluid into the pleural cavity (Box 18-2).[8] The most common cause is malignant lymphatic obstruction from intraluminal spread of tumor or transmural invasion. Lymphatic obstruction leads to rupture and spillage into the pleural cavity, which may be unilateral or bilateral. Posttraumatic chylothorax has been reported after thoracic surgery, penetrating trauma, and attempted vascular catheterization.[27,28] Many cases of "congenital" chylothorax may be caused by birth trauma rather than a congenital fistula.[29] Most fistulas close spontaneously after a course of hyperalimentation and continuous drainage (with or without pleurodesis). Some patients require thoracic duct ligation at the diaphragm or at the site of injury. Lymphography may be helpful in some cases to confirm the site of leak before repair (Fig. 18-9).[30] Percutaneous embolotherapy has been used effectively as an alternative to operative intervention.[31,32]

Chylous ascites is caused by a similar spectrum of diseases (see Box 18-2).[33-35] The leak is the result of a lymphoperitoneal fistula, rupture of an obstructed lymphatic, or engorged subserosal intestinal lymphatics. The disorder is seen more frequently in children than in adults.[35] Many patients have associated lymphedema. Imaging occasionally is required, especially in posttraumatic cases.[36] Surgical closure is necessary in many cases.

Chyluria is a rare disorder that usually is the result of malignancy, infection (particularly filariasis), or trauma.[37] The communication may be found at any site along the urinary tract. Lymphangiography and lymphoscintigraphy are used to identify the leak (Fig. 18-10).

Lymphoceles are contained lymphatic collections; most are postoperative complications (e.g., vascular surgery, kidney transplantation, lymph node dissection). Percutaneous sclerotherapy often is effective in eliminating these collections.[38-40]

Lymphocutaneous fistula is a rare complication of vascular surgical procedures, particularly groin dissections.[41] Although many of these fistulas close spontaneously with local wound care, reexploration is favored by some surgeons to hasten closure and avoid infection.

Lymphangioma

Lymphangiomas are benign congenital lymphatic tumors that can occur at many sites in the body, including soft tissue and bone. The lesions consist of enlarged lymphatic channels that usually communicate with the lymphatic system. They have been classified as simple, cavernous, or cystic.[42] The latter form includes *cystic hygromas*. Lymphangiomas usually manifest during childhood and are

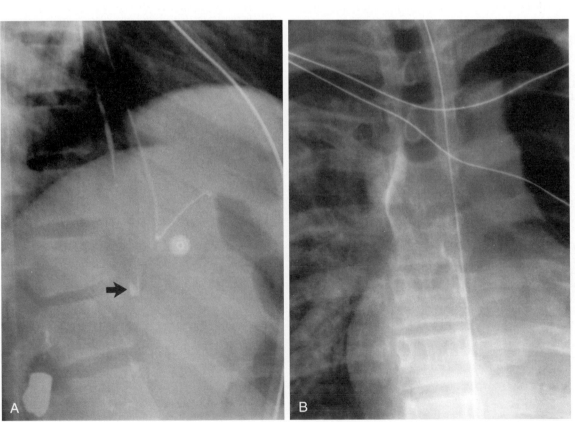

FIGURE 18-9 ■ Chylothorax after a gunshot injury. **A,** Delayed film from a pedal lymphangiogram shows the site of extravasation from the thoracic duct *(arrow).* **B,** Oily contrast opacifies the right medial pleural space.

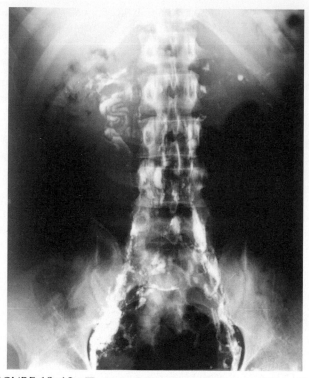

FIGURE 18-10 ■ Chyluria in a patient with filariasis. Lymphopelvic communications are identified by oily contrast in the right collecting system, and the iliac and para-aortic lymph nodes are distorted.

more common in boys than girls.[43,44] Chylothorax may be seen. Percutaneous treatment with several agents, including alcohols and Ethibloc, has been successful in selected cases.[43,45]

Lymphangiomatosis is a condition of diffuse proliferation of lymph channels.[44,46] The disease typically is seen in children and occurs more frequently in boys. Bone, soft tissue, and visceral (e.g., lung, spleen, liver, kidney) involvement are typical[47]; the latter is associated with a poor prognosis.

REFERENCES

1. Guermazi A, Brice P, Hennequin C, et al: Lymphography: an old technique retains its usefulness. Radiographics 2003;23:1541.
2. Fuchs WA: Technique and complications of lymphangiography. In: Baum S, ed. Abrams' Angiography, 4th ed. Boston, Little, Brown, 1997:1864.
3. Bruna J, Dvorakova V: Oil contrast lymphography and respiratory function. Lymphology 1988;21:178.
4. Weissleder H, Weissleder R: Interstitial lymphangiography: initial clinical experience with a dimeric nonionic contrast agent. Radiology 1989;170:371.
5. Weissleder R, Thrall JH: The lymphatic system: diagnostic imaging studies. Radiology 1989;172:315.
6. Rhoades RA, Tanner GA, eds: The microcirculation and the lymphatic system. In: Medical Physiology. Boston, Little, Brown, 1995:289.
7. Gabella G, ed: Cardiovascular system. In: Williams PL, Bannister LH, Berry MM, et al, eds. Gray's Anatomy, 38th ed. New York, Churchill Livingstone, 1995:1605.
8. Robinson CL: The management of chylothorax. Ann Thorac Surg 1985;39:90.
9. Andersson HC, Parry DM, Mulvihill JJ: Lymphangiosarcoma in late-onset hereditary lymphedema: case report and nosological implications. Am J Med Genet 1995;56:72.
10. Wright NB, Carty HML: The swollen leg and primary lymphedema. Arch Dis Child 1994;71:44.
11. Cambria RA, Gloviczki P, Naessens JM, et al: Noninvasive evaluation of the lymphatic system with lymphoscintigraphy: a prospective, semi-quantitative analysis in 386 extremities. J Vasc Surg 1993;18:773.
12. Wheatley DC, Wastie ML, Whitaker SC, et al: Lymphoscintigraphy and colour Doppler sonography in the assessment of leg oedema of unknown cause. Br J Radiol 1996;69:1117.
13. Stewart KC, Lyster DM: Interstitial lymphoscintigraphy for lymphatic mapping in surgical practice and research. J Invest Surg 1997;10:249.
14. Tiwari A, Cheng KS, Button M, et al: Differential diagnosis, investigation, and current treatment of lower limb lymphedema. Arch Surg 2003;138:152.
15. Marglin S, Castellino R: Lymphographic accuracy in 632 consecutive, previously untreated cases of Hodgkin disease and non-Hodgkin lymphoma. Radiology 1981;140:351.
16. Castellino RA, Hoppe RT, Blank N, et al: Computed tomography, lymphography, and staging laparotomy: correlations in initial staging of Hodgkin disease. AJR Am J Roentgenol 1984;143:37.
17. Castellino RA, Billingham M, Dorfman RF: Lymphographic accuracy in Hodgkin's disease and malignant lymphoma with a note on the "reactive" lymph node as a cause of most false-positive lymphograms. Invest Radiol 1974;9:155.
18. North LB, Wallace S, Lindell MM Jr, et al: Lymphography for staging lymphomas: is it still a useful procedure? AJR Am J Roentgenol 1993;161:867.
19. Libson E, Polliack A, Bloom RA: Value of lymphangiography in the staging of Hodgkin lymphoma. Radiology 1994;193:757.
20. Guermazi A, Ferme C, deKerviler E, et al: Does lymphangiography still have a place in the staging of Hodgkin's disease? Radiology 1996;199:283.
21. Fernando IN, Moskovic E, Fryatt I, et al: Is there still a role for lymphography in the management of early stage carcinoma of the cervix? Br J Radiol 1994;67:1052.
22. Stephenson NJ, Sandeman TF, McKenzie AF: Has lymphography a role in early stage testicular germ cell tumours? Australas Radiol 1995;39:54.
23. Harisinghani MG, Dixon WT, Saksena MA, et al: MR lymphangiography: imaging strategies to optimize the imaging of lymph nodes with ferumoxtran-10. Radiographics 2004;24:867.
24. Ueda K, Suga K, Kaneda Y, et al: Preoperative imaging of the lung sentinel lymphatic basin with computed tomographic lymphography: a preliminary study. Ann Thorac Surg 2004;77:1033.
25. Suga K, Yuan Y, Okada M, et al: Breast sentinel lymph node mapping at CT lymphography with iopamidol: preliminary experience. Radiology 2004;230:543.
26. Noel AA, Gloviczki P, Bender CE, et al: Treatment of symptomatic primary chylous disorders. J Vasc Surg 2001;34:785.
27. Cerfolio RJ, Allen MS, Deschamps C, et al: Postoperative chylothorax. J Thorac Cardiovasc Surg 1996;112:1361.
28. Whiteford MH, Abdullah F, Vernick JJ, et al: Thoracic duct injury in penetrating neck trauma. Am Surgeon 1995;61:1072.
29. Wasmuth-Pietzuch A, Hansmann M, Bartmann P, et al: Congenital chylothorax: lymphopenia and high risk of neonatal infections. Acta Paediatr 2004;93:220.
30. Sachs PB, Zelch MG, Rice TW, et al: Diagnosis and localization of laceration of the thoracic duct: usefulness of lymphangiography and CT. AJR Am J Roentgenol 1991;157:703.
31. Cope C, Kaiser LR: Management of unremitting chylothorax by percutaneous embolization and blockage of retroperitoneal lymphatic vessels in 42 patients. J Vasc Interv Radiol 2002;13:1139.
32. Hoffer EK, Bloch RD, Mulligan MS, et al: Treatment of chylothorax: percutaneous catheterization and embolization of the thoracic duct. AJR Am J Roentgenol 2001;176:1040.
33. Fox U, Lucani G: Disorders of the intestinal mesenteric lymphatic system. Lymphology 1993;26:61.
34. Baniel J, Foster RS, Rowland RG, et al: Management of chylous ascites after retroperitoneal lymph node dissection for testicular cancer. J Urol 1993;150:1422.
35. Browse NL, Wilson NM, Russo F, et al: Aetiology and treatment of chylous ascites. Br J Surg 1992;79:1145.
36. Andrews JT, Binder LJ: Lymphoscintigraphy pre- and post-surgical lymphatic leak repair. Australas Radiol 1996;40:19.
37. Haddad MC, Al Shahed MS, Sharif HS, et al: Investigation of chyluria. Clin Radiol 1994;49:137.

38. Zuckerman DA, Yeager TD: Percutaneous ethanol sclerotherapy of postoperative lymphoceles. AJR Am J Roentgenol 1997;169:433.

39. Sawhney R, D'Agostino HB, Zinck S, et al: Treatment of postoperative lymphoceles with percutaneous drainage and alcohol sclerotherapy. J Vasc Interv Radiol 1996;7:241.

40. Caliendo MV, Lee DE, Queiroz R, et al: Sclerotherapy with use of doxycycline after percutaneous drainage of postoperative lymphoceles. J Vasc Interv Radiol 2001;12:73.

41. Tyndall SH, Shepard AD, Wilczewski JM, et al: Groin lymphatic complications after arterial reconstruction. J Vasc Surg 1994;19:858.

42. Peh WC, Ngan H: Lymphography—still useful in the diagnosis of lymphangiomatosis. Br J Radiol 1993;66:28.

43. Herbreteau D, Riche MC, Enjolras O, et al: Percutaneous embolization with Ethibloc of lymphatic cystic malformations with a review of the experience in 70 patients. Int Angiol 1993;12:34.

44. Gomez CS, Calonje E, Ferrar DW, et al: Lymphangiomatosis of the limbs. Clinicopathologic analysis of a series with a good prognosis. Am J Surg Path 1995;19:125.

45. Dubois J, Garel L, Abela A, et al: Lymphangiomas in children: percutaneous sclerotherapy with an alcoholic solution of zein. Radiology 1997;204:651.

46. Ramani P, Shah A: Lymphangiomatosis. Histologic and immunohistochemical analysis of four cases. Am J Surg Pathol 1993;17:329.

47. Wadsworth DT, Newman B, Abramson SJ, et al: Splenic lymphangiomatosis in children. Radiology 1997;202:173.

NONVASCULAR DIAGNOSIS AND INTERVENTION

19

Percutaneous Biopsy

Thomas B. Kinney, MD

Percutaneous biopsy is a widely used interventional technique for obtaining tissue samples.[1,2] The crucial element of the procedure is image guidance, which facilitates accurate and safe needle passage. Percutaneous biopsy with image guidance is less invasive and less expensive than most surgical methods. The procedure has become safer and more effective with advances in high-resolution fluoroscopic image intensifiers; small-gauge, thin-walled needles; and specialized cytologic analyses. Cross-sectional imaging with CT, ultrasound, and MR imaging permits safe diagnosis of small, remote lesions that once were completely inaccessible in this way. The accuracy of percutaneous biopsy for the diagnosis of malignancy in the chest and abdomen is about 85% to 95%.[3] Unfortunately, definitive diagnosis of benign lesions is less accurate. Further advances in biopsy and cytopathologic methods should improve these results.

The most common indication for percutaneous biopsy is the diagnosis of malignancy, including primary neoplasms, metastatic disease, tumor staging, and recurrent disease after treatment. The procedure also is used for diagnosis of inflammatory or infectious processes, abnormal fluid collections, and diffuse organ disease. Relative contraindications include uncorrectable coagulation abnormalities, lack of a safe percutaneous pathway to the lesion, and an uncooperative patient in whom motion may increase the risk of bleeding.[4] Biopsy usually is not indicated in a patient who will undergo surgery regardless of the biopsy results.

■ TECHNIQUE

Patient Preparation

The patient's history, clinical status, and imaging studies should be reviewed and discussed with the referring physicians. Routinely performed coagulation studies include hematocrit, platelet count, prothrombin time, partial thromboplastin time, and international normalized ratio (see Chapter 1).[5] Coagulopathies should be corrected with appropriate transfusions of platelets, fresh-frozen plasma,

vitamin K, or packed red blood cells. Although institutional thresholds vary, transfusions should be considered when the prothrombin time is greater than 14.5 seconds, the international normalized ratio is greater than 1.5, or the platelet count less than 50,000/mm³. However, numerous studies have shown the relatively low predictive value of abnormal screening parameters in predicting bleeding. Surgical series also have indicated that preoperative coagulation studies correlate poorly with postoperative bleeding.[6]

Materials

A wide array of needles is available for percutaneous biopsy procedures.[7] Needles can be classified by caliber or gauge, tip configuration, and mechanism of sample acquisition. Needle sizes are divided broadly into smaller gauge (20 to 25 gauge) and larger gauge (14 to 19 gauge).[3] Thinner-gauge needles provide adequate cytologic material and often histologic material as well. Smaller-caliber needles also minimize bleeding, providing a margin of safety when multiple passes are required. Thin-gauge needles minimize complications from traversing the bowel.[4] However, they can be somewhat difficult to direct into lesions because they tend to deflect significantly, particularly in deep-seated lesions. Larger needles are easier to direct and provide better samples for cytology and histology, often with fewer needle passes. Unfortunately, the risk of hemorrhage may increase as needle size increases.[5]

Needles also are classified by tip configuration (Fig. 19-1).[7] Needles vary in the angle and bevel of the tip. The Chiba and spinal needles have bevel angles of 25 and 30 degrees, respectively. Greene, Madayag, and Franseen (or Crown) needles have 90-degree tips. Needle tips are classified also into noncutting (aspiration needles such as the Chiba or spinal) and cutting (end-cut or side-cut) types. Needles can be manual, spring-loaded, or automated.

The wide selection of needle types suggests that no design is clearly optimal and that needle selection should be based on physician preference in conjunction with consideration of the specific biopsy task at hand. In general, initial samples

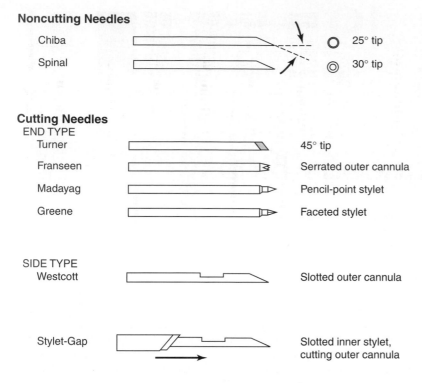

Noncutting Needles

Chiba   25° tip

Spinal   30° tip

Cutting Needles
END TYPE

Turner   45° tip

Franseen   Serrated outer cannula

Madayag   Pencil-point stylet

Greene   Faceted stylet

SIDE TYPE
Westcott   Slotted outer cannula

Stylet-Gap   Slotted inner stylet,
                 cutting outer cannula

FIGURE 19-1 ■ Standard needles used for percutaneous biopsy. All of the needles come with stylets. The spinal needle has a thicker wall than the Chiba needle. Unlike an 18-gauge spinal needle, an 18-gauge Chiba needle can accommodate a 0.035-inch guidewire. This feature is useful when aspiration yields infected fluid that requires drainage.

are obtained for cytologic analysis with fine-gauge (22-gauge) Chiba or spinal needles. If these needles do not yield satisfactory samples, a Franseen needle often yields cells for cytologic study. Superficial lesions are easy to reach; deep-seated ones may require larger-gauge needles to provide sufficient stiffness to direct the needle accurately. The vulnerability of organs along the anticipated path of the biopsy needle (e.g., pleura, bowel) may dictate needle selection, because smaller-gauge needles (>19 gauge) are relatively safe.

Preprocedure imaging characteristics also may guide needle selection. For example, smaller-gauge needles are used for metastatic disease and in patients with a known primary malignancy. In patients with no known primary malignancy at the time of biopsy or in patients with suspected lymphoma, multiple passes with fine-gauge needles or several passes with a large-gauge needle often is required to obtain adequate tissue for diagnosis. Physician experience is an important factor; automated devices yield better results if the operator is less experienced at obtaining core material by manual aspiration.

Imaging Guidance

The important factors in choosing an imaging modality for biopsy are lesion characteristics (e.g., size, location, depth), ability to visualize the abnormality, and operator experience and preference. Generally, the shortest path to the lesion is considered when planning the imaging approach, with the possible exception of peripherally located hypervascular hepatic lesions.

Fluoroscopy

Fluoroscopy is a common technique for biopsy of lung and pleural masses (Fig. 19-2). In the abdomen, fluoroscopy can be used for fine-needle biopsy of obstructing lesions of the biliary and urinary systems outlined by contrast material from percutaneously placed catheters. Disadvantages of this method include added radiation exposure to the operator and inability to visualize adjacent structures as the needle is advanced. Cross-sectional imaging studies (e.g., CT, ultrasound, MR) can be helpful in planning an approach when fluoroscopy is used.

Sonography

Ultrasound is very useful for biopsy of intra-abdominal lesions, including masses in the liver, pancreas, or kidney; bulky adenopathy in the retroperitoneum or root of the mesentery; and large adrenal masses.[8] In the chest, ultrasound is used for aspiration of pleural-based masses and fluid collections and occasionally can be used in the biopsy of peripheral pulmonary parenchymal lesions.

A complete diagnostic ultrasound study is obtained first to determine the conspicuity of the lesion, its depth, and a safe angle of approach. Ultrasound-guided biopsy can be performed with a free-hand technique or with the use of ultrasound guides. Sterilized probes or sterile probe covers allow real-time imaging while the biopsy is performed. Advantages of ultrasound include the lack of ionizing radiation, real-time imaging of needle position, and the multiplanar imaging capability that facilitates complex angled approaches often required to biopsy upper quadrant abdominal masses. Disadvantages include impaired visualization

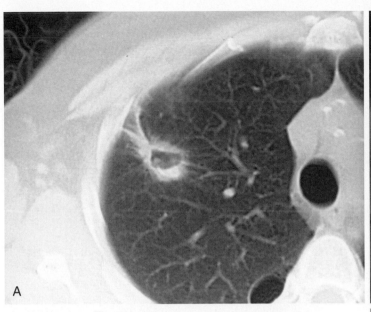

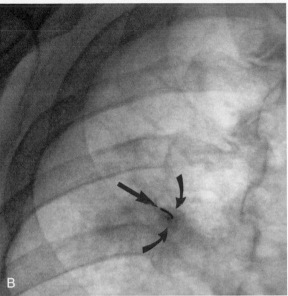

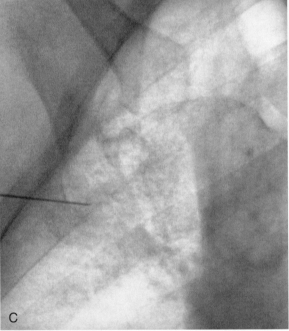

FIGURE 19-2 ■ Fluoroscopic lung biopsy. **A,** CT of the chest shows a 2-cm cavitary lesion with thickened, irregular walls and surrounding parenchymal infiltrate. **B,** Using CT to plan the approach, the needle is advanced under fluoroscopic visualization into the chest wall in the anteroposterior projection with the needle tip *(arrow)* and hub *(curved arrows)* aligned with the lesion. **C,** While the needle is still extrapleural and directly aligned with the lesion, the image intensifier is rotated, then the needle is advanced into the lesion with direct fluoroscopic visualization. The needle tip position is documented in at least two views. The biopsy is performed with fluoroscopy to ensure that the needle stays within the mass and samples different regions of the lesion. In this case, the diagnosis was coccidioidomycosis.

of deep lesions and obscuration by overlying bowel gas or bone.

Specifically designed and somewhat costly reflective needles are available. However, standard biopsy needles are visualized adequately at real-time sonography, particularly with gentle motion of the needle tip. Low-frequency transducers (e.g., 3.5-MHz sector probe) are needed for deeper lesions. Higher-frequency transducers (e.g., 7-MHz linear or phased-array probe) are used for biopsy of superficial masses such as thyroid nodules. Specifically designed probes for transvaginal and transrectal imaging have needle guides to facilitate biopsy of pelvic lesions.

The needle can be inserted perpendicular to the transducer, which may facilitate visualization by improved reflections from the needle shaft (Fig. 19-3).[8] Alternatively, the needle can be inserted in close to the ultrasound transducer.

Ideally, the entire needle should be visualized during passage through the tissues into the mass (Fig. 19-4). If the needle is not visible, misalignment between the needle path and ultrasound beam is occurring. A slight rocking motion back and forth of the ultrasound transducer may help visualize the needle. A gentle in-out motion of the needle may increase conspicuity of the needle tip as well. In every case, the needle tip should be documented as a discrete echogenic focus within the lesion in at least two views before biopsy (Fig. 19-5).

The advent of three-dimensional sonography has aided percutaneous biopsy by precise delineation of mass lesions and adjacent structures (such as blood vessels and bile ducts) in the anticipated needle pathway.[9] It also has been useful in guiding transjugular liver procedures and regional tumor ablation procedures because orthogonal images can

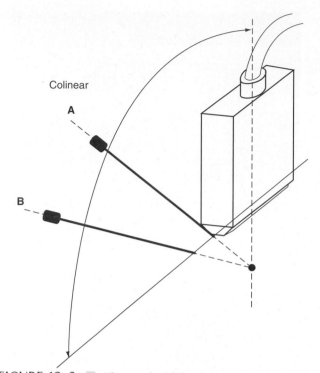

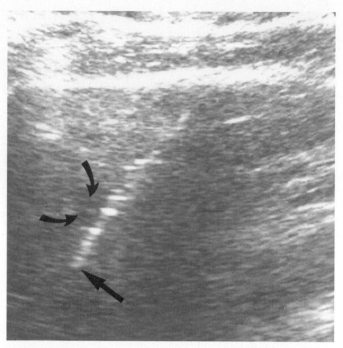

FIGURE 19-3 ■ Ultrasound-guided percutaneous biopsy. Using free-hand technique, the needle is placed at one end of the longitudinal face of the ultrasound probe **(A)**. The shaft is aligned parallel to the transducer as the needle is advanced to keep it within the sonographic field of view. If the needle is poorly seen, a more perpendicular angle **(B)** with the transducer may improve ultrasonographic reflections and make the needle more conspicuous. Needle guides are available on some ultrasound machines to simplify the biopsy.

FIGURE 19-4 ■ Ultrasound-guided percutaneous biopsy with visualization of the entire needle shaft *(straight arrow)* as it passes beyond a focal liver mass *(curved arrows)*.

be obtained in planes that are anatomically useful to the interventionalist performing the procedure.

Computed Tomography

CT is used for biopsy of smaller intra-abdominal and thoracic lesions not well seen by ultrasound or fluoroscopy. The patient is first scanned in the anticipated biopsy position (e.g., prone, supine, oblique) with images taken through the target area (Fig. 19-6). Intravenous contrast may be helpful in delineating vascular structures, in determining the vascularity of the target lesion, and for biopsy of lesions not well seen on unenhanced images (Fig. 19-7). A variety of devices is available to mark the skin during scanning and to determine the needle insertion site and angle.

A vertical needle pathway is preferable because it avoids the need for triangulation or accurate angle measurements. The needle should be visualized in the axial plane during the biopsy. Occasionally, gantry angulation may be helpful to visualize cranial-caudal angled approaches (e.g., adrenal biopsy, transthoracic biopsy with overlying ribs).

The advantages of CT include high-resolution image quality and the ability to visualize bowel. Disadvantages include additional radiation exposure for the patient, lack of real-time feedback during needle advancement and biopsy, and difficulty in using angled approaches required for targeting

abdominal masses high under the diaphragm. Spiral CT improves needle tip localization because of minimal respiratory motion artifact and fast scanning times.

CT fluoroscopy allows real-time monitoring of needle positioning during percutaneous biopsy. Since its introduction in 1996, various studies have outlined advantages and disadvantages of this technique for biopsy of various targets.[10] Advantages of CT fluoroscopy over conventional CT include the ability to time a patient's breathing to access moving lesions or to avoid ribs and other overlying structures. CT fluoroscopy allows the needle and lesion to be visualized during sampling to be sure the needle tip is properly located within the lesion. Using CT fluoroscopy in near real-time imaging requires either the operator's hands to be in the radiation beam or that special needle holders be used. The technique also is useful to perform peripheral lesional biopsy when central necrosis is present. CT fluoroscopy is not used universally, because some investigators are concerned about added radiation exposure and conflicting studies about reduced procedure times. CT fluoroscopy has been used most often for transthoracic biopsy, for which high rates of technical success have been reported with sensitivity ranging from 89% to 95% and specificity of 100%.[11] Several recent studies have shown that using intermittent "quick check" CT fluoroscopy between needle advancements instead of continuous (near real-time) fluoroscopy can reduce radiation doses significantly.

Magnetic Resonance Imaging

Several investigators have described initial experiences with MR-guided percutaneous biopsies. Potential advantages

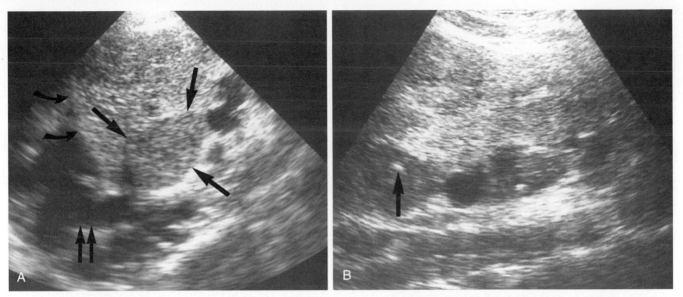

FIGURE 19-5 ▪ Ultrasound-guided percutaneous biopsy of a hepatic mass. The patient had cryptogenic cirrhosis and an incidental hypoechoic, 6-cm lesion in the medial segment of the left lobe. **A,** The sagittal image shows the lesion *(straight arrows),* pericardium *(curved arrows),* and inferior vena cava *(double arrows).* **B,** Real-time imaging shows the brightly echogenic needle tip within the lesion *(arrow).*

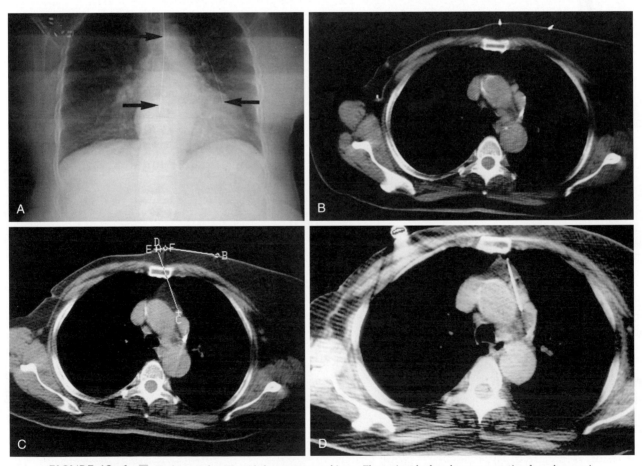

FIGURE 19-6 ▪ Technique for CT-guided percutaneous biopsy. The patient had undergone resection for colon carcinoma. Rising carcinoembryonic antigen titers were found later along with mediastinal lymphadenopathy on a CT scan. **A,** Using the initial diagnostic CT scan as a guide, the patient is positioned in the scanner with a grid marker taped to the skin *(arrows)* near the anticipated needle entry site. **B,** Scans are obtained through the lesion, and the table position that best shows the lesion is identified. Note the grid bars on the skin overlying the mass. **C,** Cursors measure the distance between grid bars (F-B), which allows determination of the cephalocaudal location of the lesion. The planned skin entry site is labeled A, and the depth of lesion is the distance from A to C. **D,** The needle is advanced in stages as serial scans follow its progress into the lesion. The needle tip is seen as a beam-hardening artifact. In this case, no malignant tissue was recovered.

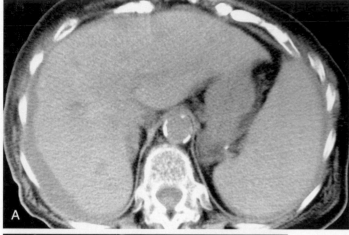

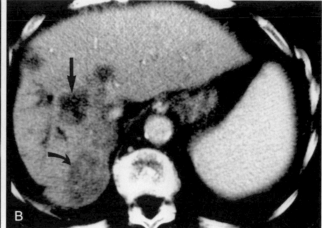

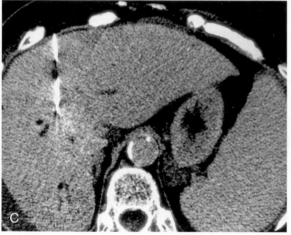

FIGURE 19-7   ■   Contrast enhancement during a CT-guided liver biopsy. The patient had a remote history of breast carcinoma and new liver masses. An earlier ultrasound-guided biopsy was nondiagnostic. **A,** The noncontrast CT scan reveals an inhomogeneous liver without clearly defined focal lesions. **B,** After contrast enhancement, the lesions become more apparent. Compare the lesion intended for biopsy *(straight arrow)* with the previous nondiagnostic lesion *(curved arrow)*. The patient also has segmental obstruction of some right lateral biliary radicals. **C,** Two needles were placed in the liver; the deeper needle is within the mass. The biopsy confirmed metastatic breast cancer.

include the ability to image lesions not readily seen by other modalities, multiplanar imaging capability, near real-time imaging during needle insertion, lack of ionizing radiation, and potential use of MR-guided tumor ablation in conjunction with biopsy.[12] Disadvantages include specially designed needles for compatibility with MR scanners, higher imaging costs, and special magnet configurations (i.e., open designs) to facilitate needle insertion.

Sampling Technique

Most biopsies are performed with the patient in a supine position, although prone and oblique positions can be used when necessary. With a few exceptions, the shortest path to the lesion is preferred. Hypervascular hepatic lesions should be approached through a sizable parenchymal track to reduce hemorrhagic complications (Fig. 19-8).[13] The likelihood of pneumothorax is reduced by minimizing the number of pleural surfaces crossed during chest and some abdominal biopsies. It is optimal to avoid traversing lung, pleura, pancreas, gallbladder, dilated or obstructed biliary ducts, and bowel during biopsy procedures. Small and large

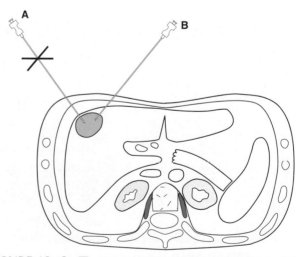

FIGURE 19-8   ■   Biopsy of suspected hypervascular peripheral hepatic lesions. Bleeding is more likely if the parenchymal track is short **(A),** With a tangential approach **(B),** a long parenchymal track should tamponade bleeding.

bowel can be crossed safely with small-gauge needles if no other pathway is available. However, sampling of intra-abdominal fluid collections through bowel loops is not advisable.

Usually it is best to start with smaller needles (e.g., 22 gauge) that can serve as localizers for subsequent needle placement. The sample is obtained by small oscillating and rotating motions of the needle hub while 5 to 10 mL of continuous suction is applied with a 10-mL syringe connected by extension tubing. During needle advancement and biopsy, the patient should suspend respiration to minimize inadvertent motion of the needle. With ultrasound, fluoroscopy, and CT fluoroscopy, the position of the needle tip can be observed continuously during biopsy so that different sectors of the lesion are sampled to increase the diagnostic yield. Before the needle is removed, the suction is released to prevent the entire sample from being aspirated into the tubing or syringe. Ideally, the biopsy is performed with a cytopathologist present.

If the sample is predominantly composed of red blood cells, a better sample may be obtained with a smaller-gauge needle (e.g., 25 gauge). A nonaspiration technique also can be used in which the needle is advanced and retracted through the lesion without suction.[14] Large lesions with necrotic centers may require biopsy of peripheral tissue to make a diagnosis (Fig. 19-9).

Single-Needle Technique

With the single-needle method, the needle is advanced into position, and its location is confirmed (Fig. 19-10). If the needle location is unsatisfactory, it is left in place to guide placement of a second needle. Each biopsy sample that is taken requires a new needle be placed into the lesion, adding to the complexity of the case and increasing risks for complications such as bleeding. This technique allows sampling of different regions of a mass, which may improve biopsy yield.

Two-Needle Technique

With the two-needle method, a needle is placed initially just superficial to the lesion to serve as a guide for subsequent needle passage and biopsy with a tandem or coaxial technique (see Fig. 19-10). Precise needle placement needs be done only once. The coaxial method is particularly useful with smaller or deep lesions that are difficult to localize. It has the further advantage that a single puncture of the visceral organ capsule (or pleura) is made, regardless of the number of biopsy needle passes that are made. The coaxial method is very commonly used for percutaneous biopsy. A disadvantage of this method is that the sampling path of the biopsy needle is limited by the direction of the outer guiding needle.

Specimen Handling

An optimal cytologic specimen consists of a small amount of soft or semiliquid material with minimal bloody contamination.[15] Smears should be composed of a thin layer of cells and fragments; blood dilutes and obscures the diagnostic material. Clotting of the specimen can be minimized by expeditious sample preparation and prerinsing the aspiration syringe and needle with a small amount of heparinized saline. Small-gauge needles (e.g., 25 gauge) also limit the blood content of the aspirate.

A small amount of aspirated material first is placed on a slide. The material is spread and then air dried or fixed in alcohol. Air-dried samples are stained with Diff-Quik (Baxter Healthcare, McGraw Park, Ill.) for prompt diagnosis.

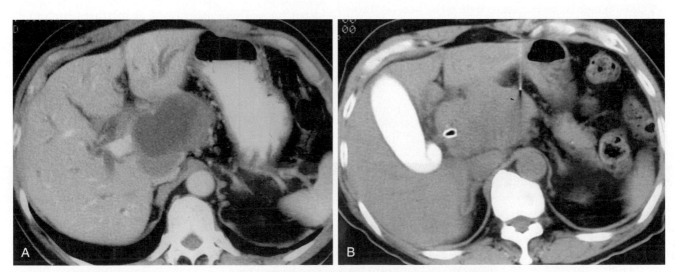

FIGURE 19-9 ■ Value of sampling multiple regions of a lesion during percutaneous biopsy. The patient had an epigastric mass, obstructive jaundice, and ascending cholangitis. **A,** CT demonstrates a large pancreatic mass encasing the hepatic artery and displacing the portal vein, with extension of the mass into the porta hepatis. The patient had undergone biliary stenting with nondiagnostic bile duct brushings. Initial samples from a CT-guided biopsy (not shown) from the center of the lesion revealed only necrotic cells. **B,** Sampling the periphery of the lesion revealed adenocarcinoma. The gallbladder contrast is residual from a recent endoscopic retrograde cholangiopancreatography.

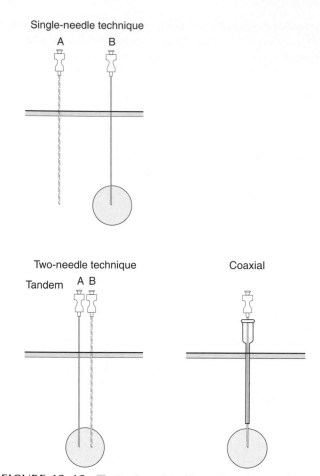

FIGURE 19-10 ■ Single- and double-needle techniques for percutaneous biopsy. **Upper panel,** Single-needle technique. If the initial pass misses the lesion, the needle (A) is used to redirect a second needle (B) into the lesion. With each attempt, a new needle is reinserted with imaging guidance. **Lower panel,** Two-needle technique. With the tandem method **(left),** a second needle (A) is slid alongside the landmark needle (B) and then used to perform the biopsy. The original needle is left in place to guide subsequent needle insertions. With the coaxial method **(right),** a larger needle (18 or 19 gauge) is inserted just up to the mass. The biopsy is performed with a longer, smaller-gauge needle (22 gauge) inside the outer guiding needle.

Larger tissue fragments or material are placed in a tube or container of 10% neutral buffered formalin for processing as a cell block. This step is particularly important if immunohistochemical staining is required for diagnosis. Occasionally, the core sample can be used to perform a "touch preparation" in which the core sample is slid onto a slide, which is then processed similarly as other cytologic samples. The remaining core sample is processed for histologic exam.

Care after Biopsy

After the biopsy is completed, imaging is performed to exclude potential complications (e.g., upright chest radiographs 1 and 4 hours after percutaneous chest biopsy or sonography of perihepatic spaces, paracolic gutters, and pelvis after percutaneous liver biopsy). The patient is monitored for 2 to 4 hours after the procedure while intravenous access is maintained and vital signs are obtained frequently.

If the patient has remained stable and no new clinical symptoms develop (e.g., chest pain, shortness of breath, abdominal pain, distention), the patient is discharged home with a family member. If vital signs are abnormal or symptoms develop, additional imaging may be required to exclude a complication.

■ SPECIFIC APPLICATIONS

Chest

Patient Selection

Percutaneous chest biopsy is performed for evaluation of nodules or masses in the lung, hilum, mediastinum, pleura, and chest wall.[16,17] In general, masses that involve lobar or segmental bronchi on chest radiography or CT suggest the presence of an endobronchial lesion, and these are best approached with bronchoscopy. On the other hand, peripherally located lesions are not that accessible with bronchoscopy and are easily reached with percutaneous biopsy. The most common indication for percutaneous chest biopsy is the diagnosis of a solitary pulmonary nodule (SPN), which is a rounded, well-defined mass of less than 3 cm that is largely surrounded by lung. Percutaneous biopsy, particularly core biopsy in conjunction with fine-needle aspiration, has been advocated for diagnosing pneumonia and mimics of pneumonia (i.e., bronchiolitis obliterans organizing pneumonia, neoplasms [lymphoma, bronchoalveolar cell carcinoma], eosinophic pneumonia, vasculitis [Wegener's granulomatosis]).[18] Percutaneous biopsy should be strictly avoided with suspected vascular lesions (e.g., arteriovenous malformation, pulmonary varix) and *Echinococcus* cysts. Relative contraindications to lung biopsy include severe obstructive pulmonary disease, moderate to severe pulmonary hypertension, contralateral pneumonectomy, ventilator dependence, and inability to cooperate with breathing instructions. These patients are at increased risk of or less able to tolerate pneumothorax after biopsy.

The workup of pulmonary lesions varies significantly among institutions with regard to the use of percutaneous needle biopsy or surgical resection for an SPN. The probability that an SPN represents a primary lung tumor rather than a metastasis from a known malignancy depends largely on the primary tumor type (e.g., 1:1.2 for colon cancer, 3.3:1 for breast cancer, 3.3:1 for bladder cancer, and 8.3:1 for head and neck cancers).[17] The false-negative rate for needle biopsy in patients with malignancy is relatively high (up to one third of procedures).[18,19] The cases in which clinical suspicion of malignancy is high require repeat biopsy and/or close follow-up. In some centers, a potentially malignant SPN in a low-risk operative patient often is resected without prior needle biopsy.

Technique

Ideally, lung nodules are visualized on posteroanterior and lateral chest radiographs. CT is helpful in planning all chest biopsies. CT can identify the most accessible lung lesion or an extrapulmonary mass that can be biopsied more safely (e.g., liver or adrenal gland). CT also outlines bullae that should be avoided to reduce the likelihood of post-biopsy pneumothorax.

Whenever possible, fluoroscopy is preferred for transthoracic biopsy. Sonography can be used for some pleural or pleural-based masses. Fluoroscopy-guided chest biopsies are greatly facilitated with the use of a C-arm (see Fig. 19-2). The needle and hub are aligned with the lesion in one view while the needle is placed initially through the skin. The tube is then rotated into the orthogonal projection as the needle is advanced to the proper depth within the lesion. Aspiration of material is performed under direct fluoroscopic visualization, with spot images documenting needle position in various projections. The technique for CT biopsy is described above. Anterior mediastinal masses can be approached through the sternum (see Fig. 19-6).[20] With very large mediastinal masses a parasternal approach can be used keeping in mind the course of the internal mammary arteries (Fig. 19-11). Artificial widening of the extrapleural (paravertebral or substernal) space by injection of saline has been used to facilitate biopsy of lesions located in the posterior or anterior mediastinum.[21] An alternative approach to mediastinal lesions avoids visceral pleural traversal by using an existing pleural effusion or an iatrogenically created pneumothorax.[22]

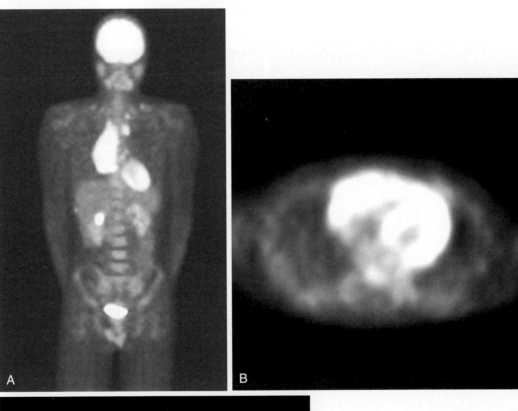

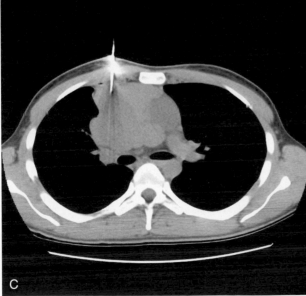

FIGURE 19-11 ■ A 20-year-old male was admitted with chest pain. A CT of the chest was obtained to exclude pulmonary embolism, but it revealed a large right anterior mediastinal mass. **A,** A whole-body positron emission tomography (PET) scan in coronal projection shows intense uptake along the right mediastinal border. **B,** Axial PET scan confirms the intense uptake of the right anterior mediastinal mass. Also note uptake in cardiac structures. **C,** CT image of biopsy procedure that was performed with coaxial 22- and 20-gauge needles for cytology and several passes with an 18-gauge coring needle. It is imperative to identify the location of the internal mammary artery using this approach so that it is not compromised. The final diagnosis was Hodgkin's lymphoma.

If a significant pneumothorax occurs, a chest tube can be placed and the biopsy procedure continued or postponed. Upright chest radiographs are obtained after the procedure (e.g., immediately and 4 hours after) to exclude a pneumothorax.

Results

Percutaneous needle biopsy of the chest is 80% to 95% accurate in the diagnosis of malignant lesions with a lower yield for benign lesions.[17-19,23] The probability of malignancy is partly a function of size (Table 19-1).[24] Patients with a

TABLE 19-1	RELATIONSHIP BETWEEN PULMONARY NODULE SIZE AND MALIGNANCY

Diameter of Solitary Pulmonary Nodule (cm)	Malignant (%)
0–1	36
1–2	51
2–3	82
>3	97

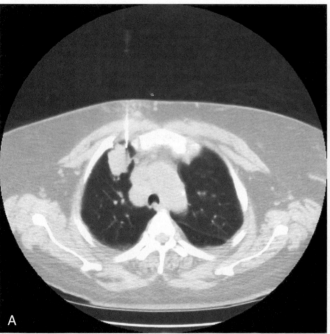

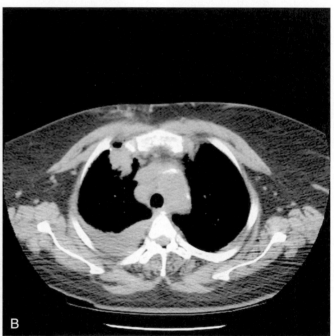

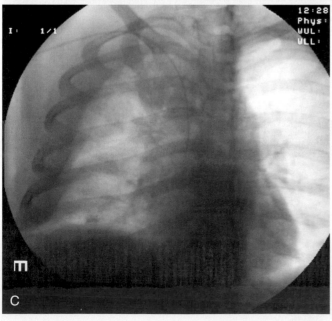

FIGURE 19-12 ■ A 54-year-old female patient with a 20-pack-year history of smoking was admitted with a right upper lobe lung mass and right hilar and mediastinal lymphadenopathy. She was sent for percutaneous lung biopsy. She had thrombocytopenia and she was given platelet transfusions. **A,** CT image shows the course of the needle, which is right parasternal and into the right upper lobe lesion. **B,** A post-biopsy CT image of the chest showed no pneumothorax, but there was interval development of pleural effusion with attenuation similar to that of muscle consistent with hemothorax. **C,** Plain chest radiograph confirms the hemothorax, which was evacuated with chest tube insertion. Treatment options at this point may include angiography to attempt to identify the bleeding site, such as an intercostal or internal mammary artery, which could be embolized. She was found to have small cell lung cancer.

nonspecific diagnosis need close follow-up, with repeat imaging and repeat percutaneous biopsy.

Complications

The most common complication of lung biopsy is pneumothorax, which occurs in 10% to 35% of cases. The risk of pneumothorax is increased with preexisting lung disease, number of needle passes, and advanced age. Nearly all pneumothoraces appear on the 1-hour postbiopsy chest film, and essentially all are detected on radiographs obtained 4 hours after biopsy.

Most cases can be managed conservatively; repeat films are obtained to document reduction or resolution of the pneumothorax. Treatment is required for about 5% to 15% of patients, based on development of symptoms, an enlarging pneumothorax, or pneumothorax that occupies over 25% of the hemithorax. Some pneumothoraces respond to simple aspiration with a plastic cannula.[25,26] In a minority of cases, however, a chest drainage tube is required.

Anterior access is gained through the second intercostal space in the mid-clavicular line. A direct trocar technique is used to place a 8- to 10-French chest tube if a large pneumothorax is present. Smaller pneumothoraces can be entered using the Seldinger method as well. Air is removed by aspiration, Pleur-evac device, or Heimlich valve. Some operators clamp the tube (or place to water seal) soon after placement and remove it if the pneumothorax does not recur soon thereafter. Otherwise, patients are admitted overnight.

Additional complications include pulmonary hemorrhage, hemothorax (Fig. 19-12), hemoptysis, malignant needle tract seeding, and systemic air embolism (Fig. 19-13).[27,28] Systemic air embolism is a rare (<0.07%), potentially fatal complication that also may result in neurologic morbidity. The formation of a communication between an airway and a pulmonary vein is one assumed mechanism of air embolism during biopsy. An uncooperative patient that coughs during the biopsy procedure may contribute to pulmonary venous air by the increased air pressure in the bronchial tree while coughing. Another mechanism may occur when the needle tip is positioned within a pulmonary vein and air enters the lumen of the needle. The last mechanism of systemic air embolism is air introduced into the pulmonary arterial circulation may advance into the pulmonary veins by traversing the pulmonary microcirculation, even without presence of an arteriovenous malformation. Very rarely, coronary air embolism may result in myocardial infarction, cardiac arrest, or dysrhythmias. Hyperbaric oxygen is one possible treatment modality for such cases.

Liver

Patient Selection

Liver biopsy may be performed by an operative, percutaneous, or transvenous route. Surgical biopsy is indicated when an abdominal operation is planned regardless of the biopsy results. Percutaneous techniques are used to obtain

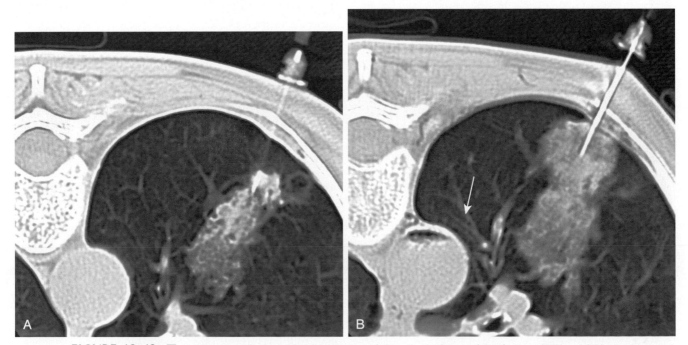

FIGURE 19-13 ■ A 77-year-old female with a long history of cigarette smoking and emphysema (FEV$_1$ < 0.9 L) on home oxygen use was found to have a left lower lobe pulmonary nodule. She was referred for percutaneous lung biopsy. **A,** CT image during the biopsy, performed with the patient in a prone position, shows the needle in the lesion with pulmonary hemorrhage extending anteriorly from the lesion. **B,** The patient had an uncontrolled episode of coughing during which air was aspirated into the needle. She had a grand mal seizure. A repeat CT of the chest demonstrates air within the thoracic aorta *(arrow)*, intercostal, and spinal arteries. She responded to supportive measures and was found to have a lung adenocarcinoma, which was treated with radiation therapy (she was not a surgical candidate).

fine-needle aspirates for cytology and core biopsy; the latter is required when architectural detail is needed for diagnosis and staging of diffuse liver diseases. Transvenous liver biopsy is used in patients with coagulation disorders, massive ascites, portal hypertension, morbid obesity, or large vascular tumors (see Chapter 10). Reports differ about the relative safety of percutaneous biopsy in patients with massive ascites.[29]

Technique

The primary indication for percutaneous liver biopsy is the diagnosis of focal liver lesions (Box 19-1). Liver biopsy is performed with image guidance to evaluate diffuse liver disease such as hepatitis and cirrhosis. Hepatic masses can be approached with ultrasound or CT, including CT fluoroscopy (see Fig. 19-7). Real-time imaging with sonography greatly facilitates the procedure (see Figs. 19-4 and 19-5). CT is necessary for lesions that are not well seen by ultrasound. CT of small liver lesions is affected by respiratory motion, although this problem is minimized with spiral techniques. Many hepatic masses that require biopsy lie deep to the lower ribs and the pleural space. Whenever possible, a subcostal approach should be chosen to avoid traversing the pleura and producing a pneumothorax. A steep subcostal approach combined with deep inspiration often is required to reach lesions high on the dome of the liver. Ultrasound is preferred in this case, because sufficient gantry angulation with CT usually is not possible. An intercostal, transpulmonary approach avoiding aerated lung can be done with CT with a small risk of pneumothorax.[30] Recognition of colonic

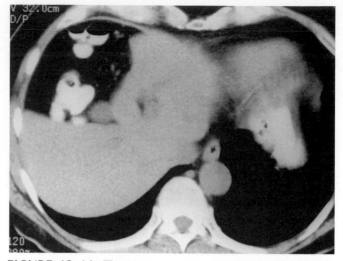

FIGURE 19-14 ■ Effect of colonic position on percutaneous liver biopsy. The initial biopsy to exclude hemochromatosis was performed without imaging guidance and was nondiagnostic. The proximal portion of the right colon is interposed between the right lobe of the liver and the hemidiaphragm. Biopsy through this route is relatively unsafe.

interposition (i.e., Chilaiditi's syndrome) also is important when planning a liver biopsy (Fig. 19-14).

Aspiration biopsy for cytologic analysis is sufficient for many focal hepatic lesions. However, core biopsy is required for the diagnosis of certain liver tumors.

Results

A retrospective study of 510 percutaneous liver biopsies using cytology alone showed a 1% frequency of nondiagnostic biopsies and a 94% sensitivity and a 93% specificity for tumor.[31] Unfortunately, false-positive results occurred in 18 cases (7% of all benign lesions) and false-negative results were obtained in 14 cases (5% of all malignant lesions). Cytologic liver biopsy may be limited for several reasons:

■ Inherent similarity of hemangioma, focal nodular hyperplasia, and hepatic adenoma to well-differentiated hepatocellular carcinoma
■ Reactive changes in hepatocytes related to acute and chronic inflammation or infection mimicking malignant cells
■ Liver cirrhosis and parasitic infections failing to provide a cytologic diagnosis

Most hemangiomas larger than 3 cm can be diagnosed with scintigraphy, MR imaging, or CT scanning. Suspected hemangiomas can be biopsied safely if small needles are used (e.g., 20 to 25 gauge) and the needle passes through a normal parenchymal track en route to the lesion.[32] Biopsy of hemangiomas most often yields blood. The presence of endothelial cells suggests hemangioma; the finding of capillary vessels in conjunction with blood and endothelial cells is diagnostic (Fig. 19-15).

Ultrasound-guided biopsy of portal venous thrombi is safe and effective.[33] The procedure is aided by color flow imaging and can stage and diagnose hepatocellular carcinoma.

BOX 19-1 ■ **Focal Lesions of the Liver**

Benign Lesions
Simple cyst*
Cavernous hemangioma*
Focal nodular hyperplasia*
Regenerating nodule
Adenoma*
Focal fatty replacement*
Amebic abscess†
Pyogenic abscess
Echinococcal cyst*†
Hematoma*
Infarct
Pseudoaneurysm*

Malignant Lesions
Hepatocellular carcinoma*†
Cholangiocarcinoma
Metastases
Lymphoma
Angiosarcoma

---

*Imaging alone may provide a diagnosis.
†Laboratory studies (e.g., serology) may aid the diagnosis.

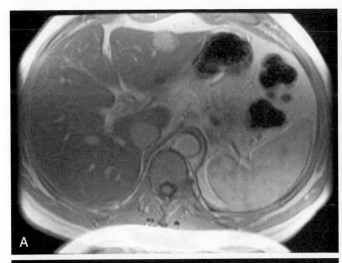

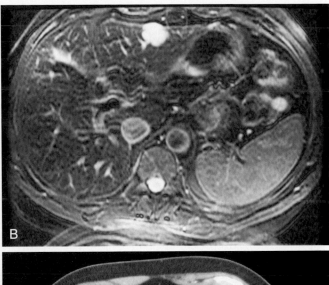

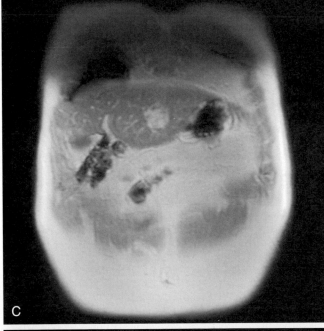

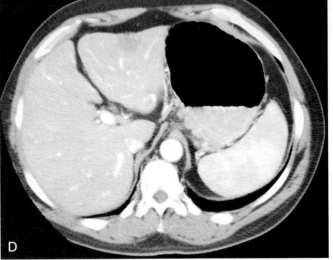

FIGURE 19-15 ■ A 67-year-old male patient with a history of colorectal cancer was found to have a lesion in the left lobe of the liver during follow-up imaging. Axial T1 and T2 and coronal T1 images of the liver (**A, B,** and **C**) were felt to be atypical for hemangioma, and biopsy was suggested. CT images in arterial and delayed phases confirm the CT findings (**D** and **E**). A biopsy was performed with ultrasound and the diagnosis was hemangioma. There was no postbiopsy bleeding.

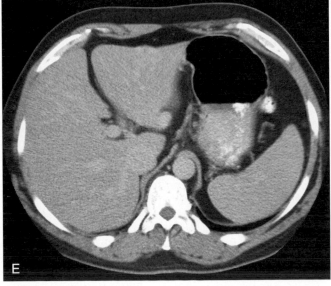

Complications

The major complications of percutaneous liver biopsy are bleeding, pneumothorax, malignant needle track seeding, and infection. Although rare, fatal hemorrhage can result, particularly after biopsy of a hemangioma or hypervascular neoplasm. Hemorrhagic complications from liver biopsy of diffuse liver diseases are less common than with biopsy of malignant lesions. Bleeding usually occurs within several hours of the procedure and often can be managed conservatively.[34] Hemorrhage may occur into the peritoneum or into the biliary system (i.e., *hematobilia*). Less than 5% of outpatient liver biopsy patients requires admission.

The most common signs of significant bleeding are abdominal or shoulder pain and hemodynamic instability. When clinical suspicion arises, serial hematocrits and CT or ultrasound imaging should be obtained. In patients who continue to bleed, angiography and transcatheter embolization may be required to control bleeding. Needle track seeding is less frequent than with biopsy of the pancreas. Fatal carcinoid crisis has been reported after biopsy of liver metastases.[35]

Adrenal Gland

Patient Selection

Percutaneous biopsy is used for diagnosing focal lesions of the adrenal gland. The most common adrenal masses are nonfunctioning adenomas and metastases (Box 19-2).[36] Adrenal adenomas are seen in as many as 5% of patients undergoing CT. In an asymptomatic patient with an adrenal mass, the size of the mass and the presence or absence of a primary malignancy must be considered in determining the need for biopsy. When adrenal lesions are larger than 3 cm,

the likelihood of malignancy is much greater than with smaller lesions. Even in patients with a known primary and an adrenal lesion, the likelihood of a positive biopsy is only about 50%. In some cases, nonfunctioning adenomas can be diagnosed confidently by CT (noncontrast CT with threshold values to detect low attenuation or contrast washout methods) or chemical shift MR imaging without the need for tissue sampling. Application of these cross-sectional methods has reduced the number of adrenal biopsies yielding benign diagnoses to less than 12% in patients with extra-adrenal malignancies.[37] When adrenal masses smaller than 1 cm are detected in patients undergoing imaging procedures for nonadrenal problems (e.g., kidney stones, trauma, and nonspecific abdominal pain), these masses are called adrenal "incidentalomas."[38] These should all be evaluated for hormonal activity, including 1-mg overnight dexamethasone suppression test; total 24-hour urinary metanephrines and fractionated catecholamines; and, in hypertensive patients, a serum potassium level and plasma aldosterone concentration–to–plasma renin activity ratio. All hormonally active tumors are resected. Inactive tumors are resected based on size, imaging characteristics, and interval growth. Percutaneous biopsy of these incidentalomas is generally unwarranted.

Technique

Adrenal masses often are best approached posteriorly, respecting the location of pleural reflections. Other routes include a transhepatic approach for right-sided lesions and an anterior approach for left-sided lesions. Unfortunately, the latter route is associated with a 6% incidence of pancreatitis.[39]

Results and Complications

In a large study of percutaneous biopsy of adrenal masses, the reported sensitivity was 93%, accuracy was 96%, and the negative predictive value was 91%.[40] Repeat biopsy was recommended in cases in which the sample did not contain benign adrenal tissue or malignant cells. Adrenal adenoma and adrenocortical carcinoma may be difficult to distinguish histopathologically. If a discrepancy exists between the imaging and pathology results, surgical intervention may be advocated.

The complication rate after adrenal biopsy is 1% to 11%. The most common complication is pneumothorax. Postprocedure chest radiographs must be obtained to exclude this possibility. Other adverse events include bleeding, pancreatitis, hemothorax, and, rarely, precipitation of a hypertensive crisis from biopsy of an unsuspected pheochromocytoma.[41] Reported complications from biopsy of pheochromocytomas have included transient headaches, labile blood pressures, abdominal pain, hemodynamic instability, uncontrolled hemorrhage, and death. An acute hypertensive crisis is treated with phentolamine (1 mg IV) followed by intravenous infusion of phentolamine (20 mg in 500 mL of 5% dextrose) titrated to the blood pressure. A nitroprusside drip (50 mg in 500 mL of 5% dextrose) is also effective. If cardiac arrhythmias occur, propranolol is given intravenously at 1 mg/minute for a total of 5 to 10 mg.

BOX 19-2   ■   Focal Lesions of the Adrenal Glands

Unilateral Lesions
Metastases
Primary adenocarcinoma
Benign adenoma*†
   Functional
   Nonfunctional
Pheochromocytoma†
Neuroblastoma
Myelolipoma*
Adrenal cyst*

Bilateral Lesions
Metastases
Hemorrhage*
Tuberculosis or histoplasmosis
Bilateral pheochromocytoma†

---

*Imaging alone may provide a diagnosis.
†Laboratory studies may aid the diagnosis.

Because pheochromocytoma has no specific imaging features, the diagnosis is based on clinical suspicion with confirmatory testing via a 24-hour urine collection for catecholamines and their breakdown products or serum catecholamines.

Pancreas

Patient Selection

Percutaneous pancreatic biopsy most often is performed for the diagnosis of suspected ductal adenocarcinoma in patients who are considered to be unsuitable for surgery by imaging studies. Operative candidates often go directly to laparotomy. The differential diagnosis of pancreatic masses is wide (Box 19-3).

Technique

Pancreatic biopsy is performed with CT or ultrasound guidance. If the stomach or small bowel lies in the anticipated needle pathway, small-caliber needles (e.g., 20 to 22 gauge) should be used. Traversal of the colon should be avoided.

Transsplenic biopsy of lesions in the tail of the pancreas (avoiding the splenic hilum) is relatively safe with small-gauge needles. A posterior transcaval approach to pancreatic biopsy of lesions in or near the head of the pancreas has recently been described.[11]

Results

Historically, the overall yield for percutaneous biopsy diagnosis of pancreatic malignancy is about 80%. It is believed that these modest results are related to the scirrhous nature of the tumor and the surrounding desmoplastic, inflammatory reaction. Later series have reported accuracies of 86% and 95% for CT and ultrasound-guided biopsy, respectively.[42] The higher rates for ultrasound may relate to the better lesional conspicuity of pancreatic lesions with ultrasound. CT with contrast may improve the accuracy of pancreatic biopsies. Results are better for larger lesions (>3 cm) with larger needles (16 to 19 gauge) and when the lesion is located in the body or tail of the gland. In addition to standard cytologic evaluation of tissue, fluid analysis for viscosity, enzymes, and tumor markers may be valuable for cystic lesions.[43]

Complications

Complications develop after approximately 3% of procedures and include hemorrhage, pancreatitis, and pancreatic duct fistulas. Pancreatitis may be more common after biopsy of a normal gland.[44] Because rapid intra-abdominal spread of disease has been described after intraoperative biopsy of pancreatic tumors, some surgeons believe that percutaneous biopsy should be avoided if curative resection is planned. Track seeding from needle biopsy has been reported, but it is rare.[45]

Kidney

Patient Selection

Renal disorders may be divided into diffuse processes that produce medical renal diseases and focal mass lesions.[46] Large-core biopsy for medical renal disease often is performed by a nephrologist, with limited imaging guidance. Occasionally, a radiologist is asked to perform such a biopsy in situations in which the nephrologist is unable to obtain adequate material. Focal, solid mass lesions in patients with no known malignancy usually undergo operative biopsy or resection. Indications for biopsy of solid renal masses include suspected lymphoma and metastatic disease. Percutaneous kidney biopsy by an interventional radiologist has several indications:

- Medical renal disease when imaging is difficult (e.g., obese patients, atrophic kidneys) or initial biopsy is inadequate
- Focal renal mass in a patient with underlying malignancy
- Focal renal mass in a nonoperative patient
- Focal renal mass in a patient with fever of unknown origin
- Evaluation of complex cysts

Technique

Biopsy of focal renal masses is performed with ultrasound guidance.[46] CT is required when the mass is difficult to visualize with sonography (Fig. 19-16). A posterior approach is used.

Biopsy for medical renal disease and transplantation complications usually is performed with ultrasound guidance. Biopsy of the lower pole is preferred to avoid vessels in the renal hilum or possible injury to the liver or spleen. Large-core biopsy (16 to 18 gauge, usually with an automated device) is required to obtain the 5 to 10 glomeruli needed for diagnosis.[47,48] Transjugular renal biopsy can be applied in patients at high risk for bleeding complications.

BOX 19-3 ■ Focal Lesions of the Pancreas

Neoplastic Lesions
Ductal adenocarcinoma
Islet cell (neuroendocrine) tumor
Cystic neoplasm
Papilloma (intraductal)
Lymphoma
Sarcoma or other mesenchymal tumor

Non-neoplastic Lesions
Focal pancreatitis
Abscess
Hemorrhage (including pseudoaneurysms)
Pseudocyst
Fluid collection
Hydatid cysts

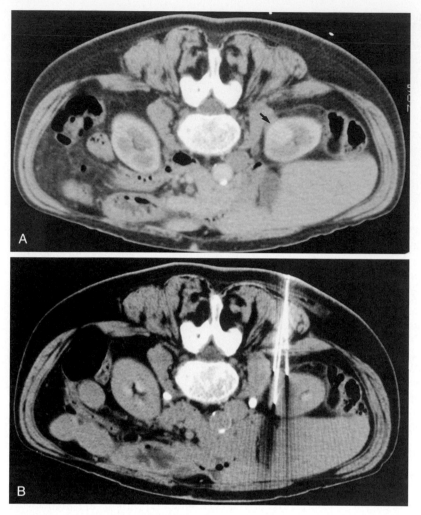

FIGURE 19-16   ■   CT-guided kidney biopsy. **A,** CT in the prone position shows a hyperdense right renal mass *(arrow)* in a patient with cutaneous melanoma. Grid bars are taped to the skin over the lesion. **B,** Three passes were made with 22-gauge Chiba needles. The outer needles missed the lesion but were left in place to assist with accurate placement of the third needle just beyond the mass.

Results and Complications

Using 18-gauge needles, a diagnosis is established in 85% to 95% of patients with medical renal disease.[49]

Complications follow about 1% to 6% of percutaneous renal biopsies.[47,50] After biopsy, small arteriovenous fistulas and pseudoaneurysms are relatively common. Many of these close spontaneously without the need for treatment. Significant hematomas with falling hematocrit levels and persistent gross hematuria are uncommon. A prospective study of medical renal biopsies in 471 patients found that 161 (34.1%) of patients experienced postbiopsy bleeding (33.3% hematomas, 0.4% gross hematuria, 0.4% arteriovenous fistula).[51] Major complications occurred in six patients (1.2%), with two requiring blood transfusions, three requiring angiograms, and one requiring nephrectomy. There were no deaths. Angiographic evaluation and transcatheter embolization are required occasionally for treatment of bleeding that does not stop with conservative measures.

Spleen

Splenic biopsies rarely are performed because focal masses are uncommon. Although there is particular concern about splenic hemorrhage, biopsy with 20- to 22-gauge Chiba or spinal needles is relatively safe.[52] Biopsy may be performed with CT or ultrasound guidance. The largest, most superficial lesion usually is chosen; the splenic hilum, colon, kidney, lung, and pleura should be avoided. Hemorrhage is the most common complication (typically 0 to 1.5% but as high as 10% of patients); other complications include pneumothorax, pleural effusion, and colonic injury.

Other Abdominal and Pelvic Sites

Retroperitoneal masses can be approached from an anterior or posterior route. The major disadvantage of the anterior approach is that bowel may be traversed. However, this route is reasonable if cytologic analysis using small-caliber needles is sufficient. If lymphoma is suspected, core biopsy may be required for immunocytochemical studies, flow cytometry, cytogenetic analysis, or molecular studies, and a posterior route is preferable. Biopsies of almost all retroperitoneal masses are conducted under CT or ultrasound guidance.

Metastatic lymphadenopathy from tumors of the gastrointestinal and genitourinary tracts can be diagnosed in about 65% to 90% of cases.[53] Historically, the diagnostic accuracy

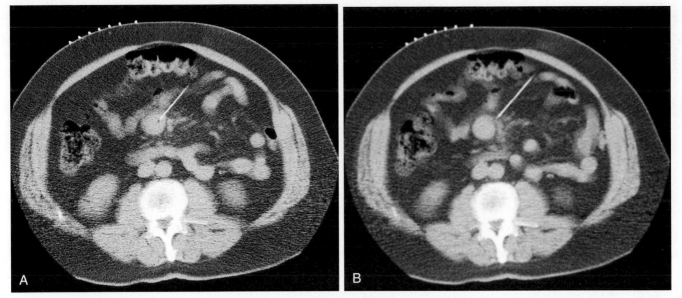

FIGURE 19-17   ■   An 80-year-old male patient with abdominal pain was found to have lymphadenopathy that slowly enlarged on follow-up serial CT scans of the abdomen. **A** and **B,** CT-guided biopsy shows percutaneous biopsy performed around surrounding, adjacent bowel loops.

of percutaneous biopsy in patients with lymphoma is about 20% lower than for nonlymphomatous retroperitoneal lesions. Later series reported higher success rates.[54] A negative percutaneous biopsy cannot entirely exclude a malignant process. If several properly performed biopsy attempts fail to provide a cytologic or histologic diagnosis, an excisional biopsy may be required. The yield for malignant forms of retroperitoneal fibrosis is relatively low, and surgical biopsy often is needed to identify the diffusely dispersed malignant cells that are characteristic of this condition.[55]

Peritoneal soft tissue masses and *mesenteric lymphadenopathy* are amenable to percutaneous biopsy techniques. Ultrasound guidance greatly facilitates biopsy of these entities.[56] Such lesions often are better visualized by external compression with the transducer to displace bowel loops overlying the mass. Deeper lesions can be approached with CT (Fig. 19-17). Biopsy of peritoneal masses poses a small risk of ileus or peritonitis (<1%).

Pelvic lymphadenopathy or *soft tissue masses* can be approached through transperitoneal (anterior or transgluteal), extraperitoneal, transvaginal, or transrectal routes. The transvaginal approach is useful especially for biopsy of primary or recurrent adnexal or ovarian masses.[57] For diagnosis of metastatic prostate cancer, CT-guided biopsy with thin section CT is accurate in up to 97% of cases.[58]

Presacral masses in patients who have undergone abdominoperineal resection can be evaluated with percutaneous biopsy. Although such masses are not uncommon in postoperative patients, a rising carcinoembryonic antigen level or asymmetric thickening of the presacral space may indicate recurrence. These lesions are accessed easily through a transgluteal approach, taking care to avoid the sciatic nerve running in the anterior third of the greater sciatic notch.

Percutaneous biopsy techniques also can be applied to a variety of uncommon intra-abdominal or intrapelvic lesions, including omental cakes, mesenteric root masses, and mucosal lesions of the stomach, bile ducts, or urinary tract (Fig. 19-18).

Thyroid

Patient Selection

Thyroid nodules are the most common pathologic finding in the thyroid gland.[59] In general, about 4% to 7% of the population of the United States has clinically palpable thyroid nodules. The incidence of thyroid nodules increases with age and is more prevalent in females of all ages. Autopsy studies indicate that clinical exam has limited ability to detect nodules, particularly smaller nodules and nodules situated deeper within the thyroid gland. Several studies also have shown that ultrasound of a patient's thyroid gland that has a normal physical exam demonstrates occult nodules in about 50% of cases. Many nodules are brought to attention as a result of other diagnostic imaging studies, such as chest CT, carotid sonography, and cervical spine MR imaging. Less than 5% of thyroid nodules are malignant. Thyroid cancer is the most common malignancy of the endocrine system, with more than 80% representing papillary thyroid carcinoma.[59] In 2005, 25,690 new cases of thyroid cancer are expected to be diagnosed in the United States, with estimated deaths from thyroid cancer at 1,490.[60]

Clearly, there is a need to differentiate the uncommon but important thyroid carcinoma from the common, insignificant thyroid nodule (Table 19-2). Unfortunately, there is much overlap in the ultrasonographic appearance of benign and malignant nodules (Fig. 19-19).[61] Ultrasonographic features suggesting malignancy include a solid, hypoechoic nodule; punctuate calcifications; a poorly defined, indistinct, or blurred lesional margin; direct invasion of the nodule through the thyroid capsule; and central rather than peripheral vascularity within the lesion.[59,62] Note that size of a nodule is not a reliable indicator of the benign or malignant nature of thyroid nodules. Hyperechoic nodules, cystic nodules, and nodules with complete halos are typically benign. In most cases, fine-needle aspiration biopsy of the thyroid can differentiate benign

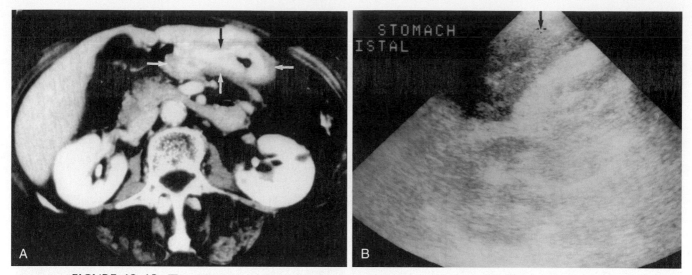

FIGURE 19-18 ■ Percutaneous gastric wall biopsy. The patient had multiple negative endoscopic gastric biopsies. The upper gastrointestinal series had a linitis plastica appearance. **A,** CT scan shows diffuse gastric wall thickening *(arrows).* **B,** The biopsy under sonographic guidance *(arrow)* revealed signet cell–positive gastric carcinoma.

nodules from thyroid neoplasms, which has reduced the number of patients undergoing surgical excision of benign nodules.

Risk factors for thyroid cancer include family history of thyroid malignancy, a history of prior head and neck radiation, age younger than 30 years or older than 60 years, and patients with multiple endocrine neoplasia type 2.

Technique

The patient is asked to lie supine on a stretcher. Neck extension aids in visualizing the thyroid gland; this can be obtained by placing a rolled towel behind the patient's lower neck. Sonography is performed with a high-frequency (8 to 15 MHz) linear array transducer to localize the nodule to be biopsied. A sterile ultrasound probe is set up and sterile gel placed on the patient's neck. The skin and subcutaneous tissues are anesthetized with 1% lidocaine. A 3-cm, 25-G needle is then placed into the lesion with continuous sonographic visualization. The needle trajectory is made parallel to the long axis of the head of the transducer to improve needle visualization (see Fig. 19-3). Specimens may be obtained by either a nonaspiration or an aspiration technique. The patient is instructed to refrain from talking, breathing, or swallowing while the biopsy is being performed. With the nonaspiration technique, cells are pulled into the needle by capillary effect. With this technique, the biopsy is performed by moving the needle back and forth vigorously through the nodule until bloody material is seen at the hub of the needle. The suction aspiration technique is

performed by connecting a 10-mL syringe to the 25-gauge needle with connecting tubing. A similar biopsy motion is used while suction is applied with 1- to 2-mL aspiration of the syringe. The samples are placed onto a slide. If the gross appearance of the smear appears scant, additional passes should be made (up to 6 to 8 passes), assessing different parts of the nodule to increase the biopsy yield. Some investigators have used 20- and 22-gauge cutting-needle biopsy guns for cases that are hypocellular, particularly if the lesion is larger than 1 cm.

Results and Complications

Reported rates of diagnostic accuracy range from 85% to 95%.[59,63] The use of thyroid fine-needle aspiration biopsy has been shown to reduce the number of thyroidectomies by approximately 50%, roughly double the surgical yield of carcinoma, and reduce the overall cost of medical care in these patients by 25%.[63] The yield from biopsy of cystic thyroid nodules is lower, with about 39% of cases yielding unsatisfactory cytologic results.[64] It is somewhat controversial about what should be done with nondiagnostic findings from thyroid biopsy. These should not be considered to be benign. Follow-up of these nondiagnostic cases is at the discretion of the referring physician, because further management might include repeated biopsy, surgery, or close imaging surveillance. One study found that repeat biopsy of such cases revealed malignant lesions in about half of the cases.[65] They suggested that operators wait at least 3 months

TABLE 19-2   DIFFERENTIAL DIAGNOSIS OF THYROID NODULES

Benign	Malignant
Hyperplastic nodule; adenomatous nodule	Primary (papillary, follicular, Hürthle, medullary, anaplastic)
Follicular or Hürthle cell adenoma	metastases (renal, breast, melanoma)
Lymphocytic thyroiditis	Lymphoma
Cyst (pure cyst is rare: <3%)	

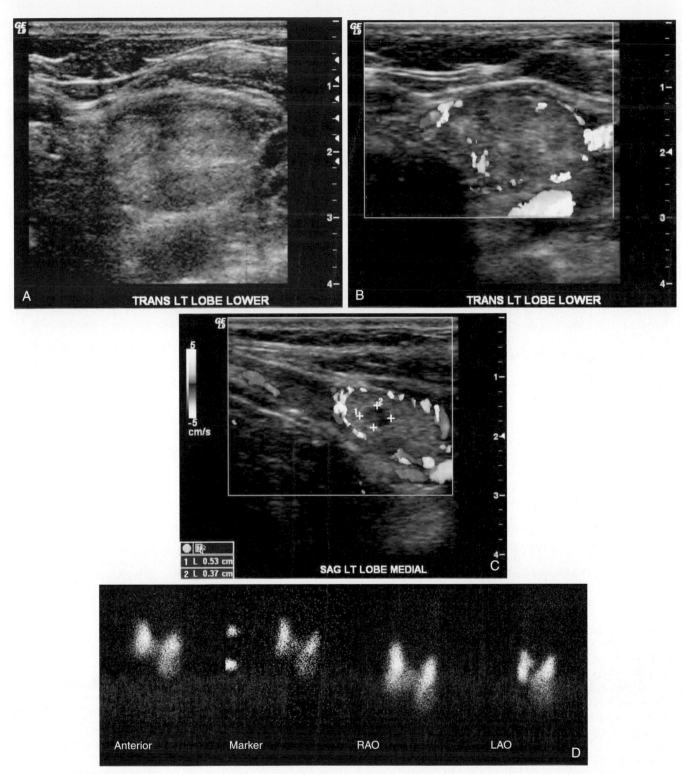

FIGURE 19-19 ■ A 62-year-old female patient developed hoarseness and had a thyroid ultrasound demonstrating a left lower pole thyroid nodule **(A, B,** and **C). D,** A nuclear medicine thyroid scan performed 6 hours after oral administration of 232 μCi I^{123} demonstrated a cold nodule in the lower left pole. A percutaneous aspiration of the left lower pole nodule with several passes with 25-gauge needles revealed a follicular neoplasm. LAO, left anterior oblique; RAO, right anterior oblique.

before repeat biopsy be performed because biopsy-induced reparative cellular atypia complicates subsequent cytologic diagnosis. It is important to recognize the overlapping cytologic features of hyperplastic/adenomatoid nodules, follicular adenoma, and follicular variant of papillary thyroid carcinoma. The complication rate from thyroid biopsy is less than 1% and most relate to small hematomas.

METHODS TO REACH INACCESSIBLE LESIONS

In general, the shortest pathway from the skin and the lesion is chosen for percutaneous biopsy, but occasionally this may not be possible because of interposed bowel, bone, lung, pleura, and major vessels. Some of techniques to overcome these problems have been described above, including transsternal biopsies, displacement of structures by injected fluid or carbon dioxide, and manual compression with an ultrasound transducer. The "triangulation method" was described by vanSonnenberg in 1981 as a method to solve cranial or caudal angled approaches to lesions.[66] This uses the Pythagorean theorem or lengths of triangles to direct in the proper cranial or caudal angles. In certain cases, angling the gantry may solve these cranial-caudal angulation problems, and this is particularly helpful with ribs overlying subpleural pulmonary masses.

A few studies have reported on using custom-made curved needles as a way of accessing lesions with interposed structures (Fig. 19-20).[67,68] The first study used 20- to 23-gauge needles to perform fluoroscopy-guided biopsy. After careful selection of the skin entry site, initial introduction of the needle is made in a direction away from the lesion to avoid the interposed structure, and gradual change is made in direction of the needle insertion when the curved part of the needle has been inserted so that the lesion is accessed. Repeat biopsies with this technique require

additional needles because this is not a coaxial method. The second study, by Sze, uses a coaxial technique with custom bent thin-walled 19-gauge needles that are then inserted with CT or MR fluoroscopy. A 21-gauge needle is advanced through the arc-shaped, outer 19-gauge needle to perform the biopsy. A variation is to use a straight 18-gauge needle through which a curved 22-gauge needle is advanced.[11]

REFERENCES

1. Bret PM, Fond A, Casola G, et al: Abdominal lesions: a prospective study of clinical effectiveness of percutaneous fine-needle biopsy. Radiology 1986;159:345.
2. Hooper KD: Percutaneous, radiographically guided biopsy: a history. Radiology 1995;196:329.
3. Reading CC, Charboneau JW, James EM, et al: Sonography guided percutaneous biopsy of small (3 cm or less) masses. AJR Am J Roentgenol 1988;151:189.
4. Charboneau JW, Reading CC, Welch TJ: CT and sonographically guided needle biopsy: current techniques and new innovations. AJR Am J Roentgenol 1990;154:1.
5. Silverman SG, Mueller PR, Pfister RC: Hemostatic evaluation before abdominal interventions: an overview and proposal. AJR Am J Roentgenol 1990;154:233.
6. Shapiro M: Approach to the patient with a coagulopathy. J Vasc Interv Radiol 1996;7(Part 2):73.
7. Gazelle GS, Haaga JR: Guided percutaneous biopsy of intraabdominal lesions. AJR Am J Roentgenol 1989;153:929.
8. Matalon TAS, Silver B: US guidance of interventional procedures. Radiology 1990;174:43.
9. Rose SC, Roberts AC, Kinney TB, et al: Three-dimensional ultrasonography for planning percutaneous drainage of complex abdominal fluid collections. J Vasc Interv Radiol 2003;14:451.
10. Katada K, Kato R, Anno H, et al: Guidance with real-time CT fluoroscopy: Early clinical experience. Radiology 1996;200:851.
11. Gupta S: New techniques in image-guided percutaneous biopsy. Cardiovasc Interv Radiol 2004;27:91.
12. Silverman SG: Percutaneous abdominal biopsy: recent advances and future directions. Semin Intervent Radiol 1996;13:3.
13. Solbiati L, Livraghi T, De Pra L, et al: Fine-needle biopsy of hepatic hemangioma with sonographic guidance. AJR Am J Roentgenol 1985;144:471.
14. Kinney TB, Lee MJ, Filomena CA, et al: Fine-needle biopsy: prospective comparison of aspiration versus nonaspiration techniques in the abdomen. Radiology 1993;186:549.
15. Dodd LG, Mooney EE, Layfield LJ, et al: Fine-needle aspiration of the liver and pancreas: a cytology primer for radiologists. Radiology 1997;203:1.
16. Quint LE, Park CH, Iannettoni MD: Solitary pulmonary nodules in patients with extrapulmonary neoplasms. Radiology 2000;217:257.
17. Thanos L, Galani P, Mylona S, et al: Percutaneous CT-guided core needle biopsy versus fine needle aspiration in diagnosing pneumonia and mimics of pneumonia. Cardiovasc Intervent Radiol 2004;27:329.
18. Permutt LM, Johnston WW, Dunnick NR: Percutaneous transthoracic needle aspiration: a review. AJR Am J Roentgenol 1989;152:451.
19. Calhoun P, Feldman PS, Armstrong P, et al: The clinical outcome of needle aspirations of the lung when cancer is not diagnosed. Ann Thorac Surg 1986;41:592.
20. D'Agostino HB, Sanchez RB, Laoide RM, et al: Anterior mediastinal lesions: transsternal biopsy with CT guidance. Radiology 1993;189:703.
21. Langen HJ, Klose KC, Keulers P, et al: Artificial widening of the mediastinum to gain access for extrapleural biopsy. Radiology 1995;196:703.
22. Bressler EL, Kirkham JA: Mediastinal masses: alternative approaches to CT-guided needle biopsy. Radiology 1994;191:391.
23. Johnston WW: Percutaneous fine needle aspiration biopsy of the lung: a study of 1015 patients. Acta Cytol 1984;28:218.
24. Zerhouni EA, Stutuk FP, Siegelman SS, et al: CT of the pulmonary nodule: a cooperative study. Radiology 1986;160:319.

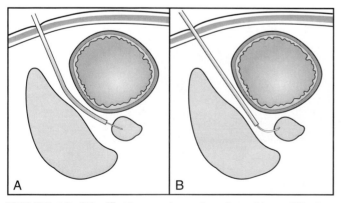

FIGURE 19-20 ▪ The use of curved needles to biopsy difficult to access lesions. A soft tissue mass is located medial to the iliac wing and posterior to the cecum. **A,** A thin-walled, curved, outer, 19-gauge needle is used to direct a thinner 21-gauge needle into the mass for biopsy. **B,** A straight 18- or 19-gauge needle is advanced proximal to the lesion. A 22-gauge needle with a bent tip is advanced through the straight needle into the lesion for biopsy. It is not possible to use a coring needle in this type of setup.

25. Yankelevitz DF, Davis SD, Henschke CI: Aspiration of a large pneumothorax resulting from transthoracic needle biopsy. Radiology 1996;200:695.

26. Yamagami T, Kato T, Iida S, et al: Efficacy of manual aspiration immediately after complicated pneumothorax in CT-guided lung biopsy. J Vasc Interv Radiol 2005;16:477.

27. Arnold B, Zwiebel WJ: Percutaneous transthoracic needle biopsy complicated by air embolism. AJR Am J Roentgenol 2002;178:1400.

28. Cardella JF, Bakal CW, Bertino RE, et al: Quality improvement guidelines for image-guided percutaneous biopsy of adults. J Vasc Interv Radiol 2003;14:S227.

29. Murphy FB, Barefield KP, Steinberg HV, et al: CT or sonography-guided biopsy of the liver in the presence of ascites: frequency of complications. AJR Am J Roentgenol 1988;151:485.

30. Gervais DA, Gazelle GS, Lu DS, et al: Percutaneous transpulmonary CT-guided liver biopsy: a safe and technically easy approach for lesions located near the diaphragm. AJR Am J Roentgenol 1996;167:482.

31. Lüning M, Schröder K, Wolff H, et al: Percutaneous biopsy of the liver. Cardiovasc Intervent Radiol 1991;14:40.

32. Cronan JJ, Esparza AR, Dorfman GS, et al: Cavernous hemangioma on the liver: role of percutaneous biopsy. Radiology 1988;166:135.

33. Withers CE, Casola G, Herba MJ, et al: Intravascular tumors: transvenous biopsy. Radiology 1988;167:713.

34. Hanes CH, Lindor KD: Outcome of patients hospitalized for complications after outpatient liver biopsy. Ann Intern Med 1993;118:96.

35. Bissonnette RT, Gibney RG, Berry BR, et al: Fatal carcinoid crisis after percutaneous fine-needle biopsy of hepatic metastases: case report and literature review. Radiology 1990;174:751.

36. Dunnick NR, Korobkin M, Francis I: Adrenal radiology: distinguishing benign from malignant adrenal masses. AJR Am J Roentgenol 1996;167:861.

37. Paulsen SD, Nghiem HV, Korobkin M, et al: Changing role of image-guided percutaneous biopsy of adrenal masses. AJR Am J Roentgenol 2004;182:1033.

38. Thompson GB, Young WF: Adrenal incidentaloma. Curr Opin Oncol 2003;15:84.

39. Kane NM, Korobkin M, Francis IR: Percutaneous biopsy of left adrenal masses: prevalence of pancreatitis after anterior approach. AJR Am J Roentgenol 1991;157:777.

40. Silverman SG, Mueller PR, Pinkney LP, et al: Predictive value of image-guided adrenal biopsy: analysis of results of 101 biopsies. Radiology 1993;187:715.

41. Casola G, Nicolet V, van Sonnenberg E, et al: Unsuspected pheochromocytoma: risk of blood-pressure alterations during percutaneous adrenal biopsy. Radiology 1986;159:733.

42. Brandt KR, Charboneau JW, Stephens DH, et al: CT- and US-guided biopsy of the pancreas. Radiology 1993;187:99.

43. Lewandrowski K, Lee J, Southern J, et al: Cyst fluid analysis in the differential diagnosis of pancreatic cysts: a new approach to the preoperative assessment of pancreatic cystic lesions. AJR Am J Roentgenol 1995;164:815.

44. Smith EH: Complications of percutaneous abdominal fine-needle biopsy. Radiology 1991;178:253.

45. Ferruci JT, Wittenberg J, Margolies MN, Carey RW: Malignant seeding of the tract after thin-needle aspiration biopsy. Radiology 1979;130:345.

46. Vassiliades VG, Bernadino ME: Percutaneous renal and adrenal biopsies. Cardiovasc Interv Radiol 1991;14:50.

47. Mostbeck GH, Wittich GR, Derflur K, et al: Optimal needle size for renal biopsy: in vitro and in vivo evaluation. Radiology 1989;173:819.

48. Cozens NJ, Murchison JT, Allan PL, Winney RJ: Conventional 15-G needle technique for renal biopsy compared with ultrasound guided spring-loaded 18-G needle biopsy. Br J Radiol 1992;65:594.

49. Nyman RS, Cappelen-Smith J, al Suhaibain H, et al: Yield and complications in percutaneous renal biopsy: comparison between ultrasound-guided gun biopsy and manual techniques in native and transplant kidneys. Acta Radiol 1997;38:431.

50. Sateriale M, Cronan JJ, Savadier LD: A 5-year experience with 307 CT-guided renal biopsies: results and complications. J Vasc Interv Radiol 1991;2:401.

51. Manno C, Strippoli FM, Arnesano L, et al: Predictors of bleeding complications in percutaneous ultrasound guided renal biopsy. Kidney Intl 2004;66:1570.

52. Quinn SF, vanSonnenberg E, Casola G, et al: Interventional radiology in the spleen. Radiology 1986;161:289.

53. Lawrence DD, Carrasco CH, Fornage B, et al: Percutaneous lymph node biopsy. Cardiovasc Intervent Radiol 1991;14:55.

54. Silverman SG, Lee BY, Mueller PR, et al: Impact of positive findings at image-guided biopsy of lymphoma on patient care: evaluation of clinical history, needle size, and pathologic findings on biopsy performance. Radiology 1994;190:759.

55. Amis ES: Retroperitoneal fibrosis. AJR Am J Roentgenol 1991;157:321.

56. Memel DS, Dodd GD, Esola CC: Efficacy of sonography as a guidance technique for biopsy of abdominal, pelvic, and retroperitoneal lymph nodes. AJR Am J Roentgenol 1996;167:957.

57. Bret PM, Guibaud L, Atri M, et al: Transvaginal US-guided aspiration of ovarian cysts and solid pelvic masses. Radiology 1992;185:377.

58. Oyen RH, Van Poppel HP, Ameye FE, et al: Lymph node staging of localized prostatic carcinoma with CT and CT-guided fine-needle aspiration biopsy: prospective study of 285 patients. Radiology 1994;190:315.

59. Lewis BD, Charboneau JW, Reading CC: Ultrasound-guided biopsy and ablation in the neck. Ultrasound Q 2002;18:3.

60. American Cancer Society. Cancer Facts and Figures 2005. Atlanta, American Cancer Society, 2005.

61. Ahuja AT, Meterweli C: Ultrasound of thyroid nodules. Ultrasound Q 2000;16:111.

62. Papini E, Guglielmi R, Bianchini A, et al: Risk of malignancy in non-palpable thyroid nodules: predictive value of ultrasound and color-Doppler features. J Clin Endocrinol Metab 2002;87:1941.

63. Hegedüs L, Bonnema SJ, Bennedbaek FN: Management of simple nodular goiter: current status and future perspectives. Endocr Rev 2003;24:102.

64. O'Malley ME, Weir MM, Hahn PF, et al: US-guided fine-needle aspiration biopsy of thyroid nodules: adequacy of cytologic material and procedure time with and without immediate cytologic analysis. Radiology 2002;222:383.

65. Baloch Z, LiVolsi VA, Jain P, et al: Role of repeat fine-needle aspiration biopsy (FNAB) in management of thyroid nodules. Diagn Cytopathol 2003;29:203.

66. vanSonnenberg E, Wittenberg J, Ferrucci JT, et al: Triangulation method for percutaneous needle guidance: the angled approach to upper abdominal masses. AJR Am J Roentgenol 1981;137:757.

67. Carrasco CH, Wallace S, Charnsangavej C: Aspiration biopsy: use of a curved needle. Radiology 1985;155:254.

68. Sze DY: Use of curved needles to perform biopsies and drainages of inaccessible targets. J Vasc Interv Radiol 2001;12:1441.

20

Transcatheter Fluid Drainage

Horacio B. D'Agostino, MD, Denisse Hurvitz, MD, Linda Nall, MD,
Eduardo Gonzalez Toledo, MD, PhD, and Guillermo P. Sangster, MD

■ TECHNIQUE

Patient Selection

Percutaneous or transorificial fluid drainage (PFD) is one of the most common interventional radiology procedures performed today.[1-5] PFD provides definitive treatment of most sterile and infected collections in the chest, abdomen, pelvis, and musculoskeletal system. It has largely replaced surgical incision and drainage as first-line treatment for these conditions. Specific indications for PFD are discussed in the following sections.

Contraindications to PFD include uncorrectable coagulopathy and lack of a safe pathway for catheter insertion, usually because of interposed bowel or large blood vessels. In some of these situations, simple aspiration of the fluid collection through a small-gauge needle may be safe and effective.[6]

Patient Preparation

Coagulopathies must be corrected before the procedure (see Chapter 1). Patients with suspected infected fluid collections usually are receiving antibiotics by the time drainage is requested. Otherwise, a broad-spectrum cephalosporin (e.g., 1 g of cefazolin IV) is given within 1 hour of the procedure. The administration of antibiotics immediately before the procedure does not interfere with cultures of fluid aspirated from the collection. PFD is performed with intravenous conscious sedation and local anesthesia. General anesthesia is indicated for children and uncooperative patients.

Imaging Guidance and Access

The most crucial steps in most percutaneous drainage procedures are selection of the access route and imaging modality for guidance of needle and catheter insertion.

Whenever possible, guidance with sonography and fluoroscopy is preferable because they allow real-time monitoring of our manipulations and less radiation to the patient than with CT. Small collections and those situated deep in the chest, abdomen, or pelvis are drained under CT guidance. Fluoroscopy alone is suitable when there is gas within the collection and a safe pathway is identified on a predrainage CT scan. Seemingly inaccessible pelvic fluid collections may be approached with sonography using a transvaginal or transrectal route.

In general, the shortest distance between the skin and the collection without interposing viscus or vessels is chosen for needle entry and catheter insertion. The selection of the skin entry site is based on previous diagnostic studies (e.g., plain radiographs, sonography, CT, MR imaging) and anatomic considerations (i.e., knowledge of the expected location of vessels and viscus that may be at risk for injury). The preselected pathway is confirmed by immediate preprocedure fluoroscopy, sonography, or a limited CT study. A wide area is sterilized, and local anesthesia is applied to the skin and soft tissues where the needle and catheter will be inserted.

Diagnostic aspiration usually is performed with small-caliber needles (e.g., 18- to 22-gauge spinal or Chiba needles) of sufficient length to easily reach the collection. Unlike the 18-gauge spinal needle, the thinner-walled, 18-gauge Chiba needle accepts a 0.035-inch guidewire. When fluoroscopy or sonography is used for guidance, the localizing needle is inserted into the collection under direct visualization (Fig. 20-1). When CT guidance is used, the needle is inserted using a technique similar to that for percutaneous biopsy (see Chapter 19). A CT scan is repeated to assess needle placement. If the needle is not positioned properly, it is left in place and used as a marker for the insertion of a second needle. Successful puncture of the collection is confirmed by CT.

Diagnostic Aspiration

Diagnostic aspiration can determine the nature of fluid collections, the ability to drain the collection percutaneously,

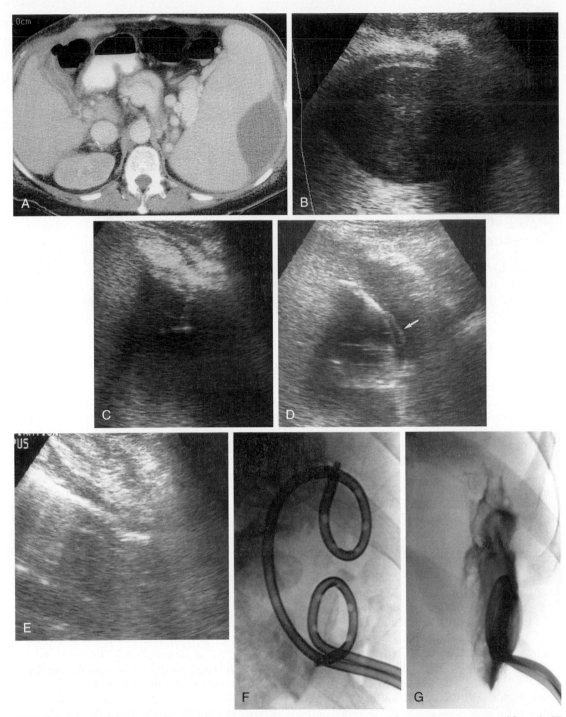

FIGURE 20-1 ▓ Ultrasound-guided drainage of a splenic abscess in a patient with portal hypertension and fever. **A,** CT shows a subcapsular splenic fluid collection. Note the enhancing varices in the splenic hilum and pericholecystic fluid around a collapsed gallbladder. **B,** Coronal sonographic image of the subcapsular cavity. **C,** A needle is inserted into the fluid collection with real-time sonographic guidance. **D,** A guidewire was advanced through the needle, over which a 10-French pigtail drainage catheter was placed *(arrow).* **E,** The cavity has completely collapsed after aspiration. **F,** A second drainage tube was placed. **G,** Follow-up tube injection 2 weeks later shows a small residual cavity.

and is of assistance in selection of the drainage catheter. Typically, a 22-gauge needle is inserted into the collection, and suction is applied with a 20- or 50-mL syringe. If no fluid is aspirated, 20-gauge and then 18-gauge needles are inserted sequentially in tandem with the first needle or into another area of the lesion. Dry aspiration from a well-positioned 18-gauge needle is proof that percutaneous drainage of the lesion is not feasible. In this situation, several biopsies are obtained and specimens sent for cytology and microbiology.

Aspiration of fluid confirms the location of the needle and allows assessment of the characteristics of the fluid (e.g., color, viscosity, turbidity, smell). The specimen is sent for Gram stain and culture. If catheter placement is indicated, only a small volume of fluid (2 to 4 mL) is removed to avoid decompressing the collection and making tube insertion more difficult.

The decision to proceed with catheter placement is based on several factors. Diagnostic or therapeutic aspiration alone is sufficient for sterile pleural fluid or ascites and for selected asymptomatic, uninfected collections elsewhere. Infected collections usually require catheter drainage. Sterile abscesses (i.e., white blood cells without organisms on Gram stain) also are treated with tube placement. Cysts and pseudocysts require catheter drainage to prevent recurrence after simple aspiration. However, there is a trend toward one-step needle aspiration without catheter placement for abscesses in certain locations expected not to have communication with the gastrointestinal tract or biliary or urinary ductal structures. This approach may be successful in up to 90% of selected cases.[6-10]

Catheter Insertion

Assessment of the type of fluid to be drained (e.g., pus, bile, lymph, urine, blood) and its characteristics (e.g., clear, viscous, particulate, clot filled) are used to select the drainage catheter size and type. Nonviscous fluid is drained with 8- to 10-French catheters. Viscous fluid and fluid with particles requires larger tubes (e.g., 12 to 24 French). Drainage catheters generally should have an inner retention mechanism (e.g., locking pigtail [Cope loop], locking Malecot type).

A scalpel is inserted along the localizing needle shaft to enlarge the skin puncture and underlying fascia enough to accommodate the catheter. Catheters may be placed by tandem-trocar, Seldinger, or direct trocar technique.

Tandem-trocar technique has been a popular method for drainage catheter insertion. The drainage catheter is loaded with the metal stiffening cannula and inner stylet. The distance between the skin and the collection (measured by ultrasound or CT) is marked on the catheter shaft with a Steri-Strip flag. The catheter is placed in the skin hole in tandem with the needle and then inserted into the collection. Catheter advancement is monitored by fluoroscopy or sonography. When CT is used for guidance, the stylet is removed and fluid is aspirated to confirm catheter position in the collection. The catheter may be fed off the metal cannula into the collection or advanced over a 0.035-inch floppy wire inserted through the cannula into the cavity. Use of a guidewire avoids perforation of the cavity by the catheter, disrupts any internal septations, and assists with smooth coiling of the catheter.

The *Seldinger technique* is the preferred method for placement of catheters in all collections and is recommended for small collections and those that are difficult to access. The Seldinger technique may be challenging for CT-guided PFD. An 0.035-inch guidewire is inserted through an 18-gauge, thin-walled needle (e.g., Chiba) and coiled in the collection (see Fig. 20-1). Under direct visualization with fluoroscopy or ultrasound, the tract is progressively enlarged with Teflon dilators and the catheter is inserted

over the guidewire with the metal stiffener but without the stylet. If CT has been required for access, the patient may be then transferred to a fluoroscopy suite with the needle and wire secured in place for catheter insertion.

Direct trocar placement of a catheter is safe only when the collection is large and superficial. After the skin entry site is selected and local anesthesia applied, a skin incision is made with a scalpel and the tissues are spread with a Kelly clamp. The catheter with the stiffening cannula and stylet is inserted directly into the collection. The tube is delivered directly over the cannula or over a protective guidewire.

After catheter insertion, the collection is completely evacuated. It is common for the initial aspirate to be relatively nonviscous, followed by thicker fluid, and then by minimally sanguinous material. The fluid often is blood tinged when the cavity is completely evacuated as suction is applied to the dry cavity wall. Ultrasound or CT images obtained immediately after drainage confirm complete fluid aspiration or demonstrate undrained collections. The drainage tube may be repositioned or additional catheters inserted if large residual collections or pockets are identified.

Catheter Care

A large-bore, three-way stopcock is attached to the catheter hub. The cavity is irrigated with 10- to 20-mL aliquots of normal saline until the aspirated fluid is clear. To prevent bacteremia and sepsis, avoid overdistention of the collection.

The catheter shaft is secured to the skin in an oblique or transverse orientation in relationship to the cephalocaudal axis of the patient to prevent catheter shaft kinking when the patient sits up. Catheters are sutured to the skin with 2 to 3/00 silk or other nonabsorbable material for external fixation. There are several adhesive retention devices that may be used in lieu of a suture. Large-bore catheters placed in the chest or abdomen also may require skin sutures. A mesentery made of adhesive tape wrapped around the catheter and applied to the skin is used as an extra precaution against accidental catheter dislodgement.

In general, catheters are connected to a collection bag for drainage by gravity. This setup is more effective when the fluid drained is nonviscous. Collections with viscous fluid or particulate material need catheter irrigation and may require intermittent low wall suction (50 mm Hg, 20 cm H_2O). Continuous low wall suction is used for thoracic collections. Chest drainage catheters are connected to a Pleur-evac that is connected to wall suction. The Pleur-evac is a water-seal device with a fluid collection chamber and a safety mechanism to prevent excessive suction. High-output collections (e.g., gastrointestinal or urinary tract fistulas) benefit from continuous low wall suction to keep the cavity dry and promote healing.

Postprocedure Care

The catheter shaft, connections, and external fixation devices are checked daily or when the patient is seen at clinic follow-up. The tube is irrigated to maintain patency.

Without irrigation, catheters occlude, regardless of their size. Proper catheter irrigation involves several steps:

■ Placement of a syringe in the stopcock and aspiration of residual fluid
■ Injection of 5 to 10 mL of normal saline
■ Aspiration of the irrigant
■ Reflushing the catheter with 5 mL of normal saline

For inpatients, catheter irrigation is done about three times each day by the floor nurses. Viscous collections may require more frequent irrigation (e.g., every 4 to 6 hours). Calculation of daily catheter output should take into account the volume of irrigant injected during the 24-hour period. t-PA instillation may be helpful for infected hematomas or loculated collections that respond poorly to simple tube drainage.

A catheter sinogram may be performed 2 to 3 days after initial drainage to visualize the residual fluid collection cavity and to assess for the presence of a fistula. By this time, the patient's acute condition should have improved. Diluted contrast is injected through the catheter slowly and under low pressure. Catheter sinograms are not required for simple collections. The study is necessary for collections in which a fistula is suspected and before cyst or lymphocele sclerosis. Fistulas also may be signaled by an increase in tube output.

Postprocedure Imaging

Cross-sectional imaging is indicated if the patient's condition fails to improve or worsens after PFD. Fevers should resolve within 3 to 5 days of tube placement. CT is preferred because it provides a complete survey of the anatomic compartment where the fluid collection has been drained and of other areas where residual or satellite collections may exist. Chest radiographs may be used to assess the drainage effectiveness of diffuse thoracic collections. CT scan of the thorax may be preferred for loculated thoracic collections. Long-term follow-up imaging may be required if the patient has a condition that is likely to recur (i.e., pancreatic pseudocysts, lymphoceles, cystic tumors).

Catheter Removal

There are five major criteria for catheter removal:

1. Improvement in the patient's clinical condition as indicated by disappearance of fever or pain or signs of intestinal, biliary, or urinary obstruction caused by the collection
2. Improvement in abnormal laboratory tests, including return of the white blood cell count to the normal range, improvement in laboratory values that were abnormal because of obstruction caused by the fluid collection, and sterilization of previously positive aspirates
3. Catheter output should return to an immeasurable amount (<10 mL/day). When drainage volume decreases to 20 to 30 mL/day, catheter irrigation is discontinued.

If catheter output remains below 10 mL/day for more than 24 hours, the catheter is removed unless a pancreatic, intestinal, or urinary fistula is present.
4. Resolution of the fluid cavity is assessed by catheter sinogram. The cavity usually shrinks immediately after drainage. When the size of the fluid collection does not resolve despite proper drainage, a necrotic or cystic tumor should be suspected.
5. Absence of fistula. Fistulas close with proper drainage unless certain conditions exist:
   The system (e.g., respiratory, gastrointestinal, urinary, biliary) is obstructed distally.
   Infection or tumor resides in the track.
   The patient has a circumstance that impairs healing (e.g., poor nutrition, steroid therapy).

Fluid collections recur if the fistula has not healed by the time the drainage catheter is removed. Sometimes a fistula is seen on catheter sinogram despite minimal drainage from the catheter because fluid can escape through another route. In this situation, the catheter is clamped for 1 to 3 days to allow reaccumulation of fluid. If no collection is identified by imaging, the catheter can be removed. Fluid collections associated with fistulas may require prolonged drainage (sometimes up to months). Persistent low-output drainage can be managed by downsizing the drainage tube and gradually removing it over 3 to 5 days. Presumably, this technique allows collapse and closure of the tract as the catheter is pulled out.

■ RESULTS AND COMPLICATIONS

The success rate of PFD combined with antibiotics and nutritional support is about 90% for simple collections (cysts, unilocular abscesses). The cure rate drops to 70% for complex collections such as infected hematomas, multilocular abscesses, abscesses complicated by bowel fistula, pancreatic abscesses, and infected necrotic pancreatic collections. Drainage failures often are attributed to residual undrained collections, early tube removal, or inadequate position (or number) of catheters. However, even when PFD is not completely curative, it often converts an emergent operation (with its attendant risks) to an elective procedure or obviates the need for a two-stage operation (e.g., diverting colostomy).

The major complications of PFD are bleeding, bowel or bladder perforation, and sepsis. Hemorrhage is more likely to occur in a patient with an uncorrected coagulopathy or when a suboptimal access route was used for catheter insertion. Inadvertent bowel perforation may take place when bowel motility is impaired by adhesions or ileus. If a loop of bowel is traversed en route to a fluid collection, a second catheter is placed in the collection. The first catheter is withdrawn until its tip is in the bowel lumen. This enterostomy catheter is removed when a mature track has formed. If an abnormally distended loop of bowel is mistaken for an abscess, aspiration yields yellow-green fluid that contains bubbles and is not foul smelling. In this situation, the catheter should *not* be removed but rather kept in place for 10 to 15 days until a track has formed. The catheter then can be removed safely, and the track closes spontaneously.

Perforation of the bladder may occur while draining lower abdomen fluid collections, regardless of the access route. Foley catheter insertion in the bladder before the procedure may avoid this complication. On recognition of bladder perforation by a drainage catheter, the catheter is removed. A Foley catheter is placed (if not already present) to ensure good bladder drainage. The Foley catheter is left in place for 5 to 7 days to allow healing of the perforation. The catheter then is clamped for 4 hours and removed if no urine leak is evident.

■ SPECIFIC APPLICATIONS

Chest

PFD is indicated for treatment of pneumothorax, empyema, malignant pleural effusion, pericardial effusion, lung abscess, and mediastinal abscess.[11] Intercostal and internal mammary vessel injury must be avoided during catheter placement. To prevent intercostal vessel laceration, needles and catheters are inserted over the upper border of the ribs. Internal mammary vessels are avoided by placing needles and catheters at least 5 cm lateral to the sternal margins. Ultrasound or CT can localize the internal mammary vessels before PFD. Catheters placed in the chest are connected to a water-seal drainage device.

Pneumothorax is a common complication of percutaneous lung biopsy and should be managed by the interventionalist.[11,12] Although not a liquid collection, its treatment has many aspects in common with abscess drainage. Indications for tube placement are large volume (>30% of the hemithorax), the appearance of symptoms (dyspnea,

decrease in blood oxygen saturation), or to re-expand a collapsed lung to continue with the biopsy. Catheter insertion is performed using anatomic landmarks or under fluoroscopic guidance. A 10-French catheter is inserted by direct trocar technique in the second or third intercostal space at the midclavicular line (Fig. 20-2). An alternative site in women and in men with bulky pectoralis muscles is the fourth or fifth intercostal space at the anterior axillary line. When the catheter enters the pleural space, the stylet is removed, and air is aspirated. The catheter with its stiffening cannula are angled cephalad toward the lung apex, and the catheter is fed off the cannula into the pleural space. The tube is connected to a Heimlich valve or a water-seal drainage device immediately after placement. Aspiration of air with a syringe is more laborious and not as effective. The catheter is left connected to drainage for at least 12 hours. It can be removed when the lung remains expanded on a follow-up chest radiograph obtained 2 hours after clamping the tube.

Empyema is an infected pleural collection usually caused by pneumonia, bronchiectasis, and/or trauma. Empyema develops in three stages[13]:

■ Acute (exudative) phase, indicated by the presence of a nonviscous, nonloculated effusion
■ Subacute phase, in which the fluid is fibrinous or purulent and the cavity may have loculations
■ Chronic (organizing) phase, when there is organization of the exudate with adhesion of the visceral and parietal pleurae (i.e., "pleural peel")

The diagnosis is made at the time of aspiration by the presence of gross pus, fluid pH 7.2 or lower, bacteria identified by the Gram stain, or a fluid glucose level less than 40 mg/dL. Acute and subacute empyema is treated successfully by PFD in greater than 80% of cases; chronic empyemas respond

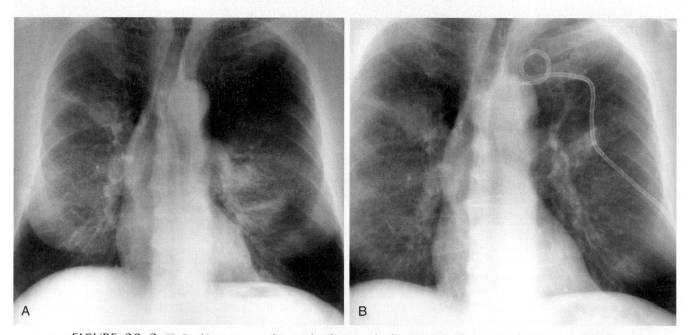

FIGURE 20-2 ■ Postbiopsy pneumothorax tube placement by direct trocar technique. **A,** The patient developed a large, symptomatic left pneumothorax after percutaneous biopsy of a lung mass with a 22-gauge Chiba needle. **B,** The pneumothorax was treated by evacuation through a 10-French pigtail catheter placed in the second intercostal space by direct trocar technique.

much less well.[14,15] Catheters are placed using ultrasound and fluoroscopy after diagnostic aspiration. CT may be used to access loculated collections, which may require multiple tubes. Catheters used vary from 12 to 24 French, depending on the viscosity of the fluid. The catheter is connected to a water-seal drainage device and continuous low wall suction after insertion. Intrapleural t-PA instillation improves drainage of residual fibrinous pleural collections.[16] In one protocol, 2 to 4 mg of t-PA in 10 to 20 mL of saline are injected every 8 hours for several days, with clamping of the tube for several hours after each instillation. Empyema catheters may be removed when there is improvement in clinical and laboratory parameters, no sign of air leak (indicating absence of a bronchocutaneous fistula), and drainage of less than 20 mL/day.

Malignant pleural effusions tend to recur rapidly after therapeutic thoracentesis. Closure of the pleural cavity with a sclerosing agent (e.g., tetracycline, doxycycline, talc, diluted sodium hydroxide, bleomycin) is an effective way to prevent recurrent effusions in more than 80% of patients.[17] Before sclerosis, the pleural fluid is drained completely. Usually, several sessions of sclerosis are needed to achieve fusion of the pleural surfaces.

Lung abscess is an infected collection of the lung parenchyma. Primary abscesses usually are the consequence of aspiration and are caused by anaerobic bacteria. Secondary abscesses arise from an adjacent infection or hematogenous spread (e.g., pneumonia, lung cyst, septic emboli). About 90% of lung abscesses respond to antibiotics, postural drainage, and bronchoscopic lavage. Those that do not resolve with the management mentioned require percutaneous drainage.[18-21] The procedure is performed with fluoroscopic or CT guidance (Fig. 20-3). A catheter pathway through abnormal lung is preferred to avoid pneumothorax and collapse of the healthy lung. Rarely, this is not possible and normal lung must be traversed by the drainage

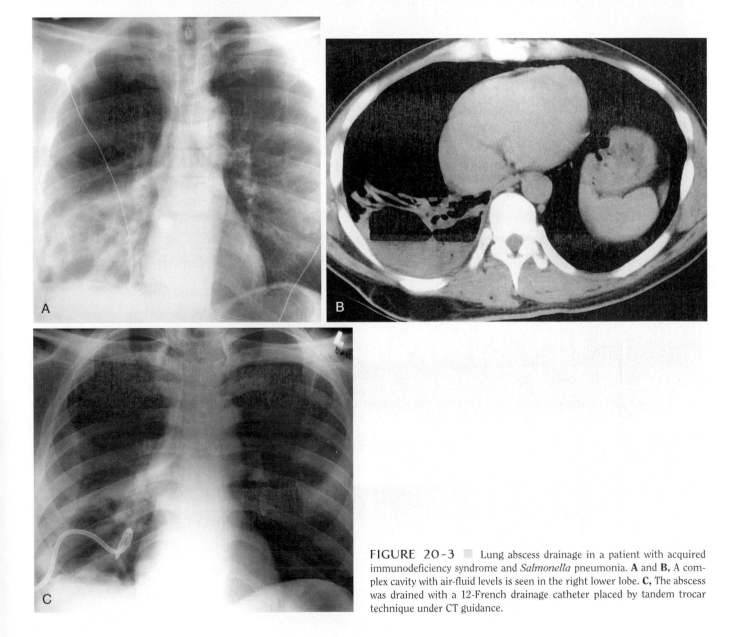

FIGURE 20-3 ■ Lung abscess drainage in a patient with acquired immunodeficiency syndrome and *Salmonella* pneumonia. **A** and **B,** A complex cavity with air-fluid levels is seen in the right lower lobe. **C,** The abscess was drained with a 12-French drainage catheter placed by tandem trocar technique under CT guidance.

catheter. The patient is positioned to keep the opposite hemithorax nondependent to avoid aspiration of the abscess fluid into the normal lung. Catheter insertion in a lung abscess establishes a controlled bronchocutaneous fistula that can be detected by air leak in the water-seal chamber of the Pleur-evac. A large air leak from a bronchocutaneous fistula can cause respiratory insufficiency in a critically ill patient. To avoid this problem, the catheter used to drain a lung abscess should be no larger than 12 to 14 French.

Mediastinal abscess is an emergent, life-threatening infection that usually occurs after thoracic surgery or endoscopy.[22] CT or sonography combined with fluoroscopy is used for image-guided tube placement with a parasternal or paraspinous approach to avoid the lung (Fig. 20-4).

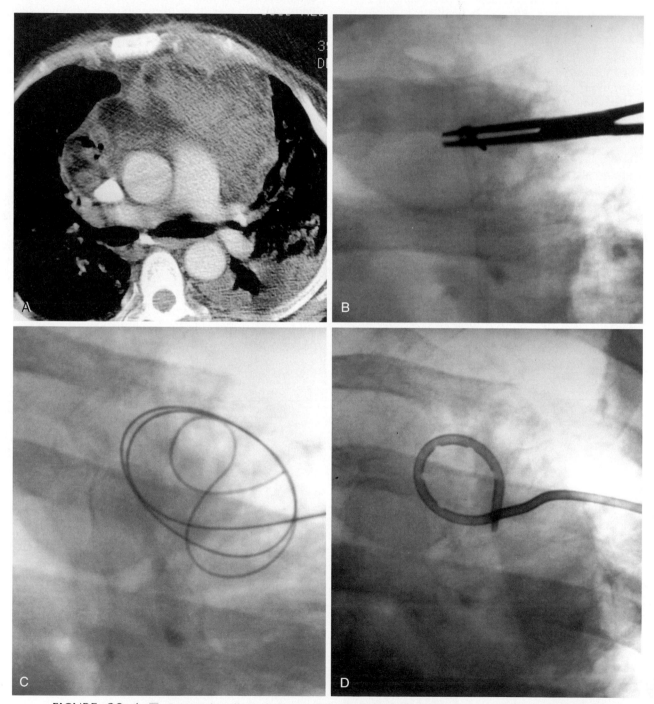

FIGURE 20-4 ■ Suspected mediastinal abscess after extravascular placement of a left subclavian central line. **A,** Inhomogeneous soft tissue density with air bubbles is present in the anterior mediastinum. Note the pleural thickening and left lower lobe infiltrate. **B,** A 16-gauge Angiocath was inserted into the collection under sonographic and fluoroscopic guidance, and serosanguineous material was aspirated. **C,** A guidewire was coiled in the cavity, over which a 10-French drainage catheter was inserted (**D**).

Pericardial effusions require drainage when there is impairment of diastolic filling of the ventricles. The cause of large symptomatic pericardial effusions include renal insufficiency, metabolic or immunologic diseases, infection, and malignancy.[23] Pericardial catheter drainage is performed under sonographic guidance with or without fluoroscopy. Malignant pericardial effusions have a high recurrence rate. Septic pericardial effusions are rare and are successfully drained percutaneously.

Liver

Pyogenic (bacterial) liver abscess may result from cholangitis, iatrogenic or criminal trauma, hematogenous septic emboli from enteric abscesses (e.g., appendicitis, diverticulitis), or tumor.[24] Acute cholangitis typically develops in patients with partial or total biliary obstruction caused by gallstones or tumor. PFD is well accepted as first-line therapy for these abscesses.[25-27] Tube insertion is done with sonographic or CT guidance. Care should be taken to avoid traversing the pleura, which may lead to empyema. Percutaneous drainage can treat the abscess and also may decompress the biliary tree if there is distal biliary obstruction. However, additional biliary drainage may be required to control sepsis. PFD is not feasible for widespread microabscesses. Single-step needle aspiration without tube placement is gaining some popularity for noncholangitic pyogenic liver abscesses.[28,29]

Hydatid cyst disease is caused by the parasite *Echinococcus granulosus.* The characteristic CT finding is multiloculated hepatic cysts with daughter collections. Medical therapy is the standard treatment.[30] Invasive procedures (PFD or surgery) are reserved for failures of drug therapy.[31-33] In the past, PFD was avoided strictly because of the fear of leakage of scolices with ensuing anaphylactic

shock or peritoneal spread. However, published series describe favorable results in controlling the disease with a combination of oral albendazole and percutaneous drainage.[34,35] Albendazole therapy begins 2 weeks before drainage and is continued until the catheter is removed. To avoid seeding the abdominal cavity at the time of drainage, aliquots of hydatid-fluid aspirate should be replaced with hypertonic (33%) saline solution. When the entire cyst is filled with saline solution, a catheter is inserted and left to gravity drainage. A catheter sinogram is performed later to assess communication with the bile ducts. If no communication is found, absolute alcohol is injected to assist in removal of the germinative layer of the cyst. Bile staining or pus in the hydatid cyst cavity is a sign that the parasites are dead.

Amebic abscess is diagnosed with serologic tests and is almost always eradicated with drug therapy such as metronidazole. Indications for amebic abscess drainage include failure of medical therapy, perforated abscess, and large collections in a peripheral location or the left lobe of the liver.[36-38] Abscesses at these sites are prone especially to rupture into the peritoneum, pericardium, or pleural space. Percutaneous drainage effectively controls symptoms from amebic abscess (Fig. 20-5). The usual duration of catheterization is less than 1 week. An alternative approach is simple aspiration with a large-bore needle or single-step catheter drainage and removal.

Congenital liver cysts usually are multiple and fall along the spectrum of polycystic kidney disease. Symptomatic dominant cysts require drainage and sclerosis.[39] However, solitary cystic liver lesions may be malignant (e.g., primary cystadenocarcinoma, metastatic disease) and are treated by surgical resection. Metastatic cystic tumors may benefit from palliative drainage to alleviate mass effect caused discomfort.

Posttraumatic biloma results from liver injury from blunt trauma, stab or gunshot wounds, or abdominal surgery.[40,41]

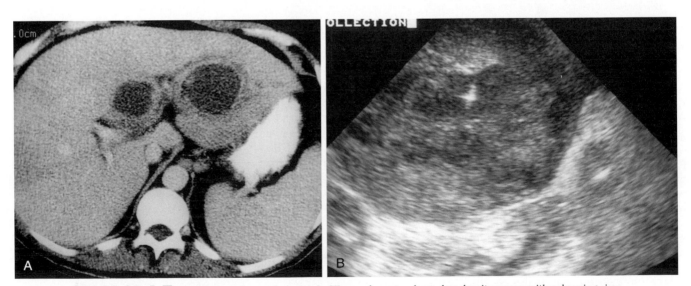

FIGURE 20-5 ■ Amebic liver abscess drainage. **A,** CT scan shows two large, low-density masses with enhancing rims and surrounding edema in the left lobe and caudate lobe. Numerous, small satellite lesions were seen throughout the liver on other images. **B,** A 22-gauge spinal needle was advanced into the left lobe cavity with sonographic guidance; frank pus was aspirated. A 12-French drainage catheter was placed by tandem trocar technique. The caudate lobe lesion was drained in a similar fashion.

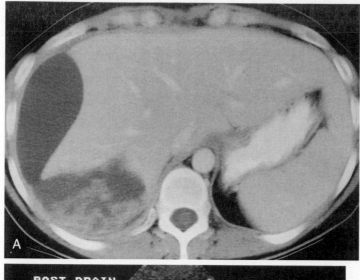

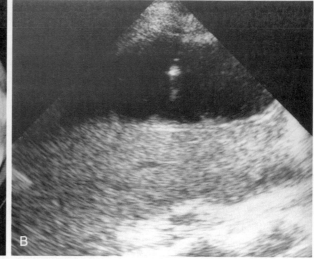

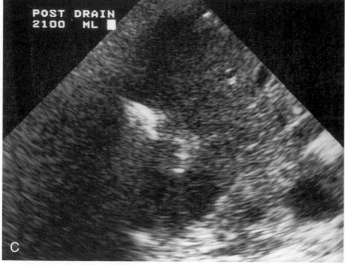

FIGURE 20-6 ■ Biloma drainage after blunt liver laceration from a motor vehicle accident. **A,** A large, subcapsular hepatic fluid collection developed days after injury to the posterior segment of the right lobe of the liver. **B,** The cavity was entered with ultrasound guidance. A vascular sheath was placed after initial guidewire insertion. Two guidewires were advanced through the sheath, allowing insertion of tandem drainage catheters into the collection. **C,** Two liters of bile were removed.

Bile accumulation from disrupted bile ducts may not require drainage if it is small, sterile, and asymptomatic. More often than not, however, bilomas become infected and require percutaneous drainage (Fig. 20-6). The presence of a biliary fistula may prolong the duration of catheterization. Biliary fistulas usually close unless there is total transection of a bile duct or distal biliary obstruction.

Ischemic fluid collections are complex bilomas caused by focal liver infarction. Liver infarcts result from severe compromise of the hepatic circulation and are seen in patients with portal vein thrombosis, occlusion of branches of the hepatic artery, or profound hypotension. Infarcts may become infected and require drainage. These collections are filled with necrotic liver parenchyma and bile. A biliary fistula is the rule after percutaneous drainage. Catheter sinograms reveal necrotic material in the bile ducts, which can cause biliary obstruction and maintain the fistula. Resolution of ischemic bilomas depends on adequate drainage, unobstructed bile ducts, and appropriate nutrition and vascular supply to allow for liver regeneration and healing of the collection cavity.

Spleen

Percutaneous drainage of splenic fluid collections is done for abscesses, liquefied infarcts, and symptomatic cysts.[42-45] Splenic abscesses are caused by hematogenous seeding (as in intravenous drug abusers) or trauma or are spread from adjacent tissue. Tube insertion is done with sonographic or CT guidance (see Fig. 20-1).[46] Care should be taken to avoid transgressing bowel, kidney, or pancreas. Transpleural drainage is not recommended but can be done safely.[47] To prevent splenic hemorrhage, the catheter is inserted by traversing the least amount of splenic parenchyma possible.

Pancreas

Basic management of all pancreatic fluid collections includes bowel rest, parenteral antibiotics, and parenteral or enteral nutrition. PFD is indicated for pancreatic pseudocysts that become infected or cause symptoms such as continued pain or bowel or biliary obstruction (Fig. 20-7).[48,49] Percutaneous drainage also plays a major role in the management of necrotic collections and pancreatic abscesses (Fig. 20-8).[50-52] Abscesses and pseudocysts may spread to the lesser sac, paracolic gutter or pararenal space, pelvis, and, occasionally, to the thorax. Pancreatic phlegmon does not respond to PFD. Because of the complex nature of pancreatic abscesses and the frequency of associated fistulas, PFD (often with multiple tubes) usually is necessary for cure. Postoperative drainage of residual infected necrosis or abscess is highly effective and used instead of reoperation. A pancreatic fluid collection in a patient without risk factors or history of pancreatitis should raise the possibility of malignancy. Drainage of pancreatic fluid collections usually is accomplished through a direct transabdominal or retroperitoneal approach. However, transhepatic, transsplenic, and transgastric drainage often can be done safely.[53,54] Complications of PFD in the pancreas occur in about 10% of cases and usually involve bleeding, infection, pneumothorax, or empyema.

A pancreatocutaneous fistula establishes when a catheter is inserted to drain a pancreatic fluid collection. With the exception of chronic pancreatic pseudocysts, most pancreatic collections have purulent, brownish or grayish fluid drainage. When the collection has resolved and debris evacuated, clear pancreatic fluid may continue to drain, causing prolonged duration of catheterization. Drainage of clear pancreatic fluid for more than 4 weeks is diagnostic of a persistent pancreatic fistula.[55] High-output pancreatic fistulas produce at least 300 mL/day. After acute inflammation has subsided, catheter drainage pancreatocutaneous fistulas can be reduced effectively by the administration of octreotide (50 to 150 μg, given subcutaneously three times daily). Octreotide (Sandostatin, Novartis Pharmaceuticals, East Hanover, NJ) is a synthetic somatostatin analogue that inhibits pancreatic fluid and enzyme secretion.[56] Octreotide has no effect while there is active pancreatitis or infection. The compound may reduce the drainage volume of pancreatic fistulas even in presence of transection or occlusion of the pancreatic duct.[57]

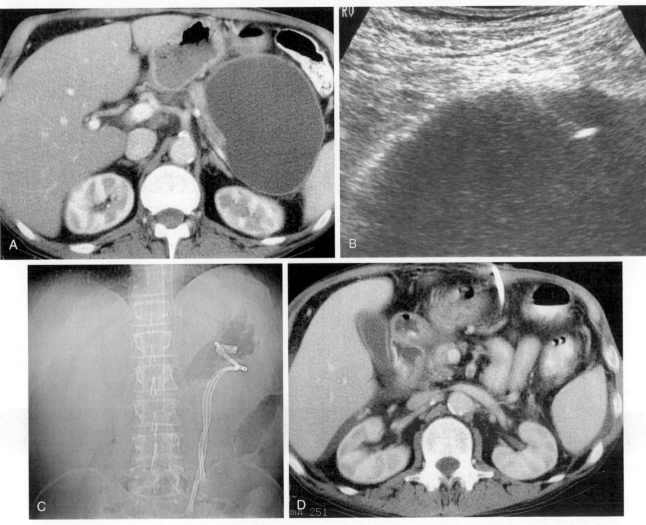

FIGURE 20-7 ■ Pancreatic pseudocyst drainage in a patient with an elevated white blood cell count and a history of pancreatitis. **A,** A large cystic mass is centered on the pancreatic tail. **B,** Using sonography, a 22-gauge Chiba needle was inserted into the collection. With the tandem trocar technique, a 10-French drainage catheter was placed. **C,** Because of persistent pain and white blood cell count elevation, a second catheter was inserted 3 days later to improve drainage. **D,** Two weeks later (with interval removal of one catheter), CT shows resolution of the pseudocyst with a persistent, strandy soft tissue density consistent with ongoing peripancreatic inflammation.

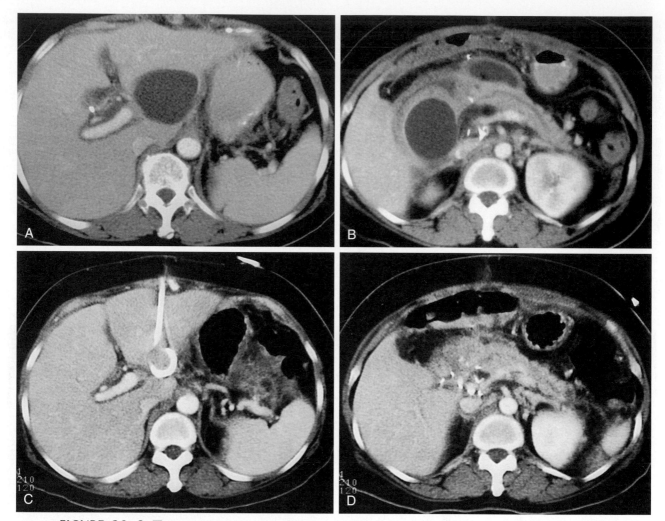

FIGURE 20-8 ■ Pancreatic abscess after a Whipple procedure for pancreatic carcinoma. **A** and **B,** Two large cystic collections with rim enhancement are found in the operative bed and the porta hepatis. An efferent bowel loop from the diversion procedure is wrapped around the lateral aspect of one cavity. The pancreatic duct is dilated. Diffuse inflammatory changes have occurred in the peripancreatic region. **C** and **D,** CT scans 10 days after drainage show resolution of the collections.

Lower Abdomen and Pelvis

A variety of disorders can produce fluid collections in the lower abdomen and pelvis (Box 20-1). PFD, along with antibiotics and bowel resection in some cases, is the primary treatment for many of these collections when they are infected, symptomatic, or produce obstruction. Percutaneous drainage often achieves a cure without surgery. After the abscess resolves, the indication for surgery depends on the nature and extent of underlying disease. PFD permits elective definitive surgery, allowing bowel resection, primary anastomosis, and wound closure. A colostomy or an open wound is therefore avoided. Patients with perforated tumors undergo surgery with the catheter in place for removal of the drainage tract en bloc with the specimen. PFD is effective for large, well-circumscribed periappendiceal abscesses without extension and for postappendectomy abscesses

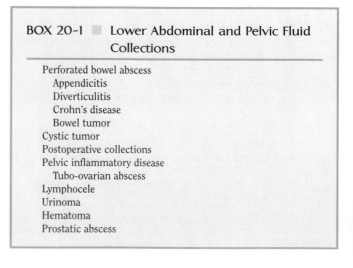

BOX 20-1 ■ Lower Abdominal and Pelvic Fluid Collections

Perforated bowel abscess
   Appendicitis
   Diverticulitis
   Crohn's disease
   Bowel tumor
Cystic tumor
Postoperative collections
Pelvic inflammatory disease
   Tubo-ovarian abscess
Lymphocele
Urinoma
Hematoma
Prostatic abscess

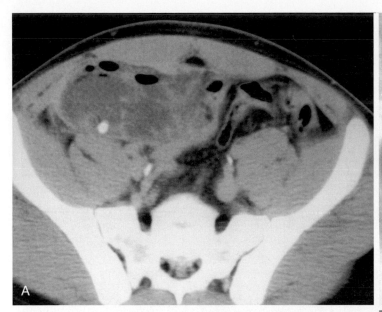

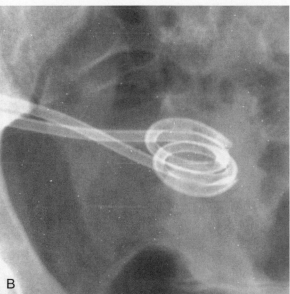

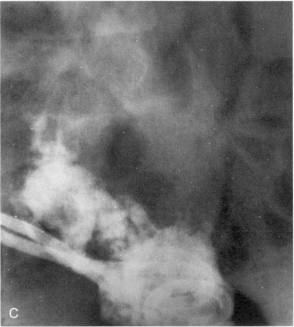

FIGURE 20-9 ■ Periappendiceal abscess drainage. **A,** A large, complex collection with gas bubbles is seen in the right lower quadrant. Note the appendicolith in the posterior aspect of the collection. **B,** Ultrasound guidance was used to place two 12-French drainage catheters. **C,** Follow-up tube injection 5 days later shows a small residual cavity but no definite communication with bowel.

(Fig. 20-9).[58-60] Diverticular abscesses localized to the pelvis or mesentery without fecal spillage respond best to PFD.[61-64] Patients with perforated bowel abscess from Crohn's disease may avoid emergent bowel resection with tube drainage.[65,66] Lymphoceles usually are secondary to pelvic operations, particularly kidney transplantation and lymph node dissection. PFD is the procedure of choice but may require protracted tube placement (>1 month).

Management of true cysts and lymphoceles often requires intracavitary injection of a sclerosing agent.[67-69] Before sclerosis is performed, a catheter sinogram is performed to exclude communication of the drained cavity with vital structures such as vessels, ductal structures, or bowel. Sclerosis is successfully achieved by multiple injections of absolute alcohol, tetracycline, or iodine solutions.

Fluid collections in the lower pelvis can be drained in several ways. The *transabdominal approach* usually is the simplest but may not be feasible because of interposed bowel. CT guidance normally is required, except for large superficial collections that can be visualized with sonography.

The *transgluteal approach* often is avoided because of the frequency of catheter-associated pain. Catheters must be inserted close to the sacral and coccygeal margins to avoid the large gluteal vessels and the sciatic nerve running through the greater sciatic foramen.[70]

The *transrectal approach* is useful for infected collections adjacent to the rectum.[71-73] Sterile collections may become infected if drained in this fashion. Access is gained using an endocavitary sonographic probe (with biopsy guide) and fluoroscopy or CT guidance with the patient in a lateral decubitus position (Fig. 20-10). A Foley catheter is inserted into the bladder prior to transrectal and transvaginal drainage to allow better visualization of the collection and to minimize the risk of bladder puncture.

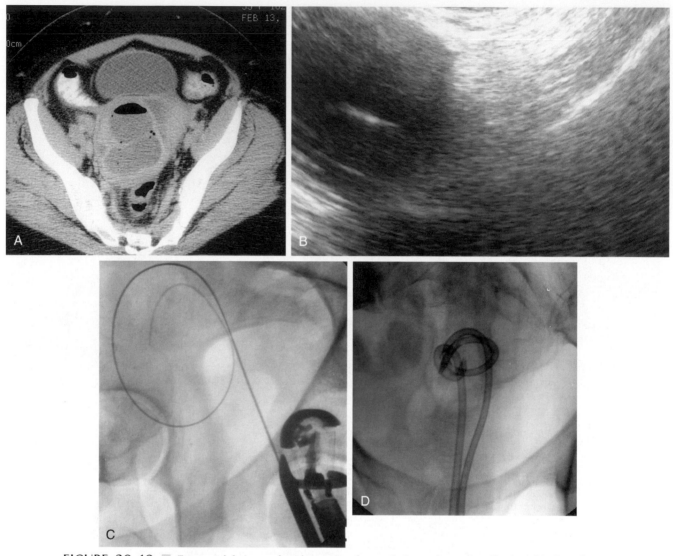

FIGURE 20-10 ■ Transrectal drainage of a tubo-ovarian abscess. **A,** A complex cystic collection with rim enhancement is seen anterior to the rectum. **B,** With the patient in the right lateral decubitus position, a sonographic probe is inserted into the rectum. The needle is advanced into the collection through a needle guide. **C,** A guidewire is coiled in the cavity. **D,** After 10- and 12-French drainage catheters were placed, 200 mL of foul-smelling exudate were aspirated.

The *transvaginal approach* is exceedingly useful in women with fluid collections in contact with the vaginal wall.[74,75] It is performed with a vaginal sonographic probe (with a biopsy guide) and fluoroscopic guidance (Fig. 20-11). Catheter insertion through the vaginal wall may be difficult.

Catheters placed transvaginally or transrectally benefit from having a locking pigtail loop (Cope) to prevent dislodgement when the patient is upright. The catheter is secured to the skin of the medial aspect of the thigh. Patients tolerate transvaginal and transrectal catheters surprisingly well.

Kidney and Retroperitoneum

Retroperitoneal collections include urinomas, perinephric abscess, renal abscess, renal cysts, iliopsoas muscle abscess, and necrotic tumors (most commonly cervical carcinoma metastases).[76] Most of these collections can be managed

successfully with PFD. Urinoma drainage usually is done after percutaneous nephrostomy to divert the urine flow that maintains the collection. Renal abscesses usually have a phlegmonous component that may not respond to percutaneous drainage. Symptomatic simple renal cysts are treated with catheter drainage and sclerosis (see Chapter 23). Iliopsoas muscle abscesses usually originate from an axial skeletal infection or other adjacent process (e.g., diverticulitis, appendicitis, infected lymph nodes).[77] Bilateral iliopsoas abscesses are usually caused by spondylitis. The offending organism is often *Mycobacterium tuberculosis*.

Musculoskeletal System

Muscular abscesses, hematomas, and lymphoceles are successfully drained percutaneously. Abscess recurrence caused by osteomyelitis depends on control of the bone infection.

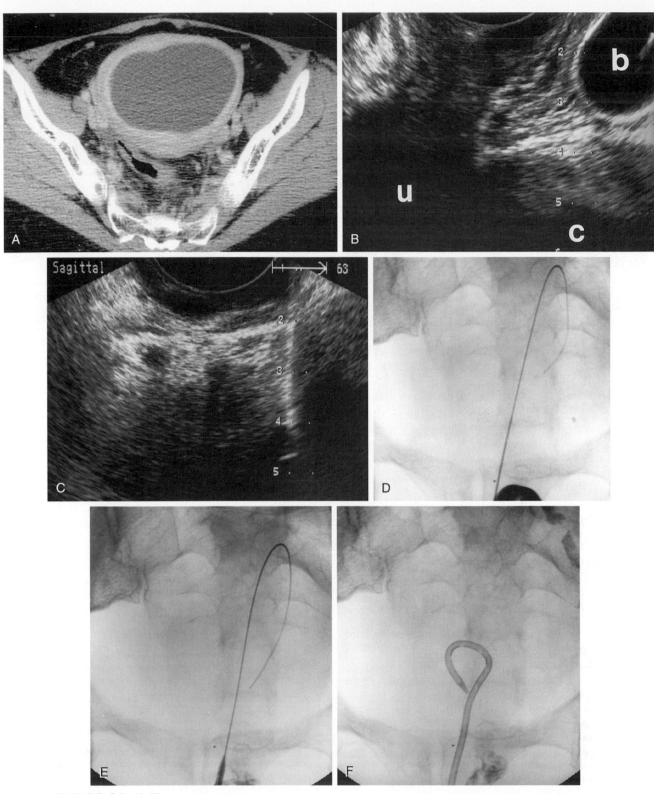

FIGURE 20-11 ■ Transvaginal drainage of pyometrium caused by cervical obstruction from carcinoma. **A,** The uterus is dilated and fluid filled. **B,** Sagittal transvaginal sonography identifies the dilated uterus (u), cervix (c), and bladder with indwelling Foley catheter (b). **C,** The transvaginal needle is advanced into the uterus. **D,** A guidewire is inserted through the needle. **E,** A 10-French drainage catheter is advanced over the guidewire. **F,** Final catheter placement in the uterine cavity.

Hip effusions also have been drained percutaneously. Few data are available on the success rate of percutaneous drainage for joint effusions.

Advanced Management for Drainage of Collections with Necrotic Debris

Complex fluid collections with debris, such as partially liquefied pancreatic necrosis and necrotic tumors, may benefit from controlled vigorous manipulations through the catheter tract. These collections are approached as it has been described previously with the difference that multiple catheters are used. Usually, at least one of them is a large-bore straight or J-shaped catheter (18 to 32 French in diameter). Hefty catheters spontaneously or with the help of energetic irrigation allow removal of large pieces of devitalized tissues. Follow-up of large diameter drainage catheters is more time consuming but rewarding regarding the results obtained.

Furthermore, catheter tracts may be used for videoendoscopy-guided grasping of residual material using baskets or forceps.[78-80] Fluoroscopy- and videoendoscopy-assisted percutaneous debridement and drainage have proven effective in clearing collections from solid debris material. These technical advancements have enhanced percutaneous drainage and broadened the scope of minimally invasive evacuation of collections without the need of open surgery.

REFERENCES

1. Mueller PR, vanSonnenberg E: Interventional radiology in the chest and abdomen. N Engl J Med 1990;322:1364.
2. vanSonnenberg E, D'Agostino HB, Casola G, et al: Percutaneous abscess drainage: current concepts. Radiology 1991;181:617.
3. Bakal CW, Sacks D, Burke DR, et al: Quality improvement guidelines for adult percutaneous abscess and fluid drainage. J Vasc Interv Radiol 1995;6:68.
4. Mueller PR, vanSonnenberg E, Ferrucci JT Jr: Percutaneous drainage of 250 abdominal abscesses and fluid collections. Part II: Current procedural concepts. Radiology 1984;151:343.
5. vanSonnenberg E, Mueller PR, Ferrucci JT Jr: Percutaneous drainage of 250 abdominal abscesses and fluid collections. Part I: Results, failures, and complications. Radiology 1984;151:337.
6. Wroblicka JT, Kuligowska E: One-step needle aspiration and lavage for the treatment of abdominal and pelvic abscesses. AJR Am J Roentgenol 1998;170:1197.
7. Kuligowska E, Keller E, Ferruci JT: Treatment of pelvic abscesses: value of one-step sonographically guided transrectal needle aspiration and lavage. AJR Am J Roentgenol 1995;164:201.
8. Miller FJ, Ahola DT, Bretzman PA, et al: Percutaneous management of hepatic abscess: a perspective by interventional radiologists. J Vasc Interv Radiol 1997;8:241.
9. Seeto RK, Rockey DC: Pyogenic liver abscess. Changes in etiology, management and outcome. Medicine (Baltimore) 1996;75:99.
10. Nielsen MB, Torp-Pedersen S: Sonographically guided transrectal or transvaginal one-step catheter placement in deep pelvic and perirectal abscesses. AJR Am J Roentgenol 2004;183:1035.
11. Klein JS, Schultz S, Heffner JE: Interventional radiology of the chest: image-guided percutaneous drainage of pleural effusions, lung abscess and pneumothorax. AJR Am J Roentgenol 1995;164:581.
12. Cantin L, Chartrand-Lefebvre C, Lepanto L, et al: Chest tube drainage under radiological guidance for pleural effusion and pneumothorax in a tertiary care university teaching hospital: review of 51 cases. Can Respir J 2005;12:29.
13. Light RW: Parapneumonic effusions and empyema. Clin Chest Med 1985;6:55.
14. Lee MJ, Saini S, Brink JA, et al: Interventional radiology of the pleural space: management of thoracic empyema with image guided catheter drainage. Semin Intervent Radiol 1991;8:29.
15. Merriam MA, Cronin JJ, Dorfman GS, et al: Radiographically guided percutaneous catheter drainage of pleural fluid collections. AJR Am J Roentgenol 1988;151:1113.
16. Lee KS, Im J-G, Kim YH, et al: Treatment of thoracic multiloculated empyemas with intracavitary urokinase: a prospective study. Radiology 1991;179:771.
17. Loutsidis A, Bellenis I, Argiriou M, et al: Tetracycline compared with mechlorethamine in the treatment of malignant pleural effusions: a randomized trial. Respir Med 1994;88:523.
18. vanSonnenberg E, D'Agostino HB, Casola G, et al: Lung abscess: CT guided drainage. Radiology 1991;178:347.
19. Moore AV, Zuger JH, Kelly MJ: Lung abscess: an interventional radiology perspective. Semin Intervent Radiol 1991;8:36.
20. Rice TW, Ginsberg RJ, Todd TR: Tube drainage of lung abscesses. Ann Thorac Surg 1987;44:356.
21. Wali SO, Shugaeri A, Samman YS, Abdelaziz M: Percutaneous drainage of pyogenic lung abscess. Scand J Infect Dis 2002;34:673.
22. Stavas J, vanSonnenberg E, Casola G, et al: Percutaneous drainage of infected and noninfected thoracic fluid collections. J Thorac Imaging 1987;2:80.
23. Kabukcu M, Demircioglu F, Yanik E, et al: Pericardial tamponade and large pericardial effusions: causal factors and efficacy of percutaneous catheter drainage in 50 patients. Tex Heart Inst J 2004;31:398.
24. Tazawa J, Sakai Y, Maekawa S, et al: Solitary and multiple pyogenic liver abscesses: characteristics of the patients and efficacy of percutaneous drainage. Am J Gastroenterol 1997;92:271.
25. Johnson RD, Mueller PF, Ferruci JT Jr, et al: Percutaneous drainage of pyogenic liver abscesses. AJR Am J Roentgenol 1985;144:463.
26. Do H, Lambiase RE, Deyoe L, et al: Percutaneous drainage of hepatic abscesses: comparison of results in abscesses with and without intrahepatic biliary communication. AJR Am J Roentgenol 1991;157:1209.
27. Gerzof SG, Johnson WC, Robbins AH, et al: Intrahepatic pyogenic abscesses: treatment by percutaneous drainage. Am J Surg 1985;149:487.
28. Rajak CL, Gupta S, Jain S, et al: Percutaneous treatment of liver abscesses: needle aspiration versus catheter drainage. AJR Am J Roentgenol 1998;170:1035.
29. Yu SC, Ho SS, Lau WY, et al: Treatment of pyogenic liver abscess: prospective randomized comparison of catheter drainage and needle aspiration. Hepatology 2004;39:932.
30. Smego RA Jr, Sebanego P: Treatment options for hepatic cystic echinococcosis. Int J Infect Dis 2005;9:69.
31. Saremi F, McNamara TO: Hydatid cysts of the liver: long-term results of percutaneous treatment using a cutting instrument. AJR Am J Roentgenol 1995;165:1163.
32. Bret PM, Fond A, Bretagnolle M, et al: Percutaneous aspiration and drainage of hydatid cysts of the liver. Radiology 1988;168:617.
33. Mueller PR, Dawson SL, Ferruci JT Jr, et al: Hepatic echinococcal cyst: successful percutaneous drainage. Radiology 1985;155:627.
34. Dziri C, Haouet K, Fingerhut A: Treatment of hydatid cyst of the liver: where is the evidence? World J Surg 2004;28:731.
35. Etlik O, Arslan H, Bay A, et al: Abdominal hydatid disease: long-term results of percutaneous treatment. Acta Radiol 2004;45:383.
36. Baijal SS, Agarwal DK, Roy S, et al: Complex ruptured amebic liver abscesses: the role of percutaneous catheter drainage. Eur J Radiol 1995;20:65.
37. vanSonnenberg E, Mueller PR, Schiffman HR, et al: Intrahepatic amebic abscesses: indications for and results of percutaneous catheter drainage. Radiology 1985;156:631.
38. Ken JG, vanSonnenberg E, Casola G, et al: Perforated amebic liver abscesses: successful percutaneous treatment. Radiology 1989;170:195.
39. vanSonnenberg E, Wroblicka JT, D'Agostino HB, et al: Symptomatic hepatic cysts: percutaneous drainage and sclerosis. Radiology 1994;190:387.
40. Pachter HL, Knudson MM, Esrig B, et al: Status of nonoperative management of blunt hepatic injuries in 1995: a multicenter experience with 404 patients. J Trauma 1996;40:31.
41. Faust TW, Reddy KR: Postoperative jaundice. Clin Liver Dis 2004;8:151.
42. Quinn SF, vanSonnenberg E, Casola G, et al: Interventional radiology in the spleen. Radiology 1986;161:289.

43. Ng KK, Lee TY, Wan YL, et al: Splenic abscess: diagnosis and management. Hepatogastroenterology 2002;49:567.
44. Thanos L, Dailiana T, Papaioannou G, et al: Percutaneous CT-guided drainage of splenic abscess. AJR Am J Roentgenol 2002;179:629.
45. Tasar M, Ugurel MS, Kocaoglu M, et al: Computed tomography-guided percutaneous drainage of splenic abscesses. Clin Imaging 2004;28:44.
46. Chou YH, Hsu CC, Tiu CM, et al: Splenic abscess: sonographic diagnosis and percutaneous drainage or aspiration. Gastrointest Radiol 1992;17:262.
47. McNicholas MM, Mueller PR, Lee MJ, et al: Percutaneous drainage of subphrenic fluid collections that occur after splenectomy: efficacy and safety of transpleural versus extrapleural approach. AJR Am J Roentgenol 1995;165:355.
48. Torres WE, Evert MB, Baumgartner BR, et al: Percutaneous aspiration and drainage of pancreatic pseudocysts. AJR Am J Roentgenol 1986;147:1007.
49. vanSonnenberg E, Wittich GR, Casola G, et al: Percutaneous drainage of infected and noninfected pancreatic pseudocysts: experience in 101 cases. Radiology 1989;170:757.
50. vanSonnenberg E, Wittich GR, Chon KS, et al: Percutaneous radiologic drainage of pancreatic abscesses. AJR Am J Roentgenol 1997;168:979.
51. D'Agostino HB, Fotoohi M, Aspron MM, et al: Percutaneous drainage of pancreatic fluid collections. Semin Intervent Radiol 1996;13:101.
52. Steiner E, Mueller PR, Hahn PF, et al: Complicated pancreatic abscesses: problems in interventional management. Radiology 1988;167:443.
53. Matzinger FR, Ho CS, Yee AC, Gray RR: Pancreatic pseudocysts drained through a percutaneous transgastric approach: further experience. Radiology 1988;167:431.
54. Mueller PF, Ferrucci JT Jr, Simeone JF, et al: Lesser sac abscesses and fluid collections: drainage by transhepatic approach. Radiology 1985;155:615.
55. Fotoohi M, D'Agostino HB, Wollman B, et al: Persistent pancreatocutaneous fistula after percutaneous drainage of pancreatic fluid collections: role of cause and severity of pancreatitis. Radiology 1999;213:573.
56. Gyr KE, Meier R: Pharmacodynamic effects of Sandostatin in the gastrointestinal tract. Digestion 1993;54(Suppl 1):14.
57. D'Agostino HB, vanSonnenberg E, Sanchez RB, et al: Treatment of pancreatic pseudocysts with percutaneous drainage and octreotide. Work in progress. Radiology 1993;187:685.
58. vanSonnenberg E, Wittich GR, Casola G, et al: Periappendiceal abscesses: percutaneous drainage. Radiology 1987;163:23.
59. Jamieson DH, Chait PG, Filler R: Interventional drainage of appendiceal abscesses in children. AJR Am J Roentgenol 1997;169:1619.
60. Jeffrey RB Jr, Federle MP, Tolentino CS: Periappendiceal inflammatory masses: CT directed management and clinical outcome in 70 patients. Radiology 1988;167:13.
61. Neff CC, vanSonnenberg E, Casola G, et al: Diverticular abscesses: percutaneous drainage. Radiology 1987;163:15.
62. Mueller PR, Saini S, Wittenberg J, et al: Sigmoid diverticular abscesses: percutaneous drainage as an adjunct to surgical resection in 24 cases. Radiology 1987;164:321.
63. Ambrosetti P, Chautems R, Soravia C, et al: Long-term outcome of mesocolic and pelvic diverticular abscesses of the left colon: a prospective study of 73 cases. Dis Colon Rectum 2005;48:787.
64. Gervais DA, Ho CH, O'Neill MJ, et al: Recurrent abdominal and pelvic abscesses: incidence, results of repeated percutaneous drainage, and underlying causes in 956 drainages. AJR Am J Roentgenol 2004;182:463.
65. Casola G, vanSonnenberg E, Neff CC, et al: Abscesses in Crohn disease: percutaneous drainage. Radiology 1987;163:19.
66. Doemeny JM, Burke DR, Meranze SG: Percutaneous drainage of abscesses in patients with Crohn's disease. Gastrointest Radiol 1988;13:237.
67. Gilliland JD, Spies JB, Brown SB, et al: Lymphoceles: percutaneous treatment with povidone-iodine sclerosis. Radiology 1989;171:227.
68. Sawhney R, D'Agostino HB, Zinck S, et al: Treatment of postoperative lymphoceles with percutaneous drainage and alcohol sclerotherapy. J Vasc Interv Radiol 1996;7:241.
69. Tasar M, Gulec B, Saglam M, et al: Posttransplant symptomatic lymphocele treatment with percutaneous drainage and ethanol sclerosis. Long-term follow-up. Clin Imaging 2005;29:109.
70. Ryan JM, Murphy BL, Boland GW: Use of the transgluteal route for percutaneous abscess drainage in acute diverticulitis to facilitate delayed surgical repair. AJR Am J Roentgenol 1998;170:1189.
71. Pereira JK, Chait PG, Miller SF: Deep pelvic abscesses in children: transrectal drainage under radiologic guidance. Radiology 1996;198:393.
72. Lomas DJ, Dixon AK, Thomson HJ, et al: CT guided drainage of pelvic abscesses: the peranal transrectal approach. Clin Radiol 1992;45:246.
73. Gazelle GS, Haaga JR, Stellato TA, et al: Pelvic abscesses: CT guided transrectal drainage. Radiology 1991;181:49.
74. vanSonnenberg E, D'Agostino HB, Casola G, et al: US-guided transvaginal drainage of pelvic abscesses and fluid collections. Radiology 1991;181:53.
75. Nosher JL, Winchman HK, Needell GS: Transvaginal pelvic abscess drainage with US guidance. Radiology 1987;165:872.
76. Paley M, Sidhu PS, Evans RA, et al: Retroperitoneal collections—aetiology and radiological implications. Clin Radiol 1997;52:290.
77. Gupta S, Suri S, Gulati M, et al: Ilio-psoas abscesses: percutaneous drainage under image guidance. Clin Radiol 1997;52:704.
78. Echenique AM, Sleeman D, and Yrizarry J: Percutaneous catheter-directed debridement of infected pancreatic necrosis: results in 20 patients. J Vasc Interv Radiol 1998;9:565.
79. D'Agostino HB, Venable D, Gimenez M, et al: Percutaneous Videoendoscopy-Assisted Removal of Necrotic Debris from Pancreatic Fluid Collections. SCVIR 27th Annual Scientific Meeting, April 6-April 11, 2002, Baltimore, Maryland; J Vasc Interv Radiol Supplement 2002;13:S104.
80. Mui LM, Wong SK, Ng EK, et al: Combined sinus tract endoscopy and endoscopic retrograde cholangiopancreatography in management of pancreatic necrosis and abscess. Surg Endosc 2005;19:393.

21

Gastrointestinal Interventions

Gerant Rivera-Sanfeliz, MD, and Gregory M. Lim, MD

ESOPHAGUS

Esophageal Stricture Dilation

Etiology and Natural History

Esophageal strictures from a variety of benign and malignant etiologies require dilation therapy when patients develop symptoms of dysphagia. For centuries, the mainstay of therapy for esophageal strictures has been dilation. Using a piece of carved whalebone for dilation in the setting of achalasia was described in the 17th century.

Benign processes such as peptic disease, surgery, Schatzki's ring, and radiation can produce esophageal strictures. Other less frequent etiologies include extrinsic compression, photodynamic therapy, caustic injury, empiric dilations, webs, and tracheostomy.

Esophageal strictures can be divided in two groups: simple and complex. Strictures that have diameters allowing the passage of an endoscope and are otherwise short, focal, and not angulated are categorized as simple. Complex strictures, however, are those that are angulated, long (>2 cm), irregular, or have a severely narrowed lumen. Often, these complex strictures are refractory to dilation therapy. Strictures caused by surgical anastomoses, radiation therapy, caustic ingestion, and photodynamic therapy represent most refractory strictures.

Although initial dilation typically results in symptomatic relief, recurrence of the stricture with return of symptoms is common. In the setting of peptic stricture, approximately 30% to 60% of patients require repeat dilations within a year.[1] Several studies have attempted to identify prognostic factors associated with increased need for multiple dilations. Patients with peptic strictures who experienced weight loss or lacked symptoms of heartburn were more likely to require multiple sessions; however, the severity of the initial stenosis or the type and size of dilator used did not have an impact on recurrence.[2]

Patient Selection

Esophageal dilation is contraindicated in the setting of recent or acute esophageal perforation, bleeding diathesis, severely compromised pulmonary function or airway obstruction, severe or unstable cardiac disease, or in patients with large thoracic aortic aneurysms.

Technique

The "rule of threes" generally is accepted and applied to dilation of esophageal strictures.[1] Specifically, after moderate resistance is encountered during dilation therapy with Savary-type dilators, no greater than three consecutive dilators should be used in a single session. There is no objective data specifically dealing with balloons; therefore, a conservative approach to dilation should be undertaken to reduce the chances of perforation. Multiple dilation sessions frequently are required to achieve a luminal diameter of at least 12 mm.

Three general types of dilators are in use currently. These include mercury- or tungsten-filled bougies, over-the-wire polyvinyl dilators, and balloon catheters. The bougie-type dilators produce both radial and longitudinal force compared with the other two types. Except for instances in which longitudinal forces should be avoided, no clear advantage has been demonstrated between the dilator types.[3]

Although the majority of these procedures is performed under endoscopic guidance only, fluoroscopy has been an instrumental aid in the setting of complex strictures. Several authors report reduced complication rates and improved therapeutic results when fluoroscopy was used.[4,5] In cases of proximal lesions in which successful intubation of the esophagus with the endoscope may be met with difficulty, fluoroscopy becomes the sole means for guidance.

Results

For benign strictures, balloon dilation is technically successful in 90% of the cases and clinical success is achieved in approximately 70% of patients at 2-year follow-up.[6] The results are not as favorable with radiation strictures, and malignant strictures only achieve transient results. Dysphagia caused by external compression of the esophagus rarely responds to dilation.

During the 1990s, several studies demonstrated a high complication rate associated with aggressive dilation of malignant esophageal strictures.[7,8] However, properly performed dilation is safe, considering the types of strictures and the debilitated patients who require this therapy.[9,10] Dilation of malignant esophageal strictures currently is performed as an adjunct to endoscopic staging of esophageal tumors or as temporary palliative treatment before considering surgery, placement of self-expanding stents (see below), or laser photoablation.

Complications

The most serious complication following dilation is esophageal perforation. The reported rate is 0.1% to 0.4%.[11,12] As expected, complex strictures have an increased risk for rupture. Mild bleeding is reported commonly following dilation and usually is self-limited. Severe bleeding occurs in 0.4% of patients.[13] Inadvertent passage of the dilator into the trachea is rarely a reported problem.

Esophageal Stricture Stent Placement

Carcinoma of the esophagus is notoriously difficult to manage with approximately 60% of patients suitable only for palliative treatment. Even after surgery, almost 20% of patients have dysphagia secondary to recurrence of the disease or anastomotic strictures.[14]

Laser therapy, radiation therapy, and placement of plastic stents have been used for palliation. Laser therapy offers effective palliation with a low rate of complications. However, it is not suitable for extrinsic compression, is difficult to perform if the narrowed region is long and tortuous, and requires repeated treatments with expensive equipment that is not readily available.[15] Radiation therapy achieves palliation of dysphagia in less than 40% of patients and may take up to 2 months until dysphagia is relieved.[16] Although rigid plastic stents are inexpensive and readily available, complication rates including perforation (8%), stent migration, tumor overgrowth, and bleeding are not infrequent.[17]

Frimberger first proposed treating malignant dysphagia with metal stents in 1983.[18] Knyrim and colleagues, in their controlled trial published in 1993, concluded that self-expanding stents were a safe and cost-effective alternative to conventional plastic endoprosthesis in the treatment of esophageal obstruction due to inoperable cancer.[19] Several additional series have used self-expanding metallic stents with low procedure-related mortality and low morbidity.[20-25]

Patient Selection

The indications for metallic stent placement in the esophagus include the following:

- Palliative treatment of malignant dysphagia
- Palliation of malignant esophageal fistulas or perforations
- Benign refractory strictures in poor surgical candidates

Technique

The stents approved by the U.S. Food and Drug Administration (FDA) are the covered/uncovered Wallstent (Boston Scientific, Natick, Mass.), covered Gianturco-Rosch z-stent (Cook, Inc., Bloomington, Ind.), and covered/uncovered Ultraflex stents (Boston Scientific). The Wallstent has excellent radiopacity, has the highest radial force (more appropriate for extrinsic compression), and is easy to deploy (Fig. 21-1). However, it foreshortens during deployment, which must be taken into consideration when choosing the length of the stent. The z-stent has good radiopacity, minimal shortening, and may have an antireflux valve. It lacks flexibility, requires a bulky sheath (up to 31 French), and is difficult to deploy. Stent shortening, poor radiopacity (nitinol), and an unprotected delivery system make the Ultraflex stent deployment more difficult than the Wallstent. The lower radial force and greater flexibility of the Ultraflex probably are responsible for less chest pain and better patient tolerance. It is the preferred stent for high esophageal lesions.

Stents should never be placed across the superior esophageal sphincter (C5-C6 level) because of patient discomfort and aspiration risk.[26] Crossing the gastroesophageal junction with the stent should, if possible, be avoided.[26] A transoral route is used and predilation is performed to facilitate rapid stent expansion and removal of the delivery system. If a fistula is present, dilation is not performed because of fear of enlarging the abnormal communication. The stent should cover the lesion and have a safety margin of at least 2 cm of normal esophagus at each end. When the stent is properly positioned, the esophageal stricture produces a waist at the center of the stent. Esophageal stent placement may further compress the trachea and precipitate respiratory distress. When significant airway compression is present, tracheobronchial stent placement should be performed first.[26]

After stent placement, patients need to modify their diets to prevent large boluses of food from becoming impacted within the stent. If a stent without a valve is used to cross the distal esophageal sphincter, the patients are placed on antireflux measures that include elevation of the head of the bed and acid suppression therapy.

Results

Esophageal stent placement is technically successful in 97% to 100% of cases.[27] Dysphagia is relieved in 90% of patients who undergo esophageal stent placement.[28] Successful closure of tracheo- or bronchoesophageal fistulas can be achieved in 70% to 100% of patients.[29] Treatment failure occurs more frequently when the esophagus is dilated, preventing stent-wall apposition, and when the fistula is in proximity to the superior esophageal sphincter. Overall, the reintervention rate is 25%.[26]

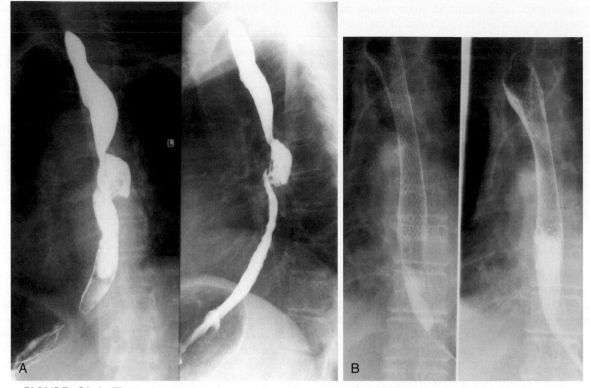

FIGURE 21-1 ◼ Esophageal stent placement for malignant stricture. **A,** Esophagogram shows narrowing of the midesophagus secondary to an excavating esophageal carcinoma. **B,** Widely patent esophagus following deployment of covered Wallstent.

Complications

Complications of esophageal stent placement are low and include chest pain (Wallstent), reflux esophagitis, aspiration, stent migration (0 to 35%), esophageal perforation or fistulization (0 to 8%), obstruction (4% to 18%), severe bleeding (0 to 6%), and tracheal compression.[30] The mortality rate associated with esophageal stent placement is approximately 0.5% to 2%.[28]

The most common complication seen in covered stents is migration, whereas the most common complication seen in uncovered stents is tumor ingrowth. To minimize migration, changes in stent design have been implemented that include covering inside the metal mesh (exoskeleton), uncovered segments at both ends (longer proximally), and larger proximal diameter (cone-shaped stent). Such an example is the Flamingo stent (Boston Scientific/Medi-tech).

◼ STOMACH

Percutaneous Gastrostomy and Gastrojejunostomy

Treatment Options

Malnutrition is a common problem affecting up to 40% of hospitalized patients, increasing their morbidity and mortality.[31] Nutritional support can be given either enterally or parenterally. Unfortunately, parenteral nutrition is costly and has high risks of complications, including sepsis, hepatic dysfunction, metabolic disturbances, vein thrombosis, and gut mucosal atrophy leading to barrier disruption and bacterial translocation.[32] Several randomized controlled studies have concluded that enteral feeding has lower complication rates when compared with its parenteral counterpart.[33,34]

Enteral feeding requires a functioning gut and can be provided in the short term via nasogastric or nasoenteral tubes. In the long term, however, these tubes have high complication rates, including mechanical failure and aspiration pneumonia. Patients with chronic swallowing disorders or obstruction to swallowing, those who are unable to ingest food due to head trauma or stroke, or those with anorexia due to underlying diseases such as cancer may benefit from more permanent accesses such as gastrostomy, gastrojejunostomy, or jejunostomy.

Egeberg and Sedillot described the first surgical gastrostomies in the early 19th century, and although the procedure is not a difficult one technically, it can be associated with significant morbidity and even mortality.[35] These findings may be related to the use of general anesthesia and poor wound healing in debilitated patients. Percutaneous techniques were introduced approximately two decades ago and have largely supplanted open surgery based on its fewer complication rates.[36]

Minimally invasive gastrostomy can be performed using endoscopic (percutaneous endoscopic gastrostomy [PEG]) or fluoroscopic (percutaneous gastrostomy [PG]) guidance. The advantage of PG over PEG is that a skilled endoscopist is not required and endoscopy may be limited in patients with an esophageal or pharyngeal obstruction. In addition, sedation can be minimized with PG. Wollman and colleagues published a comparison of surgical, endoscopic, and fluoroscopic techniques for gastrostomies that included a meta-analysis of the literature.[37] Their conclusion was that PG is associated with a higher success rate than is PEG and less morbidity than either PEG or surgery. More recently, Hoffer and colleagues performed a prospective, randomized comparison and concluded that PG had a higher success rate and fewer complications, whereas PEG took less time, cost less, and required less tube maintenance.[38] Button gastrostomy tubes typically are placed in children. A recent report describes use of this alternate device in adults.[39]

Patient Selection

The major indication for PG is nutritional support in patients with the following disorders:

- Head and neck tumors or malignant esophageal tumors
- Swallowing impairment due to cerebrovascular accident or neuromuscular disorder
- Nutritional supplementation for chronic illness or extensive surgery
- Severe gastroesophageal reflux and recurrent aspiration (percutaneous gastrojejunostomy [PGJ])
- Functional or organic gastric outlet obstruction (PGJ)

PG also may be used for gastrointestinal decompression. This indication is more common in patients with carcinomatosis causing chronic intestinal obstruction. More infrequent indications include patients with craniofacial abnormalities and patients with impaired intestinal absorption, requiring slow infusions of elemental diet into the small bowel via a gastrojejunostomy or jejunostomy.[40]

Absolute contraindications to PG include uncorrectable coagulopathy and unsatisfactory anatomy (Fig. 21-2). The presence of a ventriculoperitoneal (VP) shunt also is considered an absolute contraindication, but this notion has recently been challenged. Sane and colleagues found a 9% shunt infection rate with 23 PEGs placed 1 month following the VP shunt and concluded that patients are at a greater risk for infection.[41] Graham and colleagues performed 15

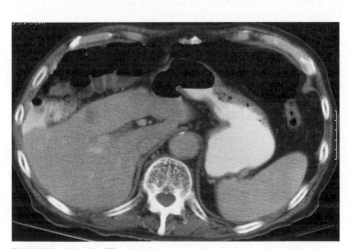

FIGURE 21-2 ■ Colon interposition between the stomach and abdominal wall precludes placement of a percutaneous gastrostomy.

PEGs for a minimum of 1 week (mean 2.2 weeks) after shunt placement and had no infections.[42] Finally, Taylor and colleagues performed 16 shunts in 13 patients requiring gastrostomies (half before PEG and half after PEG, timing otherwise unclear) and found a 50% shunt infection rate.[43] They concluded that the development of infection was not related to the sequence of or interval between shunt and gastrostomy placement and recommended avoiding simultaneous placement in the acute phase of a patient's hospital admission. These are small series that include only PEG procedures, limiting our ability to reach conclusions regarding the safety of PG in conjunction with VP shunt placement.

Other relative contraindications include massive ascites, abdominal varices, prior gastric surgery, pathology involving the anterior gastric wall, and severe gastroesophageal reflux (for PG) (Box 21-1).

Placing gastrostomies in patients with short life expectancies has been a topic of considerable interest in the medical literature. The mortality rate after PG is highly related to a patient's underlying status and predictors include age, malignancy, diabetes mellitus, and pulmonary disease.[44,45] Rising health costs and quality-of-life issues also are common concerns when placing PGs. Investigators estimate the cost of hospital visits for tube dislodgement or malfunction at almost $11 million per year in the United States.[46] Some investigators argue that if no physiologic benefit is expected or if the improvement in physiologic status has no effect on quality of life (e.g., permanent vegetative state), then the health care team has no obligation to offer or perform an intervention.[47] The issue is controversial and depends on the philosophy of the institution, the physician in charge, the individual who inserts the tube, and the wishes of the patient and the family.

There are marked differences between gastrostomy and gastrojejunostomy feedings. Stomach feedings can be given in boluses and prepared at home with a blender; the patient tolerance is excellent. Jejunal feedings, on the other hand, require nutrient solutions prepared in a pharmacy and delivered by a pump, and patient tolerance is variable. Tolerance to enteral nutrition may be improved by tailoring the solution's volume, rate, and concentration to the individual's condition.

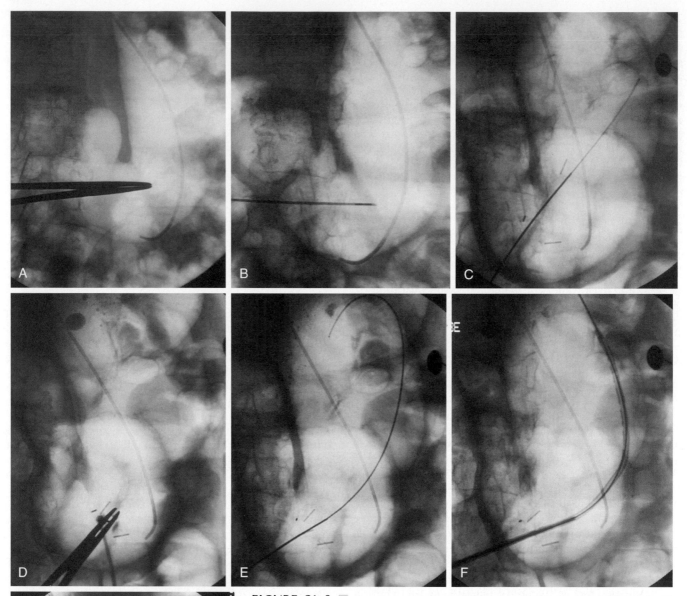

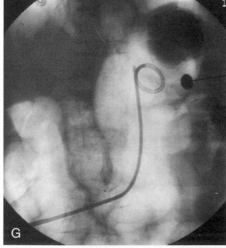

FIGURE 21-3 ■ Percutaneous gastrostomy procedure. **A,** The stomach is distended with air through a directional catheter. The skin entrance site is marked with a clamp. **B,** The stomach is entered with a 16-gauge needle loaded with a T-fastener. **C,** The T-fastener is deployed with a guidewire. **D,** A clamp is used to center the needle over the desired puncture site. **E,** After three T-tacks have been placed, the skin is punctured in the middle of the triangle, and a guidewire is coiled in the fundus of the stomach. **F,** The catheter is inserted into the stomach. **G,** The pigtail is locked and secured in the fundus of the stomach.

Technique

A fasting period of 8 hours is required prior to the procedure (Fig. 21-3). Barium frequently is administered the day before for colonic opacification, and ultrasound is used to delimit the liver contour. A nasogastric tube is inserted and used for stomach insufflations during the procedure (Fig. 21-4). Glucagon can be helpful in placing a gastrostomy if the stomach decompresses rapidly during the manipulations; however, it may increase the difficulty in crossing the pylorus when placing a gastrojejunostomy tube. Patients with prior gastric resection, upper abdomen interventions, esophageal obstruction, or a nondistensible stomach due to carcinomatosis may require CT to assist in stomach identification and puncture (Fig. 21-5).

Prophylactic antibiotics, although controversial, have been recommended recently in a randomized trial.[48] The stomach is punctured in the midbody anteriorly and care is taken to avoid the superior epigastric artery that runs beneath the rectus abdominis muscle as well as the gastric and gastroepiploic arteries located along the lesser and greater curvatures of the stomach, respectively.

Many interventionalists perform percutaneous gastropexy using T-fasteners. T-fasteners are 1-cm metallic bars that have a monofilament suture attached at their midportion, forming a "T" configuration. The need for gastropexy is most relevant during the first week after which a fibrous tract develops around the catheter.[49] In theory, gastropexy may minimize the risk of peritoneal leakage, prevent tube migration into the peritoneal cavity, and tamponade gastric bleeding (Fig. 21-6). They also may facilitate insertion of larger tubes and access to the gastric tract in cases of inadvertent tube dislodgement. Dewald and colleagues compared 1000 gastropexy and nongastropexy gastrostomies and concluded that no risk was added with gastropexy.[50] Thornton and colleagues performed a randomized comparison of gastrostomies with and without T-fasteners and concluded that fasteners should be used routinely based on a 10% incidence of serious technical complications in the nongastropexy group that included four catheters in the peritoneal cavity.[51] However, they also noted a 10% incidence of pain and 13% incidence of skin excoriation at the T-fastener sites.

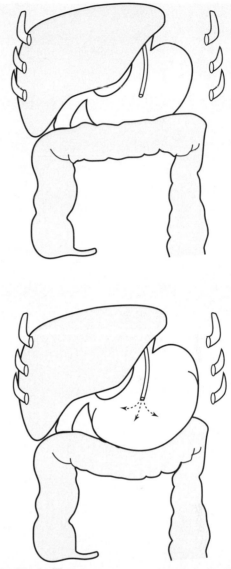

FIGURE 21-4 ■ Insufflation of the stomach provides a larger target for puncture and displaces the transverse colon inferiorly.

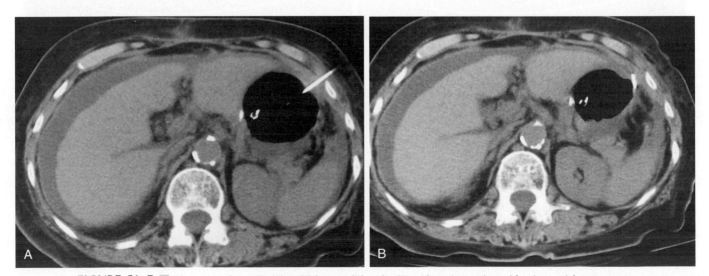

FIGURE 21-5 ■ Placement of a needle **(A)** and T-fastener **(B)** under CT guidance in a patient with prior partial gastrectomy.

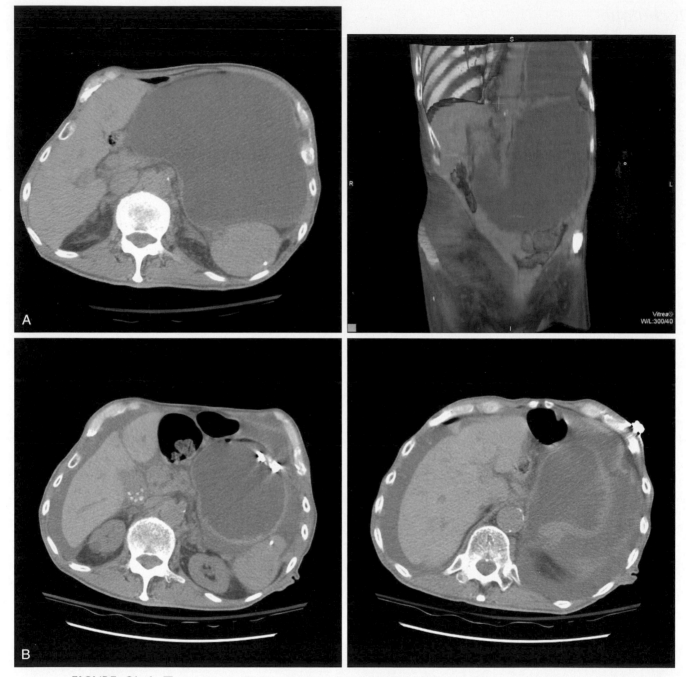

FIGURE 21-6 ■ Percutaneous gastrostomy for gastric outlet obstruction without T-fasteners. **A,** Axial (left) and coronal (right) CT images show gastric outlet obstruction. **B,** Axial CT images 12 hours after non–T-fastener gastrostomy show peritoneal leakage and associated inflammation.

The procedure is performed under fluoroscopic guidance using an over-the-guidewire technique. Most interventionalists prefer to place the tube with a retrograde technique, though antegrade techniques have been described, particularly when larger or a more PEG-like tube is needed. There is a wide variety of gastrostomy and gastrojejunostomy tubes that differ in both size and retention mechanisms. No single gastrostomy catheter is appropriate for all patients. Radiologically placed tubes tend to be smaller (12 to 14 French) and therefore are more prone to occlusions, especially when pill fragments are administered. Endoscopic tubes have better retention systems, including large internal bolsters or bulbs that prevent dislodgement, a common scenario with the radiologically placed tubes regardless of the type of retention device.

Clark and colleagues use the per oral technique to insert PEG-like tubes in patients who are deemed to be at high risk for pulling out the gastrostomy or with gastrostomies to be converted later to skin level buttons, or per physician request for a large-bore tube.[52] This technique requires retrograde catheterization of the esophagus followed by exteriorizing the wire through the mouth and delivering the catheter using an antegrade technique typical of PEG placement. Unfortunately, this carries the higher risk of stomal infections due to passage of the tube through the oral cavity. Giuliano and colleagues advocate placing large-bore tubes using the standard retrograde radiologic technique by dilating the tract with a 10-mm diameter × 12-cm-long balloon, inserting a 24- to 26-French Amplatz peel-away sheath, followed by delivery of a 20- to 24-French MIC-type gastrostomy catheter (Medical Innovations Corporation/Ballard Medical Products, Draper, Utah).[53] The MIC tube is a silicone transparent tube with an internal balloon and an external ring flange commonly used in open or laparoscopic gastrostomy procedures. They used a three-point T-fastener gastropexy in all of their 109 gastrostomies and concluded that percutaneous large-bore catheter placement is safe and has the same technical success and morbidity and mortality rates when compared with surgically or endoscopically placed tubes, as well as small-bore tubes placed under fluoroscopic guidance.

Some interventionalists prefer jejunal placement of feeding tubes, citing the high prevalence of pulmonary aspiration in chronically ill patients and that gastrostomies adversely affect gastric emptying, which may increase the risk even further.[54] When performing a gastrojejunostomy, the gastric puncture should be directed toward the pylorus. Direct puncture into the antrum should be avoided to prevent potential impairment of gastric emptying function. On occasion, clinicians may request conversion of a gastrostomy to a gastrojejunostomy due to gastroesophageal reflux or aspiration risks. In general, 1 to 2 weeks should be allowed for tract maturation prior to repeated manipulation because experimental studies show a firm gastrocutaneous tract within 7 days.[49]

Postprocedure Care

Patients are observed for 4 hours and monitored for abdominal pain, distention, and bleeding. Gastrostomy tubes are placed to gravity drainage for 24 hours to decompress the stomach and monitor for bleeding complications. Patients remain fasting for the following 24 hours. Tube feeding tolerance and progression can be monitored using residual volume measurements every 6 hours, with full nutrition generally achieved within 48 hours. T-fasteners can be removed in 7 to 10 days.

Catheter care instructions are given to the patient and relatives, including information about tube feedings, catheter maintenance, and how to recognize signs and symptoms that may herald complications.

Results

Technical success rate for PG is 95% to 100% and the procedure-related mortality rate varies between 0 and 3.2%.[40] A meta-analysis of the literature reported a technical success of 95% for PEG and 100% for surgical gastrostomies.[38] Technical failure results from lack of safe access route, most commonly from overlying transverse colon. Other causes for failure include massive ascites, gastric cancer, peritoneal carcinomatosis, overlying open abdominal wound, and previous gastric surgery. A small pneumoperitoneum immediately after the procedure is common.

Complications

Complications are rare. In a recent meta-analysis, Wollman and coworkers reported a 5.9% overall complication rate and a 0.3% mortality rate for PG.[37] By contrast, PEG was associated with a 9.4% complication rate, whereas surgery was associated with a complication rate of 19.9%.

Peritonitis is a rare but serious complication following gastrostomy and may result as a consequence of leakage or inadvertent infusion of the nutrient into the peritoneal cavity. Early detection, discontinuation of feedings, and antibiotics can control a minor leak. Contrast studies through the tube may fail to show the leak, but an enlarging pneumoperitoneum is considered to be a reliable sign of intraperitoneal leakage.[40]

Aspiration pneumonia secondary to gastroesophageal reflux has long been considered a major cause of morbidity and mortality in patients with feeding gastrostomies. Gastrostomies affect gastric emptying and, theoretically, may increase the risk for aspiration.[54] However, Olson and colleagues found no causal relationship between gastrostomy tube placement and gastroesophageal reflux in their prospective study.[55] They recommend PGJ placement only in patients with reflux or who are at high risk for aspiration pneumonia.

Bleeding following PG placement usually is self-limited but can be significant in patients with an underlying coagulopathy. If bleeding persists, direct arterial injury should be suspected. Other etiologies include gastritis or gastric ulceration.

Wound infections after PG are rare and occur within a week following tube placement. They are treated with local care and antibiotics. In this respect, PG differs from PEG, in which the latter has a higher frequency of skin infections since the tube is contaminated by oral flora as it is passed through the mouth and oropharynx on its way to the stomach.[56] Tube malfunction or dislodgement is treated with tube replacement. Vigorous tube flushing must be performed after each tube use, particularly when dealing with small-bore gastrostomies, in order to prevent frequent tube occlusion.

Stent Placement for Gastroduodenal Obstructions

Gastric outlet and duodenal obstruction in patients with inoperable cancer causes inability to tolerate food, vomiting, and cachexia. The use of self-expandable stents as a palliative tool for patients with these conditions has been reported. Published data suggest that the procedure is a safe and effective nonsurgical treatment of malignant gastric and duodenal obstructions.[57] The Wallstent endoprosthesis is the most commonly used device. Tumor ingrowth of the uncovered stent has not been of significant clinical concern because of the limited life expectancy of these patients.

■ JEJUNUM

Percutaneous Jejunostomy

Treatment Options

Patients with history of chronic aspiration, gastric or esophageal surgery, or abnormal stomach position may not be suitable candidates for PG/PGJ and may require a jejunostomy (Box 21-2). Jejunostomy can be performed using several techniques that include surgical, endoscopic, laparoscopic, and percutaneous.

There are three basic types of surgical jejunostomy: Witzel jejunostomy, Roux-en-Y jejunostomy, and needle catheter jejunostomy.[58] The latter is used most frequently and involves the placement of a thin tube into the jejunum via a seromuscular space tunnel using the Seldinger technique. The external end of the tube is exteriorized through the abdominal wall at a site distant from the laparotomy incision. However, surgical jejunostomy can be associated with significant morbidity and mortality.[59] In addition, patients usually are poor surgical candidates due to chronic illness, debilitated state, or poor nutritional status.

Direct percutaneous endoscopic jejunostomy can be performed in patients who have had gastric surgery with a gastroscope; otherwise, a long enteroscope is needed to reach the first 2 feet of jejunum.[60] In addition to access issues, it may be difficult to transilluminate the abdominal wall through a deeply seated or easily mobile bowel. The failure rate can be as high as 14% and can be associated with colonic perforation and abdominal wall abscess.[60]

Laparoscopic jejunostomy requires general anesthesia, absence of significant intra-abdominal adhesions, and a skilled operator. In two series there was an 8% to 12.5% conversion rate to open surgery and an 11% to 25% serious complication rate, including volvulus.[61,62]

Technique

Percutaneous jejunostomy can be performed through a previous jejunostomy site or de novo. Gray and colleagues were first to describe the percutaneous technique, and several technical reports have followed confirming its feasibility and safety for feeding, decompression, and the management of bilioenteric anastomotic strictures.[63,64] Fluoroscopic guidance is routinely used. CT fluoroscopy guidance recently has been suggested to facilitate the visualization and catheterization of mobile, anteriorly positioned unopacified or nondistended bowel.[65]

BOX 21-2 ■ Indications for Percutaneous Jejunostomy
Chronic aspiration
Previous gastric surgery or resection
Abnormal stomach position
Duodenal or gastric outlet obstruction

Most interventionalists agree that appropriate bowel distention and the use of T-fasteners are two important factors for the technical success of percutaneous jejunostomy. Bowel distention can be achieved with a nasogastric or nasoduodenal tube. A catheter with an occlusion balloon may be used to increase the intraluminal pressure and provide a target for the needle. Care should be taken not to create torsion during deployment of the locking tube and emphasis should be placed in correctly sizing the diameter of the loop with the traversed jejunum. Feeding can be started in 24 hours following the intervention. The technical success rate of percutaneous jejunostomy is in the vicinity of 95%.

A dislodged surgical jejunostomy can be replaced percutaneously. The attempts usually are more successful when performed fewer than 10 days after dislodgement or removal of the tube. Hietmiller and colleagues recommend marking the jejunopexy site with radiopaque markers to assist visualization at recatheterization.[66]

Nasojejunal Tube Placement

Nasojejunal tubes are used for nutritional support in patients who are unable to eat and in whom a more permanent percutaneous access is not needed or desired. Care is taken to anesthetize the oropharynx with Cetacaine spray and Xylocaine jelly is injected into the selected nostril. Using fluoroscopic guidance, a long diagnostic catheter (Kumpe, vertebral) and guidewire are manipulated through the pylorus past the ligament of Treitz. An exchange-length guidewire is advanced and a Ring-McLean nasojejunal tube (Cook, Inc.) is delivered over the guidewire.

The pylorus usually is the most difficult site to traverse when placing a nasojejunal tube. Injecting air admixed with contrast through the catheter may facilitate manipulations as well as stimulate peristalsis. Mucosal and skin erosion around the nostril caused by prolonged nasojejunal intubation can be minimized by careful tube fixation and keeping the skin dry.

■ COLON

Percutaneous Cecostomy

Percutaneous cecostomy (PC) is an alternative to open or laparoscopic surgical cecostomy for decompression of prolonged cecal dilation. The risk for colonic perforation increases when the cecal diameter exceeds 12 cm and when the distention has been present for several days.[67] In the event of perforation, the mortality rate approaches 40%.[67] In the pediatric population, PC has been used as colonic access for the administration of antegrade enemas in patients with chronic fecal incontinence.[68] PC also has been described using endoscopic techniques.[69]

Cecal dilation can occur by mechanical or functional obstruction (Ogilvie's syndrome). Contraindications to PC include severe bowel ischemia, perforation, or an uncorrectable coagulopathy. The technique is similar to placement of a gastrostomy and T-fasteners are used. The catheter is flushed frequently to prevent clogging. The procedure, although infrequent, is highly technically successful with acceptable morbidity rates in appropriately selected patients.[70-72]

Colonic Obstruction

Between 10% and 30% of patients with colorectal carcinoma have large bowel obstruction at the time of presentation.[73] Emergency colectomy carries a high morbidity (50%) and high mortality (23%) rate.[74] Surgical alternatives

include a temporizing colostomy followed, in operable candidates, by two- or three-stage surgery. Stents are indicated for palliative treatment of unresectable colonic malignancy or for temporary colonic decompression to allow bowel cleansing in preparation for single-stage colonic surgery.[75,76]

Technique

Stent placement is accomplished using fluoroscopy with the patient in a lateral or oblique position (Fig. 21-7). Available stents are the enteral Wallstent, Gianturco-Rosch z-stent, and the Ultraflex stent. The use of a long sheath may facilitate further catheter manipulations. The lesion should

FIGURE 21-7 ■ Colonic stent placement for temporary decompression in preparation for single stage surgery. **A,** Plain abdominal radiograph shows large bowel dilation secondary to obstructing distal descending colon carcinoma. **B,** Guidewires and catheters are manipulated across the obstruction. **C,** Deployment of Wallstent is initiated. **D,** Deployment is completed. **E,** Abdominal film 12 hours after the procedure shows successful relief of obstruction. Note no pre– or post–stent deployment balloon dilation.

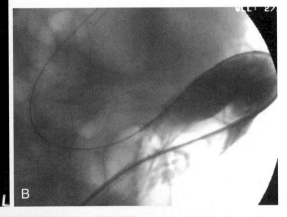

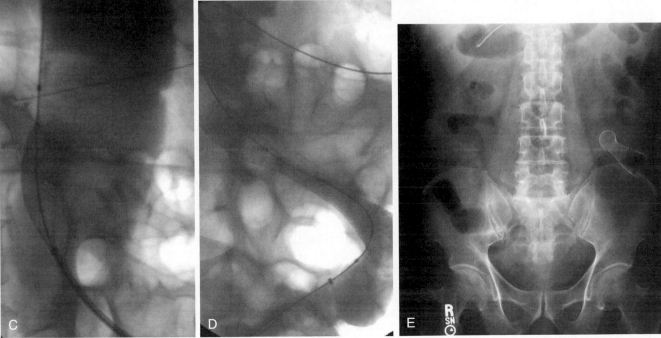

not undergo pre- or post-stent dilation because of the risk for perforation.[77] The ends of the stent should be placed in bowel segments that are straight to avoid kinks. An abdominal radiograph is obtained at 24 hours to assess for stent expansion, position, and success of decompression.

Results

The technical success rate is 78% to 100%, and the clinical success rate is 84% to 100%.[78-81] The complication rate has been reported to be from 14% to 42%, with most complications being minor.[78-81] Severe complications are rare and consist of migration, perforation, and sepsis.

Complications

Early migration is often due to small-caliber stents, fully covered stents, or stents with weak radial force. Late stent migration has been attributed to shrinkage of the tumors following adjuvant chemotherapy. Perforation may result from catheter manipulations and balloon dilation or be due to erosion of the colonic wall by the ends of the stent.

REFERENCES

1. Lew RJ, Kochman ML: A review of endoscopic methods of esophageal dilation. J Clin Gastroenterol 2002;35:117.
2. Agnew SR, Pandya SP, Reynolds RP, Preiksaitis HG: Predictors for frequent esophageal dilations of benign peptic strictures. Dig Dis Sci 1996;41:931.
3. Yamamoto H, Hughes R, Schroeder K: Treatment of benign esophageal strictures by Eder-Puestow or balloon dilators: a comparison between randomized and prospective nonrandomized trials. Mayo Clin Proc 1992;67:228.
4. Broor S, Raju TW, Catalano MF: Long term results of endoscopic dilatation for corrosive esophageal strictures. Gut 1993;34:1498.
5. McClave S, Brady P, Wright R, et al: Does fluoroscopic guidance for Maloney esophageal dilation impact on the clinical endpoint of therapy: relief of dysphagia and achievement of luminal patency. Gastrointest Endosc 1996;43:93.
6. McLean GK, Cooper GS, Hartz WH, et al: Radiologically guided balloon dilation of gastrointestinal strictures. Part I. Technique and factors influencing procedural success. Part II. Results of long-term follow-up. Radiology 1987;165:35,41.
7. Catalano MF, Van Dam J, Sivak AV, et al: Malignant esophageal strictures: staging accuracy of endoscopic ultrasonography. Gastrointest Endosc 1995;41:535.
8. Roubein LD: Endoscopic ultrasonography and the malignant esophageal stricture: implications and complications. Gastrointest Endosc 1995;41:613.
9. Pfau PR, Ginsberg GG, Lew RJ, et al: Efficacy and safety of esophageal dilations for endosonographic evaluation of malignant esophageal strictures. Am J Gastroenterol 2000;95:2813.
10. Wallace MB, Hawes RH, Sahai AV, et al: Dilation of malignant esophageal stenosis to allow EUS guided fine needle aspiration: safety and effect on patient management. Gastrointest Endosc 2000;51:309.
11. Hernandez LJ, Jacobson JW, Harris MS: Comparison among the perforation rates of Maloney, balloon, and Savary dilation of esophageal strictures. Gastrointest Endosc 2000;51:460.
12. Karnac I, Tanyel FC, Buyukpamuken N, et al: Esophageal perforations encountered during the dilation of caustic esophageal strictures. J Cardiovac Surg 1998;39:373.
13. Silvis SE, Nebel O, Rogers G, et al: Endoscopic complications: results of the 1974 American Society of Gastrointestinal Endoscopy survey. JAMA 1976;235:928.
14. Earlam R, Cunha-Melo JR: Malignant esophageal strictures: a review of techniques for palliative intubation. Br J Surg 1982;69:61.
15. Mason RC, Bright N, McColl I: Palliation of malignant dysphagia with laser therapy: predictability of results. Br J Surg 1991;78:1346.
16. Albertson M, Ewers SB, Widmark H, et al: Evaluation of the palliative effect of radiotherapy for esophageal carcinoma. Acta Oncol 1989;28:267.
17. Ogilvie AL, Dionfield MW, Percuson R, et al: Palliative intubation of esophagogastric neoplasms at fiberoptic endoscopy. Gut 1982;23:1060.
18. Frimberger E: Expanding spiral: a new type of prosthesis for the treatment of malignant esophageal stenosis. Endoscopy 1983;15:213.
19. Knyrim K, Wagner HJ, Keymling M, et al: A controlled trial of an expansile metal stent for palliation of esophageal obstruction due to inoperable cancer. N Engl J Med 1993;329:1302.
20. Song H-Y, Lee DH, Seo T-S, et al: Retrievable covered nitinol stents: experience in 108 patients with malignant esophageal strictures. J Vasc Interv Radiol 2002;13:285.
21. Acunas B, Rozanes I, Sayi I, et al: Treatment of malignant dysphagia with nitinol stents. Eur Radiol 1995;5:599.
22. Cwikiel W, Tranberg K-G, Cwikiel M, et al: Malignant dysphagia: palliation with esophageal stents—long term results in 100 patients. Radiology 1998;207:513.
23. Park HS, Do YS, Suh SW, et al: Upper gastrointestinal tract malignant obstruction: initial results of palliation with a flexible covered stent. Radiology 1999;210:865.
24. Poyanli A, Sencer S, Rozanes I, et al: Pallaitive treatment of inoperable malignant esophageal strictures with conically shaped covered seltf expanding stents. Acta Radiol 2001;42:166.
25. Sabharwal T, Hamady MS, Chui S, et al: A randomized prospective comparison of the Flamingo Wallstent and Ultraflex stent for palliation of dysphagia associated with lower third oesophageal carcinoma. Gut 2003;52:922.
26. Therasse E, Oliva VL, Lafontaine E, et al: Balloon dilation and stent placement for esophageal lesions: indications, methods, and results. Radiographics 2003;23:89.
27. Acunas B, Poyanli A, Rozanes I: Intervention in gastrointestinal tract: the treatment of esophageal, gastroduodenal and colonic obstructions with metallic stents. Eur J Radiol 2002;42:240.
28. Baron TH: Expandable metal stents for the treatment of cancerous obstruction of the gastrointestinal tract. N Engl J Med 2001;344:1681.
29. Morgan R, Adam A: Use of metallic stents and balloons in the esophagus and gastrointestinal tract. J Vasc Intervent Radiol 2001;12:283.
30. Wang MA, Sze DY, Wang ZP, et al: Delayed complications after esophageal stent placement for treatment of malignant esophageal obstructions and esophagorespiratory fistulas. J Vasc Interv Radiol 2001;12:465.
31. Pearce CB, Duncan HD: Enteral feeding. Nasogastric, nasojejunal, percutaneous endoscopic gastrostomy, or jejunostomy: its indications and limitations. Postgrad Med J 2002;78:198.
32. Waitzberg DL, Plopper C, Terra RM: Access routes for nutritional therapy. World J Surg 2000;24:1468.
33. Kudsk KA, Corce MA, Fabian TC, et al: Enteral versus parenteral feeding: effects on septic morbidity after blunt and penetrating abdominal trauma. Ann Surg 1992;215:503.
34. Moore FA, Feliciano DV, Andrassy RJ, et al: Early enteral feeding, compared with parenteral, reduces postoperative septic complications: the results of meta-analysis. Ann Surg 1992;216:172.
35. Wasiljew BK, Ujiki GT, Beal JM: Feeding gastrostomy: complications and mortality. Am J Surg 1982;143:194.
36. Cosentini EP, Sautner T, Gnant M, et al: Outcomes of surgical, percutaneous endoscopic and percutaneous radiologic gastrostomies. Arch Surg 1998;133:1076.
37. Wollman B, D'Agostino HB, Walus-Wigle JR, et al: Radiologic, endoscopic and surgical gastrostomy: an institutional evaluation and meta-analysis of the literature. Radiology 1995;197:699.
38. Hoffer EK, Cosgrove JM, Levin DQ, et al: Radiologic gastrojejunostomy and percutaneous endoscopic gastrostomy: a prospective, randomized comparison. J Vasc Interv Radiol 1999;10:413.
39. Lyon SM, Haslam PJ, Duke DM, et al: De novo placement of button gastrostomy catheters in an adult population: experience in 53 patients. J Vasc Interv Radiol 2003;14:1283.
40. Ozmen MN, Akhan O: Percutaneous radiologic gastrostomy. Eur J Radiol 2002;43:186.
41. Sane SS, Towbin A, Bergey EA, et al: Percutaneous gastrostomy tube placement in patients with ventriculoperitoneal shunts. Pediatr Radiol 1998;28:521.

42. Graham SM, Flowers JL, Scott TR, et al: Safety of percutaneous endoscopic gastrostomy in patients with vetriculoperitoneal shunt. Neurosurgery 1993;32:932.

43. Taylor AL, Carroll TA, Jakubowski J, et al: Percutaneous endoscopic gastrostomy in patients with ventriculoperitoneal shunts. Br J Surg 2001;88:724.

44. Taylor CA, Larson DE, Ballard DJ, et al: Predictors of outcome after percutaneous endoscopic gastrostomy: a community-based study. Mayo Clin Proc 1992;67:1402.

45. Stuart SP, Tiley EH, Boland JP: Feeding gastrostomy: a critical review of its indications and mortality rate. South Med J 1993;86:169.

46. Odom SR, Barone JE, Docimo S, et al: Emergency department visits by demented patients with malfunctioning feeding tubes. Surg Endosc 2003;17:651.

47. Angus F, Burakoff R: The percutaneous endoscopic gastrostomy tube: medical and ethical issues in placement. Am J Gastroenterol 2003;98:272.

48. Ahmad I, Mouncher A, Abdoolah A, et al: Antibiotic prophylaxis for percutaneous endoscopic gastrostomy—a prospective, randomized, double-blind trial. Aliment Pharmacol Ther 2003;18:209.

49. vanSonnenberg E, Wittich GR, Brown LK, et al: Percutaneous gastrostomy and gastroenterostomy: 1. Techniques derived from laboratory evaluation, AJR Am J Roentgenol 1986;146:577.

50. Dewald CL, Hiette PO, Sewall LE, et al: Percutaneous gastrostomy and gastrojejunostomy with gastropexy: experience in 701 procedures. Radiology 1999;211:651.

51. Thornton FJ, Fotheringham T, Haslam PJ, et al: Percutaneous radiologic gastrostomy with and without T-fastener gastropexy: a randomized comparison study. Cardiovasc Intervent Radiol 2002;25:467.

52. Clark JA, Pugash RA, Pantalone RR: Radiologic peroral gastrostomy. J Vasc Interv Radiol 1999;10:927.

53. Giuliano AW, Yoon HC, Lomis NN, et al: Fluoroscopically guided percutaneous placement of large-bore gastrostomy and gastrojejunostomy tubes: review of 109 cases. J Vasc Interv Radiol 2000;11:239.

54. Ho C-S, Yeung EY: Percutaneous gastrostomy and transgastric jejunostomy. AJR Am J Roentgenol 1992;158:251.

55. Olson DL, Krubsack AJ, Stewart ET: Percutaneous enteral alimentation: gastrostomy versus gastrojejunostomy. Radiology 1993;187:105.

56. Jain NK, Larson DE, Schroeder KW, et al: Antibiotic prophylaxis for percutaneous endoscopic gastrostomy: a prospective, randomized, double-blind clinical trial. Ann Intern Med 1987;107:824.

57. Park KB, Do YS, Kang WK, et al: Malignant obstruction of gastric outlet and duodenum: palliation with flexible covered metallic stents. Radiology 2001;219:679.

58. Pearce CB, Duncan HD: Enteral feeding. Nasogastric, nasojejunal, percutaneous endoscopic, or jejunostomy: its indications and limitations. Postgrad Med J 2002;78:198.

59. Tapia J, Murguia R, Garcia G, et al: Jejunostomy: techniques, indications, and complications. World J Surg 1999;23:596.

60. Mellert J, Naruhn MB, Grund KE, et al: Direct endoscopic percutaneous jejunostomy (EPJ). Clinical results. Surg Endosc 1994;8:867.

61. Duh QY, Senocozlieff-Englehart AL, Siperstein AE, et al: Prospective evaluation of the safety and efficacy of laparoscopic jejunostomy. West J Med 1995;162:117.

62. Hotozeka M, Adams RB, Miller AD, et al: Laparoscopic percutaneous jejunostomy for long term enteral access. Surg Endosc 1996;10:1008.

63. Gray RR, Ho CS, Yee A, et al: Direct percutaneous jejunostomy. AJR Am J Roentgenol 1987;174:931.

64. Perry LJ, Stokes KR, Lewis WD, et al: Biliary intervention by means of percutaneous puncture of the antecolic jejunal loop. Radiology 1995;195:163.

65. Davies RP, Kew J, West GP: Percutaneous jejunostomy using CT fluoroscopy. AJR Am J Roentgenol 2001;176:808.

66. Heitmiller RF, Venbrux AC, Osterman FA: Percutaneous replacement jejunostomy. Ann Thorac Surg 1992;53:711.

67. Saunders MD, Kimmey MB: Colonic pseudo-obstruction: the dilated colon in the ICU. Semin Gastrointest Dis 2003;14:20.

68. Chait PG, Shlomovitz E, Connolly BL, et al: Percutaneous cecostomy: update in technique and patient care. Radiology 2003;227:246.

69. Ramage JI, Baron TH: Percutaneous endoscopic cecostomy: a case series. Gastrointest Endosc 2003;57:752.

70. vanSonnenberg E, Varney RR, Casola G, et al: Percutaneous cecostomy in Ogilvie syndrome: laboratory observations and clinical experience. Radiology 1990;175:679.

71. Morrison MC, Lee MJ, Stafford SA, et al: Percutaneous cecostomy: controlled transperitoneal approach. Radiology 1990;176:574.

72. Benacci JC, Wolff BG: Cecostomy. Therapeutic indications and results. Dis Colon Rectum 1995;38:530.

73. Deans GT, Krukowski ZH, Irwin ST: Maliganant obstruction of the left colon. Br J Surg 1994;81:1270.

74. Beuchter KJ, Boustany C, Cailloutte R, et al: Surgical management of the acutely obstructed colon: a review of 127 cases. Am J Surg 1988;156:163.

75. Mainar A, Tiger E, Maynar M, et al: Colorectal obstruction: treatment with metallic stents. Radiology 1996;198:761.

76. Binkert CA, Ledermann H, Jost R, et al: Acute colonic obstruction: clinic aspects and cost-effectiveness of preoperative and palliative treatment with self-expanding metallic stents—a preliminary report. Radiology 1998;206:199.

77. Canon CL, Baron TH, Morgan DE, et al: Treatment of colonic obstruction with expandable stents: radiology features. AJR Am J Roentgenol 1997;168:199.

78. Choo IW, Do YS, Suh SW, et al: Malignant colorectal obstruction: treatment with a flexible covered stent. Radiology 1998;206:415.

79. Camunez F, Echenagosia A, Simo G, et al: Malignant colorectal obstruction treated with self-expanding metallic stents: effectiveness before scheduled surgery and in palliation. Radiology 2000;216:492.

80. Baron TH, Dean PH, Yates MR, et al: Expandable metal stents for the treatment of colonic obstruction: techniques and outcomes. Gastrointest Endosc 1998;47:277.

81. De Gregorio MA, Mainar A, Tejero E, et al: Acute colorectal obstruction: stent placement for palliative treatment—results of a multicenter study. Radiology 1998;209:117.

22

Biliary System

Steven C. Rose, MD

Percutaneous invasive procedures involving the biliary system are designed to prove, characterize, and treat suspected biliary obstruction and, occasionally, biliary leaks. Huard provided the initial description of transhepatic cholangiography (THC) in 1937.[1] Remolar and coworkers first described external percutaneous biliary drainage (PBD) in 1956.[2] Nevertheless, these procedures did not become widely accepted until the late 1970s, when skinny-needle puncture techniques and coaxial exchange systems were developed to minimize the incidence of serious procedure-related hemorrhagic complications. Since their development in the late 1980s, endoscopic retrograde cholangiopancreatography (ERCP) and subsequently transendoscopic biliary drainage have diminished the need for THC and PBD. Percutaneous therapy continues to have a role in patients with anatomy unfavorable to endoscopic procedures and in institutions without skilled interventional endoscopists.

■ NORMAL ANATOMY

The bile ducts of the posterior and anterior segments of the right hepatic lobe join near the porta hepatis to form the main right hepatic duct. The bile ducts of the medial and lateral segments of the left hepatic lobe merge to become the left main hepatic duct.[3] The right posterior and right anterior segmental bile ducts join the left main hepatic duct directly in about 25% and 6% of individuals, respectively. The right and left main hepatic ducts coalesce in the hilum to form the common hepatic duct. At the porta hepatis, the bile ducts run anterior to the hepatic artery and portal vein. The gallbladder empties into the cystic duct, which is joined by the common hepatic duct to become the common bile duct (CBD), which travels within the hepatoduodenal ligament to drain through the sphincter of Oddi into the duodenum. A number of potential aberrant communications exists between the biliary tree and the gallbladder. The complex relationship between the biliary ductal system and the Couinaud hepatic segmental nomenclature has been described by Gazelle and colleagues.[4]

■ TRANSHEPATIC CHOLANGIOGRAPHY

Patient Selection and Preparation

Given the widespread use of advanced cross-sectional imaging and ERCP, nearly all patients have THC in conjunction with PBD. The primary indication for THC is to confirm, localize, and characterize obstructive disease of the biliary system in patients with symptoms of pruritus or cholangitis who are not amenable to ERCP. Increasingly, MR cholangiography is being used to image the biliary system noninvasively.[5] Occasionally, THC and PBD are used as part of the nonoperative management of patients with biliary leaks from bile duct injuries.

In addition to establishing the presence of biliary obstruction, cholangiography can localize the obstruction and frequently determines the benign or malignant cause of the stricture. However, the cholangiographic appearance may be misleading. The final diagnosis rests on tissue analysis. In patients who are candidates for operative resection and biliary-enteric decompression, the tissue diagnosis usually is made from the operative specimen. In cases managed nonoperatively, the transhepatic access is a convenient route for obtaining the necessary material.

The relative benefits and risks of THC are weighed against those of endoscopic and operative diagnostic methods. Primary factors in the selection of patients include the suspected anatomic level, cause of biliary obstruction, and the availability of highly skilled practitioners.

Most distal (periampullary) bile duct obstructions are managed endoscopically. Middle (extrahepatic and extrapancreatic) CBD lesions typically undergo operative resection with creation of a biliary-enteric anastomosis. Proximal (hilar) hepatic duct and intrahepatic bile duct strictures usually are treated with percutaneous techniques.

Bacterial overgrowth is common with biliary obstruction, particularly when caused by malignancy. Infectious complications are one of the common sources of fatal and major nonfatal complications. Biliary colonization with enteric organisms should be assumed in all patients with obstructive jaundice, whether evidence of suppurative cholangitis exists or not. Antibiotic prophylaxis is therefore routinely recommended.[6-8] An antibiotic with appropriate coverage for gram-negative bacteria should be administered parenterally approximately 1 hour before the procedure to obtain adequate periprocedural blood levels.

The liver is a highly vascular organ, and the targeted bile ducts course adjacent to hepatic arteries and portal veins, which may be inadvertently injured. Coagulation factors (i.e., prothrombin time, partial thromboplastin time, platelet count, and, occasionally, the bleeding time) should be assessed and corrected if possible.[9] A severe uncorrectable coagulopathy is a contraindication to the procedure. Massive, circumferential ascites impedes effective tamponade of blood or bile in addition to increasing the difficulty of catheter manipulation and the likelihood of accidental catheter dislodgement. These patients should have an alternative procedure or undergo paracentesis immediately before the transhepatic intervention. Uncooperative patients are also at high risk for bleeding complications for several reasons and should undergo an alternative procedure or receive general anesthesia.

Transhepatic biliary drainage procedures are significantly more painful than most diagnostic and interventional vascular procedures. Pain management should be liberal, particularly because multistaged procedures are common. Abundant local anesthesia and heavy conscious sedation, appropriately trained personnel, and monitoring equipment are essential. Frequently, assistance from anesthesia personnel is advisable and may include monitored analgesia (e.g., propofol and nitrous oxide) or general anesthesia.[10] Intercostal nerve blocks can help with body wall pain. Most operators have found celiac plexus blocks to be cumbersome and ineffective.[11]

Technique

Skinny-needle access into the intrahepatic bile ducts is the essence of THC and the first step of PBD. Access into the biliary system is gained through the right intrahepatic bile ducts using a low right intercostal approach or through the left intrahepatic bile ducts using an anterior subxiphoid entry (Fig. 22-1). The right-sided approach often is preferred, because most interventional radiologists are comfortable

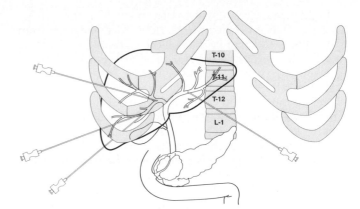

FIGURE 22-1 ■ Routes for percutaneous biliary access. Left-sided access is subcostal from the anterior abdomen. Right-sided access is subcostal or low intercostal from the right mid-axillary line, directed toward the 11th thoracic vertebral body.

with the technique, the operator's hands are not in the fluoroscopic field during guidewire and catheter manipulation, and the right lobe contains most of the hepatic parenchyma. Disadvantages include pain related to irritation of the rib periosteum, risk of crossing the parietal pleura (leading to bilothorax, empyema, and, rarely, pneumothorax), occasionally unfavorable angles for manipulation of catheters into the CBD, and the palmate-type (i.e., like a maple leaf), right-sided biliary branching pattern. This anatomic feature is more likely to result in isolated biliary segments in the setting of invasive hilar malignancy (Fig. 22-2).

Advantages to the left-sided approach include the ability to use ultrasound guidance to find a suitable bile duct while avoiding the adjacent vascular structures, the usually favorable angles for catheterization between the left-sided bile ducts and the CBD, and the more pinnate (i.e., like a feather) branching pattern typical of the left-sided bile duct (see Fig. 22-2), which is less likely to result in segmental isolation with invasive malignancy. Subxiphoid catheters avoid the pleura completely, usually are less uncomfortable than intercostal catheters, and are easier for the patient to flush. Disadvantages of left-sided access include increased radiation exposure to the radiologist's hands and less experience by many interventional radiologists with this sometimes challenging technique. In patients with hilar malignancy that has resulted in isolation of right and left bile ducts, right- and left-sided biliary procedures should be planned, particularly if evidence of suppurative cholangitis exists.

FIGURE 22-2 ■ Biliary branching pattern. Shaded surface display of a spiral CT cholangiogram performed through an indwelling, left-sided percutaneous biliary drainage catheter in a patient with pancreatic adenocarcinoma. **A,** Right anterior oblique view displays the pinnate-type (feather-like), left-sided branching pattern. **B,** Inferior view depicts palmate-type (maple leaf–like), right-sided branching pattern.

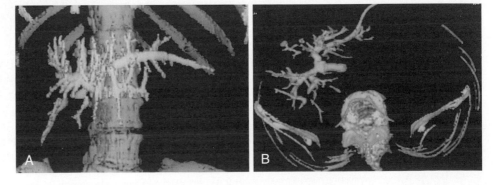

Right-sided access involves placement of a skinny (e.g., 22-gauge Chiba) needle into the right-sided bile ducts from a low intercostal approach along the right mid-axillary line (see Fig. 22-1). The needle should enter below the 10th rib to avoid the parietal pleural reflection, although a more cephalad entry point frequently is required by the position of the inferior margin of the right lobe of the liver or the anticipated location of the porta hepatis. Fluoroscopy is used to assess the costophrenic sulcus during full inspiration to guarantee that the lung does not cross the projected access route. The needle is passed over the superior aspect of a given rib to minimize the risk of injury to the intercostal arteries. Under fluoroscopic guidance, the needle is then directed along a plane parallel to the tabletop and aimed toward the 11th thoracic vertebral body. If the same access may be used for biliary drainage, the needle pass should stop at approximately the right midclavicular line to avoid inadvertent puncture of left-side bile ducts, through which it would be nearly impossible to negotiate a guidewire or catheter toward the CBD.

The needle stylet is removed, and a small-volume syringe (e.g., 1 to 5 mL) with 60% strength contrast medium is attached. Small aliquots (e.g., 0.1 to 0.2 mL) of contrast material are delivered while the needle tip is slowly retracted under fluoroscopy. If the contrast material remains as a smudge at the needle tip, the tip is located in the liver parenchyma, and it should continue to be withdrawn. If contrast medium enters a tubular structure but then flows readily away, the needle tip probably resides within a vascular structure and withdrawal is continued. If contrast material fills a tubular structure and remains in the region of the needle tip, the tip probably is within the biliary system. Injection of an additional 5 to 10 mL should confirm the intrabiliary location and determine the ductal diameter and relationship to the porta hepatis and obstructive lesions.

Left-sided access originates from the left subcostal aspect of the epigastrium. Sonographic guidance permits direct visualization of the skinny needle as it is directed into an acceptable left bile duct while minimizing the likelihood of traversing the adjacent left hepatic artery or left portal vein branch (Fig. 22-3). Aspirated bile should be sent for routine Gram stain, culture, and sensitivity tests; if infectious complications arise, informed choices can be made regarding antimicrobial therapy.

If a diagnostic THC is to be performed without subsequent PBD, removal of 5 to 10 mL of bile alternating with instillation of 5 to 10 mL of contrast material permits diagnostic cholangiographic images while minimizing the risk of bacteremia and possible gram-negative sepsis. If a biliary leak is suspected, full-strength (60%) contrast material is warranted to visualize the fistula. However, if intraluminal filling defects (e.g., stones) or disease with subtle bile duct wall abnormalities (e.g., sclerosing cholangitis) is suspected, 60% contrast medium should be diluted by one half with normal saline solution. The biliary system should be aspirated before removal of the skinny needle if drainage is not planned.

Imaging Findings

Most pathologic processes of the biliary tree are manifested in a few forms[12-18]:

■ Abnormally small-caliber bile ducts or occlusion of the bile ducts (Table 22-1)

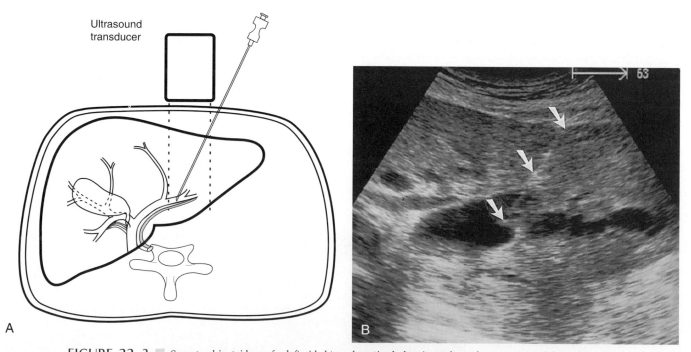

FIGURE 22-3 ■ Sonographic guidance for left-sided transhepatic cholangiography and percutaneous biliary drainage. **A,** The ultrasound probe has a transverse orientation along the axis of the left-sided bile duct and adjacent hepatic artery and portal vein. The skinny needle courses along the sonographic imaging plane to selectively enter the bile duct. **B,** The transverse sonogram depicts the needle course *(arrows)* through the liver and into the dilated left-sided bile duct.

TABLE 22-1   NARROWING OR OCCLUSION OF THE BILIARY DUCTS

Disease or Cause	Suggestive Findings
Pseudostricture due to positional underfilling of contrast material (Fig. 22-4)	Supine: narrow proximal (hilar) CBD and nonopacified left bile ducts Prone: narrow distal CBD and nonopacified right bile ducts Eliminated by positional changes
Pseudocalculus due to mucosal prolapse (Fig. 22-5)	Distal CBD meniscus Mimics stone or polyp Intermittently disappears as sphincter opens
Cholangiocarcinoma (Fig. 22-6)	Usually located near hilum or associated with sclerosing cholangitis Usually occlusive Usually abrupt margin Nodular surface
Pancreatic or ampullary carcinoma (Fig. 22-7)	Located at distal CBD Fixed lesion "Rat tail" appearance Usually occlusive
Extrinsic adenopathy	Usually hilar or suprapancreatic CBD Nonspecific May have smooth surface
Fibrosis (Fig. 22-8)	Located at biliary-enteric or biliary-biliary anastomosis, site of injury, papilla, or in proximity to stones Usually short segment Usually smooth
Sclerosing cholangitis (Fig. 22-9)	Multifocal strictures Intra- and extrahepatic May have diffuse narrowing Often mural diverticular outpouching
AIDS-related cholangitis Ischemic or chemotoxic structures (Fig. 22-10)	Similar to sclerosing cholangitis, papillary stenosis, or both Patients with liver transplant or liver malignancy and transcatheter chemoinfusion or chemoembolization Multifocal, diffuse intrahepatic strictures May have anastomotic stricture May have associated sloughed debris, leaks
Oriental cholangiohepatitis (Fig. 22-11)	Multiple intrahepatic strictures Upstream dilation, especially left lobe Usually associated with innumerable stones

AIDS, acquired immunodeficiency syndrome; CBD, common bile duct.

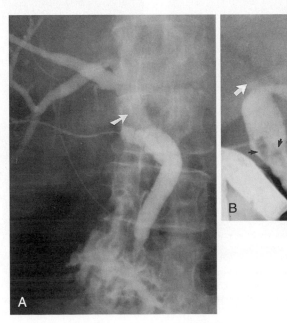
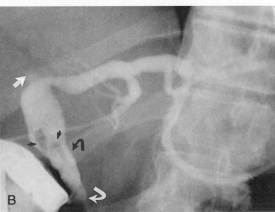

FIGURE 22-4 ■ Artifactual nonopacification of bile ducts caused by underfilling with contrast material, which has a higher specific gravity than bile. **A,** T-tube cholangiogram in a supine patient. The nondependent common hepatic duct *(arrow)* appears narrow, and the left-sided bile ducts did not fill at all. **B,** Endoscopic retrograde cholangiopancreatography in a nearly prone patient. The nondependent distal common bile duct appears narrow (between *curved arrows*). Right-sided ducts *(straight white arrow)* are not opacified. The irregular filling defect *(small black arrows)* in the distal common bile duct is viscous bile.

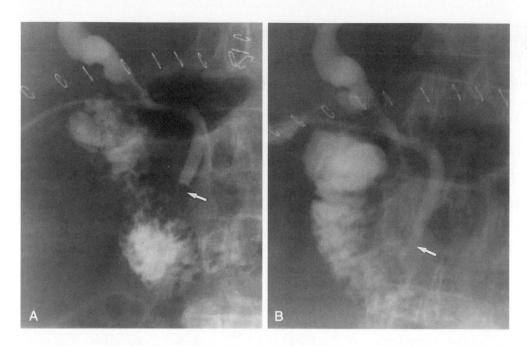

FIGURE 22-5 ■ Mucosal prolapse. **A,** A polypoid filling defect is identified in the distal common bile duct *(arrow)*. **B,** A few minutes later, the sphincter has opened *(arrow)*.

- Abnormally large-caliber bile ducts (Table 22-2)
- Filling defects within the intraluminal contrast material (Table 22-3)
- Extraluminal location of contrast material (Table 22-4)

Biliary manometry is required occasionally to establish the presence of distal obstruction. The technique is modeled on the urodynamic Whitaker test.[19,20] A baseline biliary pressure is established through the THC needle or through an external PBD catheter. A resting biliary pressure that exceeds 15 cm H_2O is diagnostic for downstream obstruction. If the resting pressure is less than 15 cm H_2O, a saline infusion challenge is indicated. Saline mixed with dilute contrast material is infused through a suitable infusion pump, initially at a rate of 2 mL/minute and then at 4, 8, and 10 mL/minute. After 5 to 10 minutes of infusion at each rate, the biliary pressure is recorded. If the biliary pressure exceeds 20 cm H_2O at any point during saline infusion, a diagnosis of a significant downstream obstruction can be made. If the pressure does not exceed 20 cm H_2O despite a saline infusion rate of 10 mL/minute, a significant downstream occlusion is excluded.

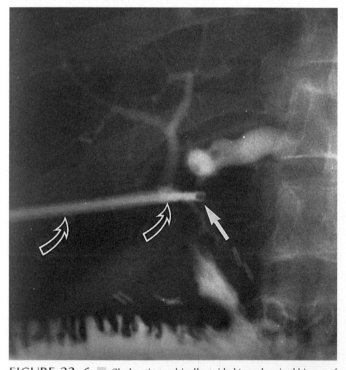

FIGURE 22-6 ■ Cholangiographically guided transluminal biopsy of hilar cholangiocarcinoma using a myocardial biopsy forceps *(straight arrow)* introduced through a vascular-type percutaneous transhepatic sheath *(curved arrows)*.

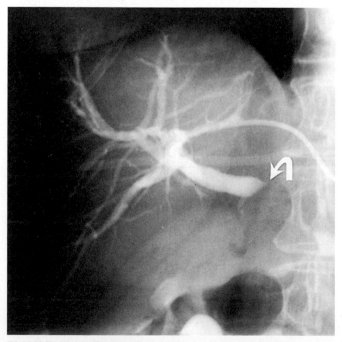

FIGURE 22-7 ■ Malignant stricture in the common bile duct caused by pancreatic carcinoma. The stricture has a "rat-tail" or beaked appearance *(curved arrow)*, typical of malignant periampullary strictures.

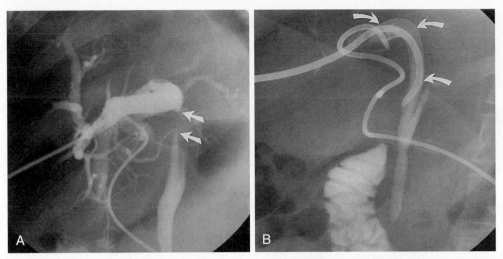

FIGURE 22-8 ■ Expandable metallic stent for a benign tuberculous stricture. Contrast-enhanced CT scan showed dilation of intrahepatic bile ducts bilaterally. The extrahepatic bile ducts were normal. **A,** Left anterior oblique view of a cholangiogram performed through a bilateral percutaneous biliary drainage catheter defined a near-occlusive eccentric stricture *(arrows)* of the hilar portion of the common bile duct, which had been retracted posteriorly, presumably because of fibrosis. **B,** After attempted percutaneous cholangioplasty, which failed because of elastic recoil, an 8-mm-diameter, 40-mm-long Wallstent *(arrows)* was deployed successfully. The left anterior oblique view documented excellent stent position and expansion.

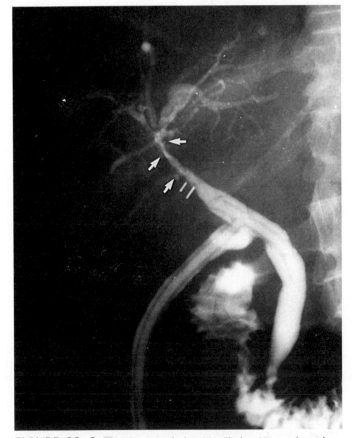

FIGURE 22-9 ■ Sclerosing cholangitis. Cholangiogram through an indwelling T-tube shows multiple strictures of intrahepatic and extrahepatic bile ducts. Scattered normal segments of intrahepatic bile ducts are seen upstream from the strictures; otherwise, intrahepatic ducts are of small caliber. Subtle diverticula *(arrows)* of the strictured common hepatic duct are detected, and the surgical clips are from a cholecystectomy.

Aspirated bile may be collected for cytologic examination. Cytologic material also can be obtained using a miniature brush biopsy device mounted on a guidewire (Fig. 22-19). The brush biopsy device is introduced through an angiographic catheter with the brush passed intraluminally to and fro across the stricture. The brush tip is then cut off and placed in a fixative solution. Another technique for obtaining cytologic material is fluoroscopically guided percutaneous skinny-needle aspiration (Fig. 22-20). Using the THC or PBD access, cholangiography is performed to localize the stricture. Through a second percutaneous approach (usually anterior subcostal), a skinny needle is advanced using fluoroscopic guidance to sample the identified stricture.

Higher diagnostic yields for proving benign or malignant disease come from histologic examination of larger tissue samples because cellular architecture can be evaluated. To accommodate the larger transluminal biopsy devices, a vascular access sheath is placed into the biliary system through the transhepatic route. The hemostatic valve permits passage of the device while contrast material is injected through the side arm port to guide the biopsy.

All transluminal biliary biopsy devices originally were developed for intravascular use and include myocardial biopsy forceps (see Fig. 22-6) and the Simpson atherectomy device (Devices for Vascular Interventions, Temecula, Calif.).[21,22] The flexible transjugular liver biopsy needle (Cook, Inc., Bloomington, Ind.) should not be used because it is designed to penetrate several centimeters beyond the lumen and may injure the adjacent hepatic artery or portal vein, possibly in an intraperitoneal location.

Results and Complications

When the bile ducts are dilated, THC can be performed in almost every case. With nondilated biliary systems, the

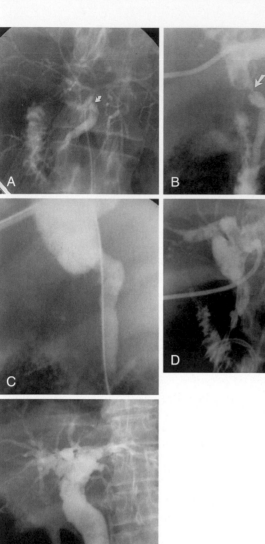

success rates range from 60% to 96%, depending on the number of passes that the operator is willing to make.[15,23-28] THC is extremely accurate (96%) in differentiating obstructive from hepatocellular causes of jaundice.[29] Bile duct dilation usually indicates biliary obstruction, although in certain diseases, such as sclerosing cholangitis and the cholangiopathy associated with hepatic arterial chemoinfusion therapy and hepatic arterial occlusive disease in liver transplant recipients, the bile ducts may not dilate significantly in response to downstream obstruction.[15,30] Alternatively, the cholangiographic appearance of the intrahepatic bile ducts may not reflect the biliary dynamics of an incompletely occlusive benign stricture (e.g., at a biliary-enteric anastomosis) or the physiologic response to an intervention (e.g., cholangioplasty or stent placement). In these occasional situations, biliary manometry may be helpful to establish the presence of downstream obstruction.[19,20] The major complications of transhepatic cholangiography are sepsis and bleeding. Serious complications occur in 3% to 8% of cases.[23-27]

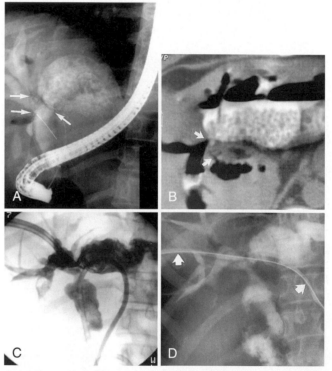

FIGURE 22-10 ■ Cholangioplasty for treatment of a benign (ischemic) biliary stricture. **A,** Initial T-tube cholangiogram in a patient 1 week after orthotopic liver transplantation that was complicated by thrombosis of the hepatic artery. A mild stricture of the choledochal anastomosis *(arrow)* coexisted with diffuse narrowing of the intrahepatic bile ducts. **B,** Five months later, left-sided percutaneous biliary drainage (PBD) was performed to treat obstructive jaundice and suppurative cholangitis. The diagnostic cholangiogram was performed several days after PBD and demonstrated a high-grade anastomotic stricture *(arrow)* with associated upstream bile duct dilation and numerous intraluminal filling defects caused by necrotic debris. **C,** The cholangiogram after dilation documented satisfactory expansion of the stricture. **D,** After balloon cholangioplasty, a 12-French internal and external PBD catheter was left to stent the anastomosis. **E,** Endoscopic retrograde cholangiopancreatography performed 5 months after the cholangioplasty confirmed that the anastomotic site was stricture free. Global dilation of the common bile duct and central portions of the intrahepatic bile ducts, the various calibers of peripheral intrahepatic bile ducts, and the copious intraluminal biliary debris are typical late findings of ischemic cholangiopathy.

FIGURE 22-11 ■ Staged multimodality management of complex biliary disease (Oriental cholangiohepatitis). **A,** Endoscopic retrograde cholangiopancreatography (ERCP) demonstrated multiple hilar biliary strictures *(arrows)*, dilation of multiple intrahepatic bile ducts, and innumerable biliary calculi located within a massively dilated left bile duct. Pneumobilia resulted from prior endoscopic papillotomy. **B,** Magnified view of the abdominal CT scan after the ERCP confirmed the hilar biliary strictures *(arrows)*, bile duct dilation, and calculi. **C,** After bilateral biliary drainage, balloon cholangioplasty of the hilar biliary strictures, multiple sessions of basket retrieval of pigmented biliary calculi, and oral administration of ursodeoxycholic acid, the cholangiogram demonstrated improvement in the hilar biliary luminal diameter, partial resolution of the intrahepatic bile duct dilation, and near-complete removal of the calculi. **D,** After successful transluminal therapy, the bilateral percutaneous biliary drainage catheters have been converted to a chronic indwelling Silastic U-tube *(arrows)* to preserve transhepatic biliary access. (Courtesy of Thomas Kinney, MD, and Horacio D'Agostino, MD, University of California, San Diego, Medical Center.)

TABLE 22-2 DILATED BILIARY DUCTS

Disease or Cause	Suggestive Findings
Obstruction (see Figs. 22-7 and 22-8)	Diffuse, though may disproportionately affect extrahepatic or left lobe bile ducts Upstream from obstructing structure (stricture, stone)
Prior obstruction	History of treated obstruction Contrast material flows to bowel May need manometry to distinguish from true obstruction
Choledochal cysts	
Type I (80% to 90%) (Fig. 22-12)	Extrahepatic CBD Fusiform, single
Type II (2%) (Fig. 22-13)	Extrahepatic CBD Saccular or diverticular, single
Type III (1% to 5%)	Intraduodenal, single
Choledochocele	
Type IV	Multiple cysts Usually intrahepatic and extrahepatic
Type V (Fig. 22-14)	Caroli's disease Single or multiple Intrahepatic or extrahepatic bile ducts Associated hepatic fibrosis, renal cysts, renal tubular ectasia
Late-phase ischemic injury (see Fig. 22-10)	History of liver transplantation Central biliary ectasia with debris[14] Peripheral pruning of intrahepatic bile ducts
Denervation	History of liver transplantation Diffuse dilation May have sphincter of Oddi dysfunction
Oriental cholangiohepatitis (see Fig. 22-11)	Listed in Table 22-1

CBD, common bile duct.

Cytologic study performed on aspirated bile may identify cells shed by bile duct malignancy. Fluid obtained from the initial puncture probably has the highest yield. Harell and coworkers collected 20 mL of bile for cytodiagnosis through THC, PBD, T-tube, or operative biliary duct aspiration in 27 patients with obstructive jaundice; malignant cells were detected in 7 of 15 patients with malignant strictures for a

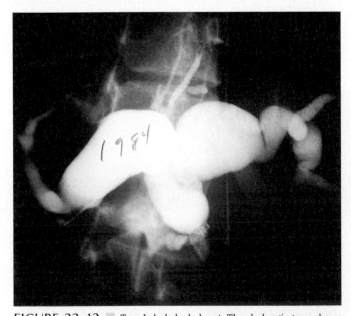

FIGURE 22-12 ■ Type I choledochal cyst. The cholangiogram shows diffuse dilation of the common hepatic duct and central portions of both left and right intrahepatic ducts. The patient previously had undergone resection of the common bile duct (high risk for cholangiocarcinoma) with creation of choledochojejunostomy drainage.

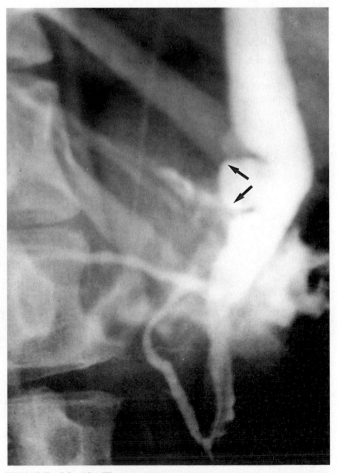

FIGURE 22-13 ■ Type II choledochal cyst. Endoscopic retrograde cholangiopancreatography (with scope removed) shows a focal eccentric outpouching (arrows) in the suprapancreatic portion of the common bile duct.

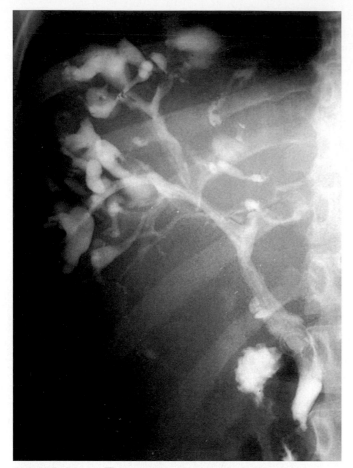

FIGURE 22-14 ■ Caroli's disease. The cholangiogram was performed by means of a right percutaneous biliary drainage catheter. Multiple intrahepatic segments of cystic dilation are evident. (From Rose SC, Kumpe DA, Weil R III: Percutaneous biliary drainage in diffuse Caroli's disease. AJR Am J Roentgenol 1986;147:159. Copyright © 1986, American Roentgen Ray Society.)

TABLE 22-3   BILIARY DUCT FILLING DEFECTS

Disease or Cause	Suggestive Findings
Air bubbles (Fig. 22-15)	Shape conforms to surrounding structures Shape changes with movement Fragmentation and coalescence May be able to be aspirated May be seen exiting catheter Usually move to nondependent bile ducts
Blood clot (Fig. 22-16)	History of invasive procedure or injury Usually forms cast of bile duct Usually disappears or shrivels within 48 hr
Stones (Fig. 22-17; see also Fig. 22-11)	Often faceted, smooth If mobile, often falls to dependent portion of bile duct Constant shape No fragmentation without manipulation No coalescence Single or multiple Frequently associated with strictures or gallstones May be impacted in distal common bile duct (meniscus) or cystic duct (Mirizzi syndrome with common hepatic duct obstruction)
Pseudocalculus	Listed in Table 22-1
Polypoid tumor	Eccentric, nonmobile Usually nodular surface
Debris (see Fig. 22-10)	Irregular, mobile Usually associated with sphincterotomy, biliary-enteric anastomosis, metallic expandable stent into bowel, or ischemic injury
Parasites	May appear curvilinear or wormlike May be associated with strictures or stones Others listed in Table 22-1

sensitivity of 47%, specificity of 100%, and accuracy of 58%.[30] Muro and colleagues reported 34% sensitivity and 100% specificity for cytologic examination of bile obtained from PBD in patients with malignant strictures.[31] Despite a relatively low sensitivity, a biliary cytologic study probably is worthwhile because it involves no additional risk, is relatively inexpensive, and may avoid more costly and invasive

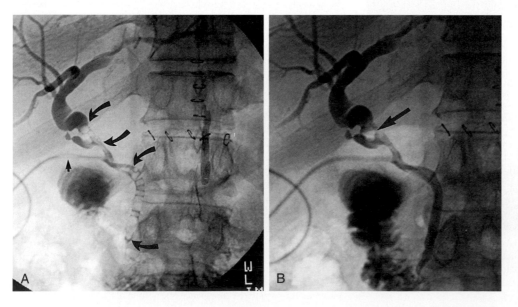

FIGURE 22-15 ■ Air bubbles at cholangiography. **A,** An air bubble is seen within the T-tube *(small arrow)*. The bubble shape conforms to the wall of the common bile duct and to other bubbles *(between curved arrows)*. **B,** Continued injection of contrast material expels the bubbles from the distal duct. The three bubbles in the common hepatic duct have coalesced into a single large bubble *(arrow)*.

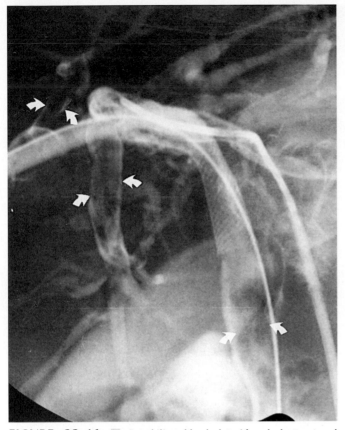

FIGURE 22-16 ▪ Intrabiliary blood clot. After deployment and expansion of a Wallstent for a tuberculous biliary stricture, a cast of the biliary system caused by the blood clot is evident *(arrows)*. A cholangiogram performed several days later showed spontaneous clearance of blood.

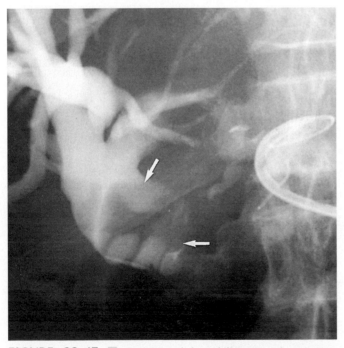

FIGURE 22-17 ▪ An impacted, large biliary stone is seen on a cholangiogram performed through the left percutaneous biliary drainage catheter. The stone *(arrows)* has a typical faceted surface and causes peripheral biliary dilation.

TABLE 22-4	BILIARY DUCT LEAKAGE
Disease or Cause	**Suggestive Findings**
Elevated intraluminal pressure (obstruction) (Fig. 22-18)	Downstream stricture Hepatic abscesses or suppurative cholangitis
Poor ductal wall integrity Bile duct injury Dehisced biliary anastomosis or cystic duct stump Ischemia Radiation therapy	History of right upper quadrant surgery or injury, hepatic artery thrombosis, or irradiation Associated with bilomas, intrahepatic or extrahepatic abscesses, ascites, and fistulas to bowel, skin, or wounds May be associated with downstream strictures

tests if results are positive for malignancy. The reported sensitivity of fluoroscopically guided skinny-needle aspiration ranges from 60% to 83%.[32,33] Savader and coinvestigators[34,35] found fluoroscopic intraductal brush biopsy to have a sensitivity of 26% and specificity of 96% for detection of malignancy. Although all of the cytologic techniques involve little risk, they are relatively insensitive in diagnosing biliary malignancy, particularly cholangiocarcinoma, and generally are of no use in excluding malignancy.

Although published reports are limited, diagnostic yields using biopsy devices seem higher than those for cytologic techniques, with sensitivities from 30% to 80% for patients who had prior negative skinny-needle aspiration or brush biopsy results.[21,22,30-35] Periprocedural morbidity is acceptably low (0 to 10% of cases).

▪ PERCUTANEOUS BILIARY DRAINAGE

Patient Selection

PBD is performed for decompression of symptomatic biliary obstruction or diversion of bile flow away from biliary leaks in patients whose anatomy (e.g., prior choledochojejunostomy) or disease location (e.g., porta hepatitis or intrahepatic bile ducts) is not favorable for endoscopic or operative drainage procedures. In addition to the contraindications for THC (including severe uncorrectable coagulopathy and massive ascites), PBD is ineffective and therefore relatively contraindicated in patients with multifocal biliary obstruction due to hepatic metastases.

Technique

Initial transhepatic access into the biliary system is identical to the technique used for THC. If the skinny needle used for the THC has entered the biliary system in a suitable location, a 0.018-inch guidewire should be advanced sufficiently far enough into the system that the stainless steel mandrel is positioned within the bile ducts (Fig. 22-21). Features favorable for use of a biliary radical for PBD include a bile duct diameter adequate to accept an 8- to 10-French drain, a system with favorable angles of approach to the porta

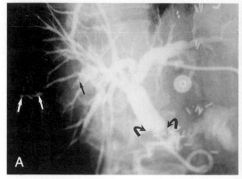

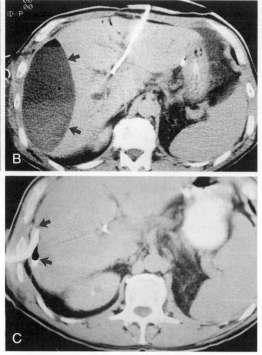

FIGURE 22-18 ■ Biliary leak. **A,** Cholangiogram performed through the left internal-external drainage catheter shows extravasation of contrast *(straight arrows)* along a prior right-sided biliary drainage track and an obstructive stricture at the choledocho-jejunostomy anastomosis *(curved arrows)*. **B,** A large subcapsular hepatic abscess *(arrows)* is identified by contrast-enhanced CT. Percutaneous drainage of the abscess was performed with initial return of thick, purulent material, which later converted to bile. **C,** Another CT scan 12 days later documents successful treatment of the abscess *(arrows)* by simultaneous diversion of bile through the left percutaneous biliary drainage catheter and drainage of the infected biloma. The biliary-enteric anastomotic stricture was treated with balloon cholangioplasty.

hepatis and CBD, and an entry point at least a couple of centimeters upstream from the biliary stricture or leak to allow a pigtail loop to form or accommodate several side holes of a drainage catheter.

If the initial biliary puncture is unsuitable, the biliary system can be opacified through the first needle to guide a second skinny needle into a more desirable location. Over the 0.018-inch guidewire, the skinny needle is replaced for a coaxial exchange set so that a 0.038-inch working guidewire can be advanced into the biliary system with the original 0.018-inch wire left as a safety guidewire. The access set can be removed and an angiographic catheter advanced over the working guidewire into the intrahepatic bile ducts.

In patients with evidence of suppurative cholangitis, manipulation (including contrast injection) should be

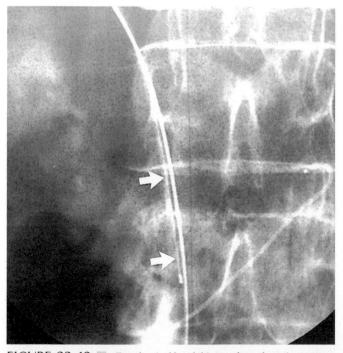

FIGURE 22-19 ■ Transluminal brush biopsy of extrahepatic common bile duct cholangiocarcinoma. Brush biopsy *(arrows)* passes adjacent to the safety guidewire.

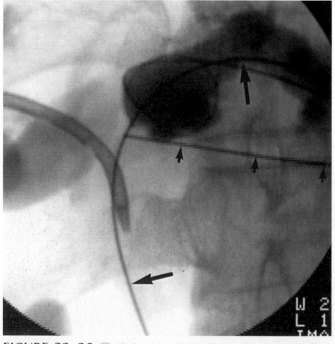

FIGURE 22-20 ■ Cholangiographic guidance of percutaneous fine-needle aspiration biopsy of cholangiocarcinoma. A fine needle *(small arrows)* was advanced under fluoroscopic guidance until it struck the left-sided biliary safety guidewire *(large arrows)* within the strictured segment.

FIGURE 22-21 ■ Steps for converting transhepatic cholangiography into percutaneous biliary drainage. **A,** The 0.018-inch guidewire is advanced well into the biliary system through the skinny needle, which is then removed. **B,** Over the 0.018-inch guidewire, a coaxial exchange set is passed into the bile ducts. **C,** After removing the metal stiffening cannula and inner small-bore coaxial dilator, a 0.038-inch working guidewire and a 5-French angiographic catheter are introduced through the sheath and negotiated across the stricture (represented by a pancreatic head mass in these diagrams). **D,** After removal of the outer exchange system sheath, the 0.018-inch safety guidewire has been secured on the drape. Over the 0.038-inch heavy-duty working guidewire, an 8- to 12-French multiple-side-hole biliary drain is passed into an appropriate position.

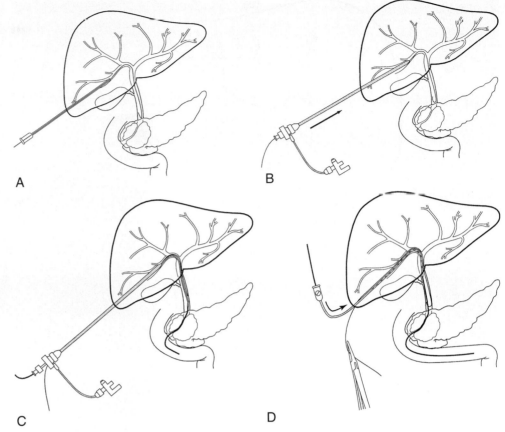

minimized and an external-type PBD placed and left to gravity drainage. In uninfected patients, 5 to 15 minutes of gentle probing with the guidewire and catheter frequently is successful in traversing the stricture or leak to pass a guidewire into the bowel. If the obstructing lesion cannot be traversed safely at the initial sitting, a repeated attempt often is successful after 2 to 3 days of decompression. The transhepatic tract is then dilated using serial fascial dilators before advancement of the biliary drain.

After the biliary drainage catheter is positioned, it is secured in two locations: intra-abdominally, using the locking pigtail tip of the catheter looped within the dilated bile duct or bowel, and at the skin, using sutures or various adhesive devices to secure the catheter to the abdominal wall. The catheter is then attached to a drainage bag for at least overnight external-type decompression. The catheter and tubing of the drainage bag need to be fluid filled and the drainage bag placed in a more dependent position than the patient's bile ducts to allow siphonage to occur effectively. The drain should be flushed with approximately 10 mL of sterile saline solution two to three times daily and the biliary output recorded.

Selection of Biliary Drainage Route

Fundamentally, three types of biliary drainage exist: external, internal-external (universal), and internal. Each option has

advantages and disadvantages. The choice of drainage mechanism should reflect the patient's clinical situation and lifestyle, the anatomy and pathology of the underlying stricture or leak, the patient's life expectancy, and planned adjunctive or operative therapy.

In *external PBD*, all catheter side holes are located upstream from the site of obstruction, usually along the inside curvature of the pigtail loop (Fig. 22-22). The catheter shaft passes out the abdominal wall. Bile, by necessity, must drain externally through the catheter lumen into a drain bag. External drainage using siphonage is the most effective transcatheter method for decompression of the biliary system and, therefore, is usually indicated in patients with evidence of suppurative cholangitis or severe liver dysfunction from long-standing biliary obstruction. An external PBD is flushed and exchanged easily. However, it is the least secure of the three drainage options, is a nuisance for the patient and caregivers because of the drain exiting the body and the required drainage bag, and is associated with the loss of biliary fluids, electrolytes, and bile salts. Serum fluid and electrolyte status need to be monitored and replaced as needed. In the malnourished patient, bile may be collected and administered orally to assist with fat and fat-soluble vitamin absorption.

Internal-external PBD involves a percutaneous transhepatic catheter that traverses the obstructive lesion and has side holes proximal and distal to the site of obstruction (Fig. 22-23). Frequently, a locking pigtail tip secures the downstream (central) portion within the bowel. When attached

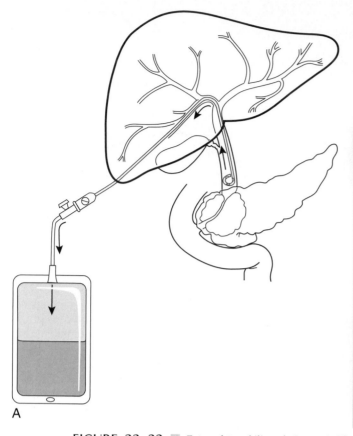

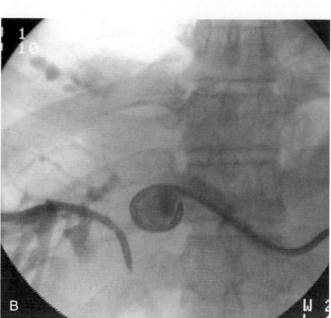

FIGURE 22-22 ■ External-type biliary drainage. **A,** The catheter position relative to the site of obstruction and the mandatory external direction of bile flow into the attached bile bag are illustrated. **B,** Right and left external biliary drains in a patient with suppurative cholangitis caused by an obstructing hilar carcinoma (i.e., Klatskin tumor).

to a drainage bag, bile is handled by entering the upstream side holes and exiting by the transhepatic catheter shaft into a drainage bag. Alternatively, when the PBD catheter is capped, bile that enters the upstream side holes is diverted across the site of obstruction to be dumped into the downstream CBD or small bowel. Advantages of internal-external PBD include improved catheter security relative to external drainage, avoidance of a drainage bag, easy catheter exchange over a guidewire, and excellent access for adjunctive treatment of benign or malignant strictures. Disadvantages include frequent occlusion of the catheter by debris (usually mucus produced by the small bowel) and the catheter shaft exiting the body, which may be distasteful or limit some patients' lifestyles.

Internal PBD involves a conduit (i.e., plastic tube or expandable metallic stent) that traverses the obstructive stricture and allows bile to flow directly into the bowel (Fig. 22-24). No drain exits the body wall. Advantages include a high degree of security (i.e., no catheter shaft to entangle passing objects or be grasped by delirious patients); physiologic use of biliary fluid, electrolytes, and bile salts; and optimized lifestyle (i.e., no exiting catheter, required flushing, or drainage bags). Significant disadvantages include the loss of access for adjunctive biliary intervention (i.e., any transcatheter adjuncts should be considered

before conversion of internal-external drainage to complete internal-type drainage) and loss of ability to exchange occluded drainage systems altogether (i.e., expandable metallic stents) or dependency on transendoscopic exchange (i.e., plastic endoprostheses).

Results and Complications

Reported technical success for external and internal-external PBD ranges from 94% to 97%.[36-38] Complications may be minor or life threatening. Major periprocedure complications primarily are caused by hemorrhage (usually hemobilia) and infection (i.e., sepsis, suppurative cholangitis, or hepatic abscesses) and occur in 4% to 8% of cases.[36-40] Massive hemobilia may be caused by fistulous connections between the hepatic artery or portal vein branches and the biliary tree. Hepatic arterial injury is diagnosed with hepatic arteriography and treated with transcatheter embolization. During arteriography, the biliary drain may need to be removed over a guidewire to identify the point of contrast extravasation. If no hepatic arterial injuries are identified, a portal vein injury is probable and is treated with placement of a second transhepatic biliary drain, followed by

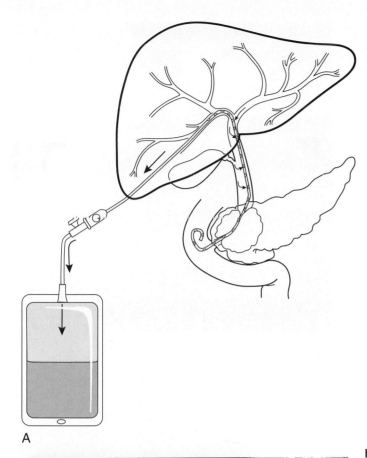

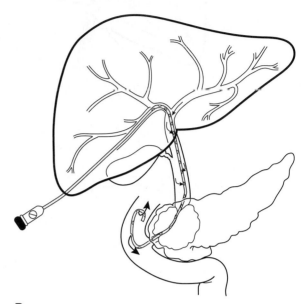

A

B

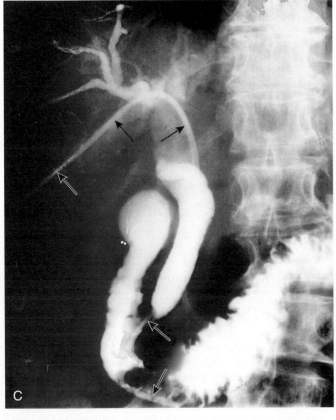

FIGURE 22-23 ▧ **A,** Internal-external percutaneous biliary drainage (PBD) with external drainage. Note the entrance of bile into the catheter side holes and delivery of bile into the dependent drainage bag. **B,** The internal-external PBD catheter has been capped so that bile is diverted into the duodenum. **C,** Cholangiogram performed through an internal-external PBD catheter *(arrows)* in a patient with ampullary carcinoma. Contrast fills the common bile duct and duodenum.

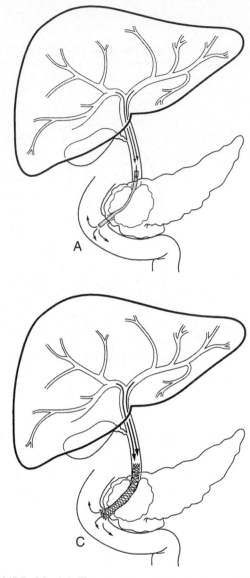

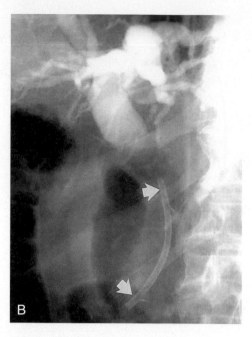

FIGURE 22-24 ■ Internal-type biliary drainage. **A,** Bile flows from the common bile duct (CBD) through the plastic internal biliary endoprosthesis into the duodenum. **B,** Radiograph of an endoscopically placed 10-French plastic endoprosthesis *(arrows)* after the endoscope has been removed in a patient with CBD obstruction by pancreatic head adenocarcinoma. **C,** Expandable metallic stent for internal biliary drainage.

embolization of the initial transhepatic tract, usually with a combination of angiographic coils and large Gelfoam "torpedoes."

Procedure-related fatality is reported in 1% to 6% of patients who undergo PBD.[36-38] In patients with malignant strictures, however, fatal and major nonfatal complications are two to three times higher than in patients with benign strictures, probably because of poorer overall health, longer duration of intubation, and the likelihood of bacterial colonization in patients with malignant biliary obstruction.[41]

Minor procedure-related complications occur in 20% to 30% of procedures. Delayed complications are probably a function of the type of PBD drainage, catheter hygiene, and duration of intubation. Complications include catheter occlusion, catheter dislodgement, and suppurative cholangitis.

■ TREATMENT OF BENIGN BILIARY STRICTURES

Patient Selection

Appropriate case selection for treatment of benign strictures centers on the likelihood of restenosis and the results of alternative methods. Most patients with periampullary benign strictures should undergo endoscopic sphincterotomy. Surgical biliary-enteric diversion provides better long-term patency than does cholangioplasty or placement of expandable metallic stents in patients with anastomotic or extrahepatic, extrapancreatic biliary strictures, particularly if the stricture has not been repaired previously and the surgeon is highly experienced. Because of the lack of viable surgical alternatives short of liver transplantation for treatment of intrahepatic biliary strictures, percutaneous treatment is warranted in patients with dominant strictures caused by sclerosing cholangitis, nonanastamotic strictures after liver transplantation, and other benign intrahepatic strictures.[42-47]

Techniques

Benign biliary strictures may be dilated with transluminal angioplasty balloons (i.e., *balloon cholangioplasty*) (see Fig. 22-10). In addition to the transhepatic route, balloon dilation catheters may be introduced into the biliary system by an operatively placed T-tube, a Hutson-Russell loop (i.e., the Roux-en-Y bowel loop used to drain the biliary system is tacked to the anterior abdominal wall), or an endoscope. The densely fibrotic nature and propensity for elastic recoil of most benign biliary strictures frequently require higher dilation pressures (e.g., 10 to 15 atm), prolonged expansion (e.g., 2 to 20 minutes), and repeated balloon expansion.[47] Because cholangioplasty is significantly more painful than most interventional radiologic procedures, deep sedation or general anesthesia is required.[10] The relatively high likelihood of stricture recurrence suggests that the preservation of access to the biliary system (e.g., chronic indwelling PBD, T-tube) is prudent in many of these patients, particularly those with sclerosing cholangitis or Oriental cholangiohepatitis, to minimize discomfort and complications associated with re-accessing the biliary system for subsequent cholangioplasty and possible stone extraction (see Fig. 22-11).

Given the long life expectancy of most patients with benign biliary strictures, stent occlusion due to epithelial hyperplasia, mucinous debris, or calculi is a serious impediment to routine use of an expandable metallic stent.[45,48-50] In benign disease, expandable biliary stents should be reserved for patients who are not operative candidates and in whom balloon dilation has failed (see Fig. 22-8), who have a limited life expectancy (e.g., obstructive cholangiopathy in a patient with advanced acquired immunodeficiency syndrome), or who have biliary strictures in a transplanted liver and require a bridge to liver retransplantation.[45,46] In such cases, use of expandable metallic stents with a relatively low metallic surface area (e.g., Gianturco-Rosch Z-stent, Cook, Inc., Bloomington, Ind.) may result in a longer primary patency than other types of stents.[46,49,50]

Recently introduced covered stents may hold promise for prolonged durability compared with bare metallic stents. The inner surface of the stent is covered with a thin layer of fabric with very small pore size (approximately 1 μm) to minimize biliary epithelial ingrowth and adherence of debris.[51,52] The outer metallic wires have extensions to prevent stent migration. Because these stents are covered with an impermeable membrane, particular care must be taken not to cover and potentially occlude the pancreatic duct (risk of pancreatitis), the cystic duct (risk of cholecystitis), or a bile duct branch (risk of biliary obstruction, cholangitis, and cholangitic abscesses). Long-term biostability of the fabric membrane is not known.

Results and Complications

After internal-external PBD has been established, the initial technical success rates for balloon cholangioplasty are typically high (88% to 100%). Complication rates vary widely (as high as 60%) and usually are caused by suppurative cholangitis.[10,15,42-44,47,53-60] Long-term patency rates depend on the location and cause of the stricture. Mueller and coworkers reported 36-month clinical primary patency rates of 76% for iatrogenic strictures, 67% for biliary-enteric anastomotic strictures, and 42% for strictures caused by sclerosing cholangitis.[55] For patients who have developed biliary strictures (usually intrahepatic) after liver transplantation, a 6-year secondary patency of 70% was by reported Zajko and colleagues.[47] However, Diamond and coworkers observed recurrence in all patients.[45] In patients with transplanted livers, primary patency is longer for nonanastomotic strictures than for anastomotic strictures.[15,47] Citron and Martin reported primary clinical patency rates (mean follow-up, 32 months) of 100% for intrahepatic CBD strictures; 92% for extrahepatic, extrapancreatic CBD strictures; 33% for intrapancreatic strictures; and 75% for biliary-enteric anastomotic strictures.[59] Most investigators leave 10- to 14-French (3.3- to 4.7-mm) soft catheters across the cholangioplasty site for several weeks or months to act as a stent, although the need for postdilation catheter stenting is undocumented.

Reported technical success and clinical response for use of metallic expandable stents to treat benign biliary strictures approaches 100%.[45,46,48-50,61,62] The rate of major nonfatal complications is 5% to 18%, although only one procedure-related fatality occurred among 174 patients so treated. Primary patency rates range from 73% to 92% at 6 months, 66% to 75% at 12 months, 40% to 59% at 24 months, 22% to 38% at 48 months, and 0 to 9% at 60 months. Depending on the duration of follow-up, 13% to 60% of patients require reintervention, with resulting secondary patency rates of 69% to 88% at 3 to 5 years. No long-term data are available regarding use of covered stents to treat benign biliary strictures.

■ TREATMENT OF MALIGNANT BILIARY STRICTURES

Patient and Stent Selection

Expandable metallic stents usually are indicated in long-term patients with malignant strictures, because the stent is likely to remain patent for a longer period (median patency, 6 to 8 months) than most patients' life expectancies (mean, 3.4 to 7.8 months, depending on tumor type) (Fig. 22-25).[48,62,63] Multiple investigators have found that *metallic* expandable stents remain patent longer, have lower complication rates, and require fewer repeat interventional procedures to maintain patency compared with *plastic* endoprostheses, particularly those delivered through the transhepatic route.[64-66] Metallic stents with a relatively tight lattice such as the Wallstent (Schneider USA, Inc., Minneapolis, Minn.) or the Strecker nitinol stent (Boston Scientific, Watertown, Mass.),

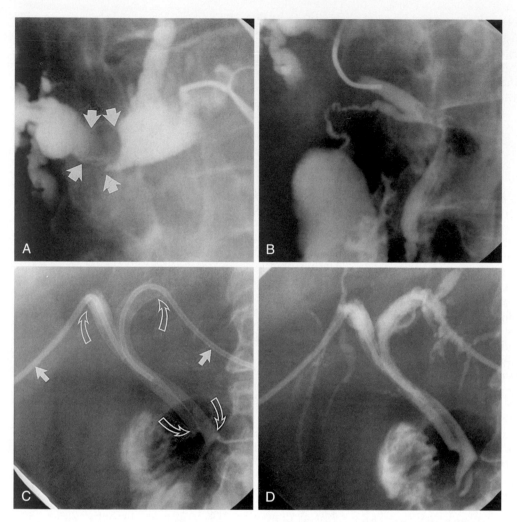

FIGURE 22-25   ▪   Expandable metallic stent for treatment of malignant stricture (hilar cholangiocarcinoma). CT (not shown) identified bilateral bile duct dilation. **A,** Transhepatic cholangiography through a left-sided approach documents hilar common bile duct (CBD) occlusion and mass *(arrows).* **B,** An angiographic catheter has been negotiated across the occlusive tumor into the CBD. **C,** Two 10-mm-diameter, 90-mm-long Wallstents *(curved arrows)* have been deployed from separate left- and right-sided biliary accesses to drain both biliary systems. Temporary external-type drainage catheters *(straight arrows)* have been left to provide overnight external biliary decompression to minimize the risk of cholangitis or sepsis and to provide transhepatic biliary access while the external drains are capped during a trial of internal drainage. The external biliary drains usually are removed after 1 to 2 days if internal drainage is successful. **D,** Cholangiogram performed through the external drains documents satisfactory stent placement and free drainage into the duodenum.

and stents that are significantly longer than the diseased segment provide optimized patency, because they resist tumor ingrowth through the stent struts and are less prone to tumor overgrowth beyond the ends of the stent. Covered stents such as the Viabil stent (WL Gore Inc., Flagstaff, Ariz.) may improve primary patency because the impermeable fabric prevents tumor ingrowth into the stent lumen.[51,52]

Results and Complications

Reported initial technical success rates range from 75% to 100%.[48,62-67] Initial clinical relief of symptoms occurs in greater than 70% of patients.[48,62,63,67-74] Reported procedure-related fatality rates range from 0 to 3%. Major nonfatal periprocedure complications range from 8% to 61% and are related primarily to the initial establishment of PBD rather than the additional deployment of a metallic stent.

Reported primary patency rates of bare stents range from 67% to 85% at 6 months, 50% to 55% at 1 year, and 10% to 37% at 2 years. Given the relatively short life expectancies of these patients, only about 7% to 29% of stents require reintervention. Thirty-day mortality rates are approximately 10% to 15%, and death results primarily from the underlying malignancy. Several investigators are studying covered, coated, and impregnated stents to preserve conduit patency.[51,52,75-77] Some investigators report improved primary patency results at 6 months (76%, 77%) and 12 months (76%, 77%) using covered stents to treat malignant strictures, though mean survival remained short (146 days and 9.2 months).[51,52] The incidence of cholecystitis (12%) and branch duct obstruction (10%) was higher than expected with bare metallic stents. The cost of the covered stents is approximately two to three times that of most bare metallic stents.

For *percutaneous brachytherapy,* the internal-external PBD catheters make ideal conduits for passage of iridium Ir 192 wires or seeds incorporated into a modified angiographic guidewire. This treatment is useful particularly for locally invasive Klatskin-type cholangiocarcinomas of the porta hepatis. A thin platinum shield absorbs beta particle emission, resulting in local intraductal delivery of pure gamma radiation. Brachytherapy may be combined with external beam irradiation. Although this treatment is not commonly used, several reports suggest modest survival improvement (i.e., 10 to 17 months versus 2 to 8 months for historical controls treated with PBD and no irradiation).[78-82] Infectious and hemorrhagic complications are common in this group of patients with or without irradiation; however, ulceration of the gastrointestinal tract is an added risk of radiation therapy.[78] After irradiation, deployment of expandable metallic stents may provide improved biliary drainage with a lower rate of infectious complications and, possibly, longer survival.[49,82]

■ TREATMENT OF BILIARY STONES

As an alternative to operative removal, *endoscopic sphincterotomy* followed by biliary stone extraction using wire retrieval baskets or occlusion balloons often is used in patients with retained CBD stones after cholecystectomy. It is used also for patients with choledocholithiasis and an intact gallbladder who are elderly (>65 years old) or are at high risk for operative CBD exploration. The procedure is associated with a high rate of technical success (i.e., successful sphincterotomy in approximately 95% in current series, with clearance of stones in approximately 85%).[83-90] The morbidity rate of approximately 4% to 16% is relatively low. Major complications usually are caused by hemorrhage from the sphincterotomy, pancreatitis, sepsis, or bowel perforation.

A mature *T-tube sinus tract* (at least 5 weeks old) can be used for stone extraction (Fig. 22-26). A guidewire is placed through the T-tube, and the T-tube is removed and replaced with a sheath, which is directed toward the stone. The guidewire is withdrawn and replaced with a wire basket (e.g., Wittich basket [Cook, Inc., Bloomington, Ind.]). The expanded diameter of the basket varies and should be selected to match the diameter of the bile duct. The basket is opened by withdrawing a protective sheath. The stone is entrapped by spinning the basket, after which the sheath is gently snuggled down over the basket. Sufficiently small stones may be removed through the T-tube sinus tract. Otherwise, a balloon occlusion catheter can be used to deliver intrahepatic calculi into the CBD and then to push them into the bowel (see Fig. 22-26). At the end of the procedure, a drainage catheter is left in place to minimize the likelihood of sepsis, provide a route for follow-up cholangiography, and preserve access in case some stones remain. Technical success rates in experienced hands range from 77% to 97%, with major complications in 4% to 9% of cases and procedure-related fatality rates of 0 to 1%.[90-94] Percutaneous stone extraction through a T-tube sinus tract may require multiple sessions, particularly if the stones are numerous, large, or impacted in intrahepatic bile ducts located peripheral to biliary strictures.

In patients with innumerable biliary calculi (e.g., Oriental cholangiohepatitis), large stones (>1.5 cm diameter), or unfavorable anatomy (e.g., prior biliary-enteric drainage procedure), stone removal may be performed by a *percutaneous transhepatic route* (see Fig. 22-11). Although some cases may be managed with fluoroscopically guided techniques similar to those employed for stone extraction through a T-tube sinus tract, many of these patients have such a large stone burden or complex biliary anatomy (dilated and strictured) that percutaneous endoscopically guided lithotripsy techniques are required for successful therapy.[95-97]

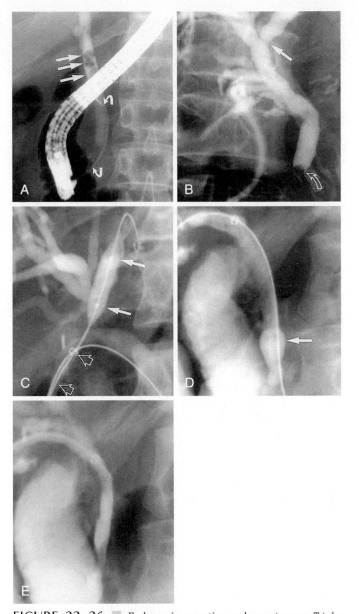

FIGURE 22-26 ■ Endoscopic, operative, and percutaneous T-tube treatment of biliary calculi. **A,** Endoscopic retrograde cholangiopancreatography shows multiple common bile duct (CBD) and intrahepatic biliary stones *(straight arrows)*. The sphincterotome *(curved arrows)* was used to perform a papillotomy; multiple CBD calculi were removed using wire stone retrieval baskets and an occlusion balloon catheter. **B,** One week after an operative cholecystectomy for cholecystolithiasis and CBD exploration, the T-tube cholangiogram detected a retained 7-mm-diameter stone in the distal CBD *(curved arrow)* and a weblike stricture of the central left bile duct *(straight arrow)*. **C,** After passage of a heavy guidewire, the T-tube was replaced with a 12-French vascular-type sheath *(open arrows)*. A 10-mm × 4-cm balloon dilation catheter *(solid arrows)* was used to dilate the left bile duct stricture. **D,** An occlusion balloon *(arrow)* was used to push the stone into the CBD and through the papilla into the duodenum. **E,** A completion cholangiogram confirmed the stone's absence.

Between 4 and 10 days after biliary drainage has been established and cholangitis or sepsis has been treated, the transhepatic tract is dilated to accommodate a large (e.g., 18-French) sheath. A small-bore endoscope (e.g., 15-French choledochoscope with a 6-French working channel) is advanced through the sheath into the biliary system, directed to the stones, and used to guide stone fragmentation with a suitable lithotriptor (e.g., electrohydraulic lithotriptor, ultrasonic lithotriptor, pulsed-dye laser). Care must be taken to avoid the surrounding bile duct walls or subjacent blood vessels.

Reported technical success for percutaneous transhepatic lithotripsy ranges from 93% to 100%, although complications can be substantial; procedure-related fatality rates are 0 to 4%, and nonfatal major morbidity rates are 0 to 24%.[95-100] Patients with large stones or innumerable stones are likely to have recurrent calculi even if the biliary tracts appear stone free, especially when strictures are present. Transhepatic endoscopy also has been used for staging and biopsy in patients with suspected cholangiocarcinoma, differentiation of cholangiographic masses or filling defects, removal of postoperative biliary foreign bodies (e.g., sutures or clips), guidance for cauterization of intraductal bleeding sites, and inspection of biliary-enteric anastomoses.[35,97,98,101,102]

■ BILIARY LEAKS

Biliary leaks usually result from biliary tract surgery. Other causes include hepatic surgery or invasive procedures, ischemia due to hepatic arterial occlusive disease (e.g., liver transplant recipients), downstream biliary obstruction, or penetrating injuries (see Fig. 22-18). Because bile can escape into the peritoneum or a localized space, the intrahepatic bile ducts usually are not dilated. The diagnosis and characterization of the biliary injury require cross-sectional imaging, preferably with CT, to assess for bilomas or abscesses, and cholangiography with or without endoscopy.

Nonoperative management of biliary fistulas includes certain features:

- Diversion of biliary flow through PBD or transendoscopically
- Placement of a catheter across the injured segments to preserve bile duct continuity
- Drainage of associated fluid collections (e.g., bilomas, abscesses)
- Relief of downstream obstruction, if present[103-108]

If downstream strictures are present, often they require operative decompression.[109] Although transcatheter embolization of biliary leaks has been described, the safety and effectiveness of this technique have yet to be proved.[110]

■ COMBINED PERCUTANEOUS, ENDOSCOPIC, AND OPERATIVE PROCEDURES

Percutaneous transhepatic access to the biliary system may be a useful adjunct to operative or transendoscopic procedures. Preoperative placement of a relatively stiff PBD catheter (e.g., Ring biliary drainage catheter [Cook, Inc., Bloomington, Ind.]) through one or both intrahepatic duct systems and then into the duodenum may assist the surgeon

during porta hepatis dissection in patients with biliary strictures who have had prior right upper quadrant surgery and in whom extensive adhesions have occurred. The time required for exposure of the bile ducts or vascular structures is reduced significantly.[111] PBD also may assist intraoperative placement of transhepatic Silastic biliary stents or U-tube drains.

In patients in whom endoscopic drainage has failed because of inability of the endoscopist to cannulate the bile ducts, the so-called *rendezvous procedure* may be performed to permit endoscopic access into the biliary systems or to provide improved guidewire tension for delivery of transluminal devices across difficult strictures.[112,113] The rendezvous procedure is performed by passing a 300- to 400-cm guidewire and 5- to 6-French angiographic catheter percutaneously through the biliary system and into the small bowel. The endoscopist then can snare the guidewire easily and withdraw it through the mouth. The through-and-through "body floss" guidewire is threaded through the working channel of the interventional endoscope, and the desired transluminal device (e.g., endoprostheses and pusher catheter, expandable metallic stent delivery system) is passed over the guidewire retrograde into the desired location in the biliary system. After the guidewire is removed, the angiographic catheter may be used for antegrade cholangiography and as a safety drain in case of infectious complications or unexpected biliary obstruction.

The primary advantage of the rendezvous procedure is the ability to place a relatively large-bore drain (3.3 to 12 mm) with a small-caliber transhepatic route (1.7 to 2 mm). However, expandable metallic stents often can be placed more simply by a transhepatic approach. Rendezvous procedures now are used less frequently than in the past.

■ PERCUTANEOUS CHOLECYSTOSTOMY

Patient Selection

Most benign disease of the gallbladder is managed by operative cholecystectomy. During the late 1980s and early 1990s, several nonoperative techniques were developed as an alternative to open cholecystectomy for treatment of calculus cholecystitis, including percutaneous cholecystostomy with percutaneous lithotripsy or stone dissolution and extracorporeal shock wave lithothripsy.[114] The rapid growth of laparoscopic cholecystectomy during the early 1990s has largely rendered these techniques obsolete.

There are two major indications for percutaneous cholecystostomy. The first is possible acalculous cholecystitis in critically ill patients with sepsis of unknown origin (Fig. 22-27). In septic patients, clinical features suggesting this diagnosis include abnormal liver function test results, right upper quadrant pain, and sonographic findings of a distended gallbladder, thickened gallbladder wall, intraluminal sludge or stones, pericholecystic fluid, or the presence of a sonographic Murphy's sign. Radionuclide studies are of little value, because most critically ill patients do not show radionuclide uptake by the gallbladder on hepatobiliary

FIGURE 22-27 ■ Percutaneous chole-cystostomy in a critically ill postoperative patient with sepsis of unknown origin. **A,** The sonogram shows thickening of the gallbladder wall and intraluminal sludge. **B,** Sonographic guidance was used to puncture the gallbladder with a 22-gauge Chiba needle *(arrows)* through a transperitoneal route. **C,** Fluoroscopic guidance permitted the Seldinger technique to be used to introduce a 12-French locking pigtail catheter *(arrows).* **D,** Repeat CT scan 3 days later confirmed the intracholecystic pigtail location adjacent to the cystic duct with adequate gallbladder decompression.

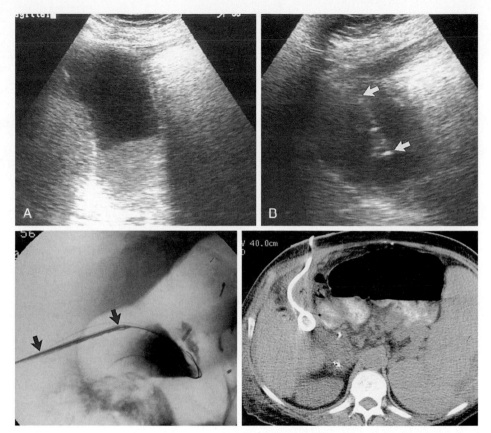

scintigraphy. The diagnosis is based on the clinical response to percutaneous cholecystostomy because neither the Gram stain nor the results of bile culture are helpful.[115]

The second indication is calculus cholecystitis in poor operative candidates (Fig. 22-28). In patients whose operative contraindication is temporary (e.g., acute myocardial infarction), percutaneous cholecystostomy permits drainage of the gallbladder so that cholecystectomy may be performed electively at a later time. In patients with a permanent contraindication to surgery (e.g., intractable congestive heart failure), the percutaneous cholecystostomy access route can be used to extract the gallstones using forceps, wire baskets, or various lithotriptors.[116] In approximately one half of patients, gallstones do not recur.[117]

Technique

Percutaneous cholecystostomy may be performed at the bedside under sonographic guidance in critically ill patients. When feasible, the procedure should be performed in an interventional radiology suite to permit manipulation of guidewires and catheters under fluoroscopy. In patients with distorted anatomy, CT may be necessary to obtain initial skinny-needle and guidewire access into the gallbladder.

Two percutaneous approaches may be used for cholecystostomy. In the *transhepatic approach,* a needle is directed from a subcostal or intercostal site in the right mid-axillary line toward the "bare area" of the gallbladder fossa, where the gallbladder is attached to the liver capsule. The primary advantages of this route are that the likelihood of bile spillage into the peritoneum is minimized and the gallbladder is relatively fixed to the liver, which facilitates puncture of the gallbladder wall. Disadvantages include the risk of hemorrhagic complications from transhepatic passage and the 90-degree angle with the long axis of the gallbladder, which makes catheter manipulations difficult.

In the *transperitoneal approach,* the needle is directed from the subcostal right anterior abdomen, beneath the liver margin into the fundus of the gallbladder along the long axis of the organ. This technique is safest in patients with a distended gallbladder, which is often adherent to the anterior abdominal wall (see Fig. 22-27). Advantages of transperitoneal access include avoidance of the hemorrhagic complications associated with the transhepatic route and pain from intercostal catheter passage and the ease of intraluminal manipulation. Disadvantages include the risk of accidental perforation of bowel (especially the colon) and peritoneal spillage of bile if the gallbladder fundus is not adherent to the abdominal wall.[118] If the gallbladder fundus is mobile, the trocar technique rather than Seldinger technique may be used to minimize peritoneal spillage.[119]

Regardless of the access route, the percutaneous cholecystostomy drain should be left in place for at least 4 weeks to allow formation of a mature fibrinous sheath or sinus tract around the catheter shaft. The percutaneous cholecystostomy catheter should not be removed from patients with persistent gallstones, because they may obstruct normal

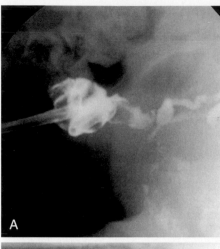

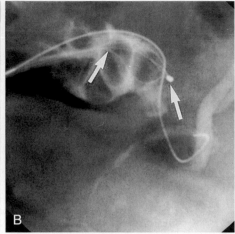

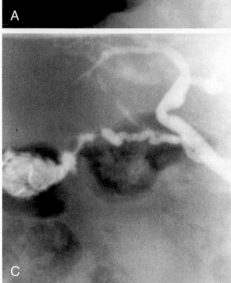

FIGURE 22-28 ■ Percutaneous chole-cystostomy for treatment of cholelithiasis and chronic cholecystitis in a 79-year-old patient with severe chronic obstructive pulmonary disease. **A,** Cholecystogram after percutaneous cholecystostomy documented multiple large gallstones. **B,** After multiple sessions of gallstone extraction using wire-stone retrieval baskets *(arrows)* and trans-catheter contact dissolution therapy using ethyl propionate, the gallstones were eliminated successfully. **C,** Termination cholecystogram documented complete removal of gallstones and satisfactory drainage through the cystic duct.

drainage through the cystic duct. In patients without gallstones, cholecystography should be performed to ensure normal drainage through the cystic duct and CBD. When catheter removal is anticipated, it should be withdrawn over a guidewire and replaced with a suitably sized vascular access sheath.[120] Contrast material can be injected through the sheath side arm while the sheath is withdrawn along the tract. If contrast material remains only within the tract and gallbladder lumen, the sheath and guidewire can be removed safely. However, if leakage is seen (indicating an immature or incomplete track), a new catheter can be placed over the guidewire.

Results and Complications

Most percutaneous cholecystostomy catheters are placed at the bedside in the intensive care unit (ICU) with a transhepatic approach using ultrasound. Even in these suboptimal conditions, percutaneous cholecystostomy is technically successful in 93% to 100% of cases.[121-127] The procedure-related mortality rate is 0 to 2%, and the nonfatal complication rate is 0 to 12%. One complication relatively unique to percutaneous cholecystostomy is intraprocedural vasovagal reaction, probably because of manipulation within the

gallbladder.[128] Minimizing intracystic manipulation may prevent this reaction, which usually responds to fluid administration and intravenous atropine.

The likelihood of clinical response to percutaneous cholecystostomy drainage depends on the patient's clinical situation. Among critically ill patients in the ICU with sepsis of an unknown cause and an abnormal gallbladder sonogram, 39% to 63% become afebrile with normalization of leukocytosis and weaning from pressor drips within 24 to 72 hours. Among patients who respond, many have the drainage tube removed after recovery and avoid cholecystectomy altogether. Percutaneous cholecystostomy in this group is diagnostic and therapeutic.[124] Most critically ill septic patients who fail to respond to percutaneous cholecystostomy die, usually of their underlying illnesses, but also commonly from biliary sepsis.[127] The diagnostic significance of a clinical failure of percutaneous cholecystostomy is less clear. It implies that sepsis originated from a different source or that the gallbladder is gangrenous.

Among stable patients with acute calculus cholecystitis and a contraindication to surgery, 93% respond clinically.[123,127] Many of these patients undergo a delayed, elective cholecystectomy, although a few are treated with stone removal and subsequent percutaneous cholecystostomy removal. A significant minority require lifelong intubation because of the critical nature of their underlying medical condition.[126,127]

Acknowledgment. I wish to express my gratitude to Pamela Rosario for her assistance in manuscript preparation.

REFERENCES

1. Huard P, Do-Xuan-Hop: La ponction transhepatique des canaux biliares. Bull Soc Med Chir Indochine 1937;15:1090.
2. Remolar J, Katz S, Rybak B, et al: Percutaneous transhepatic cholangiography. Gastroenterology 1956;31:39.
3. Shlansky-Goldberg R, Weintraub J: Cholangiography. Semin Roentgenol 1997;32:150.
4. Gazelle GS, Lee MJ, Mueller PR: Cholangiographic segmental anatomy of the liver: implications for interventional radiology. Semin Intervent Radiol 1995;12:119.
5. Lopera JE, Soto JA, Munera F: Malignant hilar and perihilar biliary obstruction: use of MR cholangiography to define the extent of biliary ductal involvement and plan percutaneous interventions. Radiology 2001;220:90.
6. Spies JB, Rosen RJ, Lebowitz AS: Antibiotic prophylaxis in vascular and interventional radiology: a rational approach. Radiology 1988;166:381.
7. Clark CD, Picus D, Dunagan WC: Bloodstream infections after interventional procedures in the biliary tract. Radiology 1994;191:495.
8. McDermott, Schuster MG, Smith TP: Antibiotic prophylaxis in vascular and interventional radiology (review). AJR Am J Roentgenol 1997;169:31.
9. Silverman SG, Coughin BF, Selzer SE, et al: Current use of screening laboratory tests before abdominal interventions: a survey of 603 radiologists. Radiology 1991;181:669.
10. Lee MJ, Mueller PR, Saini S, et al: Percutaneous dilatation of benign biliary strictures: single session therapy with general anesthesia. AJR Am J Roentgenol 1991;157:1263.
11. Savader SJ, Bourke DL, Venbrux AC, et al: Randomized double-blind clinical trial of celiac plexus block for percutaneous biliary drainage. J Vasc Interv Radiol 1993;4:539.
12. Eisenberg RL: Bile Duct Marking and Obstruction. In: Gastrointestinal Radiology: A Pattern Approach, 3rd ed. Philadelphia, Lippincott-Raven, 1996:851.
13. Chartrand-Lefebre C, Dufresne M-P, Lafortune M, et al: Iatrogenic injury to the bile duct: a working classification for radiologists. Radiology 1994;193:523.
14. Majoie CB, Reeders JW, Sanders JB, et al: Primary sclerosing cholangitis: a modified classification of cholangiographic findings. AJR Am J Roentgenol 1991;157:495.
15. Ward EM, Kiely MJ, Maus TP, et al: Hilar biliary strictures after liver transplantation: cholangiography and percutaneous treatment. Radiology 1990;177:259.
16. Eisenberg RL: Cystic dilatation of the bile ducts. In: Gastrointestinal Radiology: A Pattern Approach, 3rd ed. Philadelphia, Lippincott-Raven, 1996:872.
17. Savader SJ, Benenati JF, Venbrux AC, et al: Choledochal cysts: classification and cholangiographic appearance. AJR Am J Roentgenol 1991;156:327.
18. Eisenberg RL: Filling defects in the bile ducts. In: Gastrointestinal Radiology: A Pattern Approach, 3rd ed. Philadelphia, Lippincott-Raven, 1996:837.
19. vanSonnenberg E, Ferrucci JT, Neff CC, et al: Biliary pressure: manometric and perfusion studies at percutaneous transhepatic cholangiography and percutaneous biliary drainage. Radiology 1983;148:41.
20. Savader SJ, Cameron JL, Pitt HA, et al: Biliary manometry versus clinical trial: value as predictors of success after treatment of biliary tract strictures. J Vasc Inter Radiol 1994;5:757.
21. Terasaki K, Wittich GR, Lycke G, et al: Percutaneous transluminal biopsy of biliary strictures with a bioptome: technical note. AJR Am J Roentgenol 1981;156:77.
22. Kim D, Porter DH, Siegel JB, et al: Common bile duct biopsy with the Simpson atherectomy catheter. AJR Am J Roentgenol 1990;154:1213.
23. Pereiras R Jr, Chiprut RU, Greenward RA, et al: Percutaneous transhepatic cholangiography with a "skinny" needle: a rapid, simple, and accurate method in the diagnosis of cholestasis. Ann Intern Med 1977;86:562.
24. Okuda K, Tanikawa K, Emura T, et al: Nonsurgical percutaneous transhepatic cholangiography—diagnostic significance in medical problems of the liver. Am J Dig Dis 1974;19:21.
25. Redeker AG, Karvountzis GG, Richman RH, et al: Percutaneous transhepatic cholangiography: an improved technique. JAMA 1975;231:386.
26. Harbin WP, Mueller PR, Ferrucci JT Jr: Transhepatic cholangiography—complications and use patterns of the fine needle technique: a multi-institutional survey. Radiology 1980;135:15.
27. Gold RP, Casarella WJ, Stern G, et al: Transhepatic cholangiography: the radiological method of choice in suspected obstructive jaundice. Radiology 1979;133:39.
28. Funaki B, Zaleski GX, Straus CA, et al: Percutaneous biliary drainage in patients with nondilated intrahepatic bile ducts. AJR Am J Roengenol 1999;173:1541.
29. Shea WJ Jr, Demas BE, Goldberg HI, et al: Sclerosing cholangitis associated with hepatic arterial FUDR chemotherapy. radiographic-histologic correlation. AJR Am J Roentgenol 1986;146:717.
30. Harell GS, Anderson MF, Berry PF: Cytologic bile examination in the diagnosis of biliary duct neoplastic strictures. AJR Am J Roentgenol 1981;137:1123.
31. Muro A, Mueller PR, Ferrucci JT Jr, Taft PD: Bile cytology: a routine addition to percutaneous biliary drainage. Radiology 1983;149:846.
32. Hall-Craggs MA, Lees MR: Fine-needle aspiration biopsy: pancreatic and biliary tumors. AJR Am J Roentgenol 1986;147:399.
33. Teplick SK, Haskin PH, Kline TS, et al: Percutaneous pancreaticobiliary biopsies in 173 patients using primarily ultrasound or fluoroscopic guidance. Cardiovasc Intervent Radiol 1988;11:26.
34. Mendez G Jr, Russell E, Levi JV, et al: Percutaneous brush biopsy and internal drainage of biliary tree through endoprosthesis. AJR Am J Roentgenol 1980;134:653.
35. Savader SJ, Prescott CA, Lund GB, et al: Intraductal biliary biopsy: comparison of three techniques. J Vasc Interv Radiol 1996;7:743.
36. Mueller PR, vanSonnenberg E, Ferrucci JT Jr: Percutaneous biliary drainage: technical and catheter-related problems in 200 procedures. AJR Am J Roentgenol 1982;138:17.
37. Hamlin JA, Friedman M, Stein MG, et al: Percutaneous biliary drainage: complications of 118 consecutive catheterizations. Radiology 1986;158:199.
38. McNicholas MM, Lee MJ, Dawson SL, et al: Complications of percutaneous biliary drainage and stricture dilatation. Semin Intervent Radiol 1994;11:242.
39. Carrasco CH, Zounoza J, Bechter WJ: Malignant biliary obstruction: complications of percutaneous biliary drainage. Radiology 1984;152:343.
40. Yee AC, Ho C-S: Complications of percutaneous biliary drainage: benign vs malignant diseases. AJR Am J Roentgenol 1987;148:1207.
41. Cohan RH, Illescas FF, Saeed M, et al: Infectious complications of percutaneous biliary drainage. Invest Radiol 1986;21:705.
42. May GR, Bender CE, LaRusso NF, et al: Nonoperative dilation of dominant strictures in primary sclerosing cholangitis. AJR Am J Roentgenol 1985;145:1061.
43. Skolkin MD, Alspaugh JP, Casarella WJ, et al: Sclerosing cholangitis: palliation with percutaneous cholangioplasty. Radiology 1989;170:199.
44. Rossi P, Salvatori FM, Bezzi M, et al: Percutaneous management of benign biliary strictures with balloon dilatation and self-expanding metallic stents. Cardiovasc Intervent Radiol 1990;13:231.
45. Diamond NG, Lee SP, Niblett RL, et al: Metallic stents for the treatment of intrahepatic biliary strictures after liver transplantation. J Vasc Interv Radiol 1995;6:755.
46. Culp WC, McCowan TC, Lieberman RP, et al: Biliary strictures in liver transplant recipients: treatment with metal stents. Radiology 1996;199:339.
47. Zajko AB, Sheng R, Zetti GM, et al: Transhepatic balloon dilation of biliary strictures in liver transplant patients: a 10-year experience. J Vasc Interv Radiol 1995;6:79.
48. Tesdal IK, Adamus R, Poeckler C, et al: Therapy for biliary stenoses and occlusions with use of three different metallic stents: single center experience. J Vasc Interv Radiol 1997;8:869.
49. Coons H: Metallic stents for the treatment of biliary obstruction: a report of 100 cases. Cardiovasc Intervent Radiol 1992;15:367.
50. Hausegger KA, Kugler C, Uggowitzer M, et al: Benign biliary obstruction: is treatment with the Wallstent advisable? Radiology 1996;200:437.

51. Schoder M, Rossi P, Uflacker R, et al: Malignant biliary obstruction: treatment with ePTFE-FEP-covered endoprotheses—initial technical and clinical experiences in a multicenter trial. Radiology 2002;225:35.
52. Bezzi M, Zolovkins A, Cantisani V, et al: New ePTFE/FEP-covered stent in the palliative treatment of malignant biliary obstruction. J Vasc Intervent Radiol 2002;13:581.
53. Salomonowitz E, Castaneda-Zuniga WR, Lund G, et al: Balloon dilation of benign biliary strictures. Radiology 1984;151:613.
54. Gallacher DJ, Kadir S, Kaufman SL, et al: Nonoperative management of benign postoperative biliary strictures. Radiology 1985;156:625.
55. Mueller PR, vanSonnenberg E, Ferrucci JT Jr, et al: Biliary stricture dilatation: multicenter review of clinical management in 73 patients. Radiology 1986;160:17.
56. Williams HJ Jr, Bender CE, May GR: Benign postoperative biliary strictures: dilation with fluoroscopic guidance. Radiology 1987;163:629.
57. Moore AV Jr, Illescas FF, Mills SR, et al: Percutaneous dilation of benign biliary strictures. Radiology 1987;163:625.
58. Gibson RN, Adam A, Yeung E, et al: Percutaneous techniques in benign hilar and intrahepatic strictures. J Intervent Radiol 1988;3:125.
59. Citron SJ, Martin LG: Benign biliary strictures: treatment with percutaneous cholangioplasty. Radiology 1991;178:339.
60. Suman L, Civelli EM, Cozzi G, et al: Long-term results of balloon dilation of benign bile duct strictures. Acta Radiologica 2003;44:147.
61. Irving JD, Adam A, Dick R, et al: Gianturco expandable metallic biliary stents: results of a European clinical trial. Radiology 1989;172:321.
62. Rossi P, Bezzi M, Rossi M, et al: Metallic stents in malignant biliary observation: results of a multicenter European study of 240 patients. J Vasc Interv Radiol 1994;5:279.
63. Boguth L, Tatalovic S, Antonucci F, et al: Malignant biliary obstruction: clinical and histopathologic correlation after treatment with self-expanding metal prostheses. Radiology 1994;192:669.
64. Knyrim K, Wagner HJ, Pausch J, et al: A prospective randomized controlled trial of metal stents for malignant obstruction of the common bile duct. Endoscopy 1993;25:207.
65. Wagner H-J, Knyrim K, Vakil N, et al: Plastic endoprostheses versus metal stents in the palliative treatment of malignant hilar biliary obstruction: a prospective and randomized trial. Endoscopy 1993;25:213.
66. Lammer J, Hausegger KA, Fluckiger F, et al: Common bile duct obstruction due to malignancy: treatment with plastic versus metal stents. Radiology 1996;201:167.
67. Lameris JS, Stoker J, Nijs HG: Malignant biliary obstruction: percutaneous use of expandable stents. Radiology 1991;179:703.
68. Lee MJ, Dawson SL, Mueller PR, et al: Palliation of malignant bile duct obstruction with metallic biliary endoprostheses: technique, results and complications. J Vasc Interv Radiol 1992;3:665.
69. Salomonowitz EK, Antonucci F, Heer M, et al: Biliary obstruction: treatment with self-expanding metal prostheses. J Vasc Interv Radiol 1992;3:365.
70. Gordon RL, Ring EJ, La Berge JM, et al: Malignant biliary obstruction: treatment with expandable metallic stents—follow-up of 50 consecutive patients. Radiology 1992;182:697.
71. Becker CD, Glattli A, Malbach R, et al: Percutaneous palliation of malignant obstructive jaundice with the Wallstent endoprosthesis: follow-up and reintervention in patients with hilar and non-hilar obstruction. J Vasc Interv Radiol 1993;4:597.
72. Pinol V, Castells A, Bordas JM, et al: Percutaneous self-expanding metal stents versus endoscopic polyethylene endoprostheses for treating malignant biliary obstruction: randomized clinical trial. Radiology 2002;225:27.
73. Lee BH, Choe DH, Lee JH, et al: Metallic stents in malignant biliary obstruction: prospective long-term clinical results. AJR Am J Roentgenol 1997;168:741.
74. Inal M, Akgul E, Aksungur E, et al: Percutaneous self-expanding uncovered metallic stents in malignant biliary obstruction. Complications, follow-up, and reinterventions in 154 patients. Acta Radiologica 2003;44:139.
75. Alvarado R, Palmaz JC, Garcia OJ, et al: Evaluation of polymer-coated balloon expandable stents in the bile ducts. Radiology 1989;170:975.
76. Miyayama S, Matsui O, Terayama N, et al: Covered Gianturco stents for malignant biliary obstruction: preliminary clinical evaluation. J Vasc Interv Radiol 1997;8:641.
77. Severini A, Mantero S, Tanzi MC, et al: In vivo study of polyurethane-coated Gianturco-Rosch biliary Z-stents. Cardiovasc Intervent Radiol 1999;22:510.
78. Hayes JK Jr, Sapozink MD, Miller FJ: Definitive radiation therapy in bile duct carcinoma. Int J Radiat Oncol Biol Phys 1988;15:735.
79. Nunnerly HB, Karani JB: Intraductal radiation. Radiol Clin North Am 1990;28:1237.
80. Fritz P, Brambs H-J, Schraube P, et al: Combined external beam radiotherapy and intraductal high dose rate brachytherapy on bile duct carcinomas. Int J Radiat Oncol Biol Phys 1994;29:855.
81. Montemaggi P, Costamagna G, Dobelbower RR, et al: Intraluminal brachytherapy in the treatment of pancreas and bile duct carcinoma. Int J Radiat Oncol Biol Phys 1995;32:437.
82. Kamada T, Saitou H, Takamura A, et al: The role of radiotherapy in the management of extrahepatic bile duct cancer: an analysis of 145 consecutive patients treated with intraluminal and/or external beam radiotherapy. Int J Radiat Oncol Biol Phys 1996;34:767.
83. Allen B, Shapiro H, Way LW: Management of recurrent and residual common duct stones. Am J Surg 1981;142:41.
84. Mee AS, Vallon AG, Croker JR, et al: Non-operative removal of bile duct stones by duodenoscopic sphincterotomy in the elderly. Br Med J 1981;283:521.
85. Passi RB, Raval B: Endoscopic papillotomy. Surgery 1982;92:581.
86. Escourrou J, Cordova JA, Lazordities F, et al: Early and late complications after endoscopic sphincterostomy for biliary lithiasis with and without the gallbladder "in situ." Gut 1984;25:598.
87. Leese T, Neo PT, Lemos JP, Carr-Locke DL: Successes, failures, early complications and their management following endoscopic sphincterostomy: results in 394 consecutive patients from a single centre. Br J Surg 1985;72:215.
88. Broughan TA, Sivak MV, Hermann RE: The management of retained and recurrent bile duct stones. Surgery 1985;98:746.
89. Vaira D, D'Anna L, Ainlesy C, et al: Endoscopic sphincterotomy in 1000 consecutive patients. Lancet 1989;2:431.
90. Nussinson E, Cairns SR, Vaira D, et al: A 10 year single centre experience of percutaneous and endoscopic extraction of bile duct stones with T-tube in situ. Gut 1991;32:1040.
91. Mazzariello RM: A fourteen-year experience with nonoperative instrument of retained bile duct stones. World J Surg 1978;2:447.
92. Burhenne HJ: Percutaneous extraction of the retained biliary tract stones: 661 patients. AJR Am J Roentgenol 1980;134:888.
93. Caprini JA, Thorpe CJ, Fotopoulos JP: Results of nonsurgical treatment of retained biliary calculi. Surg Gynecol Obstet 1980;151:630.
94. Mason R: Percutaneous extraction of retained gallstones via the T-tube track—British experience of 131 cases. Clin Radiol 1980;31:497.
95. Stokes KR, Falchuk KR, Clouse ME: Biliary duct stones: update in 54 cases after percutaneous transhepatic removal. Radiology 1988;170:999.
96. Picus D, Weyman PJ, Marx MV: Role of percutaneous intracorporeal electrohydraulic lithotripsy in the treatment of biliary tract calculi: works in progress. Radiology 1989;170:989.
97. Rossi P, Bezzi M, Fiocca F, et al: Percutaneous cholangioscopy. Semin Intervent Radiol 1996;13:185.
98. Venbrux AC, Robbins KV, Savader SJ, et al: Endoscopy as an adjunct to biliary radiologic intervention. Radiology 1991;180:355.
99. Bonnel DH, Liguory CE, Cornud FE, et al: Common bile duct and intrahepatic stones: results of transhepatic electrohydraulic lithotripsy in 50 patients. Radiology 1991;180:345.
100. Harris VJ, Sherman S, Trerotola SO, et al: Complex biliary stones: treatment with a small choledochoscope and laser lithotripsy. Radiology 1961;199:71.
101. Picus D: Percutaneous biliary endoscopy. J Vasc Interv Radiol 1995;6:303.
102. Guenther RW, Vorwerk D, Klose KJ, et al: Fine-caliber cholangioscopy. Radiol Clin North Am 1990;28:1171.
103. Kaufman SL, Kadir S, Mitchell SE, et al: Percutaneous transhepatic biliary drainage for bile leaks and fistulas. AJR Am J Roentgenol 1985;144:1055.
104. Liguory C, Vitale GC, Lefebre JF, et al: Endoscopic treatment of postoperative biliary fistulae. Surgery 1991;110:779.
105. Binmoeller KF, Katon RM, Shneidman R: Endoscopic management of postoperative biliary leaks: review of 77 cases and report of two cases with biloma formation. Am J Gastroenterol 1991;86:227.
106. Trerotola SO, Savader SJ, Lund GB, et al: Biliary tract complications following laparoscopic cholecystectomy: Imaging and intervention. Radiology 1992;184:195.
107. vanSonnenberg E, D'Agostino HB, Easter DW, et al: Complications of laparoscopic cholecystectomy: coordinated radiologic and surgical management in 21 patients. Radiology 1993;188:399.

108. Ernst O, Sergent G, Mizrahi D, et al: Biliary leaks: treatment by means of percutaneous transhepatic biliary drainage. Radiology 1999;211:345.

109. Zuidema GD, Cameron JL, Sitzmann JV, et al: Percutaneous transhepatic management of complex biliary problems. Ann Surg 1983;197:584.

110. Oliva VL, Nicolet V, Soulez G, et al: Bilomas developing after laparoscopic biliary surgery: percutaneous management with embolization of biliary leaks. J Vasc Interv Radiol 1997;8:469.

111. Crist DW, Kadir S, Cameron JL: The value of preoperatively placed percutaneous biliary catheters in reconstruction of the proximal part of the biliary tract. Surg Gynecol Obstet 1987;165:421.

112. Chespak LW, Ring EJ, Shapiro HA, et al: Multidisciplinary approach to complex endoscopic biliary intervention. Radiology 1989; 170:995.

113. Gordon RL, Ring EJ: Combined radiologic and retrograde endoscopic and biliary interventions. Radiol Clin North Am 1990;28:1289.

114. Malone DE: Interventional radiologic alternatives to cholecystectomy. Radiol Clin North Am 1990;28:1145.

115. McGahan JP, Lindfors KK: Acute cholecystitis: diagnostic accuracy of percutaneous aspiration of the gallbladder. Radiology 1988; 167:669.

116. Gillams A, Curtis SC, Donald J, et al: Technical considerations in 113 percutaneous cholcystolithostomies. Radiology 1992;183:163.

117. Gibney RG, Chow K, So CB, et al: Gallstone recurrence after cholecystolithostomy. AJR Am J Roentgenol 1989;153:287.

118. Warren LP, Kadir S, Dunnick NR: Percutaneous cholecystostomy: anatomic considerations. Radiology 1988;168:615.

119. Garber SJ, Mathieson JR, Cooperberg PL, et al: Percutaneous cholecystostomy: safety of the transperitoneal route. J Vasc Interv Radiol 1994;5:295.

120. D'Agostino HB, vanSonnenberg E, Sanchez RB, et al: Imaging of the percutaneous cholecystostomy tract: observations and utility. Radiology 1991;181:675.

121. Teplick SK, Harshfield DL, Brandon JC, et al: Percutaneous cholecystostomy in critically ill patients. Gastrointest Radiol 1991;16:154.

122. Lee MJ, Saini S, Brink JA, et al: Treatment of critically ill patients with sepsis of unknown cause: value of percutaneous cholecystostomy. AJR Am J Roentgenol 1991;156:1163.

123. de Manzoni G, Furlan F, Guglielmi A, et al: Acute cholecystitis: ultrasonographic staging and percutaneous cholecystostomy. Eur J Radiol 1992;15:175.

124. Browning PD, McGahan JP, Gerscovich EO: Percutaneous cholecystostomy for suspected acute cholecystitis in the hospitalized patient. J Vasc Interv Radiol 1993;4:531.

125. Lo LD, Vogelzang RL, Braun MA, et al: Percutaneous cholecystostomy for the diagnosis and treatment of acute calculous and acalculous cholecystitis. J Vasc Interv Radiol 1995;6:629.

126. Boland GW, Lee MJ, Leung J, Mueller PR: Percutaneous cholecystomy in critically ill patients: early response and final outcome in 82 patients. AJR Am J Roentgenol 1994;163:339.

127. England RE, McDermott VG, Smith TP, et al: Percutaneous cholecystostomy: who responds? AJR Am J Roentgenol 1997;168:1247.

128. vanSonnenberg E, D'Agostino HB, Goodacre BW, et al: Percutaneous gallbladder puncture and cholecystostomy: results, complications and caveats for safety. Radiology 1992;183:167.

23

Urologic and Genital Systems

Steven B. Oglevie, MD

Revolutionary developments in the radiologic diagnosis and interventional therapy of diseases of the genitourinary tract have occurred during the past two decades. A broad spectrum of interventional radiologic procedures now are performed routinely in the genitourinary tract. Well-accepted urinary interventions include percutaneous nephrostomy, nephrostolithotomy, ureteral stent placement, and benign ureteral stricture dilation. These mainstream urinary interventions have become entrenched in contemporary clinical practice and have a substantial impact on the lives of patients with complex urinary tract diseases. Radiologically guided retrograde interventions through ileal conduits and through the urethra are gaining popularity and provide attractive alternatives to retrograde endoscopic interventions. Selective salpingography and fallopian tube recanalization have been accepted and endorsed as treatment options for infertility due to fallopian tube obstruction. No matter what clinical problem is being addressed, the patient's interests are best served by close cooperation and communication between the radiologist and the urologist or gynecologist, whose technical skills are complimentary.

▇ PERCUTANEOUS NEPHROSTOMY

Anatomy

The kidneys are retroperitoneal organs surrounded by perinephric fat and enclosed by Gerota's fascia. Their axis parallels the psoas muscle so that the upper pole is medial and slightly more posterior than the lower pole. During normal development, the kidney ascends and rotates medially about its vertical axis such that the renal hilum is directed anteromedially at an angle of approximately 30 degrees from the horizontal plane.

The main renal artery and vein lie anterior to the renal pelvis. However, a posterior branch of the renal artery courses behind the renal pelvis to supply the dorsal segments. A percutaneous nephrostomy (PCN) tract extending directly into a calyx has the least chance of causing substantial arterial

injury (Fig. 23-1). Punctures into an infundibulum or directly into the renal pelvis carry a higher risk of hemorrhagic complications, because larger arterial branches may have been traversed.

The calyces usually are arranged in anterior and posterior rows. At the upper and lower poles, fusion results in compound calyces. During urography in the anteroposterior projection, the posterior calyces generally are seen "end on," whereas the anterior calyces extend laterally (Fig. 23-2). However, substantial normal variation occurs. Oblique imaging, ultrasound, or injection of air often is required to identify posterior calyces with the patient prone. Discrimination between the anterior and posterior calyces is critical, because posterior calyces are strongly preferred for most PCN procedures.

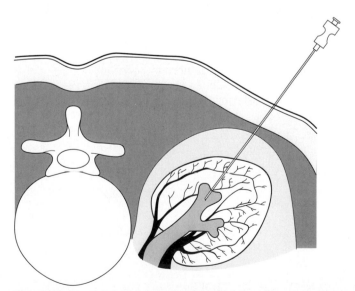

FIGURE 23-1 ▇ Ideal posterolateral approach to a posterior calyx. This approach is advantageous because it minimizes the risk of arterial injury and provides a straight vector for advancement of guidewires, dilators, and catheters into the renal pelvis. The tract is far enough lateral not to traverse paraspinal muscles but not so lateral as to risk colon perforation.

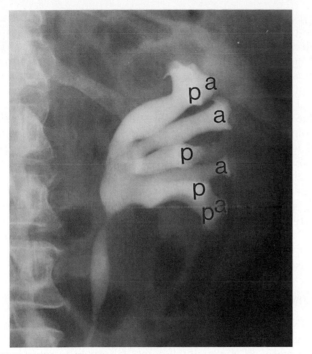

FIGURE 23-2 ■ Anterior (a) and posterior (p) calyces are differentiated on anteroposterior urography.

Understanding the normal and variant relationships of the kidneys with surrounding structures is important to safe and successful placement of a PCN.[1] The descending colon lies in the anterior pararenal space, and its relationship to the left kidney is determined by the position of the lateroconal fascia. In approximately 10% of patients, the descending colon lies behind a horizontal line at the posterior edge of the left kidney. In about 1% of cases, the descending colon extends behind the left kidney and is at risk for injury if a standard PCN approach is employed.[2] Rarely, the ascending colon lies posterolateral to the right kidney and medial to the liver.

The pleura extends posteriorly down to the 12th vertebral body and then extends laterally crossing the 12th, 11th, and 10th ribs. Although great normal variation occurs, about one half of the right kidney and one third of the left kidney lie above this posterior reflection of the pleura.

The liver is anterolateral to the upper pole of the right kidney. In some patients, a portion of the right lobe of the liver may extend posterolateral to the upper pole of the kidney. The position of the spleen is more variable. It typically lies superolateral to the kidney but often is adjacent to the lateral margin and frequently may be posterolateral to the upper pole. Because of these variants of colonic, hepatic, and splenic anatomy, review of prior cross-sectional imaging studies is strongly recommended before PCN.

Patient Selection

The indications for PCN fall into four broad categories (Box 23-1). Each patient must be considered individually, because some have both indications for and contraindications to the procedure. The decision about whether to perform PCN depends on the details of the particular situation and on the other available options.

Relief of Urinary Obstruction

The most common indication for PCN is relief of urinary obstruction. Imaging studies should be performed to demonstrate hydroureteronephrosis, and they usually delineate the anatomic level of obstruction and the cause (Fig. 23-3). The ureteral obstruction may be acute, as with obstructing ureteral calculi or traumatic ureteral injury. However, the

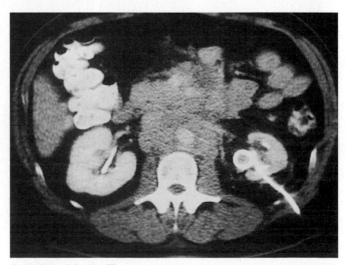

FIGURE 23-3 ■ Decompressive percutaneous nephrostomy for infected hydroureteronephrosis due to lymphoma. Marked cortical atrophy was caused by long-standing obstruction. The ideal posterolateral approach into a posterior calyx is demonstrated.

obstruction may be long-standing, as with primary urothelial neoplasms, extrinsic compression, or direct invasion by retroperitoneal or pelvic malignancies.

In patients with bilateral obstruction or with obstruction of a solitary kidney, PCN is indicated for preservation of renal function. If the degree of hydronephrosis and cortical thinning is markedly worse on one side, the contralateral side may be decompressed to preserve renal function. Alternatively, both sides may be decompressed to restore as much renal function as possible and to eliminate the chance of pyonephrosis on the undrained side. In some patients with widely disseminated malignancies and very short life expectancies, decompression may not be indicated. Many oncologists believe a uremic death is a reasonably painless way for a patient to expire. This decision must be addressed individually and tailored to the desires of the patient and his or her family.

In patients with acute unilateral ureteral obstruction, decompression is justified to preserve renal function on the affected side. Long-standing obstruction is associated with an irreversible deterioration of renal function and parenchymal atrophy. Although the patient's serum blood urea nitrogen and creatinine levels usually do not become elevated with unilateral obstruction, the damage to the ipsilateral kidney is progressive and irreversible when not addressed promptly. Decompression with PCN may allow the cause of acute ureteral obstruction to be addressed on a more elective basis without risk of losing renal function.

In any patient with hydroureteronephrosis and suspicion of infection, emergent decompression is indicated. Infection may be suggested by fever, leukocytosis, or frank sepsis with hypotension and tachycardia. Although these patients must be treated immediately with intravenous fluids and antibiotics, delay in urinary decompression is not justified. The decompressive procedures in patients with pyonephrosis must be conducted and monitored with care, because the septic condition may be worsened with the intervention.

Patients with chronic unilateral hydroureteronephrosis due to malignancy do not necessarily require decompression unless infection is suspected (see Fig. 23-3). In the absence of malignant disease, kidneys that contribute greater than 20% of overall renal function are considered to be worth salvaging. This assessment may be impossible to make in the face of obstruction. The finding of mild or moderate cortical atrophy on CT or ultrasound is not a reliable predictor of poor potential for functional recovery after a PCN. Decompressive PCN may be indicated to assess the recoverable function of a chronically occluded kidney. A substantial increase in renal plasma flow predicts recovering renal function.

Diversion of Urine

PCN is used to divert urine in cases of urinary leakage (Fig. 23-4). Injury to the urinary tract may be iatrogenic or traumatic. PCN, usually in combination with ureteral stent placement, allows most ureteral injuries to seal. The stent is thought to serve as a scaffold for ureteral healing. Percutaneous drainage of associated urinomas that accumulated before urinary diversion also may be performed. In cases of malignant or inflammatory fistulas, PCN is indicated to divert urine. PCN alone frequently does not divert urine flow enough to allow a fistula to close. In this case, ureteral

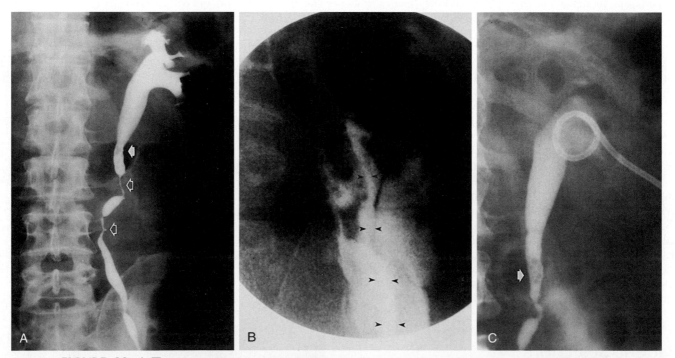

FIGURE 23-4 ■ Percutaneous nephrostomy (PCN) for diversion of urine from a ureteral injury. **A,** Retrograde urogram during attempted ureteroscopic retrieval of ureteral stone *(closed arrow)* shows two injured mid-ureter segments *(open arrows)*. **B,** This image shows further ureteral injury with extravasation of contrast material from the ureter *(arrowheads)*. **C,** Antegrade nephrostogram after PCN for urinary diversion shows ureteral stones *(arrow)* and an injured segment with leakage. A ureteral stent was placed, and this injury healed without further intervention.

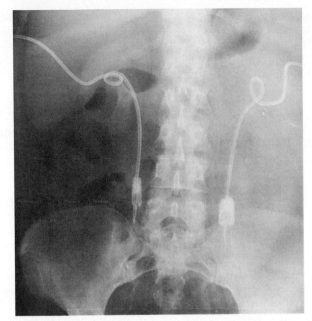

FIGURE 23-5 ▪ Diversion of urine from a malignant vesicovaginal fistula using nephroureteral occlusion balloons.

occlusion or stent placement may be required (Fig. 23-5). PCN has been used also to divert urine and treat patients successfully with hemorrhagic cystitis.[3]

Access for Diagnostic Interventions

Percutaneous access may be performed to permit antegrade pyelography. The collecting system may be better imaged with direct contrast injection than with excretory urography, particularly in cases of high-grade urinary obstruction (Fig. 23-6). Dynamic flow and pressure studies (e.g., Whitaker test) may be performed to determine the significance of urographically detected stenoses and to assess the results of interventions such as endopyelotomy or balloon ureteral dilation. Biopsies of urothelial lesions may be performed through the nephrostomy access using brushes and forceps. The nephrostomy access may be dilated to permit diagnostic nephroscopy and ureteroscopy.

Access for Therapeutic Interventions

Ureteral strictures may be dilated and ureteral stents can be placed. Foreign bodies such as encrusted or occluded ureteral stents may be retrieved through the nephrostomy access (Fig. 23-7). Stone therapy can be performed with chemodissolution or mechanical fragmentation and extraction. Antifungal agents may be infused directly through the nephrostomy tube to treat fungus balls in the upper urinary tract.[4,5] Nephroscopically guided operations can be performed, including resection of urothelial neoplasms and endopyelotomy.

Contraindications

Contraindications to PCN include uncorrectable coagulopathy and an uncooperative patient. If hyperkalemia is severe (i.e., potassium level greater than 7 mEq/L), hemodialysis should be performed to correct the electrolyte balance before the procedure.

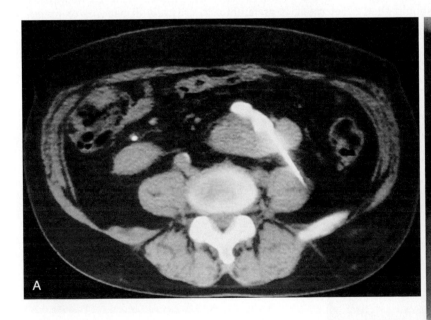

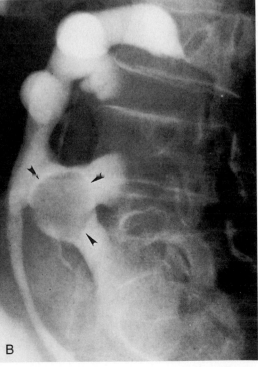

FIGURE 23-6 ▪ Antegrade pyelography in a patient with a horseshoe kidney and unexplained hematuria. **A,** CT-guided access to a calyx in a horseshoe kidney. **B,** Antegrade pyelography reveals a large mass *(arrowheads)* not detected on other imaging studies. This mass proved to be a suburothelial renal cell carcinoma.

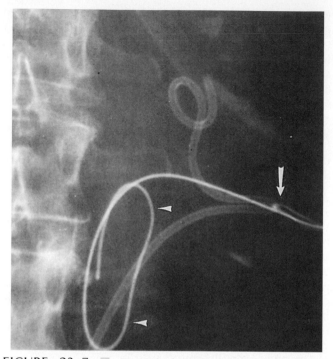

FIGURE 23-7 ■ Retrieval of occluded ureteral stent through the percutaneous nephrostomy tract. The stent is removed with a loop snare *(arrow)* while a safety guidewire remains coiled in proximal ureter *(arrowheads)*.

Surgical and Medical Alternatives

It usually is advantageous to initially consider a retrograde approach for renal drainage in patients with obstructive uropathy. This approach carries a lower risk of hemorrhagic complications but probably also carries a greater (although still very small) risk of ureteral injury. PCN should then be reserved for patients in whom retrograde attempts are unsuccessful or not feasible. A surgical nephrostomy (Fig. 23-8) may be placed directly into the renal pelvis, but this is rarely indicated because PCN can be performed safely and effectively in almost all patients. Medical therapy for obstructive uropathy is limited. In some patients with widely disseminated malignancy and obstructive uropathy, renal function may improve with the administration of corticosteroids.[6]

Technique

Preprocedure Care

Before the procedure, patients should be screened and treated for any coagulopathy. Review of any prior abdominal imaging is strongly suggested to detect variant anatomy of colon, spleen, and liver, which should be considered when selecting the nephrostomy approach.

Prophylactic antibiotics should be administered intravenously 60 minutes before the procedure. The most common urinary tract pathogens are *Escherichia coli*, *Klebsiella*, *Enterococcus*, and *Proteus* species. For prophylaxis in the absence of any overt infection, ampicillin, cefazolin, or cefoperazone may be given. When infection exists, therapy is directed toward the isolated organisms. Ticarcillin, piperacillin, and an aminoglycoside may be used to provide broader coverage.[7] The antibiotics should be continued for 24 to 48 hours in patients at low risk for urosepsis and for 48 to 72 hours in high-risk patients.

Procedure[8]

The patient is placed in the prone position when a rotating C-arm unit is available for fluoroscopy. When the procedure is carried out with a fixed fluoroscopy unit, the prone oblique position, with the side to undergo nephrostomy elevated, is preferable. In critically ill patients or pregnant patients who are unable to be placed prone, the procedure can be performed with the patient in a supine oblique position.

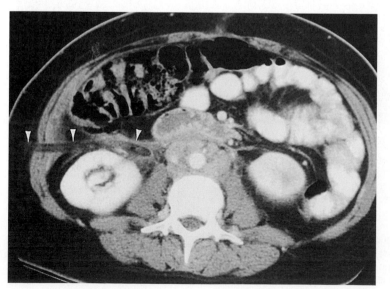

FIGURE 23-8 ■ Surgical nephrostomy. A Foley catheter *(arrowheads)* directly enters the renal pelvis. Such open surgical nephrostomies are rarely indicated unless another open procedure is being performed at the same time.

PCN is performed with fluoroscopy or with ultrasound and fluoroscopy. Fluoroscopy is used when renal function permits the intravenous administration of contrast material and results in satisfactory opacification of the collecting system. Fluoroscopy also may be used to puncture directly onto an opaque calyceal calculus. If a retrograde ureteral catheter has been placed, it may be used to opacify the collecting system.

Although many operators pass needles blindly toward the anticipated location of the renal pelvis under fluoroscopy, ultrasound-guided needle placement is safer. In patients with impaired renal function, ultrasound is useful to guide the initial puncture. A suitable calyx can be selected and

entered (Fig. 23-9A). The depth of the collecting system is determined precisely. Surrounding organs such as the colon, spleen, and liver can be avoided.

After the collecting system has been entered with ultrasound guidance, the remainder of the procedure is carried out under fluoroscopy. CT or MR guidance for puncture occasionally may be useful in patients with congenital anomalies (i.e., horseshoe or pelvic kidneys) or aberrant anatomy (e.g., severe scoliosis, morbid obesity) (see Fig. 23-6).

Planning the puncture pathway is the most crucial step in the procedure because poorly placed punctures are associated with higher complication rates and may preclude successful completion of subsequent interventions. For a

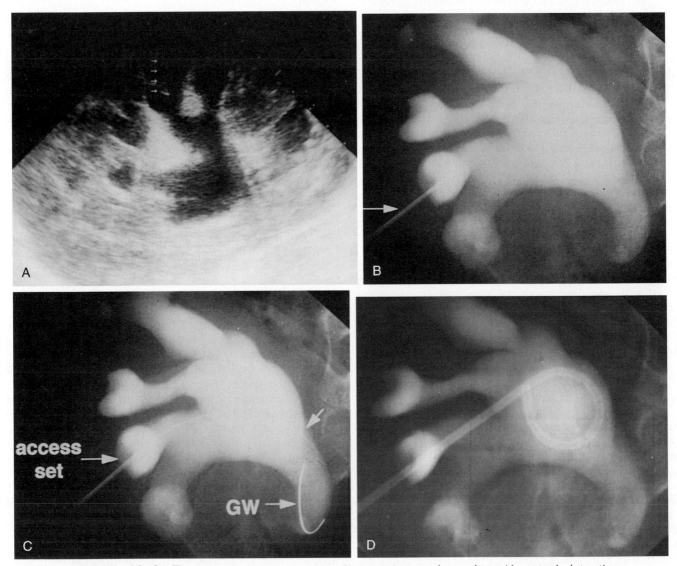

FIGURE 23-9 ■ Technique for percutaneous nephrostomy in a renal transplant with ureteral obstruction. **A,** Ultrasound-guided puncture of the selected calyx. The echogenic 22-gauge needle tip is marked with *arrows*. Urine was aspirated. **B,** The collecting system is gently opacified through the needle *(arrow)*, and the puncture site scrutinized. Because the puncture is not too central, a 0.018-inch guidewire is advanced through the needle into the obstructed ureter. **C,** The access set is then advanced over the 0.018-inch guidewire (GW). The location of the tip of the access set may be confirmed by aspirating or injecting contrast through the sidearm. A floppy-tipped, 0.035- to 0.038-inch guidewire is then advanced through the access set alongside the 0.018-inch guidewire, which is left in place as a safety guidewire. The access set is removed, and the tract may be dilated. **D,** An 8- to 10-French locking pigtail nephrostomy catheter is advanced over the larger guidewire into the renal pelvis and locked into position. The patient's creatinine level decreased from 11 to 2 mg/dL over the following 48 hours.

simple decompressive nephrostomy, puncture of a lower pole calyx is satisfactory. This approach minimizes the risk of pleural complications. If ureteral stent placement is planned, puncture of an interpolar calyx is preferable to create a gentle curve down the ureter. However, ureteral stents usually can be placed from an inferior polar approach using stiff guidewires and sheaths. Access through an upper pole calyx is required occasionally for stone extraction. In this case, the tract is intercostal, and pleural complications may occur. If an intercostal approach is required, care must be taken to avoid the intercostal vessels immediately beneath the ribs.

The ideal skin entry site is at least 12 cm lateral to the midline but medial to the posterior axillary line. If the skin entry site is too medial, the paraspinal muscles are traversed, and subsequent interventions are rendered more difficult because the guidewire and catheter must abruptly turn medially on entering the calyx. A medially placed nephrostomy also is more painful for the supine patient. If the skin entry is too lateral, the risk of colonic perforation increases.

A posterolateral approach, with the needle angled about 30 to 40 degrees from vertical, directly into a posterior calyx is favored (see Fig. 23-1). This route follows the relatively avascular posterolateral plane of the kidney (i.e., Brödel's line). Punctures generally should be made directly into a posterior calyx (see Fig. 23-1). This provides a straight vector into the renal pelvis and minimizes the amount of renal parenchyma traversed by the nephrostomy tract. Infundibular punctures or punctures directly into the renal pelvis should be avoided because large arteries may be traversed. Inadvertent puncture of anterior calyces makes subsequent interventions more difficult because of the tortuous pathway and increases the risk for significant arterial injury. Anterior calyces should be targeted only in the rare patient with an anterior calyceal stone. Oblique imaging and injection of air or carbon dioxide is helpful to determine whether a calyx punctured under fluoroscopy is posterior or anterior.

When the collecting system has been entered with a 21- to 22-gauge needle, a sample of urine should be aspirated initially for cultures. If clinical suspicion for infection is high or the urine is cloudy, opacification of the collecting system must be performed gently after evacuating an equal amount of urine. Instillation of contrast by gravity may help prevent overdistention and worsening of sepsis. Likewise, subsequent manipulations that may have been planned should be minimized until the urine has cleared.

The initial puncture site is carefully scrutinized before dilation and catheter placement (Fig. 23-9B). If instillation of contrast or air reveals the initial puncture is not into a suitable posterior calyx, the needle should be left in place to opacify the system while a new needle is guided fluoroscopically into an appropriate calyx.

After the puncture is deemed satisfactory, a 0.018-inch guidewire is advanced into the renal pelvis and ideally down the ureter. A generous skin nick is made along the needle tract. Blunt dissection of the subcutaneous tissue is performed. An 8-French access set is advanced under fluoroscopic guidance into the collecting system (Fig. 23-9C). Urine can be aspirated and contrast injected through the side arm of some access sets. A hydrostatic valve prevents leakage of urine. A 0.038-inch guidewire is advanced through

the access set into the renal pelvis or ureter. A 5-French guiding catheter may help direct the guidewire down the ureter into a secure position.

The tract is then dilated, and an 8- to 12-French locking pigtail nephrostomy catheter is placed (Fig. 23-9D). The pigtail is formed and locked while the catheter is turned. Care must be taken to avoid forming the pigtail in the ureter or in a calyceal infundibulum. The 8-French tubes are satisfactory in patients with clear urine. Larger tubes may be helpful in patients with grossly purulent urine or stone debris. Locking pigtail catheters generally are preferred over other self-retaining catheters (e.g., Malecot, accordion, Foley). The nonpigtail catheters occasionally may be useful in collecting systems not capacious enough to accommodate a pigtail.

The catheter is secured to the skin using adhesive dressings or suture. Adhesive dressings minimize catheter kinking and reduce the risk of catheter dislodgement. After the tract has matured, a simple dry dressing may be placed over the exit site. The catheter is left to gravity drainage with close monitoring of urine output. It requires irrigation only if blood clots occlude the tube. Three-way stopcocks should not be left attached, because they may inadvertently become turned the wrong way and obstruct urinary drainage.

Patients should be followed closely after the procedure for hemorrhagic or septic complications. In patients with bilateral obstructive uropathy undergoing PCN, dramatic fluid and electrolyte shifts may occur with postobstructive diuresis. In carefully selected patients, PCN may be performed safely as an outpatient procedure.[8] In this situation, however, the operator should have a low threshold for admission if there is any evidence of hemorrhage, sepsis, or severe pain during or after the procedure.

Catheter Maintenance

Chronic indwelling nephrostomy tubes usually should be exchanged every 3 to 6 months to prevent encrustation and occlusion. Some patients may require exchanges as often as every 6 weeks. It is better to err on the side of frequent catheter exchanges than to have the catheter occlude and have the patient develop sepsis or further deterioration of renal function due to obstruction. If the catheter is initially exchanged at 3 months and appears to be functioning well, the interval may be increased by 1 month at a time up to 6 months.

Patients with chronic indwelling nephrostomy tubes invariably develop colonization with bacteria, fungi, or both.[9] Asymptomatic bacteremia occurs frequently (about 10%) during routine catheter exchanges; preprocedural antibiotics are not successful at preventing bacteremia.[10] Nonetheless, many operators routinely give antibiotics for tube exchanges, particularly when the tube has been functioning poorly. For patients with cardiac valvular disease, a full course of antibiotics should be administered before catheter exchange to minimize the risk of bacteremia. Despite therapeutic levels of antibiotics during catheter exchange, a septic reaction may still occur as a reaction to endotoxin released into the vascular system.

Patients with occluded catheters can present a challenge for catheter exchange. The pigtail catheter retention string initially should be secured so that it is not pushed down the catheter into an occlusive tangle with repeated attempts at guidewire passage. Hydrophilic guidewires are preferred for negotiating an occluded catheter. If the end hole cannot be passed, a side hole is acceptable. After the guidewire is through the catheter, the string is released to allow the loop to open. If no guidewire can be passed, a sheath may be passed over the catheter, after its hub has been cut off. The catheter can then be removed and replaced through the sheath.

Catheter dislodgement represents an urgent situation, because rapid tube replacement is required to maintain tract patency. Tracts that have not had a tube replaced within 48 to 72 hours are difficult to renegotiate. All patients with PCN tubes should be educated about the urgency of this situation. After sterile preparation, the tract is probed with a dilator. Contrast may be injected to define the tract, and a hydrophilic wire is then negotiated back into the collecting system.

Results

In patients with obstructed, dilated collecting systems, a decompressive PCN can be placed successfully in almost all cases. Technical success should be expected in greater than 95% of cases.[11,12] In nondilated collecting systems or complex stone cases, technical success may decrease to 85% to 90%.

The clinical response to PCN by patients with urosepsis often is dramatic. In one series of patients with gram-negative septicemia and urinary obstruction complicated by infection, PCN reduced mortality from 40% to 8%.[13] However, PCN in patients with pyonephrosis may exacerbate or precipitate septicemia as a result of bacteria entering the bloodstream through peripapillary veins from catheter manipulation or overdistention.[13,14]

In patients with fungal urinary infections, antifungal agents can be infused directly into the collecting system (Fig. 23-10). This approach is advantageous because effective therapeutic levels can be achieved in the urinary tract without the associated systemic toxicity from intravenous administration. Fungus balls can be disrupted mechanically and extracted through the nephrostomy tract.[15]

In most patients with azotemia due to obstruction, PCN provides rapid improvement of renal function.[16] The procedure commonly is used as a temporizing measure to improve renal function while the underlying obstruction is addressed therapeutically.

In patients with terminal malignancies and azotemia due to bilateral obstruction, unilateral PCN usually suffices to preserve renal function.[17] Bilateral drainage is indicated if pyonephrosis is suspected or unilateral drainage is unsatisfactory for restoring renal function. Unfortunately, the long-term survival rate after palliative diversion for malignant ureteral obstruction is poor, with only 25% of patients surviving 1 year.[18] Even with careful patient selection, 32% of patients are unable to achieve any improvement in quality of life after PCN.[19] After an open and frank discussion about the physical, emotional, and financial burdens associated with a drainage catheter, most patients and families opt for the drainage catheter as a means to extend life for as little as a few months. Patients with hormone-responsive prostate

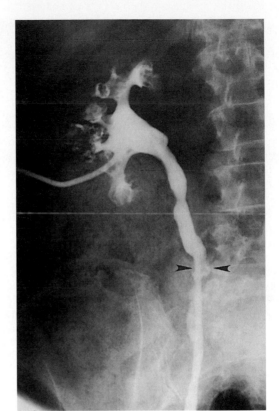

FIGURE 23-10 ■ Percutaneous nephrostomy for treatment of fungal pyelonephritis in a diabetic patient. Biopsy of a polypoid lesion in the mid-ureter *(arrowheads)* using an atherectomy device revealed a mycetoma; others are seen in the calyces and renal pelvis. Amphotericin, infused directly through the catheter, produced a good clinical response.

carcinoma usually live longer than those with hormone-resistant prostate cancer or other pelvic malignancies.[20] Preservation of renal function is more beneficial in the former group.

Complications

The mortality rate for PCN is about 0.2%, which compares favorably with the mortality rate for surgical nephrostomy (≤6%).[21,22] The major procedure-related complications are bleeding and sepsis. Hemorrhage requiring transfusion or other treatment occurs in 1% to 3% of patients undergoing PCN.[12,23,24] One series of 144 nephrostomies placed using combined CT and fluoroscopic guidance had no hemorrhagic or other major complications.[25] Most bleeding associated with PCN is transient and self-limited. It is not uncommon to have pink urine for several days after the procedure. If small clots block the catheter, the catheter should be irrigated with sterile saline.

Major arterial injury should be suspected when the urine remains grossly bloody after 3 to 5 days, when new clots are demonstrated in the collecting system on follow-up nephrostograms, or when there is a significant drop in hematocrit. These patients should undergo angiographic evaluation with embolization of injured vessels (Fig. 23-11). If the initial angiogram is negative, the nephrostomy may be

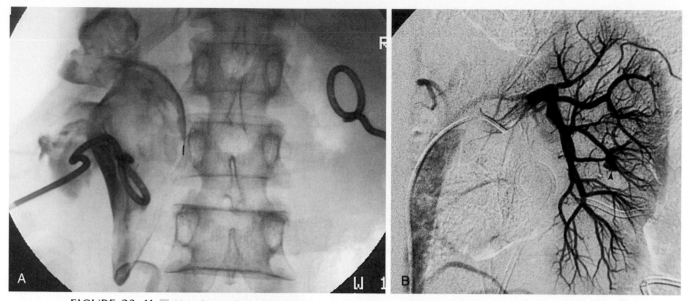

FIGURE 23-11 ■ Major hemorrhage after percutaneous nephrostomy (PCN). **A,** Persistent clot in the collecting system (seen in prone position) 3 days after PCN raised the suspicion for an arterial injury. **B,** Angiography in supine position reveals an interlobar artery pseudoaneurysm *(arrowhead)* that was embolized subsequently. The arterial injury is not in the path of the nephrostomy and was the result of a needle pass thought unsuitable for PCN placement.

removed over a guidewire to relieve the tamponading effect of the catheter, and the angiogram is repeated. If the drop in hematocrit is out of proportion to the quantity of blood in the urine, the patient may have a retroperitoneal hematoma. Retroperitoneal hemorrhage is best evaluated with CT. Unsuspected retroperitoneal hematomas not requiring treatment have been reported in up to 13% of patients.[26]

Significant hemorrhage usually is caused by laceration of lobar arteries. Pseudoaneurysm, arteriovenous fistula, arteriocaliceal fistula, or frank extravasation may be seen at arteriography. The risk of hemorrhage is minimized by using fine needles for puncture, using appropriate guidance, and avoiding puncture of the anteromedial renal vessels.

Although the reported frequency of sepsis after PCN ranges from 1% to 21%,[8,13,21,24] a review of 454 procedures revealed an incidence of serious sepsis requiring intensive care unit admission of only 1.3%.[12] Less severe septic reactions with shaking chills, fever, and tachycardia without hypotension occur more often. Fever occurs in about 15% and septic shock in 2% to 7% of patients with pyonephrosis who have been pretreated with antibiotics.[14,21] Patients with infected urine or stones are at higher risk for PCN-related sepsis.

For elective PCN for stone disease, antibiotic therapy ideally should be initiated and continued until the urine is clear. Diagnostic nephrostograms, ureteral catheterization, and stent placement should be delayed in patients with pyonephrosis until the urine has cleared.

Pleural complications include pneumothorax and empyema from infected urine entering the pleural space along the nephrostomy tract. These complications are prevented by obtaining access beneath the 12th rib. One study showed that PCN tracts above the 12th rib traverse the pleura in 29% of cases on the right and 14% of cases on the left.[27] However, most transgressions of the pleural space are silent. Pleural complications occur in only about 0.2% of decompressive nephrostomies.[12] When upper polar access is required for stone therapy, the risk of pleural complications increases to as much as 12%.[28,29]

Minor perforations of the collecting system occur in about 2% of patients. If a satisfactory drainage catheter is placed in the collecting system, these leaks usually heal spontaneously over the next 48 to 72 hours. Urinomas requiring drainage are less common and occur rarely with standard 8- to 12-French PCN tubes. After removal of larger PCN catheters used for nephrostolithotomy, urinomas are more common. Other rare complications of PCN include air embolism and puncture of the colon, spleen, liver, and gallbladder.[30-33]

Catheter dislodgement is minimized with the use of self-retaining loop catheters. Less than 1% of these devices are dislodged within the first month of placement.[12] Malecot catheters commonly used after nephrostomy tract dilation may become difficult to extract if tissue bridges grow over the catheter flanges.[34] These devices should therefore be used with caution for long-term drainage. The entrapped catheters may be safely removed using endoscopic techniques to cut the anchoring tissue bridges.

■ INTERVENTIONS FOR RENAL STONE DISEASE

Renal stone disease is seen in about 1 of 1000 hospitalized patients. Although most stones pass spontaneously, about 40% require some intervention.[35] The first PCN performed expressly for the purpose of stone removal was reported in 1976.[36] Since then, open pyelolithotomy has been replaced almost completely by minimally invasive techniques. Almost all renal calculi can be managed successfully with extracorporeal shock wave lithotripsy (ESWL) or percutaneous nephrostolithotomy (PCNL), with success rates that rival open surgery but with significantly less morbidity, recovery time, and cost.

Patient Selection

The approach to patients with urinary tract stones is summarized in Table 23-1.[37,38] ESWL is appropriate for about 80% of renal and upper ureteral stones. ESWL has limited value for stones that are large, hard (i.e., cystine), infected, tightly impacted in the ureter, or located in the lower pole of the kidney. Passage of ESWL stone fragments may be impeded by anatomic abnormalities. In these situations, PCNL is the procedure of choice (Box 23-2). PCNL has improved the success and diminished the complications of ESWL for staghorn calculi.[39]

Technique

Retrograde placement of a ureteral catheter or compliant occlusion balloon catheter is extremely helpful in many cases (Fig. 23-12). This catheter can be used to visualize the collecting system with iodinated contrast or gas. Distention of the upper urinary tract may facilitate manipulation of guidewires around larger stones.

The procedure can be performed in one or two stages. The access, tract dilation, and stone extraction may be

TABLE 23-1   MANAGEMENT OF URINARY TRACT STONES

Stone Size or Location	Therapy
<5 mm	Fluids, narcotics
Small renal (<2.5 cm)	ESWL
Large renal (>2.5 cm)	PCNL
Upper ureteral	ESWL, PCNL
Lower ureteral	Ureteroscopy

ESWL, extracorporeal shock wave lithotripsy; PCNL, percutaneous nephrostolithotomy.

BOX 23-2   Indications for Percutaneous Nephrostolithotomy

Large stones (>2.5 cm)
Staghorn calculi
Infected stones
Stones associated with compromised drainage (e.g., urinary obstruction, dependent calices, caliceal diverticula)
Cystine stones
Abnormal body habitus (e.g., scoliosis, morbid obesity)
Certain removal of all calculus material important
Failure of other treatment modalities

---

performed during the same session. Alternatively, a staged procedure may be performed in which the access is performed initially and the stone extraction is performed on a subsequent day. The tract may be dilated during the first or second session. The two-stage approach allows the access

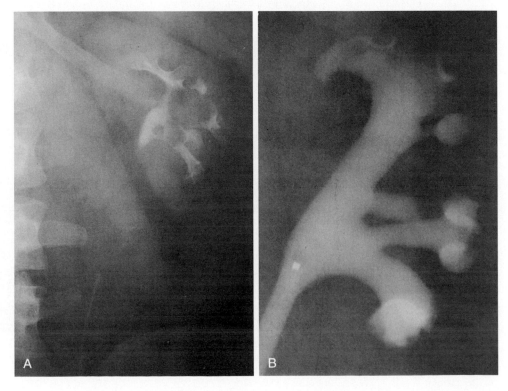

FIGURE 23-12 ▮ Placement of retrograde ureteral balloon catheter to facilitate access for percutaneous nephrostolithotomy. **A,** Excretory urography shows a large stone in the renal pelvis. **B,** Injection through a retrograde catheter placed 6 weeks later shows stone resolution.

procedure to be performed carefully using optimal fluoroscopy and without operating room time constraints. If perforation of the collecting system or hemorrhage occurs, tract dilation and stone removal can be delayed.

Access

Planning the approach and entry site is the most critical step of the PCNL procedure. The puncture site must allow the stone to be accessed and removed but not be made directly into the pelvis or infundibulum. If the initial puncture site is not ideal, it is wise to make a new puncture in a more suitable position than to proceed with tract dilation through which the stone cannot be removed.

The rationale for using a posterolateral approach at the edge of the paravertebral muscles below the 12th rib was discussed in a previous section. Puncture of a posterior calyx is preferred for most cases to provide a straight path to the renal pelvis and minimize the risk of arterial injury. For calyceal and diverticular stones, a direct puncture onto the stone is preferred.

After the approach has been determined, the collecting system must be visualized. This step may be accomplished by injecting an indwelling ureteral catheter, administering intravenous contrast, inserting a fine needle directly onto the stone using fluoroscopy, or localizing with ultrasound. Injection of carbon dioxide or room air is helpful to identify posterior calices.

For the definitive puncture of the targeted calyx, 21- or 18-gauge needles may be used. The 18-gauge needles are directed more easily and help with negotiation of a guidewire around the stone. A 0.038-inch guidewire can be advanced directly into the collecting system. The 0.018-inch guidewires used with 21-gauge needles often are difficult to negotiate around complex stones. The guidewire is then advanced down the ureter into the bladder using a curved catheter and a curved-tip hydrophilic guidewire.

If stone removal will be performed at a later date, a 5-French catheter is left in the bladder to provide quick and secure access for subsequent tract dilation. If the stone is associated with obstruction or bleeding, a nephrostomy catheter may be left in the renal pelvis.

Tract Dilation

The procedure should be performed using epidural or general anesthesia. Two stiff guidewires are advanced into the bladder using a peel-away sheath placed in the nephrostomy tract. The safety guidewire is then coiled and placed beneath a sterile towel in the event that access is lost during stone manipulation. The tract dilation may then be carried out using high-pressure balloons or sequential tapered fascial dilators.

With the balloon technique, the working Teflon sheath is backloaded onto the balloon and advanced directly over the completely expanded balloon (Fig. 23-13). Alternatively, a dilator and sheath may be backloaded onto the balloon and advanced over the deflated balloon. Occasionally, dense scar tissue at the renal capsule from prior open or percutaneous interventions precludes complete balloon expansion (Fig. 23-14). In this situation, sequential dilators may be employed, or the tissue may be spread with forceps. Sequential dilators are somewhat more traumatic and frequently displace the kidney substantially during tract dilation. Another disadvantage of sequential dilators is that the tract is detamponaded during dilator exchanges, and blood loss may be substantial.

Usually the sheath tip is advanced to the location of the stone. However, if the infundibulum leading to the stone is

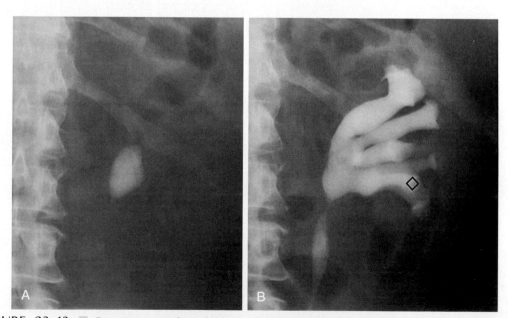

FIGURE 23-13 ■ Percutaneous nephrostolithotomy (PCNL) tract dilation using a balloon catheter. **A,** The plain radiograph shows a large calcified stone. **B,** Excretory urography shows the stone to be obscured by contrast in the renal pelvis. The ideal approach for PCNL is beneath the 12th rib, through the posterior calyx *(open diamond).*

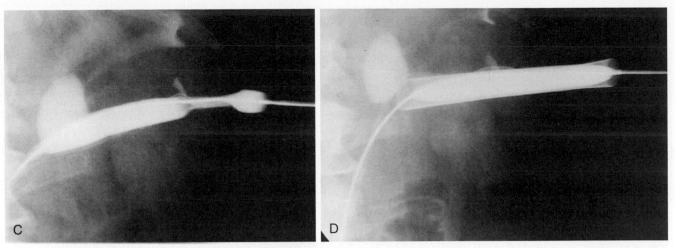

FIGURE 23-13 *Cont'd* ■ **C,** After two stiff guidewires are advanced securely down the ureter, the balloon is expanded. **D,** With the balloon completely expanded, the backloaded Teflon sheath is advanced over the balloon into the collecting system. The stone is then fragmented and removed under nephroscopic visualization.

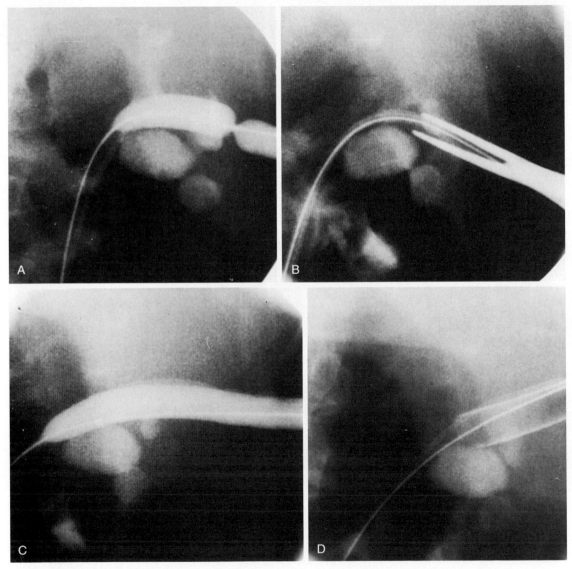

FIGURE 23-14 ■ Tract dilation is difficult because of renal capsular fibrosis from prior percutaneous nephrostolithotomy. **A,** During balloon tract dilation, a refractory waist is observed in the balloon at the renal capsule. Two balloons were ruptured without overcoming the tissue, and sequential dilators were used in an attempt to overcome capsular fibrosis without success. **B,** A surgical forceps was then advanced into the tract, and the capsular tissue was spread. **C and D,** Another balloon was completely expanded, and the 30-French sheath was advanced into the collecting system. The stones were removed successfully.

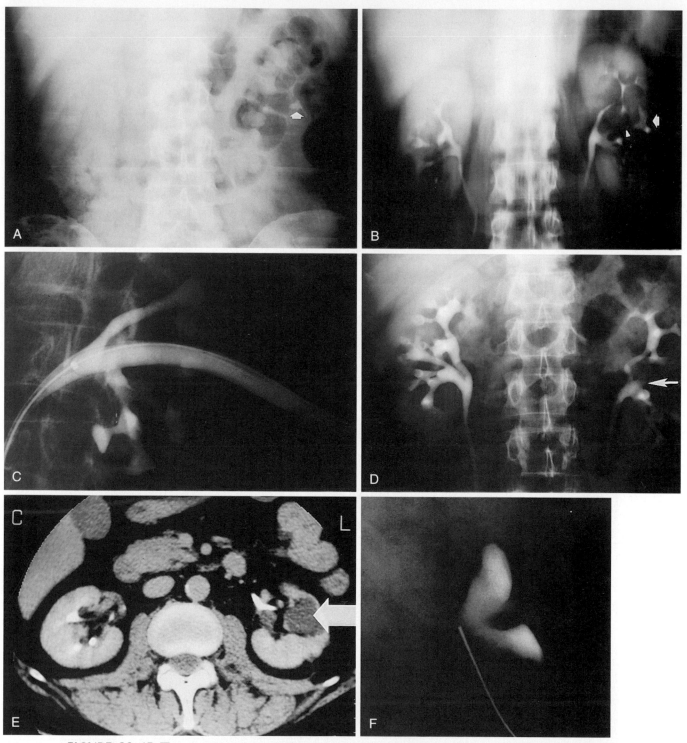

FIGURE 23-15 ▪ Sequestration of a calyx after balloon injury of infundibulum. **A,** A 1-cm calcified stone *(arrow)* was associated with flank pain and recurrent infection. **B,** Tomogram during excretory urography showed the stone to be in an anterior interpolar calyx *(arrow)*, subtended by a long, thin infundibulum *(arrowhead)*. **C,** After gaining access directly to the calyx, the tract was dilated and the balloon advanced into the renal pelvis. The stone was removed successfully. Six months later, the patient developed recurrent flank pain. **D** and **E,** Excretory urography and CT demonstrated infundibular occlusion with a sequestered calyx *(arrows)*. **F,** The sequestered calyx was punctured, and injection under pressure reproduced the patient's pain. The calyx was then completely aspirated, with resolution of symptoms.

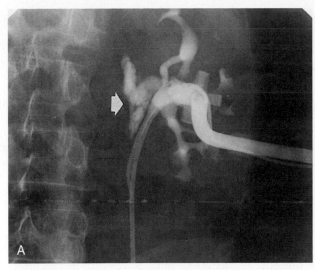

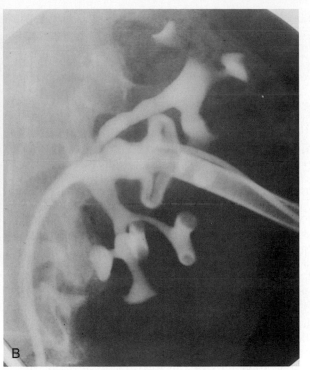

FIGURE 23-16 ■ Perforation of the collecting system during tract dilation. **A,** Immediately after tract dilation, perforation with extravasation of contrast *(arrow)* is observed. **B,** The nephroscopic stone extraction was delayed 2 days, and the perforation healed spontaneously, permitting successful stone extraction.

narrow, it may be injured during tract dilation (Fig. 23-15). In such cases, the sheath should be advanced only to the calyx. A flexible or rigid scope of narrower caliber then may be advanced through the infundibulum to reach the stone. Because of the large volumes of irrigation fluid required for endoscopic visualization of the stone and collecting system, collecting system perforation may be associated with copious retroperitoneal extravasation. When perforations are identified during the access or tract dilation procedure, the endoscopic procedure should be delayed for several days until the collecting system has sealed (Fig. 23-16).

After endoscopic stone fragmentation and removal, a 24-French Malecot nephrostomy catheter usually is left in place. This catheter usually is advanced over the safety guidewire at the termination of the procedure. The ureteral tip maintains secure access to the urinary tract in the event that the catheter pulls back. In this situation, a guidewire can be readvanced into the urinary bladder and the catheter advanced back into the collecting system. The ureteral tip also minimizes injury to the renal pelvis during catheter placement.

A nephrostogram should be performed within 24 to 48 hours to detect residual stone fragments. If the collecting system appears clear and there is brisk passage of contrast to the urinary bladder, the catheter may be removed. Residual clots may be differentiated from stone fragments using CT. If there is any question about antegrade flow of urine to the bladder, a Whitaker test may be performed. If necessary, an endopyelotomy may be performed before the catheter is removed and the tract is abandoned. Premature removal of nephrostomy tubes before confirmation of antegrade flow may lead to urinomas (Fig. 23-17).

Results

The technical success rate of PCNL varies with the complexity of stone disease and with the techniques used for stone fragmentation and extraction. Several large series have shown that the overall success rate for removal of renal

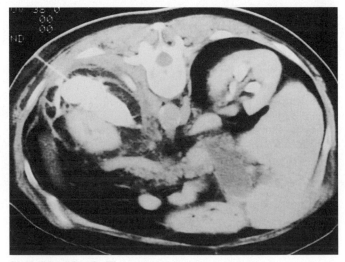

FIGURE 23-17 ■ Urinoma resulted from premature removal of a nephrostomy tube after percutaneous nephrostolithotomy (PCNL). No nephrostogram was performed after PCNL, and the nephrostomy tube was removed without confirming ureteral patency. CT with intravenous contrast shows accumulation of contrast-enhanced urine in the retroperitoneum. This urinoma was drained percutaneously (needle), and a new percutaneous tract was created to address the proximal ureteral occlusion.

pelvic stones is 96% to 99%.[40-42] The success rate for ureteral stones is somewhat lower (about 85%) because of frequent adherence and submucosal burying of ureteral stones. As more complex cases are referred only after failure of ESWL, the overall success rate probably will diminish.

Complications

In a mail survey tabulating the results of 8595 PCNL procedures from 62 institutions, Lang reported a decrease in serious complications from 15% during the first 20 cases to 1.5% with more experienced operators.[43] Hemorrhage requiring transfusion occurs in 1% to 3% of cases. Arterial injury requiring angiographic evaluation and embolization or balloon tamponade occurs in about 0.5% of cases.[44] The risk of hemorrhagic complications does not appear to be associated with tract size but does appear to be associated with stone size. Medial punctures directly into the infundibulum or renal pelvis carry a higher risk of significant arterial injury.

Collecting system perforation is not uncommon during the process of stone removal. The injury may be caused by sharp stone fragments or the instruments introduced to fragment or retrieve the stone. When perforation is recognized, the endoscopic procedure should be stopped to avoid extravasating large volumes of irrigant into the retroperitoneum (see Fig. 23-16). These perforations heal spontaneously if satisfactory drainage is provided. Follow-up nephrostograms generally show resolution of the extravasation in 24 to 48 hours, and stricture formation is rare.

Sepsis occurs in about 1% of cases. Pleural complications are higher with an intercostal approach and occur in less than 1% of cases overall. Injuries to the colon, spleen, liver, and duodenum are rare (<0.5%) complications of PCNL.

■ URETERAL STENT PLACEMENT

Patient Selection

Ureteral stent placement is indicated for a broad variety of clinical problems (Box 23-3). It is important to attempt or at least consider the retrograde approach for renal drainage before resorting to the percutaneous route. PCN with antegrade stent placement usually is reserved for patients in whom retrograde attempts are unsuccessful or not feasible.

For patients with nephroureteral obstruction, ureteral stents have distinct advantages over external drainage through a PCN tube. The drainage with stents is internalized, eliminating the need for external drainage tubing and collecting bags. The completely internalized ureteral stent is tolerated better by patients, and it decreases the risk of urosepsis from the inevitable colonization of external drainage catheters.[9,10] Ureteral stents also have several disadvantages. Stent malfunction often is initially silent and requires sonography or cystography for diagnosis. Stent patency varies with the clinical situation. Stone-forming patients tend to develop rapid stent occlusion, and stent exchange may be required as frequently as every 6 weeks. In general, stents should be exchanged every 6 months with transurethral cystoscopic or fluoroscopic guidance to prevent encrustation and occlusion. Stents may cause debilitating irritation of the bladder wall or trigone in some patients. Some patients prefer externally draining PCN tubes because function can be assessed easily and replacement is simple.

The nephroureteral stent is an alternative to externally draining PCN tubes and internally draining ureteral stents. This device differs from the standard double-J ureteral stent in that it has a locking Cope loop positioned in the renal pelvis and a short segment of catheter extending out the nephrostomy tract. The external segment of catheter may be capped to restore antegrade flow of urine from the renal pelvis, through the stent, and into the urinary bladder. The advantage of this device is that diagnosis of occlusion requires only a nephrostogram. If the patient develops flank pain or fever, she or he can open the catheter to external drainage until receiving medical attention. Likewise, catheter exchange over a guidewire is simple and does not require anesthesia, cystoscopy, or other transurethral interventions. These catheters are ideal for short-term ureteral stenting when it is advantageous to maintain access to the upper urinary tract for further evaluation with nephrostograms or a Whitaker test.

External PCN drainage is preferred over ureteral stents in several situations (Box 23-4). In the occasional patient with vesicocutaneous fistula due to advanced pelvic malignancy, diversion of urine with ureteral occlusion is beneficial to facilitate fistula closure and minimize tissue breakdown and nursing care requirements. Nephroureteral catheters are available with ureteral occlusion balloons to treat this difficult group of patients (see Fig. 23-5).

BOX 23-3 ■ Indications for Ureteral Stent Placement
Bypass ureteral obstructions
Divert urinary stream to allow leaks to heal
Maintain ureteral caliber after interventions
Facilitate stone fragment passage during extracorporeal shock wave lithotripsy
Provide palpable landmark for localization of the ureter at surgery

BOX 23-4 ■ Contraindications to Ureteral Stent Placement
Bladder outlet obstruction
Spastic or noncompliant bladder
Bladder fistula
Incontinence
Active hematuria
Active infection

Technique

For antegrade stent placement, the ideal nephrostomy access should provide a reasonably straight vector down the ureter from an interpolar or upper pole calyx. However, with available guidewires, catheters, and sheaths, antegrade stents usually can be placed even from a lower pole access.

Stent placement is facilitated by allowing the nephrostomy tract to mature for 1 to 2 weeks. By allowing any PCN-related hematuria to clear, the risk of immediate stent occlusion by clots is minimized. By allowing the ureteral caliber to decrease and edema to resolve, the ureteral obstruction is negotiated more easily with catheter and guidewire manipulation.

Almost all ureteral strictures can be traversed with a curved catheter and an angled hydrophilic guidewire (Fig. 23-18). If the catheter tends to buckle in the renal pelvis, a sheath may be advanced into the proximal ureter.

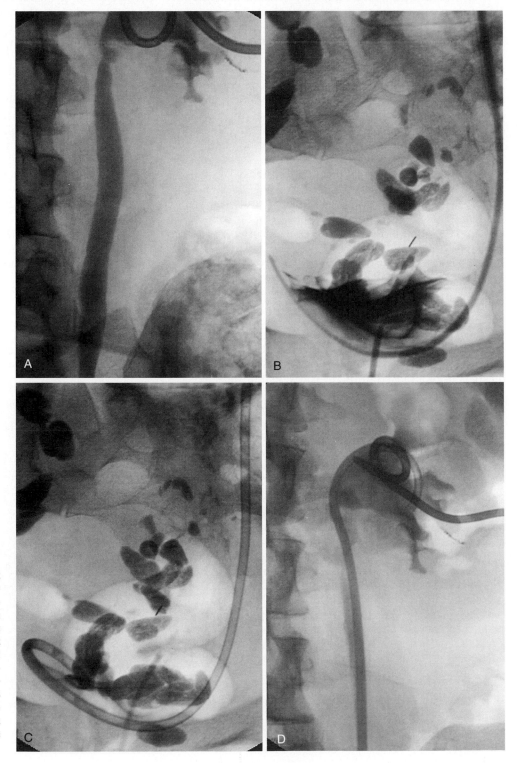

FIGURE 23-18 ■ Ureteral stent placement for a distal ureteral obstruction due to infiltrating cervical carcinoma. **A,** Contrast injection through the percutaneous nephrostomy tube showed a stagnant column of contrast in the ureter. **B,** A double-J ureteral stent was placed through the nephrostomy tract into the bladder to decompress the ureter. **C,** The distal pigtail has re-formed in the bladder. **D,** The proximal pigtail has partially re-formed in the renal pelvis after removal of the sheath.

When the guidewire has crossed the obstruction, a catheter should be advanced and injected to confirm its location in the bladder. Too vigorous manipulation of the hydrophilic guidewire may easily puncture the urothelium. A 4-French hydrophilic catheter usually follows the hydrophilic guidewire into the urinary bladder. The guidewire then may be exchanged for a stiff guidewire (Amplatz Super Stiff guidewire, Boston Scientific, Watertown, Mass.).

If necessary, the stricture is dilated to allow the ureteral stent to pass freely to the bladder. Van Andel Teflon dilators (Cook, Inc., Bloomington, Ind.) may be used to dilate to 1-French size larger than the ureteral stent. Alternatively, a 3- to 4-mm angioplasty balloon may be used.

The appropriate stent length is determined by using a guidewire to measure the distance between the mid-bladder and the renal pelvis. Most patients require a 22- to 24-cm stent. Care should be taken not to choose an overly long stent that may irritate the bladder trigone. A long peel-away sheath at least 1-French size greater than the ureteral catheter then is advanced over the stiff guidewire.

The C-Flex stent (Cook, Inc., Bloomington, Ind.) and Percuflex stent (Boston Scientific, Watertown, Mass.) appear to be most advantageous with regard to patency, flexibility, and resistance to fracture. For most cases, 6- to 8-French stents are preferred. Larger stents may cause ureteral ischemia and stricture formation but are used routinely when preservation of ureteral caliber is important, such as after stricture dilation.

The stent is then assembled with the inner stiffener and the pushing catheter.[45,46] It is advanced over the guidewire, through the Teflon sheath, and into the urinary bladder. The upper end of the stent must be identified fluoroscopically and positioned well within the collecting system, usually in the renal pelvis. The peel-away sheath then may be removed to allow the upper pigtail to be formed. Holding the pushing catheter in place, the stiffener is removed. By gently pulling on the suture attached to the proximal end of the stent, it can be positioned in the renal pelvis and the pigtail configuration formed. This usually requires withdrawal of the stiff guidewire, at least until only the floppy tip remains in the proximal end of the stent. When the proximal end of the stent is released, the guidewire may be advanced and coiled in the renal pelvis for subsequent nephrostomy placement. Alternatively, the nephrostomy may be placed over a safety guidewire introduced at the beginning of the procedure. The suture is cut and removed by pulling on one end while observing the stent fluoroscopically to ensure it remains in optimal position.

A nephrostomy tube usually is left in place for 24 hours. The catheter should be capped to force urine through the stent and prevent early stent occlusion with clot. If the patient subsequently develops flank pain or fever, the nephrostomy can be opened to gravity drainage. A nephrostogram is performed the day after stent placement to confirm stent location and patency before nephrostomy removal. The nephrostomy should be removed under fluoroscopic observation to ensure that it does not become entangled in the ureteral stent.

If there is great difficulty advancing catheters over the guidewire and through the stricture, the guidewire may be passed through the urethra to provide through-and-through access and facilitate catheter passage. A blunt Foley catheter lubricated with viscous lidocaine jelly is passed into the bladder. A guidewire then is advanced through the Foley catheter, which is exchanged for a short vascular sheath to protect the urethra during subsequent interventions. The ureteral guidewire may be captured in the bladder using a vascular snare and pulled out through the urethra to provide secure, through-and-through access.[47] With both ends of the wire held securely, a stent can be advanced through any stricture. This technique also has proven useful for replacement of ureteral stents (Fig. 23-19). After capturing the free end of the stent in the urinary bladder, it is pulled through the urethra. As soon as the stent tip is brought out of the urethra, a guidewire is advanced up the stent into the renal pelvis. Stent replacement over the guidewire is then straightforward. This fluoroscopically guided technique is successful in up to 97% of cases.[48] It is simple and well tolerated by female patients because of the short urethra.

Patients with urinary diversions into an ileal conduit who develop obstruction may be treated with retrograde, antegrade, or combined placement of ureteral stents. If contrast refluxes from the conduit into the ureter, the ureter may be fluoroscopically catheterized.[49] Alternatively, after decompressive PCN, antegrade catheterization of the occluded ureteroenteric anastomosis is usually simple. The guidewire then may be passed out the ileal loop and a locking pigtail catheter may be advanced retrograde into the renal pelvis (Fig. 23-20). The hub of the catheter is left free in the urinary collection bag. This approach minimizes the number of catheters and collection bags required for decompression.

Results

Successful antegrade placement of ureteral stents can be achieved in greater than 80% of cases. Several novel

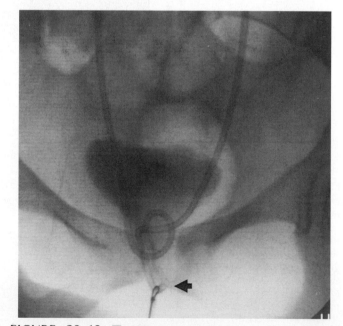

FIGURE 23-19 ■ Fluoroscopically guided exchange of ureteral stents. The left stent has been snared *(arrow)* and is being withdrawn through a sheath placed in the urethra.

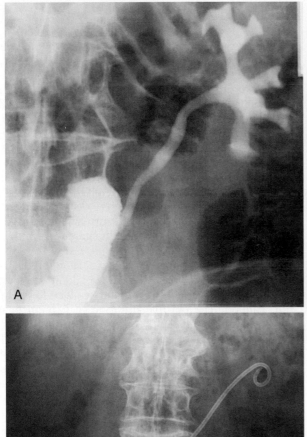

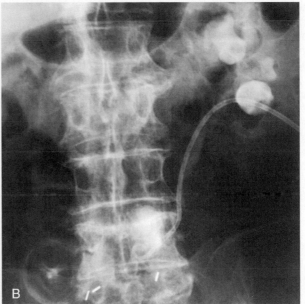

FIGURE 23-20 ■ Conversion of a percutaneous nephrostomy (PCN) to a retrograde ureteral catheter in a patient with urinary diversion into an ileal loop. **A,** Initial loopogram shows reflux into the left ureter. **B,** The ureteroenteric anastomosis subsequently became strictured and a left PCN was performed. At that time, it was easy to cross the anastomotic obstruction and place a nephroureteral catheter. **C,** To simplify the drainage, a guidewire is passed out the loop, and a locking pigtail catheter is advanced retrograde up the ureter. The catheter hub is left free in the loop drainage bag.

approaches have been described for patients with impassable strictures.[50-52] One technique uses a perforating guidewire or electrocautery to create a new tract between the distal ureter and urinary bladder. A stent is placed through the newly created tract to maintain its patency. Another approach connects percutaneous nephrostomy and suprapubic cystostomy tubes in a subcutaneous tunnel.[52]

Complications

The most frequent complication encountered with ureteral stents is occlusion due to encrustation. The rate at which encrustation develops is highly variable and depends on the degree of crystalloid supersaturation in the urine and on the presence of infection. Long-term stent patency varies from 2 to 18 months. Stent life may be optimized by encouraging patients to maintain a high fluid intake. Stents ideally should not be placed into bloody or infected collecting systems. Prophylactic antibiotics may prolong stent patency by minimizing the risk of infection and the associated acceleration of encrustation. Patients should be evaluated clinically at 3 months, and if stent occlusion is suspected, sonography or cystography should be performed. Stents should be routinely exchanged at least every 6 months.

Metallic stents do not appear to offer any advantage over conventional plastic stents for nephroureteral occlusion.[53] Early metallic stent occlusion is a frequent result of debris build-up or edema; late stent occlusion is the result of tumor overgrowth or fibrous tissue. There is a limited role for metallic stents in the treatment of ureteroenteric anastomotic strictures, which are notoriously refractory to simple balloon dilation.

Other complications of ureteral stent placement include collecting system perforation, improperly positioned stents, stent migration, stent fracture, erosive damage to the ureter with resultant ischemia and stricture formation, upper urinary tract infection due to reflux, and bladder irritation. Patients with bladder irritation present with disabling urgency and frequency caused by stents that are too long and push the bladder trigone. Symptoms may be reduced with antispasmodics and usually resolve over several days. Occasionally, symptoms are refractory to medical therapy, and the stent may have to be removed. A rare complication of ureteral stent placement is fistula formation between the iliac artery and the ureter. Predisposing factors are ureteral ischemia and iliac aneurysms.

■ BENIGN URETERAL STRICTURE DILATION

Etiology

Ureteral strictures can be benign or malignant (Box 23-5). Urologic procedures (particularly endoscopy) are the single most common cause of iatrogenic ureteral strictures, accounting for 42% of cases in one series.[54] Gynecologic and general surgical procedures account for 34% and 24% of cases, respectively. Ureteral injury occurs in about 10% of patients undergoing endoscopic manipulations in the ureter. Strictures occur at the anastomosis of ureteroenteric diversion procedures in 4% to 8% of cases. The common denominator underlying most causes of benign ureteral strictures is ischemia. A vicious cycle of ischemia and scarring is thought to be responsible for stricture formation.

Balloon dilation of malignant ureteral strictures does not provide long-term patency. Preservation of renal function in these patients depends on ureteral stent placement or external drainage through a PCN.

BOX 23-5 ■ **Causes of Ureteral Strictures**

Malignant Lesions
Primary urothelial tumor
Compression or invasion by retroperitoneal or pelvic
  malignancies

Benign Lesions
Iatrogenic
  Urologic procedures
  Gynecologic or general surgical procedures
  Ureteroenteric anastomotic strictures
Recurrent stone passage
Penetrating trauma
Radiation therapy
Infection (e.g., tuberculosis, bilharziasis)
Retroperitoneal fibrosis

Technique

A middle or upper polar access facilitates crossing the lesion with guidewires and catheters because of the straighter vector afforded. A sheath is advanced through the nephrostomy tract into the proximal ureter to straighten the path and facilitate catheter manipulation. Hydrophilic guidewires and gently curved catheters are used to cross the stricture. After the lesion has been crossed, the catheter is advanced across the lesion and injected with contrast to make sure the ureter has not been perforated. Tight strictures are easiest to cross with 4-French hydrophilic catheters. The guidewire is exchanged for a super-stiff Amplatz guidewire. If there is difficulty advancing the catheter over the guidewire, the guidewire may be snared in the urinary bladder, affording through-and-through control of the guidewire and enabling the catheter to be advanced.

Balloons with diameters of 4 to 10 mm are used for ureteral dilation. When standard balloon angioplasty is unsuccessful, consideration should be given to use of a cutting balloon. The optimal duration of balloon dilation is unknown. Stents of 8 to 10 French are generally left across the treated region for 1 to 2 months to serve as a scaffold for muscular and urothelial healing. Nephroureteral catheters are ideal for this purpose (Fig. 23-21). After 1 to 2 months, the nephroureteral catheter is exchanged for a nephrostomy tube. In 1 to 2 weeks, the treated stricture is reevaluated with a nephrostogram and a Whitaker test. There is some debate about the value of repeat dilation if recurrent stenoses are identified.[55]

Results

Although the immediate technical success of ureteral dilation exceeds 90%, long-term patency is highly variable. In one series of multiple balloon dilation procedures on 28 benign strictures, long-term patency was maintained in only 18% of treated lesions.[55] Other investigators have identified groups of patients who respond more favorably. Lang and Glorioso[56] reported that 91% of strictures less than 3 months old responded to dilation, compared with 53% of older strictures. Strictures associated with ischemia or fibrosis responded in only 21%, whereas 70% of strictures without vascular compromise responded well. Other series found no such difference in outcome based on the interval between ureteral injury and treatment.[57]

Tuberculous strictures have been treated successfully in 75% of cases and probably close to 100% for strictures less than 1.5 cm long.[58] Strictures of ureteroenteric anastomoses have been treated successfully with balloon dilation in 50% and 70% of native and transplant kidneys, respectively.[59,60] Strictures related to ureterolithotomy, ureteral endoscopy, and gynecologic surgery responded in 100%, 71%, and 62% of cases, respectively, in one series.[61] However, strictures associated with radical hysterectomy or retroperitoneal fibrosis responded poorly (33% and 0, respectively).

Interpretation of this widely varying and often contradictory literature is difficult. Unfortunately, the series with the most meticulous and rigorous follow-up also tend to report

FIGURE 23-21 ■ Balloon dilation of an iatrogenic distal ureteral stricture resulting from ureteroscopic retrieval of a stone. **A,** Retrograde pyelography shows a distal ureteral stricture. **B,** The stricture was dilated with an 8-mm balloon. The waist *(arrow)* on the balloon was overcome with higher pressure. **C,** A nephroureteral catheter was left in place for 6 weeks to allow for muscular healing. **D,** The catheter was then removed, and a follow-up nephrostogram revealed no residual stenosis. A urodynamic challenge test result was normal.

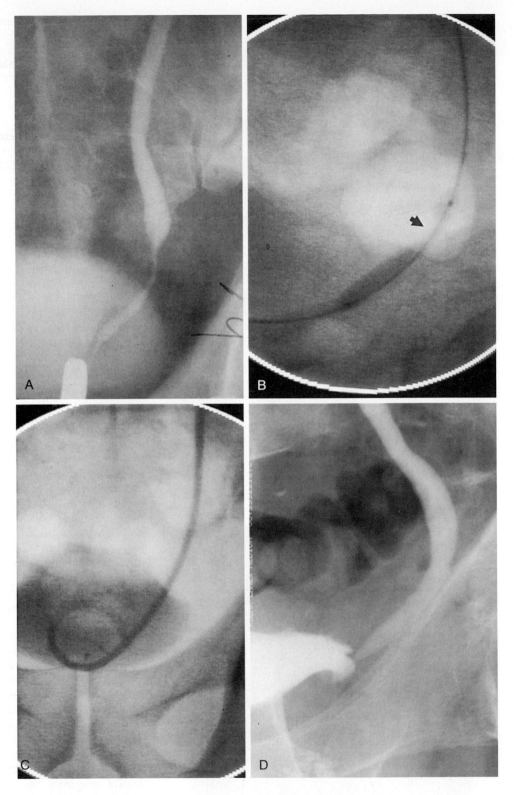

the lowest long-term patencies. Overall, the long-term patency for balloon dilation of benign ureteral strictures is about 50%. Because surgical treatment is much more invasive and has only modest results, many authorities favor an initial trial of balloon dilation for benign ureteral strictures before subjecting the patient to operative repair. The results can be assessed easily with a nephrostogram and urodynamic challenge, and about one half of patients are spared the cost and morbidity of open surgical repair.

Balloon dilation and stent placement also may be used for ureteropelvic junction (UPJ) obstruction as a primary alternative to pyeloplasty or for recurrent obstruction after pyeloplasty. The reported success rates vary from 64% to 86%.[62-64] Stents specifically designed for UPJ obstruction should be used after the dilation. These devices have a 12- to 14-French segment spanning the treated UPJ, then taper to 5 to 7 French.

URETERAL PERFUSION CHALLENGE (WHITAKER TEST)

Differentiation of a dilated but unobstructed renal collecting system from a functionally significant obstruction is a common and difficult clinical problem. A physiologic ureteral perfusion study is considered the most definitive way to make this distinction. The ureteral perfusion challenge initially was described by the English urologist Robert Whitaker.[65,66] The test measures the resistance of the ureter to fluid infusion into the renal pelvis.

Patient Selection

The Whitaker test is used most commonly in the patient with a dilated renal pelvis in whom UPJ obstruction is suspected but unconfirmed by intravenous urography, a radionuclide renogram, or a diuretic renogram. It also is indicated in children with hydroureter, urinary tract infection, and a voiding cystogram that does not demonstrate vesicoureteral reflux. The ureteral perfusion challenge is used to monitor the results of operative (Fig. 23-22) or radiologic interventions (e.g., endopyelotomy, ureteral stricture dilation.) It is helpful also in evaluating collecting system

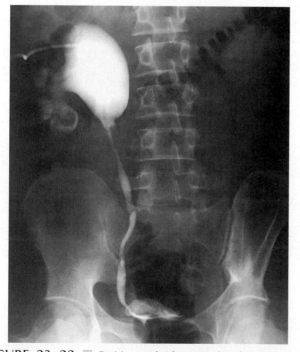

FIGURE 23-22 ■ Positive result of a ureteral perfusion challenge (Whitaker test) after pyeloplasty for ureteropelvic junction obstruction. The patient subsequently underwent endopyelotomy, which was followed by a normal perfusion challenge result and a good clinical outcome.

dilation in renal transplant recipients.[67] Because as many as 5% of patients with urinary obstruction may show no dilation of the collecting system, a Whitaker test is indicated in cases of suspected nondilated obstructive uropathy.

Technique

In the test as formulated by Whitaker, the renal pelvis is perfused with 10 mL/minute of fluid for 3 to 5 minutes, and the pressure gradient between the kidney and bladder is measured. A normal individual shows an absolute renal pelvis pressure of less than 25 cm H_2O and a pressure gradient of less than 15 cm H_2O at maximal flow challenge. The renal pelvic pressure may be measured through the infusing needle or catheter immediately after the infusion ceases. Alternatively, the pressures may be recorded simultaneously during infusion through a nephrostomy tube or through a second needle placed in the collecting system.

The examiner must be careful to avoid simultaneous pressure recordings during infusion through small needles or catheters. In this situation, the needle or catheter may be responsible for a pressure gradient. When in doubt, a trial test can be performed through an identical needle or catheter on the benchtop to confirm that no pressure head develops during infusion through the catheter or needle itself. A Foley catheter should be in place to measure the pressure in the bladder. If the Foley is left open to gravity drainage and it is confirmed fluoroscopically that no urine is accumulating in the bladder, the bladder pressure is assumed to be zero.

Before ureteral perfusion is initiated, baseline manometry is performed. If a large gradient is found at rest or the resting pressure within the kidney approaches 30 cm H_2O, no perfusion test is required. Although the normal ureteral flow is only 0.25 to 0.5 mL/minute, the unobstructed ureter can accommodate a much higher flow rate. The perfusion challenge should be performed with 30% iodinated contrast material to allow fluoroscopic visualization of upper tract dilation, the narrowed segment, and the degree of bladder distention. The perfusion challenge is begun at 5 mL/minute for 5 minutes. The perfusion rate may be doubled up to 20 mL/minute to enhance the sensitivity of the test.

The pressure gradient is normally less than 15 cm H_2O. A pressure gradient more than 22 cm H_2O is diagnostic of an obstructed upper urinary tract. Pressure gradients between 15 and 22 cm H_2O are indeterminate. Increasing the perfusion rate (up to 20 mL/minute) can resolve many of these cases. When the test result is positive, spot films should be obtained to document the site of obstruction. If the challenge test result is negative or indeterminate, it may be helpful to repeat the study with the bladder distended, because some cases of obstruction are evident only after bladder filling. Likewise, repeating the challenge in different patient positions may produce a positive result.[68]

The accuracy of the ureteral perfusion test has not been determined because there is no satisfactory standard against which the results can be compared. In Whitaker's series of 170 perfusion challenges, clinical and radiographic criteria were used to assess the results. There were only six cases in which indeterminate results were obtained.

■ RENAL TRANSPLANT INTERVENTIONS

The most common nonvascular complications of kidney transplantation are abnormal fluid collections, obstruction, and ureteral stricture. *Fluid collections* associated with renal transplants include lymphoceles, urinomas, hematomas, seromas, and abscess. Lymphoceles are caused by leakage from damaged lymphatics in the pelvis or transplanted kidney. They are seen within weeks to years of surgery. Urinomas, seromas, and hematomas usually manifest within the first few weeks after transplantation. Percutaneous drainage for diagnosis and treatment is preferred over surgery in most patients.

Obstruction may be difficult to distinguish from other causes of renal transplant dysfunction. Because the risk of PCN is low and the consequence of a delayed diagnosis of obstruction may be loss of the transplant, a low threshold for PCN as a diagnostic challenge is advocated.[60,69] The usual cause of renal transplant obstruction is stenosis at the ureterovesical anastomosis. Extrinsic compression on the collecting system by hematoma, lymphocele, or urinoma also can produce an obstruction. If obstruction coexists with a fluid collection, percutaneous drainage of the fluid may relieve the collection and the obstruction (Fig. 23-23).

When planning PCN of a transplant, it is important to avoid entry into the peritoneum by making the needle entry lateral to the transplant and skin incision. Ultrasound is ideal for imaging guidance. An anterolateral upper or middle polar calyx should be selected to facilitate ureteral catheterization. Internalized stents are preferred over catheters that project externally to minimize the risk of infection in this immunocompromised group of patients.

Ureteral strictures are treated successfully with balloon dilation in about 60% to 70% of cases (Fig. 23-24).[60,69] However, the success of balloon dilation decreases to less than 20% in patients with ureteric obstruction occurring more than 3 months after transplantation. In renal transplants with ureteral leakage, percutaneous treatment with nephroureteral stents is successful in 59% of cases.[69]

■ RENAL CYST ASPIRATION

Patient Selection

By imaging alone, simple benign renal cysts can be distinguished from cystic malignancies with greater than 90% accuracy.[70,71] Only 5% to 7% of cystic renal lesions require diagnostic cyst puncture with cytologic evaluation and cystography. Cyst aspiration also is indicated in patients with unexplained hematuria and renal cysts and in those with recurrent urinary tract infections when cyst infection is suspected. Therapeutic cyst drainage is done for renal cysts that may be responsible for pain, urinary tract obstruction, infection, or renin-dependent hypertension.

Technique

Renal cysts are aspirated easily using 21- or 22-gauge needles and sonographic guidance. CT occasionally is required for obese patients. The fluid in a benign simple cyst should be clear or slightly yellow. A small amount of blood that clears during the drainage indicates a traumatic tap. Bloody fluid that does not become more serous during aspiration suggests tumor.[72,73] When malignancy is suspected, the entire volume of aspirated fluid is sent for cytologic analysis. Although this technique is reported to be quite sensitive, a negative result does not entirely exclude malignancy.[74,75]

A cystogram is performed after the cyst has been completely drained by replacing the aspirated volume with dilute contrast material. Double-contrast techniques have

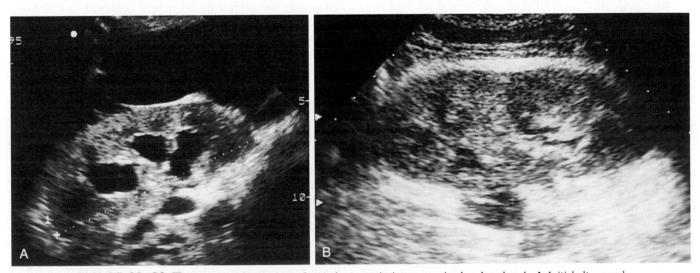

FIGURE 23-23 ■ Renal transplant hydronephrosis due to extrinsic compression by a lymphocele. **A,** Initial ultrasound scan shows a large fluid collection superficial to the hydronephrotic transplant kidney. **B,** After percutaneous drainage and alcohol sclerosis of the lymphocele, ultrasound shows that hydronephrosis has resolved.

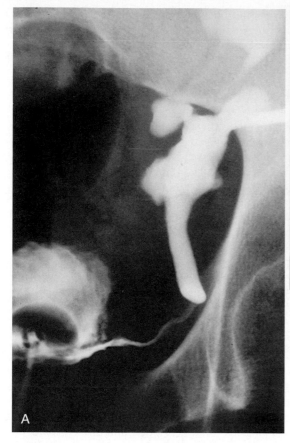

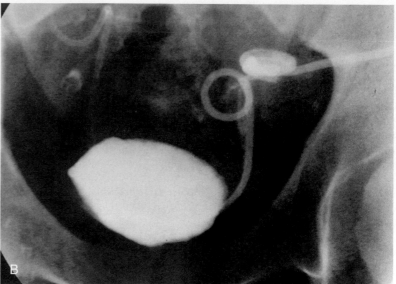

FIGURE 23-24 ■ Treatment of an ischemic transplant ureteral stricture. **A,** The antegrade nephrostogram shows a stricture of the distal ureter 6 weeks after transplantation. **B,** The stricture was dilated with an 8-mm balloon, and a short ureteral stent was left in place for 8 weeks. The stent was then removed, and stricture has not recurred.

been described but rarely improve visualization of cyst cavity. A simple benign cyst should have a perfectly smooth wall. Any wall irregularity raises the possibility of malignancy. However, incomplete distension of the cyst or adherent mural thrombus from prior hemorrhage may cause wall irregularity and can be confused with malignancy.

Results and Complications

With the combination of cyst fluid and cystogram analysis, the accuracy of cyst aspiration for exclusion of malignancy is reported to be 95% to 98%.[76] The accuracy is lower if the cyst is hemorrhagic or highly septate. Simple needle aspiration is safe, with major complications reported in less than 3% of cases.[77] The most common complication is perinephric hemorrhage, which occurs in fewer than 0.3% of cases when 20- to 22-gauge needles are used. Other reported complications include pneumothorax, arteriovenous fistula, infection, urinoma formation, and bowel puncture. Tract seeding along the needle pathway after aspiration of a cystic malignancy has been reported but is a rare event.[78]

Aspirated renal cysts often recur (30% to 100% of procedures) because the cuboidal epithelium around the cavity rapidly produces fluid and refills the cyst.[79,80] For initial symptomatic improvement followed by recurrence of symptoms, cyst sclerosis should be considered.

■ RENAL CYST SCLEROSIS

Cyst sclerosis is performed to devitalize the secreting cuboidal epithelial cells lining the cyst cavity and prevent recurrence. Absolute alcohol (the most commonly used sclerosant) destroys the cyst epithelium within 1 to 3 minutes and penetrates the cyst wall within 4 to 12 hours of exposure.[80] Other agents that have been used include glucose, phenol, Pantopaque, tetracycline, bismuth, and povidone iodine.

Technique

Cyst sclerosis generally is performed through small pigtail catheters. The cyst volume is estimated by measuring the aspirated fluid volume. Dilute contrast then is injected using a volume that exceeds the anticipated volume of sclerosant to be administered. It is critical to confirm that all contrast remains in the cyst cavity and does not communicate with the collecting system or the vascular system or extravasate into the retroperitoneum. If extravasation is observed, the cystogram is repeated in several days to document closure from tract maturation before proceeding with sclerosis. If communication with the collecting system or vascular system is seen, sclerosis should be withheld to avoid urothelial or vascular injury. Essentially all injected contrast material must be withdrawn easily to ensure that sclerosant is not sequestered.

The proper volume of sclerosant is about 50% of the estimated cyst volume. It is prudent to limit the total volume to less than 100 mL to prevent lethal systemic toxicity in the unlikely event that sclerosant leaks out of the cyst wall (e.g., patient fall with intraperitoneal spillage). Alcohol is left within the cavity for only about 5 minutes. During this time, positional maneuvers may be employed to distribute the alcohol around the walls of the cyst. The sclerosant then is aspirated completely. The catheter may be removed immediately or left in place to monitor output. If daily catheter output exceeds 10 mL, sclerosis may be repeated.

Cyst sclerosis also can be accomplished in a single step through the aspiration needle or through an 18-gauge multiple side-hole sheath and needle. This technique eliminates the need for catheter placement and the risk of cyst rupture during manipulation. The procedure is better tolerated, and there is no need for an external catheter. Positional maneuvers are avoided to prevent inadvertent needle displacement.

Results and Complications

The effectiveness of renal cyst sclerotherapy with alcohol is greater than 90%, with a reported recurrence rate of less than 3%.[80] Pain may be minimized by injection of lidocaine into the cyst immediately before cyst sclerosis. Significant complications are unusual. Microscopic hematuria is uncommon and usually self-limited. Infections occur in less than 0.5% of patients and probably are minimized with single-step sclerosis. Sclerosis of parapelvic cysts carries the additional theoretical risk of damage to the adjacent hilar structures. Pelvic-ureteric obstruction caused by sclerosis-induced fibrosis has been reported.[81]

Surgical alternatives to percutaneous cyst aspiration and sclerosis include open surgical cyst unroofing, laparoscopic cyst unroofing, and marsupialization of the cyst into the collecting system through a percutaneous 24- to 30-French tract. The success rates of surgical therapy and cyst sclerosis are comparable.

■ URETHROPLASTY AND URETHRAL STENTS

Although the urethra is easily accessible to urologic endoscopic devices, alternative techniques for treatment of benign prostatic hypertrophy and urethral strictures have been developed.[82] Balloon dilation for benign prostatic hypertrophy is performed only after cystoscopy, voiding cystourethrography, and transrectal ultrasonography. The procedure is performed with topical anesthesia and intravenous conscious sedation. Retrograde urethrography is used to mark carefully the location of the external urinary sphincter, which must be avoided to prevent incontinence. Balloons with diameters of 25 to 30 mm are used to dilate the urethra proximal to the external sphincter for 10 minutes.

Repeat urethrography is performed, and a 20- to 22-French Councill catheter balloon is placed overnight.

Prostatic urethroplasty provides symptomatic improvement in 75% to 85% of carefully selected patients.[82] The ideal patient has bilobar prostatic enlargement, less than a 50-g prostatic mass, 2.5- to 4.5-cm-long prostatic urethra, moderate symptoms of prostatism, and adequate detrusor function. Absolute contraindications include localized prostatic malignancy, obstructing median lobe, decompensated detrusor muscle, and extremely large gland size (>60 g). Relative contraindications include multiple, large prostatic calculi, chronic bacterial prostatitis, residual urine volume exceeding 50% of bladder capacity, and urethral strictures.

Balloon dilation does not permit histologic examination of prostatic fragments for carcinoma in situ. Symptomatic relief often is temporary, with most patients having recurrent complaints by 18 months.[83] Prostatic stents may offer a simple and effective alternative to prostate surgery.[82]

Most benign urethral strictures are the result of trauma or inflammation. Congenital urethral strictures are rare. Urethral strictures usually are treated by urologists with bougies, filiforms, or sounds. Balloon dilation and metallic stent placement have been used with encouraging preliminary results.[82-86]

■ SELECTIVE SALPINGOGRAPHY AND FALLOPIAN TUBE RECANALIZATION

Of the estimated 2 to 3 million infertile couples in the United States,[87] about 40% of cases are caused by factors involving the fallopian tubes. Selective salpingography and fallopian tube recanalization are endorsed by the American Society for Reproductive Medicine as primary treatment for tubal obstruction when one or both tubes fail to fill at hysterosalpingography.[88]

The intramural portion of the fallopian tube is about 1 cm long and has a diameter of about 1 mm. Infection and subsequent inflammation or fibrosis are leading causes of proximal tubal occlusion. Chlamydial or gonococcal salpingitis or postpartum endometritis are the most frequent infections responsible for proximal tubal occlusion. It is postulated that some cases of proximal tubal obstruction are caused by tubal spasm. Mucus or debris impacted in the intramural or proximal isthmic portions of the tube are commonly encountered in cases of proximal tubal obstruction. Fallopian tube occlusion in the isthmic, ampullary, or fimbriated portions of the tube usually is caused by previous pelvic infection or endometriosis.

Patient Selection

Selective salpingography is indicated for infertility attributed to unilateral or bilateral obstruction involving the first 2 cm of the fallopian tube. The "proximal" form of the disease is the most treatable. Recanalization of the distal segments is technically more difficult and less likely to be followed by a successful intrauterine pregnancy. Selective salpingography alone can establish or confirm patency in about one third of patients with apparent tubal obstruction, which is encountered in 21% to 37% of hysterosalpingograms.[89-91] When selective salpingography fails to opacify the proximal tube, efforts to recanalize the tube are indicated.

The procedure is performed under fluoroscopic guidance or combined hysteroscopic and laparoscopic guidance. If the patient has not had laparoscopy and has a history of pelvic inflammatory disease, proximal tubal obstruction is best evaluated with combined hysteroscopy and laparoscopy. If a uterine cavity mass can be removed hysteroscopically, an endoscopically guided procedure is favored. If the patient has an obstruction involving the isthmic portion of the tube or has had laparoscopy that showed absent or minimal pelvic disease, the procedure is best carried out with fluoroscopic guidance.

Contraindications to fallopian tube recanalization include active pelvic inflammatory disease, previous tubal surgery, severe tubal or peritubal pathology detected on laparoscopy, distal tubal occlusion, severe intrauterine adhesions, and an intrauterine mass.

Technique

The procedure is performed on an outpatient basis and should be scheduled during the first 10 days of the menstrual cycle (i.e., follicular phase). Prophylactic antibiotics (e.g., 100 mg of doxycycline, given twice daily) should be started on the day before the procedure and continued for 4 days afterward. The procedure is performed with sterile technique after standard scrubbing and draping of the perineum. Intravenous conscious sedation usually is sufficient for patient comfort; paracervical anesthesia usually is not required for cervical dilation.

A guiding catheter is inserted through the cervix under direct visualization. The most commonly used catheters have an intrauterine retention balloon or a vacuum cup that is placed on the cervix. These devices provide a sterile conduit through which catheters and guidewires may be introduced. Conventional hysterosalpingography should be performed with diluted water-soluble contrast to confirm proximal tubal occlusion and to localize the uterine cornua without obscuring the catheters.

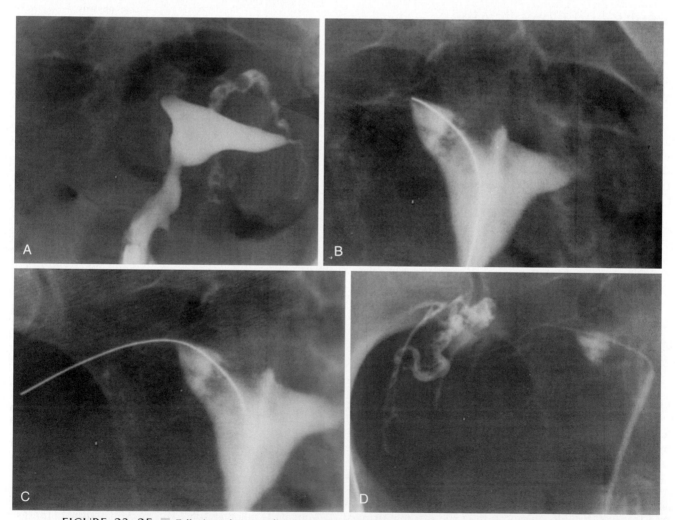

FIGURE 23-25 ▦ Fallopian tube recanalization. **A,** Hysterosalpingogram shows a left fallopian tube with intraperitoneal contrast spillage but no filling of the right tube. **B,** Selective right salpingography confirms occlusion of the right fallopian tube. **C,** A microcatheter and wire were manipulated across the occlusion. **D,** After removal of the microcatheter, repeat selective salpingography revealed patency of the right fallopian tube.

A 5-French catheter is advanced coaxially through the guiding catheter and used to selectively catheterize the tubal ostium. Full-strength contrast is then injected. If proximal tubal obstruction persists, efforts to clear the obstruction should be made (Fig. 23-25). A coaxial microcatheter system with a 3-French catheter and a 0.018-inch or smaller guidewire is advanced through the 5-French outer catheter. When the microcatheter has been advanced beyond the obstruction, the guidewire is removed, and contrast is injected to check distal tubal patency. The microcatheter is then removed, and contrast is injected through the 5-French catheter to evaluate the tube. Recanalization is then performed on the other side, if necessary. A final hysterosalpingogram is obtained to confirm and document tubal patency.

A 0.035-inch hydrophilic guidewire placed directly through the 5-French catheter may cross the obstruction more easily and eliminate the need for microcatheters.[92] After successful guidewire traversal, the wire is removed, and distal tubal patency is confirmed by ostial injection through the 5-French catheter. The patient is observed for 30 to 60 minutes after the procedure and advised that vaginal spotting may occur for 3 days or less.

Results

Reporting standards for selective salpingography and fallopian tube recanalization have not been established, which makes comparison of techniques, success rates, and treatment strategies difficult.[90] No convincing evidence indicates that any one technique is superior.

Overall, successful recanalization of at least one fallopian tube is achieved in about 80% of cases.[90,93] The subsequent intrauterine pregnancy rates average between 20% and 30%.[90,93,94] The rate of ectopic pregnancy is about 3% to 4%, which is comparable to the rate in the general population.[90,95] Fallopian tubes that require only minimal manipulation to reestablish patency are more likely to be associated with subsequent pregnancy than tubes requiring excessive guidewire and catheter manipulation. Some patients in the former category may have mucous plugs (which are flushed out by the initial selective contrast injection) without underlying mural disease. Although tubal disease does not preclude successful pregnancy, the pregnancy rates are higher when the tubes appear normal at salpingography. In one series, 95% of patients with tubal obstruction but normal tubes were successfully recanalized, and 45% became pregnant.[95]

If pregnancy has not occurred within 6 months of successful tubal recanalization, approximately 50% of evaluated patients are found to have reblockage of one or both fallopian tubes.[95] Repeat recanalization is possible, and pregnancies have resulted after the second or even third procedure.

Complications

Mild uterine cramping and vaginal bleeding are common after fallopian tube catheterization. Low-grade fevers may develop.

Tubal perforations occur in less than 5% of patients but usually are without clinical sequelae and do not require additional treatment. The radiation dose to the ovaries is generally less than 1 rad (10 mGy).[96]

REFERENCES

1. Goodwin WE, Casey WC, Woolf W: Percutaneous trocar (needle) nephrostomy in hydronephrosis. JAMA 1955;157:891.
2. Prassopoulos P, Gourtsoyiannis N, Cavouras D, Pantelidis N: A study of the variation of colonic positioning in the pararenal space as shown by computed tomography. Eur J Radiol 1990;10:44.
3. Zagoria RJ, Hodge RG, Dyer RB, Routh WD: Percutaneous nephrostomy for treatment of intractable hemorrhagic cystitis. J Urol 1993;149:1449.
4. Bell DA, Rose SC, Starr NK, et al: Percutaneous nephrostomy for nonoperative management of fungal urinary tract infections. J Vasc Interv Radiol 1993;4:311.
5. Oliver SE, Walker RJ, Woods DJ: Fluconazole infused via a nephrostomy tube: a novel and effective route of delivery. J Clin Pharm Ther 1995;20:317.
6. Hamdy FC, Williams JL: Use of dexamethasone for ureteric obstruction in advanced prostate cancer: percutaneous nephrostomies can be avoided. Br J Urol 1995;75:782.
7. Ryan JM, Ryan BM, Smith TP: Antibiotic prophylaxis in interventional radiology. J Vasc Interv Radiol 2004;15:547.
8. Millward SF: Percutaneous nephrostomy: a practical approach. J Vasc Interv Radiol 2000;11:955.
9. Cronan JJ, Marcello A, Horn DL, et al: Antibiotics and nephrostomy tube care: preliminary observations: Part I. Bacteriuria. Radiology 1989;172:1041.
10. Cronan JJ, Horn DL, Marcello A, et al: Antibiotics and nephrostomy tube care: preliminary observations: Part II. Bacteremia. Radiology 1989;172:1043.
11. Ramchandani P, Cardella JF, Grassi CJ, et al: Quality improvement guidelines for percutaneous nephrostomy. J Vasc Interv Radiol 2003;14:S277.
12. Farrel TA, Hicks ME: A review of radiologically guided percutaneous nephrostomies in 303 patients. J Vasc Interv Radiol 1997;8:769.
13. Lang EK, Price ET: Redefinitions of indications for percutaneous nephrostomy. Radiology 1983;147:419.
14. Yoder IC, Pfister RC, Lindfors KK, Newhouse JH: Pyonephrosis: imaging and intervention. AJR Am J Roentgenol 1983;141:735.
15. Bell AD, Rose SC, Starr NK, et al: Percutaneous nephrostomy for nonoperative management of fungal urinary tract infections. J Vasc Interv Radiol 1993;4:311.
16. Gadducci A, Madrigali A, Facchini V, Fioretti P: Percutaneous nephrostomy in patients with advanced or recurrent cervical cancer. Clin Exp Obstet Gynecol 1994;21:71.
17. Chapman ME, Reid JH: Use of percutaneous nephrostomy in malignant ureteric obstruction. Br J Radiol 1991;64:318.
18. Markowitz DM, Wong KT, Laffey KJ, et al: Maintaining quality of life after palliative diversion for malignant ureteral obstruction. Urol Radiol 1989;11:129.
19. Hoe JW, Tung KH, Tan EC: Reevaluation of indications for percutaneous nephrostomy and interventional uroradiologic procedures in pelvic malignancy. Br J Radiol 1993;71:469.
20. Dowling RA, Carrasco CH, Babaian RJ: Percutaneous urinary diversion in patients with hormone refractory prostate cancer. Urology 1991;37:89.
21. Stables DP, Ginsberg NJ, Johnson ML: Percutaneous nephrostomy: a series and review of literature. AJR Am J Roentgenol 1978;130:75.
22. Gonzales-Serva L, Weinnerth JL, Glenn JF: Minimal mortality of renal surgery. Urology 1977;9:253.
23. Mahaffey KG, Bolton DM, Stoller ML: Urologist directed percutaneous nephrostomy tube placement. J Urol 1994;152:1973.
24. Lee WJ, Patel U, Patel S, Pillari GP: Emergency percutaneous nephrostomy: results and complications. J Vasc Interv Radiol 1994;5:135.
25. Barbaric ZL, Hall T, Cochran ST, et al: Percutaneous nephrostomy: placement under CT and fluoroscopy guidance. AJR Am J Roentgenol 1997;169:151.

26. Cronan JJ, Dorfman GS, Amis ES, Denny DF Jr: Retroperitoneal hemorrhage after percutaneous nephrostomy. AJR Am J Roentgenol 1985;144:801.

27. Hopper KD, Yakes WF: The posterior intercostal approach for percutaneous renal procedures: risk of puncturing the lung, spleen, and liver as determined by CT. AJR Am J Roentgenol 1990;154:115.

28. Richenberg J, Kellet M, Records D: Three cases of thoracic complication of intercostal percutaneous nephrostolithotomy and a review of the literature. J Intervent Radiol 1995;10:23.

29. Picus D, Weyman PJ, Clayman RV, McClennan BL: Intercostal space nephrostomy for percutaneous stone removal. AJR Am J Roentgenol 1986;147:393.

30. Miller GL, Summa J: Transcolonic placement of a percutaneous nephrostomy tube: recognition and treatment. J Vasc Inter Radiol 1997;8:401.

31. Reinberg Y, Moore LS, Lange PH: Splenic abscess as a complication of percutaneous nephrostomy. Urology 1989;34:274.

32. Martin E, Lujan M, Paez A, et al: Puncture of the gallbladder: an unusual cause of peritonitis complicating percutaneous nephrostomy. Br J Urol 1996;77:464.

33. Cadeddu JA, Arrindell D, Moore RG: Near fatal air embolism during percutaneous nephrostomy placement. J Urol 1997;158:1519.

34. Sardina JI, Bolton DM, Stoller ML: Entrapped Malecot nephrostomy tube: etiology and management. J Urol 1995;153:1882.

35. Dretler SP. Laser lithotripsy: a review of 20 years of research and clinical applications. Lasers Surg Med 1988;8:341.

36. Fernstrom I, Johannson B: Percutaneous pyelolithotomy: a new extraction technique. Scand J Urol Nephrol 1976;10:257.

37. LeRoy AJ: Diagnosis and treatment of nephrolithiasis: current perspectives. AJR Am J Roentgenol 1994;163:1309.

38. Mindell HJ, Cochran ST: Current perspectives in the diagnosis and treatment of urinary stone disease. AJR Am J Roentgenol 1994; 163:1314.

39. Meretyk S, Gofrit ON, Gafni O, et al: Complete staghorn calculi: random prospective comparison between extracorporeal shock wave lithotripsy monotherapy and combined with percutaneous nephrostolithotomy. J Urol 1997;157:780.

40. Segura JW, Patterson DE, LeRoy AJ, et al: Percutaneous removal of kidney stones: review of 1,000 cases. Urology 1985;134:1077.

41. Reddy PK, Hulbert JC, Lange PH, et al: Percutaneous removal of renal and ureteral calculi: experience with 400 cases. Urology 1985;134:662.

42. Lee WJ, Smith AD, Cubell V, et al: Percutaneous nephrolithotomy: analysis of 500 cases. Urol Radiol 1986;8:61.

43. Lang EK: Percutaneous nephrostolithotomy and lithotripsy: a multiinstitutional survey of complications. Radiology 1987;162:25.

44. Pollack HM, Banner MP: Percutaneous extraction of renal and ureteral calculi: technical considerations. AJR Am J Roentgenol 1984;143:778.

45. D'Agostino R, Yucel EK: New method for simultaneous placement of antegrade ureteral stent and nephrostomy tube. AJR Am J Roentgenol 1994;162:879.

46. D'Agostino R, Goldberg RM: Percutaneous ureteral stents: a modified system to facilitate antegrade placement. J Vasc Interv Radiol 1996;7:427.

47. Kwok PC, Cheung JY: A radiological approach to the through and through technique for percutaneous passage of ureteric strictures. Clin Radiol 1996;51:879.

48. deBaere T, Denys A, Pappas P, et al: Ureteral stents: exchange under fluoroscopic control as an effective alternative to cystoscopy. Radiology 1994;190:887.

49. Banner MP, Amendola MA, Pollack HM: Anastomosed ureters: fluoroscopically guided transconduit retrograde catheterization. Radiology 1989;170:45.

50. Cornud FE, Casanova JP, Bonnel DH, et al: Impassable ureteral strictures: management with percutaneous ureteroneocystostomy. Radiology 1991;180:451.

51. Lang EK: Percutaneous ureterocystostomy and ureteroneocystostomy. AJR Am J Roentgenol 1988;150:1065.

52. Lingam K, Paterson PJ, Lingam MK, et al: Subcutaneous urinary diversion: an alternative to percutaneous nephrostomy. J Urol 1994;152:70.

53. vanSonnenberg E, D'Agostino HB, O'Laoide R, et al: Malignant ureteral obstruction: treatment with metal stents—technique, results and observations with percutaneous intraluminal ultrasound. Radiology 1994;191:765.

54. Selzman AA, Spirnak PJ: Iatrogenic ureteral injuries: a 20-year experience in treating 165 injuries. J Urol 1996;155:878.

55. Kwak S, Leef JA, Rosenblum JD: Percutaneous balloon catheter dilatation of benign ureteral strictures: effect of multiple dilatation procedures on long-term patency. AJR Am J Roentgenol 1995;165:97.

56. Lang EK, Glorioso LW III: Antegrade transluminal dilatation of benign ureteral strictures: long-term results. AJR Am J Roentgenol 1988; 150:131.

57. O'Brien WM, Maxted WC, Pahira JJ: Ureteral stricture: experience with 31 cases. J Urol 1988;140:737.

58. Chang R, Marshall FF, Mitchell S: Percutaneous management of benign ureteral strictures and fistulas. J Urol 1987;137:1126.

59. Bierkens AF, Oosterhaf GO, Meuleman EJ, Debruyne FM: Anterograde percutaneous treatment of ureterointestinal strictures following urinary diversion. Eur Urol 1996;30:363.

60. Benoit G, Alexandre L, Moukarzel M, et al: Percutaneous antegrade dilation of ureteral strictures in kidney transplants. J Urol 1993;150:37.

61. Van Arsdalen KN, Banner MP: The management of ureteral and anastomotic strictures. Probl Urol 1992;6:420.

62. Snow TM, Wells IP, Hammonds JC: Balloon rupture and stenting for pelviureteric junction obstruction: abolition of waisting is a prognostic marker. Clin Radiol 1994;49:708.

63. Gerber GS, Lyon ES: Endopyelotomy: patient selection, results and complications. Urology 1994;49:708.

64. McClinton S, Steyn JH, Hussey JK: Retrograde balloon dilatation for pelviureteric junction obstruction. Br J Urol 1993;71:152.

65. Whitaker RH: Methods of assessing obstruction in dilated ureters. Br J Urol 1973;45:15.

66. Whitaker RH: An evaluation of 170 diagnostic pressure flow studies of the upper urinary tract. J Urol 1979;121:602.

67. Kashi SH, Irving HC, Sadek SA: Does the Whitaker test add to antegrade pyelography in the investigation of collecting system dilatation in renal allografts? Br J Radiol 1993;66:877.

68. Ellis JH, Campo RP, Marx MV, et al: Positional variation in the Whitaker test. Radiology 1995;197:253.

69. Fontaine AB, Nijjar A, Rangaraj R: Update on the use of percutaneous nephrostomy/balloon dilation for the treatment of renal transplant leak/obstruction. J Vasc Interv Radiol 1997;8:649.

70. Sarma DP, Weilbaecher TG, Waggenspack GA: Renal cell carcinoma presenting as a single large cyst. J Surg Oncol 1986;32:30.

71. Hartman DS, Weatherby ED, Laskin WB, et al: Cystic renal cell carcinoma: CT findings simulating a benign hyperdense cyst. AJR Am J Roentgenol 1992;159:1235.

72. Newhouse JH, Pfister RC: Renal cyst puncture. In: Athanasoulis CA, Pfister RC, Greene RE, Roberson GH, eds. Interventional Radiology. Philadelphia, WB Saunders, 1982:409.

73. Sandler CM: Renal cyst puncture and percutaneous drainage of perirenal fluid. In: Kadir S, ed. Current Practice of Interventional Radiology. Philadelphia, BC Decker, 1991:662.

74. Lang EK: The differential diagnosis of renal cysts and tumors: cyst puncture, aspiration, and analysis of cyst content for fat as diagnostic criteria for renal cysts. Radiology 1966;87:883.

75. Ljunberg B, Holmberg G, Sjodin JG, et al: Renal cell carcinoma in a renal cyst: a case report and review of the literature. J Urol 1990;143:797.

76. Lang EK: Renal cyst puncture studies. Urol Clin North Am 1987;14:91.

77. Lang EK: Renal cyst puncture and aspiration: a survey of complications. AJR Am J Roentgenol 1977;128:723.

78. von Schreeb T, Arner O, Skovsted G, et al: Renal adenocarcinoma: is there a risk of spreading tumour cells in diagnostic puncture? Scand J Urol Nephrol 1967;1:270.

79. Ozgur S, Cetin S, Ilker Y: Percutaneous renal cyst aspiration and treatment with alcohol. Int Urol Nephrol 1988;20:481.

80. Bean WJ: Renal cysts: treatment with alcohol. Radiology 1981;138:329.

81. Camacho MF, Bondhus MJ, Carrion HM, et al: Ureteropelvic junction obstruction resulting from percutaneous cyst puncture and intracystic isophendylate injection: an unusual complication. J Urol 1979; 124:713.

82. Castaneda F, Hernandez-Graulau JM: The lower genitourinary tract. In: Baum S, Pentecost MJ, eds. Abrams' Angiography—Interventional Radiology. Boston, Little, Brown, 1997:614.

83. Chiou RK, Binard JE, Ebersole ME, et al: Randomized comparison of balloon dilation and transurethral incision for treatment of symptomatic benign prostatic hyperplasia. J Endourol 1994;8:221.

84. Mohammed SH, Wirima J: Balloon catheter dilatation of urethral strictures. AJR Am J Roentgenol 1988;150:327.

85. Russinovican LK, Griggs W, Jander P: Balloon dilatation of urethral strictures. Urol Radiol 1980;2:33.

86. Milroy E, Chapple C, Eldin A, et al: A new stent for the treatment of urethral strictures: preliminary report. Br J Urol 1989;63:392.
87. Mishell DR Jr: Evaluation of the infertile couple. In: Lobo RA, Mishell DR Jr, eds. Mishell's Textbook of Infertility, Contraception, and Reproductive Endocrinology, 4th ed. Malden, Mass, Blackwell Science, 1997:496.
88. American Fertility Society: Guideline for tubal disease. Am Fertil Soc 1993;6:7.
89. Hovespian DM, Bonn J, Eschelman DJ, et al: Fallopian tube recanalization in an unrestricted patient population. Radiology 1994;190:137.
90. Thurmond AS: Pregnancies after selective salpingography and tubal recanalization. Radiology 1994;190:11.
91. Woolcott R, Petchpud A, O'Donnell P, Stanger J: Differential impact on pregnancy rate of selective salpingography, tubal catheterization and wire-guided recanalization in the treatment of proximal fallopian tube obstruction. Hum Reprod 1995;10:1423.
92. Millward SF, Claman P, Leader A, Spence JE: Technical report: fallopian tube recanalization—a simplified technique. Clin Radiol 1994;49:496.
93. Flood JT, Grow DR: Transcervical tubal cannulation: a review. Obstet Gynecol Surv 1993;48:768.
94. Darcy MD, McClennan BL, Picus D, et al: Transcervical salpingoplasty: current techniques and results. Urol Radiol 1991;13:74.
95. Thurmond AS, Rösch J: Nonsurgical fallopian tube recanalization for treatment of infertility. Radiology 1990;174:371.
96. Hedgpeth PL, Thurmond AS, Fry R: Radiographic fallopian tube recanalization: absorbed ovarian radiation dose. Radiology 1991;180:121.

Index

Page numbers followed by *b*, *f*, or *t* indicate material in boxes, figures, or tables, respectively.